Mayes' Midwifery
A Textbook for Midwives
Twelfth Edition

Mayes' Midwifery
A Textbook for Midwives
Twelfth Edition

Edited by

Betty R Sweet RN, RM, MTD BEd (Hons)
*Lecturer in Midwifery at the University of Surrey and
International Consultant in Midwifery Education
Formerly Senior Lecturer in Midwifery Studies
at the Royal College of Midwives*

with

Denise Tiran RGN, RM, ADM, PGCEA
*Principal Lecturer, Complementary Therapies/Midwifery,
School of Health, University of Greenwich*

Baillière Tindall
London   Philadelphia   Toronto   Sydney   Tokyo

Baillière Tindall
WB Saunders Company Ltd
24–28 Oval Road
London NW1 7DX, UK

The Curtis Center
Independence Square West
Philadelphia, PA 19106–3399, USA

Harcourt Brace & Company
55 Horner Avenue
Toronto, Ontario M8Z 4X6, Canada

Harcourt Brace & Company, Australia
30–52 Smidmore Street
Marrickville, NSW 2204, Australia

Harcourt Brace & Company, Japan
Ichibancho Central Building, 22–1 Ichibancho
Chiyoda-ku, Tokyo 102, Japan

Twelfth edition 1997
Reprinted 1998

A catalogue record for this book is available from the British Library

ISBN 0–7020–1757–4

Typeset by J&L Composition, Filey, North Yorkshire
Printed and bound in Great Britain by Bath Press, Colour Books, Glasgow

Contents

Part Seven   Education in Preparation for Childbirth and Parenthood

Part Eight   From Pregnancy to Labour

Part Nine   The Puerperium and Midwifery Practice

Part Twelve Complications of the Puerperium

Part Thirteen Sexuality and Fertility

Part Fourteen The Newborn Baby

Part Fifteen   Health and Social Services

Part Sixteen   The Sociological Context of Childbirth

Part Seventeen   The Midwife and the Midwifery Profession

Contributors

Hazell Abbott MSc, RN, RM, ADM, PGCEA
Senior Lecturer in Midwifery, University of Luton

Gilly Andrews RGN ENB A08
Clinical Nurse Specialist in Family Planning, King's College Hospital, London; and Clinic Sister, Gynaecology and Menopause Clinic, The Lister Hospital, London

Carmel Bagness MA Medical Ethics, RGN, RM ADM, PGCEA
Wolfson School of Health Sciences, Thames Valley University, Wexham Park Hospital, Slough, Berkshire

Jean A Ball MSc, DipN(Dist), RGN, RM
Hon. Senior Teaching Fellow, Nuffield Institute for Health, University of Leeds

Christine Bewley BEd(Hons), RN, RM, ADM
Senior Lecturer and Programme Leader for Preregistration BSc(Hons) in Midwifery, Middlesex University

Debra Bick BA(Hons), RGM, RM, MMed Soc
Research Fellow in Midwifery, Department of Public Health and Epidemiology, Medical School, University of Birmingham, Edgbaston, Birmingham

Eileen Brayshaw MCSP, SRP, FETC
Superintendent Physiotherapist, St James's University Hospital, Leeds

Margaret I Brock RN, RM, ADM, PGCEA
Lecturer Practitioner, Oxford Brookes University, The Oxford Hospital, Women's Centre, Oxford

Elizabeth H Clark BA PhD
Head of Distance Learning, RCN Institute, Royal College of Nursing, 20 Cavendish Square, London

Terri Coates RN, RM, ADM, Dip Ed
Distance Learning Tutor for the South Bank University; Practising Midwife in Salisbury

Pauline Cooke MSc, RGN, RSCN, RM, ADM, PGCEA
Lecturer/Practitioner, The Centre for Midwifery Practice, Queen Charlotte's & Chelsea Hospital, Goldhawk Road, London

Iris G Cooper RN, RM
Senior Midwifery Manager, University Hospital, Queen's Medical Centre, Nottingham

Ann Cowper SRN, SCM, MTD, DN(London)
Independent Family Planning Nurse and Trainer for ENB 901 Worthing

Tandy Deane-Gray BSc, PGCEA, ADM, RM, RGN, Cert. in Counselling & Psychotherapy
PIPPIN Co-ordinator (Parents in Partnership-Parent Infant Network); Lecturer for Parenthood Education of the Midwifery Pathway BSc Honours Degree in Midwifery Studies; Senior Lecturer in Midwifery at University of Hertfordshire

Annie Harris RGN, RM
Transformation Team, King's Health Care, King's College Hospital, Denmark Hill, London

Christine Henderson MA(Warwick), RN, RM, Dip Nurs (London), MTD, DPHE (Surrey)
Senior Research Fellow, University of Central England, Family Health and Social Sciences, Westbourne Road, Edgbaston, Birmingham

Tina Heptinstall BSc(Hons), RGN, RM, ADM, PGCEA
Senior Lecturer, School of Health, University of Greenwich, Queen Mary Hospital, Sidcup, Kent

Rosemary Jenkins RGN, RM, MTD, DMS, MBIM
Consultant in Health Care Policy

Shirley R Jones SRN, SCM, ADM, Cert Ed (FE), Ma (Medical Ethics)
Route Director, BSc (Hons) in Women's Health Studies, University of Central England in Birmingham

Nicky Leap RM
Midwife, Southeast London Midwifery Group Practice, Deptford, London

Patricia Lindsay RGN, RM, ADM, PGCEA, MSc (Medical Sociology)
Senior Lecturer, Homerton School of Health Studies, Midwifery Education Department, Peterborough District Hospital

Christine MacArthur PhD, MSc, BSc
Reader in Maternal and Child Epidemiology, Department of Public Health and Epidemiology, Medical School, University of Birmingham, Edgbaston, Birmingham

Gaynor D Maclean BA, RM, RGN, MTD
International Midwifery Consultant (Safe Motherhood and Reproductive Health)

Mary McNabb BA, BSc, RN, RM, ADM, PGCEA, MSc
Senior Lecturer, School of Health and Social Care, Southbank University, Erlang House, London

The late Rosemary Methven MSc, RN, RM, MTD, DN (Part A), FETC, DANS, RCNT
Formerly Senior Manager in Post-basic Midwifery Education

Stephanie Michaelides RN, RM, PGCEA, ADM
Senior Lecturer at the School of Midwifery and Family Health, Faculty of Health Studies, Middlesex University

Joy Moore RN, RM, MTD, DN (Lond.)
Formerly Education Officer for Midwifery, English National Board for Nursing, Midwifery and Health Visiting, Victory House, London

Noreen A Morrin
Education Officer, Midwifery Specialist of the English National Board, London

Lorraine Murray BSc(Hons), RN, RM, ADM, PGCEA
Senior Lecturer, Faculty of Health Care and Social Studies, University of Luton

Wendy O'Brien RM, ADM, PCGEA
Community Midwife, Chelsea and Westminster Healthcare NHS Trust

Catherine Rowan MA Medical Ethics, RGN, RM, ADM, PGCEA
Wolfson School of Health Sciences, Thames Valley University, Wexham Park Hospital, Slough, Berkshire

Jancis M Shepherd SRN, ONC, SCM, ADM, PGCEA, MTD, MA in Health and Nursing Studies in Progress
Senior Lecturer-Midwifery, Wolfson School of Health Sciences-Berkshire, Thames Valley University

Valerie Sheridan RN, RM, ADM, PGCEA, MSc (Midwifery)
Midwifery Lecturer, Kingston University & St George's Medical School Joint Faculty of Health Care Sciences; Link Tutor Mayday Healthcare Trust

Carol Simpson RGN, RM, ENB Course 405
Family Care Midwife, St Michael's Hospital, Bristol

Catherine Siney
Coordinator of Midwifery and Gynaecology for Women who are Drug or Alcohol Dependent, HIV Positive or Hepatitis B or C Positive; Member of the Executive and Local Management Advisory Board of the Merseyside Drugs Council

Jennifer Sleep
Reader in Nursing and Midwifery Research, Wolfson School of Health Sciences, Thames Valley University, Royal Berkshire Hospital, Reading

Jane Spillman MSc, SRN, SCM
Honorary Medical Research Consultant of the Twins and Multiple Births Association

Betty R Sweet RN, RM, MTD, BEd(Hons)
Lecturer in Midwifery at the University of Surrey; International Consultant in Midwifery Education; and Formerly Senior Lecturer in Midwifery Studies at the Royal College of Midwives

Florence M Telfer BA, MSc, MA, RN, RM, MTD, Operating Theatre Technique Diploma
Senior Lecturer, School of Human and Health Sciences, University of Huddersfield

Denise Tiran RGN, RM, ADM, PGCEA
Principal Lecturer, Complementary Therapies / Midwifery, School of Health, University of Greenwich

Irene Walton BEd(Hons), MSc, RM, MTD, CMS, FETC
Principal Lecturer – Midwifery, Liverpool John Moores University

Foreword

As a midwife I value my profession and the high standards of care which midwives have sought through education and research-based practice. I was therefore delighted to accept the invitation to write the Foreword to this extensively revised 12th Edition of *Mayes' Midwifery*. Betty Sweet and her team are to be congratulated in providing such a readable, up-to-date and well-referenced book.

I feel quite breathless as I contemplate the enormity of the task undertaken in this revision; not only a new format but much additional information make this a really new textbook for midwives. It will serve the midwifery profession well because it has taken into account the fast changing world in which midwives practice today, and the detailed referencing at the end of each chapter reflects and promotes the research-minded approach that is essential for today's midwife.

There has been a notable increase in the number of books written for midwives and this new edition will make a very important contribution to the preparation and practice of midwives. I feel sure that it will be an essential textbook for both students and practising midwives and I would urge them to own a copy of this book. It provides a comprehensive picture of the nature, breadth and depth of the midwife's role on the backcloth of the needs of women and babies and will assist midwives to equip themselves to play a lead role in the provision of woman-centred care.

It is said that 'a single moment of understanding can flood a whole life with meaning' and I believe that this book has the potential to unlock the real meaning and importance of quality midwifery practice into the next milennium.

E Jane Winship RGN RM MTD DipN(Lond)
Professional Officer Midwifery and European Affairs
United Kingdom Central Council for Nursing,
Midwifery and Health Visiting

Preface

Mayes' Midwifery has undergone a radical revision and is now a multi-author book. With contributions from 41 authors, the book has been extensively revised, largely rewritten, and includes nearly 30 new chapters to meet the needs of today's students and midwives. Many of the contributors are acknowledged experts in their particular area, whereas others are new, or relatively new writers.

Since the publication of the 11th Edition of *Mayes' Midwifery* there have been major changes in midwifery education in the UK. All initial midwifery education is now university-based and is at diploma or degree level. Continuing education opportunities for registered midwives have increased greatly and now many practising midwives are also studying for a diploma or degree. An all-graduate profession is now on the horizon, perhaps early in the next century. The profession, which will celebrate the first centenary of the first *Midwives Act* in the year 2002, can be justly proud of its achievements.

Running alongside these major advances in midwifery education have been fundamental changes in the philosophy and delivery of midwifery care to women and their families. The move towards woman-centred care has accelerated and is now government policy in the UK. Midwives, and indeed other professionals, are expected to work in partnership with women, giving continuity of care, offering choice and ensuring that they feel in control of what is happening to them. To achieve these goals the midwife must ensure that women have all the information which they require to make informed choices and decisions about the care they receive. This book attempts to meet the changing educational needs of students and of practising midwives, and reflects the changing philosophy of the approach to childbirth.

A good knowledge and understanding of the physiology of reproduction aids the intelligent practice of the midwife and the physiology in this book has been extensively rewritten in far greater depth. There are many new chapters on physiology, all of which are research-based and very widely referenced. There are also new chapters on Maternal Nutrition, and Health Promotion and Education because of the increasing evidence about the far-reaching effects of maternal nutrition, health and life-style on fetal, infant and even adult health.

New chapters on Choices and Patterns of Care, Complementary Therapies, and Community Midwifery and Home Birth are included, all of which reflect the current moves to give women greater choice about place of birth and the type and patterns of care they would like during pregnancy and childbirth. There is also a new chapter written by a physiotherapist on Physical Preparation for the Ante-, Intra- and Postnatal Periods.

All the chapters on labour have been extensively updated or rewritten and there is a new chapter on Shoulder Dystocia. It is only in recent years that professionals have become aware of the extent of the morbidity associated with childbrith and two of the key researchers in this field have written a chapter on this important subject. There are also new chapters on Sexuality and Childbirth, Infertility and Assisted Conception, and The Menopause which are written by midwives or nurses who are specialists in these fields.

New chapters in the Newborn Baby section include Thermoregulation and the Neonate, Cardiac and Circulatory Disorders in the Newborn, and Neonatal Surgery and Pain. As more women choose to have home births and the midwife becomes responsible for the full physical examination of the newborn at birth and subsequently, she must be increasingly vigilant to detect signs of cardiac and other severe abnormalities and, if suspected or detected, know the correct action to take because it may be life-saving.

The new section on The Midwife and the Midwifery Profession includes new chapters on The Law and the Midwife, The Midwife and her Education, Ethics in Midwifery Practice, Management Issues in Midwifery Practice, Quality Assurance, and Midwifery in an International Context. I should like to pay particular tribute to Rosemary Methven who wrote the chapter on The Midwife and her Education and has since died. Rosemary was a well-known and highly-respected midwife teacher whose research and publications have made a valuable contribution to the midwifery profession. Her chapter in this edition of *Mayes' Midwifery* must have been one of the last things she wrote for publication and it reflects the high standard for which she was renowned.

In addition to all these new chapters, those from the 11th Edition of *Mayes' Midwifery* have been fully updated and, in many cases, completely rewritten.

The whole book is research-based where possible, extensively referenced and most chapters also include a list of further reading and, where relevant, useful addresses. The text is very well illustrated in colour with many new diagrams and most of the illustrations from the previous edition have also been redrawn.

I have tried to ensure that this new edition of *Mayes' Midwifery* is a comprehensive textbook which will meet the needs of today's students, as well as midwives in the UK and overseas who wish to extend their knowledge of research-based midwifery and related subjects. The book also reflects the philosophy of *Changing Childbirth* (Department of Health (1993) *Changing Childbirth. Report of the Expert Maternity Group*. London: HMSO) and promotes the role of the midwife as an independent professional promoting safe motherhood and a pleasurable, fulfilling experience of childbirth for women and their families at a momentous time in their lives.

Betty R Sweet

Acknowledgements

I would like to express particular thanks to my family and friends for their patience and forbearance during recent years whilst I have been working so hard revising and editing this book. It has been a mammoth task and I am very much aware that I have neglected them in many different ways.

I would also like to thank all those who have contributed chapters to this edition of *Mayes' Midwifery*. A special thank you to authors who worked so hard to complete their chapters on time. Special thanks too to other contributors who have so willingly updated or written chapters at a late stage in the project.

It is difficult to single out people for special thanks because others who have also made a valued contribu-

tion may feel neglected. During the final stage of the project, however, I have had valuable assistance from Patricia Lindsay. Another person I should like to thank is Iris Cooper who is a marvellous sleuth at tracking down obscure references!

Finally, my thanks go to Robert Langham at Baillière Tindall who has worked hard since he became involved in the project 18 months ago to move it forward. He has relieved me of much of the time-consuming task of contacting late contributors and has kept me well-informed of progress. Thanks also to David Atkins, despite the fact that he has kept me completely proof-bound in my 'spare time' for nearly four months now!

Part One

The Midwife

1

The Midwife

Definitions

In English, the word midwife means 'with woman'. In French, the midwife is called *sage femme*, meaning wise woman, and in Latin the word, *cum-mater* is used for midwife.

The midwife has a unique role which is complementary to but different from the role of other health care professionals involved in the care of mothers and babies. The definition of a midwife was jointly developed by the International Confederation of Midwives (ICM) and the International Federation of Gynaecologists and Obstetricians (FIGO). It was adopted by these bodies in 1972 and 1973 respectively and was later adopted by the World Health Organization (WHO). In 1990 it was amended by the International Confederation of Midwives Council and the amendment was ratified by the Federation of Gynaecologists and Obstetricians in 1991 and the World Health Organization in 1992. The amended definition is as follows:

A midwife is a person who, having been regularly admitted to a midwifery educational programme, duly recognized in the country in which it is located, has successfully completed the prescribed course of studies in midwifery and has acquired the requisite qualifications to be registered and/or legally licensed to practise midwifery.

She must be able to give the necessary supervision, care and advice to women during pregnancy, labour and the postpartum period, to conduct deliveries on her own responsibility and to care for the newborn and the infant. This care includes preventative measures, the detection of abnormal conditions in mother and child, the procurement of medical assistance and the execution of emergency measures in the absence of medical help. She has an important task in health counselling and education, not only for the women, but also within the family and the community. The work should involve antenatal education and preparation for parenthood and extends to certain areas of gynaecology, family planning and child care. She may practise in hospitals, clinics, health units, domiciliary conditions or in any other service.

Midwifery Education

The education of the midwife is designed to enable her to fulfil this wide and varied role. In the UK there are two modes of midwifery education leading to registration on Part 10 of the United Kingdom Central Council (UKCC) register, that is the part of the register for midwives. The pre-registration *three-year programme*, formerly known as *direct entry*, is for those who are not registered on Parts 1 or 12 of the UKCC professional register (i.e. first-level nurses). The number of pre-registration midwifery programmes (three years) has increased markedly during the late 1980s and 1990s and attracts many mature entrants as well as those who are younger. Economically it is an attractive proposition because a midwife can be educated in three rather than four and a half years and retention rates in the profession should increase.

The other mode of midwifery education in the UK is the pre-registration (shortened) *18 months programme* for those who are already registered as first-level nurses. The number of these programmes has decreased as the number of pre-registration (three-year) programmes has increased.

All midwifery education programmes in the UK, both pre-registration (three-year) and pre-registration (shortened) 18 months, are now at diploma or degree level. The length of programmes at degree level may be extended from 3 to 4 years, or from 18 months to 2 years in some institutions. In time it is envisaged that all initial midwifery education will be at degree level.

Pre-registration (shortened) 18 months midwifery education for first-level nurses registered in the UK is accepted by the European Union, providing the midwife who has undertaken such a training programme has one year's midwifery experience as a qualified midwife. Only then is she qualified to work as a midwife in member states of the European Union. This is because most European midwives follow a full three-year midwifery programme and this year's experience for British midwives was agreed as an acceptable compromise. The European Community Midwives Directives were agreed in 1980 and implemented in 1981. Directive 80/155/EEC Article 4 defines the activities of the midwife and decrees that member states shall ensure that midwives are at least entitled to take up and pursue the following activities:

1 to provide sound family planning information and advice;
2 to diagnose pregnancies and monitor normal pregnancies; to carry out examinations necessary for the monitoring of the development of normal pregnancies;
3 to prescribe or advise on the examinations necessary for the earliest possible diagnosis of pregnancies at risk;
4 to provide a programme of parenthood education and complete preparation for childbirth including advice on hygiene and nutrition;
5 to care for and assist the mother during labour and to monitor the condition of the fetus *in utero* by the appropriate clinical and technical means;
6 to conduct spontaneous deliveries including where required an episiotomy and in urgent cases a breech delivery;
7 to recognize the warning signs of abnormality in the mother or infant which necessitate referral to a doctor and to assist the latter where appropriate; to take the necessary emergency measures in the doctor's absence, in particular the manual removal of the placenta, possibly followed by manual examination of the uterus;
8 to examine and care for the newborn infant; to take all initiatives which are necessary in case of need and to carry out where necessary immediate resuscitation;
9 to care for and monitor the progress of the mother in the postnatal period and to give all necessary advice to the mother on infant care to enable her to ensure the optimum progress of the newborn infant;
10 to carry out the treatment prescribed by a doctor;
11 to maintain all necessary records.

The British midwife also practises within a framework of the *Midwives Rules* (UKCC, 1993) and *The Midwife's Code of Practice* (UKCC, 1994) of the United Kingdom Central Council (UKCC) for Nursing, Midwifery and Health Visiting (see Chapter 84). Thus the midwife, as an independent practitioner of normal midwifery (although she usually works as a member of a team), has the limits of her practice clearly defined. Rule 33 specifies the outcomes of programmes of midwifery education leading to admission to Part 10 of the UKCC register. These outcomes are the same for all initial midwifery education, whether three-year or 18 months programmes and for both diploma and degree level midwifery education. *The Midwife's Code of Practice* gives guidance in relation to her professional practice. In addition a midwife is also required to follow the UKCC *Code of Professional Conduct for the Nurse, Midwife and Health Visitor* (UKCC, 1992).

In March each year a midwife notifies here intention to practise to each local supervising authority in the area where she intends to practise. In order to be eligible to practise a midwife has to provide evidence of professional updating. In the case of practising midwives this has meant attendance at a statutory midwifery refresher course (or other approved course or study days) every five years. With the implementation, starting in April 1995, of the UKCC's requirements for Post Registration Education and Practice (PREP), the current system of statutory refresher courses for midwives will gradually be replaced by the PREP system of continuing education. This change is scheduled to be phased in over a period of six years, thus all midwives, nurses and health visitors must meet all the PREP requirements by 1 April 2001. The PREP requirements are outlined below.

Post Registration Education and Practice (PREP)

Introduction of PREP

From April 1995 all practitioners are being notified of the new requirements for continuing education by the UKCC at the time of renewal of their UKCC registration. The new requirements will have to be met for the first time in the three years between the practitioner's next renewal of registration and the subsequent date of renewal which will be three years later. All practitioners therefore have at least three years to meet the new PREP requirement for professional development.

Requirements of PREP for the maintenance of registration

There are four main requirements:

1 *Completion of a Notification of Practice form* every three years at the time of renewal of registration. Those who change their area of practice and therefore use a different registrable qualification and those returning to practice after a break of five years or more will also be required to complete a Notification of Practice form. *Midwives will con-tinue to complete a Notification of Intention to Practise form annually as well as the Notification of Practice form every three years.*

2 *Completion of a minimum of five days of study or equivalent every three years.* The period of study must be relevant to the practitioner's professional registration and role. A practising midwife therefore who is only using a midwifery qualification will be required to focus her study on midwifery or related areas. If the midwife is also using a nursing qualification, perhaps because she has a dual role as nurse/ midwife, she will be required to include both relevant nursing and midwifery in her five days of study.

3 *Maintenance of a personal professional profile* with details of professional development and career progress. This profile should include reflection on the midwife's professional experience and document the learning which ensues from this, as well as from planned learning activities.

4 *A Return to Practice programme* if a practitioner has been out of practice for five years or more. A return to practice programme is required for those who have worked less than 100 working days or 750 hours in the previous five years. It is therefore important for midwives and other practitioners to keep a record of the hours they work in their personal professional profile.

Under existing legislation, midwives who have not practised for a period of five years or more are required to complete a Return to Practice programme and they will continue to complete these statutory Return to Practice programmes until 1 April 2000. After that date they will comply with the same new legislation as nurses and health visitors.

From April 1995 to March 2001 the UKCC is to conduct pilot studies to evaluate the effectiveness of its PREP policies and to evaluate how its requirements are being achieved. A formal audit system based on the findings of the pilot studies will be established from 1 April 2001. One of the areas which will be evaluated is self-verification by practitioners that all the statutory obligations of PREP have been fulfilled. Some practitioners will be required by the UKCC to produce evidence to support their claim that they have met all the necessary requirements to renew their registration.

PREP also includes the concept of advanced practice for midwives and for nurses. Advanced midwifery practice is mainly concerned with developments in future practice and roles. It also includes contributing to health policy and management and the determination of health needs. Some nurses may also become specialist practitioners to meet the needs of patients with specialist requirements. Since midwives mainly give total care to a defined caseload of women, the concept of specialist practitioner in one aspect of midwifery would be inappropriate.

Professional Development

Continuing education is essential for every midwife if she is to keep abreast of the many changes which affect her practice. These include:

- major scientific and technological advances;
- changes in society, in the roles of men and women, in the family and in the community;
- changes in employment;
- changes in education;
- changes in the organization of resources and the management of health care; and
- changes in attitudes, beliefs and values.

Midwives have been privileged in having statutory refresher courses since their introduction in the 1940s. Now this mode of continuing education is in the process of change and midwives have to take the responsibility to:

- review their own competence;
- set their learning objectives;
- develop an action plan which will include appropriate learning activities to meet their objectives;
- implement their action plan after discussion with their manager, supervisor or a tutor;
- reflect on the learning experience and evaluate its effectiveness;
- record their learning activities in their personal professional profile (UKCC, 1995).

Unlike statutory refresher courses, there is no formal approval required for any learning activities undertaken to meet the requirements of PREP. Midwives and other practitioners therefore have the opportunity to develop creative learning schemes to meet their particular needs and promote their professional development.

Identification of learning needs

Planning professional development, including the identification of learning needs, is the responsibility of the each individual midwife (UKCC, 1995). According to Lawson (1975) 'needs are based on assessment and diagnosis of a situation in which there is thought to be – by an "expert", or by the individual, – some deficiency.' Comprehensive needs assessment may present problems as practitioners may not always be fully aware of their needs, or may be reticent about sharing them. Bradshaw (1972) identifies the four elements of need shown in Figure 1, some of which are identified by the individual and some by the 'expert'.

Self-assessment to identify 'felt' needs should be followed by discussion with the midwife's manager and/or supervisor and it may be helpful to use a structured framework for this process such as the Johari Window (Figure 2) (Bell, 1986; Sweet, 1993).

Needs recognized by the individual may be *shared* but, for a variety of reasons, the practitioner may choose not to divulge them all, thus some are *hidden*. *Blind needs* are those which are not recognized by the individual, but have been identified by her manager/supervisor. *Undiscovered needs* are not identified by either the individual or her manager/supervisor (Sweet, 1993). A comprehensive needs assessment, first by the midwife using criteria which she has formulated, followed by collaborative discussion with her manager/supervisor, is an essential first step in planning professional development. Subsequent steps, which includes setting learning objectives and the selection of appropriate learning activities, will be based on the needs assessment. Careful needs assessment also increases self-awareness and perhaps openness which aids both personal and professional development.

Learning activities

Nowadays there is a wide choice of learning activities to meet the learning needs of midwives. These include *professional programmes*, some of which are accredited, a wide range of *degree courses* and *personal study* or *research* which is relevant to the role of the midwife. Many professional programmes now include shared learning with other disciplines which for most participants in one recent research study appeared to be a positive experience (ENB, 1995).

Most National Board-approved education programmes now carry credits which may be accumulated

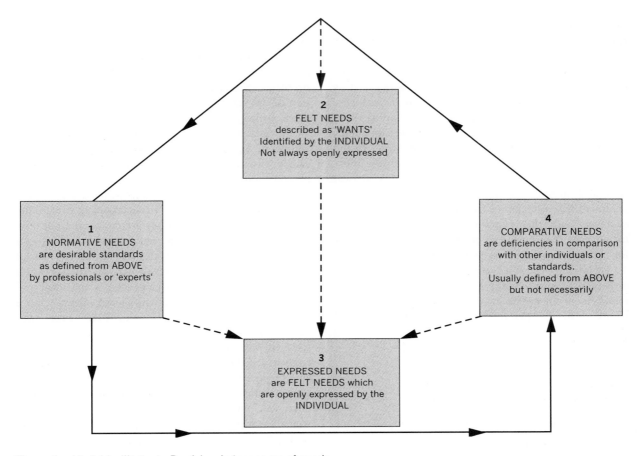

Figure 1 Model to illustrate Bradshaw's taxonomy of needs.

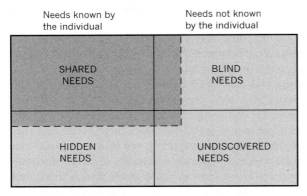

Figure 2 Johari Window: a framework for the identification of needs.

on the credit accumulation and transfer scheme (CATS). Both the pre-registration (shortened) 18 months and three-year midwifery programmes at diploma level have a total of 240 credits, 120 at level 1 and 120 at level 2. To obtain an honours degree a further 120 credits at level 3 are required, making a total of 360 credits. There are many opportunities now for midwives to continue their education after initial registration and further credits can be accumulated to achieve graduate status. Some of the Board-approved continuing education programmes which are accredited are described in Chapter 86. An encouraging development is the introduction of the scheme whereby clinical experience can be credited through a process of Accreditation of Prior Experiential Learning (APEL), and some courses which midwives have previously completed which were not credited can be assessed and recognized through Accredited Prior Learning (APL). An increasing number of midwives have now studied, or are in the process of studying at Masters or doctorate level. All midwives who wish to become teachers are now required to be graduates. This means they must either acquire a degree before they undertake a postgraduate teachers' course, or apply for entry to an undergraduate programme for teacher education.

Attendance at courses is not the only way to facilitate the continuing education of the midwife. It is equally important to read the *professional journals* regularly, to critically read *relevant reports*, including those on research, to carry out *literature searches* on topics relevant to practice and to play an *active role* in the development of the profession. The midwife must learn to develop her critical faculties, her analytical skills and the ability to present a logical, well-reasoned argument based on sound facts and supported by good evidence. Only then can she make a worthwhile contribution to the improvement of the maternity services for the benefit of mothers and babies.

All learning activities, whether a recognized course or personal research/study can contribute to the PREP requirement for professional development and must be recorded in the practitioner's personal professional profile.

Midwifery Practice

The 1990s are an exciting and challenging time for midwives with the publication and subsequent gradual implementation of the Report of the Expert Maternity Group entitled *Changing Childbirth* (DOH, 1993). This report specifies that the maternity services should be woman-centred and concentrate on meeting the needs of women using the service. For many years now women's needs and wishes have not been met as childbirth has become increasingly medicalized in hospital.

Following the Peel Report (1970) which advocated a 100% hospital confinement rate, there were major changes in the delivery of maternity care. By the 1980s 99% of women had their babies in hospital and there have been great advances in technology in an attempt to improve the outcome of pregnancy. Obstetric practice changed too, in that medical intervention in pregnancy and labour became commonplace. Increasing medical control of childbirth changed the role of the midwife, leading to less opportunity to exercise the degree of clinical responsibility for which she has been trained; hence many experienced less job satisfaction.

In recent years, however, there has been a groundswell of opposition to the medicalization of childbirth from the consumer. Many interventions have been challenged and research has now proved that some practices, such as routine induction of labour and episiotomy are unnecessary and indeed may cause problems (Sleep, 1984a, b). The evidence for promotion of delivery in hospital for safety reasons has also been challenged and is unsubstantiated (Tew, 1990).

An increasing number of women are no longer willing to be passive recipients of obstetric care, but rather wish to be active participants with more information, more control and more autonomy (DOH, 1993). Nowadays when most women have only one or two children they have high expectations of the unique experience of childbirth. They are concerned not only about their safe delivery and recovery and the birth of a normal, healthy baby, but also about the process of childbirth and their response to it. To an increasing number of women natural childbirth is the ideal and they are turning to the midwife to help them achieve the emotionally fulfilling and pleasurable experience they desire. Whether or not natural childbirth is practised, all women need a positive emotional experience from which they derive satisfaction and fulfilment and should emerge from the experience with their self-esteem intact or, indeed, enhanced. Such an experience can make an important contribution to the woman's mental health in the postpartum period (Ball, 1994).

Now that childbirth is so much safer, women are demanding more in terms of psychological and emotional fulfilment and this is still not always recognized by obstetricians and, indeed, some midwives. In a few instances this causes tension between parents and professionals which can only be resolved by good communications and a real desire on the part of professionals to meet the holistic needs of parents. This means that midwives must acquire good communication skills and learn to assess needs, plan care together with parents to meet their particular needs and then implement and subsequently evaluate the agreed care plan. Seeking to identify and meet the needs of parents presents a challenge to the midwife which she is well equipped to meet. The close relationship and trust which develops between mother and midwife helps to facilitate a positive and enriching experience of childbirth. Should complications arise and intervention become necessary, the midwife's knowledge of the couple and their needs enables her to provide appropriate help and support during what may be a difficult time for them.

The recommendations outlined in the report *Changing Childbirth* (DOH, 1993), which have been accepted by the government, should facilitate these changes in attitude and the delivery of appropriate care to women and their families. The report states that: 'purchasers and providers will need to agree in their strategic plans and contracts a range of goals and standards to be achieved and the way in which progress can be monitored.' Ten indicators of success to be achieved in five years are identified in the report and are outlined below.

1 All women should be entitled to carry their own notes.
2 Every woman should know one midwife who ensures continuity of her midwifery care – the named midwife.
3 At least 30% of women should have the midwife as the lead professional.
4 Every woman should know the lead professional who has a key role in the planning and provision of her care.
5 At least 75% of women should know the person who cares for them during their delivery.
6 Midwives should have direct access to some beds in all maternity units.
7 At least 30% of women delivered in a maternity unit should be admitted under the management of the midwife.
8 The total number of antenatal visits for women with uncomplicated pregnancies should have been reviewed in the light of the available evidence and the RCOG guidelines.
9 All front-line ambulances should have a paramedic able to support the midwife who needs to transfer a woman to hospital in an emergency.
10 All women should have access to information about the services available in their locality (DOH, 1993).

Midwives therefore have a central and very challenging role to fulfil in the fundamental changes which are at present being implemented in the maternity services.

Professional Organization for Midwives in the UK

The Royal College of Midwives supports midwives in their efforts to maintain and improve standards of care for mothers, babies and the family. It is the only professional organization and trade union in the UK which is specifically for midwives. The aim of the Royal College of Midwives is to advance the art and science of midwifery and to maintain high professional standards. The Headquarters of the College are in London and services are being regionalized by placing RCM officers in various parts of the country where they will be more easily accessible to members and be able to support the stewards more effectively (Davis, 1996). There are also over 200 local branches of the College throughout the United Kingdom. About 37 000 midwives belong to the College and enjoy the benefits of membership.

International Confederation of Midwives (ICM)

The Royal College of Midwives is a member of the International Confederation of Midwives (ICM). This is a confederation of associations of midwives from many countries in the world and the headquarters are in London. The aim of the International Confederation of Midwives is to improve the standard of care provided to women, babies and families throughout the world through the development, education and appropriate utilization of the professional midwife (ICM, 1993). The ICM is very involved in the World Health Organization Safe Motherhood Initiative which aims to reduce the number of maternal deaths in the world by half by the year 2000. Every three years the ICM holds a congress in different countries of the world. Most branches of the Royal College of Midwives try to send one or two midwives to the International Congress and these midwives then report back to their branches. It can thus be seen that midwives have the opportunity to forge links with their professional colleagues in many countries of the world as they seek to advance the art and science of midwifery and promote safe motherhood.

In 1993 at the congress in Canada the ICM presented an international code of ethics for midwives to guide the education, practice and research of the midwife. This code 'acknowledges women as persons, seeks justice for all people and equity in access to health care, and is based on mutual relationships of respect, trust, and the dignity of all members of society' (ICM, 1993).

Four times a year the ICM publishes a News-letter which enables midwives to keep in touch with midwifery developments and issues on a worldwide basis.

References

Ball, J.A. (1994) *Reactions to Motherhood*. Hale, UK: Books for Midwives Press.

Bell, E.A. (1986) Needs assessment in continuing education: designing a system that works. *J. Cont. Educ. Nurs.* 17(4): 112–114.

Bradshaw, J. (1972) A concept of social need. *New Society* 30 March: 440–443.

Davis, K. (1996) Regionalising The Royal College of Midwives. *Midwives* 109 (1296): 4–5.

DOH (Department of Health) (1993) *Changing Childbirth Part 1: Report of the Expert Maternity Group*. London: HMSO.

English National Board (1995) An evaluation of shared learning in educational programmes of preparation for nurse, midwife and health visitor teachers. Research Highlights. London: ENB.

ICM (International Confederation of Midwives) (1993) *International Code of Ethics*. London: ICM.

Lawson, K.H. (1975) *Philosophical Concepts and Values in Adult Education*. Milton Keynes: Open University Press.

Peel Report (1970) *Report of the Standing Maternity and Midwifery Advisory Committee* (Chairman Sir John Peel) *Domiciliary Midwifery and Maternity Bed Needs*. London: HMSO.

Sleep, J. (1984a) Episiotomy in normal delivery, 1. *Nursing Times* 80(47): 29–30.

Sleep, J. (1984b) Episiotomy in normal delivery, 2. *Nursing Times* 80(48): 51–54.

Sweet, B.R. (1993) *Midwifery Education*. London: Distance Learning Centre, South Bank University.

Tew, M. (1990) *Safer Childbirth – a Critical History of Maternity Care*. London: Chapman & Hall.

UKKC (United Kingdom Central Council for Nursing, Midwifery and Health Visiting) (1992) *Code of Profesional Conduct for the Nurse, Midwife and Health Visitor*. London: UKCC.

UKCC (1993) *Midwives Rules*. London: UKCC.

UKCC (1994) *The Midwife's Code of Practice*. London: UKCC.

UKCC (1995) *PREP & You*. London: UKCC.

2

The Female Pelvis

The pelvic girdle is a strong bony ring which forms an essential part of the skeletal framework. In humans it supports, through the spinal column, the weight of the upper part of the body and transmits this weight to the lower limbs. It contains and protects the reproductive organs, as well as the bladder and rectum. It is through this bony ring, moreover, that the child must pass during birth: to understand how this occurs the midwife should have a working knowledge of pelvic anatomy.

It is sometimes asked why human mothers have longer and more difficult labours than animals. It is partly because the upright posture of the human race has resulted in the development of a spine with four slight curves and a pelvis in which the birth canal is distinctly curved. Most mammals have an almost straight spine and a cylindrical birth canal. The absence of a curve allows the young to be born comparatively easily. There is no cranium to be moulded or to cause prolonged labour. By contrast the human fetus has a large head, chiefly cranium, which has to adapt itself, sometimes by moulding to the mother's curved pelvis. Labour is thus more difficult mechanically and more liable to complications. Furthermore the human brain is more highly developed, leading to a greater awareness of pain, apprehension and fear. Many women approaching labour are apprehensive and fearful and this state of mind can adversely affect uterine contractions, prolonging labour and increasing pain. Fortunately, with good antenatal preparation and understanding support during labour these effects can be minimized.

It is convenient first to consider the bones, joints and ligaments which together constitute the pelvic girdle, and then, much more importantly, to study the pelvis as a whole.

The Pelvic Bones

The pelvis is comprised of four bones: two *innominate* or unnamed bones; the *sacrum*; and the *coccyx*.

INNOMINATE BONE

Each innominate bone (Figures 1 and 2) is made up of three bones: the *ilium*, the *ischium* and the *pubis*. In childhood they are separated by cartilage; after the age of 20–25 years they are fused into one mass of bone.

Ilium

The ilium is the upper expanded part of the innominate bone. Its concave inner surface is the *iliac fossa*; its curved upper border is the *iliac crest*. This ends in front at the *anterior superior iliac spine*, both spine and crest being palpable under the skin; at the back the crest ends at the *posterior superior iliac spine*. The two posterior spines are marked by two dimples. Below

each anterior and posterior superior iliac spines lie the *inferior iliac spines*. All these spines form attachment points for muscles of the trunk, hips and thighs. Below the iliac fossa is a distinct ridge, the *iliopectineal line*, ending in front at a roughened swelling, the *iliopectineal eminence*, where ilium and pubis fuse. Below this, on the outer side of the innominate bone, is a cup-shaped depression, the *acetabulum*, where the femur articulates, forming the hip joint; here the ilium fuses with both ischium and pubis. The ilium forms two-fifths of the acetabulum.

Ischium

The ischium is roughly L-shaped and forms the posterior–inferior part of the pelvis. It has an upper

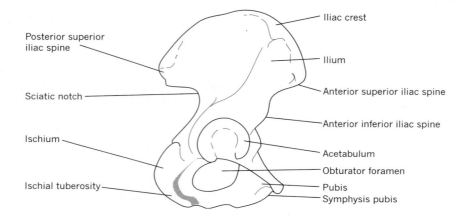

Figure 1   The outer or lateral surface of the right innominate bone.

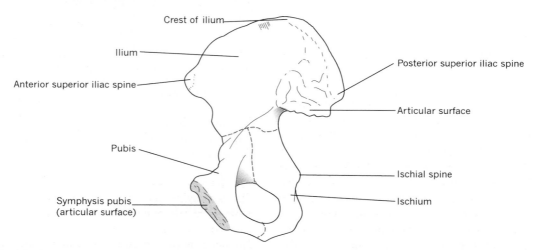

Figure 2   The inner or medial surface of the right innominate bone.

thicker body that joins the ilium and a lower, thinner portion that joins the pubis. Spines of the ischium project medially into the pelvic cavity and are used to estimate the station of the presenting part during labour. The strongest part of the pelvis is made up of the thickened inferior surface of the body of the ischium called a *tuberosity*. In the sitting position, total body weight is borne by the tuberosities. The medial surface of the ischium has attachment points for the ischiococcygeus muscle, which forms part of the pelvic floor, while the spine and tuberosity provide attachment points for the sacrospinous and sacrotuberous ligaments.

The two ischial spines may be palpated vaginally and they afford important evidence of the size of the pelvic outlet. If they project inwards too much they will significantly reduce the transverse diameter of the pelvic outlet. The ischial spine divides the greater from the lesser sciatic notch.

Pubis

The pubic bone forms the anterior portion of the pelvis. It is a small bone with a body and two *rami*. The upper ramus joins the ilium at the iliopectineal eminence and forms one-fifth of the acetabulum. The lower ramus fuses with the ramus of the ischium, forming the anterior boundary of the obturator foramen and the *subpubic arch*. The bodies of the two pubes meet at the symphysis pubis and form the apex of the *pubic arch*. In a good gynaecoid pelvis the subpubic arch should be at least 90° to allow the fetal head to emerge easily from the pelvis at delivery.

SACRUM

The sacrum (Figure 3) lies between the two ilia and forms the back of the pelvis. It is a wedge-shaped bone consisting of five fused vertebrae, the first of which has a prominent upper margin known as the *sacral promontory*. This, an important pelvic landmark, juts into the pelvic cavity, decreasing the anteroposterior diameter of the pelvic brim. If this diameter is seriously decreased it will delay or prevent the descent of the fetus into the pelvis. The smooth concave anterior surface is called the hollow of the sacrum and the areas on either side of the promontory are the *alae* or wings. The rough convex posterior surface is for the attachment of muscles. The sacrum is perforated by four sets of *foramina* through which pass the sacral nerves.

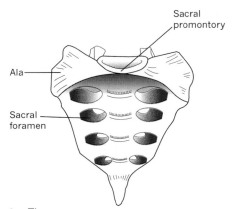

Figure 3 The sacrum.

COCCYX

The coccyx, the lowest part of the spine, is a small triangular-shaped bone. Its base is uppermost and it articulates with the lower end of the sacrum. It consists of four fused rudimentary vertebrae. The coccyx gives attachment to ligaments, to muscle fibres of the anal sphincter and, along with the sacrum, to the ischiococcygeus muscle which forms the posterior section of the pelvic floor. During labour the coccyx moves backwards to enlarge the pelvic outlet, thus allowing more space for the passage of the fetus.

Pelvic Joints

Sacroiliac joints

The sacroiliac joints are two slightly movable synovial and fibrous joints that are formed where the ilium joins with the first two sacral vertebrae on either side. Borell and Fernström (1957), using X-rays, found that mobility was greater in pregnant and puerperal women than in nulliparae and women examined one year or more after delivery. As a result of this increased mobility, there is an increase in the diameter of the pelvic brim (true conjugate) and in the sagittal diameter of the outlet.

Symphysis pubis

This is a slightly movable secondary cartilaginous joint between the two pubic bones. In the last two months of pregnancy the gap between the symphysial surfaces of the pubic bone increases from about 4 mm to 7 mm (Joseph, 1988).

Sacrococcygeal joint

This is a hinge joint between the sacrum and the coccyx which, at the end of labour, allows the coccyx to move backwards, facilitating delivery.

Pelvic Ligaments

To fulfil its supporting function, the pelvic girdle requires great strength and stability and the joints are reinforced by powerful ligaments:

▶ *Sacroiliac ligaments*: These are strong ligaments which pass in front of and behind each sacroiliac joint.
▶ *Symphysis pubis*: This is similarly strengthened by ligaments. Ligaments bridge certain spaces in the walls of the pelvis.
▶ *Sacrotuberous ligaments*: The two sacrotuberous ligaments extend from the sides of the sacrum to the ischial tuberosities, thus crossing the greater and lesser sciatic notches.
▶ *Sacrospinous ligaments*: These pass from the sides of the sacrum to the ischial spines, extending across the greater sciatic notches.

The pelvic joints and ligaments are relaxed in pregnancy due to hormonal action. This allows 'give' which fractionally increases the pelvic measurements. Where there is an element of disproportion this increase may be vitally important. On the other hand, the increased mobility of the pelvic joints may create a feeling of instability in some women and it is probably responsible for the low backache commonly experienced in late pregnancy and in the early puerperium.

The Pelvis as a Whole

When the model pelvis (Figure 4) is examined it is easily seen to be divided by a distinct bony ridge into a broad upper part and a smaller lower region. The upper division, the *false pelvis*, plays no part in the processes of labour and is of little importance to the midwife. The lower part, the *true pelvis*, is, on the other hand, of the first importance and will need to be considered in detail.

The true pelvis is bounded at the back by the sacrum, at the sides mainly by the ischia and in front by the pubes; it thus forms a complete and practically unyielding ring of bone. Because the fetus must pass through this bony girdle to be born, its size, shape and anatomical landmarks should be studied carefully.

The true pelvis consists of:

▶ a *brim* or *inlet*, the first part to be negotiated by the fetus;
▶ a curved *cavity*, traversed next; and
▶ an *outlet* through which the fetus emerges during birth.

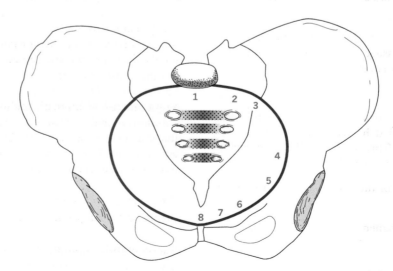

Figure 4   The pelvic brim: 1, sacral promontory; 2, sacral ala; 3, sacroiliac joint; 4, iliopectineal line; 5, iliopectineal eminence; 6, superior pubic ramus; 7, body of pubic bone; 8, symphysis pubis.

Normally, the fetus is just able to pass through this bony canal, but should the pelvis be rather small or misshapen, or should the fetus be unusually large or presenting abnormally, progress could become difficult or even impossible.

Pelvic brim or inlet

This bony ridge is seen to be almost circular, except posteriorly where the sacral promontory juts into the brim of the pelvis. The boundaries of the pelvic brim are readily traced on a model (Figure 4):

1 Promontory of the sacrum;
2 Wings or alae of the sacrum;
3 Right and left sacroiliac joints;
4 Right and left iliopectineal lines;
5 Right and left iliopectineal eminences;
6 Upper inner borders of the superior pubic rami;
7 Upper inner borders of the bodies of the pubes;
8 Upper inner border of the symphysis pubis.

Pelvic cavity

This extends from the brim to the outlet. It will be noted to be shallow in front and deeper at the back. The boundaries are:

▶ Hollow of the sacrum;
▶ Sacroiliac joints;
▶ Ischia and the sacrospinous ligaments;
▶ Right and left upper and lower pubic rami;
▶ Bodies of the pubes and the symphysis pubis.

The pelvic cavity is circular. Its anterior wall is 4.5 cm deep, whereas the posterior wall is 12 cm deep. Clearly anything passing through the cavity must move in a curved rather than a straight path.

Pelvic outlet

The outlet appears ovoid or even diamond-shaped, being partly bounded by ligaments. It is the lowest level at which the fetus is on all sides constricted by bone. It is described at two levels:

1 The boundaries of the upper obstetrical outlet are:

▶ Lower sacrum;
▶ Sacrospinous ligaments and ischial spines;
▶ Pubic arch.

2 The boundaries of the lower anatomical outlet are:

▶ Tip of the coccyx;

▶ Sacrotuberous ligaments and ischial tuberosities;
▶ Pubic arch.

The coccyx extends lower, but it is mobile and swings backwards during birth. The tuberosities, too, are lower than the spines and slightly wider apart. If the fetus can pass through the obstetric outlet, therefore, it should have no difficulty in emerging from the anatomical outlet.

DIAMETERS OF THE PELVIS

The pelvis is normally large enough for the fetal head to pass through without difficulty. However, should the head be only slightly larger than normal, or the pelvis in any direction smaller than usual, progress might become impossible. Accordingly, the normal dimensions of the pelvis (and of the infant's head) are described in detail.

The midwife should familiarize herself with these dimensions and she will then more readily appreciate any abnormality in either the size or shape of the pelvis. A simplified summary is shown in Figure 5.

Diameters of the brim

Anteroposterior diameter This diameter extends from the sacral promontory to the upper inner border of the symphysis pubis and measures approximately 11 cm. It is also called the *obstetric conjugate* and, since it is the first narrow strait the fetal head has to pass, it is the most important of the pelvic measurements.

The *anatomical* or *true conjugate* is measured from the promontory of the sacrum to the centre of the upper surface of the symphysis pubis. It is slightly longer than the obstetric conjugate but the extra space is not available for the passage of the fetus.

Right and left oblique diameters The right oblique passes from the right sacroiliac joint to the left iliopectineal eminence and the left oblique extends from the left sacroiliac joint to the right iliopectineal eminence. Each measures about 12 cm.

Transverse diameter This is between the widest points on the iliopectineal lines and measures 13 cm.

Sacrocotyloid diameter This is from the sacral promontory to the iliopectineal eminence on the same side; it measures 9 cm.

Diagonal conjugate This is measured from the

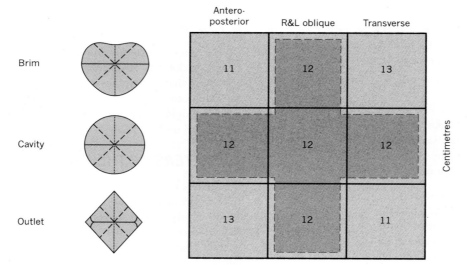

Figure 5   The pelvic measurements.

apex of the pubic arch to the sacral promontory. It measures about 1.25 cm more than the obstetric conjugate (12.25 cm). In a small pelvis where the measurement is less than 12 cm it can be assessed vaginally as the examining fingers are likely to come into contact with the bony promontory.

The pelvic brim is thus smaller from back to front than from side to side.

Diameters of the cavity

At a level half way between the brim above and the outlet below, the cavity is almost circular. The diameters, similar in direction to those of the brim, are again the anteroposterior, the right and left obliques and the transverse. All measure approximately 12 cm.

Diameters of the outlet

The anteroposterior diameter extends from the sacrococcygeal joint to the lower border of the symphysis pubis and measures 13 cm. The oblique diameters pass obliquely forwards from the sacrospinous ligaments and thus cannot be accurately measured. They are about 12 cm. The transverse diameter of the outlet, between the ischial spines, measures 10.5–11 cm.

The outlet is thus slightly smaller than the brim, but it is very unusual for a fetal head to pass through the brim and then be unable to pass through the outlet.

The outlet is clearly wider from front to back and

narrower from side to side. It is thus not surprising that the fetal head commonly enters the pelvis with its long diameter transversely across the brim, rotates in the cavity and emerges from the outlet with its long diameter anteroposterior.

AXIS OF THE BIRTH CANAL

The axis of the birth canal describes the direction in which the fetus moves in order to pass through the pelvis:

▶ An axis is a line passing through the centre of a plane.
▶ A plane is an imaginary flat surface.

Plane of the brim

When a woman stands erect the pelvis slopes quite steeply. The anterior superior iliac spines are in the same plane as the symphysis pubis. We describe the plane of the pelvic brim as sloping at an angle of 55° to the horizontal (Figure 6). The axis of the brim is thus directed backward and downward. This is the direction in which the fetal head moves in order to enter the pelvic brim.

Plane of the cavity

This plane lies across the mid-point of the sacrum and pubic bone.

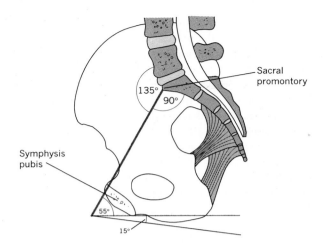

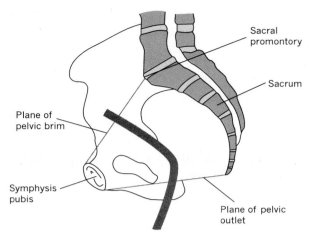

Figure 6 The pelvis, showing the degrees of inclination: inclination of the pelvic brim to the horizontal, 55°; inclination of pelvic outlet to the horizontal, 15°; angle of pelvic inclination, 135°; inclination of the sacrum, 90°.

Plane of the outlet

This slopes at an angle of 15° and is almost horizontal.

The fetal head follows the axis of each plane. It descends in a straight line through the plane of the brim and the plane of the cavity until it reaches the level of the ischial spines; here it is deflected by the pelvic floor and its course changed from downwards and backwards to downwards and forwards. The marked bend is known as the *axis of the birth canal* or the *curve of Carus* (Figures 7 and 8).

The axis of the birth canal needs to be kept in mind for the intelligent conduct of almost any obstetric

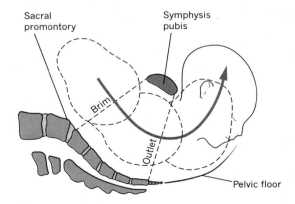

Figure 7 The axis of the birth canal.

Figure 8 The curve of the birth canal.

procedure, e.g. observation of engagement of the fetal head or testing its ability to engage; observation of progress in labour, by abdominal and vaginal examination; expulsion of the placenta, either by fundal pressure or by cord traction; and by the obstetrician when applying forceps.

ANGLES OF THE PELVIS

Angle of pelvic inclination

This is the angle between the plane of the brim and the anterior surface of the fifth lumbar vertebra. It is usually about 135°.

Sacral angle

This is the angle between the plane of the brim and the anterior surface of the first sacral vertebra. It usually measures about 90° and gives some indication of the size of the cavity in relation to the brim. If the angle is less than 90° the cavity is smaller than the brim, whereas if it is more than 90° the cavity is larger.

Subpubic angle

This is the angle between the two inferior pubic rami which form the pubic arch. In a good gynaecoid pelvis it should be 90° or more.

Angle of inclination of the pelvic brim

This is the angle the plane of the pelvic brim makes with the horizontal when the woman is in a standing position. It is about 55°. When the angle is greater than

55° there may be delay in engagement of the head in labour. This occurs quite commonly in some African races.

Angle of inclination of the pelvic outlet

This is the angle the upper border of the obstetric outlet makes with the horizontal when in a standing position. It is about 15°.

COMPARISON OF THE MALE WITH THE FEMALE PELVIS

In the female (Figure 9):

▶ Bones are lighter and smoother.
▶ Brim is rounded.
▶ Cavity is shallower and more capacious.
▶ Outlet is larger.
▶ Sacrosciatic notch is wider.
▶ Acetabula are further apart.
▶ Pubic arch is wider.
▶ Sacrum is wider and more curved.

VARIATIONS IN THE SHAPE OF THE PELVIS

Many variations have been reported in the shape and size of the bony pelvis in different study populations. From these findings, numerous overlapping classifications have been adopted and racial, sexual, hormonal and nutritional factors have been suggested to explain the predominance of particular pelvic types in different social groups. Before the advent of X-ray pelvimetry in the 1920s, most studies were carried out on dried pelves, using collections obtained by museums and departments of anatomy. The resulting classifications were presented without any data on the physique,

health or socio-economic status of the study population from which the pelves were derived.

Subsequent studies using X-ray pelvimetry gained more accurate data on pelvic dimensions (Caldwell *et al.*, 1940). Of these, comparative studies on different socio-economic groups began to identify long-term nutrition as a key determinant of the shape and size of the pelvis. In the 1950s, a study was done to compare the pelvic shapes of male medical and female nursing students with those of ward patients attending a public hospital in the United States. Data were categorized as a relative distribution of four different shapes of the pelvic brim, classified as 'elongated', 'round', 'oval' and 'flat'. Male and female students displayed a similar predominance of 'elongated' and 'round' brims, while ward patients displayed a much lower incidence of 'elongated' brims and a higher incidence of the more abnormal 'oval' and 'flat' shaped brims.

While no systematic data were included on the height and physique of the different groups, the pattern of difference in pelvic shape was thought to arise from the superior nutrition and health of students, compared to those unable to afford private medical care.

These results were confirmed and extended in a prospective study of women who gave birth in Aberdeen Maternity Hospital from 1948 to 1953. In this detailed study, data were collected on the height, physique, general health, pelvic shape and social class background of the women involved. A much higher proportion of 'flat' shaped brims were found among women of short stature whose partners were largely classified as unskilled labourers. In contrast, a predominance of 'round' shaped brims were found in taller women whose partners were classified into higher socio-economic groups.

When these results were obtained, further data were

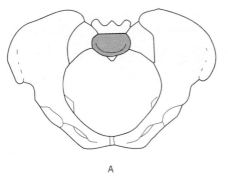

A   B

Figure 9 **A**: The female pelvis. **B**: The male pelvis.

collected to compare the pelvic shapes of men and women of average and below average height. Male medical students of average height displayed an equal predominance of 'round' shaped pelvic brims, to women of comparable height and similar social class background. In contrast, 'flat' and 'shield-shaped' pelvic brims were found to be most common in men and women of below average height from lower socioeconomic groups. Taken together, these findings indicate that long-term nutrition, rather than genetic or hormonal factors, strongly influences pelvic shape in adult life. In the latter study of men and women from a single urban setting, flatter pelves were largely associated with those of shorter stature who were found to have reduced intakes of calcium, vitamin D and protein during childhood.

In developing countries pelvic contraction resulting in cephalopelvic disproportion often leads to obstructed labour. It usually results from stunted growth of women due to malnutrition and untreated infection in childhood and adolescence (Kwast, 1992).

The four shapes of the pelvic brim are described as follows (Figure 10):

1 Gynaecoid, i.e. round.
2 Anthropoid, i.e. elongated.
3 Android, i.e. oval.
4 Platypelloid, i.e. flat.

Gynaecoid pelvis

This is the normal female pelvis. Over 50% of the patients examined by Caldwell *et al.* (1940) had a pelvis of this type.

In the gynaecoid pelvis (Figure 10):

▶ The brim is round in shape.
▶ The pelvis is shallow.

▶ The subpubic angle is wide, 90° or more.
▶ The sacrosciatic notch is wide.
▶ The transverse diameter of the outlet is 10 cm at least.

During labour, the head engages in the brim of the pelvis in the transverse diameter or in an occipitoanterior position and the mechanism of labour is normal.

Anthropoid pelvis

This type of pelvis resembles the pelvis of the ape. An alternative name is the *pithecoid pelvis*. (Anthropoid means man-like, pithecoid means ape-like.) This type was found in about 25% of those examined by Caldwell *et al.* (1940).

In the anthropoid pelvis (Figure 10):

▶ The brim is oval in shape, with an increase in the anteroposterior diameter and a corresponding decrease in the transverse diameter.
▶ The sacrum is long and narrow and may contain six vertebrae from fusion of the fifth lumbar vertebra with the sacrum. This increases the inclination of the pelvic brim and is called high assimilation. It tends to hinder engagement of the fetal head.

During labour, the head may engage in the anteroposterior diameter, sometimes with the occiput posterior. The head may descend through the pelvis persistently occipitoposterior and be born face-to-pubes. This pelvic shape has been noted in unusually tall, well-built women. Generally the pelvis is so large that labour is easy.

Android pelvis

This type of pelvis resembles the male pelvis and was found in about 20% of those examined by Caldwell *et al.* (1940).

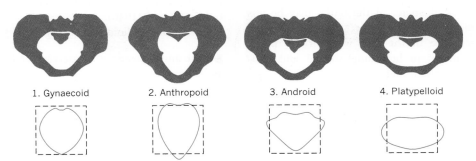

1. Gynaecoid   2. Anthropoid   3. Android   4. Platypelloid

Figure 10 Shapes of the pelvic brim.

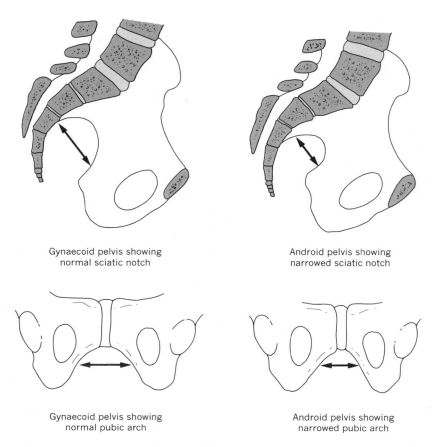

Gynaecoid pelvis showing
normal sciatic notch

Android pelvis showing
narrowed sciatic notch

Gynaecoid pelvis showing
normal pubic arch

Android pelvis showing
narrowed pubic arch

Figure 11 Comparison between a normal (gynaecoid) pelvis and an android pelvis. An android pelvis has a narrower outlet because of the narrow sciatic notch and pubic arch.

In the android pelvis (Figures 10 and 11):

▶ The brim tends to be triangular in shape, being broader at the back.
▶ The true pelvis is deep.
▶ The sacrum is straight.
▶ The subpubic angle is narrow, 60–75°.
▶ The sacrosciatic notch is narrow.
▶ The transverse diameter of the outlet may be less than 10 cm.
▶ The convergence of the side walls of the pelvis causes the pelvis to be funnel-shaped and con-tracted towards the outlet.

During labour, the available space in the forepelvis is restricted by the triangular shape of the brim. The head may engage transversely or in an occipitoposterior position. The descent of the head through the pelvis may be increasingly difficult because of the flat sacrum and outlet contraction; deep transverse arrest is likely.

Owing to the narrow subpubic angle the head is forced backwards and severe lacerations of the perineum may occur.

Platypelloid pelvis

This pelvis corresponds to the simple flat pelvis. It is rare, being found in less than 5% of those examined by Caldwell *et al.* (1940).

In the platypelloid pelvis (Figure 10):

▶ The anteroposterior diameter is short.
▶ The sacrosciatic notch is narrow.
▶ The anterposterior narrowing of the pelvis con-tinues in the cavity and outlet.

During labour, the head will engage in the transverse diameter of the brim. Rotation of the head may be restricted and deep transverse arrest of the head may occur.

CONTRACTION OF THE PELVIS

A contracted pelvis is one in which one or more diameters are so reduced as to interfere with the normal mechanism of labour. The diameter(s) may be reduced by 1 cm or more.

Types of contracted pelvis

Types of contracted pelvis include:

▶ *Rachitic flat.*
▶ *Generally contracted.*
▶ *Asymmetrical* – either associated with disease of the hip or spine, or Naegele's.

Other rare pelvic abnormalities include:

▶ Osteomalacia.
▶ Spondylolisthesis.
▶ Robert's pelvis.

Rachitic flat pelvis This pelvic deformity (Figure 12) is caused by rickets affecting a child in the second year of life. The softened bones are distorted by the weight of the body as the child sits, since walking will be delayed by the disease. The promontory of the sacrum is forced forwards towards the symphysis pubis, producing a flattened or kidney-shaped brim. The lower end of the sacrum swings backwards so that the size of the cavity and outlet is increased.

Rickets was at one time the commonest cause of gross pelvic deformity and difficult and obstructed labour, but the disease has now almost disappeared in developed countries, with the adequate diet and the addition of vitamin D for babies and children.

Effect on labour The head enters the brim with the sagittal suture in the transverse diameter. The head is incompletely flexed.

The head moves to one side of the pelvis so that the smallest diameter of the head (the bitemporal) (8 cm) can occupy the smallest diameter of the brim.

Asynclitism occurs. The head tilts sideways so that a parietal bone enters the pelvic brim; this tilt is corrected as the head enters the cavity. If the anterior parietal bone enters first with the sagittal suture lying near the sacral promontory this is called *anterior asynclitism* or *anterior parietal presentation*. If the posterior parietal presents with the sagittal suture nearer the symphysis pubis this is *posterior asynclitism* or *posterior parietal presentation* (Figure 13).

In either case given strong uterine contractions and moulding of the head by these movements the head may pass through the brim. Vaginal delivery is then possible.

Generally contracted pelvis A pelvis small in all its diameters but normal in shape may occur in women of small stature. It may be called a *justominor pelvis*. Sometimes there are in addition android characteristics, making the outlet relatively narrow.

Effect on labour If the size of the fetus is in proportion to the size of the pelvis no difficulty may be encountered. If the fetus is larger, with strong contractions, complete flexion of the head and moulding, the head may pass through the brim, but difficulty may still be encountered at the outlet. If the true conjugate is less than 8.75 cm vaginal delivery is unlikely.

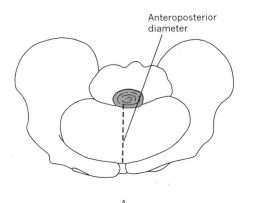

A

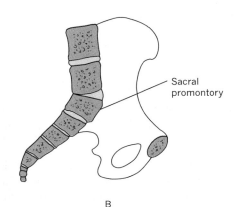

B

Figure 12 A rachitic flat pelvis. **A**: Reduced anteroposterior diameter; widened and irregular transverse diameter. **B**: Sacral promontory pushed forwards and downwards; sacrum pushed backwards.

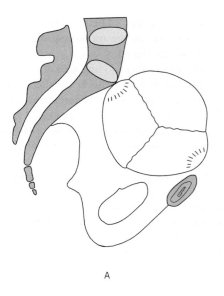 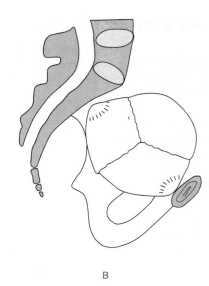

A   B

Figure 13   Posterior asynclitism.

Asymmetrical pelvis   If unequal pressure is exerted on the pelvis whilst it is growing it may become asymmetrical. This may occur in congenital dislocation of one hip or following poliomyelitis or an accident.

Deficient development of one side of the pelvis, often with bony fusion of the sacroiliac joint on the affected side, causes a rare form of asymmetrical pelvis. This is called *Naegele's pelvis*.

Robert's pelvis   In this condition there is deficient development of both sides of the pelvis with fusion of both sacroiliac joints. This may produce extreme pelvic contraction. It is extremely rare.

Osteomalacic pelvis   Osteomalacia is a disease of adults produced by deficient diet, lack of vitamin D and sunlight, as is rickets in childhood. It is rare in the UK but sometimes occurs in Asian women who do not expose their skin to sunlight. The pelvic deformity differs from that occurring in rickets because the adult walks and stands. The upward pressure of the legs on the pelvis forces the sides of the pelvis inwards. The weight of the body acting through the spine forces the promontory of the sacrum forwards. This produces the triradiate pelvis. The pelvic contraction may be very severe. In some parts of the developing world where osteomalacia is endemic it may produce secondary pelvic deformities in women who have had successful previous deliveries (Kwast, 1992).

Spondylolisthetic pelvis   In this condition the fifth lumbar vertebra slips forwards over the sacrum. It may produce extreme contraction of the true conjugate.

Detection of pelvic contraction and disproportion

Although the recognition of pelvic contraction is important, it is yet more vital to discover disproportion; that is, disparity in size between the fetus and the pelvis. If the head of the fetus has entered, or can be made to enter, the pelvic brim, vaginal delivery should be possible. The statement that the head of the fetus is the best pelvimeter will always be true.

It is possible that disproportion is present if:

▶ in a primigravida the head is not engaged and cannot be made to engage after the 37th week;
▶ in a multipara there is a history of difficult labour, forceps delivery or stillbirth.

In these circumstances the midwife should refer the woman to a doctor for further advice. A clinical examination of the pelvis will be made to determine its size and shape.

Possible outcome of labour with pelvic contraction

The outcome of labour cannot be estimated solely on the size and shape of the pelvis. The size of the fetus, the strength of the uterine contractions, the degree of moulding and flexion of the head and the position of the head will all influence labour. Normal delivery will be less likely if the fetus is large, the uterine contractions poor or the position occipitoposterior.

It is possible to subdivide cases of pelvic contraction into three groups according to the size of the true conjugate:

1 *Slight pelvic contraction*: The true conjugate is over 9.5 cm. Vaginal delivery is likely.
2 *Gross pelvic contraction*: The true conjugate is less then 8.5 cm. The delivery of a living child of normal weight at term is not usually possible. A Caesarean section at or near term and before the onset of labour is advisable.
3 *Moderate pelvic contraction*: The true conjugate is between 8.5 and 9.5 cm. With strong uterine contractions and adequate moulding of the head, vaginal delivery may be possible but, because the course of labour cannot be determined beforehand, a trial of labour is conducted.

Three possible outcomes may occur:

▶ spontaneous vaginal delivery;
▶ delay in the second stage necessitating a forceps delivery;
▶ Caesarean section if the head fails to enter the pelvis.

References

Borell, V. & Fernström, I. (1957) The movements of the sacro-iliac joints and their importance to changes in the pelvic dimensions during parturition. *Acta Obstet. Gynecol. Scand.* **36**: 42.

Caldwell, W.E., Moloy, H.C. & D'Esopo, D.A. (1940) The more recent conceptions of the pelvic architecture. *Am. J. Obstet. Gynecol.* **40**: 558.

Joseph, J. (1988) The joints of the pelvis and their relation to posture in labour. *Midwives Chronicle* March: 63–64.

Kwast, B.E. (1992) Obstructed labour: its contribution to maternal mortality. *Midwifery* 8(1): 3–7.

3

The Female Reproductive System

The female genital tract includes the *external genitalia*, collectively termed the vulva, and the *internal genitalia*, namely the vagina, the uterus, the uterine (or fallopian) tubes and the ovaries. This chapter includes the anatomy of the external genitalia, the vagina and the uterus. The anatomy of the uterine tubes can be found in Chapter 7 and the anatomy of the ovaries can be found in Chapter 5.

External Genitalia

The external genitalia (Figure 1) or vulva extend from the mons veneris anteriorly to the perineal body posteriorly.

Mons veneris (mount of Venus)
This pad of fat lies over the body of the pubic bone and is covered by skin and, after puberty, by hair.

Labia majora
The labia majora (singular, labium majus) are two thick folds of fatty tissue covered externally by skin, extending backwards from the mons veneris to the perineal area where they merge with the perineal body. The outer surface is covered with hair and the inner surface is smooth and contains sebaceous glands.

Labia minora
The labia minora (singular, labium minus) are two small folds of skin lying between and almost covered by the labia majora. They are smooth and contain a few sweat and sebaceous glands. Anteriorly they encircle the clitoris forming an upper fold, the *prepuce* or hood of the clitoris, and a small lower fold, the *frenulum*. They then divide to enclose the vestibule and, posteriorly, unite at a thin fold of skin, the *fourchette*. This is commonly torn at the birth of the first baby.

Clitoris
The clitoris is a highly sensitive, erectile structure about 2.5 cm long, situated at the anterior junction of the labia minora. It consists of two erectile bodies, the *corpora cavernosa*, which are connected to the underlying pubic bone. The anterior surface, known as the *glans clitoris*, consists of spongy, erectile tissue, similar to that of the male penis, which, in response to stimulation, becomes erect and fills with blood.

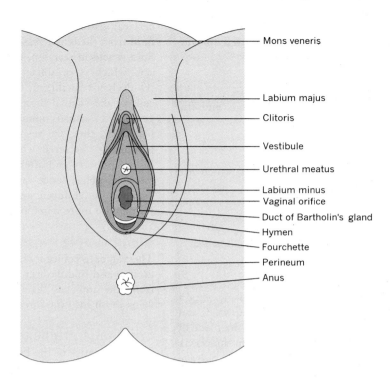

Mons veneris

Labium majus

Clitoris

Vestibule

Urethral meatus

Labium minus

Vaginal orifice

Duct of Bartholin's gland

Hymen

Fourchette

Perineum

Anus

Figure 1   The external genitalia.

Vestibule

The vestibule is the narrow space which is brought into view when the labia minora are separated. It contains the openings of the urethra and the vagina.

Urethral meatus

The meatus is a small opening about 2.5 cm below the clitoris. From here the *urethral canal* passes upwards and backwards about 3.5 cm to the neck of the bladder. To the side and slightly behind the urethral meatus are two small openings, the orifices of *Skene's ducts* from corresponding sebaecous glands. They appear as small dimples with the meatus, which has slightly raised margins, between them. A clear knowledge of these anatomical features will help the midwife in carrying out catheterization accurately and with a minimum risk of infection.

Vaginal orifice or introitus

The introitus lies betwen the labia minora and posterior to the urethra. It is partially occluded by the hymen.

Hymen

A thin membrane, the hymen, partially shuts off the vaginal introitus. In the virgin it is described as intact, having only a small opening through which the menstrual flow escapes; on the occasion of first intercourse it is ruptured and at the birth of the first child it is torn further, leaving a few tags of tissue, the *carunculae myrtiformes*, surrounding the introitus.

Bartholin's glands

These small glands lie one on either side of, and slightly posterior to, the vagina, beneath the labia. Their ducts open into the vaginal canal just external to the hymen and their secretion of mucus, together with that from Skene's glands, helps to lubricate the vulva. The secretions from both Skene's and Bartholin's glands greatly increase in response to erection of the clitoris, thereby acting as a lubricant for the external genitalia and facilitating intercourse.

Blood supply

The vulva receives its blood supply from the internal, superficial external and deep external *pudendal arteries*.

It is a very vascular structure and therefore tends to bleed heavily when lacerated, but heals well for the same reason.

Lymphatic drainage
Lymph drainage is into the inguinal glands and the external iliac glands.

Nerve supply
This is largely from the pudendal nerves which are branches of the sacral plexus.

Internal Genitalia

VAGINA

The vagina is named from the Latin word meaning a sheath. It is a fibromuscular tube directed upwards and backwards and is approximately parallel to the plane of the pelvic brim. It extends from the vulva to the cervix and is capable of great distension to allow the passage of the fetus during childbirth. The walls of the vagina normally lie in apposition except at the upper end where the cervix projects into the vagina almost at right angles, forming four recesses or *fornices*. The anterior fornix is shallow, the two lateral fornices are rather deeper and the posterior fornix is deep. Thus the anterior vaginal wall, which is 7.5 cm long, is shorter than the posterior wall, which measures about 10 cm. The lower part of the vagina is the introitus which is partially closed by the hymen in the virgin.

Structure
The wall of the vagina has four layers:

1   an inner layer of squamous epithelium which is arranged in transverse folds, known as *rugae*: this concertina-like lining allows the vagina to undergo a tremendous degree of stretching, as it must during labour to allow the passage of the fetus;
2   a vascular layer of elastic connective tissue;
3   an involuntary muscle layer consisting of outer longitudinal fibres and inner circular fibres; and
4   an outer layer of connective tissue which is part of the pelvic fascia, and which carries blood vessels, lymphatics and nerves.

The vagina has no glands, but its walls are maintained in a moist state partly by secretions from the cervical glands and partly by a transudation of serous fluid from the blood vessels to the surface. This vaginal fluid is acid in reaction, pH 4.5, since it contains lactic acid which is produced by the action of lactobacilli (Döderlein's bacilli) on the glycogen in the squamous cells of the vaginal lining. Lactobacilli are non-pathogenic and normally inhabit the vagina. The lactic acid for which they are responsible helps to destroy any pathogenic bacteria which may enter the vagina. Before puberty and after the menopause the vagina is less acid, pH 7; hence vaginal infections such as vulvo-vaginitis in children and senile vaginitis in elderly women are more common.

Blood supply
The vagina receives its blood supply from the vaginal, uterine and middle haemorrhoidal arteries which arise from the internal iliac arteries. The corresponding veins drain into the internal iliac veins.

Lymphatic drainage
The lymphatics of the lowest third of the vagina drain into the inguinal glands and those of the upper two-thirds into the internal iliac glands.

Nerve supply
Sympathetic and parasympathetic nerves from the plexus of Lee–Frankenhäuser supply the vagina. This plexus lies in the floor of the pouch of Douglas, in the region of the uterosacral ligaments. It receives branches of the second, third and fourth sacral nerves which are then distributed to the pelvic organs.

Anatomical relations

Anteriorly	Upper half	Bladder
	Lower half	Urethra
Posteriorly	Upper third	Pouch of Douglas
	Middle third	Rectum
	Lower third	Perineal body
Superiorly	Centrally	Cervix
	Above lateral	Fornices
		Ureters and uterine arteries
Inferiorly	Vaginal orifice and vestibule	
Laterally	Upper	Parametrium
	Middle	Pubococcygeus muscles
	Lower	Perineal muscle Bulbocavernosus muscles

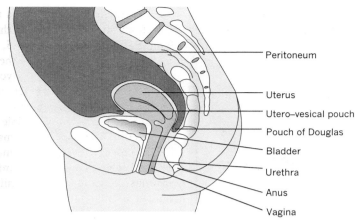

Figure 2 The pelvic organs in sagittal section.

A clear knowledge of the vagina and the adjacent structures is absolutely essential to the intelligent conduct of any midwifery procedure. Obvious examples are vaginal examinations and the conduct of deliveries.

UTERUS

The uterus is a hollow, pear-shaped, muscular organ situated in the pelvic cavity between the bladder and the rectum (Figure 2). It is anteverted, that is tilted forwards, and anteflexed, that is curved forwards on itself from the level of the internal os (Figure 3). It is 7.5 cm long, 5 cm broad at its upper part and 2.5 cm thick and weighs about 60 g. The narrow end of the uterus is inserted into the vagina, while the upper part communicates with the uterine tubes which enter one on either side (Figure 4).

Functions

The functions of the uterus are:

1 to prepare to receive the fertilized ovum;
2 to provide a suitable environment for the growth and development of the fetus throughout pregnancy; and
3 to assist in the expulsion of the fetus, placenta and membranes at term.

Structure

The uterus consists of two parts; the body or corpus, and the cervix or neck.

Body The body is the upper two-thirds of the uterus and is about 5 cm long. The cavity of the body is triangular in shape, with the apex of the triangle directed towards the cervix. The *fundus* is the upper, rounded part which lies above the insertion of the two uterine (fallopian) tubes. The upper, lateral margins where the uterine tubes enter the uterus are called the *cornua*. The *isthmus* is a slightly constricted area, approximately 7 mm long, situated at the junction of the body and cervix. During pregnancy it enlarges to form the lower uterine segment.

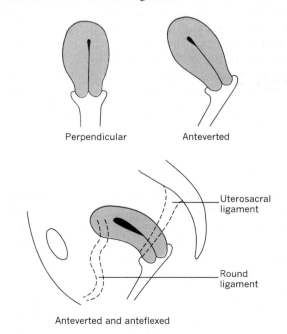

Figure 3 How the normal position of the uterus is achieved.

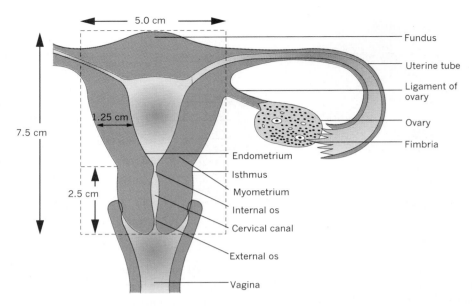

Figure 4 The uterus and the left uterine tube and ovary.

Cervix The cervix is the lowest third of the uterus and is 2.5 cm long. It is cylindrical in shape and the lower half projects at right angles into the vagina. The cavity is a spindle-shaped canal and communicates with the cavity of the body of the uterus by the *internal os* and with the vagina by the *external os*.

Uterine wall The uterine wall consists of three layers: the inner layer of *endometrium*; the middle, muscular layer called the *myometrium*; and the outer covering of peritoneum called the *perimetrium*. The endometrium of the uterus differs from that of the cervix.

Corporeal endometrium During the reproductive years the corporeal endometrium is constantly changing as its thickness and vascularity vary according to the phases of the menstrual cycle. The superficial layers are shed during the actual process of menstruation and a new endometrium is formed from the basal layer which remains unchanged throughout the cycle.

The endometrium is composed of vascular connective tissue called *stroma*, which contains many tubular glands. The stroma is covered by a layer of ciliated columnar epithelium and non-ciliated cells dip down into the stroma to the level of the myometrium to form the glands. These mucus-secreting glands open into the cavity of the uterus.

Cervical endometrium The cervical endometrium changes little during the menstrual cycle and is not shed during the process of menstruation. It is known as the *arbor vitae*, the tree of life, because it is arranged in deep folds anteriorly and posteriorly, resembling the trunk of a tree, with branches radiating off on each side. This formation is thought to facilitate the passage of the spermatozoa through the cervical canal. The upper two-thirds of the canal is lined by columnar epithelium containing deep branching glands. These are known as *compound racemose glands* and their function is to secrete an alkaline mucus. This mucus is thin at the time of ovulation to allow the spermatozoa to pass easily through the cervical canal into the uterus. A few days later it becomes thick and forms a plug in the cervical canal to prevent infection entering the uterus. If pregnancy does not occur the mucoid plug is shed.

The lower third of the cervical canal and the vaginal aspect of the cervix is covered with stratified squamous epithelium continuous with that of the vagina. It is at this *squamo-columnar junction* that carcinoma is most likely to occur.

Myometrium The myometrium is composed of plain muscle fibres (Figure 5), and forms seven-eighths of the thickness of the uterine wall. The muscle is arranged in a spiral form running from the cornua to the cervix, giving a circular effect around the uterine

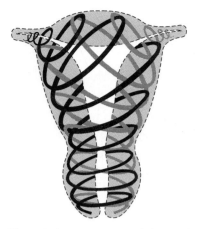

Figure 5   The spiral arrangement of the uterine muscle fibres.

(fallopian) tubes and cervix and an oblique effect over the body of the uterus. In the non-pregnant state the muscle layers are not clearly defined, but during pregnancy the myometrium becomes thicker and can be differentiated into three layers. The inner circular fibres are found mostly in the cornua and around the cervix. The middle layer of interlacing spiral fibres is thickest in the upper part of the body where the placenta is normally situated in pregnancy. The fibres contract powerfully and act as natural ligatures to the blood vessels when the placenta separates from the uterine wall in the third stage of labour. The outer layer (Figure 6) consists of longitudinal muscle fibres which extend from the cervix anteriorly, over the fundus of the uterus to the cervix posteriorly. These fibres shorten in labour when the uterus contracts and retracts, thereby facilitating the descent and expulsion of the fetus and the placenta and membranes.

Perimetrium The perimetrium is a layer of peritoneum which is draped over the uterus and uterine tubes. Anteriorly it covers the body of the uterus and is then reflected loosely on to the bladder at the level of the internal os. Posteriorly it covers the uterus and the upper third of the vagina and is then reflected back to form the pouch of Douglas. A loose double fold of perimetrium extends from the lateral borders of the uterus to the side walls of the pelvis. This is called the *broad ligament*.

Uterine ligaments

The uterus is held in its normal position of anteversion and anteflexion by the uterine ligaments (Figure 7):

1   The two *transverse cervical ligaments*, also known as the cardinal ligaments, extend from the cervix laterally to the side walls of the pelvis. These ligaments form an important support to the uterus and, if overstretched, will cause the uterus to prolapse.
2   The two *uterosacral ligaments* pass backwards from the cervix to the sacrum, encircling the rectum. These ligaments help to maintain the uterus in a position of anteversion.
3   The two *pubocervical ligaments* pass forwards from the cervix to the pubic bones. They give little support to the uterus.
4   The two *round ligaments* arise at the cornua of the uterus and descend through the broad ligament and inguinal canals to the labia majora. They help to hold the uterus in a position of anteversion.

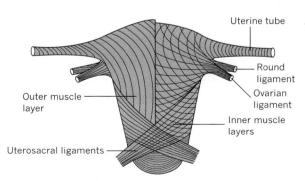

Figure 6   The outer and inner layers of uterine muscle.

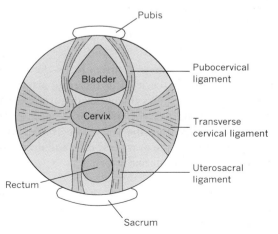

Figure 7   The uterine supports seen from above.

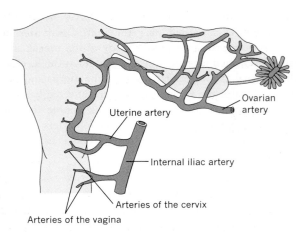

Figure 8   The blood supply to the uterus and its appendages.

5   The *broad ligament* is a double fold of peritoneum extending from the lateral borders of the uterus to the side walls of the pelvis.

Blood supply

The blood supply to the uterus (Figures 8 and 9) is derived from two pairs of arteries: the uterine and ovarian arteries.

Uterine artery   This is a branch of the internal iliac artery. It runs downwards and forwards until it reaches the parametrium where it turns inwards towards the uterus. It enters at the level of the internal os, then turns upwards at right angles and follows a spiral course along the lateral border of the uterus to anastomose with the ovarian artery. The uterine artery sends a descending branch to the cervix and vagina.

Ovarian artery   The ovarian artery leaves the abdominal aorta just below the level of the renal arteries. It passes downwards to cross the ureter then the external iliac artery passing over the pelvic brim to enter the broad ligament just below the ovary. The ovarian artery gives off branches to the ovary and tube and eventually anastomoses with the uterine artery.

Venous drainage   Blood is drained by veins accompanying the arteries. The right ovarian vein passes into the inferior vena cava and the left into the left renal vein, a distinction of some importance to the surgeon.

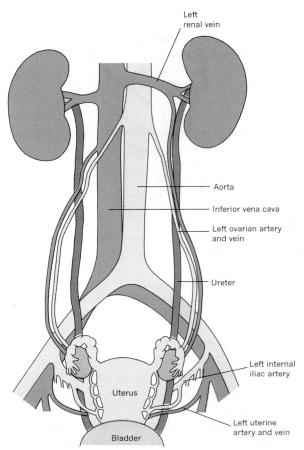

Figure 9   The blood supply to the uterus. Note where the ovarian vein terminates.

The arteries and veins of the uterus are twisted like a corkscrew. This tortuosity is lost as the uterus enlarges during pregnancy, to reform after delivery. This assists in the control of bleeding and the prevention of haemorrhage.

Lymphatic drainage

The lymphatic vessels and nodes drain off lymph from the pelvic organs. These vessels accompany the main arteries and veins, and nodes are found along the iliac vessels and aorta. Drainage from the upper portion of the uterus is to the lumbar and hypogastric nodes. From the lower portion drainage is to the hypogastric nodes.

Nerve supply

Sympathetic nerve supply   The sympathetic nerve supply to the pelvis is a continuation of a large abdominal plexus, the aortic plexus, which is continued below the level of the bifurcation of the aorta as a large network sometimes called the 'presacral nerve', lying in front of the fifth lumbar vertebra and sacral promontory. Joined by branches from the lumbar sympathetic chain, it passes downwards dividing into two branches terminating in plexuses lying on the floor of the pouch of Douglas. This network also receives fibres from the parasympathetic system and is known as the *Lee–Frankenhäuser plexus*. From here nerves pass to the uterus and other pelvic viscera.

Parasympathetic nerve supply   The parasympathetic nerves arise from the second, third and fourth sacral segments and emerge from the sacral foramina to join the plexus of Lee–Frankenhäuser.

The Menstrual Cycle

The lining of the uterus is constantly changed throughout a woman's reproductive life and, unless pregnancy occurs, is shed each menstrual cycle. These changes are under the influence of the pituitary and ovarian hormones, which are described in Chapter 6.

When menstruation occurs the endometrium is shed down to its basal layer accompanied by bleeding. Under the influence of oestrogen regeneration begins and the endometrium grows thicker. This is the proliferative phase and lasts about 10 days. Following ovulation and the production of progesterone the endometrium becomes even thicker, the glands more tortuous and full of secretions. This is the secretory phase and lasts 14 days, after which the lining is shed once more. The endometrium above the basal layer degenerates, owing to spasm in the arteries and deprivation of blood flow; necrosis occurs and the lining sloughs off to be expelled from the uterus by muscular contraction. The menstrual flow continues for about five days and the blood loss is some 50–100 ml.

The phases which are passed through by the endometrium during the 28 days of each complete cycle are as follows:

1   *Proliferative* (10 days or more): The endometrium grows thicker and the glands lengthen under the influence of oestrogens (follicular hormones).
2   *Secretory* (14 days): The glands become tortuous and produce secretion under the influence of oestrogens and progesterone (corpus luteum hormones).
3   *Menstrual* (4–6 days).

The menstrual cycle (Figure 10) recurs in most women every 28–30 days, but may vary from 21 to 42 days or more. The menstrual phase occurs 14 days after ovulation if fertilization has not occurred. In a prolonged cycle it is always the proliferative phase which is extended, not the secretory phase. The cycle continues from puberty to the menopause and in a healthy woman is interrupted only by pregnancy.

The menstrual cycle prepares the uterus for pregnancy. If conception occurs menstruation does not take place. If both ovaries are completely removed, menstruation ceases and pregnancy is impossible. Pregnancy is possible even with only a small part of one ovary.

Conception occurs shortly after ovulation, 14 days before the next period. Thus in a 35-day cycle, ovulation would occur 21 days after the period; in a 21-day cycle, only seven days after. If periods occur irregularly, the calculation of the date may prove inaccurate and in such a case more than usual care will be needed to check the date with other methods of ascertaining the expected date of confinement.

If, at the last menstrual period, the flow lasted only a few hours or one day, careful enquiries should be made before deciding on the date of expected delivery. It may be a case of 'decidual bleeding' from the lower part of the congested uterus, which is not entirely covered with the ovum until the third month of pregnancy. This slight bleeding occurs at the usual time of a menstrual period, but it should not be referred to as menstruation as it is not the result of the cycle of changes described above. It is probable that in most cases a slight loss of blood in early pregnancy is due to a threatened abortion.

The hormonal control of menstruation is described in detail in Chapter 6.

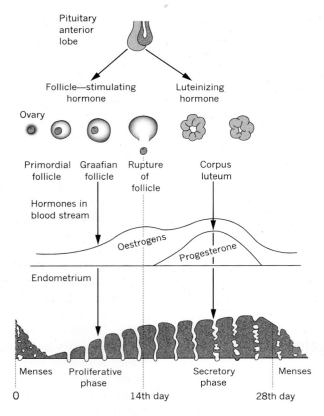

Figure 10   The menstrual cycle.

Further Reading

Anderson, M. (1979) *Anatomy and Physiology of Obstetrics*, 6th edn. London: Faber & Faber.

Armstrong, K.F. & Kidd, D.J. (1969) *Baillière's Atlas of Female Anatomy*, 7th edn. London: Baillière Tindall.

Carola, R., Harley, J.P. and Noback, C.R. (1992) *Human Anatomy and Physiology*. New York: McGraw-Hill.

Chiras, D.D. (1991) *Human Biology*. New York: West.

Johnson, M.H. and Everitt, B.J. (1995) *Essential Reproduction*. Oxford: Blackwell Scientific.

Miller, A.W.F. and Callander, R. (1989) *Obstetrics Illustrated*, 4th edn. Edinburgh: Churchill Livingstone.

Rhodes, P. (1979) *Reproductive Physiology for Medical Students*. Edinburgh: Churchill Livingstone.

Rickards, R. and Chapman, D.F. (1985) The human body and the reproductive system. *Anatomy and Physiology. A Self-instructional Course*, vol. 1, 2nd edn. Edinburgh: Churchill Livingstone.

Verralls, S. (1993) *Anatomy and Physiology Applied to Obstetrics*, 3rd edn. Edinburgh: Churchill Livingstone.

Weideger, P. (1978) *Female Cycles*. London: The Women's Press.

Williams, P.L., Warwick, R., Dyson, M. *et al.* (eds) (1989) *Gray's Anatomy*, 37th edn. Edinburgh: Churchill Livingstone.

Wilson, K.J.W. (ed.) (1990) *Ross and Wilson's Anatomy and Physiology in Health and Fitness*, 7th edn. Edinburgh: Churchill Livingstone.

4

Genetics

Genetics is a branch of biology and is concerned with two issues on inheritance traits:

1 how the traits of anatomy, physiology and behaviour are passed on to descendants; and
2 how an individual expresses those traits in their formation and throughout their life.

Individuals inherit characteristics from their genetic parents, including hair and eye colour, stature, familiar traits and susceptibility to genetic disease.

The pace of advance in our understanding of inherited traits and diseases is rapid and accelerating. These advances are making a considerable impact on the practice of obstetrics and midwifery, as elsewhere in clinical medicine. They are also making an economic impact on both developed and developing countries, both because a reduction in the incidence of inherited disease can allow the reallocation of substantial resources, and because enhanced understanding of genetic inheritance has the potential for altering the way medicine is conducted in the future, with a greater emphasis on prevention.

Initially a single cell, the fertilized ovum, contains all the inherited information which will determine the characteristics of the new individual, from the colour of hair and eyes to a possible inborn error of metabolism. The genetic material is mainly in the *cell nucleus* and is transmitted during cell division to all new cells. It is therefore present in every cell in the body. The cell nucleus contains *chromosomes*, which consist of long coils of *deoxyribonucleic acid (DNA)* in close contact with protein molecules. The *genes* are arranged in linear array along the chromosomes, with intervening sequences of uncertain function: they are responsible for virtually all inborn and inherited characteristics.

Each species has a specific number of chromosomes.

The cells of the human body carry 46; that is, 23 matching (*homologous*) pairs. Of these, 22 pairs (44 chromosomes) are similar in males and females and are called *autosomes*: the pairs are numbered by length, with chromosome 1 being the longest, and chromosome 22 being the shortest. The remaining pair are the *sex chromosomes*: in the female they consist of two X chromosomes whereas in the male there is one X and one much smaller chromosome called the Y chromosome.

Cell Division

There are two methods by which cells divide: *mitosis* and *meiosis*.

MITOSIS

Somatic cells (i.e. cells of the body) divide by a method of mitosis. This is a process by which cells repair and replace themselves. It maintains the total number of chromosomes (46) and creates an exact replica (Blackburn and Loper, 1992). Cells prepare for cell division by replicating their chromosomes, so that a cell at this stage has double the quantity of DNA found in a new cell that has just been produced. Each chromosome contracts into a dense body that is visible under the microscope, and splits lengthways to produce two identical daughter chromosomes. One new chromosome from each of the cell's 46 original chromosomes now moves to each of the two *daughter nuclei* that are being formed. The original cell is also dividing, and a nucleus is included in each of the two *daughter cells*. Each new cell has 46 chromosomes, just like the original cell (Figure 1).

MEIOSIS

Germ cells (i.e. reproductive cells or *gametes*) divide by meiosis. This is a process by which the number of chromosomes is reduced by half (23). Fertilization of an ovum by a sperm restores the cell to its full complement of 46 chromosomes (Blackburn and Loper, 1992). Meiosis consists of two nuclear divisions with only a single preparatory doubling of the genetic material. At the first meiotic division, the two members of each pair of homologous chromosomes separate into the two daughter cells. This is called a *reduction division*, because the chromosome number is reduced from 46

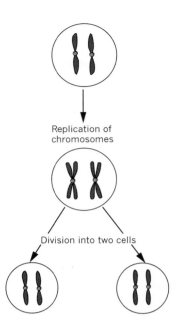

Replication of chromosomes

Division into two cells

Figure 1   In mitosis the cell splits into two genetically identical daughter cells, each of which has the same number of chromosomes as the original cell.

to 23 (i.e. the *haploid* number of chromosomes; see Figure 2). The normal cell is *diploid* – it has two of each type of chromosome. Very occasionally a child is born who is *triploid*, having three of each type of chromosome (69 in all).

The second meiotic division is just like a mitotic division, except that there are only 23 chromosomes to start with. In each cell, the 23 chromosomes split lengthways. The result is four daughter cells, each with 23 chromosomes (Figure 2). At fertilization, when ovum and spermatozoon fuse, the full diploid complement is restored.

It should be noted that meiosis differs in the two sexes, in that four spermatozoa are produced at each male meiosis, whereas only one ovum is produced by meiosis in the female. This is because the division of the cytoplasm is grossly unequal in the female, virtually all the cytoplasm being allotted to one of the four nuclei – the prospective ovum. In addition, meiosis is rapid in the male, but takes many years in the female: meiosis is begun in the female fetus, but is completed only shortly before each ovulation in the adult.

Meiosis differs from mitosis in another important respect, in that *crossing-over* can occur between chromosomes; this is not a regular feature of mitosis. Crossing-over results in a shuffling of the genes on a pair of

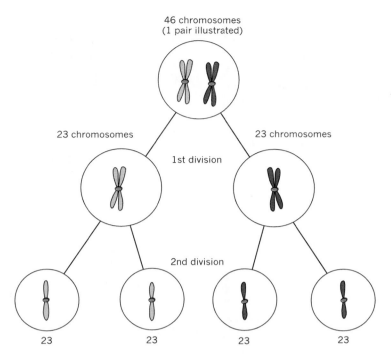

46 chromosomes
(1 pair illustrated)

23 chromosomes   23 chromosomes

1st division

2nd division

23   23   23   23

Figure 2   In meiosis the cell splits into four daughter cells, each having half the number of chromosomes as the original cell.

homologous chromosomes, so that the chromosome handed on to a child from one parent is neither the one received from the parent's mother nor the one from his/her father, but a reassortment of these (Figure 3). These recombination events can be seen under the microscope at times, and are called *chiasmata*.

Chromosomal Anomalies

The study of chromosomes is called *cytogenetics*. Chromosomes are usually studied in cells from the blood (lymphocytes), from biopsies of skin or muscle (fibroblasts), or from bone marrow. They may also be obtained from amniotic fluid or from chorionic villi, when fetal diagnosis is required. The cells are cultured

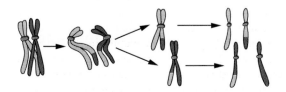

Figure 3   Crossover of genetic material during meiosis.

for some days, their cell divisions are synchronized, and then they are photographed when the chromosomes are at their most distinct. The picture of each chromosome is cut out of the photograph and matched with the other member of its pair. The process of examining the chromosomes in this way is referred to as *karyotyping* (Figure 4).

If there are too many or too few chromosomes, or there is some alteration in their structure, the pregnancy may result in abortion or an abnormal fetus. Approximately 15% of pregnancies terminate in spontaneous abortion, and about 50% of abortuses are chromosomally abnormal: nearly 7% of conceptions that implant are chromosomally abnormal.

Structural changes may result from the loss of a piece of chromosome: this is known as a *deletion*. When part of a chromosome breaks off and is added to another, it is called a *translocation*. If two chromosomes lose fragments which join back to the wrong chromosome, this is called a *reciprocal translocation*. The presence of three chromosomes of one type instead of the usual two is called *trisomy*; the presence of just one is called *monosomy*.

The commonest of the chromosomal anomalies at

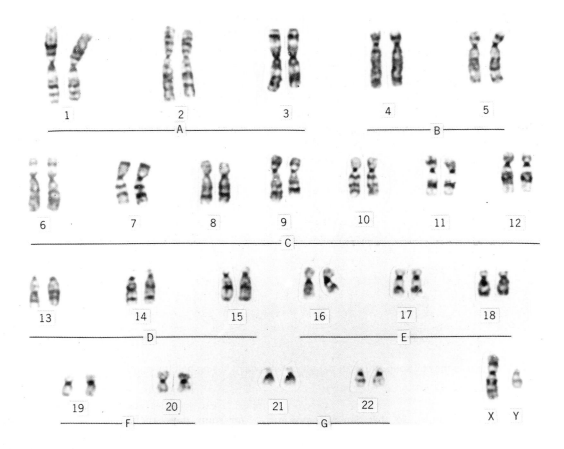

Figure 4   A normal karyotype.

birth is Down's syndrome, where there are 47 chromosomes instead of 46. This may be termed trisomy 21, because there are three of chromosome 21. The incidence is 1.5 per 1000 live births (about 1 in 650), and rises with maternal age (Harper, 1993). The risk to a woman of 44 is 25 per 1000 (1 in 34.8). Most children with Down's syndrome, however, are born to women under 30 years of age, simply because most women giving birth are aged less than 30.

A few children with Down's syndrome (1 in 20) have 46 separate chromosomes, because the extra chromosome 21 is joined to another chromosome as a translocation. In such cases, it is important to examine the parents' chromosomes because one of them may carry this translocated chromosome in a balanced fashion, having the correct amount of genetic material, but only 45 separate chromosomes, e.g. with the 21 translocated on to a chromosome 14, 22 or 21. Such a parent

is at especially high risk of having another child with Down's syndrome.

The other common chromosomal anomalies are of the sex chromosomes. 1.3% of implanted conceptions are thought to carry one X chromosome without a Y (monosomy X, Turner's syndrome). Very few of these fetuses survive to be born – about 0.4 per 1000 live-born girls. More common at birth are the other anomalies such as XXX (0.65 per 1000 girls), XXY and XYY (1.5 per 1000 boys) (Harper, 1993). These sex chromosome anomalies, however, produce fewer ill-effects than the autosomal anomalies.

Genes and Modes of Inheritance

Genetic information resides in the DNA within the cell nucleus and the genes themselves are arranged in a particular fixed manner on the chromosomes. These specific sequences of the chemical subunits (of genes) serve as the molecular code for the manufacture of particular amino acids into proteins. Any alteration of the DNA sequence may cause an abnormality or dysfunction of the resulting protein (Nairne, 1993).

Genes may be responsible, on an individual basis, for some traits and diseases, but it is now widely believed that they work together. It is therefore not only important to understand their particular role in inheritance, but also their location on the chromosomes and their relationship to other genes, as well as the sequence of their chemical subunits (Judson, 1993). Currently, there are numerous projects being conducted on an international basis to determine the entire map of the *human genome* (which is the collective term used to describe all the genes in the human cell). The Human Genome Projects hope to provide a complete picture of the structure, function and relationship of each gene (last estimated at some 50 000–100 000) or gene sequence within the next 5–10 years (Judson, 1993). The potential this knowledge promises cannot be fully appreciated yet, however it will add significantly to the current understanding of how genes are inherited from one generation to another.

Genetic disease is inherited in three different ways:

1 Autosomal dominant inheritance.
2 Autosomal recessive inheritance.
3 X-linked inheritance (also known as sex chromosome disorders).

DOMINANT AND RECESSIVE CONDITIONS

Inherited conditions are often described as being *dominant* or *recessive*. A recessive gene is expressed only if its counterpart on the homologous chromosome (the other member of the chromosome pair) is the same, while a dominant gene will be expressed whatever the other chromosome carries. Only one parent, therefore, has to have the defective gene to produce children with dominantly inherited conditions, whereas both parents must carry the defective gene to produce children with recessively inherited conditions. Most enzyme deficiencies are recessive conditions, because the body's metabolism can function adequately with reduced levels of many enzymes. Defects in structural proteins, e.g. defects in connective tissue, are often inherited as dominant conditions: their functions are too critical to allow half the gene product to be incorrect.

The terms 'recessive' and 'dominant' are abbreviations for 'autosomal recessive' and 'autosomal dominant'.

Examples of recessively inherited conditions include phenylketonuria, galactosaemia, cystic fibrosis and sickle cell disease. Examples of dominantly inherited conditions include achondroplasia, Marfan syndrome and Huntington's chorea. However, the distinction between dominant and recessive conditions is not absolute, and should not be overemphasized. Thus, carriers of the recessive condition may show some of its features in a mild form. A fetus which has received a double dose of achondroplasia is not just dwarfed like his parents, but dies soon after birth with severe respiratory difficulties: it is a matter of definition whether achondroplasia is termed a dominant condition that is lethal in double dose, or whether it is regarded as the mild manifestation in the carriers of a lethal recessive disorder.

Genes contain the information necessary to produce a particular protein molecule and, although each cell has a pair of gene locations (i.e. one from the mother and one from the father), for each characteristic there may be an alternative form of the gene. These alternatives, known as *alleles*, affect the same characteristic but produce a different expression of the characteristic. If an individual has two alleles the same at a particular gene site, or *locus*, that individual is *homozygous* at that locus for that allele. If there are two different alleles at the site on the homologous chromosomes, the individual is *heterozygous* at that locus. A dominant disorder is manifest in the heterozygous state, and a recessive disorder is manifest only in the homozygote.

INHERITANCE PATTERNS

Someone with a *dominant gene* can transmit either the normal or the abnormal gene to a child. This is a random event, so there is a 1 in 2 (50%) chance of handing on the disease gene (Figure 5). If a child is born with a dominant disorder but neither parent carries the gene, then the gene arose by mutation and the chance of recurrence is very low. When the child comes to have children, the risk will be 50% again. Problems arise if some people who carry the gene show no obvious sign, or if signs occur only later in life. For example, it is possible to carry and transmit myotonic dystrophy without suffering any ill-effects, although signs of it can be detected if they are sought. If the subtle signs are not detected on examination the parents could inadvertently be advised that the chance of recurrence in a family was very low. Again, Hunting-

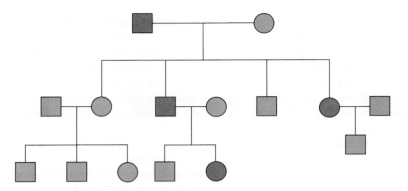

Figure 5   An autosomal dominant pedigree.

ton's chorea may not present problems until the ages of 40 or 50, after many sufferers have had their families; this constitutes the tragedy of the disease.

If a child is born with a *recessive disorder* it indicates that both parents, although unaffected themselves, must carry the abnormal gene. In this case, the concern is whether a subsequent child will be affected. The risk that either parent will hand on the abnormal gene is 1 in 2 (as for a dominant gene) so the risk that both will hand on the same gene is $\frac{1}{2} \times \frac{1}{2} = 1$ in 4 (25%) for any subsequent child (Figure 6).

In the next generation, the risk of someone with a recessive disorder transmitting it is much lower: all the children of a sufferer must carry the gene, but they will manifest the same disorder only if their partner also hands on the gene. This is most unlikely unless the carrier state is common (as for cystic fibrosis: 1 in 20 Britons carries this gene) or if the parents are close relatives. Just occasionally, two people with the same recessive disorder have children. All their children will inevitably have the same condition.

SEX-LINKED CONDITIONS

Sex-linked conditions are those carried on the X chromosome. They are more complex because the gene dosage varies between men and women, men having one X chromosome in each cell and women having two. However, only one of the two X chromosomes is active in any one cell in a woman's body. The other is inactive, and is termed a *Barr body* when it can be identified under a microscope. Which X is active is random, and differs throughout the woman's body. Thus men are affected even by a recessive disease which they carry on their X chromosome, while women are not. If a woman carries an X-linked recessive disorder, she may show

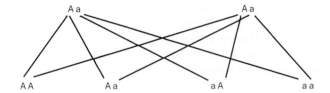

Figure 6   In an autosomal recessive disorder, the disease is only manifest if both members of a pair of chromosomes are abnormal. If both parents are carriers of the abnormal gene (a), then there is a 1 in 4 chance that a child will have the disease.

signs of it, but her normal X chromosome will prevent her suffering the same effects as a woman carrying a double dose, or a man.

Sex-linked recessive diseases are carried by women, and affect their sons. The best known such conditions are Duchenne muscular dystrophy, red–green colour-blindness and the haemophilias. A woman who carries such a disease on one of her two X chromosomes will transmit it (on average) to 1 in 2 of her children: half her sons will be affected and half her daughters will be carriers. A man who has such a condition and who has children will hand on the disease gene whenever he hands on his X chromosome. All his daughters must be carriers, and his sons cannot be affected (they receive his Y chromosome) (Figure 7).

A few diseases are X-linked dominant, affecting both sexes similarly. An example is hypophosphatae-mic (vitamin D-resistant) rickets.

MULTIFACTORIAL DEFECTS

Many conditions are influenced by several genes rather than just one or two. Such patterns of inheritance are

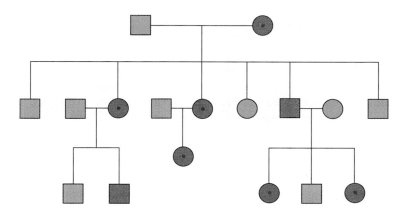

Figure 7 An X-linked pedigree.

difficult to define precisely, and are termed *polygenic*. If interaction with the environment is particularly important, as well as genes being involved, then the disorder is said to be *multifactorial* in origin. Neural tube defects and many cases of cleft lip and/or palate are multifactorial in origin.

This type of inheritance should not be confused with situations where several genes can cause the same effect, e.g. blindness. There are many different inherited conditions that cause blindness, but most of them are simple recessive or X-linked conditions. In any one case, only one mechanism will be operating. If two blind people marry and have children, their children will only be at risk if the parents have exactly the same condition causing the blindness, or if one of them is affected by a dominant gene.

In considering inherited disease, the problem arises as to why such conditions exist. New dominant diseases and sex-linked disorders can arise by a single mutation event – an error in cell division, or a mutation caused by radiation exposure or mutagenic chemicals. Recessive disorders cannot be explained so simply because both parents must carry the same aberration for the condition to occur. The rare diseases may be explained by the lack of selection against the mutation where the carrier suffers no ill-effect, but this still fails to account for the common diseases. These can sometimes be explained by some advantage accruing to the carriers (as with improved resistance to malaria conferred by a single dose of many thalassaemias and haemoglobinopathies). In other cases, such as cystic fibrosis, no such explanation has yet been established. It could be that carriers have some advantage in sexual competition, or

that gametes carrying such genes are somehow preferred, but this is speculation.

Genetic Counselling

The process of genetic counselling involves giving information to prospective parents about the risk of their having a child affected by an inherited defect, and helping them through whatever choice they decide upon. Over the past decade *genetic counselling* has become more accurate and authoritative as a result of the many developments in molecular biology. As a greater understanding of gene function and location is achieved, increased information is available to those who may be at risk of passing on abnormal traits and diseases to future generations. Counselling provides an opportunity to discuss potential risks and possible ways of planning a family for those who may be susceptible to debilitating genetically related disorders. There are several steps in this process.

Referral

Making contact comes first. Couples may be referred to a genetic counselling service for a variety of reasons. Advanced maternal age (over 35) and high serum alpha-fetoprotein levels in pregnancy are two common reasons for referral. The couple may have had a previous abnormal child and wish to know the chance of recurrence. Such a counselling visit would not usually be planned until a few months after the birth of the previous child, especially if the child had died. Counselling for future children is often inappropriate until a family has begun to come to terms with their past misfortune. In other cases, there may be a family history of a well-defined genetic condition, or there may be a history of neural tube defect, congenital heart defect or some other multifactorial condition. Such counselling may also be recommended before conception to couples who are planning a pregnancy and have a family history or specific concerns about inherited disorders.

Diagnosis

Making a precise diagnosis of the condition thought to be a risk can be very difficult and is sometimes impossible. Thus, if a previous child in a family died of suspected inherited disease some years ago, it may not be possible now to reach a precise diagnosis. Even if the affected individual is still alive, it is not always possible to make a diagnosis. New inherited metabolic disorders are still being described, and the biochemistry of previously described conditions is being clarified. Progress is also being made in the classification of *dysmorphic conditions* (patterns of malformation).

Mode of inheritance

When the diagnosis is known, it is possible to consider the mode of inheritance, if it is inherited and not acquired. Many disorders can be inherited in only one way, but this is not true of all inherited disease. Many dysmorphic syndromes can be transmitted as (autosomal) recessive or dominant conditions, or by sex-linked recessive inheritance. Examining the affected case will not distinguish these possibilities. It is necessary either to specify the mode of inheritance or to make an informed judgement as to what is most probable from considering the *pedigree* (family history) (see Chapter 19).

In considering multifactorial conditions without a clear pattern of inheritance, it is usually necessary to give recurrence risks based upon the cumulative experience of geneticists rather than upon theoretical models. These are empirical risk figures.

It is obviously important to distinguish inherited disease from similar conditions that arise for other reasons, such as congenital rubella infection.

Implications

The implications of the information for the family are discussed, and the various options open to them are presented. The natural history of the disorder is explained, along with the possibilities for treatment. If antenatal diagnosis of the disorder is possible, the methods are explained.

If the family chooses antenatal diagnosis and selective termination of pregnancy, appropriate arrangements are made. If the couple decides not to have further children, help with contraception or sterilization may be provided. Occasionally, a couple will consider other means of having children, such as artificial insemination by donor (AID) if the male partner carries a dominant disorder or if the (autosomal recessive) condition is transmitted from both parents. *In vitro* fertilization may also be considered. Some couples may wish to adopt a child, and they can be helped to contact an appropriate agency.

Family support

Whether pregnancy occurs or not, and with whatever result, family support is provided as appropriate. This may take the form of co-ordinating medical and social service support, of individual counselling, or of specific therapeutic interventions. Not all of this work is performed under the National Health Service and numerous support groups are active in this area.

The entire process is lengthy and will usually require a number of sessions. It is important to ensure that the clients understand the information they are given, so that they can make an informed decision: a written statement of the relevant facts can prove useful to the family. It is then necessary to support the family in their decision.

CASE EXAMPLES OF INHERITANCE PATTERNS

Example 1

The sister of a boy with Duchenne muscular dystrophy attends the genetic counselling clinic with her husband. Her mother's brother had the disease and died some years ago. She has a 50% chance of carrying the gene, because her mother must carry it. Since it is sex-linked, the woman would pass the disease to half her sons. There are two ways of deciding how likely this woman is to carry the abnormal gene. DNA can be extracted from blood samples from the members of her family. DNA probes are then used to see if her mother gave to her the same segment of X chromosome as she gave to her affected brother. Because the probes mark segments of chromosome close to but not at the Duchenne gene, there is always the chance that the marker and the gene have become separated by recombination at meiosis. Only occasionally can the results be 100% certain, when the absence of a length of DNA can be demonstrated.

Another method is to test the woman's blood for a muscle enzyme, creatine kinase, found in the blood of affected boys. The higher this level, the greater her chance of carrying the Duchenne gene. This is an example of how female carriers of X-linked diseases may manifest some signs of the disease. Combining the two risk figures often enables the doctor to give such a woman either a very high or a very low risk of being a carrier.

If her final risk is more than 2–5%, she may well opt for antenatal diagnosis. At present, this usually means the termination of any male fetus. Many normal males are aborted in this way. It is becoming possible in some families to determine whether or not a male fetus will be affected, and women in these families can have sons that they know will be normal.

Example 2

The daughter of a man with myotonic dystrophy attends clinic. She is eight weeks pregnant, and wishes to know the risk of her child being affected. Myotonic dystrophy is a dominant disorder characterized by muscle weakness, cataracts, baldness, some mental impairment and a typical difficulty in relaxing the grip. It is highly variable, however, so this woman may carry the gene without it being obvious. If she showed no sign, she could have an ophthalmological examination to look for early signs of cataract. It might be necessary to test her muscles electrically. The particular importance here is that her life could be endangered if she was given an anaesthetic without the diagnosis being known. Such patients are a grave anaesthetic risk.

This woman was found to carry the gene, so her risk of transmitting it to her fetus is 50%. An affected fetus born to an affected mother is at risk of the severe congenital form of myotonic dystrophy which can result in fatal respiratory problems for the infant or severe handicap. Antenatal diagnosis is possible in some families, but could not be arranged at short notice in this pregnancy. The geneticist's function in this case is to alert the woman, her obstetrician, her infant's paediatrician and their general practitioner to all the possible hazards ahead. Arrangements would also be made for antenatal diagnosis to be available in a future pregnancy, if this was the couple's wish.

Example 3

A couple attend clinic having lost a child some months before with congenital heart disease. It would be necessary to know precisely what sort of heart defect was present, and whether or not there were any other problems. Is there any other family history of congenital heart defects? No. Was there any question of rubella in early pregnancy? No – the mother had been immune when tested. Was there anything else the matter with the child? No – the child had a postmortem examination by an experienced paediatric pathologist, who had been satisfied that this was an isolated defect. (This is crucial, because heart defects can occur as one feature of dysmorphic syndromes that have a high risk of recurrence.) Photographs and X-rays were taken, and are available for review. It is important that a pathologist experienced in such work performs the post-mortem. The incidence of transposition of the great vessels (the defect in this child) is 0.4 per 1000 live births, and the risk of another child with congenital heart disease in this family is 1.7%, not very much higher than the 1% risk of congenital heart disease for all births.

Gene/DNA Probes

Each individual's DNA package is unique to them (with the exception of identical twins) and, in order to be able to recognize individual sequences of DNA, techniques have been developed to provide methods of individual DNA analysis. These techniques use *genetic probes* – labelled fragments of DNA – to determine whether a particular DNA sequence is present in a person's or a fetus's genetic material. Already this 'DNA fingerprinting' is proving important in areas of forensic science and paternity disputes.

DNA can be isolated easily from any human cell that is alive and has a nucleus, including buccal cells and skin fibroblasts. The *gene probe* or *DNA probe* is a copy of a relevant sequence that is identifiable and can be used as a 'probe' to hybridize a corresponding copy of a sample being studied. To be of use the probe has to be inserted into a 'vector' which can multiply in a host, such as a bacterium, because multiplication makes study easier.

First DNA is extracted from a patient's leucocytes (from a blood sample). Then it is digested by a *restriction endonuclease* which cuts the DNA into specific short segments by breaking it at *cleavage sites*, points at which a very specific set of four or six nucleotides occurs in a fixed order. Restriction endonuclease is a special class of bacterial enzyme which cleaves DNA wherever a very specific set of four or six nucleotides occurs in a fixed order. The resulting fragments are separated according to size in a gel by electrophoresis. The DNA is transferred from the gel to a filter (by 'Southern blotting') and the probe is applied. The probe is radioactively labelled so we can see the size of fragment to which it adheres and it can be unambiguously identified.

This technique gives us information because people differ in the pattern of cleavage sites on their chromosomes, and therefore in the size of fragment to which a probe adheres. Even a single difference in base-pair sequence can create or abolish a cleavage site, and so alter the sizes of DNA fragment that are picked out. If a patient's relatives are available for testing, it is often possible to trace how a gene has been passed down through the generations. On some occasions, however, where everyone in a family has the same pattern of cleavage sites for the relevant restriction endonuclease, it is not possible to gain any information.

The 'New' Genetics

The new genetics is a blanket term used to cover many developments in molecular biology relating to genetics. These developments include the Human Genome Projects which are working on discovering a map of the entire genome of humanity, recombinant DNA techniques, gene manipulation and therapy and genetic engineering. It is hoped that these developments will result in a decrease in the number and seriousness of inherited diseases and disorders in the future.

One option may be *genetic engineering*, through which it may become possible to replace or repair missing and defective genes with normal ones. In the early 1970s scientists at Stanford University (Nicholl, 1994) discovered procedures whereby they could alter the instructions provided by genes in bacteria. They discovered that by adding genes from other organisms to the bacterial genes it caused the bacteria to produce

proteins that they would not normally synthesize. This DNA, which comes from a variety of different sources, is called *recombinant DNA*. These techniques have recently been used with some success in plants and animals and the focus of attention is now on human beings (Nicholl, 1994). They would involve the insertion of genetic material directly into cells to alter the functioning of the cells and could be achieved either *in vitro*, prior to implantation of an embryo, or possibly on a child or adult who may be susceptible to a genetic disorder during their lifetime. At present it is possible to select the embryos to be implanted following *in vitro* fertilization in infertility treatments, but in the future the selection and implantation of healthy embryos may be an acceptable option for those who are fertile and susceptible to genetic disorders. The possibilities for the future are potentially vast and the midwife must keep up to date with these techniques in genetics as parents frequently request information following media coverage of new developments.

Prenatal Diagnosis

Prenatal sex determination and the diagnosis of an increasing number of diseases is now possible. If severe congenital anomalies or inherited diseases are diagnosed early enough, the parents have the option of having the pregnancy terminated. There is very real stress associated with antenatal diagnosis, however, and couples need unconditional support whatever their decision. The termination of fetuses at risk of malformation should never be pressed as being for the benefit of society, for it is the family who will have to live with their decision whatever it is. Also, it is false to suppose that most inherited diseases could be abolished by such methods. Many dominant and sex-linked conditions are perpetuated by mutation, while genetic disease is merely the tip of the iceberg of the defective autosomal recessive genes carried by us all.

Prenatal diagnostic procedures are screening tests either applied to all pregnant women or to all women in a particular group, or specific to a particular woman and her pregnancy. The following methods of prenatal diagnosis may be employed.

HISTORY-TAKING

A detailed family, medical and obstetric history is essential. The pedigree should highlight consanguinity (e.g. cousin marriages) and any inherited conditions or perinatal deaths. Inquiry as to racial/geographical origin may be appropriate (e.g. for haemoglobinopathies or glucose-6-phosphate dehydrogenase deficiency in those from the malarial belt, and Tay–Sachs disease in Ashkenazi Jews). Venereal diseases such as syphilis and genital herpes are also important. Further inquiry and investigation may be needed.

ROUTINE BLOOD TESTS

A number of blood tests are routinely carried out in pregnancy to aid prenatal diagnosis.

The *rhesus factor* is determined, and where it is absent the presence of rhesus antibodies is determined. Their concentration in the mother's serum indicates the severity of the rhesus disease, and amniocentesis is no longer used so widely for this purpose (see Chapter 21).

Serological tests for syphilis are also routine, because the fetus will usually escape any ill-effects if the mother is treated before 20 weeks (see Chapters 19 and 43).

Serology is used to test the mother's *immunity to rubella*: if she is not immune, it is important that she does not come into contact with the disease, particularly in the first trimester of pregnancy. Congenital rubella was a common cause of congenital deafness and blindness and of heart defects until vaccination became routine, but the immunity given by vaccination does not last indefinitely. Nor is the uptake of vaccination as high as it was hoped.

Maternal *serum alpha-fetoprotein* (AFP) may be measured at 16–18 weeks. About 80% of open neural tube defects can be detected by an increase in concentration (Kington, 1989). A raised level may also occur in cases of intrauterine death, and other fetal abnormalities (as described in Chapter 21).

Inaccurate estimation of gestational age, multiple pregnancy or diabetes may give misleading results. In about 50% of instances of raised levels no cause is found. A low level may be associated with Down's syndrome. About 30% of babies with Down's syndrome may be detected by this method.

The *triple test* is a maternal serum screening test which combines measurement of alpha-fetoprotein, unconjugated oestriol and human chorionic gonadotrophin to predict those at risk of having a baby with Down's syndrome (see Chapter 21). In some areas this test is offered to all women, and in other places only to those with identified risk factors. Amniocentesis

is offered to those with a positive result in some areas, or to those with identified risk factors in others. A screen positive result is when the risk determined by the markers is calculated to be 1 in 250 or above. A screen negative result will be a risk factor below this. About 60% of affected babies may be detected by this method (Wald *et al.*, 1994), whereas approximately 30% of affected babies are detected if amniocentesis is performed on the basis of age alone. A screen positive result will not necessarily mean that the baby has Down's syndrome, and a negative result will not exclude the possibility of an abnormality being present. The implications of the test and the meaning of results should be fully explained to the parents and counselling offered.

Maternal phenylalanine levels are checked in some areas, because a mother with elevated levels of this amino acid may have a genetically normal child who has nevertheless been damaged *in utero* by the mother's hyperphenylalaninaemia, as if the child had untreated phenylketonuria (PKU). An adult with PKU will not always adhere to the required diet, and may not appreciate the significance of this for her child, particularly if she has been affected by the condition herself to some extent.

ULTRASONOGRAPHY

In most areas of the UK women are routinely offered an ultrasound scan between 18 and 20 weeks. In addition to confirming the pregnancy, assessing gestational age, localizing the placenta and monitoring fetal growth, ultrasound has an increasingly significant role in the diagnosis of structural abnormalities in the fetus (Bernaschek *et al.*, 1994; Garmel and D'Alton, 1994).

Although equipment is becoming more sophisticated and operators more skilled, prediction of outcome may be uncertain in some instances, such as a diagnosis of choroid plexus cysts, or mild dilatation of the renal pelvis (Chitty *et al.*, 1991).

An ultrasound scan between 11 and 14 weeks may be used to predict the risk of having a chromosomally abnormal baby by measuring the amount of fluid behind the neck of the fetus. The nuchal fold thickness is measured in millimetres and is recorded by a computer in conjunction with the mother's age and period of gestation when giving an assessment of risk. The sensitivity of the test is about 85% (that is the test will show a risk of 1:250 or more if the baby has Down's syndrome). This test compares favourably with screening based on maternal age alone, or a combination of maternal age and serum biochemistry. There is a risk of a falsely elevated positive result of 5% (Nicolaides *et al.*, 1994a).

The use of ultrasound has not been found to produce any problems to date, but the effect of routine sonography on perinatal outcome has not been established, therefore the role of ultrasound in routine screening remains controversial.

AMNIOCENTESIS

This is the technique of sampling the liquor, which yields the fluid itself and the amniotic fluid cells. About 20 ml of amniotic fluid are aspirated after localization of the placenta by ultrasound. The biochemical constituents of the liquor may be tested for the accumulation of metabolites in suspected inborn errors, or for tests of fetal well-being (see Chapter 21). The cells may be used to test for an enzyme deficiency directly, or they may be grown in culture. If grown in culture, they may be used to determine the fetal karyotype, for DNA probe analysis, or for other enzyme assays. Fetal sex can be determined by karyotyping or by DNA analysis.

Traditionally, amniocentesis has been performed between 16 and 18 weeks' gestation, when the history, maternal age or other tests have indicated that there is an increased risk of abnormality. Today, however, it is becoming increasingly common to perform the test in the first trimester between 9 and 13 weeks (see Chapter 21). Small studies on amniocentesis in the first trimester have suggested that this is a relatively safe diagnostic test as an alternative to chorionic villus sampling and later amniocentesis. Crandall *et al.* (1994) studied 693 consecutive women who had amniocentesis prior to 15 weeks and found a miscarriage rate of 1.5% compared to a control group who had a standard amniocentesis and a miscarriage rate of 0.6% in the same period. A prospective study comparing early amniocentesis with chorionic villus sampling indicated that the spontaneous loss rate was higher after early amniocentesis than after chorionic villus sampling (Nicolaides *et al.*, 1994b). Randomized studies are needed to determine safety and accuracy.

A karyotype is usually obtained whenever amniocentesis is performed on a pregnancy, and it must be explained to the parents beforehand that a chromosomal anomaly may be found even when the procedure is undertaken for some other reason. They should have considered this beforehand, and should know that the sex chromosome anomalies are usually compatible with a normal life, except for infertility.

Results may occasionally be ambiguous, and there is a small risk of maternal cell contamination, or of cells failing to grow. The risk of miscarriage following amniocentesis performed between 16 and 18 weeks is commonly quoted as 1% over the spontaneous abortion rate (Tabor *et al.*, 1986).

CHORIONIC VILLUS BIOPSY

A fine catheter can be passed through the cervix or the abdominal wall into chorionic tissue, and a small sample of a few villi removed. The villi are used to detect chromosomal disorders, inborn errors of metabolism, haematological disorders or conditions amenable to DNA analysis, where single gene defects may be diagnosed by gene probes.

Chorionic villus biopsy seems to be associated with a higher rate of subsequent miscarriage than amniocentesis. For some, chorionic villus sampling is preferable to amniocentesis performed at 16 weeks because a diagnosis can be made earlier in pregnancy, thus giving the opportunity for an earlier, less traumatic termination of pregnancy, if required.

It is difficult to assess the risks of this procedure largely because of the high spontaneous miscarriage rate in the first trimester. There is also some risk of infection, intrauterine death, haematoma, placental abruption and perforation of the uterus. The incidence of limb defects has been shown to be increased following chorionic villus sampling (Hsieh *et al.*, 1995). It is therefore not recommended before 10 weeks' gestation. For further discussion see Chapter 21. Amniocentesis performed at 16 weeks is said to be more accurate than chorionic villus sampling (MRC, 1991).

FETOSCOPY

The fetus is observed through a fine fibre-optic telescope, and samples of fetal tissue may be obtained under direction vision. This can be used to diagnose haemophilia or haemoglobinopathy by fetal blood sampling, and skin diseases such as epidermolysis bullosa letalis by skin biopsy. Malformations may be diagnosed by inspection, and therapeutic interventions are a possibility, as in fetal blood transfusions for rhesus disease, and catheterization for the relief of urethral obstruction that would otherwise cause renal damage.

References

Bernaschek, G., Stuempfen, I. & Deutinger, J. (1994) The value of sonographic diagnosis of fetal malformations; indication based and screening based investigations. *Prenatal Diagnosis* **14**(9): 807–812.

Blackburn, S.T. & Loper, D.L. (1992) *Maternal, Fetal and Neonatal Physiology: A Clinical Perspective*. Philadelphia: W.B. Saunders Co.

Chitty, L.S., Hunt, G.H., Moore, J. & Lobb, M. (1991) Effectiveness of routine ultrasonography in detecting fetal structural abnormalities in a low risk population. *Br. Med. J.* **303**(6811): 1165–1169.

Crandall, B.F., Kulsh, P. & Tabsh, K. (1994) Risk assessment of amniocentesis between 11 and 15 weeks, comparison to later amniocentesis controls. *Prenatal Diagnosis* **14**(10): 913–919.

Garmel, S.H. & D'Alton (1994) Diagnostic ultrasound in pregnancy an overview. *Seminars Perinatol.* **1**(3): 117–132.

Harper, P.S. (1993) *Practical Genetic Counselling*, 4th edn. Oxford: Butterworth Heinemann.

Hsieh, F.S., Shya, M.K. & Sheu, B.C. (1995) Limb defects after chorionic villus sampling. *Obstet. Gynecol.* **85**(1): 84–88.

Judson, H.F. (1993) A history of the science and technology behind gene mapping and sequencing. In Kevles, D.J. & Hood, L. (eds) *The Code of Codes: Scientific and Social Issues in the Human Genome Project*. London: Harvard University Press.

Kington, H. (1989) Prenatal diagnosis. *Br. Med. J.* **298**(6684): 1368–1371.

MRC (Medical Research Council) (1991) Report of the Working Party on the Evaluation of CVS. *Lancet* **337**(8756): 1491–1498.

Nairne, Sir P. (1993) *Genetic Screening: Ethical Issues*. London: Nuffield Council on Bioethics.

Nicholl, D.S.T. (1994) *An Introduction to Genetic Engineering*. Cambridge: Cambridge University Press.

Nicolaides, K., Brizot, M. & Snijers, R.M.J. (1994a) Fetal nuchal translucency ultrasound screening for fetal trisomy in the first trimester of pregnancy. *Br. J. Obstet. Gynaecol.* **101**(9): 782–786.

Nicolaides, K., Brizot, M. & Patel, F. (1994b) Comparison of CVS and amniocentesis for fetal karyotyping at 10–13 weeks gestation. *Lancet* **343**(8920): 435–439.

Tabor, A., Masden, M., Obel, E.B., Philip, J., Bang, J. & Noorgaard-Pederson, B. (1986) Randomised controlled trial of genetic amniocentesis in 4606 low risk women. *Lancet* **1**: 1287–1289.

Wald, N.J., Kennard, A., Watt, H.C. & Smith, D. (1994) Value of maternal serum unconjugated oestriol measurement in prenatal screening for Down's syndrome. *Prenatal Diagnosis* **14**(18): 699–706.

5

Male and Female Reproduction – Early Development

Reproduction is the essential component of the human life cycle. In contrast to cellular reproduction or *mitosis* that goes on continually in most tissues, the *re-production* of a new individual involves the fusion of two specialized germ cells. These cells take distinctive male and female forms and are made in specific organs of reproduction, known as testes in men and ovaries in women. Like other important bodily activities, the capacity for sexual reproduction involves separate phases and complex patterns of growth and development that are regulated by neuroendocrine systems.

The capacity for sexual reproduction is initiated during early embryonic life. Cells that give rise to germs are first distinguished within the wall of the yolk sac (Figure 1). Between 4 and 6 weeks, these cells migrate to the developing sex organs or gonads. During the first six weeks following fertilization, male and female gonads undergo identical forms of development. Following this phase of organ formation, male

gonads develop distinct structures under genetic and hormonal influences. Essentially, this involves the proliferation of previously undifferentiated sex cords, leading to the formation of definitive testis cords that contain the primordial germ cells. In contrast, female gonads retain their original form; the sex cords gradually disappear and small clusters of follicular cells surround the germ cells. These structural differences explain why, in adult life, female germ cells are simply shed from the surface of the ovary while male germ cells need to travel through very long, tightly coiled tubules to leave the testis (Johnson and Everitt, 1995).

Male germ cells are called *spermatogonia* and those of the female are called *oogonia*. Within the newly differentiated testis and ovary, these cells rapidly increase in number by mitosis (Chapter 4). In the female fetus, only a few hundred germ cells are present three weeks following conception but by the fifth month, this number has reached a peak of around

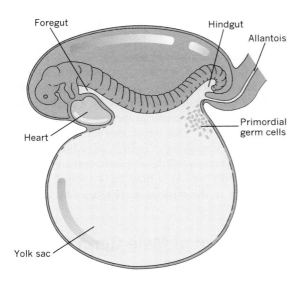

Figure 1   Schematic drawing of a 3-week-old embryo showing the primordial germ cells in the wall of the yolk sac, close to the attachment of the allantois. (Reproduced with permission from Sadler, 1990, p. 272.)

seven million cells. Once this point has been reached, male and female germ cells behave quite differently.

Development of Female Germ Cells (Oogonia)

From the third month of gestation in females, the large population of oogonia gradually embark on a new sequence of cell divisions called *meiosis* (Chapter 4), that brings to an end the simple increase by mitotic division in the overall population of germ cells. During these events, developing oocytes do not change as independent units but remain connected to one another by cytoplasmic bridges that are thought to account for the highly synchronized pattern of oogenesis (Austin, 1982). In this distinct series of events, maternal and paternal chromosomes are randomly segregated and recombined to create new and unique associations between their genetic material. In addition, total chromosomal numbers are halved, producing just

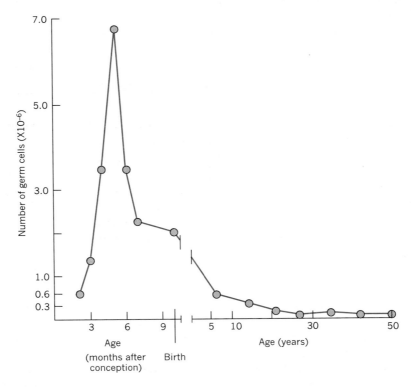

Figure 2   Changes in the total population of germ cells in the human ovary with increasing age. (Reproduced with permission from Austin, 1982, p. 25.)

one member of each of the 23 pairs of chromosomes within the cell nucleus (Johnson and Everitt, 1995).

In contrast to mitosis, this pattern of cell division is associated with the elimination of a large number of germ cells. From seven million at mid-gestation, these cells are reduced to approximately 1.5 million at birth. This is thought to happen because the complex crossing-over of chromosomes increases the likelihood of breaks and other errors. As a result of these developments, females are born with a finite number of germ cells (Austin and Short, 1982) (Figure 2).

As oocytes enter meiosis, they attract different types of ingrowing cells to form *primordial follicles*. Within these emerging cell clusters, *mesenchymal cells*, that later give rise to *granulosa cells*, secrete an outer basement membrane called the *membrane propria*. Taken together, these specialized cells provide nutrients for the developing oocyte and prevent its indiscriminate exposure to the general constituents of vascular and interstitial fluids (Byskov, 1982). With the formation of these units, meiosis is halted and further phases are only resumed following ovulation, that may occur at any time between puberty and the menopause. This prolonged pause in the process of meiosis is thought to be induced by the secretion of inhibitory factors within the surrounding follicle (Byskov, 1982; Johnson and Everitt, 1995).

During the remainder of fetal life, a few follicle cells undergo further differentiation and growth, creating several layers around the oocyte. These are called *primary follicles*. From birth to puberty, a small percentage of these follicles undergo further limited growth, followed by atresia. This leaves approximately 400 000 follicles by the beginning of reproductive life. Of these, only about 400 reach full development and are ovulated or shed, usually one at a time, in a cyclical fashion, from puberty to the menopause (Figure 3A).

Development of Male Germ Cells (Spermatogonia)

In contrast to the pattern of development in females, male cells do not begin the process of meiosis until puberty. Instead, they retain a population of resting stem cells that have the capacity for meiotic division. Although the more hazardous process of meiosis is not initiated during fetal life, male germ cells show a similar decrease in number during the second half of

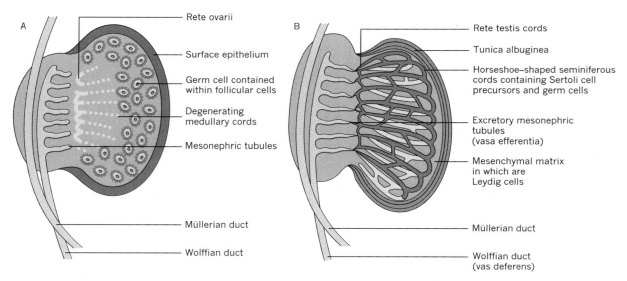

Figure 3   (A) Ovarian development around 20–24 weeks of development. In the absence of medullary cords and a true persistent rete ovarii, no communication is established with the mesonephric tubules. Hence, in the adult, ova are shed from the surface of the ovary and are not transported by tubules to the oviduct. (B) Testicular development around 16–20 weeks of development. The horseshoe shape of the seminiferous cords and their continuity with the rete testis cords is clearly illustrated. The vasa efferentia, derived from the excretory mesonephric tubules, link the seminiferous cords with the Wolffian duct. (Reproduced with permission from Johnson and Everitt (1990), p. 9.)

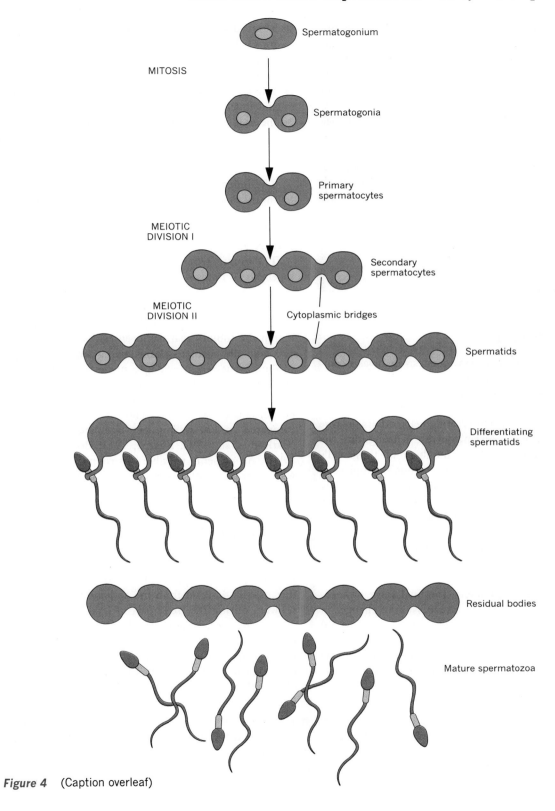

MITOSIS

MEIOTIC
DIVISION I

MEIOTIC
DIVISION II

Spermatogonium

Spermatogonia

Primary
spermatocytes

Secondary
spermatocytes

Cytoplasmic bridges

Spermatids

Differentiating
spermatids

Residual bodies

Mature spermatozoa

Figure 4   (Caption overleaf)

gestation. This parallel is thought to occur because male germ cells are simultaneously exposed to stimulators and inhibitors of meiosis. The dominant forces opposing meiosis may lead to the degeneration of cells that prematurely respond to meiotic stimulation (Johnson and Everitt, 1995).

Between birth and puberty both male and female germ cells enter a period of inactivity. From puberty onwards, male germ cells normally *begin* meiosis whereas female cells *resume* it. As males retain a population of stem cells, spermatozoa are continually formed by meiotic division throughout adult life. This implies that both types of cell division occur sequentially within the testis (Figure 3B).

Generation of Life Inside the Testes

SPERMATOGENESIS

The overall process of spermatogenesis involves a complex sequence of changes that begins with mitotic proliferation to produce large numbers of cells. While some of these continue to divide mitotically, to ensure a constant supply of sperm-creating cells, others enlarge to become primary spermatocytes. Throughout the period of maturation, large numbers of these cells remain connected to one another through cytoplasmic bridges. In this form of organization, they subsequently proceed through the various phases of meiotic divisions. This interesting feature of spermatogenesis allows the developing cells to have recourse to extra copies of each pair of chromosomes, allowing them to replace any defective gene copy with a good copy from other nuclei (Alberts *et al.*, 1994) (Figure 4).

When meiosis is complete, the final stage of spermatogenesis occurs through a succession of changes in the overall shape and organization of the nucleus and cytoplasm, as both are extensively reshaped into a more streamlined form for swift, long-distance travel. In its finished form the spermatozoon has a number of distinct features:

▶ a well-defined *tail*, of contractile microtubules, for forward movement;

▶ a *middle-piece* containing mitochondria, providing energy for cell movement;

▶ a *residual body* that disposes of excess cytoplasm; and finally

▶ the *head* enclosing the nucleus which is surrounded by an *acrosomal cap* of enzymes that are important in fertilization.

The inner membrane of the acrosome lies adjacent to the nuclear membrane of the cell while the outer membrane lies immediately beneath the plasma membrane (Chiras, 1991; Johnson and Everitt, 1995) (Figure 5).

The overall series of events that constitute spermatogenesis – mitosis, meiosis and remodelling – take place over 60–74 days in the human testes. Adult males can produce 200–300 million of these cells every day. This implies a very high concentration of activity within the tubules that has been estimated at between 300 and 600 mature sperms per gram of testis per second. Some recent evidence suggests that this biological capacity has declined significantly over the last 60 years. During the 1990s, sperm counts of 60 million per ejaculate have been reported in normal males compared to 120 million per ejaculate in the 1950s (Carlsen *et al.*, 1992; Sharpe, 1993; Bromwich *et al.*, 1994). At present, possible environmental chemicals with oestrogenic effects are being investigated (Irvine *et al.*, 1996).

STRUCTURE OF THE TESTIS

The prolific and highly complex organization of cell production in males takes place within a pair of organs that usually descend from the abdominal cavity to the scrotum during the latter part of fetal life. Composed of skin that contains large numbers of sweat glands and lined with smooth muscle and fascia, this outer covering is structured to maintain the temperature within the testes at 4–7°C lower than the abdomen. The layer of smooth muscle called the *dartos* helps to regulate the

Figure 4   The progeny of a single maturing spermatogonium remain connected to one another by cytoplasmic bridges throughout their differentiation into mature sperm. For the sake of simplicity, only two spermatogonia are shown entering meiosis to eventually form eight connected haploid spermatids. In fact, the number of connected cells that go through two meiotic divisions and differentiate together is very much larger. (Reproduced with permission from Alberts *et al.*, 1994, p. 867.)

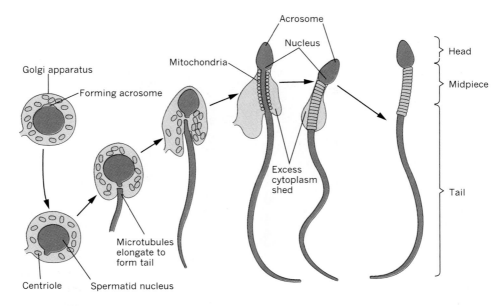

Figure 5 Sperm formation. Sperm form from spermatids in the germinal epithelium. Note the following changes: nuclear condensation, loss of cytoplasm, tail formation, alignment of the mitochondria and acrosome formation. (Reproduced with permission from Chiras, 1991, p. 438).

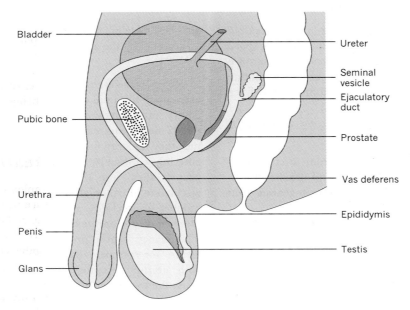

Figure 6 The male reproductive system.

internal temperature by contracting in response to cold and relaxing in response to heat (Figure 6).

The gross structure of the adult testis is composed of approximately 250 lobules that contain almost 200 m

of seminiferous tubules. These are surrounded by a distinct interstitial compartment made up of freely connecting blood and lymph vessels, nerve fibres and Leydig cells that secrete steroid hormones. The mitotic

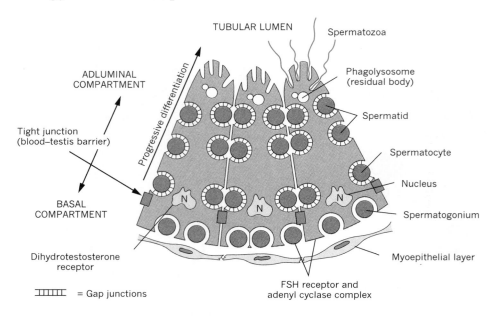

TUBULAR LUMEN

Spermatozoa

ADLUMINAL COMPARTMENT

Phagolysosome (residual body)

Progressive differentiation

Spermatid

Tight junction (blood–testis barrier)

Spermatocyte

Nucleus

BASAL COMPARTMENT

Spermatogonium

Dihydrotestosterone receptor

Myoepithelial layer

⊓⊓⊓⊓ = Gap junctions

FSH receptor and adenyl cyclase complex

BLOOD

Figure 7 Sertoli cells with developing germ cells. (Reproduced with permission from Tepperman and Tepperman, 1987, p. 119.)

phase of spermatogenesis takes place in the *Sertoli cells* that line the seminiferous tubules. The maturing sperm cells then move into a distinct *adluminal compartment* where they enter meiosis, before gradually finding their way into the tubular lumen (Johnson and Everitt, 1995) (Figure 7).

This organization of *Sertoli cells* has a number of important effects:

▶ It protects the maturing cells from direct contact with intracellular, intravascular and tubular fluids.
▶ It prevents later phases of spermatogenesis from affecting earlier ones.
▶ It provides high local concentrations of steroid hormones that are essential for spermatogenesis.

Besides their direct involvement in spermatogenesis, Sertoli cells also carry out other auxiliary activities:

▶ They phagocytose the residual bodies left behind by maturing spermatozoa.
▶ They secrete a distinct alkaline fluid into the tubular lumen.

▶ They develop receptors for the steroid hormones secreted by the adjacent Leydig cells (Alberts *et al.*, 1994).

Spermatozoa are released into the tubular lumen and carried by the fluid along the tubules that eventually empty into a single duct called the *epididymis*. During the 12 days required for transit through the epididymis, they undergo further maturational changes, before entering a muscular duct called the *vas deferens* that propels them into the ejaculatory duct. Just before ejaculation, further alkaline fluids are added from a number of accessory glands. Seminal fluid contains a number of glycoprotein and prostaglandin molecules. The former seem to provide nutritional and protective factors for spermatozoa while the latter may interact with uterine receptors that initiate contractions to assist the movement of spermatozoa within the genital tract (Drobnis and Overstreet, 1992). The overall content of a typical ejaculate contains 200–400 million spermatozoa in a volume of 3–4 ml of fluid (Chiras, 1991; Alberts *et al.*, 1994).

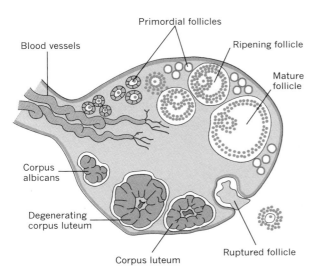

Figure 8   The sequence of changes occurring in the ovum during each menstrual cycle.

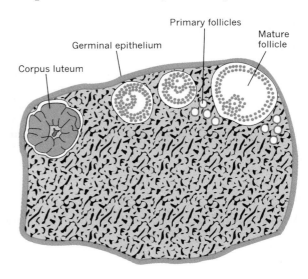

Figure 9   Diagrammatic section of an ovary. (Reproduced with permission from Williams *et al.* (1989), p. 1436.)

Generation of Life Inside the Ovary

OVARIES

Structure

The ovaries (Figures 8 and 9) are two glandular structures lying on the posterior surface of the broad ligament just below the pelvic brim and near to the infundibulum of the uterine tube. They develop in the germinal ridges of the posterior abdominal wall and during fetal life they descend into the pelvis in the same manner as the testes. They vary considerably in structure and function according to the age of the woman.

The ovaries are almond-shaped, a dull white in colour and corrugated on the surface. During the childbearing years they measure 3 cm in length, 2 cm in width and 1 cm in thickness; their weight is between 5 and 8 g. Later in life they atrophy. The ovary is attached at the back to the broad ligament by a thin mesentery, the *mesovarian*. The area is called the hilum and is the point at which ovarian vessels, nerves and lymphatics enter and leave. Each ovary is also attached to the cornu of the uterus by an ovarian ligament and to the side wall of the pelvis by the infundibulopelvic ligament.

The adult ovary resembles the testis in that each divides into two very distinct compartments. In the ovary they are the *cortex* and the *medulla*. In both organs, specialized tissue protects the enclosed germ cells and is surrounded by a more varied compartment, made up of blood and lymph vessels, nerve fibres and cells that secrete steroid hormones. But in spite of these parallels, ovarian tissue is organized very differently from that of the testis. In place of lobes of densely coiled tubules that continually generate and release vast numbers of spermatozoa, the ovary stores an ever changing population of oocytes in individual *follicles*. Following a series of complex changes involving recruitment from the pool of primordial follicles and entry into a small cohort of growing follicles, a single follicle is usually selected and released, as part of a cycle of events that takes approximately 28 days to complete.

In this constantly changing state, follicles at all phases of development and regression cluster within a thick outer cortex that forms the largest part of the gland. They are embedded in dense stroma of reticular fibres that provide supportive connective tissue and interstitial cells that are thought to contribute to growth of the outer *thecal layer* of developing follicles during the cycle. The medulla or innermost part of the ovary consists of looser connective tissue, smooth muscle cells, numerous blood vessels and a scattered group of steroid-secreting cells that resemble the Leydig cells of the testes (Williams *et al.*, 1989; Findlay, 1991).

BLOOD SUPPLY, LYMPHATIC DRAINAGE AND NERVE SUPPLY

The blood supply is from the ovarian artery, a branch of the aorta, and venous drainage to the ovarian veins. The left drains into the left renal vein and the right directly into the inferior vena cava.

The lymphatic drainage is to the posterior abdominal nodes.

The nerve supply is from the ovarian plexus.

The ovaries produce *ova* for fertilization during the childbearing years. They also produce the hormones *oestrogen* and *progesterone*. Under the influence of these hormones the endometrium of the uterus is prepared each month to receive a fertilized ovum and is subsequently shed if pregnancy fails to occur.

References

Alberts, B., Bray, D., Lewis, J. *et al.* (1994) *Molecular Biology of the Cell.* New York: Garland.

Austin, C.R. (1982) The egg. In Austin, C.R. & Short, R.V. (eds) *Reproduction in mammals*, Book 1, *Germ Cells and Fertilization*, pp. 46–62. Cambridge: Cambridge University Press.

Austin, C.R. and Short, R.V. (eds) (1982) *Reproduction in Mammals*, Book 1, *Germ Cells and Fertilization*. Cambridge: Cambridge University Press.

Bromwich, P., Cohen, J., Stewart, I. *et al.* (1994) Decline in sperm counts: an artifact of changed-reference range of 'normal'. *Br. Med. J.* **309**: 19–22.

Byskov, A.G. (1982) Primordial germ cells and regulation of meitosis. In Austin, C.R. & Short, R.V. (eds) *Reproduction in Mammals*. Book 1, *Germ Cells and Fertilization*, pp. 1–16. Cambridge: Cambridge University Press.

Carlsen, E., Giwercman, A., Keiding, N. *et al.* (1992) Evidence for decreasing quality of semen during the past 50 years. *Br. Med. J.* **305**: 609–613.

Chiras, D.D. (1991) *Human Biology.* New York: West.

Drobnis, E.Z. & Overstreet, J.W. (1992) *Oxford Rev. Reprod. Biol.* **14**: 1–45.

Findlay, J.K. (1991) The ovary. *Baillière's Clin. Endocrinol. Metab.* **5**(4): 755–769.

Irvine, S., Cawood, E., Richardson, D. *et al.* (1996) Evidence of deteriorating semen quality in the United Kingdom: birth cohort study in 577 men in Scotland over 11 years. *Br. Med. J.* **312**: 467–471.

Johnson, M.H. & Everitt, B.J. (1995) *Essential Reproduction.* Oxford: Blackwell Scientific.

Sadler, T.W. (1990) *Langhan's Medical Embryology.* Baltimore: Williams and Wilkins.

Sharpe, R.M. (1993) Declining sperm counts in men – is there an endocrine cause? *J. Endocrinol.* **136**: 357–360.

Tepperman, J. & Tepperman, H.N. (1987) *Metabolic and Endocrine Physiology.* Chicago: Year Book Medical Publishers.

Williams, P.L., Warwick, R., Dyson, M. *et al.* (eds) (1989) *Gray's Anatomy.* Edinburgh: Churchill Livingstone.

Wynn, M. & Wynn, A. (1991a) *The Case for Preconception Care of Men and Women.* Oxford: A B Academic Publishers.

Wynn, M. & Wynn, A. (1991b) The menstrual cycle as indicator in prepregnancy care. *J. Nutr. Med.* **2**: 387–398.

6

Neurohormonal Regulation of Female Reproduction

During different phases of the menstrual cycle, characteristic changes occur in many organs and all of these are very sensitive to a wide range of nutritional and emotional influences. The scope and diversity of these developments are much greater than those that occur during spermatogenesis. The events of each cycle prepare an oocyte for ovulation, fertilization and implantation, while the whole body is simultaneously prepared for major adaptations required for both pregnancy *and* lactation (Russo and Russo, 1987; Yen and Jaffe, 1991; Wynn and Wynn, 1991a,b).

Distinct alterations occur in primary and secondary organs of reproduction, while more subtle variations emerge in other parts of the body. Distinct changes include:

► recruitment, selection, growth and ovulation of the dominant follicle;

► marked proliferation and glandular changes in the endometrial lining of the uterus; and
► variations in the composition of breast tissue and cervical and vaginal secretions.

These changes are tightly controlled by the *hypothalamic–pituitary–ovarian axis* that is known to be highly sensitive to a variety of stresses and nutritional deficiencies (Wynn and Wynn, 1991b). Changes that tend to be of a more subtle character include:

► slight variations in energy and nutrient intake;
► changing levels of interstitial fluid;
► alterations in core temperature, breathing patterns, sexual interest; and
► expressions of varying neuronal activity, such as alterations in temperament and in perceptual and motor activities (Machida, 1981; Parker *et al.*, 1981; Martini *et al.*, 1994).

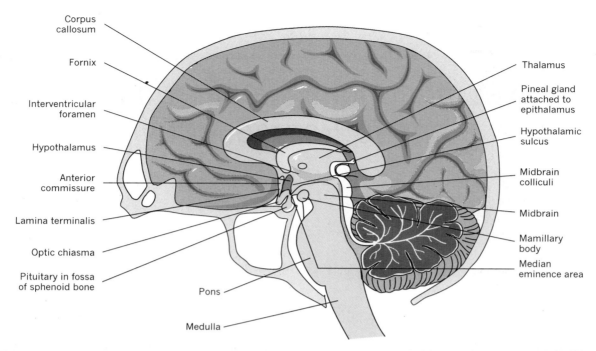

Figure 1   Sagittal section of the human brain with the pituitary and pineal glands attached. Note the comparatively small size of the hypothalamus and its rather compressed dimensions ventrally. The pineal is attached by its stalk to the epithalamus (habenula region) and lies above the midbrain colliculi. The thalamus (above) and the hypothalamus (below) form one wall (the right in this view) of the third ventricle. (Reproduced with permission from Johnson and Everitt, 1995, p. 102.)

These characteristic fluctuations of the menstrual cycle are synchronized by complex networks of central neurosecretory cells that operate in connection with central and local hormone-secreting glands. The major neurohormonal region involved is the *hypothalamo-pituitary unit*. The *hypothalamus* is a small area at the base of the brain located below the thalamus (Figure 1) and surrounding the third ventricle which divides it into a left and right section. Anteroposteriorly, it extends from the optic chiasma to behind the mamillary body. The basal portion of the hypothalamus, forming the floor of the third ventricle is the median eminence that is connected to the *pituitary gland* by the infundibular stem (Figure 2). This region provides a major meeting point between neurosecretory nerve terminals from hypothalamic and extrahypothalamic regions and the capillary network of the portal system. Hormonal secretions from these terminals are released into particular groups of capillaries. These drain into the long portal veins that travel through the infundibular stem and then break up again into capillaries within the anterior lobe of the pituitary gland (Johnson and Everitt, 1995; Krusemann, 1992; Page, 1994).

Within the Hypothalamus

The hypothalamus is largely made up of cell bodies, axons and terminals of its own neurones, together with axons and terminals of neurones with cell bodies located in other areas of the brain, including the thalamus and the medulla. Cell bodies within the hypothalamus are organized as dense bundles of individual neurones called nuclei. The cell bodies of these different nuclei make numerous axonal connections. These are formed with other cell bodies within particular nuclei and between different nuclei throughout the hypothalamus. Specific hypothalamic nuclei also connect with neurones in other regions of the brain while others have axons that terminate within the posterior lobe of the pituitary gland. All these interactions

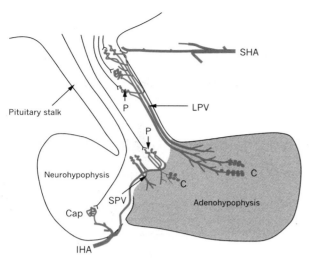

Figure 2   Sagittal section of the human pituitary gland to illustrate the neurovascular pathways by which nerve cells in certain hypothalamic nuclei control the output of anterior and posterior pituitary hormones. The axon on the left ends on the capillary bed (Cap) in the infundibular process and represents the tract from the large nerve cells of the supraoptic and paraventricular nuclei which are concerned with posterior pituitary function. The other hypothalamic axons terminate on the capillary bed (P) feeding the portal vessels which supply the adenohypophysis. Here they transmit their neurohormones into the bloodstream and the latter are then carried through the long and the short portal vessels (LPV, SPV) to the epithelial cells (C) to control the output of hormones from these cells. SHA, superior hypophysial artery; IHA, inferior hypophysial artery. (Reproduced with permission from Daniel, P. and Prichard, M.M.L. (1975) *Acta Endocrinol.* **80**: 67.)

involve the pulsatile secretion of distinct hormonal substances that are synthesized within the cell bodies. These include peptides, catecholamines and opioids that exert direct and indirect influences on specific groups of hormone-secreting cells that make up the anterior pituitary gland (Krusemann, 1992; Page, 1994).

Hypothalamic–Pituitary Connections

The hormonal interactions that occur between the hypothalamus and the pituitary gland are mediated by distinct vascular and neuronal pathways. These develop from the different morphological origins of the two lobes of the pituitary gland. The larger anterior lobe, the *adenohypophysis*, originates from an evagination of the oropharynx and has no direct neuronal connections with the hypothalamus. During embryonic life, it migrates to join with the *neurohypophysis*, or posterior lobe. This lobe develops from the hypothalamus and is a continuation of the median eminence and the pituitary stalk. In keeping with its neuronal character, the posterior lobe is largely composed of axons that project from cell bodies located in two large bundles of nuclei within the hypothalamus. In humans, an estimated 100 000 of these axons pass down through the basal hypothalamus and infundibular stalk to enter the posterior pituitary where they exhibit repeated dilatations and divisions, before terminating in capillary networks that supply the general circulation (Page, 1994).

The intermediate lobe of the pituitary constitutes a well-defined tissue in many species and has morphological features of both anterior and posterior lobes. While it originates from non-neuronal tissue, it contains a number of axon terminals connected to cell bodies in the hypothalamus. In humans, this lobe is prominent in fetal life, in pregnancy and possibly during lactation. At other times, it is recognized as scattered intermediate lobe tissue that is located in both anterior and posterior lobes (Hill *et al.*, 1993; Murburg *et al.*, 1993).

Pituitary Hormones

The *anterior lobe* of the pituitary is composed of at least five interconnected groups of hormone-secreting cells that are regulated by one or more neuronal substances from the hypothalamus (Jones *et al.*, 1990). These are released in a pulsatile manner from the median eminence of the hypothalamus and taken up by the portal system that transports them to target cells within the anterior pituitary. This rich vascular system provides the gland with very high levels of regulatory hypothalamic peptides. Distinct groups of cells within the anterior pituitary secrete peptide hormones with a range of metabolic actions that are mediated by a variety of organs and tissues throughout the body. Those most closely associated with reproduction include the following:

▶ *Follicle-stimulating hormone* (FSH) binds to receptors in the primary follicles.

▶ Luteinizing hormone (LH) binds to receptors in primary follicles and the corpus luteum.

▶ *Adrenocorticotrophic hormone* (ACTH) processed from a larger peptide, pro-opiomelanocortin (POMC) binds to receptors in the adrenal cortex.

▶ *Prolactin* binds mainly to alveolar cells in the mammary gland (Greenspan and Baxter, 1994).

The major hormones released from nerve terminals in the *posterior lobe* are vasopressin, oxytocin, opioids and dopamine. Release of *vasopressin* is stimulated by central and hypothalamic neuronal responses to water deprivation, pain and emotional anxiety. It functions in conjunction with other hypothalamic and extrahypothalamic neurones that are sensitive to different forms of stress. *Oxytocin* release is stimulated by the activation of sensory receptors in the nipple and the uterine cervix. Following its pulsatile release into the general circulation, it acts in both organs to induce the rhythmic contraction of smooth muscle (Knobil *et al.*, 1994). *Opioids* exert a tonic inhibitory control on stimulated oxytocin release from nerve terminals in the posterior pituitary (Douglas *et al.*, 1993). The *dopaminergic* nerve terminals in the posterior lobe are currently thought to be inhibited by central neuronal impulses that are generated by suckling. Since dopamine from the posterior lobe circulates to the anterior pituitary via the short portal vessels, this mechanism may also be involved in mediating the enhanced release of prolactin during suckling (Ben-Jonathan, 1991).

The intermediate lobe is composed of secretory cells that process POMC to melanocyte-stimulating hormone (MSH) and β-endorphin, together with a smaller number of nerve terminals that release dopamine and serotonin. MSH is known to stimulate specialized epithelial cells that synthesize the pigment melanin. The presence of the intermediate lobe during pregnancy may explain the enhanced pigmentation that develops during this period. It is particularly apparent as darker patches on the face, as a dark line stretching from the pubis to the umbilicus and as a darkening of the areola, nipple and perineum. Experimental studies on rats have also found that the release of both MSH and β-endorphin from the intermediate lobe is stimulated by neuronal impulses that are generated during suckling (Murburg *et al.*, 1993). These may be mediated by a central inhibition of dopamine or by stimulation of serotonin neurones. Following their release, these hormones are transported to the anterior pituitary via the short portal vessels where they are thought to directly influence the response of prolactin-releasing cells to dopamine (Barofsky *et al.*, 1983; Hill *et al.*, 1991; Porter *et al.*, 1994).

Hypothalamic–Pituitary–Ovarian Connections

The central generating neurohormonal regulator of the menstrual cycle is *gonadotrophin-releasing hormone* (GnRH) (Figure 3). This neuropeptide is released in a pulsatile manner from two groups of neurones within the hypothalamus. One group within the arcuate nucleus is located in the basal hypothalamic region, with axons projecting to the median eminence. The second, larger group is situated within the pre-optic area and adjacent anterior hypothalamus. Half of these axons project to the median eminence and the remainder go to other areas of the central nervous system including the hippocampus that is associated with sexual activity, short-term memory and motivational activities (Johnson and Everitt, 1995).

The pulsatile secretion of GnRH is regulated within the brain by complex connections with other neuronal secretions. Present evidence suggests that GnRH neurones in the arcuate nucleus are stimulated by ascending adrenergic neurones and inhibited by neurones that release dopamine. The inhibitory actions of the ovarian hormones *oestradiol* and *progesterone* are also thought to be partly mediated by adjacent dopaminergic neurones. The other group of GnRH neurones in the pre-optic area are thought to be inhibited directly by oestrogen sensitive γ-*aminobutyric acid* (GABA) neurones and indirectly by adjacent neurones that secrete *corticotrophin-releasing hormone* (CRH) in response to stress. This last group of neurones stimulates self-regulating opioid neurones that in turn directly suppress GnRH activity. All of these neurohormonal influences on GnRH in the hypothalamus are known to mediate a variety of factors, including body weight, nutritional status and different forms of stress (Wynn and Wynn, 1991a). At present, detailed evidence exists on the interactions between GnRH and ovarian steroid hormones but knowledge of the dynamic interplay between GnRH and other neuronal secretions remains to be fully identified (Johnson and Everitt, 1995).

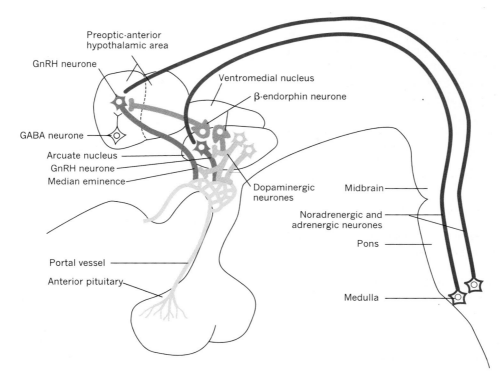

Figure 3   Schematic diagram to show some of the postulated neurochemical reactions which may control GnRH secretion. GnRH neurones lie mainly in the medial pre-optic area, but also in the arcuate nucleus. They project to the portal vessels in the median eminence. Dopamine neurones in the arcuate nucleus may modulate GnRH release. Neurones within the hypothalamus which contain β-endorphin also modulate anterior pituitary secretion, perhaps by modulating GnRH neurone activity in the pre-optic area, but perhaps also by altering dopamine neurone activity and hence GnRH (and dopamine) neurosecretion. Noradrenergic and adrenergic neurones in the medulla project to the hypothalamus and pre-optic area and have been seen by pharmacological techniques to enhance GnRH secretion. GABA-containing neurones have been shown to accumulate oestradiol and may exert local control over GnRH neurone activity. (Reproduced with permission from Johnson and Everitt, 1995, p. 132.)

The Menstrual Cycle (see Chapter 3)

NEUROHORMONAL REGULATION

Each menstrual cycle begins with the first day of menstruation. This event coincides with regression of the *corpus luteum* and a fall in the secretion of oestrogen and progesterone. Within the uterus, withdrawal of steroid support leads to shedding of the endometrial lining, while in the ovary, declining levels of progesterone are thought to have a permissive role in relaxing the inhibition of follicular growth that is evident in the luteal phase of the cycle. During menses, a new cohort of approximately 12 growing follicles appears from the trickle of growing follicles that emerge continually

from the resting pool of primordial follicles that formed during fetal life (Espey and Ben-Halim 1990; Baird, 1990) (Figures 4 and 5).

The fall in circulating levels of ovarian steroids during menses relaxes their inhibitory actions on both GnRH activity and on the release of FSH and LH from the anterior pituitary gland. During the early follicular phase of the cycle, secretion of GnRH increases slightly. This induces a small increase in circulating levels of FSH, followed after a day or so, by a similar increase in levels of LH. Within the cohort of growing follicles, this changing hormonal profile stimulates the emergence of FSH receptors on granulosa cells that form non-vascularized layers immediately surrounding the oocyte. This is followed by the

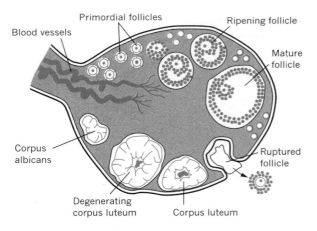

Figure 4   The sequence of changes occurring in the ovum during each menstrual cycle.

development of LH receptors on the surrounding vascularized layers of thecal cells (Figure 6).

OOCYTE–FOLLICLE CELL INTERACTIONS – OOCYTE GROWTH

The precise significance of the pituitary–ovarian axis in the early stage of follicular growth remains debatable. Earlier work tends to stress the role of changes in circulating hormone levels and the formation of specific receptors on the follicle cells, while more recent research has focused on a variety of intra-ovarian regulators (Baird, 1990; Espey and Ben-Halim, 1990; Moor *et al.*, 1990).

During the first phase of growth, varying degrees of cell proliferation and differentiation occurs in *granulosa* and *theca cells* within the cohort of growing follicles. Granulosa cells divide to become several layers thick and gap junctions form between adjacent cells. At the same time theca cells condense to form the outer compartment of the follicle. Meanwhile, the enclosed oocyte increases 300 fold in size while meiosis remains in arrest. Glycoproteins are secreted from the cell surface of the oocyte and these coalesce to form a transparent, acellular envelope called the *zona pellucida* (Austin, 1982; Baker, 1982) (Figure 6).

With further growth, theca cells enlarge to form an outer fibrous coat and an inner layer that is highly vascularized. The granulosa compartment enlarges further and fluid droplets formed from granulosa cell secretions and serum transudate accumulate between the cells. This fluid gradually forms a single pool

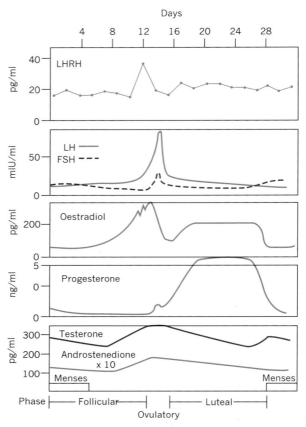

Figure 5   Profile of plasma hormone levels throughout the menstrual cycle. Note ovulatory surges of luteinizing hormone (LH) and follicle-stimulating hormone (FSH) preceded by increases in oestradiol and gonadotropin-releasing hormone (GnRH). The broad peaks of progesterone and oestradiol in the luteal phase result from secretion by the corpus luteum. (Reproduced with permission from Berne and Levy, 1993, p. 602.)

creating distinct layers of granulosa cells. A dense layer called the *cumulus* surrounds the oocyte while the remaining cells are connected by a thin stream that traverses the antrum. By cycle day seven, a single follicle grows in advance of the rest of the cohort and is called the *Graafian follicle* (Johnson and Everitt, 1995) (Figure 7).

Considerable evidence suggests that the nutrient requirements of the oocyte are met by intercellular transport systems that connect it to the surrounding follicle. The avascular granulosa cells have highly developed gap junctions that allow the passage of ions and small molecules. Those nearest the zona

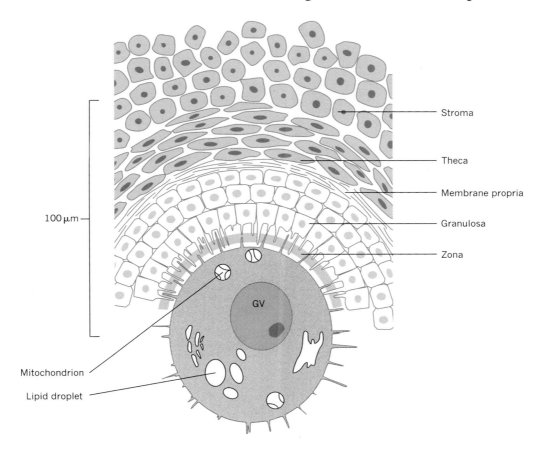

Stroma

Theca

Membrane propria

Granulosa

Zona

100 μm

GV

Mitochondrion

Lipid droplet

Figure 6

develop fine cytoplasmic processes that form permeable junctions with the oocyte membrane. These transfer maternal metabolites directly into the cytoplasm of the enclosed oocyte. At the same time, numerous microvilli on the oocyte membrane form small canals within the zona. Some evidence suggests that these may provide a means by which the oocyte can influence the organizational structure of the surrounding follicle cells (Moor *et al.*, 1990; Salustri *et al.*, 1993) (Figure 8).

HORMONAL ACTIVITIES WITHIN THE FOLLICLES

As follicular growth proceeds, LH stimulates the theca cells to produce increasing amounts of androstenedione and testosterone, with very limited amounts of oestrogen. Although granulosa cells cannot form androstenedione, this is transported from the neighbouring theca cells and enzymes within the granulosa readily convert it to oestrogen. This hormonal activity within the granulosa compartment is stimulated by FSH. Under the influence of oestrogen, granulosa and theca cells proliferate, resulting in a further increase in the size of the growing follicles (Johnson and Everitt, 1995).

From the onset of these developments, follicles grow at varying speeds. The largest of these are thought to possess a greater capacity for the production of oestrogen that becomes sufficiently high to inhibit further release of FSH from the anterior pituitary. This effect on FSH diminishes its stimulating hormonal actions within the remaining follicles. In addition, the appearance of LH receptors on granulosa cells within the dominant follicle are thought to be most accurately timed to coincide with the brief surge of LH and FSH that is stimulated by the earlier surge in oestradiol from the growing follicles (Espey and Ben-Halim, 1990)

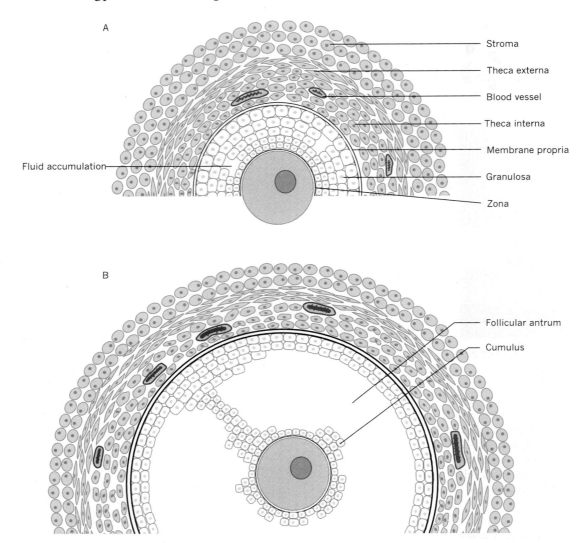

Figure 7   **A**: Early anteral follicle. **B**: Expanded anteral follicle.

PREPARING FOR OVULATION

As the follicle increases in size, synthesis of oestrogen rises and is released into the general circulation, culminating in the surge of oestradiol that precedes ovulation. Within the growing follicle, the combined actions of oestrogen and FSH stimulate the formation of LH receptors on the outer layers of granulosa cells. The dramatic pre-ovulatory surge of FSH and LH is brought about by the action of ovarian hormones on the anterior pituitary and on GnRH neurones within the hypothalamus. These co-ordinated hormonal interactions bring about a cascade of events within the ovary. The surge in FSH and LH increases thecal capillary networks that descend into the underlying layers of granulosa cells. The increasing size and vascularization of the follicle is accompanied by the local release of the prostaglandin PGE_2 and of vasodilatory substances like histamine and bradykinin. PGE_2 initiates the breakdown of collagen within the follicle wall while the other molecules set up an inflammatory reaction inside the follicle. FSH and progesterone also initiate proteolytic enzyme activity that loosen, distend and finally break down the follicular wall (Johnson and Everitt, 1995).

At the same time LH triggers a brief resumption of

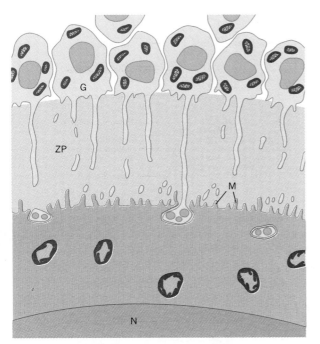

Figure 8 Fully formed zona pellucida surrounding an oocyte. G, granulosa cells; ZP, zona pellucida; M, microvilli; N, nucleus.

meiosis. Some evidence suggests that the oocyte is released from the meiotic block by an action of LH on the granulosa cells. LH is thought to disrupt an inhibitory signal that is continually transmitted by the surrounding granulosa cells (Moor *et al.*, 1990; Salustri *et al.*, 1993). During this phase of meiosis, a *secondary oocyte* is formed containing 23 chromosomes surrounded by the largest concentration of cytoplasm. The remaining 23 chromosomes are discarded to the *first polar body*, in a small enclosure of cytoplasm, on the cell periphery. At the same time, new enzymes are synthesized and formed into *granules* within the main body of cytoplasm. These gradually move towards the cell surface where they subsequently play an important role in regulating fertilization (Johnson and Everitt, 1995) (Figure 9).

Within 12 hours of the LH surge, *progesterone* replaces oestrogen as the dominant steroid hormone (see Figure 5) that is synthesized by theca and granulosa cells. This shift in steroid hormone production is accompanied by a rise in prostaglandin output that in turn leads to the activation of a number of enzymes that weaken and distend the follicle wall. The growing follicle begins to bulge under the surface of the gland and ruptures at its weakest point, allowing follicular fluid to gush out into the peritoneal cavity, carrying the oocyte, zona pellucida, and the surrounding mass of granulosa cells, into the uterine tube.

Cyclical Changes in Related Tissues

UTERUS

During the first and second half of the cycle, a complementary series of changes takes place within the endometrial lining of the uterus, the mucosal secretions of the cervix and the structure and secretions of vaginal tissue. By the end of menses, the mucous membrane lining the uterus is reduced to a thin layer of basal endometrial tissue containing few secretory glands. During the follicular phase of the ovarian cycle, endometrial and myometrial receptors for oestrogen are stimulated by rising levels of this hormone in the circulation. Within the uterus, oestrogen receptors enhance the frequency of myometrial contractions and both produce marked proliferation of the endometrial lining. In this process, epithelial cells from the endometrial glands multiply and cover the raw stromal surface with layer of simple columnar epithelium. The glandular epithelium undergoes increased mitotic activity and the highly specialized endometrial blood supply begins to regenerate (Espey and Ben-Halim 1990; Greenspan and Baxter, 1994; Johnson and Everitt, 1995) (Figure 10).

With the subsequent surge in oestrogen, a three- to five-fold increase occurs in the thickness of the endometrium and intracellular receptors for progesterone are synthesized. The secretory glands become thicker and more convoluted and the spiral arteries increase in length. The cyclical changes that occur in these blood vessels are limited to the sections that supply the active layers of the endometrium. These arteries arise within the myometrium from branches of the uterine artery. They supply blood to the basal unchanging portion of the endometrium, as basal or straight arteries and only adopt the characteristic spiral appearance when they enter the innermost layers of the endometrium (Figure 11). (See also Chapter 3 for menstrual cycle.)

Following ovulation, the rise in circulating levels of progesterone stimulates the endometrial glands to synthesize secretory substances that are rich in glycoproteins, sugars and amino acids. Meanwhile, the surrounding stromal tissue undergoes further proliferation and individual cells become larger and oedematous. Within the myometrium, progesterone induces

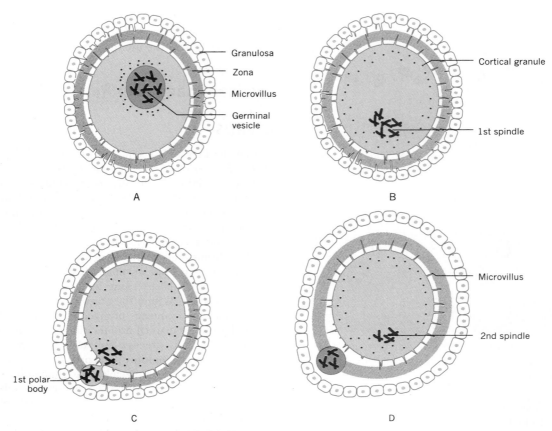

Figure 9   Reactivation of meiosis in the pre-ovulatory oocyte. A few hours after LH stimulation of the follicle (A to B), the germinal vesicle breaks down, and the chromosomes complete prophase and arrange themselves on the first meiotic spindle. Meanwhile, cytoplasmic contact between oocyte and granulosa cells ceases and cortical granules made by the Golgi apparatus migrate to the surface. Subsequently, the first meiotic division is completed with expulsion of the first polar body (B to C). The chromosomes immediately enter the second meiotic division but stop at second metaphase. The cytoplasm around the eccentrically placed spindle is devoid of cortical granules and the overlying membrane lacks microvilli (C to D). The oocyte is ovulated in this arrested state. (Reproduced with permission from Johnson and Everitt, 1995, p. 86.)

cellular enlargement and depresses the excitability of uterine muscle. During this phase, endometrial receptors for both oestradiol and progesterone decline.

CERVIX AND VAGINA

The cervix and vagina undergo cyclical changes that vary the receptiveness of these tissues to the presence of spermatozoa. Under the influence of oestradiol, in the follicular phase of the cycle, the muscles of the cervix relax. This creates a progressive widening of the external os which reaches a maximum width of 3–4 mm around the period of ovulation. At the same time the secretory capacity of the epithelial cells inceases. These cells produce up to 600 mg/day of clear watery, alkaline, mucus mid-cycle which falls to 20–60 mg at other periods of the cycle. Experiments have shown that following the pre-ovulatory surge in oestradiol, the mucus becomes very stretchable and greatly facilitates the movement of spermatozoa (Greenspan and Baxter, 1994).

The vaginal canal is lined by a stratified squamous epithelium identical to that covering the external os. Like the cervix, the vagina is highly responsive to oestrogen and progesterone. As the follicular phase progresses, epithelial cells proliferate under the influence of oestrogen and accumulate intracellular glyco-

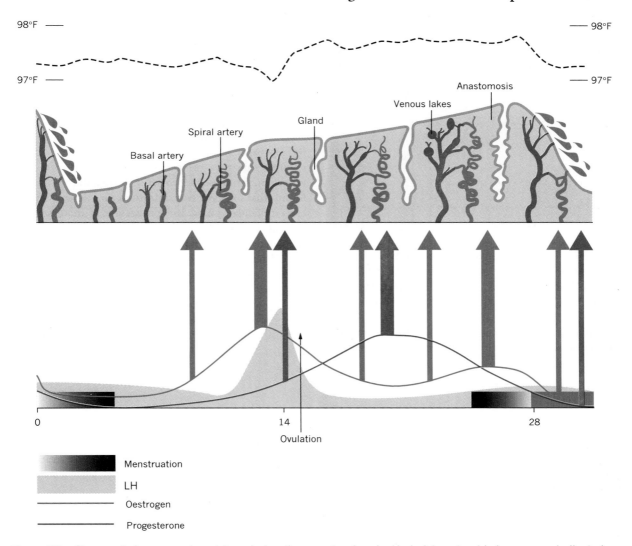

Figure 10   Changes in human endometrium during the menstrual cycle. Underlying steroid changes are indicated below and basal body temperature is indicated above. Thickness of arrows indicates strength of action. (Reproduced with permission from Johnson and Everitt, 1995, p. 176.)

gen that is fermented to lactic acid by the normal bacterial flora. This gives vaginal fluid its mildly acidic character which may protect the area against infection. During periods of sexual excitation, the acidity of vaginal fluid is partially neutralized by increased blood flow that alters the electrolyte balance of vaginal fluid. By increasing the surface pH of the vaginal wall, these events protect the ejaculated sperm from the acid environment of the unstimulated vagina (Greenspan and Baxter 1994).

MAMMARY GLAND

Cyclical changes also occur in the mammary gland. From puberty onwards, these develop in a cumulative manner until approximately 35 years. In each successive cycle during this period, hormonal-induced changes do not return to the starting point of the previous cycle. During each cycle, cellular changes in breast tissue follow a contrasting pattern to those in the endometrium. Mammary epithelium shows decreased DNA synthesis and mitotic divisions in the first half of the cycle, followed by maximal proliferation after

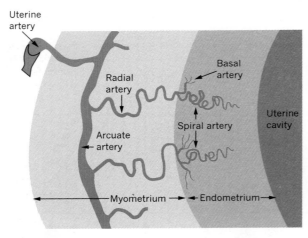

Figure 11   The arterial supply to the uterine endometrium. (Reproduced with permission from Studd, J. (ed.) (1989) *Progress in Obstetrics and Gynaecology*, vol. 7, p. 28. Edinburgh: Churchill Livingstone.)

ovulation (Russo and Russo, 1987). The contrasting pattern of cellular activity in uterine and mammary epithelium is reflected in cyclical differences in steroid hormone receptor concentrations in the two organs. In mammary tissue receptors for oestrogen, like those in the endometrium, decline during the second half of the cycle. But in contrast to the endometrium, those for progesterone remain fairly constant throughout both phases of the cycle (Soderqvist *et al.*, 1993).

During the second half of the cycle, secretory activity may also occur together with increases in breast volume, due to a prolactin-induced increase in fluid retention. Studies on prolactin during the cycle have found that plasma concentrations are lowest in the early follicular phase and progressively increase during the rest of the cycle. This pattern seems to be regulated by an indirect stimulatory influence of GnRH on prolactin-releasing cells and rising levels of ovarian steroid hormones, beginning with the pre-ovulatory surge in oestradiol. Maximal prolactin release in response to GnRH has been found during the peri-ovulatory period and the luteal phase of the cycle (Carandente *et al.*, 1989; Brumsted and Riddick, 1992).

References

Austin, C.R. (1982) The egg. In Austin, C.R. & Short, R.V. (eds) *Reproduction in Mammals*, Book I, *Germ Cells and Fertilization*, pp 46–62. Cambridge: Cambridge University Press.

Baird, D.T. (1990) The selection of the follicle of the month. In Evers, J.L.H. & Heineman, M.J. (eds) *From Ovulation to Implantation*, pp. 3–19. Amsterdam: Excerpta Medica.

Baker, T.G. (1982) Oogenesis and ovulation. In Austin, C.R. & Short, R.V. (eds) *Reproduction in Mammals*, Book I, *Germ Cells and Fertilization*, pp. 17–45. Cambridge: Cambridge University Press.

Barofsky, A.-L., Taylor, J. & Massari, J. (1983) Dorsal raphe-hypothalamic projections provide the stimulatory serotonergic input to suckling-induced prolactin release. *Endocrinology* 113 (5): 1894–1983.

Ben-Jonathan, N. (1991) Prolactin releasing and inhibiting factors in the posterior pituitary. In MacLeod, R.M. *et al.* (eds) *Neuroendocrine Perspectives*, pp. 1–38. New York: Springer-Verlag.

Berne, R.M. & Levy, M.N. (eds) (1993) *Principles of Physiology*. St Louis: Mosby Year Book.

Brumsted, J.R. & Riddick, D.H. (1992) Prolactin and the human menstrual cycle. *Seminars Reprod. Endocrinol.* 10(3): 220–227.

Carandente, F., Angeli, A., Battista, G *et al.* (1989) Rhythms in the ovulatory cycle: 1st: prolactin. *Chronobiologica* 16: 35–44.

Douglas, A.J., Dye, S., Leng, G. *et al.* (1993) Endogenous opioid regulation of oxytocin secretion through pregnancy in the rat. *J. Neuroendocrinol.* 5: 307–314.

Espey, L.L. & Ben-Halim, I.A. (1990) Characteristics and control of the normal menstrual cycle. *Obstet. Gynaecol. Clin. North Am.* 17(2): 275–298.

Greenspan, F.S. & Baxter, J.D. (eds) (1994) *Basic and Clinical Endocrinology*. London: Prentice Hall.

Hill, J.B., Nagy, G.M. & Frawley, L.S. (1991) Suckling unmasks the stimulatory effect of dopamine on prolactin release: possible role for ax-melanocyte-stimulating hormone as a mamotrope responsiveness factor. *Endocrinology* 129(2): 843–847.

Hill J.B., Lacy, E.R., Nagy, G.M. *et al.* (1993) Does ax-melanocyte-stimulating hormone from the pars intermedia regulate suckling-induced prolactin release? Supportive evidence from morphological and funcional studies. *Endocrinology* 133(6): 2991–2997.

Johnson M.H. & Everitt, B.J. (1995) *Essential Reproduction*. Oxford: Blackwell Scientific.

Jones, T.H., Brown B.L. & Dobson, P.R.M. (1990) Paracrine control of anterior pituitary hormone secretion. *J. Endocrinol.* 127: 5–13.

Knobil, E., Neill, J.D., Greenwald, G.S. *et al.* (eds) (1994) *The Physiology of Reproduction*. New York: Raven Press.

Kruseman, A.C.N. (1992) Structure and function of the hypothalamopituitary axis. In Grossman, A. (ed.) *Clinical Endocrinology*, pp. 67–73. Oxford: Blackwell Scientific.

Machida, H. (1981) Influence of progesterone on arterial

blood and CSF acid–base balance in women. *J. Appl. Physiol.* **51**(6): 1433–1436.

Martini, M.C., Lampe, J.W., Slavin, J.L. *et al* (1994) Effect of the menstrual cycle on energy and nutrient intake. *Am. J. Clin. Nutr.* **60**: 895–899.

Moor, R.M., Nagai, T. & Gandolfi, F. (1990) Somatic cell interactions in early mammalian development. In Evers, J.L.H. & Heineman, M.J. (eds) *From Ovulation to Implantation*, 177–191. Amsterdam: Excerpta Medica.

Murburg, M.M., Wilkinson, C.W., Raskind, M.A. *et al.* (1993) Evidence of two differentially regulated populations of peripheral β-endorphin-releasing cells in humans. *J. Clin. Endocrinol. Metab.* **77**(4): 1033–1040.

Page, R.B. (1994) The anatomy of the hypothalamo-hypophysial complex. In Knobil, E., Neill, J.D., Greenwald, G.S. *et al.* (eds) *The Physiology of Reproduction*, pp. 1527–1619. New York: Raven Press.

Parker, C.R., Winkel, C.A., Rush, A.J. *et al.* (1981) Plasma concentrations of 11-deoxycorticosterone in women during the menstrual cycle. *Obstet. Gynecol.* **58**(1): 26–30.

Porter, T.E., Grandy, D., Bunzow, J. *et al.* (1994) Evidence that stimulatory dopamine receptors may be involved in the regulation of prolactin secretion. *Endocrinology* **134**(3): 1263–1268.

Russo, J. & Russo, I.H. (1987) Development of the human mammary gland. In Neville, M.C. & Daniel, C.W. (eds) *The Mammary Gland*, pp. 67–78. New York: Plenum Press.

Russo, J. & Russo, I.H. (1987) Development of the human mammary gland. In Neville, M.C. & Daniel, C.W. (eds) *The Mammary Gland*, pp. 67–93. New York: Plenum Press.

Salustri, A., Hascall, V.C., Camaioni, A. *et al.* (1993) Oocyte–granulosa interactions. In Adashi, E. Y. & Leung, P.C.K. (eds) *The Ovary*, pp. 209–225. New York: Raven Press.

Soderqvist, G., Schoultz, B., Tani, E. *et al.* (1993) Estrogen and progesterone receptor content in breast epithelial cells from healthy women during the menstrual cycle. *Am. J. Obstet. Gynecol.* **169**(3): 874–879

Wynn, M & Wynn, A. (1991a) *The Case for Preconception Care of Men and Women.* Oxford: A B Academic Publishers.

Wynn, M & Wynn, A. (1991b) The menstrual cycle as indicator in prepregnancy care. *J. Nutr. Med.* **2**: 387–398.

Yen, S.S.C. and Jaffe, R.B. (eds) (1991) *Reproductive Endocrinology.* Philadelphia: W.B. Saunders.

Further Reading

Kruseman, A.C.N. (1992) Structure and function of the hypothalamopituitary axis. In Grossman, A. (ed.) *Clinical Endocrinology*, pp. 67–73. Oxford: Blackwell Scientific.

Parker C.R., Winkel, C.A., Rush, J. *et al.* (1980) Plasma concentrations of 11-deoxycorticosterone in women during the menstrual cycle. *Obstet. Gynecol.* **58**(1): 26–30.

7

Fertilization

Fertilization – the fusion of spermatozoon and ovum – usually occurs within the uterine (fallopian) tube. Each uterine tube is approximately 10 cm long and extends laterally from the cornua of the uterus. Around the time of ovulation, smooth muscle fibres within the tube display characteristic movements that bring the distal portion of the tube into apposition with the ovary containing the dominant follicle. As the oocyte is shed from the ovarian surface, it is picked up by finger-like extensions from the terminal end of the tube. These involute to draw the oocyte from the peritoneal cavity, towards the site of fertilization within the uterine tube.

The Uterine Tubes

The uterine tubes are composed of three distinct strata:

1 an external covering of peritoneum and connective tissue;

2 intermediate layers of smooth muscle; and
3 an internal mucosa largely composed of ciliated and secretory epithelium.

Both muscular and epithelial tissues display large variations in their pattern of organization and degrees of thickness in different sections of the tube. Significant variation also occurs in the autonomic nerve supply to different sections of the tube. In the *isthmus*, which contains the greatest concentration of muscle fibres, longitudinal and circular layers are richly innervated with high densities of adrenergic nerve terminals. In contrast, the terminal end of the tube is poorly innervated and adrenergic endings are usually restricted to the walls of the blood vessels, rather than the muscle fibres (Figure 1) (Pauerstein and Eddy, 1979).

ANATOMICAL REGIONS

Along its length, the uterine tube has been divided into four distinct regions:

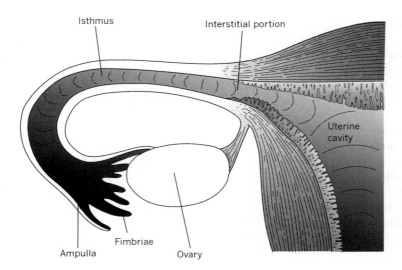

Figure 1   The divisions of the uterine tube.

1   The *infundibulum* is the trumpet-shaped distal portion that terminates as a fimbriated end. This portion is lined with a dense layer of ciliated epithelium. One fimbria is slightly longer than the rest and is applied to the tubal pole of the ovary. Around the time of ovulation, the tube is brought into apposition with the ovary by a change in orientation of muscles surrounding this *ovarian fimbria* which is thought to be essential for the normal mechanisms of oocyte pick-up (Pauerstein and Eddy, 1979; Hunter, 1988).

2   The adjacent *ampulla* forms the longest portion of the tube and is the meeting place for the oocyte and spermatozoa. This section is characterized by thick mucosal folds and poorly defined muscle layers. The ampullary diameter varies from 1–2 mm at its junction with the isthmus to more than 1 cm at its distal end.

3   The *isthmus* begins at the uterotubular junction and extends distally for 2–3 cm. This portion contains the largest concentration of muscle fibres within the tube. Along this segment, the lumen reaches its narrowest diameter, ranging from 100 μm to 1 mm.

4   The *interstitial portion* is continuous with the uterine cavity. The transition between the tubular lumen and the uterine cavity is characterized by a marked increase in the number of ciliated cells and by alterations in the shape of secretory cells. Muscles at the uterotubal junction are formed from four bundles characterized by interlacing spiral fibres that allow strong constriction of the interstitial portion of the tube. Together with the high con-

centration of muscle in the adjacent isthmus, this arrangement is thought to regulate sperm transport and storage and the movement of the oocyte following fertilization (Hunter, 1988).

BLOOD SUPPLY, LYMPHATIC DRAINAGE AND INNERVATION

The uterine tubes receive blood from ovarian and uterine arteries and venous drainage follows the arterial supply. The lymph vessels drain to the aortic and lumbar nodes. Extrinsic innervation is derived from both sympathetic and parasympathetic fibres (Pauerstein and Eddy, 1979).

UTERINE TUBES AS A TRANSITIONAL ENVIRONMENT FOR THE DEVELOPING OOCYTE

During the menstrual cycle, the tubular mucosa undergoes cyclical alterations similar to those in the endometrial lining of the uterus. In the first half of the cycle, both secretory and ciliated cells become larger, under the influence of oestrogen. Around ovulation, ciliated cells become broader and lower while secretory cells become more distended with fluid and protrude above the ciliated cells to form dome-like structures within the tubular lumen. Following ovulation, microscopic holes appear in secretory cell membranes and these coalesce to allow the release of intracellular secretions that have accumulated during the first half of the cycle (Hunter, 1988).

Studies on the changing volume of tubular fluid during the cycle suggest that production increases significantly during the late proliferative phase. Larger volumes have been consistently reported around the time of ovulation than at other phases of the cycle. These hormone-dependent changes in fluid volume may influence oocyte preparation for fertilization. Experiments on animals have found that during its passage through the uterine tubes, the zona pellucida surrounding the oocyte loses certain molecules, in exchange for ones that originate in the surrounding tubular fluid (Brown and Cheng, 1986; Leese, 1995).

The rates of ciliary movements are also influenced by ovarian hormones. Around ovulation, beating of the dense concentration of cilia in the fimbriated portion is closely synchronized, allowing the oocyte to be propelled into the ampulla. During this period, cilia in the ampulla also beat in the direction of the isthmus, suggesting that they act to further propel the oocyte towards the site of fertilization. Increased ciliary activity occurs in conjunction with raised concentrations of noradrenaline, particularly in the isthmus where it acts to contract the large muscular layers for a limited period around ovulation. This activity is thought to play an important role in regulating oocyte movement from the ampulla and subsequent movements of the newly formed *zygote* towards the site of implantation in the uterus (Hunter, 1988).

To understand the tubular environment in relation to the changing metabolic needs of the developing oocyte, recent research has focused on variations in chemical and nutritive factors within the uterine tubes following ovulation. This work has provided extensive data showing that precisely timed modulations occur in oxygen tension, nutrient concentrations, electrolytes and macromolecules in different parts of the tube that complement the changing metabolic capacity of the developing oocyte. Findings on specific molecules indicate that during the greater part of its journey through the uterine tubes, the early embryo is an undifferentiated, non-vascularized structure that utilizes exogenous sources of energy and shows optimal development in an alkaline environment with low concentrations of glucose and oxygen and a plentiful supply of albumen. Experimental evidence suggests that the nutritive environment of the tubular lumen is regulated by hormonal-induced secretions of the tubular mucosa and metabolic activities of the cumu-lus cells surrounding the oocyte (Gardner and Leese, 1990, Leese, 1991, 1995).

Fertilization of the Oocyte

The series of events leading to fertilization involve the co-ordinated transport of one oocyte and a much larger number of spermatozoa, during their brief period of survival within the genital tract. Once the oocyte enters the uterine tube, it has an estimated lifespan of 6–24 hours, while spermatozoa have been estimated to remain in a viable state for 30–80 hours, following their arrival in the vaginal cavity. During this brief period, both sets of cells are subject to a number of physiological changes designed to ensure that only one of the 2–4 million spermatozoa that arrive in the vagina following sexual intercourse or insemination is allowed to fuse with the oocyte membrane and enter the cell cytoplasm.

SPERM TRANSPORT AND CAPACITATION

Spermatozoa enter the genital tract in approximately 3–4 ml of seminal fluid that is thought to buffer the acidity of vaginal secretions. Of these, over 99% are immediately lost by leakage from the vagina. Those that remain behave as a heterogeneous population of cells that spend variable times in the cervix and show differential rates of transport through the uterus. This arrangement is thought to enhance the chances of fertilization, by creating a reservoir of spermatozoa in the cervix that trickle gradually to the uterine tube (Drobnis and Overstreet, 1992).

During their passage through the genital tract, spermatozoa undergo a final series of changes before they are ready for fertilization. The first of these is called *capacitation*. In this process the composition of the cell membrane undergoes a number of modifications that are thought to include the removal of certain molecules added during ejaculation. A great deal of evidence suggests that these alterations are brought about by interactions between spermatozoa and the secretions they encounter during their transport through the cervix, uterus and uterine tubes. Spermatozoa that have undergone capacitation exhibit hyperactive motility that provides them with increased thrusting power thought to be essential for penetration through the zona pellucida surrounding the oocyte

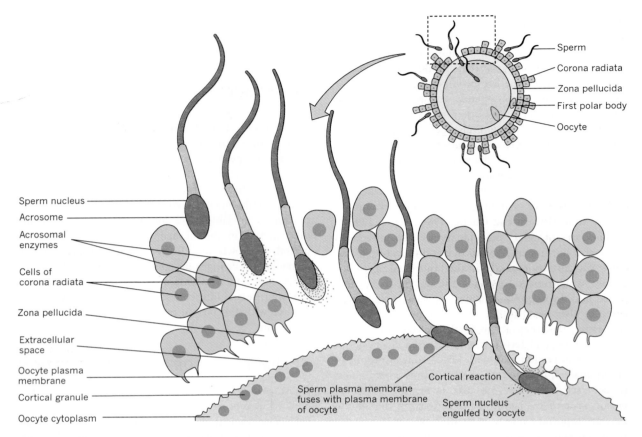

Figure 2 Fertilization and cortical reaction. After capacitation, the plasma membrane of the sperm and the outer membrane of the acrosome fuse and the membranes break down, releasing enzymes that allow the sperm to penetrate the corona radiata. Sperm digest their way through the zona pellucida via enzymes associated with the inner acrosomal membrane. Sperm are engulfed by the oocyte plasma membrane. Cortical granules are released when the sperm cell contacts the membrane. These granules cause other sperm in contact with the membrane to detach. (Reproduced with permission from Chiras, 1991, p. 471).

membrane (Drobnis *et al.*, 1992; Alberts *et al.*, 1994) (Figure 2).

FUSION OF OOCYTE AND SPERMATOZOON

Unlike the process of capacitation, which can occur at a number of sites within the genital tract, the final set of transformations in spermatozoa only occurs as a result of binding with the zona pellucida. Initially, the attachment is very loose and involves a number of spermatozoa. Firmer bonding follows as an oocyte-binding protein on the sperm surface is recognized by sperm receptors on the zona pellucida. During this phase, the inner plasma membrane at the apical end of the sper-

matozoa fuses with the outer membrane of the acrosome and forms a series of membrane-bound vesicles. As these attach to the zona pellucida, the membrane is removed, inducing the previously enclosed enzymes to be externalized. These proteolytic enzymes digest sections of the zona pellucida that surround the sperm head. Subsequent movement through the zona occurs very rapidly, creating immediate access to the oocyte membrane. Only spermatozoa that have undergone this *acrosome reaction* are capable of fusing with the oocyte. Usually, the spermatozoon that makes first contact with the oocyte proceeds to fertilization. In the process of fusion, the plasma membrane of the sperm head is phagocytosed by the oocyte (Alberts *et al.*, 1994).

Immediately after the oocyte and spermatozoon

have fused, a series of ionic changes occur in the oocyte cytoplasm. As a result of these changes, the *cortical granules* that were formed following ovulation bind to the oocyte membrane, which releases their content into the space between the surface of the oocyte and the surrounding zona pellucida. This event is called the *cortical reaction*. The vesicles contain enzymes that modify the structure of the plasma membrane providing a block to the entry of further spermatozoa.

The Zygote

The newly formed cell containing maternal and paternal chromosomes is called a *zygote*. Within 2–3 hours of fertilization, the zygote proceeds with the final phase of meiosis that was halted immediately following ovulation. In this phase, female chromosomes divide mitotically, yielding one haploid set of female chromosomes within the main body of the cytoplasm and the remaining set which are discarded to a second *polar body* on the cell periphery. This later disintegrates, along with the first polar body that was formed at ovulation (Figure 3).

During the same period, the cytoplasmic content of the sperm cell membrane combines with that of the ovum and over the next 2–3 hours the sperm nuclear membrane gradually breaks down. Between 4 and 7 hours following cell fusion, the two sets of haploid chromosomes are formed into male and female *pronuclei*, as each become surrounded by distinct membranes, in opposite poles of the cell. During this period, the chromosomes synthesize DNA in preparation for the first mitotic division. As chromosomal content increases, the pronuclear membranes break down, bringing together the two sets of male and female chromosomes. These events form the diploid complement of a new individual. The fully equipped cell immediately proceeds with a first mitotic division that transforms the zygote into a two-cell *conceptus*. Current evidence suggests that the initial division is regulated by maternal mRNAs stored within the oocyte cytoplasm. But following the two-cell stage, the pre-embryonic genome is activated and begins to synthesize new proteins for subsequent cell divisions (Alberts *et al.*, 1994).

Within the uterine tube, a further series of *undifferentiated* divisions follow at approximately 12-hour intervals until 8–16 increasingly smaller cells have

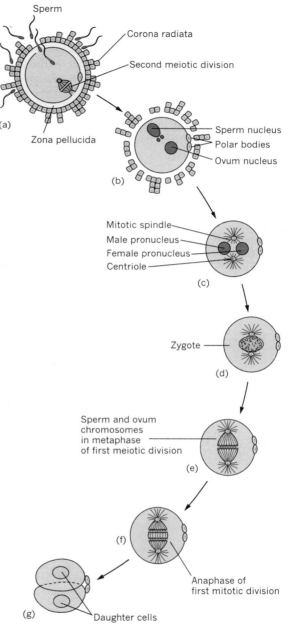

Figure 3 The zygote prepares for division. (a) The sperm contacts the plasma membrane of the oocyte, second meiotic division takes place. (b) Sperm and oocyte pronuclei form. (c) The pronuclei migrate toward the centre of the cell. Chromosomes condense and a mitotic spindle forms. (d) Chromosomes condense and nuclear membrane breaks down. (e) Metaphase plate is formed. (f) Anaphase of the first meiotic division. (g) Two daughter cells form. (Reproduced with permission from Chiras, 1991, p. 472.)

been formed within the zona pellucida. At this point, the conceptus reaches the uterine cavity, where it prepares to embark on a new *differentiated* process of cell division that is marked by net growth in the overall structure. Preparation begins, as the cells nudge closer together and form gap junctions to regulate the flow of molecules between the centre and the periphery. This initiates a process of making the outer cells morphologically distinct from those located in the centre, allowing the embryo to create its own specialized environment.

Morula

At this point the conceptus is called a *morula* (because it resembles a mulberry). During this initial phase of cell division, the conceptus remains within the zona pellucida. This smooth outer covering is thought to provide an overall structure for the inner mass of cells which also prevents their premature adhesion to the uterine epithelium. From the morula stage onwards, metabolic activity is sharply increased. Glucose is consumed in increasing quantities and the embryo appears to require hormones and growth factors for development (Leese, 1995) (Figure 4).

Blastocyst

Over the next 24 hours the morula begins to accumulate fluid within the centre, forming it into a thin layer of outside cells that develop a distinct epithelial polarity and surround a discrete cluster of cells within the cavity. Now known as a *blastocyst* and composed of 34–64 cells, the conceptus utilizes metabolic substrates from endometrial fluids for a further 24 hours, before the outer cells digest their way out of the zona pellucida and come into direct contact with uterine epithelium. At this point the outer rim of cells begins to synthesize a glycoprotein hormone, chorionic gonadotrophin (hCG) that is similar in structure to luteinizing

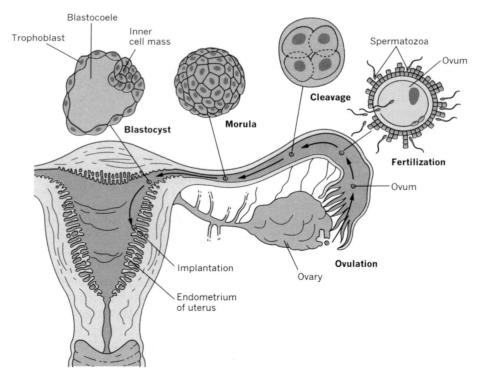

Figure 4   Fertilization and early embryonic development. Fertilization usually occurs in the upper third of the uterine tube. The zygote begins to divide (this is known as cleavage), but remains in the uterine tube for about three days. (Reproduced with permission from Chiras, 1991, p. 470.)

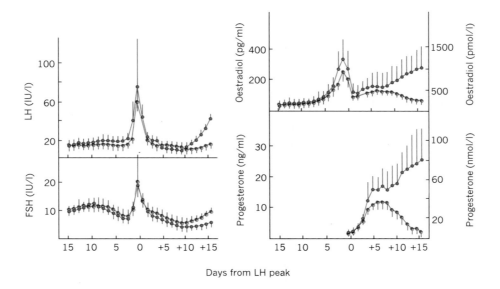

Figure 5   Mean (± SD) log concentrations of LH, FSH, oestradiol and progesterone in 27 control (non-conception cycles) (●—●) and 26 conception cycles (●—●). (Reproduced with permission from Lenton, 1982, p. 136.)

hormone (LH). Because of this similarity, hCG acts on LH receptors in thecal and granulosa cells of the corpus luteum. This provides a continuous stimulus for increased secretion of progesterone and oestrogen, that allows these hormones to maintain the endometrium in an optimum state for implantation (Figure 5).

The Corpus Luteum

When the oocyte leaves the ovary with its surrounding layers of cumulus cells, the remaining follicle collapses around the central cavity that undergoes fibrosis over several days. Following the surge of LH at ovulation, both thecal and granulosa cells have the capacity to synthesize progesterone. During this phase of the cycle, thecal cells are thought to synthesize oestrogen and some progesterone, although the major increase in progesterone output occurs in the granulosa cells that undergo distinct alterations following ovulation. During the luteal phase, these cells cease to proliferate. Instead they grow in size as they develop an increasing number of cytoplasmic organelles which are required for steroid hormone production. In this process of

transformation, granulosa cells become vascularized and in the cow they also acquire a yellow-orange pigment called *lutein*. The term *corpus luteum* derives its name from the study of this species (Gibori, 1993; Johnson and Everitt, 1995).

The rising level of circulating progesterone during the luteal phase initiates a number of changes within the genital tract that facilitate implantation. Under the influence of progesterone, the cervix becomes firmer and more tightly closed and cervical secretions become scant, viscous and cellular, making it more difficult for spermatozoa to enter the uterus. Within the lining of the uterus and uterine tubes, progesterone stimulates copious glandular secretions. Following ovulation, these secretions supply the conceptus with essential nutrients prior to implantation. In addition, this hormone relaxes muscle layers in the isthmus portion of the tube that assists the movement of the conceptus towards the uterine cavity. In the late luteal phase, further changes occur within the uterus. The endometrial stroma undergoes a process of *decidualization*, as it synthesizes a number of hormones and other molecules that are essential for initial growth and immunoprotection of the embryo (Yen and Jaffe, 1991).

References

Alberts, B., Bray, D., Lewis, J. *et al.* (1994) *Molecular Biology of The Cell.* New York: Garland.

Brown, C.R. & Cheng, W.K.T. (1986) Changes in composition of porcine zona pellucida during development of oocyte to the 2- to 4-cell embryo. *J. Embryol. Exp. Morphol.* **92**: 183–191.

Chiras, D.D. (1991) *Human Biology.* St Paul: West Publishing.

Drobnis, E.Z. & Overstreet, J.W. (1992) Natural history of mammalian spermatozoa in the female reproductive tract. *Oxford Rev. Reprod. Biol.* **14**: 1–45.

Gardner, D.K. & Leese, H.J. (1990) Concentration of nutrients in mouse oviduct fluid and their effects on embryo development and metabolism *in vitro. J. Reprod. Fertil.* **88**: 361–368.

Gibori, G. (1993) The corpus luteum of pregnancy. In Adashi, E.Y. & Leung, P.C.K. (eds) *The Ovary*, pp. 261–317. New York: Raven Press.

Hunter, R.H.F. (1988) *The Fallopian Tubes.* Berlin: Springer-Verlag.

Johnson, M. & Everitt, B.J. (1995) *Essential Reproduction.* Oxford: Blackwell Scientific.

Leese, H.J. (1991) Metabolism of the preimplantation mammalian embryo. *Oxford Rev. Reprod. Endocrinol.* **13**: 35–72.

Leese, H.J. (1995) Metabolic control during preimplantation mammalian development. *Human Reprod.* **1**(1): 63–72.

Leese, M.J. (1990) The energy metabolism of the preimplantation embryo. In Wiley, L.M. & Heyner, S. (eds) *Early Embryo Development and Paracrine Relationships*, pp. 67–78. New York: Alan R. Liss.

Lenton, E.A., Sulaiman, R., Sobowale, O. *et al.* (1982) The human menstrual cycle: plasma concentrations of prolactin, LH, FSH, oestradiol and progesterone in conceiving and nonconceiving women. *J. Reprodn Fertility* **65**: 131–139.

Pauerstein, C.J. & Eddy, C.A. (1979) Morphology of the fallopian tube. In Beller, F.K. & Schumacher, G.F.B. (eds) *The Biology of the Fluids of the Female Genital Tract.* New York: Elsevier.

Yen, S.S.C. & Jaffe, R.B. (eds) (1991) *Reproductive Endocrinology.* Philadelphia: WB Saunders.

8

Implantation and Development of the Placenta

The First Phase

Between five and seven days following ovulation, the endometrium displays transient support for the attachment and implantation of the embryo. Growing evidence suggests that these initial processes are regulated in different ways by the inner cell mass, the outer trophectodermal layers of the blastocyst and by hormonal-induced changes in the endometrium.

Trophoblast cells covering the inner cell mass make initial contact with the endometrium by proliferating and forming junctional complexes with the surface epithelium. At the same time, the apical membranes of the epithelial cells display a variety of oestrogen-induced changes that are thought to facilitate cell recognition and interaction with the trophectoderm. These include a progressive shortening of the microvilli, creating a flatter surface, and reduced thickness of the normally dense coating of glycoproteins. During the period of implantation, the cell surface molecules have been characterized as a range of hormone-depen-

dent residues known to regulate cell-adhesion (Hustin, 1992; Wegner and Carson, 1994). Infiltration follows as trophoblast cells displace the epithelium by sending long, slender intercellular protrusions that disrupt the tight junctions between the epithelial cells. In this way trophoblast cells establish contact with glandular and decidual cells lying beneath the surface, by forming a labyrinthic structure, from which the more elaborate villi will later emerge (Hustin and Franchimont, 1992).

During this phase, trophoblast cells rapidly differentiate into two layers that form the origins of the *chorion* and the *fetal portion* of the placenta. The chorion forms the wall of the chorionic sac within which the inner cell mass and the amniotic and yolk sacs are suspended by the connecting stalk. Trophoblast cells in contact with the decidua become cuboidal. These *cytotrophoblast cells* contain a single nucleus and a well-defined plasma membrane. They continually divide to form an outer layer of multinucleated *syncytiotrophoblast (or plasmoditrophoblast) tissue* that ceases to have distinguishable cell membranes. This arrangement creates a continuous common cytoplasm across the whole surface of the developing placenta. At the same time, the inner cell mass differentiates to form an extra-embryonic mesoderm that lines the entire inner surface of the blastocyst.

DEVELOPMENT OF THE CYTOTROPHOBLAST SHELL

The early villi are composed only of cytotrophoblast cells. Once these have formed, they are gradually supported by ingrowth of the underlying mesoderm. Proliferating cytotrophoblast cells extend laterally from one villi to the next and form a continuous shell around the conceptus (Figure 1). Contact between the decidual layer and the cytotrophoblast becomes less direct as a layer of fibrinoid material develops between the shell and maternal tissue (Hustin, 1992).

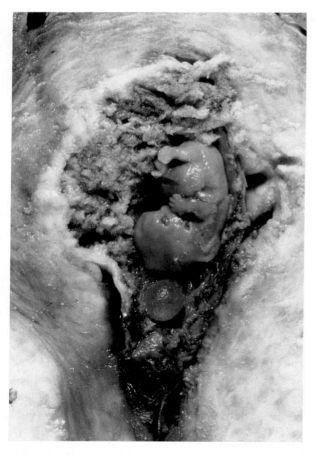

Figure 1   The trophoblast shell. (Photograph courtesy of Dr J. Hustin.)

ENDOMETRIAL RESPONSES TO IMPLANTATION

The surface epithelium and underlying decidua show distinct responses to implantation. Epithelial cells around the implantation site multiply rapidly to form a complete cover for the growing blastocyst which is enveloped in a thick layer of syncytiotrophoblast by approximately nine days following fertilization. During the early weeks of pregnancy the epithelial gland cells show a dramatic rise in the secretion of specific glycoproteins. One of these has been identified as a progesterone-dependent retinol-binding protein that seems to be involved in transporting retinol to the trophoblast and embryo for cell growth and differentiation (Bell, 1988).

More extensive hormone-induced changes occur within the underlying decidua. Decidual cells produce a range of *matrix proteins*, which form a loose lattice-type network that allows free passage of water, ions and large molecules between the decidua and the embryo. Following fertilization, a thickened fibrous network is formed that subsequently undergoes a degree of dissolution at the site of the implanting blastocyst. This may result from the action of trophoblast enzymes or from a progesterone-induced release of *relaxin* by the decidua (Starkey, 1993). Like the epithelial glands, decidual cells also synthesize and release specific glycoproteins. One of these molecules has been identified as a growth factor binding protein that may participate in regulating the pace and extent of trophoblast implantation (Bell, 1988; Hustin and Franchimont, 1992). Decidual cells that release relaxin have also been found to contain *prolactin*, which is regulated by a number of factors from adjoining cells in the decidua, placenta and membranes. The physiological activity of prolactin within the decidua remains unclear but experimental findings suggest that it promotes blastocyst growth, suppresses specific aspects of the immune response and inhibits myometrial contractility, thus creating a smooth local environment for implantation (Yohkaichiya *et al.*, 1988; Healy, 1991; Handwerger *et al.*, 1992).

IMMUNOSUPPRESSIVE AND ANTI-INFLAMMATORY ACTIVITIES

Trophoblast and decidual cells express modified forms of various components of the immune system. The transplantation antigens are absent from trophoblast cells and other antigens present are found in all human tissues and therefore tolerated by the maternal immune system. First trimester studies also indicate that the syncytiotrophoblast – situated at the maternal embryonic interface – expresses high levels of PGE, which modulates many immune system activities. Local maternal tissue seems to be the target of PGE, as the underlying cytotrophoblast contains high concentrations of prostaglandin dehydrogenase (PGDH), an enzyme that inactivates prostaglandins and thereby protects embryonic and fetal tissues from prostaglandins produced by maternal endometrial cells (Eriwch and Keirse, 1992; Kelly, 1994).

While the decidua contains all the cells necessary to produce both an immune and an inflammatory response, evidence suggests that many of these activities are selectively compromised in pregnancy. This phenomenon has been demonstrated in T cells and in small and large lymphocytes. Current research indicates that locally released growth factors and PGE_2 may operate in different ways to modulate immune responses to placentation and promote trophoblast proliferation (Dudley *et al.*, 1990; Starkey, 1993; Kelly, 1994).

OPTIMAL ENVIRONMENT FOR ORGANOGENESIS

Recent animal studies suggest that the optimal conditions for early embryonic development are characterized by low oxygen tensions. In *in vitro* conditions, early embryos have been found to exhibit increased glycogen metabolism and maximum survival rates when oxygen tension was maintained between 2.5 and 5% (Khurana and Wales, 1989; Fisher and Bavister, 1993). This unusual environment is thought to be peculiarly suited to organ formation. Embryonic haemoglobins which last for the first eight weeks of gestation are able to combine with oxygen at the very low tension found in interstitial fluids. In keeping with these results, oxygen tension in the surrounding trophoblast has also been found to be lower than that in the underlying endometrium during the first 12 weeks of gestation (Rodesch *et al.*, 1992).

These findings have led to suggestions that the early embryo derives its external nutritional support from the secretory products of epithelial glands and decidual cells. Developments within the endometrium fully complement this notion. From the moment of implantation, glandular cells secrete rapidly increasing amounts of glycoproteins that promote cell growth and organ differentiation. At the same time the underlying decidua undergoes considerable reorganization, as it forms an array of matrix proteins and differentiated secretory cells that provide growth-promoting factors for the embryo and immunoprotection for trophoblast infiltration (Hustin and Franchimont, 1992; Starkey, 1993).

Evidence suggesting that the early embryo utilizes local nutrients from the endometrium has also been supported by a number of studies on the characteristic features of early trophoblast infiltration. Ultrasound images using a vaginal probe have been obtained for chorionic villous sampling during the first 12 weeks of pregnancy. These pictures have demonstrated that over this period of organ formation, trophoblast infiltration forms a thick undulating layer of actively growing cells called the cytotrophoblastic shell, with primitive villi that sprout extravillous columns of cytotrophoblast cells on the maternal surface. Many of these enter and plug the walls of spiral arterioles while others remain mobile around the intervillous spaces (Hustin, 1992).

During the first 12 weeks, trophoblast migration into the spiral arteries occurs primarily within the decidual segments. First the distal tips of these blood vessels are plugged with cytotrophoblast cells that are continuous with the trophoblastic shell or with the proliferating tips of the emerging villi. Sheets of these endovascular trophoblasts migrate along the capillary walls against maternal blood flow and accumulate within the lumen when they reach the spiral arteries. During the subsequent process of vascular infiltration, cells strip away sections of the endothelium and burrow beneath this layer, to replace elastic tissue and smooth muscle with cytotrophoblast cells that appear to surround themselves with large quantities of fibrinoid material. Later, surface endothelial cells grow over the new underlying tissues. By this process, convoluted arterial walls are converted into tubes of fibrinoid material with no elastic tissue or smooth muscle fibres. As a result of these changes, segments of the spiral arteries become more dilated and lose their capacity to respond to the vasomotor influences of continued autonomic innervation (Hustin *et al.*, 1988; Pijnenborg, 1990) (Figure 2).

During the first 12 weeks of pregnancy, ultrasound studies suggest that decidual blood vessels do not reach the intervillous space. While small amounts of plasma can percolate through the plugs from these

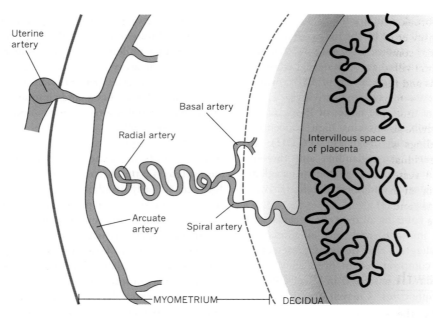

Figure 2   The arterial supply to the placenta in normal pregnancy. (Reproduced with permission from *Progress in Obstetrics and Gynaecology* (1989) **7**: 28.)

low-pressure vessels, chorionic villous sampling has rarely demonstrated the presence of maternal blood. This evidence suggests that during the first 12 weeks, the intervillous space is not immediately connected with the maternal circulation and is not yet bathed by maternal blood (Hustin and Schaaps, 1987). Earlier estimates on uterine blood flow also support this concept. In non-pregnant women, uterine blood flow is approximately 40 ml/min which rises by around 10 ml/min during the first trimester. In contrast, much larger increases occur during the second and third trimester, to reach over 800 ml/min by the end of pregnancy (De Sweit, 1991) (Figure 3).

The Second Phase

From 14 weeks onwards, a second wave of trophoblast infiltration extends into the myometrial segments of many spiral arteries. As in decidual segments, this activity replaces muscular and elastic tissue with unidentified fibrinoid material that converts them into widened, funnel-like tubes that have lost their capacity to respond to the vasomotor influences of continued autonomic innervation. At the same time the tropho-blast shell becomes thinner and more irregular as fetal

growths enlarges its internal volume. An increasing number of extravillous cells become distinct from the shell surface and these gradually open up low-pressure flow of maternal blood within the intervillous space. Experimental evidence on humans and monkeys suggests that the velocity of blood flow from the spiral arterioles to the intervillous space is similar to that of

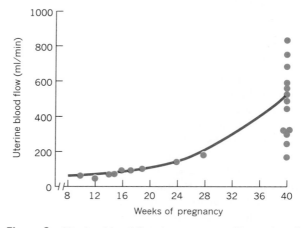

Figure 3   Uterine blood flow in pregnancy. (Reproduced with permission from Hytten F & Chamberlain G (1991) *Clinical Physiology in Obstetrics*, p. 20. Oxford: Blackwell Scientific.)

an actively flowing brook entering a reed-filled marsh (Ramsey, 1963; Ramsey *et al.*, 1976).

The onset of direct communication between maternal blood and placental villi coincides with the completion of organogenesis and the onset of fetal life. During this phase, the roughly formed organs undergo progressive development and rapid growth that requires large increases in uterine size and blood volume. Taken together, these findings suggest that the structural alterations in the decidual and myometrial segments of the uterine blood vessels are set in place to allow for the emergence of an expanding low-pressure system that optimizes gas and nutritional exchange across the placental surface.

Placental Growth and Development

Chorionic villi cover the entire chorionic sac until approximately eight weeks' gestation. As the sac subsequently grows into the endometrial cavity, this portion of the chorion gradually becomes compressed against the *decidua capsularis* – the area of decidual lining that surrounds the site of implantation. With continued growth, the blood supply is reduced and

these villi slowly degenerate, although the trophoblast cells between them remain viable for the remainder of pregnancy. This portion of the chorion, known as *chorion laeve*, forms an interface between fetal amnion and areas of maternal decidua that are not occupied by the placenta. Despite the absence of a direct blood supply, the chorion laeve has diverse layers of metabolically active tissue. It is composed of a layer of fibroblast cells that are contiguous with the amnion, a reticular layer, a type of basement membrane and 2–10 layers of trophoblast cells that are closely applied to the decidua capsularis. Taken together, these cells produce a number of enzymes that degrade locally synthesized substances including prostaglandins, oxytocin and platelet-activating factor, all of which have a capacity to stimulate myometrial contractility (Erwich and Keirse, 1992) (Figure 4).

As villi of the chorion laeve disappear, those attached to the *decidua basalis* rapidly develop to form the mature placenta. The cytotrophoblast shell extends laterally and penetrates deeper into maternal tissue, between the *anchoring villi*, and increasingly complex *branching villi* formed in the intervillous space. Each stem villus forms the centre of the villous tree. Fetal arterioles carrying poorly oxygenated blood enter the villi and break up into an extensive arterio-

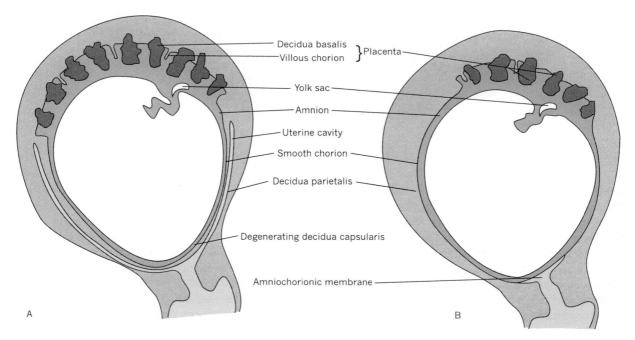

Figure 4 Development of the fetal placenta and fetal membranes. (Reproduced with permission from Moore and Persaud, 1993, p. 114.)

capillary–venous network. The 60–70 branching villi that make up the mature placenta provide a large surface area for gaseous and metabolic exchange between fetal blood within the villi and maternal blood circulating around the external surface from the inter-villous space (Sheppard and Bowwar, 1989) (Figure 5).

Summary of Placental Function

The placenta is a complex organ capable of fulfilling all the requirements of the fetus *in utero*. It selects the

substances required by the fetus from the maternal blood. Many of these substances are used immediately but some are stored and others are changed by the placenta to render them suitable for fetal use. The placenta has five main functions.

Respiratory

Oxygen in the form of oxyhaemoglobin is carried to the uterine sinuses by branches of the uterine and ovarian arteries. In the intervillous spaces the oxyhaemoglobin separates into haemoglobin and oxygen. The oxygen diffuses through the walls of the villi and combines

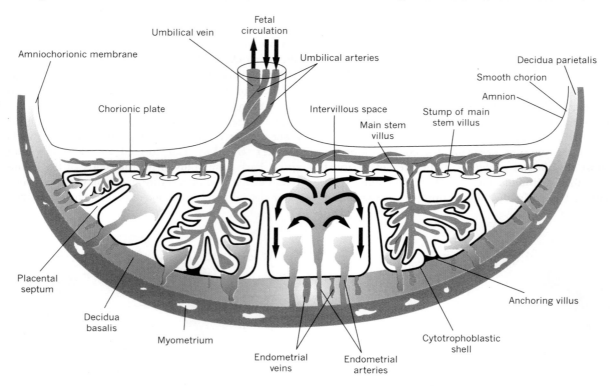

Figure 5   Schematic drawing of a section through a full-term placenta showing: (1) the relation of the villous chorion (fetal part of the placenta) to the decidua basalis (maternal part of the placenta), (2) the fetal placental circulation, and (3) the maternal placental circulation. Maternal blood flows into the intervillous space in funnel-shaped spurts, and exchanges occur with the fetal blood as the maternal blood flows around the branch villi (branches of stem villi). It is through the branch villi that the main exchange of material between the mother and embryo/fetus occurs. The inflowing arterial blood pushes venous blood out into the endometrial veins, which are scattered over the entire surface of the decidua basalis. Note that the umbilical arteries carry poorly oxygenated fetal blood to the placenta and that the umbilical vein carries oxygenated blood to the fetus. Note that the cotyledons are separated from each other by decidual septa, projections of the maternal portion of the placenta (decidua basalis). Each cotyledon consists of two or more main stem villi and their many branches. In this drawing, only one stem villus is shown in each cotyledon, but the stumps of those that have been removed are indicated. (Reproduced with permission from Moore and Persaud, 1993, p. 117.)

with the reduced fetal haemoglobin to form fetal oxy-haemoglobin. This is carried via the umbilical vein to the fetal tissues where the oxygen is given up. The reduced fetal haemoglobin then returns via the umbilical arteries to the placenta for re-oxygenation.

Carbon dioxide from the fetus diffuses through the walls of the villi into the maternal circulation for excretion.

Nutritive

The placenta is the essential intermediary in the transport of vital nutrients. The nutritive capacity of this organ is a function of the syncytiotrophoblast layer which is covered with prominent microvilli. Through a number of nutrient-specific mechanisms the placenta selects and modifies essential nutrients from the maternal circulation to supply them, in appropriate forms and concentrations, to meet fetal requirements for structural growth and energy. Proteins for growth in tissue mass are supplied by an amino acid transport system while those that circulate as part of the immune system are supplied in their original form. Glucose, a primary substrate for fetal energy metabolism, is supplied in increasing quantities by facilitated carrier-mediated diffusion. Lipids, which are essential for structural formation of the brain and vascular system as well as for building fat stores, are transported at a very rapid rate particularly in the latter half of pregnancy (Coleman, 1989; Crawford, 1993; Jansson et al., 1993).

Excretory

The waste products of metabolism, in addition to carbon dioxide, are excreted into the maternal blood by diffusion. They are then excreted by the mother.

Protective

The placenta acts as a barrier to the passage of most bacteria. Thus cocci or bacilli in the maternal blood do not pass into the fetal blood and infect the fetus. Certain smaller organisms, such as the spirochaete of syphilis or viruses, for instance the rubella virus, are able to pass through the walls of the chorionic villi.

The placenta allows the transfer of the antibody IgG from the mother to the fetus, thus giving the baby a certain immunity to infection for its first few months of life. However, the passage of Rhesus antibodies from the mother to the fetus leads to haemolytic disease of the newborn. Most drugs and anaesthetic agents cross the placenta to the fetus and some have a teratogenic effect. Similarly, carbon monoxide from cigarette smoking crosses the placenta and is bound by fetal haemoglobin; this means that there is less fetal haemoglobin available for oxygen transport.

Endocrine

Please see Chapter 11.

References

Bell, S.C. (1988) Secretory endometrial/decidual proteins and their function in early pregnancy. *J. Reprod. Fertil. Suppl.* **36**: 109–125.

Coleman, R.A. (1989) The role of the placenta in lipid metabolism and transport. *Sem. Perinatol.* **13**(3): 180–191.

Crawford, M.A. (1993) The role of essential fatty acids in neural development: implications for perinatal nutrition. *Am. J Clin. Nutrit.* **507**(Suppl.): 703S–710S.

De Swiet (1991) The cardiovascular system. In: Hytten, F. & Chamberlain, G. (eds) *Clinical Physiology in Obstetrics*, pp. 3–38. Oxford: Blackwell Scientific.

Dudley, D.J., Mitchell, M.D. & Creighton, K. et al. (1990) Lymphokine production during term human pregnancy: Differences between peripheral leukocytes and decidual cells. *Am. J. Obstet. Gynecol.* **163**(6): 1890–1893.

Ewrich, J.J.H.M. & Keirse M.J.N.C. (1992) Placental localization of 15-hydroxyprostaglandin dehydrogenase in early and term human pregnancy. *Placenta* **13**: 223–229.

Fisher, B. & Bavister, B.D. (1993) Oxygen tension in the oviduct and uterus of rhesus monkeys, hamsters and rabbits. *J. Reprod. Fertil.* **99**: 673–679.

Handwerger, S., Richards, R.G. & Markoff, E. (1992) The physiology of decidual prolactin and other decidual protein hormones. *Trends Endocrinol. Metab.* **3**(3): 91–95.

Hustin, J. & Schaaps, J-P. (1987) Ecocardiographic and anatomic studies of the maternotrophoblast border during the first trimester of pregnancy. *Am. J. Obstet. Gynecol.* **157**(1): 162–168.

Hustin, J., Schaaps, J-P. & Lambotte, R. (1988) Anatomical studies of the utero-placental vascularization in the first trimester of pregnancy. *Trophoblast Res.* **3**: 49–60.

Hustin, J. (1992) The maternotrophoblast interface: utero-placental blood flow. In Barnea, E.R., Hustin, J. & Jauniaux, E. (eds) *The First Twelve Weeks of Gestation.* pp. 97–110. Berlin: Springer-Verlag.

Hustin, J. & Franchimont, P. (1992) The endometrium and implantation. In Barnea, E.R., Hustin, J. & Jauniaux, E.

(eds) *The First Twelve Weeks of Gestation*, pp. 26–42. Berlin: Springer-Verlag.

Jansson, T., Wennergren, M. & Illsley N.P. (1993) Glucose transporter protein expression in human placenta throughout gestation and in intrauterine growth retardation. *J. Clin. Endocrinol. Metab.* 77(6): 1554–1562.

Kelly, R.W. (1994) Pregnancy maintenance and parturition: the role of prostaglandin in manipulating the immune and inflammatory response. *Endocrine Rev.* 15(5): pp. 684–706.

Khurana, N.K. & Wales, R.G. (1989) Effects of oxygen concentration on the metabolism of [U-^{14}C]glucose by mouse morula and early blastocysts *in vitro. Reprod. Fertil. Devel.* 1: 99–106.

Moore, K.L. & Persaud, T.V.N. (1993) *The Developing Human.* Philadelphia: WB Saunders.

Pijnenborg, R. (1990) Trophoblast invasion and placentation in the human: morphological aspects. *Trophoblast Res.* 4: 33–47.

Ramsey, E.M. (1963) Serial and cineradioangiographic visualization of maternal circulation in the primate (hemochorial) placenta. *Am. J. Obstet. Gynecol.* 86(2): 213–225.

Ramsey, E.M. *et al.* (1976) Interaction of the trophoblast and maternal tissues in three closely related primate species. *Am. J. Obstet. Gynecol.* 124(6): 647–652.

Rodesch, F., Simon, P. & Donner, C. *et al.* (1992) Oxygen measurements in endometrial and trophoblastic tissues during early pregnancy. *Obstet. Gynaecol.* 80(2): 283–285.

Sheppard, B.I. & Bowwar, J. (1989) The maternal blood supply to the placenta. *Prog. Obstet. Gynaecol.* 7: 27–30.

Starkey, P.M. (1993) The decidua and factors controlling placentation. In Redman, C.W.G., Sargent, I.L. & Starkey, P.M. (eds) *The Human Placenta*, pp. 362–413. Oxford: Blackwell Scientific.

Wegner, C.C. & Carson, D.D. (1994) Cell adhesion processes in implantation. *Oxford Rev. Reproduct. Biol.* 16: 89–137.

Yohkaichiya, T., Fukaya, T. & Hoshiai, H. *et al.* (1988) Effect of prolactin on the *in vitro* cultured mouse embryo. In Mizuno, Mori, Taketani (eds) *Role of Prolactin in Human Reproduction*, pp. 210–218. Basel: Karger.

Further Reading

Healy, D.L. (1991) Endometrial prolactin and implantation. *Clin. Obstet. Gynecol.* 5(1): 95–105.

Leese, H.J. (1990) The energy metabolism of the preimplantation embryo. In Wiley, L.M. & Heyner, S. (eds) *Early Embryo Development and Paracrine Relationships*, pp. 67–78. New York: Alan R. Liss.

9

Embryonic and Fetal Developments

The transformations that occur within the inner cell mass during the first trimester are characterized by successive waves of *mitotic division, cell differentiation, tissue migration* and *reorganization*. At present the cellular mechanisms that co-ordinate these movements are not fully understood. The inner cell mass is composed of cells with varying genetic backgrounds that constantly interact with each other and have access to a variety of molecules from surrounding uterine tissues. While increasing knowledge has been gained about the sequence of events that unfold within different layers of the inner cell mass, current understanding of human embryology remains largely descriptive in character.

During the first three weeks of gestation, most changes within the inner cell mass are directed towards the formation of extra-embryonic structures in preparation for organogenesis. These changes begin with a differentiation of the inner cell mass into a bilaminar disc, composed of a distinct external layer called the *primary ectoderm* and an inner layer called the *primary endoderm*. A layer of *ectoderm* is gradually displaced by accumulating extracellular fluid. Some of these cells differentiate into amnioblasts that later

form the *amniotic membrane*, separating the cavity from the surrounding cytotrophoblast cells (Figure 1).

At the same time *endoderm cells* proliferate and migrate on to the inner surface of the cytotrophoblast, to form *Heuser's membrane*. By this migration, the blastocyst cavity is transformed into a primary and then into a definitive yolk sac. As soon as the primary yolk sac forms, a thick acellular material is secreted between Heuser's membrane and the cytotrophoblast called the *extra-embryonic mesoderm*. Over the next couple of days this tissue divides to form a second chorionic cavity, between the primary yolk sac and the cytotrophoblast. On day 12, a second wave of proliferation of the endoderm forms a new membrane that migrates over the inside of the extra-embryonic mesoderm, pushing the primary yolk sac as it moves forward. As a result of this reorganization, a smaller definitive yolk sac is formed within a larger chorionic cavity filled with extracellular fluid. Distinct layers of the yolk sac give rise to blood cells, endothelial cells and germ cells. Fusion of the endothelial cells gives rise to small capillary networks. At the same time, blood cells and capillaries develop within the placental villi. At approximately 19 days, the two sets of vessels

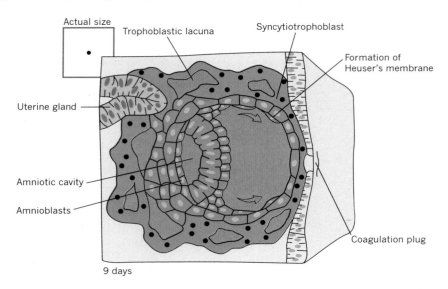

Actual size
Trophoblastic lacuna
Syncytiotrophoblast
Formation of Heuser's membrane
Uterine gland
Amniotic cavity
Amnioblasts
Coagulation plug
9 days

Figure 1   By 9 days, the embryo is completely implanted in the uterine endometrium. The amniotic cavity is expanding, and the hypoblast has begun to proliferate and migrate out over the cytotrophoblast to form Heuser's membrane. Trophoblastic lacunae appear in the syncytiotrophoblast, which now completely surrounds the embryo. The point of implantation is marked by a transient coagulation plug in the endometrial surface. (Reproduced with permission from Larsen, 1993, p. 36.)

establish contact, thereby creating a vascular connection between the embryo and the placenta (Moore and Persaud, 1993) (Figure 2).

Having formed a surrounding cavity of extracellular fluid and the rudiments of a vascular system, the bilaminal disc embarks on a period of extensive reorganization during the third week of gestation, that prepares the way for organogenesis. This process involves the simultaneous migration, contraction and expansion of different cell types all over the embryo. The longitudinal axis and bilateral symmetry of the future embryo is established as a result of these transformations.

During this critical stage of development, a primary structure called the *primitive streak* is formed along the longitudinal midline of the disc. This structure seems to provide an organizing centre for all cellular activities. Following its formation, subsets of cells within the ectoderm transform into a third *mesodermal* layer. These migrate widely to form a variety of connective tissues and stromal components of individual glands (Braude and Johnson, 1990).

The formation of this trilaminal disc allows specific precursor cells for different bodily tissues to be laid down in their correct spatial positions. Over the next 6–8 weeks, each layer of the disc undergoes cell divisions and further differentiation and folding that gives rise to

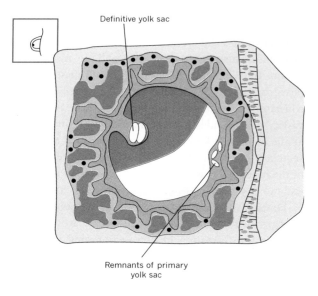

Definitive yolk sac

Remnants of primary yolk sac

Figure 2   The primary yolk sac breaks up and is reduced to a collection of vesicles at the embryonic end of the chorionic cavity. (Reproduced with permission from Larsen, 1993, p. 39.)

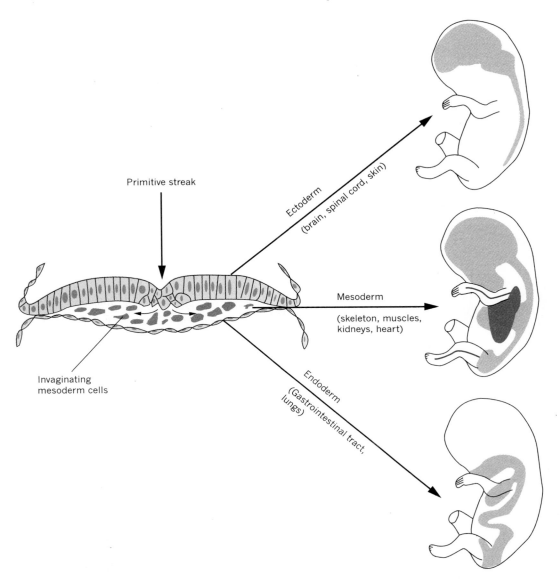

Primitive streak

Ectoderm
(brain, spinal cord, skin)

Mesoderm

(skeleton, muscles,
kidneys, heart)

Endoderm
(Gastrointestinal tract,
lungs)

Invaginating
mesoderm cells

Figure 3   The trilaminar disk (reproduced with permission from Dunstan (1990) p. 214.)

basic organs and definitive body structures. Once the conceptus has entered this phase of organ formation, it becomes an *embryo*, as it has developed the distinct tissues that will constitute the fetus (Figure 3).

Amniotic Fluid

As the embryo forms and grows, the amniotic membrane also expands until it encloses the entire embryo, except for the umbilical area. The amniotic membrane is composed of a single layer of cuboidal epithelial cells on a loose connective tissue matrix. Between the fourth and eighth weeks of gestation, the production of amniotic fluid increases, to reach approximately 20 ml. This causes the amnion to swell, until it takes over the chorionic space, thus bringing the amnion and chorion in contact with each other. From this point onwards, amniotic fluid volume increases from approximately 350–450 ml at 20 weeks, to 800–1000 ml at 36–39 weeks and then begins to decline (Moore and Persaud, 1993; Johnson and Everitt, 1995) (Figure 4).

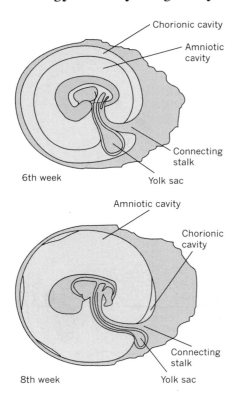

Chorionic cavity

Amniotic cavity

Connecting stalk

6th week   Yolk sac

Amniotic cavity

Chorionic cavity

Connecting stalk

8th week   Yolk sac

Figure 4   The rapidly expanding amniotic cavity fills with fluid and obliterates the chorionic cavity between the sixth and eighth weeks. (Reproduced with permission from Larsen, 1993, p. 124.)

REGULATION OF FLUID VOLUME

During the first half of pregnancy, the composition of amniotic fluid is similar to fetal or maternal plasma and its volume increases are closely related to fetal weight. Until about 20 weeks, the dynamics of amniotic fluid volume are thought to involve a transmembrane pathway from maternal blood via the placenta and movement of fluid and other molecules across the fetal skin, which offers no impediment to the flow of fluid into the amniotic sac. From 17 to 25 weeks' gestation, this pattern of flow diminishes, as the fetal skin begins to to keratinize. During the second half of pregnancy, the fetal kidneys and lungs make a growing contribution to amniotic fluid, while the gastrointestinal tract becomes a major pathway for its removal. Estimates of daily volumes near term suggest that fetal urine contributes

800–1200 ml, lung fluid 170 ml and 500–1000 ml is removed by fetal swallowing (Gilbert, 1991).

At present the mechanisms regulating amniotic fluid volume are poorly understood. During the second half of pregnancy amniotic fluid is hypo-osmolar as compared with maternal and fetal plasma. This osmotic gradient would be expected to drive water from the amniotic cavity into the maternal and fetal circulations via the umbilical cord, placenta and membranes. However, the precise volumes that move through these pathways remain to be confirmed (Gilbert, 1991; Brace, 1995).

Other evidence suggests that decidual prolactin and PGE_2 from the amniotic membrane and umbilical cord may be involved along with other hormones in regulating amniotic fluid volume. Concentrations of prolactin in amniotic fluid are 5- to 10-fold higher than in the maternal circulation. Levels increase sharply in the second trimester, reaching mean values of about 3500 ng/ml around 20 weeks, before declining significantly to a second plateau of about 500 ng/ml by 34 weeks. This pattern is thought to result from a fall in decidual production and a simultaneous rise in degradation by the fetal kidneys. Prolactin may regulate the volume of amniotic fluid by controlling electrolyte exchange across the chorio-amniotic membranes (Kletzky, 1992; Handwerger et al., 1992).

In a variety of epithelial-related cells PGE_2 has been found to actively regulate ion flow. Because it is the predominant prostaglandin in the amnion, it seems possible that it may be involved in absorbing fluid across the growing amniotic membrane. The action of PGE_2 and other placental peptides like atrial natriuretic peptide (ANP) may regulate the removal of fluid into the maternal circulation and help to counterbalance the large inflow of fetal urine during the latter part of pregnancy (Gilbert, 1991; Demir et al., 1992; Kelly, 1994) (Figure 5).

This dynamic volume of fluid provides essential space for fetal growth and movements, particularly during the second half of pregnancy. In late pregnancy and labour, it equalizes the pressure exerted by uterine contractions and creates a cushion for the umbilical cord, preventing compression of the umbilical vessels between the fetus and the uterine wall during fetal movements and contractions. At the same time, liquor volume also modulates excessive overriding of the bones of the fetal skull which protects the underlying cerebral membranes and blood vessels as the head is moulded during descent and rotation in the pelvis.

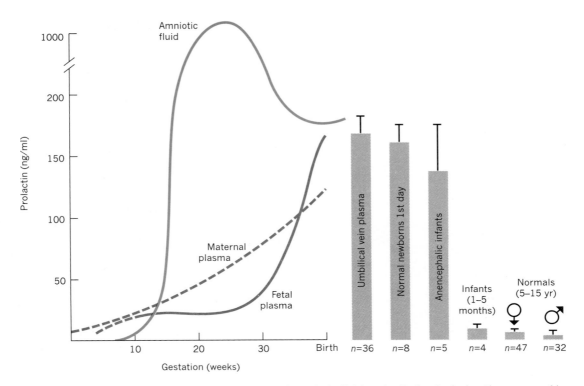

Figure 5   Comparisons of patterns of maternal, fetal and amniotic fluid prolactin levels during the course of human pregnancy. On the right, plasma levels of prolactin in normal and anencephalic newborns are compared with those of normal infants, children and adolescents. (Aubert *et al.*, 1975; Schenker *et al.*, 1975.)

Organ Formation

BRAIN AND CENTRAL NERVOUS SYSTEM

The human nervous system begins to form at approximately 18 days after fertilization, making it the first organ system to initiate development. A specific area of the ectodermal layer thickens to produce an oval-shaped portion called the *neural plate*. On either side of the midline of this plate, two longitudinal neural folds grow in size and curve towards each other and subsequently fuse to form the first outline of the *neural tube*. As the neural tube is formed, some neuroectodermal cells lying along the crest of each neural fold lose their attachment to neighbouring cells. These *crest cells* migrate and form an irregular mass on either side of the neural tube. Later, they give rise to the sensory ganglia of the spinal and cranial nerves and contribute to the specialized chromaffin cells of the adrenal medulla. During the fetal phase of development, the fully formed tube gives rise to the central nervous system, while the tubular lumen gives rise to the spinal canal and the brain ventricles (Figure 6).

By 19 days' gestation, the three major divisions – *forebrain*, *midbrain* and *hindbrain* – are demarcated by indentations in the neural folds and a diverticulum called the *infundibulum* begins to grow downwards from the forebrain division, giving rise to the posterior section of the *pituitary gland*. At the same time an ectodermal evagination of the oropharynx begins to grow towards the infundibulum. It subsequently loses its connections with the oral cavity and forms a discrete sac known as the *anterior pituitary gland*.

From four weeks' gestation, major regions of the brain emerge and neurones start to differentiate from the epithelium of the neural tube, creating a very active phase of brain cell division. The thalamus and hypothalamus become demarcated by the end of week 5 and differentiation continues throughout embryonic development. At the end of the first eight weeks, the head makes up almost half of the embryo and directs the first movements of the limbs.

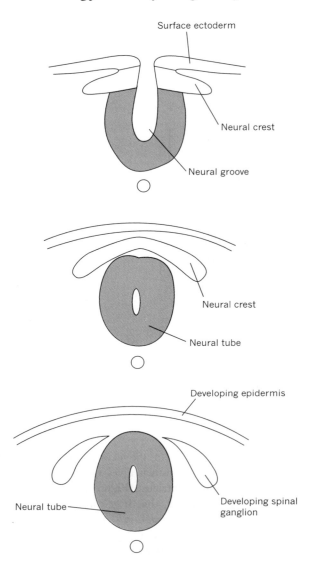

Figure 6 Portions of diagrammatic transverse sections through progressively older embryos illustrating formation of the neural groove, the neural tube and the neural crest up to the end of the fourth week. (Reproduced with permission from Moore and Persaud, 1993, p. 62.)

Eyes and ears

From five weeks' gestation, two *neuroectodermal pockets* expand laterally from the hollow forebrain. These optic vesicles go through successive phases of differentiation and re-modelling to form the eye cup. Mesoderm surrounding the optic cup forms the inner vascular choroid and the fibrous outer sclera while mesenchymal tissue gives rise to the lens. At the same time the inner ear begins to form in a similar manner. Small diverticula bud from hollow otic vessels that continue to grow and reshape to gradually form the series of interconnected structures that make up the inner ear.

Nutritional requirements

Growth of neural and retinal membranes is determined by the availability of essential and non-essential fatty acids. Humans depend on dietary sources for an adequate supply of essential fatty acids. During pregnancy, maternal lipid metabolism is altered substantially to increase lipid stores and provide increasing levels of circulating lipids for uptake by the placenta and mammary gland. Recent research has focused on the important role of the placenta in producing, modifying and transporting preformed long-chain essential fatty acids. The fetal brain and retina can only use this variety to form their highly specialized cell membranes which are involved in signal transmission. Brain growth occurs at a very fast rate *in utero*, particularly during the last trimester. After birth, maternal transfer of these lipids continues during suckling. During this period, brain and retinal cell division declines while the rate of synaptic connections increases dramatically as the newborn interacts with the new environment (Carlson, 1992; Herrera *et al.*, 1992; Crawford, 1993; Makrides *et al.*, 1995).

CARDIOVASCULAR DEVELOPMENT

The cardiovascular system is essential for fetal growth and development, as it supplies nutrients and facilitates gaseous exchange in all parts of the body. Like the brain, the vascular system is largely composed of membranes that use essential fatty acids for structural formation and as precursors for a variety of prostaglandins that regulate dilation, constriction and other thrombogenic activities. Recent evidence indicates that the formation of a healthy vasculature is critically dependent on the absence of cortisol. Disruption of these conditions is associated with poor fetal growth and may be secondary to long-term problems in maternal nutrition arising from social deprivation (Wynn *et al.*, 1991; Edwards *et al.*, 1993; Seckl, 1994; Wynn *et al.*, 1994; Barker, 1995).

The heart

Cells that are destined to form the primitive heart tube begin as two oval clusters of mesoderm on either side

of the midline of the embryo. This precardiac mesoderm migrates towards the head and fuses in the midline, creating two parallel cords of cells. These soon
enlarge and develop internal canals that become the
endocardial tubes. These fold over and fuse to create
the primitive *cardiac tube*, which is composed of one
atrium and one ventricle. Primitive blood vessels begin
to form during the third week of development and
pulsation of the primary cardiac tube can be detected
at approximately five weeks' gestation. Between 5 and 8
weeks, septa are formed within the heart, which partition it into four chambers (Moore and Persaud, 1993).

Intrauterine (fetal) circulation

In utero the fetus relies on the placenta to carry out its
respiratory, nutritional and excretory functions. It has
no need of lungs and is mostly concerned with pumping blood to the placenta so that the necessary gaseous
exchange can take place.

The fetal circulation has adapted for this purpose. It
differs from the adult circulation in that blood is
oxygenated in the placenta and not in the lungs. This
is a less efficient method and, therefore, requires
several modifications:

Larger and more numerous red cells (6–7 million/
mm^3)

Higher haemoglobin content (20.7 g/dl) to pick up the
maximum amount of oxygen

Modified form of haemoglobin (HbF) which is active
in the slightly more acid blood

Certain additional structures:
Ductus arteriosus
Ductus venosus
Foramen ovale
Two hypogastric arteries

The basic organization of intrauterine circulation is
established during early embryonic life: *Umbilical
veins* bring oxygenated blood to the heart, from the
chorion frondosum; the *vitelline veins* return blood
from the yolk sac; and the *cardinal veins* return blood
from various parts of the body. Blood enters the heart
via the sinus venous and flows through a single atrium
and ventricle. When the ventricle contracts, blood is
pumped through the bulbus cordis, passes into the
dorsal aorta and eventually returns to deliver waste
products to the chorion (Moore and Persaud, 1993)
(Figure 7).

During fetal life the vascular system becomes more

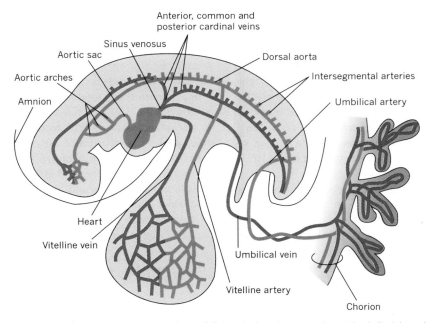

Figure 7 Diagram of the cardiovascular system (about 26 days) showing vessels on the left side only. The umbilical vein
carries well-oxygenated blood and nutrients from the chorion (embryonic part of the placenta) to the embryo. The
umbilical arteries carry poorly oxygenated blood and waste products to the chorion. (Reproduced with permission from
Moore and Persaud, 1993, p. 306.)

extensive as it parallels the increasing size and complexity of individual organs and tissues. Oxygenated blood returns from a greatly enlarged placenta, via the umbilical vein. Approximately 50% of this blood enters a hepatic microcirculation and later joins the inferior vena cava via the hepatic veins. The remaining blood passes directly to the inferior vena cava, through a shunt called the *ductus venosus*. Blood flow through this vascular bypass is thought to be regulated by a physiological sphincter that responds to changing volume in the umbilical vein. This mechanism helps to protect the fetus from erratic fluctuations in blood pressure (Walker, 1993).

In addition to well-oxygenated blood from the placenta, the inferior vena cava also receives less oxygenated blood from the abdomen, pelvis and lower limbs, representing more than 66% of total venous return. Before entering the heart, the inferior vena cava bifurcates into two channels: the *foramen ovale* links it to the left atrium and a small inlet links it to the right atrium. In the left atrium, the foramen ovale ends in a one-way valve that only permits blood flow from right to left. Flow patterns in the right atrium allow 50% of oxygenated blood returning from the placenta to be shunted to the left atrium. This right-to-left flow through the foramen ovale is maintained by the larger quantity and greater speed of blood flow from the inferior vena cava on the right, compared to that entering the left atrium via the pulmonary veins from the lungs. During fetal life, lung tissue extracts oxygen from the low circulating blood volume that enters from the right ventricle and returns poorly oxygenated blood to the left atrium. Low venous return from the lungs is actively maintained by the exposure of pulmonary vessels to blood Po_2, which keeps them in a state of hypoxic vasoconstriction (Moore and Persaud, 1993; Walker, 1993).

A small amount of well-oxygenated blood from the inferior vena cava enters the right atrium. This is mixed with poorly oxygenated blood returning from the head via the superior vena cava which mainly enters the right ventricle through the tricuspid valve. From the right ventricle, only 10% of blood enters the lungs via pulmonary arteries. The remaining 90% is diverted into the descending aorta via a muscular artery called the *ductus arteriosus*, which connects the main pulmonary artery with the aorta. Throughout fetal life, patency and therefore relaxation of this muscular artery is actively maintained by high circulating levels of PGE_2 and by the local release of PGI_2. As a result of

this shunt, most blood leaving the right ventricle is responsible for perfusing the lower body and the placenta (Moore and Persaud, 1993; Walker, 1993).

In the left atrium, the pulmonary component combines with a much larger volume of more highly oxygenated blood from the inferior vena cava. From the left atrium, blood passes into the left ventricle. A small amount of this blood supplies the heart, two-thirds leaves via the ascending aorta to perfuse the upper part of the body with highly oxygenated blood, while the remaining one-third flows through the aortic isthmus to the descending aorta and then to the lower body and placenta (Walker, 1993). The two *hypogastric arteries* convey deoxygenated blood to the placenta.

The shunting of blood on the venous side by the foramen ovale and on the arterial side by the ductus arteriosus are structural devices designed to organize the circulation so that most blood bypasses the lungs and is directed to the placenta. This large volume of poorly oxygenated blood returning to the placenta also flows much more rapidly than the more highly oxygenated blood that supplies the upper part of the body. The rate of flow tends to be most rapid in the descending aorta. From this vessel, blood is directly pumped into the umbilical arteries and returns for gaseous exchange in the placenta (Walker, 1993) (Figure 8).

During intrauterine life, the fetal–placental circulation operates as a single unit. This organization provides a low-resistance, high-capacity reservoir in the vascular bed of the placenta, which is maintained by the absence of valves in the umbilical veins. From animal experiments, total fetal–placental blood volume is estimated at 100–120 ml/kg body weight, with 80–90 ml/kg representing fetal blood volume at any given time while the remainder is contained within the umbilical–placental circulation. This additional capacity helps to protect the fetal circulation from fluctuations in blood pressure and blood flow distribution at a time when autoregulation of regional blood flow is not fully developed. The major changes that take place in the fetal circulation at birth are described in Chapter 63.

UROGENITAL SYSTEM

Variations of mesodermal tissue give rise to the urinary and genital organs and to the outer cortex of the adrenal gland. The urinary and genital systems are very closely interwoven. They arise largely from the same type of tissue and the excretory ducts of both systems initially enter a common cavity, the *cloaca*.

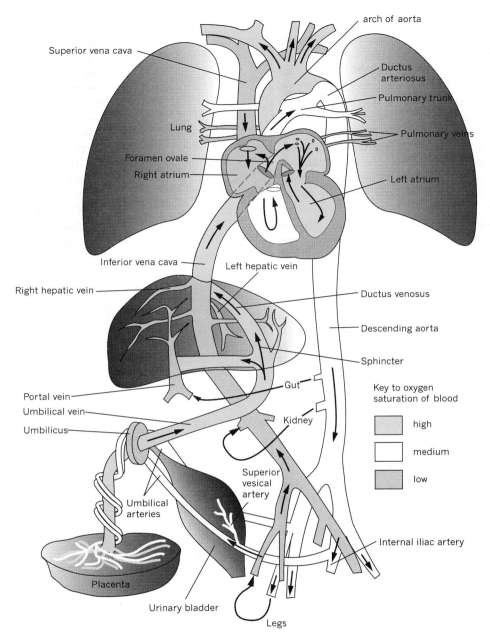

Figure 8   Schematic illustration of fetal circulation. The colours indicate the oxygen saturation of the blood and the arrows show the course of the blood. The organs are not drawn to scale. Observe that three shunts permit most of the blood to bypass the liver and lungs: (1) the ductus venosus, (2) the foramen ovale, and (3) the ductus arteriosus. (Reproduced with permission from Moore and Persaud, 1993, p. 344.)

With further development, the interconnections between the two systems remain more evident in males. During fetal life, primitive urinary ducts are transformed into the main genital duct, while in the adult, urine and semen are discharged through a common duct, the penile urethra.

In humans, formation of the definitive kidneys is preceded by a rudimentary development of a pair of nephritic vesicles and *mesonephric ducts*. The vesicles remain non-functional and disappear by the end of the fourth week, while the ducts produce small amounts of urine between 6 and 10 weeks' gestation. These subsequently regress in females, while in males they persist to form elements of the genital system.

Early in the fifth week a pair of *ureteric buds* sprout from the distal portion of the mesonephric ducts. These grow into a pouch of mesodermal tissue on either side of the sacral region – the *metanephric blastema* – which forms the definitive kidneys. The ureters and collecting ducts differentiate from the ureteric bud, while the nephrons or definitive urine-forming units differentiate from the metanephric blastema. Between 6 and 9 weeks' gestation, the kidneys ascend from the sacral region, to a lumbar site just below the adrenal glands (Moore and Persaud, 1993) (Figure 9).

From 5 to 14 weeks' gestation, the two distinct structures forming the kidneys undergo successive phases of bifurcations and extensions, as the system develops its elaborate network of calyces and tubules. When the ureteric bud first contacts the metanephric blastema, its tips extend to form an ampulla that subsequently gives rise to the renal pelvis. From 6 to 32 weeks' gestation, the ureteric bud undergoes numerous bifurcations that subsequently coalesce to form both major and minor calyces and collecting ducts. Meanwhile the nephrons emerge from metanephric tissue surrounding the ampulla, which differentiates to form a Bowman's capsule, the distal convoluted tubule and the loop of Henle. At the same time a dense capillary network forms within the capsule and extends in a parallel fashion alongside the remaining sections of the tubules. During the tenth week, the distal convoluted tubules join on to the collecting ducts and the system starts to produce urine (Moore and Persaud, 1993).

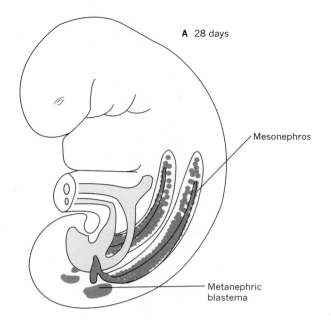

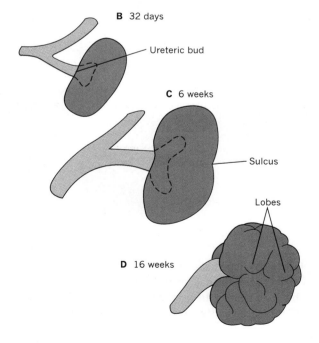

Figure 9   Origin of the metanephric kidneys. (A) A metanephric blastema develops from intermediate mesoderm on each side of the body's axis early in the fifth week. (B) Simultaneously, the metanephric ducts sprout ureteric buds that grow into each metanephric blastema. (C) By the sixth week, the ureteric bid bifurcates and the two growing tips (ampullae) induce superior and inferior lobes in the metanephros. (D) Additional lobules form during the next 10 weeks in response to further bifurcation of the ureteric buds. (Reproduced with permission from Larsen, 1993, p. 241.)

Urine is formed as plasma from the glomerular capillaries and is filtered to produce a dilute filtrate which is then concentrated by the convoluted tubules and the loop of Henle. From there it passes into the bladder and out into the surrounding amniotic fluid. During fetal life the formation of urine is not used to clear waste products from the blood, as this activity is carried out by the placenta. Instead urine serves to supplement the production of amniotic fluid. During the second half of pregnancy, urine is formed at the rate of 800–1200 ml per day, making it the largest single contributor to the volume of amniotic fluid (Gilbert, 1991).

Adrenal cortex

During intrauterine life, the adrenal cortex works in conjunction with the placenta to establish interdependent hormonal interactions that cross fetal, placental and maternal compartments to provide a variety of conditions needed for fetal and neonatal development. Specific activities of this feto-placental unit include:

▶ regulating placental synthesis of oestrogen, stimulating the synthesis and release of placental progesterone and maternal prolactin;
▶ initiating a cascade of events that increases maternal plasma and red cell volume;
▶ regulating placental metabolism of cortisol;
▶ promoting growth of the mammary gland and stimulating its uptake of lipids during the third trimester, in preparation for lactation (Longo, 1993; Skinner, 1993; Winter, 1992; Pepe and Albrecht, 1990, 1995).

Development of the adrenal glands

The central regulatory role of the adrenals is indicated by their spectacular growth and secretory capacity during intrauterine life. Cells forming the adrenal cortex appear at 3–4 weeks' gestation and enlarge rapidly to equal the size of the kidneys by the end of the first trimester. By 6–8 weeks' gestation, the cortex forms a distinct *fetal zone*, beneath an outer subcapsular rim of immature cells that resemble those in the outer zone of the adult gland. During the second trimester, the adrenals enlarge in direct proportion to the increase in total body weight. At this time their relative weight is 35 times the adult value. In the third trimester, gland weights continue to increase but at a slower rate than the rest of the body. At term, the fetal adrenals are similar in size to those in the adult (Seron-Ferre and Jaffe, 1981; Pearson Murphy and Branchaud, 1994).

Most of the increased weight of the adrenals is associated with growth of an inner fetal zone that comprises approximately 80–90% of its overall volume at term. Until late in gestation, cells of the outer *adult zones* remain small and are less well vascularized than the larger cells of the fetal zone. The overall steroid-producing capacity of the adrenal glands also exceeds that in the adult. It is estimated that near term, the glands produce a minimum of 100–200 mg of steroids per day, compared to 20–30 mg in resting adults (Seron-Ferre and Jaffe, 1981; Winter, 1992; Pearson Murphy and Branchaud, 1994) (Figure 10).

In the first half of pregnancy, adrenal growth seems to be largely regulated by growth factors derived from within the glands, along with those from other fetal organs, including the placenta, liver and kidneys. Until the latter part of pregnancy, the active steroid-producing fetal zone is predominantly involved in the synthesis of an androgen called dehydroepiandrosterone sulphate (DHEAS). This hormone provides placental tissue with an essential substrate for the synthesis of oestrogens (Pepe and Albrecht, 1990, 1995).

Placental hypothalamic–pituitary regulation

During the first half of pregnancy, the synthesis of DHEAS is largely stimulated by placental hCG and by ACTH-related peptides and prolactin from the fetal pituitary gland. Since hCG first appears in the maternal circulation at the beginning of implantation and reaches highest concentrations during the first trimester, placental tissue must provide the initial stimulatory influence on the fetal adrenals. Within the fetal pituitary, cells containing ACTH-related peptides and prolactin appear between 5 and 10 weeks' gestation and are followed by the emergence of neurovascular links between the hypothalamus and the pituitary gland. By 12 weeks' gestation, corticotrophin-releasing hormone (CRH) and arginine vasopressin (AVP) are present within the hypothalamus. Together, these hormones provide essential stimulation for the development and secretory activity of ACTH-releasing cells in the pituitary (Pepe and Albrecht, 1990).

ACTH is first detectable in fetal plasma at approximately 12 weeks and shows a slight increase along with

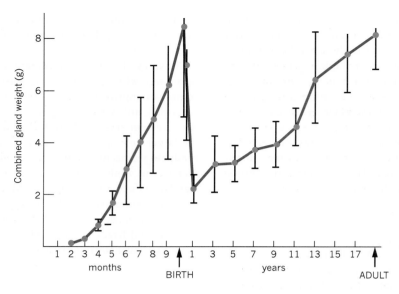

Figure 10　Adrenal gland weights during development. The means ± SD of prenatal gland weights are shown. (From Munro and Neville 1982, p. 12.)

gestational age. But unlike the situation in adults, ACTH does not form the principle corticotroph during most of fetal life. Instead two other related peptides, melanocyte-stimulating hormone (MSH) and corticotrophin-like intermediate lobe peptide (CLIP), have been found in higher concentrations within the pituitary. This pattern continues until late in gestation when the proportion of ACTH increases, until it becomes the dominant hormone at term. Since ACTH has been found to stimulate growth of the adult but not the fetal zone of the adrenal gland, its low concentration throughout gestation is thought to facilitate the continued dominance of the fetal zone. At the low concentrations that characterize most of pregnancy, ACTH is centrally involved in regulating fetal zone utilization of LDL-cholesterol, for the production of DHEAS. Near term, its increased concentration stimulates proliferation of the adult cortisol-producing zone of the gland (Pepe and Albrecht, 1990).

In contrast to ACTH, prolactin seems to be released in the absence of hypothalamic regulation. From approximately 14 weeks onwards, fetal serum concentrations of prolactin show a linear increase with advancing gestation. In addition to its stimulatory influence on steroid hormone production in the fetal zone of the adrenal gland, prolactin enhances the process of lung maturation during the last trimester (Buster, 1984; Thorpe-Beeston *et al.*, 1992).

Adrenal medulla

In contrast to the cortex, the chromaffin cells of the medulla are formed from adjacent sympathetic ganglia that are derived from the neural crest. Unlike the cortex, this part of the gland enlarges at a slow rate during fetal life. For most of this period, larger and much more active islets of chromaffin cells form independently of the medulla, along the outside of the aorta. Immature chromaffin cells have been observed from approximately eight weeks and significant concentrations of noradrenaline have been found from 15 weeks' gestation. No degeneration has been found to occur in these cells until the postnatal period (Phillippe, 1983).

Within the medulla, small groups of cells containing measurable amounts of noradrenaline have been observed at nine weeks but their content remains low until the third trimester. From this point onwards, the medulla becomes innervated by autonomic fibres containing noradrenaline and simultaneously receives increased plasma concentrations of cortisol from the surrounding cortex. The neuronal developments increase the medullary capacity to produce noradrenaline in response to stress while the local increases in cortisol stimulate production of an enzyme that converts noradrenaline to adrenaline. While noradrenaline remains predominant in the fetal response to stress, the rising capacity for cortisol production near term produces a sharp increase in the medullary capacity to produce adrenaline. The proportion of adrenaline increases progressively from approximately 28 weeks to term, when it constitutes around 50% of total catecholamine content of the medulla. As measured in amniotic fluid, catecholamine metabolites increase between the second and third trimester and plasma catecholamine concentrations rise progressively during the course of labour. These changes mediate a range of cardiovascular, metabolic and respiratory responses to labour and delivery (Phillippe, 1983; Lagercrantz and Slotkin, 1986; Lagercrantz and Marcus, 1992).

GASTROINTESTINAL SYSTEM

Through a process of midline folding during week 4, the endodermal layer gives rise to the gastrointestinal and respiratory systems. By the fifth week of gestation, the primitive gastrointestinal tube differentiates into a *foregut*, *midgut* and *hindgut*. Meanwhile, hepatic, cystic and pancreatic diverticula bud from the foregut, giving rise to the *liver*, *gall bladder* and *pancreas*. During the sixth week, the endodermal epithelium proliferates until it fills the gut lumen. Over the next three weeks, the tube is recanalized and lined with definitive mucosal epithelium that differentiates from the endoderm. Soon afterwards, the gastrointestinal tract becomes involved in regulating the circulation of amniotic fluid. At 16 weeks' gestation, the fetus has been estimated to swallow 7 ml of amniotic fluid per hour, rising to approximately 120 per hour by 28 weeks. This fluid has been found to accumulate in the stomach where it is absorbed into the underlying tissues (Gilbert 1991; Moore and Persaud, 1993) (Figure 11).

The liver

The liver is a major haematopoietic organ during embryonic and fetal life. When it initially appears, blood-forming cells have already begun to collect between hepatic cells and vessel walls. This growing activity contributes to the rapid increase in the weight of the liver, which reaches approximately 10% of body weight by 10 weeks' gestation. During the last eight weeks of gestation, this activity declines and at birth the liver is approximately 5% of total body weight.

In contrast to the early capacity for red cell produc-

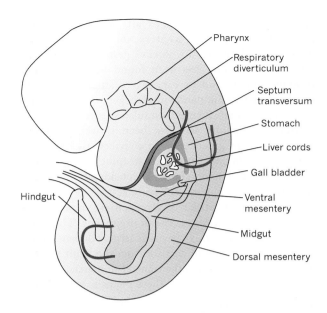

Figure 11 Structure of the gut tube. The foregut consists of the pharynx, located superior to the respiratory diverticulum, the thoracic oesophagus, and the abdominal foregut inferior to the diaphragm. The abdominal foregut forms the abdominal oesophagus, stomach and about half of the duodenum and gives rise to the liver, the gall bladder, the pancreas and their associated ducts. The midgut forms half the duodenum, the jejunum and ileum, the ascending colon and about two-thirds of the transverse colon. The hindgut forms one-third of the transverse colon, the descending and sigmoid colons, and the upper two-thirds of the anorectal canal. The abdominal oesophagus, stomach and superior part of the duodenum are suspended by dorsal and ventral mesenteries; the abdominal gut tube excluding the rectum is suspended in the abdominal cavity by a dorsal mesentery only. (Reproduced with permission from Larsen, 1993, p. 209.)

tion, hepatic regulation of carbohydrate metabolism does not emerge until the latter part of pregnancy and shows considerably different regulatory features than the adult. Under basal non-stressed conditions, fetal glucose is largely supplied from the maternal circulation via the placenta. The fetal liver displays a high glucose uptake and a large capacity for glycolysis but gluconeogenic enzyme activity remains low until after birth. Glucose uptake is stimulated by raised maternal glucose concentrations and is inhibited by physiological concentrations of fatty acids, amino acids and lactate. Hepatic receptors for insulin can be demonstrated by 12–15 weeks' gestation. Although no clear association has been found between insulin receptor activity and its capacity to stimulate glucose uptake or the accumulation of glycogen, *in vitro* studies have shown that insulin stimulates glycogenesis in hepatocytes. Insulin has also been shown to inhibit the synthesis of gluconeogenic enzymes, thereby promoting anabolic metabolism. In keeping with this tendency, the fetal liver shows a considerably reduced sensitivity to the glucose-releasing actions of glucagon.

Substantial quantities of glycogen are deposited in the liver during the latter part of pregnancy. The onset and maintenance of this activity is largely dependent on the enhanced release of cortisol from the adult zone of the adrenal gland. When the transfer of maternal fuel is acutely interrupted at birth, these deposits are utilized, during the first 24 hours after birth, to maintain blood glucose (Jones, 1989).

Nutritional requirements

During the latter part of pregnancy, an adequate maternal supply of nutrients is particularly important for appropriate growth and development of the liver and endocrine pancreas. Experimental evidence suggests that prolonged hypoglycaemia lowers fetal concentrations of growth factors that promote B cell proliferation and permanently alters the pattern of enzyme activity in the liver. Both of these findings have been associated with the emergence of impaired glucose tolerance and disturbed lipid metabolism in adult life (Barker, 1995).

RESPIRATORY SYSTEM

The laryngotracheal tube arises as a small protrusion from an area of the foregut, close to that which becomes the stomach. Once formed, the foregut elongates rapidly, separating the emerging stomach from the section that gives rise to the lungs. From the initial small protrusion, the lungs take shape through a series of bifurcations which begin with the emergence of right and left lobular buds that correspond in number to those in the mature organ. Between 5 and 26 weeks' gestation, these branch a further 16 times, to generate the *respiratory trees*. By 16 weeks, all bronchial airways have been formed and further growth proceeds by elongation and widening of existing airways. Towards the end of this phase, each terminal bronchiole divides into two or more *respiratory bronchioles*, while the mesodermal tissues surrounding them become highly vascularized. From 26 weeks onwards, the respiratory bronchioles continually subdivide to produce approximately 20–70 million primitive alveoli that are vascularized by a dense network of capillaries (Moore and Persaud, 1993) (Figure 12).

During fetal life, these potential air spaces are filled with liquid that is actively formed by the pulmonary epithelium from the surrounding circulation. Experiments on fetal lambs have found that the volume of liquid increases from 4–6 ml/kg body weight, at mid-

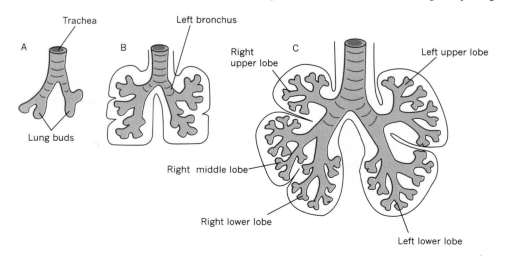

Figure 12   Successive stages in the development of the trachea and lungs. (A) At 5 weeks. (B) At 6 weeks. (C) At 8 weeks. (Reproduced with permission from Sadler, 1990, p. 231.)

gestation, to more than 20 ml/kg body weight, near term. This liquid expansion of the potential air space maintains a small distending pressure in the lumen that approximates the functional residual capacity of the aerated lung in the newborn. In addition to this functional role in lung development, lung fluid has also been found to assist in the emergence of surfactant-producing epithelial cells that can be identified from approximately 24 weeks' gestation.

During these successive phases of lung development, a number of different cellular changes occur in pulmonary tissues. Until approximately 17 weeks, cuboidal epithelium contains abundant amounts of glycogen. The gradual decrease that subsequently occurs is thought to represent use of glycogen in the formation of surfactant. Some cuboidal epithelial cells of the respiratory bronchioli also differentiate into thin flat cells that become more closely associated with the surrounding capillaries. During the last eight weeks, cells lining the terminal sacs become thinner, allowing the capillaries to surround their entire surface gradually. In addition, a second type of cuboidal epithelial cell begins to differentiate within the alveoli. Under the stimulatory influence of a number of different hor-

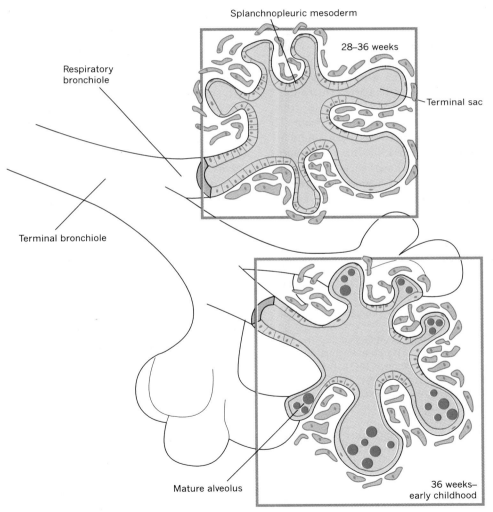

Figure 13   Maturation of the lung tissue. Terminal sacs (primitive alveoli) begin to form between weeks 28 and 36 and begin to mature between 36 weeks and birth. Only 5–20% of all terminal sacs produced by the age of 8, however, are formed prior to birth. (Reproduced with permission from Larsen, 1993, p. 123.)

mones, including cortisol, catecholamines and prolactin, these cells synthesize, store and secrete a complex substance called *surfactant*, which is composed of a number of different glycerophospholipid and protein molecules. As secretion rates increase, this substance forms a lipid monolayer that lines the lumen of the alveoli. The lipid properties of surfactant reduces surface tension of the terminal sacs, and prevents them from collapsing following the onset of respiration (Figures 12 and 13).

While lung tissue extracts rather than supplies oxygen to the circulation *in utero*, intermittent breathing activity occurs from approximately 11 weeks' gestation. Results of longitudinal studies from 24 weeks suggest that the pattern of this activity is integrated with sleep cycles, fetal movements and circadian rhythms. In general, breathing activity only occurs during periods of rapid eye movement sleep. Episodes of fetal movements are associated with a reduction or absence of breathing. This is particularly evident during nightly periods of gross body movements that coincide with lowest levels of breathing. From 22 weeks onwards breathing activity has been found to reach minimum levels between 1900 and 2400 hours. Episodic breathing *in utero* is thought to stimulate the development of lung tissue and respiratory muscles and some experimental evidence suggests that it may increase cardiac output and blood flow to vital organs including the heart, brain and placenta. Its presence is generally taken as an indicator of fetal well-being, since periods of hypoxia have been shown to depress fetal breathing.

THE MAMMARY GLAND

During the fourth week of gestation, the mammary gland emerges as thickened ridges of ectoderm that initially extend from the axilla to the inguinal regions. Over the next four weeks, mammary ridges thicken in the pectoral area and progressively invade the underlying mesenchyme. Between 10 and 12 weeks' gestation, epithelial buds begin to form and from approximately 15 weeks onwards, these divide into secondary buds that subsequently subdivide into a growing number of *lactiferous ducts*, with some primitive lobular branches. Cells destined to become myoepithelial cells emerge as differentiated ectodermal cells that are localized around the developing ducts. In males and females, development continues in an identical manner until term, when 15–20 primitive lobes have formed. At birth, cells lining both ducts and alveoli demonstrate a transient capacity for secretory activity that is stimulated by the transplacental passage of maternal hormones. This may produce slight glandular enlargement that subsides within 3–4 weeks (Russo and Russo, 1987).

References

Aubert, M.L., Grumbach, M.M. & Kaplan, S.L. (1975) The autogenesis of human fetal hormones. *J. Clin. Invest.* **56**: 155.

Barker, D.J.P. (1995) Fetal origins of coronary heart disease. *Br. Med. J.* **311**: 171–174.

Brace, R.A. (1995) Progress toward understanding the regulation of amniotic fluid volume. Water and solute fluxes in and through fetal membranes. *Placenta* **16**(1): 1–18.

Braude, P.R. and Johnson, M.H. (1990) The embryo in contemporary medical science. In Dunstan, G.R. (ed.) *The Human Embryo*, pp. 208–221. Exeter: University of Exeter Press.

Buster, J.E. (1984) Fetal, placental, and maternal hormones. In Beard, R.W. & Nathaniesz, P.W. (eds) *Fetal Physiology and Medicine*, pp. 559–599. New York: Butterworths.

Carlson, S.E. (1992) Very long chain fatty acids in the developing retina and brain. In Polin, R.A. & Fox, W.W. (eds) *Fetal and Neonatal Physiology*, pp. 341–346. Philadelphia: W.B. Saunders.

Crawford, M.A. (1993) The role of essential fatty acids in neural development: implications for perinatal nutrition. *Am. J. Clin. Nutr.* **57**(Suppl.): 703S–710S.

Demir, N., Celiloglu, M. & Thomassen, P.A.B. (1992) Prolactin and amniotic fluid electrolytes. *Acta Obstet. Gynecol. Scand.* **71**: 197–200.

Dunstan, G.R. (ed) (1990) *The Human Embryo*. Exeter: University of Exeter Press.

Edwards, C.R., Benediktsson, R., Lindsay, R.S. *et al.* (1993) Dysfunction of placental glucocorticoid barrier: link between fetal environment and adult hypertension. *Lancet* **341**: 355–357.

Gilbert, S.F. (1991) *Developmental Biology*. Massachusetts: Sinauer.

Handwerger, S., Richards, R.G. & Markoff, E. (1992) The physiology of decidual prolactin and other decidual protein hormones. *Trends Endocrinol. Metab.* **3**(3): 91–95.

Herrera, E., Lasuncion, M.A. & Asuncion, M. (1992) Placental transport of free fatty acids, glycerol, and ketone bodies. In Polin, R.A. & Fox, W.W. (eds) *Fetal and Neonatal Physiology*, pp. 291–298. Philadelphia: W.B. Saunders.

Johnson, M. & Everitt, B.J. (1995) *Essential Reproduction*. Oxford: Blackwell Scientific.

Jones, C.T. (1989) Fetal maturation in late pregnancy. In

Turnbull, A. & Chamberlain, G. (eds) *Obstetrics*, pp. 119–127. Edinburgh: Churchill Livingstone.

Kelly, R.W. (1994) Pregnancy maintenance and parturition: the role of prostaglandin in manipulating the immune and inflammatory response. *Endocrine Rev.* **15**(5): 684–706.

Kletzky, O.A. (1992) Maternal and fetal prolactin. *Semin. Reprod. Endocrinol.* **10**(3): 282–286.

Lagercrantz, H. & Slotkin, T.A. (1986) The 'stress' of being born. *Sci. Am.* **254**: 92–102.

Lagercrantz, H. & Marcus, C. (1992) Sympathoadrenal mechanisms during development. In Polin, R.A. & Fox, W.W. (eds) *Fetal and Neonatal Physiology*, pp. 160–169. Philadelphia: WB Saunders.

Larsen, W.J. (1993) *Human Embryology*. New York: Churchill Livingstone.

Longo, L.D. (1993) Maternal blood volume and cardiac output during pregnancy: an hypothesis of endocrinologic control. *Am. J. Physiol.* **245**: R720–729.

Makrides, M., Neumann, M., Simmer, K. *et al.* (1995) Are long-chain polyunsaturated fatty acids essential nutrients in infancy? *Lancet* **345**: 1463–1468.

Moore, K.L. & Persaud, T.V.N. (1993) *The Developing Human*. Philadelphia: W.B. Saunders.

Pearson Murphy, B.E. & Branchaud, C.L. (1994) The fetal adrenal. In Tulchinsky, D. & Little, B.A. (eds) *Maternal–Fetal Endocrinology*, pp. 276–286. Philadelphia: W.B. Saunders.

Pepe, G.J. & Albrecht, E.D. (1990) Regulation of the primate fetal adrenal cortex. *Endocrine Rev.* **11**(1): 151–176.

Pepe, G.J. & Albrecht, E.D. (1995) Actions of placental and fetal adrenal steroid-hormones in primate pregnancy. *Endocrine Rev.* **16**(5): 608–648.

Phillippe, M. (1983) Fetal catecholamines. *Am. J. Obstet. Gynecol.* **146**(7): 840–855.

Russo, J. & Russo, I.H. (1987) Development of the human mammary gland. In Neville, M.C. & Daniel, C.W. (eds) *The Mammary Gland*, pp. 67–78. New York: Plenum Press.

Sadler, T.W. (1990) *Langhan's Medical Embryology*. Baltimore: Williams and Wilkins.

Seckl, J.R. (1994) Glucocorticoids and small babies. *Q. J. Med.* **87**: 259–262.

Seron-Ferre, M. & Jaffe, R.B. (1981) The fetal adrenal gland. *Ann. Rev. Physiol.* **43**: 141–162.

Schenker, J.G., Ben-David, M. & Polishuk, W.Z. (1975) *Am. J. Obstet. Gynecol.* **123**: 834.

Skinner, S.L. (1993) The renin system in fertility and normal human pregnancy. In Robertson, J.I.S. & Nicholls, M.G. (eds) *The Renin-Angiotensin System*, Vol. 1, pp. 50.1–50.14. London: Gower Medical.

Thorpe-Beeston, J.G., Snijders, R.J.M., Felton, C.V. *et al.* (1992) Serum prolactin concentration in normal and small for gestational age fetuses. *Br. J. Obstet. Gynaecol.* **99**: 981–984.

Walker, A.M. (1993) Circulatory transitions at birth and the control of neonatal circulation. In Hanson, M.A., Spencer, J.A.D. & Rodeck, C.H. (eds) *Fetus and Neonate: Physiology and Clinical Applications*, Vol. 1, *The Circulation*, pp. 160–196. Cambridge: Cambridge University Press.

Winter, J.S.D. (1992) Fetal and neonatal adrenocortical physiology. In Polin, R.A. & Fox, W.W. (eds) *Fetal and Neonatal Physiology*, pp. 1829–1841. Philadelphia: W.B. Saunders.

Wynn, A.H.A., Crawford, M.A., Doyle, W. *et al.* (1991) Nutrition of women in anticipation of pregnancy. *Nutr. Health* **7**: 69–88.

Wynn, S.W., Wyn, A.H., Doyle, W. & Crawford, M.A. (1994) The association of maternal diet and the dimensions of babies in a population of London women. *Nutr. Health* **9**(4): 303–315.

10

The Fetal Skull

The fetal skull is ovoid or egg-shaped and corresponds to the shape of the brain. It differs from that of an adult in the large size of the vault in relation to the face.

Divisions of the Fetal Skull

For the purpose of obstetrics, the fetal skull (Figure 1) may be considered as divided into three sections:

1 The *vault*, containing the cerebral hemispheres.
2 The *base*.
3 The *face*.

The bones of the base and the face are firmly united and, therefore, incompressible. The vault extends from the orbital ridges to the nape of the neck and is compressible.

Regions of the Fetal Skull

The fetal skull is subdivided into the following regions which are related to the degree of flexion or extension and presentation of the fetal head.

The *vertex* is the area bounded in front by the anterior fontanelle, behind by the posterior fontanelle and laterally by the parietal eminences.

The *brow*, or sinciput, is the area over the frontal bone.

The *occiput* is the area over the occipital bone.

The *face* extends from the supraorbital ridges to the chin.

The *vault* is composed of thin sheets of bone separated, at the sutures, by membrane. This arrangement permits considerable moulding and overlapping during labour and allows for the progressive development of

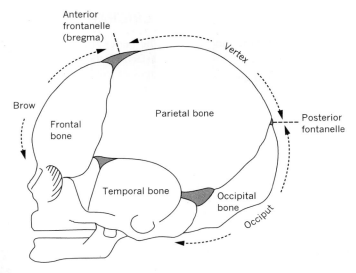

Figure 1   The bones, fontanelles and regions of the fetal skull.

the brain during childhood. The vault of the skull is composed entirely of membrane in early fetal life. Later, ossification begins at centres in the membranous vault and the bones are formed. At birth the membrane still remains between the bones at the sutures and fontanelles. The points from which ossification spreads in the fetal skull are the occipital protuberance, the parietal eminences and the frontal bosses.

The *vault* of the fetal skull is made up of:

▶ Two frontal bones.
▶ Two parietal bones.
▶ Two temporal bones.
▶ One occipital bone.

These bones are joined to each other and to the bones of the face and the base of the skull by sutures (Figure 2).

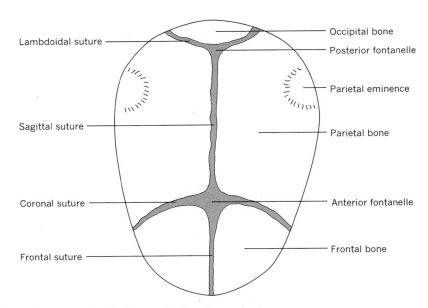

Figure 2   The fetal skull, showing the bones, fontanelles and sutures.

SUTURES

The sutures of the vault are four in number and are composed of soft, fibrous tissue.

1 The *frontal* suture unites the frontal bones; this suture is fused in an adult.
2 The *sagittal* suture, so called from its resemblance to an arrow, unites the two parietal bones.
3 The *lambdoidal* suture, named from its resemblance to the Greek letter lambda (λ), unites the posterior margins of the parietal bones to the occipital bone.
4 The *coronal* suture, the part of the head where the crown of victory was placed in Olympian days, unites the frontal bones to the anterior margins of the parietal bones.

The *temporal* sutures have no obstetric importance.

FONTANELLES

A fontanelle is a membranous, non-ossified area of the skull found where three or more sutures meet. There are two fontanelles of importance in obstetrics – anterior and posterior.

Anterior fontanelle

The anterior fontanelle or bregma is the meeting place of four sutures. It is kite-shaped, 2–2.5 cm across and 2.5–3 cm in length. It may be palpated on vaginal examination when the head is deflexed as in an occipitoposterior position. In this region the skull is not fully ossified until the child is 16–18 months old.

Posterior fontanelle

This is triradiate in shape and is the meeting place of three sutures. It is a useful guiding point when making a vaginal examination as, by locating its position, one can determine the relationship of the head to a particular part of the maternal pelvis. It closes soon after birth, but may remain slightly open for a time in a preterm infant.

The sutures and fontanelles allow moulding of the fetal head during labour with temporary alteration in its shape. This moulding naturally puts some strain upon the internal structures, namely the folds of dura mater, the falx cerebri and the tentorium cerebelli.

FORAMEN MAGNUM

The base of the skull is perforated by a circular opening called the foramen magnum, through which the spinal cord passes.

PERICRANIUM

The pericranium is the periosteum covering the outer surface of the bones of the skull and attached at the edges of the bones. In the centre of the bone it is less firmly attached.

SCALP

The scalp is the thick, soft, movable part over the pericranium; its loose tissues are composed of skin, roots of hair, certain muscle fibres, blood vessels and connective tissue.

Diameters of the Fetal Skull

The position adopted by the presenting part, in relation to the pelvic brim, simultaneously determines the degree of flexion or extension of the fetal head and the precise realignment of the skull bones during labour and delivery. To assess the size of the fetal skull in relation to various diameters of the maternal pelvis, diameters have been measured which correspond to common postures adopted by the fetal head as it enters the pelvic brim.

Longitudinal diameters

The size of the fetal skull can be estimated by measuring the distances between certain points (Figure 3). The diameters of the head can best be understood by learning them according to the posture of the fetal head, that is the degree of flexion or extension (Figure 4):

1 *Suboccipitobregmatic*, 9.5 cm, measured from the junction of the head with the neck behind to the centre of the anterior fontanelle. This diameter presents when the head is fully flexed and engages in a normal presentation.
2 *Suboccipitofrontal*, 10 cm, measured from the junction of the head with the neck behind to the centre of the frontal suture. This diameter presents when the head is almost completely flexed. It stretches the soft parts of the birth canal as the forehead emerges at the outlet and in the after-coming head in a breech delivery.
3 *Occipitofrontal*, 11.5 cm, measured from the glabella (bridge of the nose) to the occipital protuberance. This diameter lies across the pelvis in an occipito-

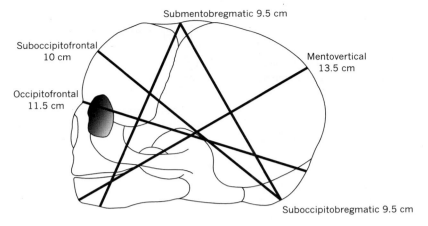

Figure 3   The diameters of the fetal skull.

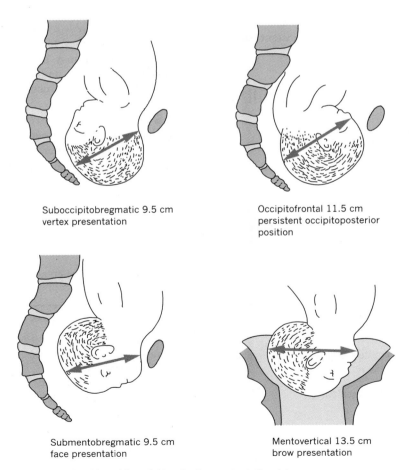

Suboccipitobregmatic 9.5 cm
vertex presentation

Occipitofrontal 11.5 cm
persistent occipitoposterior
position

Submentobregmatic 9.5 cm
face presentation

Mentovertical 13.5 cm
brow presentation

Figure 4   The diameters of the fetal head in relation to the maternal pelvis.

posterior or occipitolateral position with deficient flexion.

4   *Mentovertical*, 13.5 cm, measured from the point of the chin to the highest point on the vertex. The head is midway between flexion and extension. It presents in a brow presentation.

5   *Submentovertical*, 11 cm, measured from the junction of the chin with the neck in front to the highest point on the vertex. This diameter presents in a face presentation when the head is not fully extended.

6   *Submentobregmatic*, 9.5 cm, measured from the junction of the chin with the neck in front to the centre of the anterior fontanelle. This diameter engages when the head is fully extended in a face presentation.

Transverse diameters

1   *Biparietal*, 9.5 cm, measured between the parietal eminences.

2   *Bitemporal*, 8 cm, between the most distant parts of the coronal suture.

Circumference of the Fetal Skull

The circumferences of the fetal skull are:

▶ *Suboccipitobregmatic*, 33 cm.
▶ *Occipitofrontal*, 35 cm.
▶ *Mentovertical*, 39 cm.

The importance of knowing the circumference of the fetal head is that when the head is well flexed the suboccipitobregmatic circumference (33 cm) fits into the lower uterine segment, and also enters the pelvic brim more easily than when deflexed. The circumference of a deflexed head is about 35 cm (occipitofrontal), which does not fit well into the lower uterine segment and is often delayed in its entrance in the pelvic brim. This may result in early rupture of the membranes and, in some cases, a prolonged and possibly difficult labour.

Moulding

As the measurements of the fetal head correspond very closely to those of the maternal pelvis, it is necessary to understand their relationship to each other, and also the effect of pressure and moulding of the head. The result of moulding is a diminution of the diameters which are most compressed, compensated for by the elongation of those which are not compressed. This process is made possible by the sutures and fontanelles, which allow the bones to overlap; the reduction in presenting diameter may be more than 0.5 cm. The frontal bone is pushed under the anterior portion of the parietal bone and the occiput under the posterior part.

It is possible to recognize the way in which the baby's head has passed through the pelvis by examining the moulding soon after birth. The alterations due to moulding which occur with the various presentations are shown in Figure 5 and Table 1.

Moulding which is extreme in degree, or too rapid, or in which the head is compressed in abnormal diameters may cause a tear of the falx cerebri or the tentorium cerebelli. If the tear involves the contained

Table 1   Variations in the diameters of the fetal skull due to compression and moulding (see also Figure 5)

(a)	Vertex presentation with good flexion	Suboccipitobregmatic decreased Biparietal decreased Mentovertical increased
(b)	Persistent occipitoposterior position of the vertex	Occipitofrontal decreased Biparietal decreased Submentobregmatic increased
(c)	Face presentation	Submentobregmatic decreased Biparietal decreased Occipitofrontal increased
(d)	Brow presentation	Mentovertical decreased Biparietal probably decreased Suboccipitobregmatic increased

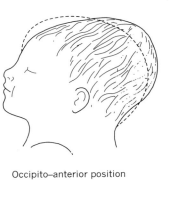
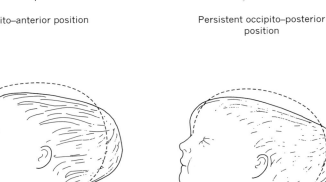

Occipito–anterior position

Persistent occipito–posterior position

Face presentation

Brow presentation

Figure 5   Moulding of the fetal head.

or adjacent blood vessels an intracranial haemorrhage results.

Caput Succedaneum in Cephalic Presentations

During labour and after rupture of the membranes the head is pressed against the ring formed by the dilating cervix. This impedes circulation in the scalp and a swelling due to congestion and oedema forms in the loose tissues of the scalp. The swelling or caput succedaneum forms on the unsupported presenting area which projects through the cervix (Figure 6). The area covered by the caput depends on the degree of dilatation of the cervix and after full dilatation could cover the whole presenting area. The size of the swelling varies greatly. If the labour is easy little caput may form, but if the contractions are strong and advance of the fetal head is slow the caput will become much larger. The size of the caput and the degree of moulding are indications of the compression the head sustains in labour. In a left occipitoanterior position the caput forms on the posterior part of the right parietal bone. In a right occipitoanterior position the caput forms on the left parietal bone. In an occipitoposterior position with deficient flexion the caput forms on the anterior part of the anterior parietal bone, near the bregma. A secondary caput may form over the occiput in a prolonged second stage of labour by pressure of the head against the partially dilated vulva.

Internal Structures of the Fetal Skull

DURA MATER

The dura mater is a tough fibrous membrane which covers the outer surface of the brain and dips down between the brain substance to form partitions, thus

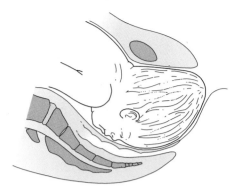

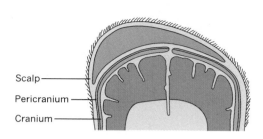

Figure 6   Caput succedaneum.

dividing the brain into compartments. There are two main partitions (Figure 7):

▶ *Falx cerebri*: This is a double fold of dura mater which forms a partition between the two cerebral hemispheres. It is attached to the inside of the skull starting at the root of the nose, follows the line of the frontal and sagittal sutures and continues to the internal occipital protuberance. The lower edge of the falx cerebri is unattached and is sickle-shaped.

▶ *Tentorium cerebelli*: This is a fold of dura mater which lies horizontally and at right angles to the falx cerebri. It is shaped like a horseshoe and is attached at the sphenoid bone on each side, along the petrous portion of the temporal bone to the internal occipital protuberance. It separates the cerebrum from the cerebellum.

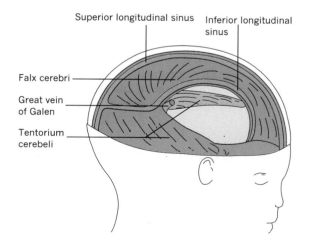

Figure 7   Internal structures of the fetal skull.

The posterior part of the falx cerebri is attached to the midline of the tentorium cerebelli. The brainstem passes just in front of this junction before it leaves the cerebral hemispheres.

SINUSES

The cerebral membranes contain four large sinuses which drain blood from the brain:

1 *Superior longitudinal sinus*: This runs along the upper border of the falx from the bridge of the nose to the occipital protuberance.
2 *Inferior longitudinal sinus*: This runs along the lower border of the falx to its junction with the tentorium cerebelli.
3 *Straight sinus*: A continuation of the inferior longitudinal sinus, this runs in a posterior direction along the junction of the falx cerebri until it joins the superior longitudinal sinus.
4 *Great vein of Galen*: This is made up of many vessels from the brain substance. It joins the straight sinus at its junction with the inferior longitudinal sinus.

When moulding occurs in labour the cerebral membranes and the sinuses contained within them are subjected to stretching. In normal labour these structures can usually withstand such stress, but where moulding is excessive or occurs too rapidly or in an unfavourable direction, the membranes and sinuses may be torn and haemorrhage ensures. Tentorial tears are the most likely. The tear occurs in the tentorium cerebelli near its attachment to the falx and therefore may involve the great vein of Galen, the straight sinus and the inferior longitudinal sinus.

Further Reading

Beck, F. (1985) *Human Embryology: The Development of Structure and Function*, 2nd edn. London: Blackwell Scientific.

England, M.A. (1990) *A Colour Atlas of Life before Birth. Normal Fetal Development*. London: Wolfe Medical.

Larsen, W.J. (1993) *Human Embryology*. New York: Churchill Livingstone.

Moore, K.L. (1988) *Essentials of Human Embryology*, 4th edn. Philadelphia: BC Decker.

Moore, K.L. and Persaud, T.V.N. (1993) *The Developing Human*, 5th edn. Philadelphia: WB Saunders.

Part Four

Biological Adaptations to Pregnancy

11

Placental Hormones in Pregnancy

Current research findings suggest that the placenta plays a strategic endocrine–paracrine role during pregnancy and labour. This unique organ synthesizes a number of hormones of hypothalamic and pituitary origin and selectively releases them into maternal and fetal compartments through a variety of interactions with both neuroendocrine systems. In this way, a range of maternal activities are augmented and modified to actively support embryonic and fetal development within the uterine cavity (Pepe and Alberecht, 1995).

Human Chorionic Gonadotrophin

Trophoblast tissue first synthesizes and secretes human chorionic gonadotrophin (hCG), a glycoprotein hormone that has chemical and biological similarities to luteinizing hormone (LH), follicule-stimulating hormone (FSH) and thryoid-stimulating hormone (TSH) from the pituitary gland. The complete hCG molecule is secreted by the syncytiotrophoblast, under the stimulatory influence of gonadotrophin-releasing hormone (GnRH) which has been identified in adjacent cytotrophoblast cells. The pattern of hCG secretion is markedly different from other placental hormones. Rising production by human blastocysts has been demonstrated *in vivo* six days after fertilization and it is detectable in the maternal circulation as implantation begins. Over the next 5–6 weeks, circulating levels rise in a linear fashion, reaching maximum concentrations by 8–10 weeks' gestation. Between approximately 11 and 13 weeks, hCG declines rapidly to reach a plateau by 20 weeks that continues for the remainder of pregnancy (Figure 1) (Kaplan *et al.*, 1991; Ogren and Talamantes, 1994).

In the *maternal compartment*, hCG has been found to:

▶ stimulate ovarian and thyroid hormone secretion;
▶ decrease the osmotic thresholds for thirst and release of vasopressin; and
▶ inhibit the production of lymphocytes.

Within the *uterus*, *in vitro* evidence suggests that hCG:

▶ modulates the invasion of trophoblast cells;
▶ promotes growth in the number and size of smooth muscle cells; and
▶ inhibits myometrial contractility.

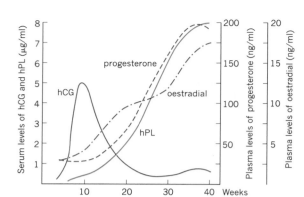

Figure 1 Changes in serum and plasma levels of main peptide and steroid hormones during pregnancy. (Reproduced with permission from Rosso, 1990, p. 139.)

In *placental tissue*, hCG stimulates synthesis and secretion of oestrogen and progesterone, while in the *decidua* it has been shown to augment the secretion of prolactin and relaxin (Adcock *et al.*, 1973; Davison *et al.*, 1988; Ballabio *et al.*, 1991; Buster and Carson, 1991; Ren and Braunstein, 1992; Kornyei *et al.*, 1993; Yagel *et al.*, 1993; How *et al.*, 1995).

The stimulatory effect of hCG on ovarian hormonal activity is essential for the establishment of pregnancy. During the first 7–8 weeks of gestation, hCG acts on LH/hCG receptors in the corpus luteum to maintain secretion of progesterone and oestrogen until synthesis of these hormones can be taken over by the placenta. Secretion of progesterone by the ovary reaches maximum levels about four weeks following conception and then rapidly declines. From eight weeks onwards, the absence of ovarian progesterone has little impact on the conceptus or on urinary levels of pregnanediol. This means that maximum hCG concentrations in maternal plasma are reached at a time when placental tissue is producing sufficient progesterone for the continuation of pregnancy. The sustained increase in hCG levels for a further four weeks appears to induce some refractoriness in LH/hCG receptors in the corpus luteum, as they gradually respond by producing lower levels of oestrogen and progesterone (Ogren and Talamantes, 1994).

The thyrotrophic influences of hCG within the *maternal compartment* have not been fully investigated. However, many metabolic changes of early pregnancy can be explained by an increased level of thyroid activity. During the first trimester:

▶ maternal appetite increases;
▶ glucose sensitivity improves;
▶ oxygen consumption is significantly raised; and
▶ levels of body fat and overall weight are substantially increased (Clapp *et al.*, 1988; Fraser, 1991).

Within the *embryonic compartment*, hCG has a range of regulatory influences on neuroendocrine development. The stimulatory influence of hCG on maternal thyroid activity seems to be directed towards making thyroxine available to the embryo and fetus for development of the brain and other neuronal tissues. Both thyroxine and its nuclear receptors have been identified in the human brain several weeks before the onset of active secretion, during the phase of rapid neuroblast division in the forebrain (Morreale de Escobar *et al.*, 1988; Ballabio *et al.*, 1991).

In *in vitro* experiments on human fetal adrenal tissue at 12–18 weeks gestation, hCG stimulates the production of dehydroepiandrosterone sulphate (DHEAS) which provides placental tissue with an essential prerequisite for the synthesis of oestrogen. In the male testes, hCG also stimulates testosterone production that promotes the development of sexual differentiation (Pepe and Albrecht, 1990).

REGULATION OF hCG SECRETION

The specific pattern of hCG secretion in early pregnancy is largely determined by the stimulatory actions of placental GnRH and growth factors, the overall inhibitory actions of progesterone and oestrogen and less well-defined influences of a number of embryonic organs. GnRH stimulates the synthesis and pulsatile secretion of hCG in early placental tissue and this action has been confirmed by the presence of GnRH receptors in the syncytiotrophoblast. Levels of GnRH within the maternal circulation have also been shown to parallel those of hCG, with concentrations in the first half of pregnancy nearly double those in the second. Between 6 and 12 weeks' gestation, placental growth factors also have a stimulatory influence on the secretion of hCG (Siler-Khodr *et al.*, 1991; Maruo *et al.*, 1992; Lin *et al.*, 1995).

Current evidence suggests that the progressive rise in progesterone concentration during the first trimester is largely responsible for the fall in hCG that occurs from approximately 11 weeks' gestation. While oestrogen has a stimulatory influence on hCG, this seems to be blocked by progesterone. *In vitro* studies have found that high levels of progesterone inhibit GnRH-stimulated hCG in placental tissue at 7–10 weeks. This pattern of negative feedback regulation is very similar to the interactions that occur between these steroid hormones and LH and GnRH during the luteal phase of the cycle (Wilson *et al.*, 1984; Ogren and Talamantes, 1994).

Additional embryonic influences on the pattern of hCG secretion have also been suggested. In *in vitro* experiments, a variety of organ tissues at successive periods in the first trimester have demonstrated both stimulatory and inhibitory effects on hCG and progesterone. While no clear pattern has yet emerged, some form of regulation seems likely, since completion of the embryonic phase of development coincides with the hCG plateau which is followed by much lower levels during the subsequent period of fetal growth. Experiments on fetal tissues have also shown that placental supplies of hCG are likely to be supplemented by active local synthesis. *In vitro* experiments have demonstrated that fetal kidney, lung and liver tissues synthesize and secrete hCG (Barnea *et al.*, 1989; Barnea and Shurtz-Swirski, 1992; Shurtz-Swirski *et al.*, 1991).

Human Placental Lactogen

Human placental lactogen (hPL) is a polypeptide hormone produced by the syncytiotrophoblast with chemical and biological similarities to growth hormone and prolactin from the pituitary gland. This hormone is present in placental tissue 18 days postconception and can be detected in the maternal circulation during the fifth week of gestation. Plasma concentrations increase linearly until 30–34 weeks' gestation, to reach peak concentrations of 5–10 µg/ml. Near term, the secretion rate of hPL is approximately 1.0 g/day which is considerably greater than any other protein hormone (Handwerger, 1991; Ogren and Talamantes, 1994).

Considerable research findings indicate that hPL is involved in a wide range of growth and metabolic activities in maternal and fetal compartments. Within the decidua, hPL seems to be involved with hCG and prolactin in modulating trophoblast invasion. Several maternal adaptations in carbohydrate and lipid metabolism are also influenced by hPL. Recent *in vitro* experiments have found that hPL stimulates cell proliferation and insulin secretion in human islet cells. In early pregnancy the threshold of glucose-stimulated insulin secretion is lowered and insulin sensitivity improves. This adaptation enhances overall metabolic efficiency and increases maternal uptake and storage of available nutrients, in preparation for increased placental uptake of glucose, lipids and proteins and mammary uptake of lipids in the second half of pregnancy (Herrera *et al.*, 1988; Fraser, 1991; Clarke Brelje *et al*, 1993; Freemark *et al.*, 1993; Sorenson *et al.*, 1993).

Recent experiments suggest that hPL has a direct growth-promoting influence on a number of fetal tissues. Detailed experiments on rats suggest that the appearance of hPL receptors is regulated in a tissue-specific manner. They appear at mid-gestation in adrenal tissue, followed by the renal tubules and small intestine and present slightly later in the pancreas and liver (Freemark *et al.*, 1993). These findings on the fetal adrenals have also been confirmed in humans, where evidence suggests that hPL may participate with hCG and prolactin in stimulating the production of DHEAS. Receptor binding within the small intestine and kidneys suggests that hPL stimulates growth and differentiation of the villous surface and the renal tubules. In the fetal liver, hPL stimulates enzyme activity that is critical for regulating protein, RNA and DNA synthesis and for stimulating the storage of glycogen that is particularly important in the latter part of gestation, in preparation for extrauterine life (Handwerger, 1991).

REGULATION OF hPL SECRETION

Secretion of hPL seems to be regulated by a number of metabolites, hormones and growth factors. Studies on the effects of varying concentrations of metabolites suggest that hPL secretion increases between meals when nutrient availability is low and declines following food intake when nutrient availability is high. Experimental studies have demonstrated that hPL concentrations increase 30–40% in women fasted for 84–90 hours between 16–22 weeks' gestation (Handwerger, 1991; Ogren and Talamantes, 1994).

Recent experiments on the mechanisms involved in synthesis and release of hPL suggest that it is regulated by Apo A-I, the major protein constituent of high-density lipoprotein (HDL). In support of these findings, trophoblast cells contain specific receptors for HDL and maternal plasma HDL concentrations rise from 14 weeks' gestation. Recent experiments have demonstrated a direct stimulatory effect of Apo A-I on hPL gene expression from trophoblast cells in culture. Other *in vitro* experiments suggest that placental growth factors, angiotensin II, dopamine and a chorionic protein factor may also be involved in paracrine regulation of hPL production within the placenta (Fahraeus *et al.*, 1985; Handwerger *et al.*, 1987, 1995; Alsat and Malassine, 1991; Handwerger, 1991; Maruo *et al.*, 1992; Petit *et al.*, 1993).

The Fetal Adreno-Placental Unit

OESTROGEN

The placenta operates in conjunction with the fetal zone of the adrenal gland to produce oestrogen and progesterone and metabolize corticosteroids. Together, the placenta and fetal adrenal glands contain the full complement of enzymes needed to synthesize steroid hormones from low-density lipoprotein cholesterol. Because of the functional interactions between them, these relatively small organs exchange, metabolize and release more steroids than any other human endocrine tissue.

Throughout most of gestation, DHEAS is the major hormone released by the fetal zone of the adrenals. While some cortisol is synthesized by the smaller outer zones, the necessary enzyme remains inactive until the second half of pregnancy and the fetus is supplied with low concentrations of glucocorticoids via the placenta. Within the fetal compartment, these operate to suppress fetal pituitary production of adrenocorticotrophic hormone (ACTH) which limits growth and maturation of the adult zone of the adrenal gland. In contrast, DHEAS is synthesized in increasing quantities from fetal sources of cholesterol within the larger fetal zone of the gland. Mean umbilical cord plasma concentrations range from 1131 to 1517 ng/ml until approximately 34 weeks' gestation and then increase steadily to 2463 ng/ml at term (Figure 2) (Pepe and Albrecht, 1990, 1995).

DHEAS provides the principal substrate that is used by the placenta for the synthesis of oestrogen and most is supplied by the fetus. By approximately seven weeks' gestation, more than 50% of oestrogen entering the maternal circulation is synthesized by the placenta. Thereafter, plasma concentrations increase in a linear manner until term. Very large quantities of different variants of oestrogen are produced. Compared to non-pregnant values, the production rate of oestradiol increases from 0.1–0.6 mg to 15–20 mg/24 hours near term while that of oestriol increases from 0.02–0.1 mg to 50–150 mg/24 hours near term. It has been estimated that daily oestrogen production by one

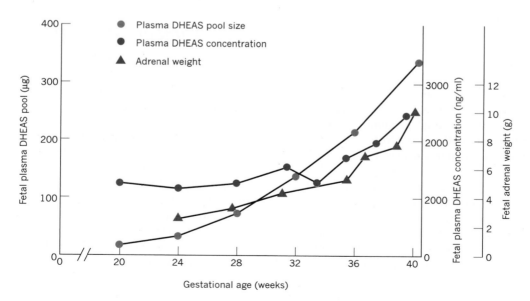

Figure 2   Relationships among estimated plasma DHEAS pool size, umbilical cord plasma concentration and adrenal weight. (Reproduced with permission from Parker *et al.*, 1992, p. 1218.)

woman at term is equivalent to the daily production of 1000 women during the menstrual cycle (Casey and MacDonald, 1993).

PROGESTERONE

Serum progesterone concentrations rise in a linear manner with advancing gestation. During the first two weeks, values rise to around 25 ng/ml which is double that in the non-pregnant cycle. Until 10 weeks they remain fairly constant; then placental secretion fully replaces that of the corpus luteum. Thereafter, plasma levels increase gradually and then more steeply, to reach 150–175 ng/ml at term. During the third trimester, production rates are approximately 250 mg/day, which is nearly 10-fold greater than those in the luteal phase of the cycle. In humans and other primates, there is no significant change in the relative concentrations of progesterone and oestrogen in the peripheral circulation in the latter part of pregnancy.

Fetal membranes at term have the capacity to increase local tissue concentrations of oestrogen and progesterone. Receptors in the myometrium seem to decrease towards term (Mitchell *et al.*, 1984; Yen, 1991; How *et al.*, 1995).

Current evidence suggests that low-density lipoprotein cholesterol is taken up from the maternal circulation and used by the placenta to synthesize progesterone. Trophoblast cells contain low-density lipoprotein receptors that have been shown to increase in response to oestrogen. Subsequent enzyme activity in the placental conversion of cholesterol to pregnenolone have also been shown to be stimulated by oestrogen. Since placental oestrogen formation is highly dependent on fetal adrenal production of DHEAS, these findings point to the central importance of the fetal adrenals in regulating key points in the pathway that synthesizes progesterone (Albrecht and Pepe, 1990; Pepe and Albrecht, 1995).

References

Adcock, E.W., Teasdale, E., August, C.S. *et al.* (1973) Human chorionic gonadotrophin: its possible role in maternal lymphocyte suppression. *Science* 181: 845–847.

Albrecht, E. & Pepe, G.J. (1990) Placental steroid hormone biosynthesis in primate pregnancy. *Endocrine Rev.* 11(1): 124–150.

Alsat, E. & Malassine, A. (1991) High density lipoprotein interaction with human placenta: Biochemical and ultrastructural characterization of binding to microvillous receptor and lack of internalisation. *Molec. Cell. Endocrinol.* 77: 97–108.

Ballabio, M., Poshyachinda, M. & Ekins, R.P. (1991) Pregnancy-induced changes in thyroid function: role of human chorionic gonadotrophin as putative regulator of maternal thyroid. *J. Clin. Endocrinol. Metab.* 73(4): 824–831.

Barnea, E.R. & Shurtz-Swirsky, R. (1992) Endocrinology of the placenta and embryo-placental interaction. In Barnea, E.R. *et al.* (eds) *The First Twelve Weeks of Gestation*, pp. 128–153. Berlin: Springer-Verlag.

Barnea, E.R., Simon, R.J. & Kol, S. (1989) Human embryonic extracts modulate placental function in the first trimester: effects of visceral tissues upon chorionic gonadotrophin and progesterone secretion. *Placenta* 10: 331–344.

Buster, J.E. & Carson, S.A. (1991) Placental endocrinology and diagnosis of pregnancy. In Gabbe, S.G., Niebyl, J.R., Simpson, J.L. (eds) *Obstetrics, Normal and Problem Pregnancies*, pp. 59–91. New York: Churchill Livingstone.

Casey, M.L. & MacDonald, P. (1993) Placental endocrinology. In Redman, C.W.G., Sargent, I.L., Starkey, P.M. *The Human Placenta*, pp. 237–272. Oxford: Blackwell Scientific.

Clapp, J.F., Seaward, B.L., Sleamaker, R.H. *et al.* (1988)

Maternal physiological adaptations to early pregnancy. *Am. J. Obstet. Gynecol.* 159(6): 1456–1460.

Clarke Brelje, T., Scharp, D.W., Lacy, P.E. *et al.* (1993) Effect of homologous placental lactogens, prolactins, and growth hormones on islet *B*-cell division and insulin secretion in rat, mouse, and human islets: implications for placental lactogen regulation of islet function during pregnancy. *Endocrinology* 132(2): 879–887.

Davison, J.M., Shiells, E.A., Philips, P.R. *et al.* (1988) Serial evaluation of vasopressin release and thirst in pregnancy: The role of chorionic gonadotrophin in the osmoregulatory changes of gestation. *J. Clin. Invest.* 81: 798–801.

Fahraeus, L., Larsson-Cohn, L. & Wallentin, L. (1985) Plasma lipoproteins including high density lipoprotein subfractions during normal pregnancy. *Obstet. Gynaecol* 66(4): 468–472.

Fraser, R.B. (1991) Carbohydrate metabolism. In Hytten, F., Chamberlain, G. (eds) *Clinical Physiology in Obstetrics*, pp. 204–212. Oxford: Blackwell Scientific.

Freemark, M., Kirk, K., Pihoker, C. *et al.* (1993) Pregnancy lactogens in the rat conceptus and fetus: Circulating levels, distribution of binding, and expression of receptor messenger ribonucleic acid. *Endocrinology* 133(4): 1830–1842.

Handwerger, S. (1991) Clinical counterpoint: The physiology of placental lactogen in human pregnancy. *Endocrine Rev.* 12(4): 329–336.

Handwerger, S., Quarfordt, S., Barret, J. *et al.* (1987) Apolipoproteins AI, AII, and CI stimulate placental lactogen release from human placental tissue. *J. Clin. Invest.* 79: 625–628.

Handwerger, S., Myers, S., Richards, R. *et al.* (1995) Apo-lipoprotein A-1 stimulates placental lactogen expression by human trophoblast cells. *Endocrinology* **136**(12): 5555–5560.

Herrera, E., Lasuncion, M. A., Gomez-Coronado, D. (1988) Role of lipoprotein lipase activity on lipoprotein metabolism and the fate of circulating triglycerides in pregnancy. *J. Clin. Endocrinol. Metab.* **158**(6): 1575–1583.

How, H., Huang, Z-H., Zuo, J. *et al.* (1995) Myometrial estradiol and progesterone receptor changes in preterm and term pregnancies. *Obstet. Gynaecol.* **86**(6): 936–940.

Kaplan, M., Barnea, E.R., Bersinger, N.A. (1991) Patterns of spontaneous pulsatile secretion of human chorionic gonadotrophin and pregnancy specific β1 glycoprotein by superfused placental explants in first and last trimester. Lack of episodic human placental lactogen secretion. *Acta Endocrinol. (Copenhagen)* **124**: 331–337.

Kofinas, A.D. (1990) Progesterone and estradiol concentrations in nonpregnant and pregnant human myometrium. *J. Reprod. Med.* **35**: 1045–1050.

Kornyei, J.L., Lei, Z.M. & Rao, C.V. (1993) Human myometrial smooth muscle cells are a novel target of direct regulation by human chorionic gonadotrophin. *Biol. Reprod.* **49**: 1149–1157.

Lin, L.-S., Roberts, V.J. & Yen, S.S. (1995) Expression of human gonadotrophin-releasing hormone receptor gene in the placenta and its functional relationship to human chorionic gonadotrophin. *J. Clin. Endocrinol. Metab.* **80**(2): 580–585.

Maruo, T., Matsuo, H., Murato, K. *et al.* (1992) Gestational age-dependent dual action of epidermal growth factor on human placenta early in gestation. *J. Clin. Endocrinol. Metab.* **75**(5): 1362–1367.

McGregor, W.G. *et al.* (1981) Fetal tissue can synthesize a placental hormone: Evidence for chorionic gonadotrophin *b*-subunit synthesis by human fetal kidney. *J. Clin. Invest.* **68**: 306–309.

Mitchell, B.F., Cross, J., Hobkirk, R. *et al.* (1984) Formation of unconjugated estrogens from estrone sulfate by dispersed cells from human fetal membranes and decidua. *J. Clin. Endocrinol. Metab.* **58**: 845.

Morreale de Escobar, G., Obregon, M.J. & Escobar del Rey, F. (1988) Transfer of thyroid hormones from mother to fetus. In Delange, F., Fisher, D.A., Glinoer, D. (eds) *Research in Congenital Hypothyroidism*, pp. 15–28. New York: Plenum Press.

Ogren, L. & Talamantes, F. (1994) The placenta as an endocrine organ: Polypeptides. In Knobil, E. & Neill, J.D. (eds) *The Physiology of Reproduction*, pp. 875–945. New York: Raven Press.

Pepe, G.J. & Albrecht, E.D. (1990) Regulation of the primate fetal adrenal cortex. *Endocrine Rev.* **11**(1): 151–176.

Pepe, G.J. & Albrecht, E.D. (1995) Actions of placental and fetal adrenal steroid hormones in primate pregnancy. *Endocrine Rev.* **16**(5): 608–648.

Petit, A., Gallo-Payet, N., Vaillancourt, C. *et al.* (1993) A role of extracellular calcium in the regulation of placental lactogen release by angiotensin-II and dopamine in human term trophoblastic cells. *J. Clin. Endocrinol. Metab.* **77**(3): 670–676.

Ren, S-G. & Braunstein, G.D. (1992) Human chorionic gonadotrophin. *Seminars Reprod. Endocrinol.* **10**(2): 95–105.

Schuler, L.A. (1993) The placental lactogen/prolactin/growth hormone activities of the placental and fetal membranes. In Rice, G.E. *et al.* (eds) *Molecular Aspects of Placental and Fetal Membrane Autoacoids*, pp. 303–338. Boca Raton: CRC Press.

Shurtz-Swirski, R., Simon, R.J., Cohen, Y. *et al.* (1991) Human embryo modulates placental function in the first trimester: Effect of neural tissues upon chorionic gonadotrophin and progesterone secretion. *Placenta* **12**: 521–523.

Siler-Khodr, T.M., Kang, I.A. & Khodr, G.S. (1991) Current topic: Symposium on placental endocrinology 1. Effects of chorionic GNRH on intrauterine tissues and pregnancy. *Placenta* **12**: 91–103.

Sorenson, R.L., Clarke Brelje, T. & Roth, C. (1993) Effect of steroid and lactogenic hormones on islets of Langerhans: A new hypothesis for the role of pregnancy steroids in the adaptation of islets to pregnancy. *Endocrinology* **133**(5): 2227–2234.

Wilson, E.A., Jawad, M.J. & Powell, D.E. (1984) Effect of estradiol and progesterone on human chorionic gonadotrophin secretion *in vitro*. *Am. J. Obstet. Gynecol.* **149**(2): 143–148.

Yagel, S., Geva, T.E., Solomon, H. *et al.* (1993) High levels of chorionic gonadotrophin retard first trimester trophoblast invasion *in vitro* by decreasing urokinase plasminogen activator and collagenase activities. *J. Clin. Endocrinol. Metab.* **77**(6): 1506–1511.

Yen, S.S.C. (1991) Endocrine metabolic adaptations in pregnancy. In Yen, S.S.C., Jaffe, R.B. (eds) *Reproductive Endocrinology*, pp. 936–981. Philadelphia: W.B. Saunders Company.

12

Maternal and Fetal Physiological Responses to Pregnancy

In healthy, well-nourished women, extensive modifications occur in all bodily systems in response to the varying requirements of pregnancy. These changes begin to emerge during the luteal phase of the cycle, largely facilitated by rising levels of oestrogen, progesterone and deoxycorticosterone (DOC). In addition to the steroid-induced changes in the inner linings of the reproductive tract, oestrogen stimulates an increased retention of intravascular fluid and increases the capacity of intercellular connective tissues to retain water. The resulting fall in plasma osmolality stimulates a compensatory retention of sodium and water by the kidneys and the slight increase in intravascular fluid may also explain the rise in measures of glomerular filtration rate. At the same time, some of the increased progesterone is converted to DOC, a glucocorticoid hormone that acts on the distal tubule of the kidney to promote the reabsorption of sodium from the urine. The resulting shifts in fluid produce the slight tendency towards oedema that characterizes the second half of the cycle (Davison and Noble, 1981; Davison and Lindheimer, 1989; Schrier and Briner, 1991) (Figure 1).

Premenstrual *engorgement of breast tissue* also results from local oedema and cell proliferation due to the activation of oestrogen and progesterone receptors in different sections of the mammary gland. A slight *hyperventilation* also develops during the luteal phase

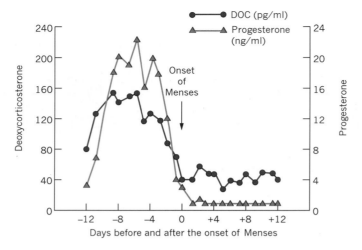

Figure 1   Relationship between mean plasma concentrations of deoxycorticosterone (DOC) and progesterone in women during the menstrual cycle. (Reproduced with permission from Parker *et al.*, 1981, p. 28.)

of the cycle and alveolar and arterial tensions of carbon dioxide are lower than those observed prior to ovulation. Present evidence indicates that this occurs through the combined neuronal actions of oestrogen and progesterone within the respiratory centre in the medulla. Rising oestrogen levels during the luteal phase stimulate the synthesis of progesterone receptors in these neurones while the simultaneous increase in progesterone activates them by increasing their sensitivity to PCO_2.

Following fertilization, these luteal changes are accentuated and gradually merge with others that arise in response to the complex patterns of hormonal interactions that characterize early pregnancy. In very early pregnancy, many women experience a heightened *sense of smell*, particularly of noxious substances like nicotine; a distaste for coffee and sugary foods; varying degrees of nausea and increased saliva and an overwhelming *desire for sleep*. Changes in smell, taste and saliva closely follow the pattern of human chorionic gonadotrophin (hCG) secretion and tend to diminish as levels of this hormone decline. The increased desire for sleep during the first trimester has been attributed to the predominant influence of progesterone on neuronal activity in the brain. Experiments on animals have demonstrated that progesterone diminishes excitatory neuronal transmitters while oestrogen increases brain receptors for progesterone as well as for other inhibitory and stimulatory neurotransmitter substances (Smith, 1991).

Cardiovascular Adaptations

Rise in cardiac output

The maternal cardiovascular system undergoes extensive changes in response to pregnancy. It is generally agreed that cardiac output rises by about 40% during pregnancy but uncertainty remains about the exact timing and pattern of the component changes and the underlying factors that bring them about (deSwiet, 1991b; Duvekot *et al.*, 1995).

Early studies using various invasive methods suggested that cardiac output increased gradually until the end of the second trimester and then declined towards non-pregnant values during the third trimester. This view was subsequently modified with the use of improved equipment and by taking measurements of women lying in a lateral rather than supine position in the third trimester. In general, these cross-sectional studies reported that cardiac output peaked before 30 weeks and plateaued over the remainder of pregnancy (deSwiet, 1991b).

More recent data have come from longitudinal studies using improved non-invasive techniques. While values for cardiac output vary considerably in different population groups, these studies generally suggest that it rises significantly during the first trimester, either peaks at 32 weeks with no significant changes thereafter, or continues to show further small rises until term (Mabie *et al.*, 1994). Measures of the pattern and relative contribution of heart rate and stroke volume to increased cardiac output suggest that heart rate is the more variable component in different population groups (Robson *et al.*, 1989; Capeless and Clapp, 1989; Duvekot *et al.*, 1993).

Recent studies have found that *stroke volume* increases significantly by 8 weeks; peaks at 16–22 weeks and plateaus or shows further small increases during the third trimester. This represents a rise of 21–22% over pre-pregnant values. In different studies, *heart rate* has been found to increase significantly above pre-pregnant values by 5 and 16 weeks' gestation. Data on the remainder of pregnancy suggest that the increase peaks at 31–32 weeks and shows no significant change thereafter. Until more longitudinal studies are available, current evidence indicates that heart rate may increase by between 11 and 17% over pre-pregnant values (Robson *et al.*, 1989; Capeless and Clapp, 1989; Duvekot *et al.*, 1993).

Peripheral arterial vasodilation

Recent findings suggest that cardiac output rises in early pregnancy in response to a fall in systemic vascular resistance that produces a reduced afterload in the myocardial fibres during left ventricular ejection. Decreases in both *mean arterial pressure* and total *peripheral resistance* are evident at eight weeks' gestation and reach their lowest point by the middle of pregnancy, before returning to similar or slightly above pre-pregnant values at term. The decline in peripheral vascular resistance seems to be brought about by early relaxation in systemic, renal and pulmonary vascular tone and by the later development of new vascular beds in the placenta (Schrier and Briner, 1991).

The initial fall may be induced during the luteal phase of the cycle by rising levels of oestrogen and progesterone. Experimental studies in non-pregnant ovariectomized sheep have reproduced the characteristic sequence of changes in vascular and fluid dynamics in early pregnancy by a gradual infusion of oestrogen into the systemic circulation. In addition, progesterone has been shown to reduce muscle tone in the vasculature (Magness and Rosenfeld, 1989; Omar *et al.*, 1995).

The current hypothesis suggests that when fertilization occurs, the further fall in peripheral vascular resistance creates a state of *relative hypovolaemia* that the heart attempts to modify by an increase in stroke volume and heart rate (Davison and Noble, 1981;

Clapp *et al.*, 1988; Schrier and Briner, 1991; Duvekot *et al.*, 1993). This compensatory increase in cardiac output produces a rise in vascular filling state that is characterized by a rise in left atrial diameter, a rise in glomerular filtration rate and a fall in plasma renin, between the fifth and eighth week of gestation (Duvekot *et al.*, 1993). Recent studies on humans and animals have demonstrated that the fall in vascular resistance precedes the rise in circulating blood volume during pregnancy. This suggests that systemic vasodilation may be a primary adaptation to pregnancy that initiates a rise in cardiac output and maintains overall tissue perfusion and blood pressure, prior to significant increases in circulating blood volume (Phippard *et al.*, 1986; Capeless and Clapp, 1989) (Figure 2).

Blood volume

The increase in blood volume is composed of a maximum rise of *50% in plasma volume* and a *20% rise in red cell volume*. The time course of the increase in plasma volume is quite different from that which occurs in red cell mass. Plasma volume begins to increase in the first trimester, increases more rapidly in the second and only slightly during the remainder of pregnancy. In contrast, expansion in red cell mass only begins in the second trimester and achieves highest increases in the third. Because of the different pace at which these changes proceed, haemoglobin concentration and haematocrit decline progressively until about 30 weeks' gestation. From then onwards, this trend is reversed, since increases in red cell volume outstrip those of plasma volume during the last trimester (Figure 3).

ERYTHROPOIESIS

The increase in red cell mass during pregnancy is stimulated by erythropoietin. This glycoprotein hormone is synthesized in ground tissue, in the kidneys and to a lesser extent in the liver. Levels of serum immunoreactive erythropoietin remain at non-pregnant values during the first trimester, begin to rise during the second and reach maximum levels during the third trimester. Within the bone marrow, erythropoietin acts on erythrocyte colony-forming cells. These give rise to increasing numbers of mature erythrocytes within two days of increased levels of erythropoietin within the circulation.

At present, the precise mechanisms involved in stimulating erythropoietin during pregnancy remain

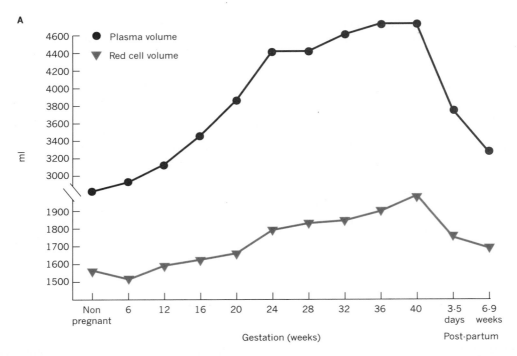

Figure 2 **A**: Mean total plasma and red cell volume during normal pregnancy. (Reproduced with permission from Lund *et al.*, 1967, p. 399.)

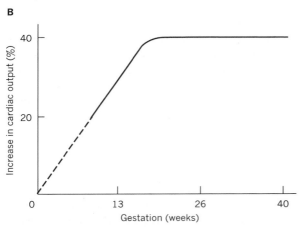

Figure 2 **B**: Changes in cardiac output through pregnancy. (Reproduced with permission from Hytten *et al.*, 1991, p. 8.)

unclear. Recent evidence suggests that components of the maternal plasma renin–angiotensin system may be involved. Angiotensinogen and erythropoietin share a number of similarities. Both compete for specific binding to erythropoietin receptors on human bone-marrow cells and bone-marrow cells show binding of angiotensinogen that is inhibited by erythropoietin.

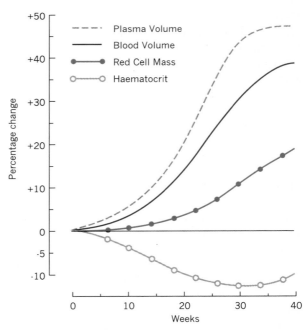

Figure 3   Changes in plasma volume, blood volume, red cell mass and haematocrit during normal pregnancy, expressed as a percentage of pre-pregnancy levels. (Reproduced with permission from Rosso, 1990, p. 25.)

This evidence suggests that angiotensinogen is a precursor for erythropoietin. In addition, animal experiments indicate that angiotensin II exhibits significant renal and extrarenal erythropoietin-stimulating activity. But while both components are increased in the maternal circulation during pregnancy, the timing and possible interactions between these components and erythropoietin remain to be clarified. A number of pregnancy hormones have both stimulatory and inhibitory influences on the actions of erythropoietin. Progesterone partly prevents the inhibitory influence of oestrogen on stem cell utilization of erythropoietin, while both placental lactogen and prolactin enhance the stimulatory action of erythropoietin on red cell production. At present, however, the precise significance of these hormonal actions remains unclear (Cotes *et al.*, 1983; Beguin *et al.*, 1990; Neng Lai and Fai Lui, 1993).

RENIN–ANGIOTENSIN SYSTEM

Current evidence suggests that plasma volume expansion is primarily regulated by an oestrogen-stimulated rise in angiotensin II that activates the maternal vascular renin–angiotensin system as a result of the progressive rise of oestrogen in the maternal circulation (Skinner, 1993).

Evidence is accumulating to suggest that renin–angiotensin systems operate in a number of fetal and maternal sites during pregnancy. In embryonic and fetal tissues, components of the system have been found to accelerate cell growth and division and to stimulate the formation of blood vessels and tissue vascularization. In uteroplacental tissues, components of the system are thought to be involved in regulating local blood flow and liquor volume. Although many aspects of these recent findings remain uncertain, the emerging picture suggests that renin–angiotensin systems play an important role in creating conditions that enhance fetal growth (Broughton Pipkin, 1993; Downing *et al.*, 1995).

To date, greatest understanding has been gained of the vascular renin–angiotensin system. Its increased activity during pregnancy is initiated by the release of dehydroepiandrosterone (DHEAS) from the fetal zone of the adrenals. When it reaches the placenta, DHEAS is efficiently converted to a form that serves as substrate for the synthesis of oestrogen. Rising levels of oestrogen in the maternal circulation provide the main stimuli for the hepatic production of a specific globulin that circulates in plasma and acts as a substrate for

renin. Angiotensinogen or renin substrate increases very early in pregnancy and closely mirrors oestrogen levels in individual women (Skinner, 1993).

Renin Renin is a proteolytic enzyme that is synthesized and released mainly by specialized smooth muscle cells of afferent arterioles entering the glomeruli of the kidney. On reaching the blood stream, renin cleaves off part of angiotensinogen, triggering an enzymatic cascade that initially forms a biologically inactive peptide called *angiotensin I*. The next phase requires the action of angiotensin-converting enzyme that circulates in plasma and is found in most tissues, but particularly high activities of the enzyme have been found in the lungs. This glycoprotein cleaves off part of angiotensin I to form the biologically active peptide angiotensin II that acts directly on the proximal tubules to enhance fluid reabsorption, and on the adrenal cortex to stimulate increased production of aldosterone.

Angiotensin II By the second week of pregnancy, plasma levels of angiotensin II are double those in the non-pregnant state. Within the kidneys, angiotensin II stimulates increased fluid reabsorption in the proximal tubular cells, by enhancing the reabsorption of bicarbonate. Within the adrenals, angiotensin II stimulates cells in the outer zone of the cortex to secrete aldosterone. In the non-pregnant state, angiotensin II also acts on peripheral arterioles as a potent vasoconstrictor. During pregnancy, this pressor effect is thought to be counteracted by the vasodilatory activity of progesterone and oestrogen and by the vascular release of dilatory prostaglandins (Skinner, 1993; Cook and Trundinger, 1993).

ALDOSTERONE

In situations of hypovolaemia, aldosterone acts mainly on the distal tubules to enhance the reabsorption of sodium. Plasma levels of aldosterone increase significantly by 12 weeks' gestation and reach a plateau at 30 weeks which is 3–5 times higher than non-pregnant values. During the first half of pregnancy, effective renal plasma flow increases by 70–80% and then declines slightly in the third trimester, but still remains 50–60% above non-pregnant values, which is greater than occurs in any other physiological state. The resulting increase in glomerular filtration rate increases the sodium load from 20 000 to 30 000 mmol/day. Current evidence suggests that in these conditions, neither progesterone or aldosterone have a major role in fluid regulation. Instead, fetal provision of increasing substrate for placental synthesis of oestrogen brings about adaptative changes in maternal cardiovascular and renal capacity that provide the conditions needed to promote fetal growth and nutrition (Longo, 1983; Romen *et al.*, 1991; Skinner, 1993; Pepe and Albrecht, 1995; Duvekot *et al.*, 1995; Steer *et al.*, 1995).

Progesterone and deoxycorticosterone

Within the kidneys, progesterone acts to enhance the excretion of sodium by decreasing its reabsorption in the proximal sections of the tubules and by blocking the increased reabsorption of sodium by aldosterone in the distal tubules. At present it is not clear to what extent this progesterone action operates as a negative feedback element of the maternal plasma renin–angiotensin system during pregnancy. Some of the large increase in progesterone is converted to DOC, which acts on the distal tubules to promote the reabsorption of sodium. Rising levels of DOC occur by approximately eight weeks' gestation and increase 10–15-fold, to a peak of approximately 100 µg/dl at term, which is higher than that of aldosterone. However, the salt-retaining properties of this hormone are 30–50

times less potent than those of aldosterone (Nolten and Rueckert, 1981; Skinner, 1993) (Figure 4).

ATRIAL NATRIURETIC PEPTIDE

The other main hormone that may influence renal handling of sodium during pregnancy is atrial natriuretic peptide (ANP). ANP is a peptide hormone produced in the atrial chambers of the heart. Outside of pregnancy, secretion is primarily stimulated by stretching of the atrial wall that accompanies increases in blood pressure. ANP has been found to act in a number of ways to promote diuresis. Within the kidney, it directly inhibits both renin production and the tubular reabsorption of sodium and also acts on the adrenal glands to inhibit the production of aldosterone. *In vitro* studies have also shown that it produces marked relaxation of vascular smooth muscle.

Conflicting evidence currently exists on the pattern of ANP secretion during normal pregnancy. Plasma levels have been reported to decline from 20 weeks' gestation, reach lowest levels at 36 weeks and return to non-pregnant values by 12 weeks' postpartum. Another study has reported a gradual increase during the course of pregnancy to reach peak values at placental separation before declining significantly by

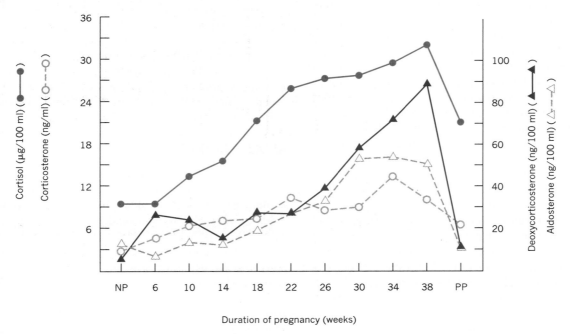

Figure 4 Mean steroid level in 11 women throughout pregnancy and postpartum (PP) compared to levels in non-pregnant (NP) women. (Reproduced with permission from Wintour *et al.*, 1978, p. 399.)

72 hours postpartum. Until more consistent data are obtained, it is not possible to identify the way in which this hormone participates in regulating fluid volume during pregnancy and the early postpartum period (Thomsen *et al.*, 1993; Yoshimura *et al.*, 1994; Mukaddam-Daher *et al.*, 1995).

Anatomical Renal Adaptations

All parts of the renal system are altered by a variety of different changes in pregnancy. The kidneys enlarge in response to increased vascular volume and the calyces, renal pelvis and ureters dilate. Dilatation occurs during the first trimester and is always more prominent on the right. The common dilatory changes seem to occur in response to increased vascular volume and are not accompanied by reduced muscle tone. In recent studies, progesterone has not been found to induce dilatation or to reduce peristalsis of the ureters. The more distinct dilatory changes on the right side have been explained by specific pressure on the ureter. A degree of obstruction seems to occur in the right ureter, as it crosses the enlarged iliac artery and ovarian vein almost at right angles, while the left ureter

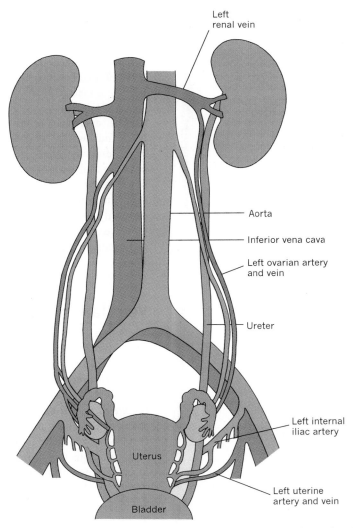

Left renal vein

Aorta

Inferior vena cava

Left ovarian artery and vein

Ureter

Left internal iliac artery

Left uterine artery and vein

Uterus

Bladder

Figure 5 Obstruction of the right ureter at the pelvic brim by an enlarged ovarian vein. Note that the ovarian vein enters the vena cava by several trunks and that the pelvic portion of the ureter is normal.

runs parallel to these vessels (Marchant, 1978; Baylis and Davison, 1991).

Real-time ultrasound studies on the kidney suggest that dilatation of the pelvis and calyces is accompanied by a progressive increase in urinary stasis. However, recent studies have found no evidence that this persists in the ureters. In contrast to earlier reports of their reduced tone and motility, recent studies have found hypertrophy of ureteric muscle and no changes in the intensity, frequency and tone of ureteral contractions during pregnancy (Cietak and Newton, 1985) (Figure 5).

During pregnancy, the bladder is progressively elevated into the abdomen and the ureteral orifices are displaced laterally by the growing uterus. These changes may produce frequency of micturition and a degree of ureteral reflux. In early pregnancy, as the uterus occupies more space in the pelvic cavity, it may compress the bladder and cause frequency. Lateral displacement of the ureteral orifices is most pronounced during late pregnancy. It is thought to reduce intraureteral pressure, predisposing to back flow of urine through the ureteral orifice. Near term, engagement of the fetus within the pelvis may also exert upward pressure on the bladder, leading to increased frequency of micturition and discomfort (Marchant, 1978; Mattingly and Borkowf, 1978) (Figure 6).

Tubular reabsorption of nutrients

The increased glomerular filtration rate also increases the load of other plasma constituents besides sodium. Urinary excretion of most amino acids increases by 200–700% above non-pregnant values, representing a loss of up to 2 g/day. In well-nourished women, this level of excretion is amply substituted by increased dietary intake (Romen et al., 1991; Baylis and Davison, 1991).

The excretion of glucose increases progressively from four weeks' gestation until term. Serial studies have demonstrated that marked variations occur between and within individuals that are not related to blood sugar concentrations or to the length of gestation. In healthy women, glycosuria seems to occur primarily as a consequence of the 50% increase in glomerular filtration rate that is maintained throughout pregnancy (Romen et al., 1991; Lind and Hytten, 1972).

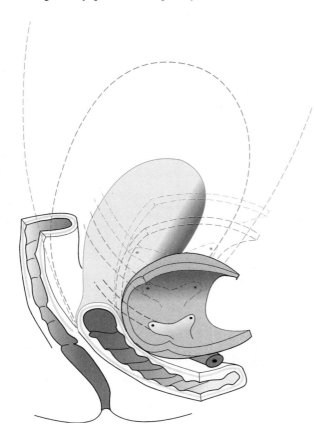

Figure 6 Anatomic changes of the bladder base with advancing pregnancy, showing elevation of the trigone and lateral displacement of the ureteral orifices. (Reproduced with permission from Mattingly and Borkowf, 1978, p. 869.)

Ventilation

Extensive anatomical and functional changes occur in the respiratory system. These accommodate both the *progressive increase in gas exchange* required by the rising blood volume and the *growing space occupied by the uterus*. From early pregnancy onwards, the overall shape of the chest alters, by a flaring of the lower ribs that seems to occur independently of any mechanical pressure from the growing uterus. This progressively increases the subcostal angle, from 68° in early pregnancy to 103° at term and increases the transverse diameter of the chest by approximately 2 cm. Because of the flaring of the lower ribs, the diaphragm rises by a maximum of 4 cm while its contribution to the respiratory effort increases and shows no evidence of being

Table 1   Pulmonary adaptations in pregnancy

Volumes/capacities	Definition	Changes
Respiratory rate	Number of breaths per minute	Unchanged
Vital capacity	Maximum amount of air that can be forcibly expired after maximum inspiration	Increases from mid-pregnancy by 100–200 ml
Inspiratory capacity	Maximum amount of air that can be inspired from resting expiratory level	Increases by 300 ml throughout pregnancy
Tidal volume	Amount of air inspired and expired with normal breath	Increases by 200 ml throughout pregnancy
Functional residual capacity	Amount of air in lungs at resting expiratory level	Decreases by 500 ml
Expiratory reserve volume	Maximum amount of air that can be expired from resting	Decreases by 200 ml throughout pregnancy
Residual volume	Amount of air in lungs after maximum expiration	Decreases by 300 ml throughout pregnancy
Total lung capacity	Total amount of air in lungs at maximum inspiration	Decreases by 300 ml throughout pregnancy

Source: from Gabbe *et al.*, 1991, p. 129.

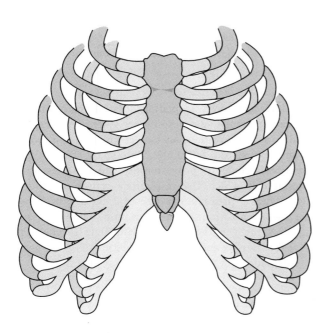

Figure 7   The ribcage in pregnancy (red) and the non-pregnancy state (blue) showing the increased subcostal angle, the increased transverse diameter and the raised diaphragm in pregnancy. (Reproduced with permission from deSwiet, 1991a, p. 88.)

impeded by the uterus. Studies on diaphragmatic movements during respiration either sitting or lying down have found them to be larger than in the non-pregnant state. This implies that breathing during pregnancy is more diaphragmatic than costal (deSwiet, 1991a; Romen *et al.*, 1991) (Figure 7).

The main functional change that occurs within the lungs is the gradual increase in the amount of air that is inspired or expired with a normal breath. This functional capacity, called *tidal volume*, increases from 500 ml in the non-pregnant state to approximately 700 ml at term. As a result of this change, women breathe more deeply during pregnancy than in the non-pregnant state (Table 1).

Since the maximum amount of air that can be expired forcibly after maximum inspiration only increases by 100–200 ml, the increase in tidal volume is produced at the expense of the expiratory reserve volume. This means that a smaller amount of air remains in the lungs at the end of quiet expiration. As less residual air is mixed with the next inspiration of fresh air, this results in lower levels of $P\text{CO}_2$ that brings about a reciprocal rise in $P\text{O}_2$. $P\text{CO}_2$ declines from approximately 39 mmHg in the non-pregnant state to 31 mmHg during pregnancy, while $P\text{O}_2$ increases from 93.4 to 101.8 mmHg, over the same period (deSwiet, 1991a) (Figure 8).

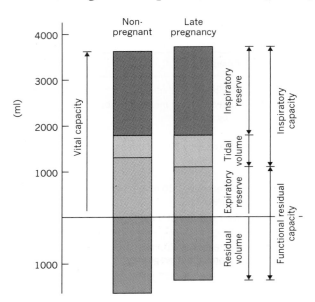

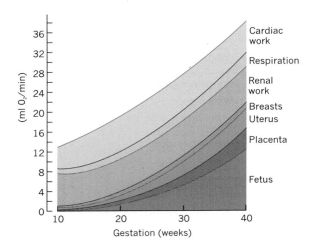

Figure 9   Partition of the increased oxygen consumption in pregnancy among the organs concerned. (Reproduced with permission from deSwiet, 1991a, p. 91.)

Figure 8   Subdivisions of the lung volume and their alterations in pregnancy. (Reproduced with permission from deSwiet, 1991a, p. 84.)

Oxygen consumption

The progressive increases in cardiac output and pulmonary ventilation are proportionately greater than those occurring in maternal and fetal oxygen consumption during pregnancy. Oxygen consumption shows a linear increase with body weight as pregnancy advances. It is composed of the overall increase in tissue mass, the higher metabolic rate of fetal and placental tissue, along with that of some maternal organs, particularly the heart, lungs and kidneys. The maximum increase in oxygen consumption of 38 ml/min is 15% above average values in the non-pregnant state (deSwiet, 1991a) (Figure 9).

This increase in oxygen consumption is facilitated by a 40–50% increase in ventilation and by an 18% increase in the oxygen-carrying capacity of the blood. Because of this relative oversupply of oxygen, higher concentrations are returned to the heart from the venous circulation, making the arteriovenous oxygen difference significantly smaller than in the non-pregnant state. The extent of the arteriovenous oxygen difference is smallest in early pregnancy and does not reach average non-pregnant values until term (deSwiet, 1991a).

The increase in ventilation during pregnancy reduces alveolar and plasma concentrations of carbon dioxide. Studies have demonstrated that arterial partial pressure of carbon dioxide (P_{CO_2}) is about 30 mmHg in late pregnancy, compared to 39 mmHg during the follicular phase of the cycle. Since fetal P_{CO_2} remains at approximately 41 mmHg, the lower levels in the maternal circulation encourage the diffusion of CO_2 from fetal blood, across the placental membranes.

Hormonal regulation

The interdependent adaptations that develop within the cardiovascular and respiratory systems are regulated by a complex interplay between maternal, placental and fetal steroid hormones. Pulmonary changes are largely effected by progesterone which resets the threshold at which the respiratory centre is stimulated. During pregnancy, a rise of 1 mmHg in P_{CO_2} increases ventilation by 6 litres/min, compared to 1.5 litres/min, in the non-pregnant state (Romen *et al.*, 1991; Bayliss and Millhorn, 1992).

Adaptations of the cardiovascular system include:

▶ enlargement of the heart;
▶ peripheral vasodilation;
▶ development of new vascular beds in the placenta;
▶ an increase in circulating blood volume; and
▶ a fall in plasma osmolality which is accompanied by a generalized oedema.

The increased size of the heart primarily affects the left ventricle. In animal experiments, this change has been shown to be stimulated by oestrogen. The accompanying changes in general systemic and uteroplacental vascular tone seem to be brought about by oestrogen and progesterone in conjunction with local vasodilatory agents (Morton, 1991; Romen et al., 1991; Pepe and Albrecht, 1995).

Peripheral vasodilation is a very striking feature of pregnancy. Dilated veins appear on the surface of the breasts as well as on the hands, face and nasal mucous membrane. Experimental evidence suggests that this generalized tendency towards vasodilation is brought about by a number of counteracting forces. These include the increased release of vasodilatory substances, prostacyclin and prostaglandin E2 (PGE_2), by vascular endothelial cells. The combined actions of oestrogen and progesterone also depress vascular responses to the pressor effects of rising levels of angiotensin II which may also be involved in stimulating the release of prostaglandins. In addition, oestrogen has been found to depress the effects of sympathetic innervation, which tends to increase the general tone of the vascular system (Broughton Pipkin et al., 1982; Friedman, 1988; Pepe and Albrecht, 1995).

Fetal Adreno-Placental Hormonal Regulation of Cortisol

For most of intrauterine life, the fetus has a limited capacity to produce cortisol as the adult zone of the adrenal gland displays minimal activity until late in gestation. During the first half of pregnancy, the fetus is supplied with low levels of cortisol via the placenta. Cortisol metabolism within the placenta and in a variety of fetal tissues seems to be mediated by oestrogen through its regulation of two distinct isoforms of 11β-hydroxysteroid dehydrogenase (11βHSD). Experimental findings suggest that up to mid-gestation, the predominant form of corticosteroid metabolism within the placenta is the reduction of cortisone to cortisol, which exceeds the oxidation of cortisol to inactive cortisone. This pattern of metabolism allows low quantities of biologically active maternal cortisol to enter the fetal compartment. Current evidence suggests that oestrogen regulates the latter but not the former reaction. Experiments have also shown that oestrogen increases the oxidation of cortisol to inactive cortisone in a variety of fetal organs. Together, these activities ensure that biologically active cortisol remains very

low in fetal tissues and largely acts on the hypothalamus to suppress corticotrophin-releasing hormone (CRH). This in turn limits pituitary capacity for ACTH production, preventing growth and maturation of the adult cortisol-producing zone of the adrenal glands (Pepe and Albrecht, 1990, 1995; Stewart et al., 1995).

As oestrogen synthesis increases with advancing gestation, oxidation of cortisol to cortisone becomes the predominant placental reaction. Research on the human placenta near term suggests that its capacity to convert cortisol to cortisone is four times higher than that required to inactivate its estimated exposure to 70 nmol maternal free cortisol/min. This shift in placental metabolism of maternal glucocorticoids has two major effects on the fetus. From mid-gestation onwards, cortisol of maternal origin decreases within the fetal compartment. Consequently, the earlier inhibitory action of maternal cortisol on growth and maturation of the adult zone is removed, while at the same time oestrogen activity within fetal tissues ensures that all organs are protected from the growth-retarding effects of cortisol. These conditions allow for the gradual maturation of the hypothalamic–pituitary–adrenal axis and the synthesis and release of fetal cortisol. Alongside the increasing capacity of the lungs and liver to convert cortisone to cortisol, production of cortisol by the fetal adrenals plays an important role in stimulating maturational changes in these organs in preparation for extrauterine life (Pepe et al., 1988; Brown et al., 1993; Pepe and Albrecht, 1995).

Recent research findings suggest that placental 11βHSD activity plays a crucial role in facilitating fetal growth and development during the second half of pregnancy. A variety of studies on humans and rats suggests that inappropriate exposure of fetal tissues to cortisol during their formative period of development creates a range of problems associated with impaired fetal growth and preterm labour. Increased release of maternal cortisol in response to social stress or poor nutrition may impose excessive demands on the capacity of 11βHSD to protect the fetal compartment from the growth-retarding effects of cortisol. Reduced growth implies lower levels of adrenal precursors for placental oestrogen, which in turn lowers its stimulatory effect on 11βHSD, thus further reducing the capacity of the placenta to inactivate cortisol (Blasco et al., 1986; Pepe and Albrecht, 1990; Tangalakis et al., 1992; Brown et al,. 1993; Edwards et al., 1993; Hedegaard *et al.*, 1993; Seckl, 1994; Challis *et al.*, 1995; Godfrey and Barker, 1995).

Maternal Hypothalamic–Pituitary–Placental Axis

Gonadotrophin-releasing hormone, follicle-stimulating hormone and luteinizing hormone

The anterior pituitary undergoes significant anatomical adaptations during pregnancy. The gland increases in size by 30–50% and a redistribution occurs in the number and relative secretory activities of its distinct cell populations. In studies on women during the first and second trimester, basal concentrations of follicular-stimulating hormone (FSH) and luteinizing hormone (LH) are undetectable and significant short-term increases only occur in response to exogenous gonadotrophin-releasing hormone (GnRH) stimulation during the first trimester. Experiments on pituitary tissue from a variety of animal species have shown that these low concentrations of FSH and LH are accompanied by a progressive fall in the number, size and functional capacity of gonadotrophs during pregnancy (Shoupe and Kletzky, 1984; Wise *et al.*, 1986; Jacobs, 1991).

Prolactin

At the same time a significant increase occurs in the number, size and secretory activity of prolactin-releasing cells. From 10 to 25% of the total population in the non-pregnant state, they grow to reach more than 50% during late pregnancy and lactation. Changes in this cell population are responsible for the overall increase in the size of the gland during pregnancy. Maternal serum levels are significantly elevated from early in the first trimester and continue rising progressively, reaching up to 20 times non-pregnant values at term (Yen, 1991).

These distinct changes appear to be regulated by the increased placental release of oestrogen and progesterone. Prolonged elevation of oestrogen has been found to inhibit GnRH activity within the hypothalamus. This mode of action seems to be predominant in the first trimester. From the second trimester onwards, the higher levels of oestrogen may also act directly to inhibit FSH and LH secretion from the anterior pituitary gland. The cellular changes that proceed simulta-neously in lactotrophs are induced by steady increases in both oestrogen and progesterone while the increased synthesis, storage and secretion of prolactin is stimulated by separate mechanisms that involve direct and indirect actions of oestrogen. Data from a number of experimental studies on animals suggest that synthesis and storage of prolactin is stimulated by a direct genomic action that takes place over 2–3 days, while prolactin secretion occurs within 2–3 hours and is mediated by oestrogen stimulation of a prolactin-releasing factor, either in the hypothalamus or the posterior pituitary gland (Murai *et al.*, 1990; Tong *et al.*, 1990).

Hypothalamic–Pituitary–Adrenal–Placental Axis

Maternal cortisol

Maternal levels of cortisol rise during the second half of pregnancy. In studies on plasma and saliva, total cortisol concentrations retain the daily variations that characterize production in the non-pregnant state. During pregnancy, daily patterns are largely similar to non-pregnant values, until approximately 25 weeks, when they began to show a higher profile (Nolten *et al.*, 1981; Allolio *et al.*, 1990; Goland *et al.*, 1992) (Figure 10).

The continued daily variation of cortisol during pregnancy indicates its overall regulation by the hypothalamic–pituitary axis. At present, it is thought that cardiovascular, metabolic and hormonal changes stimulate increasing concentrations of cortisol during pregnancy. Animal studies have also found that cortisol levels rise in response to acute stress in late pregnancy and that this rise is associated with an accelerated pattern of labour (Lawrence *et al.*, 1994, Waddell and Atkinson, 1994).

Placental steroids

Oestrogen has been found to enhance the production of a corticosteroid-binding globulin (CBG) that increases three-fold in the maternal circulation during pregnancy. While this increase in CBG could be expected to inactivate the higher levels of cortisol by increasing its binding capacity, a number of studies have demonstrated that unbound, biologically active cortisol levels rise during the third trimester (Jones *et*

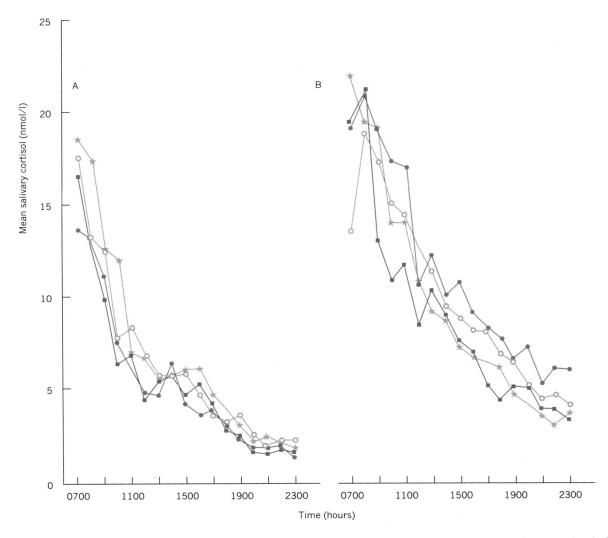

Figure 10   Salivary cortisol profiles throughout pregnancy in 10 healthy women (for clarity mean values are given). **A**: ■–■, 9–12; ●–●, 13–16; ★–★, 17–20; ○–○, 21–24; **B**: ■–■, 25–28; ●–●, 29–32; ★–★, 33–36; ○–○, 37–40 weeks of gestation. (Reproduced with permission from Allolio *et al.*, 1990, p. 281.)

al., 1989; Jones and Challis, 1990; Allolio *et al.*, 1990) (Figure 11).

Recent evidence suggests that this trend is influenced by the progressive increase in progesterone that has been found to compete with circulating cortisol for CBG-binding sites. This action is further confirmed by studies demonstrating that progesterone displays circadian variations during the second half of pregnancy that are inversely related to cortisol. In contrast to cortisol, lowest levels of progesterone have been found at 08.00 and highest levels between 16.00 and 20.00 (Junkermann *et al.*, 1982; Allolio *et al.*, 1990) (Figure 12).

This evidence of competitive binding between cortisol and progesterone has been used to explain increased tissue resistance to cortisol during pregnancy. If progesterone diminishes cortisol binding to specific glucocorticoid receptors, then higher levels of free cortisol may be stimulated to maintain its metabolic effects. In addition, the sustained increase in cardiac output and the lower levels of fasting glucose that characterize the latter half of pregnancy may also stimulate increased adrenal secretion of cortisol. Current evidence suggests that this is achieved by the increased release of placental corticotrophin-releasing

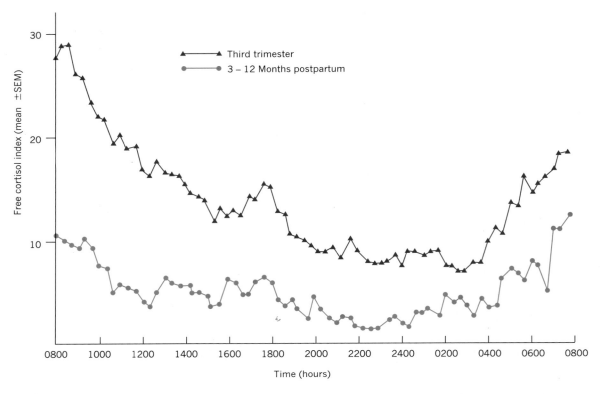

Figure 11 Patterns of mean free cortisol indexes measured at 20-minute intervals during a 24-hour period in seven third-trimester gravid women and in three women who were 3–12 months postpartum. (Reproduced with permission from Nolten and Rueckert, 1981, p. 494.)

hormone (CRH) and adrenocorticotrophic hormone (ACTH) into the maternal circulation. Rising levels of CRH from the placenta seem to downregulate pituitary CRH receptors, reducing its stimulatory influence on ACTH. At the same time placental ACTH may act as an additional stimulatory influence on maternal production of cortisol (Goland *et al.*, 1990, 1992, 1994; Fraser, 1991; Waddell and Burton, 1993; Waddell and Atkinson, 1994).

Corticotrophin-releasing hormone

Corticotrophin-releasing hormone is a neuropeptide synthesized mainly in the hypothalamus and released in response to different forms of physical and emotional stress. Its major site of action is the anterior pituitary, where it stimulates the release of ACTH, β-endorphin and other related peptides. Until the middle of the second trimester, plasma CRH remains at low or undetectable levels, similar to those in the non-pregnant state. Concentrations display a marked increase

from 28 weeks and peak during labour. Present evidence strongly indicates that this rise is of placental rather than hypothalamic origin. In contrast to circulating ACTH, no diurnal changes have been observed in plasma CRH. A low but detectable amount is present in the placenta and membranes until approximately 35 weeks, when it increases more than 20-fold during the remainder of pregnancy. Unlike that released from the hypothalamus, placental CRH is not subject to inhibition by glucocorticoids. *In vitro* findings suggest that glucocorticoids and oestrogen stimulate gene expression for CRH, while progesterone decreases levels of CRH and messenger ribonucleic acid (mRNA) in human placental tissue in culture (Frim *et al.*, 1988; Robinson *et al.*, 1988; Goland *et al.*, 1992, 1994; Chan *et al.*, 1993; Vamvakopoulos and Chrousos, 1993; Perkins and Linton, 1995; Warren and Silverman, 1995) (Figures 13 and 14).

Not all of the increase in circulating CRH is biologically active. A binding protein for CRH has been identified in plasma and found to inhibit its stimula-

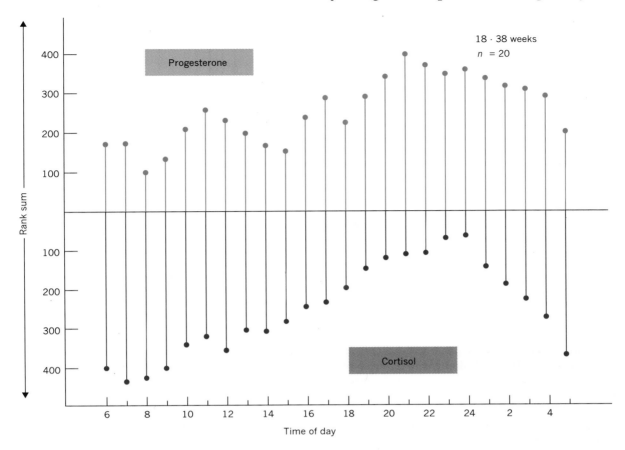

Figure 12   Inverse relation between serum progesterone and cortisol in 20 women between 18 and 38 weeks of pregnancy. Rank sums of cortisol and progesterone values are shown. (Reproduced with permission from Junkermann *et al.*, 1982, p. 102.)

tory effect on pituitary ACTH. During the first 25 weeks of pregnancy, maternal levels of CRH-binding protein remain similar to those in the non-pregnant state. Plasma concentrations decrease slightly from 26 to 30 weeks, then more rapidly, particularly over the last five weeks of gestation, to reach 33% of control values by term. This implies that concentrations of biologically active CRH rise significantly during the last trimester (Challis *et al.*, 1995; Perkins and Linton, 1995).

Adrenocorticotrophic hormone

Most studies have found that plasma ACTH remains fairly constant during pregnancy at a similar or slightly lower concentration than in the non-pregnant state. Like cortisol, the pattern of circulating ACTH shows daily variations indicating its regulation by the pitui-

tary gland. However, between 20 and 40 weeks' gestation, afternoon values of ACTH are less suppressed than in the non-pregnant state, suggesting an additional non-pituitary source of secretion (Goland *et al.*, 1992).

During pregnancy, placental CRH stimulates the synthesis of ACTH alongside other related peptides, notably melanocyte-stimulating hormone (MSH) and β-endorphin. Unlike that released from the pituitary, placental ACTH is not subject to inhibition by glucocorticoids. Evidence suggests that this additional, independent source of ACTH may also act on the maternal adrenals. Despite the higher levels of free cortisol during the third trimester, there is no indication of a simultaneous decline in ACTH within the maternal circulation. At the same time the continued rise in placental CRH during the second half of pregnancy

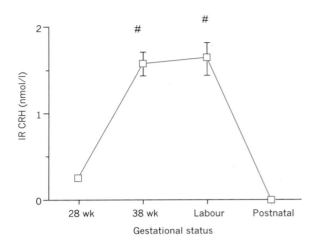

Figure 13   Profiles of immunoreactive maternal plasma corticotrophin-releasing hormone (IR CRH) during pregnancy and parturition. (Reproduced with permission from Chan *et al.*, 1993, p. 341.)

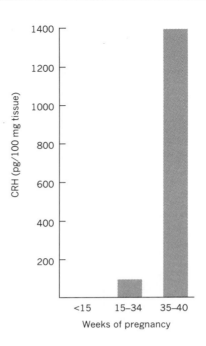

Figure 14   Changes in placental corticotrophin-releasing hormone peptide during pregnancy. (Reproduced with permisson from Frim *et al.*, 1988, p. 290.)

is not associated with a rising pattern of ACTH, suggesting a downregulation of pituitary CRH receptors. This hypothesis has been confirmed in experiments on baboons who showed a diminished response to exogenous CRH during the second half of pregnancy. Overall, these findings indicate that maternal cortisol production is regulated by placental and pituitary ACTH (Goland *et al.*, 1990; Waddell, 1993; Challis *et al.*, 1995).

Maternal and fetal significance

Current evidence suggests that these changes in the hypothalamic–pituitary–adrenal axis have a range of influences within the maternal, placental and fetal compartments during the second half of pregnancy. The rising pattern of cortisol in the maternal circulation coincides with the sustained mobilization of energy stores that is characterized by glucose resistance and hyperlipidaemia during the latter half of pregnancy. This suggests that placental CRH and ACTH may enhance the capacity of the maternal hypothalamic–pituitary–adrenal axis to meet the increased cardiorespiratory and metabolic activities that support fetal growth in the second half of pregnancy (Waddell, 1993; Waddell and Atkinson, 1994).

Within the placenta CRH, MSH and ACTH are involved in promoting different aspects of fetal growth. *In vitro* experiments on placental tissue have

shown that CRH has a potent vasodilatory action on the fetal–placental vasculature. MSH directly stimulates fetal adrenal production of DHEAS and ACTH which does not cross into the fetal compartment and increases placental production of oestrogen and progesterone (Dupouy *et al.*, 1980; Barnea *et al.*, 1986; Pepe and Albrecht, 1990; Waddell, 1993; Clifton *et al.*, 1995).

Outside of these trophic influences, CRH has a range of activities within both placental and fetal compartments that may prepare a number of organs and tissues for the onset of labour. Placental CRH is secreted into the fetal circulation reaching approximately 10% of maternal values at term. CRH-binding protein is also present in fetal plasma and follows a similar pattern to that found in the maternal circulation. The current hypothesis suggests that increased CRH in the fetal compartment assists in maturing the hypothalamic–pituitary–adrenal axis which stimulates cortisol production from the adult zone of the adrenal gland.

In the placenta, CRH is part of a number of positive feedback loops with factors that contribute towards the onset of labour. *In vitro* experiments have shown that

CRH upregulates the production of prostaglandins from the placenta and membranes while prostaglandins and other pro-inflammatory agents like interleukin-1 (IL-1) have a stimulatory influence on placental CRH. However, the significance of these and other similar findings remain to be identified *in vivo*, to take into account the modifying influences of the CRH-binding protein, the distribution of CRH receptors and the activity of hydroxyprostaglandin dehydrogenase (PGDH) which inactivates prostaglandins (Kelly, 1994; Petragalia *et al.*, 1995; Perkins and Linton, 1995; Wu *et al.*, 1995).

ENDOGENOUS OPIOIDS

Most recent studies have found that plasma concentrations of β-endorphin remain similar or lower than nonpregnant values until the third trimester, when concentrations increase significantly. During pregnancy, distinct pituitary and placental forms of β-endorphin have been identified. The pituitary source is mainly in an opioid active form, whereas that from the placenta contains little opioid activity. The pituitary form is predominant in the maternal circulation during pregnancy and its pattern of release maintains a daily rhythm that characterizes all hormones regulated by the hypothalamus. At the same time, significant correlations have been found between plasma CRH and β-endorphin during the third trimester. This suggests that the enhanced release of pituitary β-endorphin may be influenced by placental CRH (Chan and Smith, 1992; Chan *et al.*, 1993) (Figure 15).

At present the specific opiate effects of increased pituitary β-endorphin during pregnancy remains to be identified. Little is known about relations between peripheral plasma concentrations of β-endorphin and those in areas of the brain where some diffusion can occur across the blood–brain barrier. Recent attempts to explore associations between hormonal changes and maternal experiences during pregnancy have found that mood disturbances peak during the third trimester and are independent of changes in stress-related hormones. At the same time, women who experience deterioration in mood between late pregnancy and the second postnatal day have been found to show larger falls in plasma β-endorphin than those who report no such deterioration. From these findings, it has been suggested that central neurones may become dependent on β-endorphin during pregnancy (Hung, 1987; Smith *et al.*, 1990).

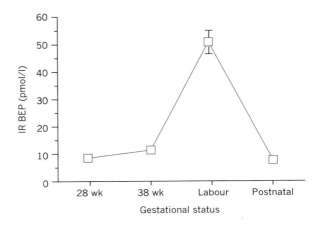

Figure 15 Profile of immunoreactive maternal plasma β-endorphin (IR BEP). (Reproduced with permission from Chan *et al.*, 1993, p. 341.)

Endogenous opioids and maternal pain threshold in late pregnancy

More recent findings in humans and other animals suggest that a distinct opioid pathway is activated in late pregnancy and labour that increases the maternal threshold for pain and discomfort. Observational studies on humans have reported a progressive rise in the pressure-induced pain threshold during the last 16 days of pregnancy. In daily tests on pregnant and non-pregnant women, discomfort thresholds also increased during the last 11 days of pregnancy and were higher than in those for non-pregnant women whose responses remained unchanged throughout the course of the study. In experiments on rats, more direct evidence suggests that this analgesia of pregnancy may be mediated by a specific opioid system in the lumbar spine which is only activated during the latter part of pregnancy. Studies that have simulated the blood concentration profiles of oestradiol and progesterone during pregnancy have demonstrated that the spinal cord concentration of the opioid peptide dynorphin rises at steroid concentrations which correspond to the last week of pregnancy (Cogan and Spinnato, 1986; Sander *et al.*, 1988, 1989; Medina, 1993).

Endogenous opioids and oxytocin

From extensive studies on rats, an endogenous opioid input on oxytocin neurones has been found to be activated during the latter half of pregnancy. In this species there is evidence of a steroid-mediated increase in the synthesis of oxytocin during pregnancy and stores accumulate in the posterior lobe of the pituitary gland. From mid-pregnancy onwards, animals receiving intravenous injections of naloxone produce significantly higher plasma concentrations of oxytocin, compared to those receiving saline alone. This evidence of a restraining influence of opioids is peculiar to periods of enhanced production of oxytocin. During pregnancy, this action is thought to be exerted by the depressive influence of opioids on the electrical activity of oxytocin neurones in the hypothalamus and by the co-release of opioids at oxytocin terminals in the posterior pituitary gland (Broad *et al.*, 1993; Douglas *et al.*, 1993).

In women, studies on plasma concentrations of β-endorphin suggest that the peripheral opioid system is activated during the third trimester. But evidence of an inhibitory opioid influence on oxytocin is indirect and associated with specific forms of stress during pregnancy and labour. In some studies, increased anxiety in late pregnancy is associated with prolonged duration of labour, uterine inertia and the higher use of oxytocin for augmentation. Both human and animal studies on acute stress during established labour have also reported a reduction or temporary halt in uterine contractions and a delay in the process of birth. Taken together, these findings suggest that endogenous opioids may act centrally to inhibit the accumulation of oxytocin during pregnancy and its release during labour (Haddad and Morris, 1985; Haddad, 1989; Peled, 1993).

The Mammary Gland

PRE-LACTATIONAL ADAPTATIONS

Maximum development of the mammary gland occurs during pregnancy. Blood flow starts to increase very soon after conception, as indicated by the early appearance of enlarged and distended veins beneath the skin. Estimates of mammary blood flow suggest that it rises from 1 to 2% of cardiac output, as pregnancy advances. The first 20 weeks are characterized by an intensification of the cell proliferation that begins during the luteal phase of the cycle. Growth of the ductal system is a predominant feature of the first half of pregnancy and is followed by enlargement and growth in the number of lobules from mid-pregnancy onwards. In this phase, new ducts are formed along with prolifera-

tion of adjoining clusters of alveoli. Towards the end of the first trimester, epithelial cells lining the alveoli also begin to differentiate from a double to a single layer of tissue. This change marks the emergence of secretory activity in the alveoli and is followed by the accumulation of secretory substances within the lumen of the alveoli during the second trimester (Russo and Russo, 1987; Fuchs, 1991).

In the third trimester, the secretory cells display an increased accumulation of lipids that are made available because of high levels of triglycerides in the maternal circulation. The process occurs through a tissue-specific increase in enzyme activity that augments the uptake of lipids from the circulation. As a result of this activity, an abundant supply of fat droplets accumulate in the secretory cells in preparation for lactation. By the end of pregnancy, the secretory alveoli form the largest part of the gland. Connective and adipose tissue progressively diminishes to form thin layers separating large, fully formed lobes of secretory cells (Russo and Russo, 1987).

The myoepithelial cells surrounding the alveoli also increase in size and number and form an open network around the epithelial cells. In rats, oxytocin receptors appear on the myoepithelial cells towards the end of pregnancy but functional capacity only develops with the onset of lactation. At this point the cytoplasm becomes packed with microfilaments that facilitate contractile activity within the cells (Fuchs, 1991).

HORMONAL REGULATION

At present, most research has focused on the response of the mammary gland to a wide variety of external hormones. However there is evidence from a variety of species for the synthesis of a range of hormones and growth factors within the gland. Current experimental findings suggest that the mammary gland operates as an endocrine organ in the luteal phase of the menstrual cycle as well as during pregnancy and lactation. While wide species variation is to be expected, some of these findings help to illuminate the complexity of hormonal interactions that have been identified in humans during pregnancy and lactation (Peaker, 1995).

In the presence of the anterior pituitary, placental steroids have been found to enhance cell proliferation, while growth hormone and prolactin have been shown to stimulate the uptake of lipids into mammary epithelial cells. Oestrogen specifically promotes elongation of the ductal system and simultaneously increases receptor concentrations for progesterone which stimulates ductal branching and development of lobes and alveoli (Haslam, 1987; Thordarson *et al.*, 1987; Fuchs, 1991; Pepe and Albrecht, 1995).

In addition to these influences on mammary development, oestrogen stimulates the synthesis and release of increasing levels of prolactin from the anterior pituitary, while rising levels of progesterone inhibit the induction of lactose, lactalbumen and casein synthesis in the alveolar cells. Progesterone is thought to exert this effect by competing with cortisol for binding to alveolar receptors. In the presence of the high levels of progesterone that persist during pregnancy, prolactin seems to act within the mammary gland in conjunction with placental steroids to promote lobular and alveolar development and to stimulate the accumulation of lipid molecules in the secretory cells (Martin *et al.*, 1980; Goodman *et al.*, 1983; Vonderhaar, 1987; Lee and Oks, 1992).

Besides these hormones, human placental lactogen (hPL) may also be involved in mammary development during pregnancy. In *in vitro* studies in humans, hPL has been found to induce substantial growth in ductal tissue that is independent of steroid hormones. However, it is not certain to what extent this occurs *in vivo*, as mammary development does not seem to be inhibited in women with very low levels of hPL during pregnancy. Uncertainties also exist on the timing of increased oxytocin receptor concentrations in the myoepithelial cells. Most studies in humans have found no increased sensitivity to exogenous oxytocin in pregnancy but marked increases have been reported in a number of studies following delivery (Wiederman *et al.*, 1964; Thordarson *et al.*, 1987; Fuchs, 1991).

Uterine Adaptations

Before pregnancy, the uterus is a small pelvic organ, with a cavity of around 10 ml and weighs approximately 50 g. By around 36 weeks, it is in contact with the anterior abdominal wall and extends as far as the xiphisternum. At this point, its weight has increased to an estimated 1100 g, representing almost a 20-fold increase in mass and its average volume is 5 litres. During pregnancy, the uterus is a central recipient of the increases in circulating blood volume. In the non-pregnant state, uterine blood flow is approximately 10 ml/min. This changes very little during early preg-

nancy but rises sharply from about 20 weeks to reach 600–800 ml/min at term, when it receives nearly 20% of total cardiac output (Steer, 1991).

Myometrial changes

The bundles of smooth muscle fibres within the uterus are arranged in three or four layers embedded in a matrix of connective tissue which acts as intramuscular tendons. Two outer layers contain longitudinal and circular fibres that are partly continuous with the supporting ligaments. The middle layers that hold the vascular supply have a criss-cross pattern of fibres that run in all directions. Finally, the inner layer is composed of longitudinal fibres and covers the decidua (Steer, 1991).

Uterine growth occurs partly by cell division, particularly in early pregnancy and by hypertrophy of existing cells during the remainder of pregnancy. Growth is stimulated by hCG and oestrogen and by the progressive distension exerted by the growing fetus. Both factors have been found to promote the synthesis of the contractile proteins, actin and myosin. During the first few months, growth is accompanied by increasing thickness of the myometrium in the corpus and the fundus. As the organ increases in length from around 12 weeks, the isthmus is gradually formed as an area containing a reduced density of muscle fibres (Steer, 1991).

The smooth muscle forming the myometrium does not have the precise transverse alignment of thick and thin filaments that characterizes the organization of skeletal fibres. Filaments of smooth muscle are situated in random bundles throughout the cells and myosin filaments are arranged alongside actin in uninterrupted unidirectional order. In addition to these main contractile filaments, smooth muscle also contains intermediate filaments. These are attached to all areas of cell membrane which allows them to form networks across the cell. As a result of this organization, contractions can generate force in any direction and also produce a much greater degree of shortening than in skeletal muscle. For most of pregnancy, however, this action remains a local event, as few intracellular connections are formed until the last few weeks (Huszar and Roberts, 1982) (Figure 16).

Influences of placental steroids

In addition to its structural differences with skeletal muscle, the myometrium has a number of additional

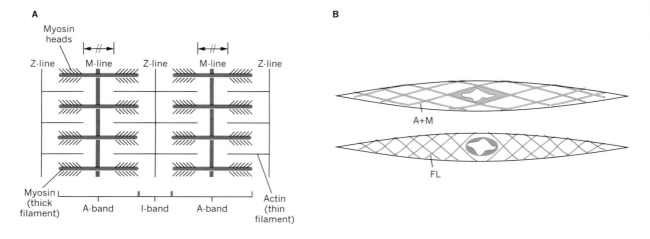

Figure 16   Diagrammatic picture of **A**: striated and **B**: smooth muscle fibres. A, actin; M, myosin; FL, filaments. (Reproduced with permission from Huszar and Roberts, 1982, p. 226.)

features that distinguish it from smooth muscle in other parts of the body. Myometrial cells are uniquely regulated by oestrogen and progesterone. During pregnancy, oestrogen induces synthesis of structural and contractile proteins and enzymes that supply energy for the process of contraction. Oestrogen also influences molecules within the plasma membrane that control its permeability for ions like sodium, potassium, calcium and chloride. These ion fluxes determine the resting potential and electrical excitability of myometrial cells (Fuchs and Fuchs, 1984; Pepe and Albrecht, 1995).

Besides having a direct effect on the structure of myometrial cells, oestrogen also regulates the formation of oxytocic and α-adrenergic receptors, both of which promote uterine contraction. During pregnancy, myometrial and decidual receptors for oxytocin increase from 27.6 fmol/mg DNA in the non-pregnant state, to 171.6 fmol/mg DNA, at mid-gestation and to 1391 fmol/mg DNA at term. Over the whole of pregnancy, this represents an 80–100-fold increase within the uterus. Some studies on women have reported an increase in α_1 receptors at term. β-Adrenergic receptor formation is also stimulated by oestrogen. While static and decreasing concentrations have been reported at term, they do not appear to be activated prior to the onset of labour (Fuchs and Fuchs, 1991; Dahle *et al.*, 1992; Wray, 1993; Pepe and Albrecht, 1995).

Some, but not all, of the actions of oestrogen are modulated by progesterone. This hormone stimulates

the synthesis of distinct and overlapping proteins and inhibits the production of oestrogen receptors and certain oestrogen-stimulated enzymes within myometrial cells. In direct contrast to oestrogens, progesterone stimulates the formation of β-adrenergic receptors which induce myometrial relaxation. But like the α-adrenergic receptors influenced by oestrogens, these are not activated before the onset of labour (Fuchs and Fuchs, 1991; Wray, 1993; Pepe and Albrecht, 1995).

In humans and other primates, no strong evidence currently exists for a local increase in the ratio of oestrogen to progesterone before the onset of labour. Plasma concentrations of progesterone progressively increase throughout pregnancy and no significant change is evident in the relative concentrations of progesterone and oestrogen in the peripheral circulation during the latter part of pregnancy. Within the myometrium at term, the ratio of progesterone to oestradiol is higher than in the general circulation and the intracellular concentration of progesterone in the myometrium is also significantly higher following labour than at elective Caesarean section. However, fetal membranes at term have the capacity to increase local tissue concentrations of oestrogen and progesterone receptors in the myometrium have been found to decrease towards term. More clear-cut answers may emerge from exploring the molecular influences of both steroids on the changing pattern of myometrial relaxation and contraction during pregnancy and labour (Khan-Dawood and Dawood, 1984; Mitchell *et al.*, 1984; Huszar and Walsh, 1991; Fu *et al.*, 1993;

Leslie *et al.*, 1994; How *et al.*, 1995; Wu *et al.*, 1995; Xuan *et al.*, 1995).

CERVICAL CHANGES

In nulliparous women, the cervix is largely composed of dense fibrous connective tissue, formed by thick, cross-linked collagen fibrils that are invested in a ground substance, composed of core proteins attached to large numbers of unbranched polysaccharide chains. These form an interconnecting lattice that actively binds to collagen fibrils, in a way that positions them to provide maximal mechanical strength. The smaller muscle content is organized as a continuous external layer and scattered bundles are located internally. Few structural changes occur in the cervix until the latter part of pregnancy. There is an overall increase in the size of the cervix which is accompanied by a rise in total collagen content, some hypertrophy of external muscle fibres and a progressive rise in vascularity. As pregnancy advances, some biopsy studies have reported a gradual reduction in collagen density, a rise in polysaccharide chains and a possible redistribution of core proteins in favour of those that are highly absorbent. In addition to the increased vascularity, these findings may explain the increasing water content and the slightly softer consistency of the cervix during pregnancy (Hughesdon, 1952; Uldbjerg *et al.*, 1983; Huszar and Walsh, 1991; Jeffrey, 1991) (see Chapter 27).

Musculoskeletal Adaptations

Considerable alterations occur in the musculoskeletal system during pregnancy. From the first trimester onwards, rising levels of oestrogens and relaxin reduce the density of connective tissue, cartilage and ligaments and increase the quantity of synovial fluid. Taken together, these changes produce a greater degree of mobility and flexibility in the joints. During the second half of pregnancy, joint mobility may be reduced, particularly in ankle and wrist joints, by increasing fluid retention in the surrounding connective tissue. At the same time, the woman's centre of gravity is displaced by the increasing size, weight and anterior orientation of the uterus as it expands into the abdominal cavity and, to a lesser extent, by the growing weight of the breasts. To compensate for the increased likelihood of tilting forward, the woman's centre of gravity is simultaneously displaced back over the pelvis, which tends to produce a progressive lordosis of the lumbar spine.

PELVIS – BONES AND LIGAMENTS

The pelvic girdle is uniquely formed to respond to hormonal and postural influences in pregnancy and labour. At birth, the bony pelvis is composed of a pair of coxal or hip bones which form the anterior and lateral walls of the pelvic cavity. The remaining wall is shaped by vertebrae which gradually fuse to form the sacrum and coccyx. Each coxal bone is made up of three adjoining bones. At birth, parts of these bones, together with their adjoining areas, are still composed of cartilage. Bone growth and ossification, together with joint fusion, continues throughout childhood, puberty and early adult life. Joint fusion is thought to be complete by approximately 25 years.

References

Allolio, B., Hoffmann, J., Linton, E.A. *et al.* (1990) Diurnal salivary cortisol patterns during pregnancy and after delivery: relationships to plasma corticotrophin-releasing-hormone. *Clin. Endocrinol.* 33: 279–289.

Barnea, E.R., Lavy, G., Fakih, H. *et al.* (1986) The role of ACTH in placental steroidogenesis. *Placenta* 7: 307–313.

Baylis, C. & Davison, J. (1991) The urinary system. In Hytten, F. & Chamberlain, G. (eds) *Clinical Physiology in Obstetrics*, pp. 245–302. Oxford: Blackwell Scientific.

Bayliss, D.A. & Millhorn, D.E. (1992) Central neural mechanisms of progesterone action: application to the respiratory system. *J. Appl. Physiol.* 73(2): 393–404.

Beguin, Y., Lipscei, G., Oris, R. *et al.* (1990) Serum immunoreactive erythropoietin during pregnancy and in the early postpartum. *Br. J. Haematol.* 76: 545–549.

Blasco, M.J., Lopez Bernal, A. & Turnbull, A.C. (1986) 11β-Hydroxysteroid dehydrogenase activity of the human placenta during pregnancy. *Hormone Metab. Res.* 18: 638–641.

Broad, K., Kendrick, K.M., Sirinathsinghji, D.J.S. & Keverne, E.B. (1993) Changes in oxytocin immunoreactivity and mRNA expression in the sheep brain during pregnancy, parturition and lactation and in response to oestrogen and progesterone. *J. Neuroendocrinol.* 5: 435–444.

Broughton Pipkin, F. (1993) The fetal renin-angiotensin

system. In Robertson, J.I.S. & Nicholls, M.G. (eds) *The Renin–Angiotensin System*, Vol. 1, pp. 51.1–51.10. London: Gower Medical Publishers.

Broughton Pipkin, F., Hunter, J.C. & Turner, S.R. (1982) Prostaglandin attenuates the pressor response to angiotensin II in pregnant subjects but not in nonpregnant subjects. *Am. J. Obstet. Gynecol.* **142**(2): 168–176.

Brown, R.W. & Chapman Edwards, C.R.W. (1993) Human placental 11β–Hydroxysteroid dehydrogenase: evidence for and partial purification of a distinct NAD-dependent isoform. *Endocrinology* **132**(6): 2614–2621.

Capeless, E.L. & Clapp, J.F. (1989) Cardiovascular changes in early pregnancy. *Am. J. Obstet. Gynecol.* **161**(6): 1449–1452.

Challis, J.R.G., Matthews, S.G. & Van Meir, C. (1995) Current topic: the placental corticotrophin-releasing hormone–adrenocorticotrophin axis. *Placenta* **16**: 481–502.

Chan, E-C. & Smith, R. (1992) β-Endorphin immunoreactivity during human pregnancy. *J. Clin. Endocrinol. Metab.* **75**(6): 1453–1458.

Chan, E-C., Smith, R., Lewin, T. *et al.* (1993) Plasma corticotrophin-releasing hormone, β-endorphin and cortisol inter-relationships during human pregnancy. *Acta Endocrinol.* **128**: 339–344.

Cietak, K.A. & Newton, J.R. (1985) Serial qualitative maternal nephrosonography in pregnancy. *Br. J. Radiol.* **58**(689): 399–404.

Clapp, J.F., Seaward, B.L., Sleamaker, R.H. *et al.* (1988) Maternal physiologic adaptations to early pregnancy. *Am. J. Obstet. Gynecol.* **159**(6): 1456–1460.

Clifton, V.L., Read, M.A. & Leitch, I.M. (1995) Corticotrophin-releasing hormone-induced vasodilatation in the human fetal–placental circulation: involvement of the nitric oxide-cycle guanosine 3′,5′-monophosphate-mediated pathway. *J. Clin. Endocrinol. Metab.* **80**(10): 2888–2893.

Cogan, R. & Spinnato, J.A. (1986) Pain and discomfort thresholds in late pregnancy. *Pain* **27**: 63–68.

Cook, C. & Trundinger, B. (1993) Angiotensin sensitivity predicts aspirin benefit in placental insufficiency. *Br. J. Obstet. Gynaecol.* **100**: 46–50.

Cotes, M.P., Camnning, C.E. & Lind, T. (1983) Changes in serum immunoreactive erythropoietin during the menstrual cycle and normal pregnancy. *Br. J. Obstet. Gynaecol.* **90**: 304–311.

Dahle, L.O., Anderson, R.G.G., Berg, G. *et al.* (1993) Alpha-adrenergic receptors in human myometrium: changes during pregnancy. *Gynaecol. Obstet. Invest.* **36**: 75–80.

Davison, J.M. & Lindheimer, M.D. (1989) Volume homeostasis and osmoregulation in human pregnancy. *Baillière's Clin. Endocrinol. Metab.* **3**(2): 451–472.

Davison, J.M. & Noble, M.C.B. (1981) Serial changes in 24 hour creatinine clearance during normal menstrual cycles and the first trimester of pregnancy. *Br. J. Obstet. Gynaecol.* **88**: 10–17.

deSwiet, M. (1991a) The respiratory system. In Hytten, F. & Chamberlain, G. (eds) *Clinical Physiology in Obstetrics*, pp. 83–100. Oxford: Blackwell Scientific.

deSwiet, M. (1991b) The cardiovascular system. In Hytten, F. & Chamberlain, G. (eds) *Clinical Physiology in Obstetrics*, pp. 3–38. Oxford: Blackwell Scientific.

Douglas, A.J., Dye, S., Leng, G. *et al.* (1993) Endogenous

opioid regulation of oxytocin secretion through pregnancy in the rat. *J. Neuroendocrinol.* **5**: 307–314.

Downing, G.J., Poisner, A.M. & Barnea, E.R. (1995) First-trimester villous placenta has high prorenin and active renin concentrations. *Am. J. Obstet. Gynecol.* **172**(3): 864–867.

Dupouy, J-P., Chatelain, A. & Allaume, P. (1980) Absence of transplacental passage of ACTH in the rat: direct experimental proof. *Biol. Neonate* **37**: 96–102.

Duvekot, J.J., Cheriex, E.C. & Pieters, F.A.A. (1993) Early pregnancy changes in hemodynamics and volume homeostasis are consecutive adjustments triggered by a primary fall in systemic vascular tone. *Am. J. Obstet. Gynecol.* **169**(6): 1382–1392.

Duvekot, J.J., Cheriex, E.C., Pieters, F.A.A. *et al.* (1995) Maternal volume homeostasis in early pregnancy in relation to fetal growth restriction. *Obstet. Gynecol.* **85**(3): 361–367.

Edwards, C.R.W., Benediktsson, R., Lindsay, R.S. *et al.* (1993) Dysfunction of placental glucocorticoid barrier: link between fetal environment and adult hypertension. *Lancet* **341**: 355–357.

Fraser, R.B. (1991) Carbohydrate metabolism. In Hytten, F. & Chamberlain, G. (eds) *Clinical Physiology in Obstetrics*, pp. 204–212. Oxford: Blackwell Scientific.

Friedman, S.A. (1988) Preeclampsia: a review of the role of prostaglandins. *Obstet. Gynecol.* **71**(1): 122–137.

Frim, D.M., Emanuel, R.L., Robinson, B.G. *et al.* (1988) Characterisation of gestational regulation of corticotrophin-releasing hormone messenger RNA in human placenta. *J. Clin. Invest.* **82**: 287–292.

Fu, X., Rexapour, M., Lofgren, M. *et al.* (1993) Unexpected stimulatory effect of progesterone on human myometrial contractile activity in vitro. *Obstet. Gynecol.* **82**(1): 23–28.

Fuchs, A-F. (1991) Physiology and endocrinology of lactation. In Gabbe, S.G., Niebyl, J.R. & Simpson, J.L. (eds) *Obstetrics, Normal and Problem Pregnancies*, pp. 175–205. New York: Churchill Livingstone.

Fuchs, A-F. & Fuchs, F. (1984) Endocrinology of human parturition: a review. *Br. J. Obstet. Gynaecol.* **91**: 948–967.

Fuchs, A-F. & Fuchs, F. (1991) Physiology of parturition. In Gabbe, S.G., Niebyl, J.R. & Simpson, J.L. (eds) *Obstetrics, Normal and Problem Pregnancies*, pp. 147–174. New York: Churchill Livingstone.

Gabbe, S.G., Niebyl, J.R. & Simpson, J.L. (eds) (1991) *Obstetrics, Normal and Problem Pregnancies*. New York: Churchill Livingstone.

Godfrey, K. & Barker, D.J.B. (1995) Maternal nutrition in relation to fetal and placental growth. *Eur. J. Obstet. Gynaecol. Repro. Med.* **61**: 15–22.

Goland, R.S., Stark, R.I. & Wardlaw, S.L. (1990) Response of corticotrophin-releasing hormone during pregnancy in the baboon. *J. Clin. Endocrinol. Metab.* **70**(4): 925–929.

Goland, R.S., Conwell, I.M., Warren, W.B. *et al.* (1992) Placental corticotrophin-releasing hormone and pituitary-adrenal function during pregnancy. *Neuroendocrinology* **56**: 742–749.

Goland, R.S., Jozak, R.N. & Conwell, I. (1994) Placental corticotrophin-releasing hormone and the hypercortisolism of pregnancy. *Am. J. Obstet. Gynecol.* **171**(4): 1287–1291.

Goodman, G.T., Akers, R.M., Friderici, H. *et al.* (1983) Hormonal regulation of *ax*-lactalbumen secretion from bovine mammary tissue cultured *in vitro*. *Endocrinology* 112(4): 1324–1330.

Haddad, F. (1989) Effect of anxiety in pregnancy. *Contemp. Rev. Obstet. Gynaecol.* 1: 123–132.

Haddad, P.F. & Morris, N.F. (1985) Anxiety in pregnancy and its relation to use of oxytocin and analgesia in labour. *J. Obstet. Gynaecol.* 6(2): 77–81.

Haslam, S.Z. (1987) Role of sex steroid hormones in normal mammary gland function. In Neville, M.C. & Daniel, C.W. (eds) *The Mammary Gland*, pp. 499–533. New York: Plenum Press.

Hedegaard, M., Henriksen, T.B., Sabroe, S. *et al.* (1993) Psychological distress in pregnancy and preterm delivery. *Br. Med. J.* 307: 234–239.

How, H., Huang, Z-H., Zuo, J. *et al.* (1995) Myometrial estradiol and progesterone receptor changes in preterm and term pregnancies. *Obstet. Gynecol.* 86(6): 936–940.

Hughesdon, P.E. (1952) The fibromuscular structure of the cervix and its changes during pregnancy and labour. *J. Obstet. Gynaecol. Br. Empire* 59: 763–776.

Hung, T.T. (1987) The role of endogenous opioids in pregnancy and anaesthesia. *Seminars Reprod. Endocrinol.* 5(2): 161–169.

Huszar, G. & Roberts, J.M. (1982) Biochemistry and pharmacology of the myometrium and labour: regulation at the cellular and molecular levels. *Am. J. Obstet. Gynecol.* 142(2): 225–237.

Huszar, G.B. & Walsh, M.P. (1991) Relationship between myometrial and cervical functions in pregnancy and labour. *Seminars Perinatol.* 15(2): 97–117.

Hytten, F. *et al.* (eds) (1991) *Clinical Physiology in Obstetrics.* Oxford: Blackwell Scientific.

Jacobs, H.S. (1991) The hypothalamus and pituitary gland. In Hytten, F. & Chamberlain, G. (eds) *Clinical Physiology in Obstetrics*, pp. 345–356. Oxford: Blackwell Scientific.

Jeffrey, J.J. (1991) Collagen and collagenase: pregnancy and parturition. *Seminars Perinatol.* 15(2): 118–126.

Jones, S.A. & Challis, J.R.G. (1990) Steroid, corticotrophin-releasing hormone, ACTH and prostaglandin interactions in the amnion and placenta of early pregnancy in man. *J. Endocrinol.* 125: 153–159.

Jones, S.A., Brooks, A.N. & Challis, J.R.G. (1989) Steroids modulate corticotrophin-releasing hormone production in human fetal membranes and placenta. *J. Clin. Endocrinol. Metab.* 68(4): 825–830.

Junkermann, H., Mangold, H., Vecsei, P. *et al.* (1982) Circadian rhythm of serum progesterone levels in human pregnancy and its relation to the rhythm of cortisol. *Acta Endocrinol.* 101: 98–104.

Kelly, R.W. (1994) Pregnancy maintenance and parturition: the role of prostaglandin in manipulating the immune and inflammatory response. *Endo. Rev.* 15(5): 684–706.

Khan-Dawood, F.S. & Dawood, M.Y. (1984) Estrogen and progesterone receptor and hormone levels in human myometrium and placenta in term pregnancy. *Am. J. Obstet. Gynecol.* 150(5): 501–505.

Lawrence, A.B., Petherick, J.C. & McLean, K.A. (1994) The effect of environment on behaviour, plasma cortisol and prolactin in parturient sows. *Appl. Animal Behav. Sci.* 39: 313–330.

Lee, C.S. & Oks, T. (1992) Progesterone regulation of a pregnancy-specific transcription repressor to β–casein gene promoter in mouse mammary gland. *Endocrinology* 131(5): 2257–2262.

Leslie, K.K., Zuckerman, D.J., Schrueffer, J. *et al.* (1994) Oestrogen modulation with parturition in the human placenta. *Placenta* 15: 79–88.

Lind, T. & Hytten, F.E. (1972) The excretion of glucose during normal pregnancy. *J. Obstet. Gynaecol. Br. Commonwealth* 79(11): 961–965.

Longo, L.F. (1983) Maternal blood volume and cardiac output during pregnancy: a hypothesis of endocrine control. *Am. J. Physiol.* 245: R720–R729.

Lund, C.J. & Donovan, J.C. (1967) Blood volume during pregnancy. *Am. J. Obstet. Gynecol.* 98(3): 393–403.

Mabie, W., DiSessa, T.G., Crocker, L.G. *et al.* (1994) A longitudinal study of cardiac output in normal human pregnancy. *Am. J. Obstet. Gynecol.* 170(3): 849–856.

Magness, R.R. & Rosenfeld, C.R. (1989) Local and systemic estradiol-17B: effects on uterine and systemic vasodilation. *Am. J. Physiol.* 256: E536–E542.

Marchant, D.J. (1978) Alterations in anatomy and function of the urinary tract during pregnancy. *Clin. Obstet. Gynaecol.* 21(3): 855–861.

Martin, R.H., Glass, M.R., Chapman, C. *et al.* (1980) Human α–lactalbumen and hormonal factors in pregnancy and lactation. *Clin. Endocrinol.* 13: 223–230.

Mattingly, R.F. & Borkowf, H.I. (1978) Clinical implications of ureteral reflux in pregnancy. *Clin. Obstet. Gynaecol.* 21(3): 863–873.

Medina, V.M. (1993) 17β–estradiol and progesterone positively modulate spinal cord dynorphin: relevance to the analgesia of pregnancy. *Neuroendocrinology* 58: 310–315.

Mitchell, B.F., Cross, J. Hobkirk, R. *et al.* (1984) Formation of unconjugated estrogens from estrone sulfate by dispersed cells from human fetal membranes and decidua. *J. Clin. Endocrinol. Metab.* 58(5): 845–849.

Morton, M.J. (1991) Maternal hemodynamics in pregnancy. In Mittelmark, R.A. & Wiswell, R.A. (eds) *Exercise in Pregnancy*, pp. 61–70. Baltimore: Williams & Wilkins.

Mukaddam-Daher, S., Gutkowska, J. & Tremblay, J. (1995) Regulation of renal atrial natriuretic peptide receptors in pregnant sheep. *Endocrinology* 136(10): 4565–4571.

Murai, I. & Ben-Jonathon, N. (1990) Acute stimulation of prolactin by estradiol: mediation by the posterior pituitary. *Endocrinology* 126(6): 3179–3184.

Neng Lai, K. & Fai Lui, S. (1993) Renin and erythropoietin. In Robertson, J.I.S. & Nicholls, M.G. (eds) *The Renin–Angiotensin System*, Vol. 1, pp. 39.1–39.8. London: Gower Medical Publishers.

Nolten, W.E. & Rueckert, P.A. (1981) Elevated free cortisol index in pregnancy: Possible regulatory mechanisms. *Am. J. Obstet. Gynecol.* 139(4): 492–498.

Nolten, W.E., Holt, L.H. & Rueckert, P.A. (1981) Deoxycorticosterone in normal pregnancy: III. Evidence of a fetal source of deoxycorticosterone. *Am. J. Obstet. Gynecol.* 139(4): 477–482.

Omar, H.A., Ramirez, R. & Gibson, M. (1995) Properties of a progesterone-induced relaxation in human placental arteries and veins. *J. Clin. Endocrinol. Metab.* 80(2): 370–373.

Parker, C.R., Winkel, C.A., Rush, J.A. *et al.* (1981) Plasma concentrations of 11-deoxycorticosterone in women during the menstrual cycle. *Obstet. Gynecol.* **58**(1): 26–30.

Peaker, M. (1995) Endocrine signals form the mammary gland. *J. Endocrinol.* **147**: 189–193.

Peled, G. (1993) Birth and the Gulf War. *MIDIRS Midwifery Digest* **3**(1): 54.

Pepe, G.J. & Albrecht, E.D. (1990) Regulation of the primate fetal adrenal cortex. *Endocrine Rev.* **11**(1): 151–176.

Pepe, G.J. & Albrecht, E.D. (1995) Actions of placental and fetal adrenal steroid hormones in primate pregnancy. *Endocrine Rev.* **16**(5): 608–648.

Pepe, G.J., Brendan, J. & Waddell, S.J. (1988) The regulation of transplacental cortisol-cortisone metabolism by estrogen in pregnant baboons. *Endocrinology* **122**(1): 78–83.

Perkins, A.V. & Linton, E.A. (1995) Placental corticotrophin-releasing hormone: there by accident or design? *J. Endocrinol.* **147**: 377–381.

Petraglia, F., Benedetto, C., Florio, P. *et al.* (1995) Effect of corticotrophin-releasing factor-binding protein on prostaglandin release from cultured maternal decidua and on contractile activity of human myometerium *in vitro. J. Clin. Endocrinol. Metab.* **80**(10): 3073–3076.

Phippard, A.F., Horvath, J.S. & Glynn, E.M. (1986) Circulatory adaptations to pregnancy – serial studies of haemodynamics, blood volume, renin, and aldosterone in the baboon. *J. Hypertension* **4**: 773–779.

Robinson, B.G., Emanuel, R.L., Frim, D.M. *et al.* (1988) Glucocorticoid stimulates expression of corticotrophin-releasing hormone gene in human placenta. *Proc. Natl Acad. Sci. USA* **85**: 5244–5248.

Robson, S.C., Hunter, S. & Boys, R.J. *et al.* (1989) Serial study of factors influencing changes in cardiac output during human pregnancy. *Am. J. Physiol.* **256**: H1060–H1065.

Romen, Y., Masaki, D.I. & Mittelmark, R.A. (1991) Physiological and endocrine adjustments to pregnancy. In Mittelmark, R.A. & Wiswell, R.A. (eds) *Exercise in Pregnancy*, pp. 9–29. Baltimore: Williams & Wilkins.

Rosso, P. (1990) *Nutrition and Metabolism in Pregnancy*. New York: Oxford University Press.

Russo, J. & Russo, I.H. (1987) Development of the human mammary gland. In Neville, M.C. & Daniel, C.W. (eds) *The Mammary Gland*, pp. 67–93. New York: Plenum Press.

Sander, H.W., Portoghese, P.S. & Gintzler, A.R. (1988) Spinal κ-opiate receptor involvement in the analgesia of pregnancy: effects of intrathecal nor-binaltorphimine, a κ-selective antagonist. *Brain Res.* **474**: 343–347.

Sander, H.W., Kream, R.M. & Gintzler, A.R. (1989) Spinal dynorphin involvement in the analgesia of pregnancy: effects of intrathecal dynorphin antisera. *Eur. J. Pharmacol.* **159**: 105–109.

Schrier, R.W. & Briner, V.A. (1991) Peripheral arterial vasodilation hypothesis of sodium and water retention in pregnancy: implications for pathogenesis of pre-eclampsia. *Obstet. Gynecol.* **77**(4): 632–639.

Seckl, J.R. (1994) Glucocorticoids and small babies. *Quart. J. Med.* **87**: 259–262.

Shoupe, D. & Kletzky, O.A. (1984) Priming with gonadotrophin-releasing hormone restores gonadotrophin secretion during first but not second trimester of pregnancy. *Am. J. Obstet. Gynecol.* **150**(5): 460–464.

Skinner, S.L. (1993) The renin system in fertility and normal human pregnancy. In Robertson, J.I.S. & Nicholls, M.G. (eds) *The Renin–Angiotensin System*, Vol. 1, pp. 50.1–50.16. London: Gower Medical Publishers.

Smith, R., Cubis, J., Brinsmead, M. *et al.* (1990) Mood changes, obstetric experience and alterations in plasma cortisol, beta-endorphin and corticotrophin releasing hormone during pregnancy and the puerperium. *J. Psychosom. Res.* **34**(1): 53–69.

Smith, S.S. (1991) Progesterone administration attenuates excitatory amino acid responses of cerebellar Purkinje cells. *Neuroscience* **42**(2): 309–320.

Steer, P.J. (1991) The genital system. In Hytten, F. *et al.* (eds) *Clinical Physiology in Obstetrics*, pp. 303–344. Oxford: Blackwell Scientific.

Steer, P., Ash Alam, M., Wadsworth, J. *et al.* (1995) Relation between maternal haemoglobin concentration and birth weight in different ethnic groups. *Br. Med. J.* **310**: 489–491.

Stewart, P.M., Fraser, M.R. & Mason, J. (1995) Type 2 11β-hydroxysteroid dehydrogenase messenger ribonucleic acid and activity in human placenta and fetal membranes: its relationship to birth weight and putative role in fetal steroidogenesis. *J. Clin. Endocrinol. Metab.* **80**(3): 885–890.

Tangalakis, K., Lumbers, E.R. & Moritz, K.M. (1992) Effect of cortisol on blood pressure and vascular reactivity in the ovine fetus. *Exp. Physiol.* **77**: 709–717.

Thordarson, G. *et al.* (1987) Role of the placenta in mammary gland development and function. In Neville, M.C. & Daniel, C.W. (eds) *The Mammary Gland*, pp. 459–489. New York: Plenum Press.

Thomsen, J.K., Fogh-Andersen, N., Jaszczak, P. *et al.* (1993) Atrial natriuretic peptide (ANP) decrease during normal pregnancy as related to hemodynamic changes and volume regulation. *Acta Obstet. Gynaecol. Scand.* **72**: 103–110.

Tong, Y., Zhao, H.L. & Abrie, F. (1990) Effects of estrogens on the ultrastructural characteristics of female rat prolactin cells as evaluated by *in situ* hybridization in combination with immunogold staining technique. *Neuroendocrinology* **52**: 309–315.

Uldbjerg, N., Ulmsten, U. & Ekman, G. (1983) The ripening of the human uterine cervix in terms of connective tissue biochemistry. *Clin. Obstet. Gynaecol.* **26**(1): 14–26.

Vamvakopoulos, N.C. & Chrousos, G.P. (1993) Evidence of direct estrogen regulation of human corticotrophin-releasing hormone gene expression. *J. Clin. Invest.* **92**: 1896–1902.

Vonderhaar, B.K. (1987) Prolactin, transport, function, and receptors in mammary gland development and differentiation. In Neville, M.C. & Daniel, C.W. (eds) *The Mammary Gland*, pp. 383–438. New York: Plenum Press.

Waddell, B.J. (1993) The placenta as hypothalamus and pituitary: possible impact on maternal and fetal adrenal function. *Reprod. Fertility Develop* **5**: 479–497.

Waddell, B.J. & Burton, P.J. (1993) Release of bioactive ACTH by perfused human placenta at early and late gestation. *J. Endocrinol.* **136**: 345–353.

Waddell, B.J. & Atkinson, H.C. (1994) Production rate,

metabolic clearance rate and uterine extraction of corticosterone during rat pregnancy. *J. Endocrinol.* **143**: 183–190.

Warren, W.B. & Silverman, A.J. (1995) Cellular localization of corticotrophin releasing hormone in the human placenta, fetal membranes and decidua. *Placenta,* **16**: 147–156.

Wiederman, J., Freund, M. & Stone, M.L. (1964) Oxytocin effect on myoepithelium of the breast throughout pregnancy. *J. Appl. Physiol.* **19**(2): 310–315.

Wintour, E.M., Coghlan, J.P., Oddie, C.J. *et al.* (1978) A sequential study of adrenocorticosteroid level in human pregnancy *Clin. Exp. Pharmacol. Physiol.* **5**: 399–403.

Wise, M.E., Sawyer, H.R. & Nett, T.M. (1986) Functional changes in luteinizing hormone-secreting cells from pre- and postpartum ewes. *Am. J. Physiol.* **250**: E282–E287.

Wray, S. (1993) Uterine contraction and physiological mechanisms of modulation. *Am. J. Physiol.* **264**: C1–C18.

Wu, W.X., Unno, S. & Giussani, D.A. (1995) Corticotrophin-releasing hormone and its receptor distribution in fetal membranes and placenta of the rhesus monkey in late gestation and labour. *Endocrinology* **136**(10): 4621–4628.

Xuan, W., Myers, D.A. & Nathanielsz, P.W. (1995) Changes in estrogen receptor messenger ribonucleic acid in sheep fetal and maternal tissue during late gestation and labour. *Am. J. Obstet. Gynecol.* **172**(3): 844–850.

Yen, S.S.C. (1991) Endocrine metabolic adaptations in pregnancy. In Yen, S.S.C. & Jaffe, R.B. (eds) *Reproductive Endocrinology,* pp. 936–981. Philadelphia: W.B. Saunders Company.

Yoshimura, T., Yoshimura, M., Yasue, H. *et al.* (1994) Plasma concentration of atrial natriuretic peptide and brain natriuretic peptide during normal human pregnancy and the postpartum period. *J. Endocrinol.* **140**: 393–397.

Part Five

Psychological Adaptations to Childbirth

13

The Psychology of Childbirth

It is important that the midwife has a good understanding of the psychological aspects of midwifery if she is to meet the holistic needs of parents and families today. Such a knowledge and understanding increases the sensitivity and perception of the midwife to the emotional changes and needs of women during pregnancy, labour and the postnatal period. It also increases her awareness of sociocultural factors, the variants in family life and relationships and different child-rearing patterns.

The midwife has an important role to play in the prevention of mental illness associated with childbirth. A knowledge of psychology helps her to understand and identify the vulnerable population during the antenatal period and the particular risk factors in individual women. It should also help her to provide more effective education for parents in both the ante- and the postnatal period.

The midwife needs to evaluate current midwifery practices critically and identify areas where improvements in care are needed for the promotion of mental health. An understanding of the normal process of grief and its problems, particularly in relation to perinatal death and the birth of a handicapped child, is essential if the midwife is to fulfil her role effectively in meeting the needs of grieving parents (see Chapter 78). She should also be able to identify and, in broad terms, diagnose mental illness in the postnatal period and understand her role in the prevention and management of these conditions.

The Transition to Parenthood

The news of a pregnancy may be received in many ways. When the pregnancy is planned, and often when it is unplanned, most couples are delighted. It is a momentous event in their lives. For the woman the birth of the first child is the transition from childhood to adulthood. It is part of her feminity, her sexuality, and she has now entered a new and important phase of her life. The father will undoubtedly be proud at this evidence of his virility. At the same time will come the realization that his responsibilities are about to increase. If he is sufficiently mature he will be ready to accept this; if not, his immaturity may exhibit itself in many changes in behaviour.

A high proportion of pregnancies are unplanned,

the couple using no form of contraception, or depending on unreliable methods. They are often unprepared for the reality of pregnancy as a normal result of intercourse. Although most couples happily accept the pregnancy, for some it is considered to be a disaster, an unwelcome intrusion into their lives, and may cause conflict between the couple, especially if wanted by one of them and not the other. Some reluctantly allow the pregnancy to continue, whereas others seek to have it terminated. An unstable relationship may break up following the discovery of an unplanned pregnancy, further adding to the distress of the expectant mother.

Childbirth is a uniquely female experience which in some ways alienates women from the opposite sex. Female relationships tend to become more important in pregnancy; thus closer ties may develop between mother and daughter and with other relatives and friends who have experienced childbirth. The woman's partner may feel left out and become jealous, especially as pregnancy advances and the woman becomes increasingly involved in her baby.

Although childbirth is now physically safer than ever before, psychological problems still abound. To some extent these are caused by the very developments and technological advances which make childbirth safer. The increase in investigations and tests carried out in pregnancy, the move from home to hospital births and the marked increase in intervention has led to the 'medicalization' of pregnancy and childbirth (Oakley, 1975). As a result, women feel that they have lost control over their bodies and the birth and this can cause great distress.

Today's parents are better informed about pregnancy and childbirth than hitherto and demand not only physical safety, but also emotional fulfilment culminating in a pleasurable, meaningful experience of birth and motherhood. They expect appropriate information which is communicated in an open, straightforward way so that they can make informed choices about their care and retain control during pregnancy, labour and the postnatal period. Midwives who appreciate the feelings and needs of parents and make every effort to form a partnership with them so that their needs and aspirations are met, make a great contribution to their emotional fulfilment and subsequent mental health.

The process of childbearing involves profound physiological and psychological changes. It is a developmental or maturational crisis and involves one of the greatest transitions in a woman's life. This transition is very rapid and involves not only major social, economic and emotional changes, but also the acquisition of a new identity, a new role and new skills. Conflict between the roles of wife, employee and career woman, daughter, mother and between independence and dependence is a common experience of women in pregnancy and can lead to an identity crisis which for some may continue until after the baby is born (Prince and Adams, 1987). As the woman begins to adapt to her new situation the crisis resolves. These changes, however, result in a reorganization of the personality.

Two contrasting views of pregnancy are held by women: some view it as a 'hurdle' to get through, whereas others consider it a developmental process. The *'hurdle' concept* is held by women who regard pregnancy as a stage to get through, a deviation from normality and think that, once over, they will return to their former state (Breen, 1975). For them pregnancy is not recognized as a developmental process. Those who consider pregnancy as a time of *development* regard it as a maturation process and recognize that change will lead to a reorganization of their personality. Breen (1975) concluded in her study that the women who best adjusted to pregnancy perceived themselves to be autonomous, in control and able to make their own decisions to deal with their problems.

Fundamental changes in relationships occur in pregnancy. Although normally long since independent of her own family, the pregnant woman usually discovers a need to re-establish close emotional ties with her parents. Family relationships and childhood events are re-appraised as the woman herself faces the prospect of motherhood. This may lead to unresolved conflicts in her own upbringing being re-awakened. The relationship between husband and wife changes from an intense, romantic affair to the complex relationship of parenthood with its new priorities and needs. For most women pregnancy involves giving up a job, even if only temporarily, and this results in a reduction in income and social contacts outside the home, thus the woman becomes more dependent on her partner. First-time parenthood is a demanding test of the couple's personal resources and maturity and of the strength of their relationship. In the majority of cases couples draw closer together and their relationship is strengthened. For a few couples, however, conflicts arise and the relationship deteriorates, often because of immaturity and sometimes because there are already problems, although they may not have been openly acknowledged.

All developmental crises require time for adjustment to the new role. During this time of transition, the individual feels some degree of emotional disturbance and turbulence. This is particularly true of a woman undergoing the process of childbearing. Like all those going through a developmental crisis, she needs much support from those around her at a time when she is particularly vulnerable to stress. It is essential for all midwives to be fully aware of the range of normal emotional changes which occur during pregnancy and the postnatal period. Only then can they sensitively meet the needs of expectant and postnatal mothers and be better able to recognize the few who develop signs and symptoms of mental illness.

Psychological Changes in Pregnancy

During pregnancy the woman's emotional state is different to that of her pre-pregnant condition. Women tend to become more 'neurotic' as pregnancy advances. This 'neurotic' state reaches a peak at about two weeks postnatally and gradually subsides to a normal level between 6 and 8 weeks after delivery (Breen, 1975). The baseline of normality is therefore altered. During this time the woman is more emotional than usual and more prone to anxiety and worry.

Attending the antenatal clinic may be the woman's first experience of hospital as a 'patient'. She may find the concept that pregnancy is a normal physiological event difficult to equate with being a hospital patient, since she associates such a role with ill-health (Prince and Adams, 1987). The emphasis of antenatal care tends to be on the physical aspects of pregnancy and feelings experienced by the woman having a baby are often neglected, although to her they may be of paramount importance and she becomes preoccupied with making sense of them (Breen, 1981). Many women feel that their needs and feelings are disregarded at antenatal clinics and that the emphasis is all on the care of the fetus. Early in pregnancy they may be advised to change their dietary habits, stop smoking and reduce alcohol intake, all for the benefit of the fetus. Although most women are anxious to do what is best for their baby, some may feel resentful if their own needs and feelings receive insufficient attention. Although this feeling may be experienced by all pregnant women, it may be exacerbated in those experiencing unfavourable environmental and social conditions, or those with inadequate emotional support from those around them. A careful history and assessment by the midwife in early pregnancy should elicit the woman's individual circumstances and psychological as well as physical needs. Midwifery care, including social and emotional support, can then be tailored to meet the woman's individual needs (Oakley, 1994; Clement, 1995).

EARLY PREGNANCY

The woman is now in a state of 'being pregnant'. Her mood is related to the delight or distress she feels at being pregnant, and is also affected by the common problems of fatigue, nausea and frequency of micturition which many women experience during these early weeks of pregnancy. The changes which are occurring in the woman's emotional state are often revealed by episodes of tearfulness and irritability at this time. For those women who have had a previous miscarriage, or if such problems arise in the present pregnancy, this may be a particularly anxious time. Such anxieties or complications lead to women feeling insecure about their pregnancies until they are well established. Hence they may refrain from telling other people and from making preparations for their baby until they are convinced that the pregnancy is going to continue.

The incidence of mental illness in the first trimester of pregnancy is as high as 15%, and for most of these women this will be their first episode of such illness. With the tiredness and discomforts of early pregnancy, it is often difficult to distinguish between normal emotional reactions and mental illness. Kumar and Robson (1978) found that 12% of women attending antenatal clinic were suffering from depression, and this figure was higher in those who had had a previous termination. Some women fear punishment for a variety of reasons, including previous terminations, and are very worried that such retribution may adversely affect the baby, causing it to die or be abnormal. These women need the opportunity to express their fears and require reassurance and support. Social support has been shown to have a beneficial effect for women with social and obstetric problems and may be offered, where possible (Hodnett, 1994a,b; Oakley, 1994).

Women may also experience other fears and fantasies throughout pregnancy, especially about what is going on inside their body. They often worry about normal physical and physiological changes and, if they are multigravidae, invariably compare the present pregnancy with their past experience. Many pregnant women also have vivid dreams which may be very disturbing. The dreams frequently involve the baby and may be interpreted by the mother as a premonition, often of something unpleasant.

SECOND TRIMESTER

During this phase of pregnancy the woman begins to 'expect a baby'. The recognition of fetal movements, her increasing abdominal growth and seeing her baby move around when she has a scan makes the developing baby a reality. Some women, however, find it difficult to believe that they are really carrying a baby right up to the time of its birth. For others it becomes a personalized being at this stage in pregnancy and many women name and talk to their fetus and are concerned about its well-being. All women are anxious and worried to a greater or lesser extent about the well-being of their developing fetus and have to rely on professionals to keep them informed of its progress. Some women find this loss of personal control difficult to accept, especially when attending a busy antenatal clinic where they may see many different doctors and midwives during the course of their pregnancy. This system gives them little opportunity to build up a relationship and develop confidence in the professionals caring for them, but with the implementation of the recommendations of the Department of Health's report called *Changing Childbirth*, which supports the concept of continuity of carer and named lead professional, this should change in the foreseeable future (DOH, 1993). With the midwife as lead professional, it should be possible for the mother and midwife to build up a relationship of trust where concerns and issues can be freely and openly discussed and the mother retains her autonomy, making well-informed choices and decisions related to her care. Instead of disempowering the mother, she retains the locus of control in pregnancy and childbirth, and this is extremely important to the mental and emotional health of the majority of women.

Some of the examinations and investigations carried out during the antenatal period can be uncomfortable and particularly stressful. It is essential that the woman and, where possible, her partner are given all necessary information about such examinations and tests to enable them to make an informed decision about whether or not they wish to have them performed. The mother who considers that termination of pregnancy is morally wrong may refuse tests to diagnose fetal abnormalities as she would wish to continue the pregnancy whatever the outcome. This is her right, thus her views should be respected and she should be supported in her decision. Others may be unsure about how to proceed should a fetal abnormality be diagnosed and may need considerable counselling with their doctor and midwife, and perhaps with a minister of religion. The woman who has a raised serum alphafetoprotein (AFP) and subsequently has amniocentesis may go through an agonizing period of waiting until the liquor AFP result is available. If the level is raised, the couple may suffer anguish whatever decision they make about their pregnancy. Even if the liquor AFP is normal, doubts about whether the baby is really normal or not may persist throughout pregnancy.

In general, women feel both physically and emotionally well during this stage of their pregnancy. In the event of any problems arising with their pregnancy, however, they easily feel guilty and upset and may attribute the problem to their lifestyle, behaviour or emotional state. Towards the end of the second trimester women tend to become increasingly emotional and are easily upset and moved to tears.

THIRD TRIMESTER

This is a crucial time for some women and their identity crisis may be accentuated when they have to give up their job and hence lose daily contact with friends and colleagues (Oakley, 1975). This may be the first time since early childhood that the woman has been free from schooling or a job. Although she may appreciate the rest and time to prepare for her baby, she may also feel lonely and isolated at home. A reduction in income may further reduce the couple's social life and independence.

Adjustment to new roles such as housewife, instead of career woman and mother, as well as wife, becomes more of a reality and it takes time before the woman is able to resolve the ensuing conflict by integrating these roles both in her thoughts and her behaviour. The woman also becomes preoccupied by her approaching labour and another source of role conflict at this time may be the medicalization of childbirth. On the one hand, the woman may have high hopes and expectations of childbirth as a momentous life experience under her control when she fulfils her role as a woman, yet the reality may be that it is managed by professionals like a medical condition which may well culminate in an obstetric operation. Such role conflict may lead to confusion, indecision and, in some cases, to depression (Kumar and Robson, 1978). Ball (1989) likens the loss of control felt by so many women during pregnancy and childbirth to that associated with the process of dying, because birth and death cannot be avoided, but must be accepted and coped with.

Changing body image can have a powerful effect on a woman and her partner in pregnancy. Some women enjoy their pregnant state until perhaps the latter weeks when they feel too heavy and cumbersome, whereas others feel unattractive and fear that they will no longer be appealing to their partner. Men, too, react in different ways, some finding the bodily changes of pregnancy attractive, while others do not find it appealing.

During this phase of pregnancy the woman's coping resources are diminished and most find it more difficult to manage major upheavals in life. Holmes and Rahe (1967) produced a list of 42 life events which people find particularly stressful and assigned a score to each one. Pregnancy has a score of 40 and a new family member 39. (The maximum score for one event is 100.) Many of the changes which women have to cope with in pregnancy and over which they have little or no control are included in the list, such as stopping work, changes in financial status, social activities and sleeping patterns. Additional events over which they do have some control, such as moving house, can be particularly stressful at this time. People vary in their ability to cope with stress. Lazarus (1966) describes the factors which influence the processes of coping and readjustment. These include factors which already exist such as personality and the individual's previous experience and confidence in their ability to cope and adjust. Other factors are the degree of stress experienced and the quality of support which is available. Although the midwife cannot change the mother's personality or her previous experience, she can make a careful assessment of the amount of stress the woman is under, assess her coping ability and offer a high level of support.

Stressful events in pregnancy are associated with the onset of preterm labour (Newton *et al.*, 1979). Psychosocial support for women in pregnancy, however, may reduce the incidence of this complication. During the last few weeks of pregnancy the series of antenatal classes usually finish and for some women this is a significant cause of stress, as they miss the peer support which has developed within the group. Encouragement by the midwife for members of the group to keep in touch and build up their own network of support can be helpful both for the latter stages of pregnancy and for the early months and, indeed, years of parenthood.

Anxieties and fears about the pregnancy begin to subside, however, especially if all seems to be progressing normally and the survival of the baby seems assured. Women now tend to become increasingly impatient with their pregnancy and long for the delivery of their baby.

Towards the end of pregnancy women slow down emotionally, although they remain easily moved to tears. They tend to withdraw socially and become increasingly absorbed in preparations for the baby. In the latter 2–4 weeks of pregnancy, concentration, short-term memory and new learning ability declines and this, together with daydreaming and an increasing preoccupation with the approaching birth, results in diminished intellectual ability. Women who work in intellectually demanding positions right up to term or who expect to pursue intellectual work soon after delivery, often find it considerably more difficult than anticipated.

Pregnancy and Libido

Sexual activity and enjoyment diminish markedly in pregnancy, especially during the first and third trimesters. In early pregnancy many couples are concerned about causing miscarriage, especially if there is a history of such problems. During the third trimester sexual activity tends to decrease, largely because it is physically uncomfortable. Most couples find other ways of expressing their loving relationship. Towards the end of pregnancy, however, there is often a sudden increase in libido (see Chapter 59).

Delivery

Women's perceptions and experiences of childbirth are so varied that it is difficult to consider all aspects. The woman's *experience* of having a baby is often neglected by professionals, the emphasis being placed on physical care and monitoring progress in order to detect any deviations from the normal which may require intervention. Safety, of course, is of paramount importance, but women also have high emotional expectations of this momentous event in their lives. When these expectations are fulfilled, and the woman can look back on her unique experience of childbirth with pride and a sense of achievement, her confidence and self-esteem are increased and she may be less likely to suffer from postnatal depression.

No matter how well prepared the woman is, the reality is usually something of a shock. The contractions are strange, uncomfortable and increasingly powerful. At a time when the expectant mother feels particularly vulnerable, she is usually in strange, often uncomfortable surroundings and may be attended by strangers. It may be the middle of the night and this adds to the sense of unreality. All women in such circumstances will be in a high state of arousal and it is very common for them to feel depersonalized, as if it were all happening to somebody else. There is a sense of loss of control because labour is a powerful and irrevocable process and there is no turning back (Ball, 1994). This can be frightening and a cause of panic in some women. In the transitional stage the woman has the alarming sensation of wanting to evacuate her bowels and bear down and this often produces a transient episode of panic and fear of losing control. For some women the actual moments of birth are thrilling, especially if they are well prepared and in control.

Immediate Post-Delivery Period

When the mother receives her baby into her arms immediately after delivery the commonest reaction is one of ecstasy and relief. The father is usually present and shares this joyful experience with his partner. There is a culture-constant pattern of behaviour at this time which starts with the mother greeting her baby and engaging in eye-to-eye contact with him. The baby is usually awake, alert and responsive during this time immediately after birth. Then the mother begins to explore her infant, peripherally first, then all over (Klaus and Kennell, 1970). Most mothers also talk to their baby during this time of exploration. The baby may then begin to indicate a desire to suck and the mother who wishes to breastfeed responds by suckling her child. The midwife should observe these clues and be available to give the mother assistance at this first feed so that she learns how to position her baby correctly on the breast, as this is the key to

successful breastfeeding. In Ball's study (1994) mothers who fed their babies within the first hour of delivery recalled more positive feelings at that time and the highest levels of satisfaction with motherhood six weeks later. A successful first feed also builds up the mother's confidence in her ability to breastfeed and she continues to feed for longer (Salariya et al., 1978). Mothers who do not wish to breastfeed should be offered the opportunity to bottlefeed their infant in response to his sucking movements.

The physical contact between the mother and baby during the first hour after birth has a beneficial effect on developing the maternal–child relationship. It has also been shown to have a positive influence on the mother's satisfaction with motherhood and her emotional well-being (Ball, 1994). It should be relaxed and unhurried and include the father too so that he can share with the mother in the joy of the birth and start getting to know his baby. Midwives therefore have the responsibility to ensure that all mothers have this enriching time of close contact with their baby during the hour after birth. Ball (1994) refers to it as the fourth stage of labour and stresses that it needs the same degree of attention and care as the other three stages.

Although it is an important and pleasurable time for mother–infant attachment, it is thought not to be absolutely crucial for human beings since the majority of mothers deprived of this early experience form good attachments to their babies at a later stage and develop close relationships with them (Ross, 1980; Svejda et al., 1980). Omission of this time, however, does have an adverse effect on the mother's satisfaction with the experience of motherhood and emotional fulfilment and this is still evident at six weeks after delivery. If this time of close contact after delivery has to be delayed because the mother is anaesthetized or ill, the midwife should ensure that the mother has the opportunity later to have a period of uninterrupted time with her baby, together with her partner. Sometimes it is not possible at birth because the baby is ill and is transferred to the neonatal unit, but the mother should always be given the opportunity to see and touch her baby, even if only briefly, and then have an uninterrupted time together with her partner so that they can share their distress and support each other. As soon as possible, usually at the time of transfer from the delivery suite to the postnatal ward, she should be taken to see her baby.

Sometimes conditions, such as birth asphyxia,

which require immediate treatment prevent the mother from holding her baby immediately after birth and she will be extremely distressed and anxious at her baby's failure to breathe at birth. Any concern for the baby, no matter how trivial, will be extremely alarming for the mother. Her perception of time will be altered so that attention to the baby lasting only a few seconds or minutes will seem like hours to her. The mother and her partner should be kept well informed about what is happening to their baby, reassured if appropriate and given the opportunity to see and hold their infant as soon as possible.

For a minority of women their immediate response to their babies is flat and unemotive. Some may be disappointed about the sex of their child. Others may feel real distaste, especially if the baby is very blood-stained or soiled with meconium. Sometimes an unfavourable response follows a distressing labour and delivery, or the mother may be too sedated to respond to the birth of her child. Most of these mothers gradually accept their baby during the next 24–48 hours. Only a small minority will have difficulty in establishing a relationship with their newborn child.

During the postnatal period many women have problems adapting to their new role. Adjustments also have to be made in family relationships to make room for the baby and this sometimes causes disharmony with siblings and/or the father. The demands of caring for a newborn baby far exceed most mothers' expectations. Disturbed nights lead to extreme tiredness and affect the mother's ability to cope with everyday situations. She feels guilty that she is an imperfect mother who is unable to cope and feels isolated in the home with her baby, often experiencing a loss of identity. A supportive and understanding partner and family, and the support of the midwife can do much to help the mother through the early weeks of motherhood. A network of support, usually built up during pregnancy, has proved to be very helpful to many women struggling to cope during the first few weeks after the birth of their baby.

Most mothers gradually adjust to their new role and resume an active and fulfilling life, but a significant number develop postnatal depression which, if not recognized and treated, can continue for many months and mar their enjoyment of the early months of motherhood (see Chapter 58).

References

Ball, J.A. (1989) Postnatal care and adjustment to motherhood. In *Midwives, Research and Childbirth*, pp. 154–175. London: Chapman & Hall.

Ball, J.A. (ed.) (1994) *Reactions to Motherhood*. Hale: Books for Midwives Press.

Breen, D. (1975) *Birth of a First Child*. London: Tavistock.

Breen, D. (1981) *Talking With Mothers*. London: Jill Norman.

Clement, S. (1995) Listening visits in pregnancy: a strategy for preventing postnatal depression? *Midwifery* 11: 75–80.

DOH (Department of Health) (1993) *Changing Childbirth*. Report of the Expert Maternity Group. London: HMSO.

Hodnett, E.D. (1994a) Support from caregivers during at-risk pregnancy. In Enkin, M.W., Keirse, M.J.N.C., Renfrew, M.J. *et al.* (eds) *Pregnancy and Childbirth Module, Cochrane Database of Systematic Reviews*. Review no. 04169. April, disk issue 1. Oxford: Update Software.

Hodnett, E.D. (1994b) Support from caregivers for socially disadvantaged women. In Enkin, M.W., Keirse, M.J.N.C., Renfrew, M.J. *et al.* (eds) *Pregnancy and Childbirth Module, Cochrane Database of Systematic Reviews*. Review no. 07674. April, disk issue 1. Oxford: Update Software.

Holmes, T.H. & Rahe, R.H. (1967) Social readjustment rating scale. *J. Psychosomatic Res.* 11: 219.

Klaus, M.H. & Kennell, J.H. (1970) Human maternal behaviour at first contact with her young. *Pediatrics* 46(2): 187–192.

Kumar, R. & Robson, K. (1978) Neurotic disturbance during pregnancy and the puerperium. In Sandler, M. (ed.) *Mental Illness in Pregnancy and the Puerperium*, pp. 40–51. Oxford: Oxford University Press.

Lazarus, R.S. (1966) Psychological stress and coping process. Quoted in Ball, J.A. (ed.) (1994) *Reactions to Motherhood*. Hale: Books for Midwives Press.

Newton, R.W., Webster, P.A.C., Binu, P.S., Naskrey, N. & Phillips, A.B. (1979) Psychosocial stress in pregnancy and its relation to the onset of premature labour *Br. Med. J.* 2: 411–413.

Oakley, A. (1975) The trap of medicalised motherhood. *New Society* 34(689): 639–664.

Oakley, A. (1994) Giving support in pregnancy: the role of research midwives in a randomised controlled trial. In Robinson, S. & Thomson, A.M. (eds) *Midwives, Research and Childbirth*, Vol. 3. London: Chapman & Hall.

Prince, J. & Adams, M.E. (1987) *Minds, Mothers and Midwives*. Edinburgh: Churchill Livingstone.

Ross, G.S. (1980) Parental responses to infants in intensive care; a separation issue re-evaluation. *Clin. Perinatol.* 7: 47–61.

Salariya, E.M., Easton, P.M. & Cater, J.L. (1978) Duration of breast feeding after early initiation and frequent feeding. *Lancet* ii: 1141–1143.

Svejda, M.J., Campos, J.J. & Emde, R.N. (1980) Mother-infant bonding: failure to generalise. *Child Develop.* 51: 775–779.

Further Reading

Argyle, M. (1978) *The Psychology of Interpersonal Behaviour*. Harmondsworth: Penguin.

Burnard, P. (1985) *Learning Human Skills*. London: Heinemann.

DeVries, R.G. (1989) Care givers in pregnancy and childbirth. In Chalmers, I., Enkin, M. & Keirse, M.J.N.C. (eds) *Effective Care in Pregnancy and Childbirth*. Oxford: Oxford University Press.

Egan, G. (1980) *The Skilled Helper*. Monterey, California: Brooks Cole.

Feher, L. (1980) *The Psychology of Childbirth*. London: Souvenir Press.

Lake, T. (1981) *Relationships*. London: Michael Joseph.

Laryea, M. (1989) Midwives and mothers perceptions of motherhood. In Robinson, S. & Thomson, A.M. (eds) *Midwives, Research and Childbirth*. London: Chapman & Hall.

Macfarlane, A. (1977) *The Psychology of Childbirth*. London: Fontana.

Rachel-Leff, J. (1992) *Psychological Processes of Childbearing*. London: Chapman & Hall.

Tschudin, V. (1982) *Counselling Skills for Nurses*. London: Baillière Tindall.

Weinmann, J. (1981) *An Outline of Psychology as Applied to Medicine*. Bristol: John Wright.

14

Communications and Counselling

Communications

The midwife's role could be said to be largely one of communication between herself and the mother. Communication is a two-way process involving all five senses – sight, sound, touch, taste and smell, although in midwifery it is the first three which are most commonly used.

One of the comments often made by new student midwives undertaking the shortened training programme, who are accustomed to the fast pace of physical work within their former nursing practice, is that midwives are not 'busy'. This is because they have not yet recognized that while midwives may not be physically busy carrying out 'nursing' tasks, they may be actively engaged in communicating with mothers – listening, discussing, questioning, advising, educating and, where necessary, counselling.

Communication is vital to the provision of both an effective and a satisfying experience for the mother and for the midwife. The advent of team midwifery and continuity of carer in 'Know your Midwife' and other schemes may have contributed to an improvement in communication (Flint, 1991), although conversely, heavy workloads and increased computerization to improve record-keeping, may reduce opportunities for interaction between mothers and midwives.

Expectant and newly delivered mothers clearly wish to receive as much information as possible, and for that information and advice to be offered in a comprehensive and comprehensible manner (Green, *et al.*, 1988). Read and Garcia (1989) found that women tend to be far less anxious and much more satisfied with their care if they receive adequate information, and they went on to make practical suggestions for improving communication. This desire for information and support is evident throughout the childbearing episode (Department of Health, 1993): antenatally (Porter and Macintyre, 1989); during hospital inpatient care (Kirkham, 1989), and postnatally in hospital and the community (Ball, 1994).

Although midwives may have relatively well-developed communications skills, factors relating to the management and organization of maternity care, such as time constraints and pressure of heavy workloads, coupled with staff shortages, may adversely affect their communication with women (Methven, 1989).

Communication consists of *verbal* and *non-verbal* elements, with the latter, especially facial expression and body position, having been shown to be often more significant than verbal interaction (Argyle *et al.*, 1970).

NON-VERBAL COMMUNICATION

Non-verbal communication includes all forms of communication except the spoken word:

▶ Facial expression, eye contact and head nodding.
▶ Gestures.
▶ Posture.
▶ Physical relationship to others.
▶ Touch.
▶ Physical appearance.
▶ Written records.

Facial expression

This is usually a most potent form of non-verbal communication, the eyes, brows and mouth being the most expressive parts of the face. Facial expressions are thought to be a combination of innate and socially learned behaviour (Knapp, 1978). However, facial expressions and speech do not always convey the same message and in these cases it is the expression rather than speech which is likely to be more convincing, especially with young people. The ability to recognize and interpret facial expressions is an essential skill for the midwife to acquire.

The midwife needs to be alert to discrepancies between what the mother says and what she actually means. For example, when conducting parent education classes which include relaxation periods, a mother may say she is comfortable in order not to delay the class or risk embarrassment by drawing attention to herself. However her facial expression (and body posture) may indicate that she is uncomfortable, and if the midwife identifies this she is then able to help the mother to achieve the best from her class. Suggestions for improving communication in antenatal classes have been made by Murphy Black and Faulkner (1988).

The midwife also has to use facial expressions appropriately. A smiling face (however fraught the midwife may feel) will go a long way towards making a mother feel welcome and special. On the other hand, a sympathetic expression will show the human, caring side of the midwife, rather than merely the professional but impersonal approach, when dealing with a family that is grieving.

Eye contact

Eye-to-eye contact is an important form of interaction between two people. Signals are received and feedback is given. People who are listening generally achieve more eye contact than those who are speaking. The speaker tends to look away from the listener when starting to speak but eye contact is established briefly at the end of a sentence and again for a longer period as that part of the conversation is completed. At these times feedback is sought and the listener receives the cue to respond. This pattern of eye contact helps the synchronization and flow of conversation. Longer periods of eye contact from the speaker tend to convey concern about the listener as a person, rather than with the subject of the conversation.

The midwife can use this knowledge to convey her care and concern to mothers at times of stress. It is often more potent than words. She also needs to acquire the skill to pick up cues, however indirect, and to respond to them. For example, during the booking history when the midwife is attempting to obtain a large amount of sensitive and intimate details about the mother, she may observe that the mother avoids eye contact. This may be due to embarrassment, or it may be because the mother is either omitting facts or not answering a question truthfully. There may be many reasons for this behaviour such as trying to conceal the fact of a previous termination of pregnancy, or that she has been abused.

In some cultures limited eye contact is the norm, and the midwife should be aware of and respect these cultural differences.

Head nodding

Head nodding is used to signify reinforcement and encouragement, and to indicate that the speaker should continue. Moving the head from side to side to denote 'no' has been related to the baby suckling at the breast. When the baby has had sufficient milk he moves his head from side to side to remove himself from the breast.

Gestures

Gestures are used to add emphasis to speech, relieve tension, for example by hand wringing, or to reveal other emotional states. These include shame when the hand is placed over the eyes, embarrassment when the hand covers the mouth, anxiety which is displayed by face touching, and aggression which is revealed by a clenched fist. The interpretation of these and other gestures often reveals far more than words.

Posture

Posture can also reveal the emotional state of a person. 'We speak with our vocal organs, but we converse with our whole body' (Abercrombie, 1969). Four main postures may be described – warm, cold, dominant and submissive. A posture which denotes *warmth* is attentive and the body leans forward, whereas one which conveys a *cold* attitude expresses withdrawal by drawing back or turning away. A *dominant* attitude is communicated by an expanded chest, a trunk which is upright or leaning back and head and shoulders held high. The *submissive* person has a dejected attitude, leans forward with bowed head and drooping shoulders and appears downcast and depressed. Anxiety can be seen in someone who is tense, stiff and upright.

Physical relationship to others

Orientation gives an indication of interpersonal attitudes. It refers to the position of the body and the angle at which one person interacts with another. It should be considered together with physical proximity since when direct face-to-face orientation occurs there is greater distance between people than with sideways orientation. For instance, it is preferable to sit at 90 degrees to the mother when taking a history or discussing aspects of care. A face-to-face position can be considered confrontational, especially when the barrier of a desk is present. If the midwife needs access to a computer she should attempt to keep the equipment as unobtrusive as possible so that the interaction takes place between the mother and midwife – and not between the mother and the computer!

When the midwife is higher than the mother, this gives a feeling of domination which is not conducive to a partnership in care. When seeing mothers in the antenatal clinic the mother should be invited to remain seated until it is necessary for her to lie on the couch to be examined. In the postnatal ward or at home the midwife should sit on a chair next to the mother when talking to her, or assisting with breastfeeding.

Personal space is important and may differ according to cultures – the British are renowned for 'keeping their distance' while the Italians frequently indulge in physical displays of affection. *Personal space* extends from about 45 cm to just over a metre, while one's *intimate space*, normally reserved only for those with whom there is a very close relationship, is less than 45 cm.

Much of the midwife's close contact with a mother may constitute an invasion of her intimate space, but the majority of our physical touch has become functional and impersonal. This may be a subconscious strategy on the part of the midwife to overcome both her own and the mother's embarrassment; it may have evolved in response to ever-increasing workloads; or it may be a means of maintaining 'professional' distance.

Touch

Midwives must be sensitive to the needs of women and learn to use touch appropriately. Sometimes, simply reaching for a mother's hand or putting an arm around her shoulders can be more effective than any spoken word. Massage and other complementary therapies are increasingly being used in an attempt to return to the nurturing so necessary to pregnant and newly delivered women at this vulnerable time of their lives.

However, it must be acknowledged that not all women wish to be touched, especially in labour. Midwives will observe women who need 'mothering' with constant physical and emotional attention, whereas others would choose to retreat into an isolated corner to labour and deliver, in much the same way that many animals do. People often treat pregnant women as objects of public property, invading their intimate space to pat their abdomens. Midwives should recognize that many women dislike this and should not develop the habit as part of their repertoire of professional gestures.

Touch is also open to various interpretations and midwives will need to use it with sensitivity. Male midwives will need to exercise exceptional discretion in the ways in which they use touch, for it would be easy for either a mother or her partner to misinterpret a gesture of kindness.

Physical appearance

Physical appearance conveys much information to others. Before even talking to an individual we are beginning to make judgements on the basis of physical appearance. As soon as the mother and the midwife meet, each will be assessing the other from the information available to them at this early stage, although it must be remembered that it is easy to make assumptions. This initial assessment will be made not only on what the person is wearing, but also on the posture, facial expression, orientation and gestures.

Women in the antenatal clinic should be respected as people and not treated as objects in which clothes are irrelevant. Fortunately, the practice of routinely asking women to change into gowns has been largely discontinued. It is good practice to uncover only those parts of the mother's body which are required to be examined. In the maternity unit mothers should be encouraged to dress in their own day wear to avoid the loss of expression, identity and status which comes from wearing night attire.

The move towards midwives abandoning uniform and wearing mufti has brought its own benefits and disadvantages. Midwives may seem more approachable to mothers and are perhaps viewed less as nurses; the hierarchical system associated with wearing uniforms is diluted; confidentiality can be maintained when visiting mothers at home. On the other hand the signals obtained from the clothes worn by the midwife must be clear – she should be clean and tidily dressed in clothes which are considered by convention to be smart. Managers may need to specify types of clothing which are not allowed to be worn, such as jeans and trainers, or leggings and tee shirts. Name badges are mandatory with clear, easily readable printing on them.

The midwife will also be able to assess, in part, the mother's physical and emotional well-being from observing her appearance and demeanour. The mother may look anxious or worried, and the midwife should explore this sensitively. A pale, tired-looking mother could be anaemic, suffering hyperemesis gravidarum, or be 'worn down' by a large family or a demanding job. The midwife should be alert to the underlying messages obtained from a mother's appearance. For example, a woman who is overly cheerful, jovial or perhaps aggressive, may be trying to hide extreme nervousness.

Written communication

Communication may be in the form of the written word, which can be either handwritten or, increasingly these days, via computerized records.

It is essential that all written communications are legible, including signatures, not only to promote effective client care, but also because of the number of legal cases which abound. Professional records must be comprehensive and completed as contemporaneously as possible. Any written information given to mothers must be comprehensible using plain language; it may be necessary to provide leaflets and other information in several languages depending on the local clientele.

Computerized records may offer a means of recording the main medical and obstetric details but can inhibit the documentation of social and psychological information: midwives must ensure that their records are not limited by the format of the computer program, or indeed, the format of the medical records.

VERBAL COMMUNICATION

The essence of good communication is to consider each person as an individual. *Culture*, *education* and *social class* are some of the factors which affect the use of language and should be considered when making an assessment of each mother. Bernstein (1971, 1972) suggested that working-class people have a more restricted language than those in the middle class. They have a more limited vocabulary, rarely use adjectives, and usually construct short, simple sentences. These restrictions may inhibit communications; especially in an unfamiliar environment. More time and encouragement may be required to promote effective communications and the midwife must listen carefully to pick up cues and respond appropriately. She should give frequent simple, clear explanations in terms which can be easily understood. Abbreviations and the use of jargon should be avoided as they may lead to confusion. It is also important to remember that intonation has a marked effect on meaning and that changes in pitch and emphasis help to clarify the spoken word.

There are many families in the UK now for whom English is not their first language. Hayes (1991) found that non-English speaking women are often given less information than other women, and this prevents them from making informed decisions about their care. This greatly increases the problems of communications and the midwife should know how to obtain suitable help. Sometimes there is a member of the family who can interpret; otherwise a member of staff or a volunteer may be available to help. Explanatory and health education leaflets in various languages are now published by some organizations and local groups and these can help to give information. Mothers who speak little or no English can feel very lost and isolated, especially in hospital, and staff need to make a special effort to communicate their care and empathy non-verbally as well as verbally.

LISTENING

Listening attentively is an active rather than a passive skill and needs considerable effort and practice to acquire and use effectively. A good listener holds their total concentration on the speaker so that she feels valued as an individual and not just another person. All distractions must be blocked out to allow good listening to continue and be effective.

A relaxed, attentive attitude and encouragement in the form of a nod or smile will encourage the speaker to continue. Meanwhile the listener carefully notes the non-verbal cues. Do they support the spoken word? Does the speaker appear anxious or is she relaxed and at ease? What does the speaker's appearance tell you about her? Does she look well? Is she clean and well cared for or does she appear ill or unkempt with poor hygiene?

Even when the midwife cannot see the mother, she may be able to detect cues in the mother's non-verbal communications. For example, sometimes the midwife can recognize the onset of the second stage of labour simply by listening to the altered sounds of a mother's breathing in a labour room (McKay and Roberts, 1990).

Attentive listening and the close observation which is part of it enables the midwife to assess the woman carefully and identify her real needs and requirements. Care can then be tailored to meet the specific needs of that individual. Only then can the mother receive the highest quality of midwifery care possible.

QUESTIONING TECHNIQUES

Skilled questioning techniques are essential for good communications. Questions may be asked in a variety of ways and midwives should know how to select the appropriate type of question since this will greatly influence the information obtained in response.

Types of questions

Closed questions Closed questions restrict the reply to a yes or no answer or to a limited factual reply. Most people find them easy to answer but they give the interviewer a high degree of control, hence the respondent has limited freedom to participate fully in the interaction. Examples of closed questions are:

Midwife: What was the date of the first day of your last normal menstrual period?
Expectant mother: 5th July 1995

or

Midwife: Do you want to breastfeed?
Expectant mother: No.

The first example illustrates the appropriate use of closed questions. They can also be used to check information such as name or address and to elicit other suitable factual information. A closed question is not appropriate in the second example, however, as the mother has not been given the opportunity to express her feelings about breastfeeding. This is an example of the misuse of closed questions and how they discourage communication.

Open questions Open questions give the respondent the opportunity to answer in a number of ways, allowing a greater degree of freedom. They encourage respondents to express their thoughts and feelings, opinions and attitudes. Mothers who are questioned in this way are more likely to voice their anxieties, reveal problems and seek information. The midwife therefore obtains greater insight into the woman as an individual and can plan care tailored to meet her specific needs. An example of an open question is as follows:

Midwife: How do you feel about breastfeeding your baby?
Mother: Well, I know it is best for the baby and I should like to give it a try, but my husband is not very keen on the idea.

This answer gives the midwife considerable information about the couple's attitude to breastfeeding. Other openings for open questions are:

Tell me about . . .
What do you . . .
How are you . . .

Leading questions Leading questions are questions which are worded in such a way that they lead the respondent towards an expected response. They can therefore elicit misleading and incorrect information. Examples of leading questions are:

The pain is better now, isn't it?

or

You slept well, didn't you?

In both examples open questions, as illustrated below, would normally be more appropriate:

How is the pain now?

and

How did you sleep?

Probing questions Probing questions are questions which encourage the respondent to expand on the information already given. They can be used for a variety of reasons, for instance to obtain more detailed information, clarify meaning or justify an earlier response. An example of a probing question to clarify meaning is:

Are you saying that your baby is sleeping more now?

Reflection or mirroring

Reflecting or mirroring is a technique whereby the interviewer picks up significant words or feelings expressed by the interviewee and repeats them back in such a way that the interviewee enlarges upon them. For example, a mother might say, 'I feel so inadequate,' and the midwife could reply, 'You feel inadequate?' This usually effectively encourages the mother to continue talking.

There are two integral parts to reflecting: *paraphrasing* and *reflection of feeling*. Paraphrasing is chiefly concerned with mirroring back the factual content of information received, whereas reflection of feeling focuses on the affective aspects. Reflection of feeling requires considerable skill since the interviewer has to identify accurately and put a name to the feelings expressed by the interviewee. Sometimes feelings are clearly stated by the interviewee, but often they are only implied or are inferred from non-verbal and other cues.

Cues

Cues are oblique references to situations, often anxieties, which may be revealed in hints or questions, or non-verbally. It is important that midwives learn to recognize cues and respond appropriately to them. Repeated cues usually indicate that the mother is asking for a response, but for some reason cannot broach the subject openly. Encouraging skills include attentive listening and picking up cues followed by appropriate responding skills. These include suitable questioning techniques, reflection and other forms of encouragement which prompt the person to feel comfortable and continue talking.

Counselling

Counselling has been described by Bond (1993) as 'a method of relating and responding to other people with the aim of providing them with opportunities to explore, to clarify and to work towards living in a more satisfying and resourceful way.' Often the midwife's work involves offering advice, information and guidance to mothers and their families. This is called *directive counselling*, although care must be taken that it does not become prescriptive and authoritative. Whenever possible the midwife should help the mother to make her own decisions, with the midwife being facilitative rather than offering solutions – this is *non-directive counselling* (Burnard, 1992).

Midwifery practice involves a combination of both directive and non-directive counselling, using all the communication skills discussed previously. Therapeutic counselling, however, requires specialized training and application, and it would not be practical or appropriate for all midwives to be fully trained counsellors; rather it is an area which some midwives choose to develop as their speciality within the profession, with some trusts employing midwife–counsellors who can concentrate on those families with specific needs such as those affected by bereavement or fetal abnormality (Lawrence, 1994).

Mack (1995) suggests that midwives can learn to offer a 'counselling approach' in their practice, in which focused and purposeful discussion is facilitated with mothers when necessary.

QUALITIES OF A COUNSELLOR

To be able to offer counselling help to others the midwife must have some insight into her own personality and needs. She should be relaxed and approachable, develop a genuine empathy with those who need help and learn to accept them as they are. Then a good relationship is likely to develop between the client and the midwife as counsellor which is essential if worthwhile interaction is to take place between them.

Many qualities are desirable in a good counsellor but the three which Rogers (1983) considers most important are:

Empathy
Acceptance
Genuineness

Empathy

Rogers defines empathy as the 'capacity to gain entry into the experience of another person, and to be able to see the world as it were through their eyes, and to communicate this understanding to him.' Great gentleness, sensitivity and skill are required to be able to empathize with another person. At intervals during the counselling process the counsellor shares her perception of the client with the client to check out the accuracy of her interpretation.

Acceptance

In counselling it is important to accept the client just as she is. The client who feels secure in the knowledge that she is meeting with understanding and acceptance is more likely to talk freely and openly about her situation and difficulties. Acceptance of the individual as she is may also be called non-possessive warmth or unconditional positive regard.

Genuineness

Genuine interest in the client is an essential component of the counselling relationship. A client will soon sense any lack of genuine interest and respond in a negative manner. The counsellor must also be true to her own values and beliefs, although she will not attempt to impose them on her client. Part of the acceptance discussed earlier is not only the ability to accept the client as she is, but also to respect her right to follow her own conscience (Nurse, 1975).

The midwife needs to recognize her own limitations as well as those situations with which it may be inappropriate to deal, for example if the midwife has recently suffered a similar experience to that of the mother (Saunders, 1994).

A 'therapeutic distance' needs to be maintained to avoid the midwife becoming too emotionally involved with the mother, but not so great as to interfere with the relationship that has been developed. The midwife should not offer solutions nor should she endeavour to seek reasons for or interpret the meaning of the individual's problem.

A MODEL OF COUNSELLING

There are many approaches to the helping process but only one (Egan, 1982) will be described here. It is a general model, which can be used in a variety of interpersonal situations, including counselling.

Egan uses a skills approach and describes three stages:

▶ Identification and clarification.
▶ Goal-setting.
▶ Action.

Identification and clarification   This is the first stage in counselling when the counsellor assists the client to explore the situation and express her feelings. A good rapport is established and the counsellor listens actively and responds with respect and empathy.

Acting as facilitator the counsellor enables the client to understand and accept her own part in the situation. In some circumstances an understanding of the problem may be sufficient to allow the client to cope with it. The counsellor uses appropriate responding skills during the interview to facilitate understanding.

Goal-setting and action   The way forward is planned by the client. Goals are set and methods of achieving them are formulated. Goals should be achievable and may be progressive. Progress is then evaluated at subsequent interviews.

Helping skills

Egan (1982) suggests that there are three essential skills for the helping process:

▶ Attending.
▶ Listening.
▶ Responding.

Attending   This is the pre-helping stage when the counsellor focuses on the client and becomes totally involved in working with her.

Listening   Listening has already been discussed but the importance of active listening cannot be overemphasized. Whilst the client is talking the midwife must be able to focus her whole attention on her and listen to and hear what she is saying. There may be an underlying meaning which becomes apparent only when the counsellor really listens and analyses what is being said. It is often very tempting for the midwife to interrupt and recount her own experiences, or to make judgements and give advice, but such interruptions must be resisted. Instead she should concentrate on enabling the client to help herself by talking through her problem and coming to the right decision. In cases of bereavement or the birth of a malformed child, skilled counselling helps the couple to come to terms with their situation.

Responding skills These are many and varied and the counsellor must select the response most appropriate to the situation. Examples of some of the possible responses are:

▶ *Questioning*, using open rather than closed questions, and sometimes probing questions.
▶ *Exploratory*, e.g. 'Can you enlarge on that?'
▶ *Empathic*, e.g. 'It seems as if you feel . . .'
▶ *Clarifying*, e.g. 'Do you mean . . . ?'
▶ *Interpreting*, e.g. 'Are you really saying . . . ?'
▶ *Making concrete*, concentrating on concrete situations, feelings, actions.
▶ *Confronting*, challenging discrepancies.
▶ *Reflective*, repeating statements in a reflective way.
▶ *Supportive*, encouraging, reassuring.

▶ *Silence*, allowed to continue for a while: periods of silence in a relaxed, trusting atmosphere can be very beneficial and productive.

When offering clients the opportunity to talk over their situation or difficulties, it is important not to allow them to become too dependent on the counsellor. The art of counselling is rather to enable the client to find her own solution and thus become more independent.

In the long term the client who has been through an experience which led to the need for counselling usually has a better insight into herself and others. This enables her to develop her own potential more fully and thus, should a similar situation recur, she should find that she is able to cope without further help.

Occasionally the midwife will perceive that her client requires more skilled help than she is able to provide and then referral to an appropriate expert is necessary.

Further information about counselling can be obtained from the British Association for Counselling, 1 Regent Place, Rugby, CV21 2PJ, UK.

References

Abercrombie, M.L.J. (1969) *The Anatomy of Judgement*. Harmondsworth: Penguin.

Argyle, M., Salter, V., Nicholson, H., Williams, M. & Burgess, P. (1970) The communication of inferior and superior attitudes by verbal and non-verbal signals. *Br. J. Soc. Clin. Psychol.* **9**: 222–231.

Ball, J. (1994) *Reactions to Motherhood*. Hale: Books for Midwives Press.

Bernstein, B. (1971, 1972) *Class Codes and Control*, Vols 1 & 2. London: Routledge & Kegan Paul.

Bond, T. (1993) *Standards and Ethics for Counselling in Action*. London: Sage Publications.

Burnard, P. (1992) *Effective Communication for Health Professionals*. London: Chapman & Hall.

Department of Health (1993) *Changing Childbirth*. Report of the Expert Maternity Group. London: HMSO.

Egan, G. (1982) *The Skilled Helper*. Belmont, California: Wadsworth.

Flint, C. (1991) Continuity of care provided by a team of midwives – the Know Your Midwife Scheme. In Robinson, S. & Thomson, A.M. (eds) *Midwives, Research and Childbirth*, Vol. 2. London: Chapman & Hall.

Green, J.M., Coupland, V.A. & Kitzinger, J.V. (1988) *Great Expectations: A Prospective Study of Women's Expectations and Experiences of Childbirth*. Cambridge: Child Care and Development Group, University of Cambridge.

Hayes, L. (1991) Communications in the maternity services. *Maternity Action* **50**: 6–7.

Kirkham, M. (1989) Midwives and information-giving during labour. In Robinson, S. & Thomson, A.M. (eds) *Midwives, Research and Childbirth*, Vol. 1, pp. 117–138. London: Chapman & Hall.

Knapp, M.L. (1978) *Nonverbal Communication in Human Interaction*. New York: Holt, Rinehart & Winston.

Lawrence, S. (1994) Prenatal grief. *MIDIRS Midwifery Digest* **4**(4): 415–417.

Mack, S. (1995) Complementary therapies for the relief of stress. In Tiran, D. & Mack, S. (eds) *Complementary Therapies for Pregnancy and Childbirth*. London: Baillière Tindall.

McKay, S. & Roberts, J. (1990) Obstetrics by ear: maternal and caregiver perceptions of the meaning of maternal sounds during second stage labour. *J Nurse Midwif.* **35**: 266–273.

Methven, R. (1989) Recording an obstetric history or relating to a pregnant woman? A study of the antenatal booking interview. In Robinson, S. & Thomson, A.M. (eds) *Midwives, Research and Childbirth*, Vol. 1, pp. 42–71. London: Chapman & Hall.

Murphy Black, T. & Faulkner, A. (1988) *Antenatal Group Skills Training: A Manual of Guidelines*. Chichester: John Wiley & Sons.

Nurse, G. (1975) *Counselling and the Nurse*. Aylesbury: HM & M.

Porter, M. & Macintyre, S. (1989) Psychosocial effectiveness of antenatal and postnatal care. In Robinson, S. & Thomson, A.M. (eds) *Midwives, Research and Childbirth*, Vol. 1, pp. 72–94. London: Chapman & Hall.

Read, M. & Garcia, J. (1989) Women's views of care during pregnancy and childbirth. In Enkin, M.W., Keirse, M.J.N.C. & Chalmers, I. (eds) *Effective Care in Pregnancy and Childbirth*, pp. 131–142. Oxford: Oxford University Press.

Rogers, C.R. (1983) *On Becoming a Person*. Boston, Mass.: Houghton Mifflin.

Saunders, P. (1994) *First Steps in Counselling*. Manchester: PCCS Books.

Part Six

Midwifery Care Before and During Pregnancy

15

Preconception Care

Preconception care is aimed at ensuring that prospective parents are in optimum health at the time of conception. Wise advice given to such couples may well enhance fetal growth and avoid fetal abnormality, which are the two main concerns regarding the outcome of any pregnancy. Health education and preconception advice and care should commence during school days. Healthy living should then become a way of life, ensuring that each person's optimum health is achieved.

Nutrition

Diet may be one of the factors in early, even intrauterine life which has an influence on health in adult life. The importance of an adequate diet at the time of conception and during pregnancy becomes clear when it is realized that the nutritional state of the mother can affect the health of her children in their adult lives, and even that of their children.

The maintenance of a normal pregnancy requires energy. The apparent extra energy requirement is about 70 000 kcal (298 MJ). Seldom, however, is this matched by an equivalent increase in food intake; evidence shows that an average increase in intake of energy of less than 0.42 MJ/day (100 kcal/day) occurs in the third trimester and virtually no change before then (COMA Report, 1991). Hytten (1990) suggests that the addition of 200 kcal daily to the usual non-pregnant diet is an appropriate amount. The average healthy, well-nourished woman probably has little need of an increase in her energy intake preconception, but the thin or poorly nourished woman needs supplementation.

Calculation of weight in relation to height is an important part of investigative care which is given in the preconception clinic. The average weight for height can be assessed by using the generally accepted, although imperfect, Body Mass Index (BMI). This is calculated using the formula:

$$BMI = \frac{weight\ (kg)}{height\ (m)^2}$$

A BMI of between 20 and 25 is considered to be within the normal range; under 20 indicates underweight and over 30 is recognized as obesity (Morgan, 1994).

Grossly *underweight* women, such as those with anorexia nervosa, are usually infertile (menstruation usually recommences when the body weight reaches 47 kg (Sutherland and Smith, 1990)). Women with a BMI under 20 have a higher frequency of intrauterine growth retardation (Rosso, 1985). The aim, ideally, should be for weight gain before the onset of pregnancy. In times of famine babies are born with much lower birthweights than normal. This can be seen in the parts of the world where there has been famine, often accentuated by wars, such as Ethiopia and South East Africa, and also occurs episodically in countries where food energy availability is marginal, as in West Africa. Retrospective research carried out in Holland on the Dutch Hunger Winter of 1944–45 showed that famine, particularly in the last trimester of pregnancy, resulted in low birthweight and early perinatal mortality (Stein *et al.*, 1975).

Obesity has undoubted associations with obstetric complications, such as hypertension, diabetes and the need for a Caesarean section. Attempts should therefore be made to correct overweight before pregnancy. Dieting should not be undertaken during pregnancy. In the first trimester it may lead to lack of essential micronutrients for the forming fetus, which during the period of organogenesis may lead to fetal malformation; and during the last trimester it may cause intrauterine growth retardation.

Diets which may be advised for overweight women can be similar to those which any woman, and indeed her family, should be consuming. Diets which are low in fat are recommended as healthier than those which contain high fat levels (COMA Report, 1991; Doyle, 1992). Fat provides more calories per gram than other dietary constituents which increases the energy density of the diet. Low-fat diets tend to be bulkier than high-fat diets and give the feeling of being full up with a smaller intake.

Food should be chosen from the *four main food groups*. If women are advised before pregnancy to eat something from each of these groups every day they will develop healthy eating habits for themselves and their families, by providing their fetuses with the best possible nutrition at the crucial time of organogenesis and have less likelihood of producing low birthweight babies. The four main food groups are:

▶ Bread, cereals and potatoes, 4–5 portions daily.
▶ Fruit and vegetables, 4–5 portions daily.
▶ Meat, fish and alternatives, 2 portions daily.
▶ Milk, cheese and yoghurt, 3 portions daily (Doyle 1992).

Foods such as biscuits, sweets, cakes, crisps, pastry and soft drinks tend to be high in fat and sugar and should be eaten only in moderation.

In a study undertaken at the Salvation Army Hospital in Hackney, London, in the late 1970s, just under 200 mothers kept diaries of everything they ate and drank for one week in each trimester. The main findings of the study were that there were serious nutrient deficits in the diets of many pregnant women living in that inner city area, and that these deficits were greatest in those mothers who had low birthweight babies (less than 2500 g) (Doyle, 1992). The strongest correlation between nutrient intake and birthweight was during the first trimester, which again indicates that adaptation of diet should take place *before* pregnancy. The major differences between the diets of the two groups of women (those producing babies of optimum birthweight (3500–4500 g) and those producing low birthweight babies) were that the optimum birthweight mothers ate substantially more cereals, muesli, oats, nuts, seeds, wholemeal bread, egg and egg dishes, dairy produce, fruit and vegetables. Their overall intake was also significantly higher (Wynn and Wynn, 1991). Doyle (1992) states that the assumption can be made that the mothers of optimum birthweight babies were more likely to have three meals a day, including breakfast, and as most breakfast cereals are fortified with vitamins and minerals, this gave them an overall much healthier diet. The BMI of these women was 23.7 kg/m^2 (Wynn and Wynn, 1991).

The COMA Report (1991) advises that for the whole population of the UK a maximum of 35% of food energy should be obtained from fat and 50% from carbohydrate in daily total energy intakes. This is also good advice to give preconception as recommended in the fourth report from the DOH Health Committee on Preconception Care (1992a). Protein intakes average 15% of total energy (COMA, 1991), and Hytten (1990) advises that, for the average European woman eating a normal diet, the extra dietary protein requirement in pregnancy is about 8.5 g per day.

When giving specific advice to women about what to eat and what not to eat it is well to remember that most people, unless highly motivated, are not prepared to make radical changes in their eating habits, and some underweight women will have poor appetites. For these latter women, vitamin and mineral supplementation may be required. Routine supplementation with iron and vitamins, however, is unnecessary (Montgomery, 1994). Particular care should be taken to avoid vitamin A supplementation in pregnancy (DHSS, 1990). Women who are anxious and feel a particular responsibility about what they eat and its consequent effects on their fetuses may appreciate being referred to the organization known as Foresight, the Association for the Promotion of Preconceptual Care, as this organization puts particular emphasis on nutrient intake (Barnes and Bradley, 1992).

See Chapter 16 for more information on maternal nutrition.

FOLIC ACID

Folic acid is one of the vitamins in the B group and is the parent molecule for a large number of derivatives known collectively as folates. They are involved in a large number of single-carbon transfer reactions.

Since the early 1960s it has been recognized that a woman's folate status might affect her risk of having a baby with a neural tube defect. The evidence was, however, inconclusive until the results of a Medical Research Council (MRC) study commenced in 1983, were known. A randomized, double-blind prevention trial with a factorial design was conducted at 33 centres in seven countries (including the UK) to determine whether supplementation with folic acid, or a mixture of seven other vitamins, around the time of conception can prevent neural tube defects (anencephaly, spina bifida, encephalocele). Over 1800 women who were at high risk of having a pregnancy with a neural tube defect, because of a previously affected pregnancy, were involved in the trial. The results suggested that

folic acid offered a protective effect of 72% (relative risk 0.28, 95% confidence interval 0.12–0.71). The researchers concluded that folic acid supplementation starting before pregnancy can be firmly recommended for all women who have had an affected pregnancy (MRC, 1991).

In 1992 an Expert Advisory Group which had been set up by the Department of Health to consider the relationship of folic acid to neural tube defects made the following recommendations:

1   For the prevention of recurrence of neural tube defect women should take folic acid supplements of 4 mg prior to, and until, the 12th week of pregnancy.
2   For the prevention of a first occurrence of neural tube defect women should have extra folate in their diets by eating more folate-rich foods, which include green leaf vegetables, black eye beans, parsnips, kidneys, yeast and beef extracts and take 0.4 mg folic acid from the time a pregnancy is planned until 12 weeks gestation (DOH Expert Advisory Group Report, 1992).

The exceptions to these recommendations are women with epilepsy as folic acid supplements may adversely affect their treatment.

Wald and Bower (1995) recommend that food such as flour should be fortified with folic acid to ensure all women have extra folate.

Infections

Any maternal infection may adversely affect the fetoplacental unit. During preconception care any residual infection should be treated and advice given about avoiding infection as far as possible during the periconceptual period. Common infections such as urinary or genital infection may cause preterm labour and influenza can lead to miscarriage (Wynn and Wynn, 1991). Gastrointestinal infections can usually be avoided by good hygiene and by cooking poultry and meat well.

LISTERIOSIS

Listeriosis is caused by a Gram-positive cocco bacillus, *Listeria monocytogenes*, which is widely distributed in the environment. It can be found in the soil, in water and in vegetation, as well as in some foods, so some exposure to the bacterium is inevitable. Unlike most bacteria that can cause food-related illness, *Listeria monocytogenes* has the unusual property of being able to multiply at temperatures which may be found in refrigerators (6°C or above). In most foods where it is present as a contaminant, it is in very low bacterial counts and is killed by adequate cooking. In some soft, ripened cheeses, however, the method of preparation may allow *Listeria* to multiply.

Although listeriosis is a rare disease, and presents in most cases as a non-specific flu-like febrile illness, it can have dire effects during pregnancy. Miscarriages, stillbirths and neonatal deaths, caused by septicaemia, have been reported as associated with listeriosis. On the basis of these reported cases the rate of miscarriage and stillbirth related to listeriosis in pregnancy is one in 7000 conceptions (Chief Medical Officer, 1989). Advice should therefore be given to women both planning a pregnancy and pregnant, to avoid eating soft, ripened cheeses such as Brie, Camembert and blue vein types. Hard cheeses such as Cheddar or Cheshire are considered safe. *Listeria* has also been found in cook-chilled meals and ready-to-eat poultry, so the advice given for these foods is to reheat them until they are piping hot rather than eat them cold (Chief Medical Officer, 1989). A survey carried out in England and Wales in 1989 showed that pâté frequently contained *Listeria* (McLauchlin *et al.*, 1991). Women should also be advised, therefore, not to eat pâté or liver sausage. As the *Listeria* bacterium is so widespread, it may contaminate salad and other foods, so women should be reminded to take general hygiene precautions when handling food.

TOXOPLASMOSIS

Toxoplasmosis is caused by a parasite, an obligate intracellular protozoan, called *Toxoplasma candii*. It causes symptoms similar to influenza. Members of the cat family are the definitive host for sexual reproduction of the parasite. Infection may occur by ingestion of raw or undercooked meat, particularly lamb or pork, or by contact with cat faeces which contain sporulated oocysts.

The rate of infection in pregnant women is 2 per 1000 (Joynson and Payne, 1988). Infection may cross the placenta and the effect on the fetus appears to depend on gestational age. If infected in early fetal life, miscarriage or stillbirth may occur. Other congenital manifestations may be hydrocephalus,

microcephaly, brain lesions, jaundice, fever, anaemia, pneumonia or chorioretinitis. About 40% of babies of infected mothers who are untreated will be congenitally infected (Pope, 1992) although only about 10% will be seriously affected (Thompson, 1993).

Treatment of acute maternal infection, or indeed of a woman infected periconceptually, may be given as a prophylactic measure to reduce the incidence of placental transfer and subsequent congenital infection (Holliman, 1992).

Women planning a pregnancy should be advised not to empty cat litter trays unless they have to, in which case they should wear gloves, always to well-cook meat, especially lamb and pork, and to observe basic hygiene rules after handling raw meat, to wash fruit and vegetables thoroughly and to wear gloves when gardening.

CHLAMYDIA PSITTACI

The organism *Chlamydia psittaci* causes the condition of enzootic abortion in ewes, and if the infection is transmitted to a pregnant woman its effects can be severe or even fatal.

Chlamydia psittaci must be differentiated from *Chlamydia trachomatis*. This latter is a common sexually transmitted disease which can lead to infertility in women, but causes only minor symptoms.

Parry (1990) gives the signs and symptoms, and outcome for six women (one of whom was a vet) who became infected with *Chlamydia psittaci*, and in all cases the condition proved fatal to the baby, and in one case the mother too.

Advice should be given, therefore, preconception to all women who may have contact with sheep not to have any contact during lambing or even during a ewe's pregnancy. The advice should also include the avoidance of any contact with orphan or weak lambs especially, with postnatal sheep, and with clothing that has been worn during lambing (Parry, 1990).

RUBELLA

Rubella is typically a mild viral childhood illness, but maternal infection occurring in early pregnancy can lead to abortion or stillbirth, low birthweight, deafness, cataracts, jaundice, purpura, hepatosplenomegaly, congenital heart disease and mental retardation (Enkin *et al.*, 1989).

In the UK, girls and boys aged 10–14 years are routinely given the rubella vaccination. The object of this is to reduce the incidence of the disease and prevent fetal infection and the congenital rubella syndrome. In a preconception clinic, screening to test for rubella antibodies should be undertaken and the women should be immunized if necessary. Women should be advised not to become pregnant for at least three months following immunization.

HUMAN IMMUNODEFICIENCY VIRUS (HIV)

The first reported case of acquired immunodeficiency syndrome (AIDS) in the UK was in 1981 (Dixon, 1987). Since that time there has been a marked increase in the number of HIV infections reported, which has included women during pregnancy and neonates. The fear that this virus has generated is caused mainly by its unpredictability and the fact that it may eventually lead to illness and death because there is no known cure.

The virus enters the bloodstream through

▶ sexual contact;
▶ blood-to-blood spread, as in intravenous drug abusers and sharing of needles;
▶ from mother to fetus;
▶ during delivery of the baby from secretions around the cervix and vagina; and
▶ through breast milk (Sutherland and Smith, 1990).

It may be months before the virus causes its first illness, which is usually an influenza-type illness, and only at this stage does the body produce antibodies. These antibodies do not, however, have any effect on the virus. A blood test will probably be positive at this point as it will show up the antibodies. The individual will usually recover fully from this first illness but has a substantial risk of developing further problems which may lead to death in the ensuing 10–15 years as the immune system breaks down (Dixon, 1987).

At a preconception clinic women who are at risk are those who are intravenous drug abusers and those who have had unprotected sexual intercourse with a sero-positive partner, who could be bisexual, a man with Central African connections, or a drug abuser. Some haemophiliac sufferers may have contracted the virus through contaminated blood transfusions. Anonymized testing for HIV antibodies in pregnant women was commenced in the UK in 1990 and results have shown that the overall prevalence of women who are HIV

positive is much greater in inner London antenatal clinics than in the rest of the country.

If a woman is thought to be at risk when seen preconception, she should be encouraged to undergo HIV testing. She must, however, be referred for both pre- and post-test counselling from counsellors especially trained for the purpose. A positive result may merit contraceptive advice, particularly if the woman has any symptoms. Evidence regarding the effect of pregnancy on the progression of HIV disease is contradictory, but Roberts (1992) suggests that it seems unlikely that there will be any significant adverse effect in asymptomatic women. If the result is negative the woman should be counselled in terms of avoidance of future exposure to the virus or at least of using a safe form of contraception (even if she is pregnant) such as a latex condom which, if intact, is an effective mechanical barrier to HIV.

The Fourth Health Committee report on preconception care concludes that all men, women and schoolchildren need to be made aware of how HIV and AIDS can be contracted and avoided, and it states that the adoption of safer sex methods can help reduce the spread of HIV (DOH, 1992a).

Medical Conditions

Any woman with a medical disorder should attend for preconception care and her treatment should be shared between her physician and the obstetric team.

DIABETES MELLITUS

Diabetes mellitus is an endocrine disorder in which there is an absolute or partial lack of the hormone insulin which leads to a disturbance of multiple metabolic pathways, although the main effect is on the metabolism of glucose. Without insulin hyperglycaemia occurs and before the discovery of insulin, in the 1920s, women with this condition were infertile.

Even since the discovery of insulin, however, the effect of diabetes on the outcome of pregnancy is significant. Although perinatal mortality is nearly down to the levels for infants of non-diabetic mothers, the risk of congenital abnormalities is up to three times as high (Enkin et al., 1989). Macrosomia is also more common than in babies born to non-diabetic mothers with its concomitant risk of shoulder dystocia. Women with vascular complications of diabetes, such as retinopathy or nephropathy, particularly if associated with hypertension, are at risk of their conditions worsening during pregnancy, and therefore need particular guidance and counselling preconception.

The aim of preconception care of the diabetic woman is to achieve normoglycaemia at the time of conception and in early pregnancy. Within the last two decades a method of gaining retrospective information about diabetic control has been developed, and this can be a most valuable tool in giving the woman advice about when to stop her contraception and start trying for a baby. The method involves a blood test to measure the glycosylated haemoglobin (HbA$_1$) and gives information about the average blood glucose levels over the previous 4–6 weeks. There is said to be an association between high HbA$_1$ levels in early pregnancy and congenital abnormalities (Ylinen et al., 1981).

A recent study undertaken in Edinburgh came to the conclusion that tight control of maternal blood glucose concentration in the early weeks of pregnancy can be achieved by the prepregnancy clinic approach and is associated with a highly significant reduction in the risk of serious (causing death or serious handicap or requiring major surgical correction) congenital abnormalities in the offspring. They also commented that hypoglycaemic episodes do not seem to lead to fetal malformation even when they occur during the period of organogenesis (Steel et al., 1990). As this study implies, tight control of diabetes often results in episodes of hypoglycaemia; it is wise, therefore, to teach the woman's partner and/or a friend how to recognize and treat a hypoglycaemic attack. Education of women with diabetes about preparation for pregnancy should begin with teenagers; the attitude and motivation of the woman is a major determinant for a successful outcome of pregnancy.

Non-insulin-dependent diabetes usually occurs in overweight, middle-aged or elderly people, but can occur in younger women. There is some evidence to suggest that gestational diabetes may be non-insulin-dependent diabetes (Sutherland and Smith, 1990). Preconception care should be similar to that given to insulin-dependent women and should include advice on diet and encouragement to achieve an optimum weight for height prior to conception.

EPILEPSY

Epilepsy is the most common neurological condition liable to affect pregnant women. The main factor in

preconception care is to modify treatment so as to, as far as possible, reduce the likelihood of fetal malformations. Many authorities state that there is a two- to four-fold increase in the incidence of fetal malformations in epileptic women, independent of treatment (Sutherland and Smith, 1990).

It is generally thought that all anticonvulsant drugs have some teratogenic effect. Malformations include oro-facial clefts, cardiac abnormalities, talipes, hip dislocations and neural tube defects (Sutherland and Smith, 1990). If drug therapy cannot be withdrawn without the woman having seizures, monotherapy should be given, and this should be commenced at least three months prior to pregnancy. A six-year prospective study undertaken in Plymouth demonstrated particularly good results in pregnancy outcome (incidence of major congenital malformations 1.1 per 100 live births and for minor malformations 8.7 per 100 live births), and gave the explanation for these results as the fact that the greater proportion of the women were controlled on a single anticonvulsant drug (Hunter and Allen, 1990).

Preconception care of epileptic women should include the prescription of extra folic acid periconceptually to avoid the development of megaloblastic anaemia.

PHENYLKETONURIA

Phenylketonuria is one of the commoner inborn errors of metabolism; it is a monogenic, autosomal recessive abnormality affecting phenylalanine metabolism. If started early enough a low phenylalanine diet will prevent the accumulation of toxic levels and so prevent mental retardation. The low phenylalanine diet can be abandoned in late childhood, when the risk of brain damage is much less.

During pregnancy high levels of phenylalanine are associated with abortion, intrauterine growth retardation, congenital heart disease, microcephaly and mental retardation (Chamberlain and Lumley, 1986). Prior to conception, therefore, the low phenylalanine diet must be recommended. When this is so, and the plasma phenylalanine concentration is maintained within the normal range, a normal baby should be born (Thompson et al., 1991).

HYPERTENSION

Hypertensive disorders in pregnancy comprise at least two distinct groups: *pregnancy-induced hypertension*, usually known as pre-eclampsia and pre-existing or *chronic hypertension*. Pre-existing hypertension may be diagnosed for the first time in pregnancy and, along with pre-eclampsia or proteinuria, may be associated with underlying renal disease (Kincaid-Smith and Fairley, 1989) (see Chapter 41).

Women attending preconception clinics who have known hypertension or who have had pre-eclampsia in a previous pregnancy can be reassured that hypotensive drugs are not teratogenic. If they have renal disease they can also be reassured that, at present, there is no evidence with moderately severe disease that pregnancy adversely affects renal function (Chamberlain and Lumley, 1986). The fetal outcome depends on the level of the blood pressure and the adequacy of renal function. Hypertension is an important cause of neonatal morbidity and mortality as it can lead to placental dysfunction, intrauterine growth retardation and preterm labour. The effect of hypertension on the woman during pregnancy can also be severe, especially if pre-eclampsia is superimposed on pre-existing hypertension. Preconception the woman should be advised to attend for antenatal care as soon as she suspects that she may be pregnant, so that careful monitoring can take place from an early stage.

Genetic Counselling

As a factor which can reduce fetal abnormalities, genetic counselling has become more important because other causes of neonatal morbidity and mortality have been overcome. For couples who require such counselling it is essential that this is undertaken preconception.

Genetic counselling assesses the risk of a baby inheriting an abnormality and seeks to advise potential parents of the ways in which this abnormality can be prevented or reduced in severity. It is essential that as full a family history as possible is taken, along with a medical and reproductive history, and that, if possible, an accurate diagnosis is made. A family pedigree is constructed.

During preconception genetic counselling it may be necessary for the clinical geneticist to give advice about physical and chemical substances which may be mutagenic. There is a large number of these substances which may be encountered in everyday life, although some more than others in certain occupations. As

previously discussed, therefore, some occupations may need to be changed. Also encountered on a regular basis are mutagens in food. Mutagens become evident in protein foods when cooked at high temperatures such as grilling, roasting or frying in fats and oils (Wynn and Wynn, 1991). Counteracting this, however, other foods are antimutagenic. These foods mainly consist of fresh vegetables, fruit and unsaturated fatty acids, which include olive oil. It is thought that the antimutagens may act by preventing absorption of mutagens (Wynn and Wynn, 1991). It may be necessary, therefore, during genetic counselling to ask questions and give advice about diet and occupation. If mutagens have been encountered, the International Commission of the Mutagen Societies (1983, cited in Wynn and Wynn, 1991) have concluded that exposed individuals should refrain from conception for three months.

Work and Lifestyle

Many women work outside the home during pregnancy and for many this may be a financial necessity. It may also confer a certain status on the woman and will normally put her in contact with friends and work colleagues, without whom she might feel a degree of boredom and loneliness. Some feel that working during a normal pregnancy has a more positive than negative effect for the healthy woman (Bishop, 1991).

When giving preconception care it is important to take as full as possible an occupational history. There may be changes in occupation which the woman would be advised to make. Jobs which involve long periods of standing, work on a vibrating machine, contact with toxic substances and excess heat, cold, noise or heavy lifting should be avoided, and the employer should be approached to provide an alternative. Toxic substances include solvents, which are found in a variety of occupations, including printing, dry cleaning, painting and areas where degreasers are used, such as the petrochemical, plastic, rubber or leather industries; also anaesthetic gases, pesticides, herbicides and some heavy metals such as lead. Radiation, particularly ionizing radiation, is known to cause microcephaly and other abnormalities (Chamberlain and Lumley, 1986). In some occupations there may be exposure to biological hazards, such as in nursing, school teaching, veterinary surgery and microbiology laboratories.

Pharmacists and nurses may be at risk in their handling of pharmaceuticals.

Recent discussion on possible physical hazards to the unborn child has focused on the effects of working with visual display units. Research reports have proved inconclusive and, at present, the advice seems to be that, as far as is known, pregnancy will not be harmed by using a visual display unit (Blackwell and Chang, 1988). Safety shields are supplied by most employers, however, and it would be wise to use one.

Potential fathers must not be forgotten when discussing possible and actual hazards to the proposed pregnancy related to type of occupation. It is likely that many of the substances, including radiation, that are thought to be embryotoxic may also cause low sperm counts and abnormal sperm (Elkington, 1985). It has been shown that abnormal sperm can lead to miscarriage (Wynn and Wynn, 1991) and it has been suggested that leukaemia in children living near nuclear plants may be caused by their father's exposure to radiation resulting in germ cell mutations (Gardner *et al.*, 1990). Recently, however, this claim has been disputed.

Work in the home can also be hazardous. There may be exposure to toxic substances, such as solvents, long periods of standing, such as when ironing, and heavy lifting which may involve lifting and carrying toddlers, or older handicapped children.

Preconception advice related to occupation should be given sensitively. It may not be possible for a man or woman to change their type of work and discussion may need to ensue, therefore, on how to minimize the potential hazards within that work, for example checking the rubella status of a school teacher and immunizing her if necessary.

The Fourth Health Committee Report on Preconception Care (DOH, 1992a) recommended that steps are taken to reduce or eliminate exposure of women and men planning pregnancy to radiation and certain chemical hazards. There is in existence a legal framework for controlling exposure to hazardous chemical substances arising from work activities (Control of Substances Hazardous to Health Regulations 1988), and in addition particular control applied to exposure to lead (Control of Lead at Work Regulations 1980). Further legislation to identify all substances which may harm the fetus is being discussed in the European Community. Although the list of possible reproductive hazards is very long, questions such as which agents and how much exposure have not been answered, and

with over 25 000 individual chemicals being used in industry (Chamberlain, 1991) it is impossible to test them all on pregnant animals, and much of the evidence about safety depends on retrospective reports of damage to human beings.

There are some substances within the general environment that are either known, or highly suspected, to be embryotoxic and an excess of which can, on the whole, be avoided. Some of these substances are included as follows.

Lead

It has long been known that exposure to high levels of inorganic lead can cause miscarriage, stillbirth and congenital abnormalities. Exposure can occur from contact with exhaust fumes from lead in petrol; from water carried in lead piping; and in certain industries. Using a water filter will remove at least a proportion of the lead in tap water, and if occupational exposure is known then the woman planning a pregnancy should ask her employer for a temporary move, if possible, into a lead-free environment.

Cadmium

This is a common pollutant, found in cigarette smoke and manufacturing industries, particularly those dealing with paint, batteries and fertilizers. Active and passive smoking should be discouraged and a change of occupation should be made if possible for pre- and periconception women.

Aluminium

There are some suspicions that this metal could be embryotoxic, so avoidance of ingestion or absorption is advised pre- and periconception. The main sources are antacids, some food additives, aluminium saucepans, covering food with foil and antiperspirants.

Mercury

This has long been recognized as a poison, and passes readily through the placenta. It can on the whole be avoided by not having contact with pesticides, fungicides and any industrial processes that use mercury. If any dental fillings are required women should ask for a non-mercury-containing amalgam, and as some fish may contain mercury, particularly tuna fish, it would be wise to avoid eating tuna fish when planning a pregnancy. A dramatic and distressing example of mercury poisoning occurred in 1956 in Minamata

Bay in Japan, where over 700 poisonings were reported and over 20 babies were born with, or quickly developed, a disease like infantile cerebral palsy. The cause was found to be methyl mercury which was released in effluents from a local manufacturing plant (Elkington, 1985).

STRESS

Pregnancy is a normal, physiological event, but when a woman's lifestyle is stressful, pregnancy can add to that stress, and pregnancy itself can be a causative factor of stress and anxiety. An origin of stress can be fear, and fear – of an abnormal baby, of pain, of loss of control – might for some women be a marked feature of pregnancy.

Advice given and investigations undertaken at a preconception clinic must therefore aim to reduce stress and fear. Some advice needs to be given with greater sensitivity than others. For example, in relation to smoking habits, clear and unequivocal advice to stop smoking must be given, but the way in which this advice is given, the attitude of the care-giver and whether or not help is offered to give up smoking can leave the woman either feeling guilty and condemned, or feeling that there is hope for her to give up the habit. Three randomized trials of interventions to reduce smoking in pregnancy, all of which included a self-help smoking cessation manual, have demonstrated a substantial reduction in smoking (Lumley, 1991), so advice on how to give up smoking can be effective.

A variety of tests have been developed to measure anxiety and a number of researchers have attempted to study stress and anxiety in pregnancy. Haddad (1989) has shown an association between maternal anxiety and oxytocin augmentation and the use of analgesia. She postulates that it is possible that high maternal anxiety interferes with normal uterine activity, thereby increasing the need for oxytocin. The augmented uterine contractions may be more painful so increasing the demand for more analgesia, or high maternal anxiety may enhance pain perception, so increasing the demand for pain relief. One of the major functions of preconception care must be to allow time for in-depth discussion of the reasons for fear and anxiety so that some alleviation can take place. Previous induced abortions, stillbirths, neonatal deaths or other unhappy obstetric experiences may need to be discussed in detail, preferably with reference to previous obstetric records.

Stressful life events such as marital breakdown, unemployment or death of a family member will markedly increase anxiety levels, and Norbeck and Tilden (1986) have reported an increase in complications of pregnancy after life stress in the year preceding pregnancy. Chronic stress, such as inadequate housing and domestic violence, must also be taken into account, as must stressful occupations and long travelling times. Fetal response to maternal stress has been documented comparatively recently.

EXERCISE

Moderate exercise, such as walking, swimming and cycling on a regular basis, is more likely to benefit a healthy woman during normal pregnancy than lead to any problems, and Huch and Erkkola (1990) state that such exercise is likely to lead to an improved course of pregnancy when compared to that of a sedentary lifestyle.

There are certain sports which should be discouraged during pregnancy, however, and preconception advice should be given about these. Women in pregnancy should be advised not to participate in team and contact sports, water skiing, scuba diving and activities involving falling. Marathon running should be strongly discouraged as this leads to an increase in core temperature (values of up to 41°C have been recorded) and hyperthermia can have teratogenic effects (Huch and Erkkola, 1990). Sports at high altitudes should also be advised against, as should regular vigorous exercise such as that carried out by top-class athletes. It has been shown that the latter can lead to a variety of complications, some of which are infertility, reduced birthweight, preterm labour and prolonged labour (Chamberlain and Lumley, 1986). Infertility is particularly evident among those who are highly motivated to maintain a low body weight, such as ballet dancers.

Work-related high physical exertion can also be deleterious to pregnancy. A report studying women in North Carolina showed that those in jobs characterized by high levels of physical exertion experienced a higher rate of preterm labour and low birthweight (under 2500 g) babies (Homer et al., 1990). Chamberlain (1991) states that, in hard physical work, the blood supply to the leg muscles can be increased 20-fold and that to the uterus halved.

Regular moderate exercise, in addition to benefiting

healthy women, may also benefit women with non-insulin-dependent diabetes mellitus. A study by Horton (1991) showed that exercise benefits women with non-insulin-dependent diabetes by increasing sensitivity to insulin in skeletal muscle and adipose tissues, and could also be applied to reversing the insulin resistance associated with gestational diabetes (see Chapter 42).

SMOKING

Tobacco smoke contains, among other things, carbon monoxide and nicotine. Carbon monoxide combines with haemoglobin in almost the same manner as oxygen, so producing carboxyhaemoglobin and reducing the normal amount of oxyhaemoglobin. Thus, in pregnant women the oxygen supply to the fetus is reduced. Nicotine is absorbed via the lungs into the bloodstream and is said to cause vasoconstriction of the spiral arterioles in the placenta, so further reducing the oxygen and also the nutrient supply to the fetus.

The main and most frequently demonstrated effect of smoking on the baby is low birthweight. A smoker has nearly twice the risk of a non-smoker in delivering a baby who weighs less than 2500 g, in fact the whole distribution curve appears to be shifted downwards (MacMahon et al., 1986). Conter et al. (1995) found that deficits in birthweight due to mothers who smoked are overcome by six months of age. They conclude that if there are no other adverse variables, such as lower socio-economic status, deficits in weight may not be permanent. It can be hypothesized that the lower birthweight is due to hypoxia secondary to the increase in maternal and fetal carboxyhaemoglobin levels, although the precise mechanism is not fully known.

It has been shown that there is a strong dose–response relationship between the number and yield (carbon monoxide, nicotine, tar) of cigarettes smoked per day and the reduction in birthweight. In a study carried out by Peacock et al. (1991b), women smoking a low quantity of low-yield cigarettes delivered babies of similar mean birthweight to those of non-smokers. Smokers of high-yield cigarettes who smoked a low quantity had babies whose birthweight was reduced to the same degree (6% or more) as those of mothers who smoked higher quantities. The threshold was said to be 13 cigarettes a day and 15 mg per cigarette of carbon monoxide.

Other reported effects of smoking on pregnancy are an association with an increased risk of miscarriage, stillbirth, preterm delivery and perinatal death, including sudden infant death (Chamberlain and Lumley, 1986).

The Fourth Report on Preconception Care (DOH, 1992a) states that smoking prevalence among women has fallen to 29%, but that there is no evidence of a reduction in smoking among younger women or teenage girls. The report states that government controls on tobacco advertising and promotion, along with health education and other factors, have led to a fall in smoking in the population as a whole from 40% in 1978 to 30% in 1992. Tobacco smoking is often linked with high alcohol and caffeine intake and poor nutritional status.

A study by Fried and Makin (1987) on the comparison of the effects of prenatal exposure to tobacco, alcohol and marihuana on birth size and subsequent growth and behaviour demonstrated that, of the soft drugs used, nicotine had the most pronounced effect. After adjustment for other relevant variables, nicotine use prior to and during pregnancy was negatively related to weight and head circumference at birth. The Black Report (Townsend et al., 1990) indicates that certain styles of living, such as cigarette smoking, are related to social class, and shows that the percentage of smokers is increased the lower the social class.

The emphasis in preconception care therefore needs to be on giving assistance to women to help them give up smoking, and particularly to the younger women, teenagers and those in the lower social classes, especially those whose nutrition is poor. It is unlikely that these women will attend preconception clinics, therefore their health education must be given either at school, in the family planning clinic, or by occupational health staff. Help to give up smoking should be given to both men and women; if only the woman's partner smokes, there still may be some adverse effect on the fetus from maternal passive smoking. The Health Education Authority has produced some training materials for health professionals to help them assist women to stop smoking during pregnancy (HEA, 1994). There is some evidence, also, that male smokers have a significantly higher percentage of morphologically abnormal sperm compared to non-smokers (Evans et al., 1981).

Advice on how to stop smoking needs to be given alongside the risks to the baby of smoking. Some couples may think that having a smaller baby may mean not much more than just having an easier birth, but the information needs to be given that birthweight is important, because of the strength of evidence which indicates that it is a good marker of the baby's postnatal health.

ALCOHOL INTAKE

Alcohol is firmly established as a fetal teratogen. Absorption of alcohol occurs rapidly and the rate of absorption is related to the amount of absolute alcohol in the drink. After ingestion, alcohol is distributed in the body according to the water content of the body parts, and during pregnancy the placenta rapidly reaches the same alcohol level as the bloodstream. Alcohol crosses the placenta easily and the fetus is particularly affected in early pregnancy during organogenesis and when its water retention is high. The fetus develops its own alcohol metabolism only after maturation of liver enzymes, which occurs in the last half of pregnancy.

The effect of heavy drinking of alcohol on the fetus has been known for many years and the term *fetal alcohol syndrome* was coined to describe the multitude of abnormal features that these babies have. They have many typical facial features, some of which are microcephaly, small eyes, flattened nasal bridge, maxillary hypoplasia, absent or poorly developed philtrum and a thin vermilion line of the upper lip; and they may also be growth and mentally retarded, of short length and have heart and urinary tract defects (Chamberlain and Lumley, 1986). What is not known is how much alcohol may cause fetal alcohol syndrome, nor what amount of alcohol is safe.

In the Bible it is stated of Samson's mother that preconception an Angel of the Lord appeared to her and instructed her 'not to drink wine or similar drink' during her pregnancy (Judges 13:3, 4, 14). Hytten (1990) states that alcohol may cause subtle damage to the fetus and that it therefore seems wise to advise pregnant women to restrict alcohol consumption as much as possible. Other researchers state that the evidence against low levels of alcohol intake, such as in social drinking, is inconsistent and inconclusive. Forrest *et al.* (1991) recommends that pregnant women should drink no more than 8 units (1 unit = 10 g absolute alcohol) of alcohol a week, or the equivalent of about one drink a day. Peacock *et al.* (1991a,b) found that women who drank more than 100 g of alcohol a week, smoked more than 13 cigarettes a day and had high caffeine intakes (more than 2801 mg a

week) had a predicted reduction in mean birthweight of 18% (95% confidence interval 11% to 24%).

Advice to women before and during pregnancy should be given with knowledge of their individual drinking habits and suggestions made to abstain or reduce levels of alcohol intake accordingly. Both partners should be made aware that excess alcohol, including a single heavy drinking episode (binge drinking), especially during the period of organogenesis is likely to cause fetal abnormalities. They should also be informed that lower levels of drinking may cause less obvious effects in the baby, such as irritability, sleeplessness or poor feeding (Chamberlain and Lumley, 1986). The White Paper (DOH, 1992b) has set a target to reduce the proportion of women drinking more than 14 units of alcohol a week from 11% to 7% by the year 2005.

DRUG ABUSE

It is possible that some women who are dependent on drugs of addiction may attend for preconception care. There are many addictive drugs, which include marihuana (cannabis), heroin, morphia, cocaine, lysergic acid diethylamide (LSD), ecstasy and some horrific concoctions of drugs. The addict may abuse a drug orally, intravenously, in which case she is at risk of contracting AIDS, or by sniffing, as in glue-sniffing.

Few reports have shown consistent problems arising from drug abuse in pregnancy, although some link opiate abuse with anaemia, premature rupture of membranes, haemorrhage, multiple pregnancy and intrauterine growth retardation (Chamberlain and Lumley, 1986).

Drug abuse is often associated with malnutrition, cigarette smoking, alcohol consumption and poor socio-economic conditions. If a woman attends for preconception care she may be motivated enough to attempt to stop abusing drugs, or at least to accept an alternative drug such as methadone before and during her pregnancy, and it may be possible to encourage her to improve her general health before conception.

Family Planning

Planning a pregnancy is obviously better than becoming pregnant unexpectedly as optimum health can be achieved prior to a planned pregnancy.

Preconception advice in relation to family planning

should take account of maternal and paternal age, maternal health and birth spacing, in addition to contraceptive methods. It is well known that some chromosomal abnormalities increase in incidence in relation to the age of the mother; Down's syndrome (trisomy 21) is said to have reached an incidence of as much as 1% by the age of 40 years (Sutherland and Smith, 1990). Increasing maternal age is also related to a higher incidence of fetal abnormalities (Wynn and Wynn, 1991). Illness, severe or chronic, may lead to premature ageing, which can also be a contributory cause of fetal abnormality. In healthy, young prospective parents the advice is normally given that the desirable time for birth spacing is about 2–4 years, and that under 2 years increases the risk of fetal malformations (Wynn and Wynn, 1991).

Contraceptive advice given at a preconception clinic would be mainly to stop certain methods of contraception and use others for a period of at least three months before conception. It is advisable to stop taking either the combined (oestrogen and progesterone) or the progesterone-only oral contraceptive pill for this period prior to conception. The cessation of these introduced hormones allows the body to regulate its own hormones and resume a regular ovulatory and menstrual cycle. The expected date of delivery can be estimated more accurately too. It may be necessary for the body to readjust its levels of some minerals and vitamins following taking oral contraceptives; the contraceptive pill can cause an upset in the zinc and copper balance in the body and may lead to a deficiency of zinc and possibly other minerals and vitamins (Smith and Brown, 1976). Use of the intrauterine contraceptive device should also be discontinued at least three months before conception, especially if one containing copper has been used. Copper has been shown to interfere with the absorption of zinc, so causing zinc deficiency (Hurley, 1981).

Couples planning some form of assisted conception may also seek preconception advice. Their reasons for seeking assisted conception may be subfertility, infertility or as a result of diagnosis of a genetic defect which could be transmitted to their baby. The latter possibility might be able to be prevented by pre-implantation diagnosis and the placement of only normal embryos in the uterus. Genetic manipulation may also be undertaken, whereby the abnormal gene may be replaced by a healthy gene and the resulting embryo placed in the woman's uterus. Preconception care should be given with sensitivity and wisdom to these couples (see Chapters 4 and 61).

Clinic Procedures

Sufficient time should be given at a preconception clinic to allow for all the necessary investigations to be undertaken, appropriate advice to be given and, above all, to listen to what the prospective parents have to say. It is likely that they will have specific reasons for attending such a clinic and they need time to discuss their thoughts, ask questions and assimilate the answers.

During the course of the clinic visit, information should be obtained from both partners about the following:

▶ Family history.
▶ Medical history.
▶ Past obstetric history – particularly preterm labour, stillbirth or small baby.
▶ Menstrual history.
▶ Method of contraception.
▶ Occupation.
▶ Dietary habits.
▶ Smoking, alcohol and any drugs taken.

Questions should be asked about any hereditary conditions, any allergies, and opportunity given to discuss any other problems or difficulties. If either of the partners do not wish to volunteer information then their decision must be respected.

Investigations undertaken will include a medical examination, testing for heart action, blood pressure, thyroid function, respiratory function, gastrointestinal normality and the presence or absence of any sexually transmitted diseases. Blood will be taken for any evidence of anaemia or haemoglobinopathies, and tests may be made for vitamin and zinc or lead levels. Hair analysis may be undertaken to assess nutritional state or exposure to toxic metals, although some authorities are of the opinion that this is not worth investigating because of its inaccuracy. If there is any history of hereditary conditions, blood will also be taken for karyotyping. Tests may also be made for the presence of rubella antibodies.

Urinalysis will be performed, particularly for the presence of protein, glucose or ketones. The former may be an indication of urinary tract infection and a midstream specimen of urine will be taken for bacteriuria. Between 4 and 15% of women have bacteriuria in pregnancy and 40% of these develop acute pyelonephritis (Kincaid-Smith and Fairley, 1989), so it is essential to treat any bacteriuria, asymptomatic or otherwise, in the preconception period. The latter two abnormal findings in the urine may indicate diabetes, and if this is present the woman should be cared for in conjunction with the physician, as with other medical conditions.

The woman should be encouraged to attend for dental treatment. A chest X-ray may be advised if there is any history of tuberculosis in the family, and if there is a history of subfertility or repeated miscarriages the partner may be advised to attend for semen analysis. If the woman has not recently had a cervical smear, this should be carried out and a full genitourinary examination may be undertaken. The woman will be weighed and her weight for height calculated if she appears over- or underweight.

If the woman or her partner are disabled they may require specific advice according to their disability, and if the woman does not speak or understand the language, she will need an interpreter with her. If the woman's culture is very different from that of her interviewer, it may be necessary to ask a colleague of the same or similar culture to assist or take over the care.

Conclusion

The Health Committee Report on the Maternity Services (DOH, 1992c) states that becoming a mother is a normal process and can indeed be seen as a manifestation of health. Preconception care can give a life-enhancing start to family life.

Preconception care can, and should, be given by a variety of people. Prospective parents in the lower socio-economic groups are less likely to attend formal preconception clinics, but the care and advice offered at such a clinic can and should be given in other settings. Health education and preconception care should start in school; the Fourth Report on Preconception Care (DOH, 1992a) recommended that all schools designate a teacher to co-ordinate health education, and that this teacher should have specialist training in sex education. A midwife or health visitor may also be called upon to teach schoolchildren about preconception care (Johnson, 1984). Parents and youth leaders should also give advice in relation to healthy living. Well-women clinics and occupational health nurses may hold specific sessions for prospective parents.

The family planning clinic nurse and doctor are in an ideal position to give specific preconception care and advice, and have three distinct roles: that of a health educator, identifier of potential problems and resource person for information (Rands, 1984). The primary health care team should give preconception care and general practitioners may do so, particularly when giving women advice about contraception (Jewell, 1990). Some hospitals have 'phone-in' services for preconception advice (Shorney, 1985) and an Open University pack has been developed for prospective parents.

As more schoolchildren, and men and women, are exposed to health education, so the value of preconception care will be recognized and the health of future generations will be improved.

References

Barnes, B. & Bradley, S.G. (1992) *Planning for a Healthy Baby*. Foresight, The Association For the Promotion of Preconceptual Care. London: Ebury Press.

Bishop, J. (1991) Work and pregnancy. *Nursing Times* 87(35): 58.

Blackwell, R. & Chang, A. (1988) Video display terminals and pregnancy. *Br. J. Obstet. Gynaecol.* 95: 446.

Chamberlain, G. (1991) Work in pregnancy. *Br. Med. J.* 302: 1070.

Chamberlain, G. & Lumley, J. (1986) *Prepregnancy Care, A Manual for Practice*. Chichester: John Wiley & Sons.

Chief Medical Officer (1989) Letter on listeriosis and food. *Midwives Chronicle and Nursing Notes* 129.

Chief Medical Officer (1990) Vitamin A intake in pregnancy. *Lancet* 336: 1063.

COMA (1991) Dietary Reference Values for Food Energy and Nutrients for the United Kingdom. Report on Health and Social Subjects 41. London: HMSO.

Conter, V., Cortinovis, I., Rogari, P. & Riva, L. (1995) Weight growth in infants born to mothers who smoked during pregnancy. *Br. Med. J.* 310: 768–771.

DHSS (1990) *Vitamin A and Pregnancy*. PL/CMO (90)11. PL/C NO. (90)10. London: DHSS.

Dixon, P. (1987) *The Truth About AIDS*. London: Kingsway Publications.

DOH (Department of Health) (1992a) *Preconception Care: Government Response to the Fourth Report from the Health Committee Session 1990–91*. London: HMSO.

DOH (1992b) *The Health of the Nation. A Summary of the Strategy for Health in England*. London: HMSO.

DOH (1992c) *House of Commons Health Committee Report on Maternity Services*. London: HMSO.

DOH Expert Advisory Group (1992) *Folic Acid and the Prevention of Neural Tube Defects. Report from an Expert Advisory Group.* London: HMSO.

Doyle, W. (1992) Preconceptional care – who needs it? *Modern Midwife* January/February: 18.

Elkington, J. (1985) *The Poisoned Womb.* London: Pelican Books.

Enkin, M., Keirse, M.J.N.C. & Chalmers, I. (eds) (1989) *A Guide to Effective Care in Pregnancy and Childbirth.* Oxford: Oxford University Press.

Evans, H.J., Fletcher, J., Torrance, M. & Hargreave, T.B. (1981) Sperm abnormalities and cigarette smoking. *Lancet* 627.

Forrest, F., du V. Florey, C., Taylor, D., McPherson, F. & Young, J.A. (1991) Reported social alcohol consumption during pregnancy and infants' development at 18 months. *Br. Med. J.* **303**: 22.

Fried, P.A. & Makin, J.E. (1987) Neonatal behavioural correlates of prenatal exposure to marihuana, cigarettes and alcohol in a low-risk population. *Neurotoxical. Teratol.* **9**(1): 1–7.

Gardner, M.J., Snee, M.P., Hall, A.J., Powell, C.A., Downs, S. & Terrel, J.D. (1990) Results of case-control study of leukaemia and lymphoma among young people near Sellafield Nuclear Plant in West Cumbria. *Br. Med. J.* **300**: 423.

Haddad, F. (1989) Effect of anxiety in pregnancy. *Contemp. Rev. Obstet. Gynaecol.* 1: 123.

HEA (Health Education Authority) (1994) *Helping Pregnant Smokers Quit: Training for Health Professionals.* London: HEA.

Holliman, R. (1992) Toxocariasis and cryptosporidiosis. *Prescribers J.* 32(3): 127.

Homer, C.J., Beresford, S.A.A., James, S.A., Siegel, E. & Wilcox, S. (1990) Work related physical exertion and risk of preterm low birthweight delivery. *Paediat. Perinatal Epidemiol.* 4: 161.

Horton, E.S. (1991) Exercise in the treatment of NIDDM. Applications for GDM? *Diabetes* 40: 175.

Huch, R. & Erkkola, R. (1990) Pregnancy and exercise – exercise and pregnancy. A short review. *Br J. Obstet. Gynaecol.* 97: 208.

Hunter, R.W. & Allen, E.M. (1990) The course and outcome of pregnancy in women with epilepsy – a 6 year prospective study. *J. Obstet. Gynaecol.* 10: 483.

Hurley, L.S. (1981) Teratogenic aspects of manganese, zinc and copper nutrition. *Physiol. Rev.* 61: 249.

Hytten, F. (1990) Nutritional requirements in pregnancy: what should the pregnant woman be eating? *Midwifery* 6: 93.

Jewell, D. (1990) Preconception clinics. *The Practitioner* **234**: 349.

Johnson, E. (1984) Pre-conceptual care: a course for school-girls. *Midwife, Health Visitor & Community Nurse* 20: 122.

Joynson, D.H.M. & Payne, R. (1988) Letter: Screening for toxoplasmosis. *Lancet* 2: 795–796.

Kincaid-Smith, P. & Fairley, K. (1989) Renal disease in pregnancy. *Fetal Med.* 1: 177.

Lumley, J. (1991) Stopping smoking – again. *Br. J. Obstet. Gynaecol.* 98: 847.

McLauchlin, J., Hall, S.M., Velani, S.K. & Gilbert, R.J. (1991) Human listeriosis and paté: a possible association. *Br. Med. J.* **303**: 773.

MacMahon, B., Alpert, M. & Salbert, E.J. (1986) Infant weight and parental smoking habits. *Am. J. Epidemiol.* 82: 247.

Morgan, J. (1994) Nutrition and pregnancy: problems and solutions. *Nursing Times* 90(46): 31–38.

MRC (Medical Research Council) Vitamin Study Research Group (1991) Prevention of neural tube defects: results of the Medical Research Council Vitamin Study. *Lancet* 338: 131.

Norbeck, J.S. & Tilden, V.P. (1986) Life stress, social support and emotional disequilibrium in complications of pregnancy: a prospective, multivariate study. *J. Health Soc. Behav.* 24: 30.

Parry, A. (1990) *Chlamydia psittaci* of ovine origin. *Midwives Chronicle & Nursing Notes* February: 50.

Peacock, J.L., Bland, J.M. & Anderson, H.R. (1991a) Effects on birthweight of alcohol and caffeine consumption in smoking women. *J. Epidemiol. Community Health* 45(2): 159.

Peacock, J.L., Bland, J.M., Anderson, H.R. *et al.* (1991b) Cigarette smoking and birthweight: type of cigarette smoked and a possible threshold effect. *Int. J. Epidemiol.* 20(2): 405.

Pope, E. (1992) Toxoplasmosis. *Midwives Chronicle and Nursing Notes* October: 300.

Rands, G. (1984) Prepregnancy care – the role of the FP nurse. *Mat. Action* May/June: 11.

Roberts, R. (1992) Sexually transmitted diseases in pregnancy. *Br. J. Hosp. Med.* 47(9): 674.

Rosso, P. (1985) A new chart to monitor weight gain during pregnancy. *Am. J. Obstet. Gynecol.* 41: 644.

Shorney, J. (1985) Exeter midwives' advisory centre. *Midwives Chronicle & Nursing Notes* January: 14.

Smith, J.C. & Brown, E. (1976) The effects of oral contraceptive action on trace element metabolism – a review. In: *Trace Elements in Human Health and Disease,* vol. 11, Essential and Toxic Elements. New York: Academic Press.

Steel, J.M., Johnstone, F.D., Hepburn, D.A. & Smith, A.F. (1990) Can prepregnancy care of diabetic women reduce the risk of abnormal babies? *Br. Med. J.* 301: 1070.

Stein, Z., Susser, M., Saenger, G. & Marolla, F. (1975) *Famine and Human Development.* Oxford: Oxford University Press.

Sutherland, H.W. & Smith, N.C. (1990) *Perspectives in Pre-Pregnancy Counselling and Care.* London: Smith-Gordon and Co.

Thompson, G.N., Francis, D.E., Kirby, D.M. & Compton, R. (1991) Pregnancy in phenylketonuria: dietary treatment aimed at normalising maternal plasma phenylalanine concentration. *Arch. Dis. Child.* 66(11): 1346.

Thompson, J. (1993) Nutrition in pregnancy. *Nursing Times* 89(2): 38.

Townsend, P., Davidson, N. & Whitehead, M. (1990) *Inequalities in Health. The Black Report and The Health Divide.* Harmondsworth: Penguin Books.

Wald, N.J. & Bower, C. (1995) Folic acid and the prevention of neural tube defects. *Br. Med. J.* 310: 1019–1020.

Wynn, M. & Wynn, A. (1991) *The Case for Preconception Care of Men and Women.* London: A B Academic Publishers.

Ylinen, K., Raivio, K. & Teramo, K. (1981) Haemoglobin A_{1C} predicts the perinatal outcome in insulin-dependent diabetic pregnancies. *Br. J. Obstet. Gynaecol.* 88: 961.

16

Maternal Nutrition

In the UK, the government has become increasingly concerned about the health of the population and the consequent costs of morbidity as a result of factors such as poor diet, smoking and alcohol intake. In the *Health of the Nation* document (DOH, 1992) the government set out its strategy for achieving several key targets for health by the year 2000, and focuses on diet as a means of reducing coronary heart disease in particular. The general recommendations include a reduction in fat, saturated fatty acids, salt and alcohol, and an increase in the amount of bread, other cereals and potatoes, fresh fruit and vegetables in the diet of individuals. The 1993 document (DOH, 1993) provided an update on progress with the various targets, and showed some small improvement in diet and alcohol consumption.

It is recognized that poor long-term eating habits and subsequent ill-health can result from inadequate nutrition during childhood. Midwives are in an invaluable position to influence the eating habits of the next generation by facilitating mothers to consider optimum nutrition. Expectant parents are usually receptive to

suggestions and are keen to adapt their lifestyle in the best interests of their baby; indeed, Anderson *et al.* (1993) confirmed that pregnant women do pay more attention to their diet than non-pregnant women. Odent (1994) stresses the need for midwives to help women to improve their diet so that healthy, full-term babies can be delivered. However, Mulliner *et al.* (1995) found, in one regional health authority, that a large proportion of midwives felt unprepared to give appropriate advice on nutrition, despite education on the subject during their initial training.

Why is Good Maternal Nutrition Important?

Much research has been carried out in recent years about the effects of inadequate maternal nutrition on the fetus. Poor dietary intake of essential nutrients can result in a higher than normal perinatal mortality and morbidity. Poor nutrition in the mother may also affect fetal growth, resulting in low-birthweight babies or preterm delivery, possibly due to low placental weight (Luke, 1994), or other obstetric complications such as maternal pregnancy-induced hypertension (Giotta, 1993; Herrera, 1993).

There is increasing concern that, as well as adversely affecting fetal growth and development, impaired maternal nutrition may influence disease programming of the fetus in adult life, such as increasing the tendency to hypertension (Godfrey *et al.*, 1994), cardiovascular disease (Barker, 1993), diabetes mellitus (Wilkin, 1993) and other conditions (Gray, 1994). Certainly, the eating habits of a mother and her family will most probably be adopted by the child, at least in the early years, and maternal nutritional status is likely to be a reliable determinant of child health (Rahman *et al.*, 1993).

Ideally, dietary advice should be given prior to conception, for it has been known since the famines of the Second World War that fetal outcome is worse if the mother is malnourished at the time of conception rather than at the time of delivery (Wynn and Wynn, 1981). A thorough investigation into the mother's diet and other aspects of her lifestyle could perhaps be better use of time at the booking history appointment, rather than focusing on the medical history, which could be obtained via alternative means, such as a questionnaire sent to the woman in advance of her appointment. Time could then be spent by the midwife in discussing the concerns of the woman and offering her information and advice. Sujitor's paper (1994) discusses the need for standard procedures to incorporate nutritional assessment into the care of all expectant mothers.

What is Nutrition?

Nutrition is the sum of the processes involved in taking in nutrients, assimilating and utilizing them. Nutrients such as proteins, carbohydrates, fats, vitamins and minerals are necessary for development, growth, normal functioning and maintenance of life and, because the body cannot produce them, they need to be obtained from a variety of food sources.

Nutritional status is affected by the amount and quality of food eaten, the digestion, absorption and utilization of food nutrients, and by biochemical individuality. In Westernized countries, eating enough food is not normally a problem. Nevertheless, many people do not eat the correct balance of nutrients, and mal-

nourishment may be a problem, although for different reasons than in developing countries, where food is scarce. Food quality may be affected by nutrient-deficient soil in which crops are grown, or by the use of pesticides. The addition of chemical preservatives, colourings and flavourings to ready-prepared food, and of antibiotics to meat, will also adversely influence nutrient absorption.

Digestion and absorption may be affected by a person's general health status or the combination of foods eaten. On the other hand, impaired absorption of certain nutrients may be iatrogenic, as when someone is taking specific drugs. Overindulgence in some foods can affect the body's ability to absorb essential nutrients; for instance, coffee and tea interfere with the absorption of zinc and iron from food (Davies and Stewart, 1987: xvi). Similarly, abuse with other substances such as alcohol, cigarettes or recreational drugs will, for a variety of reasons, result in malnourishment. Environmental factors, including lead pollution, may predispose to nutritional inadequacies. Biochemical individuality means that each person has unique nutritional requirements, which will alter according to their age, gender, general health, level of activity, genetic influences and stressors, such as pregnancy.

Weight in Pregnancy

Most mothers are expected to gain between 11 and 13 kg in weight during pregnancy, but this is dependent on maternal diet, activity, food availability (especially in the developing world), and gestation factors such as physiological sickness or multiple pregnancy. Attention to a balanced diet in the mother is more significant than concern about her weight gain, and is more likely to result in full-term babies of adequate birthweight (Susser, 1991). Conversely, Aaronson and Macnee (1989) suggest that weight gain during pregnancy is not a reliable indicator of nutritional status, for some additional weight may be due to the presence of oedema, but that total maternal weight gain is influential on fetal outcome. Nutritional counselling during pregnancy for undernourished or malnourished women has been shown to have a positive outcome for both maternal and, ultimately, fetal weight gain (Bruce and Tchabo, 1989).

There has also been some discussion regarding *restriction of energy intake* during pregnancy. Dewey and McCrory (1994) suggest that, while dieting to lose weight is not recommended during pregnancy, even for obese women, they may wish to restrict calories moderately to achieve some weight loss, particularly as the decrease in physical activity in the third trimester must be accounted for. In societies where energy intake is forcefully restricted due to lack of food, maternal metabolic adaptations are made to spare energy for fetal growth (King *et al.*, 1994). However, care must be taken when advising immigrant women, such as those from the Indian subcontinent, who may, for a variety of genetic and diet-related factors, traditionally produce small babies. Encouraging them to consume a British type of diet and increase their weight beyond that which is culturally the norm could result in large babies and consequent cephalopelvic disproportion, with all its related problems.

Muslim women are required to *fast* during Ramadan and, although some exceptions are made, pregnancy is a normal physiological event and therefore women are normally expected to comply with total fasting, i.e. no food or drink from dawn till dusk. Midwives should be aware of current teachings regarding Ramadan, and they should ask Muslim women if they are fasting (Reeves, 1992). Athar (1990) recommends that women are advised to fast only if Ramadan falls in the second trimester of pregnancy and then only if the woman is fit and healthy.

Silverton (1993) cites research by Kaplan *et al.* (1983) in which orthodox Jewish women were found to have a higher than average delivery rate immediately after fasting for 24 hours during Yom Kippur.

Essential Nutrients

PROTEINS AND AMINO ACIDS

Proteins are required for development, growth and the formation of cells and essential body secretions and fluids, including enzymes, hormones, antibodies and haemoglobin. Proteins also act as buffers, helping to regulate acid–base balance and, in the form of plasma proteins, control osmotic pressure between body fluids. They assist in the transport of lipids as lipoproteins, and of free fatty acids and bilirubin.

Proteins are necessary to maintain health, and are required in larger quantities during pregnancy to account for the extra maternal uterine and breast tissues, and for fetal development, although Maher *et*

al. (1993) found no correlation between maternal serum protein levels and fetal weight. Normal daily requirements of proteins in non-pregnant women are 29 g (World Health Organization's recommendations cited by Davies and Stewart, 1987: 107). Protein requirements rise to 39 g during late pregnancy and 46 g per day during the period of lactation. In America, recommendations for protein intake tend to be higher: Quillman (1994: 233) advocates a rise from the normal 50 g per day to 60 g during pregnancy. Hytten's (1990) British recommendation is, however, noticeably different, for he suggests an extra gestational intake of only 8.5 g per day.

It is certainly increasingly recognized that, in the West, most (non-pregnant) people consume excess amounts of animal proteins and could reduce, by half, their daily intake. Kramer's (1993) review of several clinical trials highlights the fact that there appear to be no long-term benefits to the babies of mothers who are advised to increase their protein intake significantly above their normal non-pregnant amount, or who are given supplements, and that this latter practice may even impair fetal growth. This is supported by Rush (1989). When pregnant women have a protein intake of more than 50 g daily, creatinine clearance has been found to be higher, although Shiffman *et al.* (1989) admit that they are unclear about the significance of this finding.

Proteins are composed of chains of *amino acids*, which are broken down during digestion into the individual constituents; incomplete digestion may result in amino acids being absorbed into the bloodstream, and may result in symptoms of intolerance, such as low or high blood sugar. *Essential amino acids* cannot be formed in the body and must be obtained from food, whereas *non-essential amino acids* can be synthesized in the body. Animal proteins contain all the essential amino acids, and are found in meat, poultry, fish, eggs and dairy products. However, vegetable proteins do not contain all the amino acids required for health, so those which are missing from one source must be obtained from either animal proteins or different vegetable proteins.

One third of a litre of milk, or one egg, or 60 g of meat, or 90 g of wholegrain cereal will provide normal daily protein allowances in a non-pregnant woman, so it should be relatively easy to increase this amount during pregnancy. It is, however, important that the pregnant and lactating mother eats sufficient quantities of non-protein calories to prevent the protein being used for energy.

Essential amino acids include leucine, lysine, methionine, cystine, phenylalanine, tryptophan and valine; non-essential amino acids include alanine, glutamic acid, glycine and tyrosine. Proteins are digested by being broken down into the amino acids and transported to the liver, where enzymes called amino acid transferases convert them into a more usable form. This process requires vitamin B_6; consequently, a high protein intake will require an increase in vitamin B_6 intake. For example, pregnant women are known to have higher blood levels of tryptophan, an amino acid which is converted to serotonin and which acts as a calming and antidepressive agent. A woman who has recently discontinued the contraceptive pill, which inhibits the effects of vitamin B_6, may require vitamin B_6 supplements.

Arginine, another amino acid, is usually found in large quantities in seminal fluid, but supplementation with arginine may be required in subfertile and infertile men.

Certain protein foods may become sources of potential infection for pregnant women. Meat, in particular, may be contaminated and advice regarding attention to cooking may help to prevent gastrointestinal disorders. In addition, raw meat may be contaminated by the *Listeria monocytogenes* bacterium or the parasite *Toxoplasma gondii*, so mothers should be advised against consuming raw or undercooked meat. The *Listeria monocytogenes* bacterium may also be present in unpasteurized milk (Knuppel and Drukker, 1993: 119, 133) and women are advised to refrain from eating soft cheeses, such as Brie, for this reason.

Vegetarian and vegan mothers

An adequate intake of protein is particularly significant for pregnant vegetarians and women who are vegans, i.e. those who do not eat meat, fish or dairy produce. Vegetable proteins are found in beans, peas, corn, wheat products, bread, rice, brewer's yeast, nuts, seeds and soya. For those women who eat some animal produce, milk, eggs, cheese and yogurt also contain protein. In order to eat a diet which contains sufficient protein, pregnant vegetarians should consume a variety of vegetable proteins, but vegans may need help from a dietician to ensure their intake is satisfactory. In practice, most dedicated vegans are fully aware of how to fulfil their nutritional requirements, especially those who have consciously decided to follow this practice. However, help may be needed for women whose cultural traditions require them to be vegetarians or vegans, particularly those who are newly arrived immigrants, because they may find difficulty in purchasing specific food items to which they are accustomed.

LIPIDS

Lipids, or fats, in various forms, are needed as energy (1 g of fat supplies 9 calories of energy), heat insulation and as a store of readily available food when supply fails to meet demand. More importantly, however, fats produce active biological substances essential for normal body functioning: for example, fat is the only substance to stimulate gall bladder activity, without which gallstones could form. They also facilitate the proper absorption of fat-soluble vitamins and calcium, and form a structural part of each cell wall throughout the body.

Fats are composed of *triglycerides* – three fatty acids with a unit of glycerol – and are broken down into these components during digestion. Most fatty acids can be synthesized by the body, with the exception of three essential fatty acids: linoleic acid, linolenic acid and arachidonic acid, which must be obtained from food. Essential fatty acids assist in prostaglandin production and in preventing arterial thromboses.

Fatty acids are composed of a chain of carbon atoms, with each atom having one or more free 'arms' or bonds to link with other atoms. Where one or more 'arm' is unattached, the fatty acid is unsaturated: if only one 'arm' is free it is *mono-unsaturated*; if more than one 'arm' is free it is *poly-unsaturated*. The unsaturated fatty acids are found in vegetable oils, especially safflower and sunflower, but excluding coconut and palm oil, which are saturated. Unsaturated fats are also found in fish oils. *Saturated* fats are mainly animal fats such as butter and lard, plus margarines and vegetable shortening, which have been saturated by forcing hydrogen gas through the oil (hydrogenized). Unsaturated fatty acids are preferable to saturated ones, and poly-unsaturated are the most favourable as they are more readily converted into energy; however, a balance of each type is needed for adequate nutrition.

Fatty acids depend on certain other nutrients for their metabolism, including zinc, magnesium, selenium, and vitamins B_3, C and E. There is a need for small additional quantities of fats during pregnancy, particularly for extra energy, to avoid protein calories being misused. An American investigation by Hachey (1994) explored the maternal and fetal outcomes related to fat consumption during pregnancy. The conclusion was drawn that while middle-aged multiparous mothers may be at increased risk of later developing angina or cholesterol gallstones due to the hypercholesterolaemia of normal pregnancy, this does not support a practice of low-fat diets during pregnancy. This is because serum lipids are reduced by poly-unsaturated fatty acids, some obstetric complications may be improved by n-3 fatty acids, and arachidonic acid may help visual and psychomotor development in the child. Villar *et al.* (1992) found that fetal growth may be related to the mother's nutritional status at the beginning of pregnancy and the rate at which fat is deposited, with babies being significantly lighter in mothers whose fat gain before 30 weeks' gestation was low.

CARBOHYDRATES

Carbohydrates are the main source of calories in almost all diets throughout the world. One gram of carbohydrate provides 4 calories of energy. Carbohydrates are classified as sugars (*mono-* and *disaccharides*) or starches and fibre (*polysaccharides*), and are found in plentiful supply in plants such as fruits, vegetables, legumes, grains and sugar. Some are also found in milk and other dairy products, and in honey. They are the most easily digested of all nutrients, and can be stored in the body and released as energy when required, thereby preventing excessive oxidation of fats for energy. They are the only energy source used by the lens of the eye and, under normal conditions, the central nervous system. Furthermore, carbohydrates help to regulate gastrointestinal functions by balancing the growth of normal bacterial flora against undesirable flora.

All carbohydrates are broken down partly in the mouth and mainly in the small intestine to the simplest compound, *glucose*; excess glucose is converted into glycogen to be stored by the liver. It is generally considered that, in the West, carbohydrate intake should equate to approximately half of all food consumed, which in many people would indicate a need to increase starches and fibre and decrease fats and proteins. However, it is important to advise mothers that an increase in carbohydrates should not be obtained from sweets, cakes and biscuits, but from bread, potatoes (without added fat), rice and from fruit sugars.

Indeed, mothers on low incomes would be able to eat a well-balanced diet by consuming these food items, together with vegetable proteins such as beans. On the other hand, women who have a tendency to obesity should be made aware of some of the sources of hidden sugars in savoury foods – such as baked beans, tomato sauce and many ready-prepared meals. They can be advised that there are many low-sugar alternatives available.

Additional *fibre* in the diet is also recommended in an attempt to prevent constipation, obesity, irritable bowel syndrome, gallstones, diabetes mellitus and coronary heart disease; the amount needed daily is thought to be about 30 g, whereas most people consume only about 20 g (Davies and Stewart, 1987: 128). Expectant and newly delivered mothers should be advised to have a high intake of fruit, vegetables, especially green, leafy ones, and of cereals, all of which provide essential vitamins and minerals as well as fibre. However, care should be taken to monitor the mother's iron levels, as high-fibre diets can inhibit the absorption of iron from food. This is particularly important in vegetarians, whose diets may lack sufficient iron, and in women who drink a lot of tea, which further restricts iron absorption. Jewish and other women who eat unleavened bread may be deficient in zinc, as phytates in the bread block the absorption of zinc from the diet (Davies and Stewart, 1987: 132).

VITAMINS AND MINERALS

Vitamin A

Vitamin A is required for growth and repair of cells, fighting infection and the synthesis of ribonucleic acid (RNA). It is needed for the eyes, especially night vision, for protein metabolism and aids in detoxification processes; it is also an antioxidant. Vitamin A is found in liver and kidneys, fish oils, eggs and dairy produce. It is also in apricots, broccoli, carrots, parsley, green leafy vegetables and other yellow vegetables. Deficiency of vitamin A may cause anaemias, blindness, skin disorders, tooth decay, allergies and gastrointestinal disorders. Absorption of vitamin A from the diet can be impeded by vitamin D deficiency, alcohol, coffee, mineral oil, nitrate fertilizers and strong glaring sunlight. While there is a need for adequate intake of vitamin A during pregnancy, birth defects have been found to occur in women taking supplements, or eating excessive amounts of vitamin A-containing foods such as liver during the first trimester, due to the presence of retinol (Ranjan, 1991). In 1990 the Department of Health and Social Security issued a widely publicized letter stating that the recommended daily amount (RDA) of vitamin A in pregnancy (i.e. 2500 IU) should not be exceeded because higher intakes may pose a teratogenic risk in humans. Pregnant women and those intending to become pregnant should therefore be advised not to take supplements containing vitamin A, and also to avoid liver, liver paté and liver sausage which may contain between 4 and 12 times the RDA (DHSS, 1990).

Thiamin

Thiamin, or vitamin B_1, is an antioxidant, required for the synthesis of acetylcholine within the cells. It helps to maintain healthy nerves, cardiac muscle and digestive tissues, and is necessary for the digestion of carbohydrates. Thiamin is found in whole grains, nuts and seeds, such as sunflower, brewer's yeast, fruit and green vegetables, as well as liver, kidneys, fish, eggs and milk. Absorption of available thiamin from food will be impaired by stress, food additives, alcohol, coffee, excessive sugar consumption, overcooking of vegetables, especially boiling at high temperatures, and by some antibiotics. The need for thiamin increases during pregnancy and lactation, and long-term deficiency could lead to irritability, insomnia, weight loss, oedema, poor reflexes, and ultimately to impairment of the cardiovascular, nervous and gastrointestinal systems.

Riboflavin

Riboflavin, vitamin B_2, helps to metabolize fats, proteins and carbohydrates, facilitates wound healing and regulates hormones and the growth and development of the fetus. Vitamin B_2 is found in foods which also contain thiamin, and absorption is adversely affected by antibiotics and the contraceptive pill. Deficiency may cause various external lesions, fatigue, personality disturbance, anaemia, digestive upset and hypertension.

Niacin

Niacin, vitamin B_3, helps to convert food to energy and is necessary for the metabolism of fats, proteins and carbohydrates; it regulates hormonal and enzymal actions and acts as a vasodilator. Niacin is found in liver, lean meat, poultry, fish, grains, yeast, butter and nuts, and is antagonized by alcohol, stress, coffee, high carbohydrate intake, antibiotics and antitubercular

drugs. A variety of skin and gastrointestinal disturbances may result from inadequte intake, as well as headache, memory loss, insomnia and poor appetite. If a mother is deficient in vitamin B_6 her needs for niacin will also increase.

Pyridoxine

Pyridoxine, vitamin B_6, is essential for the synthesis of proteins, antibodies, erythrocytes, and for enzyme reactions and development of the nervous system. It is also needed for healthy teeth and gums and for the release of stored glycogen. Pyridoxine is found in foods which contain other B vitamins, plus bananas, prunes and raisins, but its absorption is affected by many drugs, including the contraceptive pill, cortisone, penicillamine and antitubercular treatments. Pyridoxine requirements increase during pregnancy and lactation, with insufficient intake leading to anaemia, neuritis, convulsions, depression, dermatitis and possibly renal calculi.

Vitamin B_{12}

Vitamin B_{12}, also called cobalamin, is essential for proper functioning of the bone marrow, erythrocytes, nervous system, including myelin formation, and for the development of RNA and DNA. It also helps to regulate normal blood ascorbic levels and is important for carbohydrate metabolism. It is found in liver, kidney, fish and shellfish, and levels may be adversely affected by aspirin, the contraceptive pill, codeine, alcohol and nitrous oxide.

Deficiency can result in pernicious anaemia, poor growth, memory loss, nervous disorders and ataxia. Although requirements do not increase significantly during pregnancy, certain women are at risk of deficiency, including vegetarians, epileptics, those who have recently discontinued the contraceptive pill, and women with tapeworms. Neurological damage in the infants of vitamin B_{12}-deficient vegetarian mothers has been reported (Specker, 1994a).

Folic acid

Folic acid, a mineral, works with vitamin B_{12} for the production of erythrocytes; it is also necessary to maintain the nervous system, gastrointestinal tract and leucocytes, is involved in the production of choline and methionine and is essential for development of the fetus. The incidence of neural tube defects is increased when women are deficient in folic acid, both before and during pregnancy. Original research by Smithells *et al.* (1981) and by Laurence *et al.* (1981) highlighted this. Following further investigations by the Medical Research Council in the late 1980s (Wald *et al.*, 1990), the Department of Health (1992) recommended folate/folic acid supplementation for all women prior to conception and also during the first 12 weeks of pregnancy. This should include folic acid supplements of 0.4 mg daily. To prevent recurrence of neural tube defects the dose of folic acid supplements should be increased to 4–5 mg daily. Clark and Fisk (1994) found that there seems to be minimal compliance with this advice. Czeizei (1995) suggests that folate supplementation may also reduce the incidence of other major congenital malformations, such as in the cardiovascular system and urinary tract, as well as limb abnormalities and congenital hypertrophic pyloric stenosis. In the mother, folic acid deficiency can lead to some anaemias, depression, nervousness, cell and tissue disruptions and premature greying or loss of hair.

Food sources of folic acid include leafy greens, whole grains, nuts, oranges, broccoli, tuna, liver and kidney, but impaired absorption and utilization may occur if the woman is stressed, drinks alcohol, has recently discontinued the contraceptive pill, or is taking certain drugs such as aspirin, sulphonamides or anticonvulsants.

Vitamin C

Vitamin C is important for cell, tissue, nerve, tooth and bone health, wound healing, metabolism of amino acids, and to facilitate iron absorption. It is readily available in all citrus fruits, berries, melons, tomatoes, potatoes, parsley, green vegetables (although cooking will destroy it) and blackcurrants. Inadequate levels of vitamin C can lead to bacterial infections, bruising, oedema, haemorrhage, anaemia, poor digestion, tooth and gum disease and scurvy. Certain drugs, especially aspirin, anticoagulants, antibiotics, diuretics, cortisone, the contraceptive pill and antidepressants, can interfere with absorption, as can also pollution, industrial toxins and overcooking or poor storage of food sources. It is possible that pregnant women with low vitamin C levels, who are consequently at greater risk of infection, may also be more prone to prelabour rupture of the membranes (Casanueva *et al.*, 1991).

Vitamin D

Vitamin D helps calcium absorption and is essential for healthy bones and teeth, for the renal, cardiac and nervous systems and for blood clotting. The main source of vitamin D is the sunshine, so women who are longstay antenatal inpatients should be given the opportunity to sit outside as much as possible. It is also found in fish liver oils, liver, brewer's yeast, tuna and avocados. Drugs such as laxatives and antacids inhibit absorption so care must be taken not to overuse these for women with physiological constipation or heartburn. The mother and fetus both require additional vitamin D to prevent skeletal malformations, rickets, osteoporosis, poor muscle tone, and reduced function of the kidneys and parathyroid glands.

Specker (1994b) states that poor maternal vitamin D levels result in low breast milk levels of vitamin D, but where babies are exposed to sunshine regularly this should not be a problem. Routine vitamin D supplementation during pregnancy is not advocated, although it is postulated that women at risk of deficiency include those who avoid dairy products, or who live in northern latitudes where sunshine exposure is more limited. Specker also suggests that, theoretically, dark-skinned women are more prone to vitamin D deficiency, especially if they are new immigrants.

Vitamin E

Vitamin E, an antioxidant, is required to maintain erythrocytes, and for major bodily functions, including reproduction. It assists in retarding ageing, and helps the body to respond to stress. Whole grains, eggs, leafy greens, avocados, broccoli, cabbage, nuts, liver, kidneys and cold-pressed vegetable oils contain vitamin E, but it is destroyed by food processing, rancid fats and oils and by inorganic iron. Absorption is adversely affected by mineral oil, the contraceptive pill, chlorine and thyroid hormone. Requirements for vitamin E increase during pregnancy: indeed, what was originally called vitamin E is now known to be a group of compounds called tocopherols, a name derived from two Greek words *tocos* (childbirth) and *pheros* (to bring forth), due to the finding that animals deficient in vitamin E were unable to attain successful pregnancies. In humans deficiencies are known to result in spontaneous abortion, preterm labour and stillbirths, as well as possible anaemia and muscular or cardiovascular diseases (Davies and Stewart, 1987: 39; Kamen and Fraley, 1987).

Calcium

Calcium is necessary for the formation of bones and teeth; it helps to utilize iron, aids coagulation and regulates cardiac rhythm. It is found in milk and milk products such as yogurt, egg yolk, sardines and salmon with bones, green beans, bone marrow, tofu and soybeans. High protein or high phosphorus diets will antagonize absorption, as will either an excess or a deficit of physical activity, or stress. Drugs which affect absorption or utilization of calcium include antacids, laxatives, diuretics and anticonvulsants. Deficiencies may lead to bone disorders such as osteoporosis or osteoarthritis, dental problems, palpitations, hypertension, insomnia or muscle cramps.

Canadian research by Marcoux *et al.* (1990) suggests that dietary calcium intake during pregnancy may be inversely related to the risk of gestational hypertension, which supported the earlier findings of Lopez-Jaramillo *et al.* (1989; Lopez-Jaramillo and De Felix, 1991). Calcium supplementation during pregnancy is also considered to be of potential value in reducing the incidence of preterm delivery in high-risk groups, although Villar and Repke (1990) recognize the need for further research. However, Prentice (1994) advocates further research to determine exactly what advice should be given to pregnant women regarding calcium intakes, and points out that, while calcium intakes vary considerably around the world, no specific conditions associated with calcium deficiency have been demonstrated.

Zinc

Zinc is possibly the most important mineral for a successful outcome to pregnancy. It is necessary for cell development in the brain, thyroid gland, liver, kidneys, lungs and prostate gland, as well as normal skeletal growth, skin, hair and the repair of body tissues. Zinc is needed for metabolism of proteins and carbohydrates and of phosphorus; it also facilitates the release of stored vitamin A.

A typical list of foods containing zinc always commences with oysters, which have the highest level, but they are probably an impractical source of dietary zinc for most pregnant women. Zinc is also found in herrings, liver, eggs, milk, bones (fish or meat), nuts, whole grains, mushrooms, leafy green vegetables and paprika.

Zinc requirements rise by approximately 30% during pregnancy, to provide for the development of the fetal central nervous system, and by 40% in lactating women (Kamen and Fraley, 1987: 33). This is quoted as being anything from 15 mg daily in pregnancy (Quillman, 1994: 234) to 200 mg during lactation (Sharon, 1989: 65), but is generally thought to be about 20 mg throughout the childbearing period. Absorption is enhanced by adequate intakes of calcium, copper, vitamins A, B_6, B_{12} and C and certain amino acids. On the other hand, absorption and utilization is antagonized by alcohol, unleavened bread, processed grains, the contraceptive pill, and by excess levels of phytates and calcium. Zinc neutralizes the toxic effects of cadmium, a contributory factor in hypertension, but high levels of cadmium will inhibit the action of zinc (Sharon, 1989: 64). It is thought that excessive sweating can cause a loss of up to 3 mg of zinc per day (Sharon, 1989: 65).

Inadequate zinc levels can lead to retarded growth and mental development, delayed sexual maturity or sterility (normal semen contains large quantities of zinc), slow healing of wounds, fatigue and impaired alertness. It is reportedly also responsible for striae gravidarum. Women who are zinc deficient may have white spots on their fingernails and experience a metallic taste in the mouth. There is a risk of poor outcomes to pregnancy when mothers take in less than 6 mg daily, including low-birthweight, preterm and very preterm delivery (Scholl *et al.*, 1993) and impaired infant immune systems (Davies and Stewart, 1987: 68). The value of zinc supplements in pregnancy is still debatable, especially as it is known that gestational factors alter considerably the metabolism of zinc (Aggett, 1989). Indeed, Mahomed *et al.* (1989) found no significant maternal or fetal differences between women given supplements and those who received no additional zinc.

Iron

Iron, which is required for the manufacture of haemoglobin for oxygenation of the blood, is also important in protein metabolism, bone growth, resistance to disease and in preventing fatigue. However, although iron requirements increase during pregnancy, delivery and lactation, less emphasis is placed on routine supplementation than previously, with most authorities believing that it is an unnecessary and expensive, outmoded practice (Steer *et al.*, 1995). An inadequate iron level will lead to anaemia, fatigue, headache, palpitations and heartburn and supplementation will be required to treat iron-deficiency anaemia.

Dietary iron consumption will normally achieve sufficient serum levels of iron, although a high zinc intake, tea, coffee, intestinal parasites, antacids and tetracycline will interfere with absorption. Women who consume adequate amounts of foods containing vitamins C, E, B_6, B_{12}, folic acid, calcium, copper and other trace elements will normally be able to utilize efficiently the iron from dietary intake. Iron is found in red meats, whole grains, potatoes, eggs, leafy green vegetables, dried fruits, seaweed, nuts and cherries.

Various other trace elements are required during pregnancy, but, as with all other dietary needs, they can be obtained from eating a well-balanced diet.

The Good Food Guide

Following publication of the *Health of the Nation* White Paper (DOH, 1992), the Nutrition Task Force was established by the government to implement the nutritional targets in the White Paper. One of the many recommendations made by the Task Force is that there should be a nutritional component in the training of all health care professionals which should be based on a core curriculum.

The overall advice for good nutrition is to eat less fatty foods and more starchy foods and fruit and vegetables. Foods are divided into five main groups as follows:

▶ Bread, other cereals and potatoes.
▶ Fruit and vegetables.
▶ Milk and dairy foods.
▶ Meat and fish.
▶ Fatty and sugary foods.

Figure 1 illustrates the good food guide. The biggest section at the base of the figure represents the recommended increased consumption of bread, cereals and

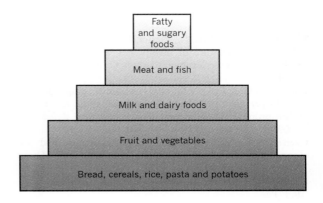

Figure 1 The 'good food guide', showing the five main groups of food.

potatoes, whereas the small section at the top indicates the need to reduce fats, in particular. This advice applies to women in pregnancy as well as the rest of the population, and should be included in health education so that both the woman and her family enjoy the benefits of good nutrition.

Conclusion

Adequate nutrition during pregnancy and lactation is vital for the continued good health of the mother and the fetus. This chapter has discussed the needs of normal women and no mention has been made of the special requirements of some mothers, for example, diabetics. Midwives should have a basic knowledge of the main dietary needs of mothers, and be able to advise women accordingly. However, it is also important that midwives are able to identify those women more at risk of poor nutrition, so that they can be referred to a specialist dietician for the most appropriate information.

References

Aaronson, L.S. & Macnee, C.L. (1989) The relationship between weight gain and nutrition in pregnancy. *Nursing Res.* 38(4): 223–227.

Aggett, P.J. (1989) Extra zinc in pregnancy. *Contemp. Rev. Obstet. Gynaecol.* 1(3): 181–189.

Anderson, A.S., Campbell, D. & Shepherd, R. (1993) Nutrition knowledge, attitude to healthier eating and dietary intake in pregnant compared to non-pregnant women. *J. Human Nutr. Dietetics* 6(4): 335–353.

Athar, S. (1990) Medical aspects of Islamic fasting. *Midwives Chronicle* 103(1227): 106.

Barker, D.J. (1993) Maternal nutrition and cardiovascular disease. *Nutr. Health* 9(2): 99–106.

Bruce, L. & Tchabo, J-G. (1989) Nutrition intervention

program in a prenatal clinic. *Obstet. Gynaecol.* **74**(3): 310–312.

Casanueva, E., Magana, L., Pfeffer, F. *et al.* (1991) Incidence of premature rupture of membranes in pregnant women with low leucocyte levels of vitamin C. *Eur. J. Clin. Nutr.* **45**: 401–405.

Clark, N.A.C. & Fisk, N.M. (1994) Minimal compliance with the Department of Health recommendation for routine folate prophylaxis to prevent fetal neural tube defects. *Br. J. Obstet. Gynaecol.* **101**(8): 709–710.

Czeizei, A.E. (1995) Nutritional supplementation and prevention of congenital abnormalities. *Curr. Opin. Obstet. Gynecol.* **7**(2): 88–94.

Davies, S. & Stewart, A. (1987) *Nutritional Medicine.* London: Pan.

Dewey, K.G. & McCrory, M.A. (1994) Effects of dieting and physical activity on pregnancy and lactation. *Am. J. Clin. Nutr.* **59**(2): 446–453.

DHSS (Department of Health and Social Security) (1990) *Vitamin A and Pregnancy.* PL/CMO (90) 11/PL/CNO (90) 10. London: DHSS.

DOH (Department of Health) (1992) *The Health of the Nation. A Strategy for Health in England.* London: HMSO.

DOH (1993) *The Health of the Nation. One Year on . . . A Report on the Progress of the Health of the Nation.* London: HMSO.

Giotta, M.P. (1993) Nutrition during pregnancy: reducing obstetric risk. *J. Perinatal Neonatal Nursing* **6**(4): 1–12.

Godfrey, K.M., Forrester, T., Barker, D.J. *et al.* (1994) Maternal nutrition status in pregnancy and blood pressure in childhood. *Br. J. Obstet. Gynaecol.* **101**(5): 398–403.

Gray, J. (1994) Maternal nutrition, fetal environment and adult disease. *Modern Midwife* **4**(8): 13–16.

Hachey, D.L. (1994) Benefits and risks of modifying maternal fat intake in pregnancy and lactation. *Am. J. Clin. Nutr.* **59**(2): 454–464.

Herrera, J.A. (1993) Nutritional factors and rest reduce pregnancy-induced hypertension and pre-eclampsia in positive roll-over test primigravidae. *Int. J. Gynecol. Obstet.* **41**(1): 31–35.

Hytten, F. (1990) Nutritional requirements in pregnancy. What happens if they are not met? *Midwifery* **6**(3): 140–145.

Kamen & Fraley (1987) *Nutrition in Nursing: the New Approach.* New Canaan, Connecticut: Keats Publishing.

Kaplan, M., Eidelman, A.I. & Aboulafia (1983) Fasting and the precipitation of labour: the Yom Kippur effect. *JAMA* **250**: 1317.

King, J.C., Butte, N.F., Bronstein, M.N. *et al.* (1994) Energy metabolism during pregnancy: influence of maternal energy status. *Am. J. Clin. Nutr.* **59**(2): 439–445.

Knuppel, R.A. & Drukker, J.E. (1993) *High Risk Pregnancy. A Team Approach,* 2nd edn. Philadelphia, WB Saunders & Co.

Kramer, M.S. (1993) Effects of energy and protein intakes on pregnancy outcome: an overview of the research evidence from controlled clinical trials. *Am. J. Clin. Nutr.* **58**(5): 627–635.

Laurence, K.M., James, N., Miller, M.H., Tennant, G.B. & Campbell, H. (1981) Double-blind randomised controlled trial of folate treatment before conception to prevent recurrence of neural tube defects. *Br. Med. J.* **282**: 1509–1511.

Lopez-Jaramillo, P. & De Felix, M. (1991) Prevention of toxaemia of pregnancy in Ecuadorian Andean women: experience with dietary calcium supplementation. *Bull. Pan Am. Health Organization* **25**(2): 109–117.

Lopez-Jaramillo, P., Naravaez, M. & Weigel, R.M. (1989) Calcium supplementation reduces the risk of pregnancy-induced hypertension in an Andean population. *Br. J. Obstet. Gynaecol.* **96**(6): 648–655.

Luke, B. (1994) Nutrition during pregnancy. *Curr. Opin. Obstet. Gynaecol.* **6**(5): 402–407.

Maher, J.E., Goldenberg, R.L., Tamura, T. *et al.* (1993) Indicators of maternal nutritional status and birth weight in term deliveries. *Obstet. Gynecol.* **81**(2): 165–169.

Mahomed, K., James, D.K., Golding, J. *et al.* (1989) Zinc supplementation during pregnancy: a double blind randomised controlled trial. *Br. Med. J.* **299**(6703): 826–830.

Marcoux, S., Brisson, J. & Fabia, J. (1990) Calcium intake from dairy products and supplements and the risks of pre-eclampsia and gestational hypertension. *Am. J. Epidemiol.* **133**(12): 1266–1272.

Mulliner, C.M., Spiby, H. & Fraser, R.B. (1995) A study exploring midwives' education in, knowledge of and attitudes to nutrition in pregnancy. *Midwifery* **11**(1): 37–41.

Odent, M. (1994) Fetal growth and the future of midwifery. *MIDIRS Midwifery Digest* **4**(1): 27–30.

Prentice, A. (1994) Maternal calcium requirements during pregnancy and lactation. *Am. J. Clin. Nutr.* **59**(2): 477–483.

Quillman, S. (1994) *Nutrition and Diet Therapy.* Pennsylvania: Springhouse Corporation.

Rahman, M., Roy, S.K., Ali, M. *et al.* (1993) Maternal nutrition status as a determinant of child health. *J. Tropical Pediat.* **39**(2): 86–88.

Ranjan, V. (1991) Vitamin A and birth defects. *Professional Care of Mother and Child* **1**(1): 3–4.

Reeves, J. (1992) Pregnancy and fasting during Ramadan. *Br. Med. J.* **304**(6830): 843–844.

Rush, D. (1989) Effects of changes in protein and calorie intake during pregnancy on the growth of the human fetus. In: Chalmers, I., Enkin, M. & Keirse, M.J. (eds) (1989) *Effective Care in Pregnancy and Childbirth.* Oxford: Oxford University Press, pp. 255–280.

Scholl, T.O., Hediger, M.L., Schall, J.I. *et al.* (1993) Low zinc intake during pregnancy: its association with very preterm and preterm delivery. Abstract of paper presented at 5th Annual Meeting of Society for Pediatric Epidemiologic Research, Minneapolis, 1992. *Paediat. Perinatal Epidemiol.* **7**(1): A2.

Sharon, M. (1989) *Complete Nutrition.* London: Prion.

Shiffman, R.L., Tejana, N., Verma, U. & McNerney, R. (1989) Effect of dietary protein on glomerular filtration rate in pregnancy. *Obstet. Gynecol.* **73**(1): 47–51.

Silverton, L. (1993) *The Art and Science of Midwifery.* London: Prentice Hall.

Smithells, R.W., Sheppard, S., Schorar, C.J., Sellar, M.J., Nevin, N.C., Harris, R., Read, A.P. & Fielding, D.W. (1981) Apparent prevention of neural tube defects by periconceptual vitamin supplementation. *Arch. Dis. Childh.* **56**: 911–918.

Specker, B.L. (1994a) Nutritional concerns of lactating women consuming vegetarian diets. *Am. J. Clin. Nutr.* **59**(4): 1182–1186.

Specker, B.L. (1994b) Do North American women need supplemental vitamin D during pregnancy or lactation? *Am. J. Clin. Nutr.* **59**(2): 484–491.

Steer, P., Alam, M.A., Wadsworth, J. *et al.* (1995) Relationship between maternal haemoglobin concentration and birth weight in different ethnic groups. *Br. Med. J.* **310**(6978): 489–491.

Sujitor, C.W. (1994) Nutritional assessment of the pregnant woman. *Clin. Obstet. Gynecol.* **37**(3): 501–514.

Susser, M. (1991) Maternal weight gain, infant birth weight and diet: causal sequences 1.2. *Am. J. Clin. Nutr.* **53**(6): 1384–1396.

Villar, J. & Repke, J.T. (1990) Calcium supplementation during pregnancy may reduce preterm delivery in high risk populations. *Am. J. Obstet. Gynecol.* **163**(4, part 1): 1124–1131.

Villar, J., Cogswell, M., Kestler, E. *et al.* (1992) Effect of fat and fat-free mass deposition during pregnancy on birthweight. *Am. J. Obstet. Gynecol.* **167**(5): 1344–1352.

Wald, N., Sneddon, J., Densem, J., Frost, C. & Stone, R. (1991) Prevention of neural tube defects: Results of the Medical Research Council vitamin study. *Lancet* **338**: 1331–1337.

Wilkin, T.J. (1993) Early nutrition and diabetes mellitus. *Br. Med. J.* **306**(6873): 283–284.

Wynn, M. & Wynn, A. (1981) *The Prevention of Handicap of Early Pregnancy*. London: Foundation for Education and Research in Childbearing.

17

Confirming Pregnancy

Pregnancy may be suspected by the woman based on her knowledge of her menstrual cycle, sexual activity and the signs and symptoms of pregnancy. As routine pregnancy testing may not be available from the general practitioner or in many NHS trusts, women may confirm their pregnancy using a home pregnancy test. Confirmation of pregnancy may also be sought from the midwife or doctor. This would be established by a detailed history and relevant clinical examination based on the signs and symptoms of pregnancy.

Signs and Symptoms of Pregnancy

The signs and symptoms of pregnancy are:

▶ Amenorrhoea.
▶ Breast changes.
▶ Nausea and vomiting.
▶ Increased frequency of micturition.
▶ Enlargement of the uterus.
▶ Skin changes.
▶ Quickening.

They appear in chronological order, as shown below.

First four weeks
Amenorrhoea Following implantation of the fertilized ovum, the endometrium undergoes decidual change and menstruation does not occur throughout pregnancy. Amenorrhoea almost invariably accompanies pregnancy and, in a sexually active woman who has previously menstruated regularly, should be considered to be due to pregnancy unless this is disproved.

Breast changes Discomfort, tingling and a feeling of fullness of the breasts may be noticed as early as the third or fourth week of pregnancy.

Nausea and vomiting This occurs in about 70% of pregnant women (Weigel and Weigel, 1989). Those affected may feel nauseated and/or vomit in the morning or at other times in the day.

Around eight weeks
Nausea and vomiting usually persists in those women who are affected.

Frequency of micturition   Frequency of micturition increases due to pressure from the enlarging uterus and increased vascularity of the bladder.

Breast changes   The breasts enlarge and the superficial veins on both the chest and breasts dilate. The enlarged breasts may be painful.

Around 12 weeks
Nausea and vomiting decrease and may now cease altogether.

Enlarged uterus   At 12 weeks the enlarged uterus is just palpable above the symphysis pubis.

Skin changes   Pigmentation of the skin occurs and is especially pronounced in brunettes. Areas of pigmentation include the nipples and areola, the linea nigra and, rarely, the chloasma. The nipples become more prominent and Montgomery's tubercles are visible on the areola.

Around 16 weeks
Nausea and vomiting have normally ceased.

Pressure on the bladder is relieved because the enlarging uterus has risen out of the pelvis. The fundus of the uterus is midway between the upper border of the symphysis pubis and the umbilicus.

The breasts start to secrete a little clear fluid called colostrum. This persists throughout pregnancy and for the first three days after delivery until milk is produced. A secondary areola may appear in brunettes.

Quickening   The first fetal movements may be felt by primigravidae at 19+ weeks and by multigravidae at 17+ weeks. The time scale of fetal movements felt by the mother ranges from 15 to 22 weeks in primigravidae and 14–22 weeks in multigravidae (O'Dowd and O'Dowd, 1985). Quickening is an unreliable indicator of gestational age.

Around 20 weeks
The secondary areola, if not already present, may appear.

The fundus of the uterus is just below the umbilicus.

Around 24 weeks
The fundus is just above the umbilicus.

Fetal parts and movements may be felt on abdominal palpation.

Fetal heart sounds may be heard with a fetal stethoscope.

At 24 weeks the fetus is considered to be capable of an independent existence.

From 28 to 40 weeks
The fundus continues to rise until at 36 weeks it reaches the xiphisternum and remains at that level until the fetal head engages. This may be accompanied by Braxton Hicks contractions. When engagement occurs the fundus descends slightly and the relief of pressure the mother experiences is called *lightening*. It may not occur in multigravidae as the head often does not engage until labour is established. With lightening the mother may breathe with more comfort but the descent of the head may cause pressure on the bladder resulting in increased frequency of micturition.

EXAMINATION PER VAGINAM

It is not now usual practice to make a vaginal examination in early pregnancy, but if an examination is made the following signs of pregnancy may be observed:

1   The *softening* of the vagina and cervix is noted. This softness, together with the elongated isthmus, makes it possible to elicit Hegar's sign between 6 and 10 weeks. On bimanual examination, the fingers in the anterior fornix and those on the abdomen almost seem to meet because the isthmus is impalpable in contrast to the enlarged upper uterine segment and the cervix.

2   *Pulsation* of the uterine arteries through the lateral fornices can be detected. This is called Osiander's sign.

3   The *lilac discolouration* of the vagina and cervix is observed. This is due to increased vascularity and is known as Jacquemier's sign.

4   *Enlargement* of the uterus is noted and compared with the period of gestation.

5   *Internal ballottement* may be elicited from 16 weeks. With two fingers in the anterior fornix the uterus is given a sharp tap. The fetus is pushed upwards and a slight impact on the fingers may be felt when the fetus returns to its original position.

6   *Braxton Hicks* contractions may be palpated from about 16 weeks. These are painless irregular uterine contractions which persist until the end of

pregnancy. A cervical smear may be performed at the same time as a vaginal examination.

POSITIVE SIGNS OF PREGNANCY

The positive signs of pregnancy are:

1 *Fetal heart sounds* may be detected at 10 weeks using Sonicaid ultrasonic equipment. At 24 weeks' gestation these sounds can be heard with the Pinard's fetal stethoscope.
2 *Fetal movements* felt by the examiner.
3 Palpation of *fetal parts*.
4 *Radiology* would show the fetal skeleton at 14–16 weeks. X-Rays should be avoided, however, as irradiation can damage the developing fetus.
5 *Ultrasonography*. A gestational sac may be visualized at 5 weeks. At 6 weeks the fetal heart may be seen pulsating, using abdominal ultrasound. Vaginal ultrasound scanning may detect these a week earlier (Chudleigh and Pearce, 1994). A viable intrauterine pregnancy is confirmed when fetal heart pulsations can be seen in the gestational sac in the uterus.

Laboratory Diagnosis of Pregnancy

Chorionic tissue which later forms the placenta starts producing a hormone, chorionic gonadotrophin (hCG), which is excreted in the urine. This hormone is usually detected in the urine within a week of the first missed period. Immunological tests depend on the detection of human chorionic gonadotrophin in the urine. Pregnancy tests are positive if 50 IU/1 hCG are detected in urine (Wasley 1988).

Home pregnancy tests have a 99% accuracy rate, take 3–5 minutes to obtain a result and are easy to use. Women are increasingly using these to confirm pregnancy in the privacy of their own homes. The market for home pregnancy tests reached £15.25 million in 1994 (Anon., 1995). The average cost is £10 for two tests. Following confirmation of pregnancy women need to contact their midwife or doctor to commence their antenatal care.

HOME OVULATION PREDICTION TESTS

Women who are planning a pregnancy may wish to use a home ovulation kit to identify the most fertile time in their menstrual cycle. Ovulation usually occurs within 72 hours of the peak of luteinizing hormone (LH) in the menstrual cycle; this is the most likely time for a pregnancy to occur. LH is produced by the pituitary gland and peaks at around day 14 in a 28-day menstrual cycle. The presence of LH may be detected in urine by using an ovulation detection kit, the dipstick changing colour if LH is present. Home ovulation kits are now available with folic acid supplements. Ideally these should be used with advice about preconception care and folic acid supplements for the first 12 weeks of pregnancy (DOH, 1992).

IMMUNOLOGICAL TESTS

Immunological pregnancy testing depends on the fact that human chorionic gonadotrophin has antigenic properties. If tanned red cells or latex particles are coated with human chorionic gonadotrophin and then exposed to the corresponding antigen they agglutinate. However, if the antiserum is added to urine containing the chorionic gonadotrophin before the sensitized cells are added, agglutination does not take place as the urine and antiserum have already reacted. In the test therefore:

1 antiserum is added to the woman's urine;
2 sensitized red cells or latex particles are added.

If agglutination does not occur, gonadotrophin is present and the test is positive. The procedures and reactions are summarized in Table 1.

Tests using latex-coated particles and a drop of urine can be read in 2 minutes. Tests using tanned red cells give a result in two hours. Both false positives and false negatives can occur. The most commonly used test in hospital laboratories now is the Hybritech test which is 99.5–99.8% accurate.

Table 1 Immunological test for pregnancy

Pregnant	Not pregnant
hCG antiserum added to urine containing hCG	hCG antiserum added to urine without hCG
↓	↓
hCG antibodies neutralized	hCG antibodies *not* neutralized
↓	↓
Add	Add
red cells or latex particles covered with hCG	red cells or latex particles covered with hCG
↓	↓
No agglutination	*Agglutination*

Differential Diagnosis of Pregnancy

Some of the pregnancy symptoms may be found in other conditions not associated with pregnancy.

Amenorrhoea

A change of environment, emotional disturbance or general illness such as tuberculosis and thyrotoxicosis can cause amenorrhoea. Hyperprolactinaemia is another cause of amenorrhoea. Amenorrhoea occurring around the menopause or after discontinuing the contraceptive pill can cause difficulties in diagnosis.

Vomiting

Vomiting may occur in a variety of conditions. It may occur in gastroenteritis or it may be a prominent feature in urinary tract infection.

Enlarged abdomen

Tumours such as ovarian cysts or fibroids and ascites may be mistaken for a pregnant uterus. Obesity may make the diagnosis of pregnancy difficult.

Fetal movements

Flatulence may be mistaken for fetal movements.

PSEUDOCYESIS

This is a phantom or false pregnancy. It may occur in women with an intense desire to become pregnant. Amenorrhoea will be present. The woman will complain of all the subjective symptoms of pregnancy, usually in a bizarre order; the abdomen may be distended and the breasts may secrete a cloudy liquid. However, she is not pregnant. The signs on which a certain diagnosis of pregnancy can be made, namely palpation of the fetus or hearing the fetal heart, are not present. Referral to a psychologist or psychiatrist may be required.

References

Anon. (1995) Diagnostic testing. Add value to grow business. *Independent Community Pharmacist* March: 24.

Chudleigh, P. & Pearce, M. (1994) *Obstetric Ultrasound*, 2nd edn. Edinburgh: Churchill Livingstone.

DOH (Department of Health) (1992) *Folic Acid and the Prevention of Neural Tube Defects*. Report from the Expert Advisory Group. London: HMSO.

O'Dowd, M. & O'Dowd, T. (1985) Quickening – a re-evaluation. *Br. J. Obstet. Gynaecol.* 92: 1037–1039.

Wasley, G. (1988) Urinary pregnancy testing. *Nursing Times* 84(36): 42–43.

Weigel, M. & Weigel, R. (1989) Nausea and vomiting of early pregnancy and pregnancy outcome. An epidemiological study. *Br. J. Obstet. Gynaecol.* 96: 1304–1311.

18

Choices and Patterns of Care

The following statements are taken from the list of recommendations and conclusions of the Health Committee review of the maternity services chaired by Sir Nicholas Winterton (House of Commons, 1992: vol. 1, p. xciv):

> Given the absence of conclusive evidence, it is no longer acceptable that the pattern of maternity care provision should be driven by presumptions about the applicability of a medical model of care based on unproved assumptions (para 43).
>
> We conclude that there is a *strong desire among women for the provision of continuity of care and carer* throughout pregnancy and childbirth, and that the majority of them regard midwives as the group best placed and equipped to provide this (para 49).
>
> We conclude that there is a widespread *demand among women for greater choice* in the type of maternity care they receive, and that the present structure of the maternity services frustrates, rather than facilitates, those who wish to exercise this choice (para 52).

A recent account of one woman's experience of the care received in the National Health Service on becoming pregnant led her to 'opt out' of the system and to seek the services of independently practising midwives (Taylor, 1994). She was fortunate enough to be able to choose who looked after her and decide the type of care she wanted and remain in control of the situation. But this can happen within the NHS as illustrated by Belbin (1996) in her account of her experience where she had choice and control within the NHS. However, for the majority of women there is limited choice. Many are satisfied with the care received, but it is clear that for a large number of women there continues to be problems relating to:

▶ who controls childbirth;
▶ who the main providers of care should be; and
▶ how and when care is delivered.

These issues give rise to heated debate as was experienced by the health committee when receiving evidence on the Maternity Services (House of Commons, 1992). The Winterton Report concentrated on 'how the NHS provides for healthy women giving birth to healthy normal children' and the above statements are taken from the list of recommendations and conclusions. So why are there such problems today?

This chapter will put the present and future situation regarding aspects of care into context by briefly reflecting upon how the main developments in the maternity services have affected and led to the current patterns of care and how they have affected those who are the receivers and providers of care at present and in the future.

The patterns of care in existence today have been greatly influenced by those who believe that pregnancy is an illness (Comaroff, 1977), that birth is only normal in retrospect, and subscribe to the view that the only way forward is to actively manage and control childbirth (Beazley, 1975; O'Driscoll and Meagher, 1993). It is considered a potentially dangerous occurrence and controlling the process concentrates on the physical aspects. This is often referred to as the 'medical model' of care, which many believe supports a continuation of a task-orientated approach to care. Before concentrating on recent developments it might be relevant to review briefly the reasons leading up to the current provision of care.

Historical Review of Midwifery Care

There is no doubt that the current complexities surrounding the organization of care are inextricably linked to the changing place of birth. Oakley (1980) in her book *Women Confined* points out that birth is a biological event taking place within a social world and how society defines reproduction is closely linked with the position of women within society. She claims that the change from female control within the community to male control in hospital was brought about by false claims that male practitioners created safer childbirth. There are a number of histories giving alternative accounts of what care was like, the place of women, perceptions of childbirth, how midwives worked and the rivalries that developed (Oakley, 1976; Cowell and Wainwright, 1981; Towler and Bramall, 1986; Donnison, 1988). The following is a very brief résumé and readers are asked to refer to these and other accounts in order to get a balanced in-depth view.

In pre-industrial society midwifery skills were learnt in practice with other women and passed on within families. There were some formal training programmes but these were expensive. Midwives attended women in their own homes and many were highly respected within society, being responsible for all aspects of childbirth. Care though was variable and depended upon the individual midwife, her values and

circumstances. The rich had the ability to choose a midwife, whilst others were very much at the mercy of sometimes disreputable handywomen/midwives.

From the fourteenth to seventeenth centuries in Europe, medicine emerged as a predominantly male professional discipline and the role of the female lay healer was suppressed. Men played only an occasional role in midwifery, when called in for difficult deliveries. By the eighteenth century men had greatly enhanced their status by the use of forceps (available by the 1720s) irrespective of their competence. In the nineteenth and twentieth centuries the female control of reproduction, which had largely persisted despite the rise of male medicine, was eroded with the inclusion of obstetrics in the curricula of professional medical training (Oakley, 1976: 23). According to Oakley (1976: 41) it was the 'Movement for Infant and Maternal Welfare' that created the final takeover in childbirth, with attention being addressed to the physical state of women as the reason for high infant mortality, rather than poor social conditions. Funds for building maternity hospitals were forthcoming (Versluysen, 1981) and the move towards hospitalization progressed. In the publications of the 'lying-in' hospitals it is clear that the process of birth had started to become a medical procedure.

An account of other policy developments at this time are included in the Winterton Report (House of Commons, 1992) and include the extra provision of clinics and beds. By 1936 the provision of a salaried domiciliary midwifery service by local authorities became compulsory. With the introduction of government-funded maternity care, differences of opinion arose as to how it should be organized; should it be midwifery-based for normal births, who should manage childbirth – obstetricians or GPs? (Figure 1).

Meanwhile the percentage of births taking place in institutions continued to rise, based on the premise of safety, from 'one per cent prior to the first world war to fifteen per cent in 1927, 24 per cent in 1933, 54 per cent in 1946, 64 per cent in 1952 and by 1968 80 per

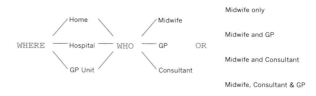

Figure 1 Complexities of the organization of care.

cent' (Campbell and Macfarlane, 1987). A national survey of midwifery practice by the English National Board (1994) put the figure at 98.7% in 1991–92.

Effect of the NHS on Midwifery Care

The National Health Service Act 1946 contributed significantly to the move to hospital and with the introduction of new technologies, medicalization of childbirth became the norm, with many procedures being introduced without systematic evaluation of their effectiveness (Oakley, 1979: 18), creating, in some instances, physical trauma and great discomfort. Emotional and social distress were products of the new childbirth and were largely neglected by many obstetricians, GPs and midwives. Various government enquiries criticized how the maternity services were administered (Ministry of Health, 1955, 1959), leading to an uncoordinated, fragmented system, with duplication and lack of continuity of care. A review of the maternity services in 1970 (DHSS Welsh Office, 1970) also reported a lack of continuity of care, duplication of roles and recommended unification of the maternity services, a multidisciplinary team approach to care and 100% hospital confinement, the latter based on no reliable evidence that this was the best or even the safest place. Hospitals became synonymous with patients and illness and therefore pregnancy became something to be treated and cured rather than a natural physiological process of great significance through which women need to be supported and assisted.

Although the system of care was more sophisticated, criticisms were made concerning hospital routines, inflexibility and poor attitudes creating a de-humanized service (Standing Maternity and Midwifery Advisory Committee, 1961; DHSS, 1976). Riley (1977: 69) pointed out that there are structural obstacles implicit within hospitals, a rigid hierarchy and division of labour militating against a humane service with continuity of care, but that some women complained of too little intervention, preferring to give control to the professional (Comaroff, 1977; Beech, 1987: 72).

Initially the dissatisfactions of women were dismissed as a 'minority group of middle class women' (Editorial, 1975; Chalmers, 1976), but research has demonstrated that this was not the case (Cartwright, 1979; Oakley, 1979; Garcia, 1982).

This dissatisfaction regarding care and lack of choice led to the formation and strengthening of various groups within the context of the social movements in the 1970s, for example the Association for the Improvement of the Maternity Services (AIMS), the National Childbirth Trust (NCT), the Maternity Alliance and the Society to Support Home Confinements (SSHC). Women were not the only ones to react: some midwives were also dissatisfied with the system, the way in which women were being treated and the erosion of their role, and the Association of Radical Midwives was established. The National Health Service Act 1973 went some way towards integrating the maternity services with one manager co-ordinating community and hospital midwifery; however, in the majority of authorities care remained compartmentalized, with midwives functioning in specific areas developing specialist skills.

With the reduction in mortality rates, removal of the fear of death in childbirth, and the improved socioeconomic situation, mothers and their babies were healthier and having a baby started to be viewed again as a normal physiological process to be enjoyed, not just a medical disorder to be endured (Figure 2). Many women began to speak out about wishing to be consulted and participate in decisions (Rantzen, 1981; Garcia, 1982) and continue to do so (NCT, 1989; House of Commons, 1992).

Choice and involvement in decisions about care and where to give birth became particular issues due to increasing pressure towards hospital confinement, leading to a reduction of community midwifery services, although the Social Services Committee (1980) pointed out that health authorities were required to maintain a community service and help mothers to make an informed choice regarding place of birth (p. 11). This committee established a Maternity Services Advisory Committee to review patterns of care and they set out a framework for maternity care. The recommendations are contained in the *Maternity Care in Action* reports (MSAC, 1982, 1984, 1985). All of the reports commented on the importance of social and psychological support, sensitivity towards a woman's feelings during childbirth as well as her physical needs. They highlight the basis for good care, emphasize flexibility and choice and that good practice involves allowing women to participate in their care, and go on to identify how organizations

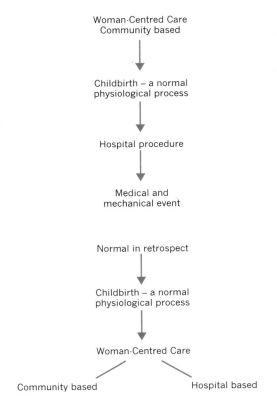

Woman-Centred Care
Community based

↓

Childbirth – a normal
physiological process

↓

Hospital procedure

↓

Medical and
mechanical event

Normal in retrospect

↓

Childbirth – a normal
physiological process

↓

Woman-Centred Care

Community based   Hospital based

Figure 2   The cycle of change in how childbirth has been viewed.

and professionals might achieve any necessary changes. The Government's response to the recent review of the maternity services reinforced the relevance of the reports in providing a framework for maternity care in the 1990s (House of Commons, 1992: 32; DOH, 1993). A working example of good practice is, of course, reflected in the work of independently practising midwives, which is a pattern of working becoming a reality in the NHS with other innovative schemes in existence (MacVicar *et al.*, 1993) and being developed (Stock and Wraight, 1993; Ball, 1993: 184; Page *et al.*, 1994).

A Return to Individualized Care?

The Social Services Committee (1980) made recommendations concerning continuity of care, humanizing the maternity service and called for better organization of care. To redress the balance the 1980s might be referred to as the drive to move from a task-oriented approach to a more individualized approach to care allowing choice, an approach implicit in the 'model/process' movement. Individualized care is not a concept unfamiliar to midwives even working within a task-focused service, the conclusion reached by Metcalf (1981) in her study.

The process of providing effective care in midwifery involves assessing, planning, implementing and evaluating, a problem-solving approach which was the essence of the 'nursing process', criticized by many midwives as an inappropriate approach to care. However models utilizing the 'process' were seen by some as useful in helping to clarify values and beliefs underpinning care (Bryar, 1988), assisting continuity, improving decision-making and enhancing the midwife's autonomy; women are seen as individuals so that care is women-centred. Models are frameworks that provide the link between theory and practice:

> Practice should be based on midwifery theory which, in turn should be based on a sound evaluation of practice.
>
> (Henderson, 1990)

Crucial to the success of individualized care is that the midwife should have a defined caseload, a specific group of women and their babies to whom she gives total care.

During the late 1980s and particularly in the 1990s following the publication of two government reports (House of Commons, 1992; DOH, 1993) many schemes have been introduced by midwives to improve continuity of care and carer. These schemes are based on a philosophy of care which is clearly recorded.

PHILOSOPHY OF CARE

Midwives need to be clear about their underlying beliefs regarding care in order to plan care effectively with women. Bertrand Russell in 1961 wrote: 'Ever since men became capable of free speculation, their actions in innumerable important respects have depended upon their theories as to the world and human life, as to what is good and what is evil.' The implication of these words is that our behaviour is determined by our beliefs about people, life and society. Statements of beliefs and ideologies are used in the health service as the basis for the provision of care, including the type of care, how it is organized, and they reflect the degree to which clients may or may not be involved in the care they receive. It is important for midwives to be involved in the development of these statements to ensure that they are realistic, achievable and appropriate to women's needs and expectations.

Downe *et al.* (1993: 4) argue that statements should reflect consumer expectations and knowledge and should be written accordingly. They use the example of a statement often included in philosophies of care in maternity units: 'The midwife and the mother are equal partners in care'. By implication the midwife and mother both participate in decisions relating to care. However, is there always equality of power in that relationship today? Are mothers allowed real choice and are they able to choose who gives care, what form it takes and where care is undertaken? Is what actually happens in reality in many instances decided by those in control of resources, and in positions of power, with both mothers and midwives failing to influence the process and the outcome?

In order for midwives to be involved in the formulation of such statements, it is important that they have a clear understanding of their own philosophy of care, and the philosophy held by women who use the services. As pointed out by Popkin and Stroll (1988: xvii):

Philosophy makes a person think . . . think about the basic foundation of his/her outlook . . . knowledge . . . beliefs. It makes one inquire into the reasons for what one accepts and does, and into the importance of one's ideas and ideals, in the hope that one's final convictions, whether they remain the same, or whether they change as a result of this examination, will at least be rationally held ones.

Determination of a philosophy of care is important to midwives because it determines the whole basis of practice, the very way in which care is organized and given, and, even more importantly, how professionals view the role of women in determining their care. Views of midwifery, of childbirth, of those receiving care all contribute towards a midwifery framework (model) by which midwives practise and will assist in decision-making. Figure 3 summarizes the influencing factors relating to the organization and type of care that will be given.

Team Midwifery – Is This the Answer?

The most successful forms of care relate to midwives holding commonly held beliefs regarding midwifery and being able to communicate with women in such a way as to know truly their wishes regarding care.

These are perhaps factors that contribute towards successful teams. In many authorities teams of midwives are being established to address the issue of continuity of care. In 1983 Flint (1991) set up the 'Know Your Midwife' (KYM) scheme to look at the feasibility of providing total care by a team of midwives. Four midwives cared for 500 women over a two-year period providing continuity of care. It resulted in fewer interventions, with women feeling higher satisfaction rates and more in control than with normal standard hospital care.

Since that time similar schemes have been set up in other parts of England and Wales and a survey commissioned by the Department of Health in 1991 was undertaken to identify how team midwifery was being implemented (Wraight *et al.*, 1993). However, as this survey reported, a team approach is not always successful in providing continuity, a concern expressed by Bower (1993: 145) and Hobbs (1993: 148) who also puts forward the view that the 'essential nature of midwifery is not in a team', and teams may not be the best way forward. The Royal College of Midwives

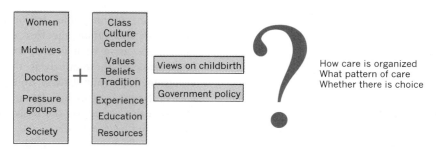

Figure 3   Influences on organization and type of care.

commissioned an in-depth look at continuity of care (Stock and Wraight, 1993), particularly issues of team midwifery in terms of key professional and industrial relations. The conclusions were that there was greater autonomy, better utilization of the skills of midwives, leading to increased satisfaction and higher status. However, working patterns were affected with the need for flexibility and a review of the grading system. Continuity was not always possible and was dependent on the size of the team and hours worked.

In the drive towards a 'women-centred' approach to care, the organizational and cultural changes that are required in some authorities will require a revolution; in others it has been evolving gradually and it is this latter approach that perhaps is more successful because involvement of the key players and careful planning are the key to success involving any change. These points were reiterated by Stock and Wraight (1993: 13–15) in their report. Many examples of good practice are contained within the literature, particularly as a result of the government initiatives following the Health Committee Report on the Maternity Services (House of Commons, 1992) and the report of the Expert Maternity Services Group (DOH, 1993). Ball (1993) reports that there are new patterns of care emerging, to create a more woman-focused system of caring, with two Midwifery Group Practices being introduced in South East Thames and ten in Riverside Health Authority. Page *et al.* (1994) give an account of a one-to-one midwifery service which has been implemented in a part of west London.

The evaluation of caseload and midwifery led schemes may point the way towards how care will be organized but evidence so far indicates that these schemes are more costly (Hundley *et al*, 1995; Spurgeon, 1996).

What Do Women Want?

What many women want is summed up in the following quote from the published proceedings of a forum established to look at choice, continuity of care and change in the maternity services in 1993.

All women want from their maternity care . . . [is] a service that offers safety, that is flexible and responsive to their individual needs, which communicates effectively, and provides the information that allows informed choices . . . a service that is respectful,

personalized . . . kind . . . gives them control . . . having confidence in the care that is being given.

(King's Fund, 1993: 4)

This echoes evidence received by the Health Committee Review on the Maternity Services in 1992, is reflected in the Expert Maternity Group's report *Changing Childbirth* (1993) and in *The Vision*, a document produced by the Association of Radical Midwives in 1986 on the possible future of the maternity services. *Changing Childbirth* is accepted government policy, and is a 'manifesto for change in the way maternity services are to be planned and provided' (DOH, 1993: 71), setting out targets to be achieved, some within the next five years. Ball (1993) identifies some of the problems to be faced if these changes are implemented within an organization being radically altered by the NHS reforms. These are altering the culture of the NHS, with market forces prevailing and jobs and systems are constantly under review. These changes may require moving from a specialist to a multiskilled workforce but care must be taken not to lose those things that are good in the present approach to care, a caution reiterated in *Changing Childbirth* and by Jamieson (1994) in an editorial on midwife empowerment.

Care must also be taken not to overgeneralize when investigating what women want and as Reid (1994) states 'to continue to ask whose voice are we listening to.' How, when and who to consult as users of maternity services was the focus of a series of conferences in 1994, 1995 and the published proceedings give an insight into the experiences of those involved in finding out what women want (Dodds *et al.*, 1996).

Conclusion

Whatever system is introduced the importance of the individual encounter must not be forgotten, a point stressed by Currell (1990) who refers to the most successful kind of care being that where the aim is known and the care is valued.

Sharing information and good communication contribute substantially to women's satisfaction and those providing care have great influence not only during the immediate period but in the future. As Oakley and Houd (1990) write: 'what they [midwives/obstetricians] do, what they say, and how they behave toward her, her baby, and her family may be unforgettable influences on her experience of becoming a mother' (p. 133). They go on to discuss the question 'What is good care?' The answer is that opinions and practices differ. There is evidence that certain practices are beneficial whilst others are harmful (Chalmers *et al.*, 1989). What we must ensure is that care is acceptable, accessible, effective and appropriate, with the woman and her baby at the centre and in as much control as she wishes to be.

In the development of the maternity services, con-stantly recurring themes relating to care have been *control*, *choice* and *continuity*. Today the Government, more than at any other time, is changing the structure and culture of the NHS, and in theory providing midwives and women with an opportunity to choose and significantly affect care. Those who have already taken up the challenge are involving themselves in the processes of purchasing care and are making possible what has seemed to some an impossible dream come true – a truly woman-centred maternity service.

References

Association of Radical Midwives (1986) *The Vision*. Ormskirk, Lancashire: ARM.

Ball, J. (1993) The Winterton Report: difficulties of implementation. *Br. J. Midwifery* 1(4): 183–185.

Beazley, J. (1975) The active management of labour. *Am. J. Obstet. Gynecol.* **122**: 162–168.

Beech, B. (1987) *Who's Having Your Baby?* London: Camden Press.

Belbin, A. (1996) Power and choice in birthgiving: a case study. *Br. J. Midwifery* 4(5): 264–272.

Bower, H. (1993) Team midwifery in Oxford. *MIDIRS Midwifery Digest* 3(2): 143–145.

Bryar, R. (1988) Midwifery and models of care. *Midwifery* 4: 111–117.

Campbell, R. & Macfarlane, J. (1987) *Where to be Born? The Debate and the Evidence*. Oxford: NEPU.

Cartwright, A. (1979) *Dignity of Labour*. London: Tavistock.

Chalmers, I. (1976) British debate on obstetric practice. *Paediatric* 3: 308–312.

Chalmers, I., Enkin, M. & Kierse, M. (eds) (1989) *Effective Care in Pregnancy and Childbirth*. Oxford: Oxford University Press.

Comaroff, J. (1977) Conflicting paradigms of pregnancy. In Davies, A. & Horobin, G. (eds) *Medical Encounters. The Experience of Illness and Treatment*. London: Croom Helm.

Cowell, B. & Wainwright, D. (1981) *Behind the Blue Door*. London: Royal College of Midwives.

Currell, R. (1990) The organisation of midwifery care. In: Alexander, J., Levy, V. & Roch, S. (eds) *Antenatal Care*. London: Macmillan.

Davies, A. & Horobin, G. (eds) *Medical Encounters: The Experience of Illness and Treatment*. London: Croom Helm.

DHSS (Department of Health and Social Security) (1976) *Organisation of the Hospital In-patient's Day*. London: HMSO.

DHSS Welsh Office (1970) *Domiciliary Midwifery and Maternity Bed Needs*. Central Health Services Council. London: HMSO.

Dodds, R., Goodman, M. & Tyler, S. (1996) *Listen with Mother*. Hale: Books for Midwives Press.

DOH (Department of Health) (1993) *Changing Childbirth*, Report of the Expert Maternity Group. London: HMSO.

Donnison, J. (1988) *Midwives and Medical Men: The History of the Struggle for the Control of Childbirth*. London: Historical Publishers.

Downe, S., Henderson, C., Methven, R. & Midgley, C. (1993) *Approaches to Care: Frameworks for Midwifery Practice*. London: Distance Learning Centre, South Bank University.

Editorial (1975) *Br. Med. J.* 539(1).

ENB (English National Board) (1994) *Report of the National Survey of Midwifery Practice 1991–1992*. London: ENB.

Flint, C. (1991) Continuity of care provided by a team of midwives. In Robinson, S. & Thomson, A. (eds) *Midwives, Research and Childbirth*, Vol. 11. London: Chapman & Hall.

Garcia, J. (1982) Women's view of antenatal care. In Enkin, M. & Chalmers, I. (eds) *Effectiveness and Satisfaction in Antenatal Care*. London: Spastics International, Heinemann.

Henderson, C. (1990) Models and midwifery. In Kershaw, B. & Salvage, J. (eds) *Models for Nursing*. London: Scutari Press.

Hobbs, L. (1993) Team midwifery – the other view. *MIDIRS Midwifery Digest* 3(2): 146–147.

House of Commons (1992) *Maternity Services Second Report* (Winterton Report) (Chaired by Sir Nicholas Winterton). London: HMSO.

House of Commons Social Services Committee (1980) *Report on Perinatal and Neonatal Mortality* (Short Report). London: HMSO.

Hundley, V., Donaldson, C., Lang, G. *et al.* (1995) Cost of intrapartum care in a midwife managed delivery unit and a consultant led labour ward. *Midwifery* II: 103–109, 12–18.

Jamieson, L. (1994) Midwife empowerment through education. *Br. J. Midwifery* 2(2): 47–48.

King's Fund (1993) *Maternity Care: Choice, Continuity and Change*. Consensus statement, April, p. 4. London: King's Fund Centre.

MacVicar, J., Dobbie, G., Owen-Johnstone, L. *et al.* (1993) Simulated home delivery in hospital: a randomised controlled trial. *Br. J. Obstet. Gynaecol.* 100: 316–323.

MSAC (Maternity Services Advisory Committee) (1982) *Maternity Care in Action*, Part 1. *Antenatal Care*. London: HMSO.

MSAC (1984) *Maternity Care in Action*, Part II. *Care During Childbirth (Intrapartum Care)*. London: HMSO.

MSAC (1985) *Maternity Care in Action*, Part III. *Care of the Mother and Baby (Postnatal and Neonatal Care)*. London: HMSO.

Metcalf, C. (1981) Patient education on a maternity ward. *Research and the Midwife, Conference Proceedings*, London.

Ministry of Health (1955) *Report of the Committee of Enquiry into the Cost of the NHS* (Guillebaud Report). London: HMSO.

Ministry of Health (1959) *Report of the Maternity Services Committee* (Cranbrook Report). London: HMSO.

NCT (National Childbirth Trust) (1989) *Rupture of the Membranes*. London: NCT.

Oakley, A. (1976) Wisewoman and medicine man: changes in the management of childbirth. In Mitchell, J. & Oakley, A. (eds) *The Rights and Wrongs of Women*. Harmondsworth: Penguin.

Oakley, A. (1979) *From Here to Maternity*. Harmondsworth: Penguin.

Oakley, A. (1980) *Women Confined*. London: Robertson.

Oakley, A. & Houd, S. (1990) *Helpers in Childbirth: Midwifery Today*. New York: WHO, Hemisphere Publishing Corporation.

O'Driscoll, K. & Meagher, D. (1993) *Active Management of Labour*, 3rd edn. London: Wolfe/Mosby.

Page, L., Jones, B., Bentley, R. *et al.* (1994) One-to-one midwifery practice. *Br. J. Mid.* 2(9): 444–447.

Popkin, R.H. & Stroll, A. (1988) *Philosophy Made Simple*. London: Heinemann Nursing.

Rantzen, E. (1981) Questionnaire to mothers. *That's Life* programme. BBC1.

Reid, M. (1994) What are the consumer views of maternity care. In Chamberlain, G. & Patel, N. (eds) *The Future of the Maternity Services*. London: RCOG Press.

Riley, E. (1977) What do women want? The question of choice in the conduct of labour. In Chard, T. & Richards, M. (eds) *Benefits and Hazards of the New Obstetrics*. London: Heinemann Medical.

Social Services Committee (1980) *Perinatal and Neonatal Mortality* (Second Report). London: HMSO.

Spurgeon, P. (1996) *Changing Childbirth: Pilot Project Evaluation Report* (unpublished). University of Birmingham: Health Services Management Centre.

Standing Maternity and Midwifery Advisory Committee (1961) *Central Health Services Council: Human Relations in Obstetrics*. London: HMSO.

Stock, J. & Wraight, A. (1993) *Developing Continuity of Care in Maternity Services*. Brighton: Institute of Manpower Studies.

Taylor, A. (1994) Opting out. *Nursing Times* 89(47): 46–47.

Towler, J. & Brammall, J. (1986) *Midwives in History and Society*. London: Croom Helm.

Versluysen, M. (1981) Midwives, medical men and poor women labouring of child. In Roberts, H. (ed.) *Women Health and Reproduction*. London: Routledge, Kegan, Paul.

Wraight, A., Ball, J. Secombe, I. *et al.* (1993) *Mapping Team Midwifery*. IMS Report series 242. Brighton: Institute of Manpower Studies.

Further Reading

Reports influencing the direction of maternity services are produced by each of the four home countries and readers are recommended to find out which are currently relevant to where they practise. The RCM supplements mentioned below refer to all of those produced prior to 1995.

English National Board (1995) *The Challenge of 'Changing Childbirth'*. Midwifery Educational Resource pack. London: ENB.
The purpose of the pack is to help midwives to reflect upon their practice. It explores many of the issues facing midwives in these challenging times. Of particular interest with this supplement is book 2 of the pack sections 2.3 Communication and negotiation. The consumer's view. 2.6 Building partnerships with women and their families. Obtainable from the English National Board.

Changing Childbirth Implementation Team Newsletter. Update.
A quarterly newsletter from the Changing Childbirth Implementation Team, free of charge. The newsletter is a means of sharing with others successes and difficulties, developments happening in trusts/health boards throughout the UK. Contact Nikki Ruffles 01223 218756.

Midwifery Development Unit (1995) *A Resource Manual*. Glasgow Maternity Unit.
A manual produced by Glasgow supported by the Scotland Board of the Royal College of Midwives. The manual contains descriptions of the processes worked through in setting up and developing a midwifery-led unit. Manuals have been distributed free of charge to all units and education institutions in Scotland. For others the cost is £35.

Royal College of Midwives supplement series. Woman centred care.
A short series on aspects of woman centred care. Number 1 January 1996. Number 2 April 1996. Obtainable from the Royal College of Midwives, London.

19

Antenatal Care

The first hospital antenatal clinic was opened in 1915 by Doctor Ferguson in Edinburgh, and was later supervised by Ballantyne who also opened the first antenatal bed for inpatients. Until then most women had no routine antenatal care from midwives or doctors during pregnancy and were rarely seen by one of these professionals until they went into labour. By that time there were often complications which may have responded to earlier diagnosis and treatment if it had been available and so improved the outcome for both mother and baby. In 1935 it was estimated that 80% of women in the UK were receiving some antenatal care and the recommended intervals were similar to those of today, namely 16, 24, 28, 32, 34 and 36 weeks and then weekly until the onset of labour (Currell, 1990; Oakley, 1982). By 1946 the estimated figure for women receiving antenatal care had risen to 91% (Charles, 1992). Now most women in the UK seek regular antenatal care and accept that it is important for their own health and that of their baby. Unfortunately those who are least likely to attend an antenatal clinic tend to be those who are most at risk of developing complications, for example, women from the lower socio-economic classes, young teenagers and women of high parity (Parsons and Perkins, 1982).

Aims of Antenatal Care

The aims of antenatal care may be summarized thus:

▶ The establishment of good communications and a relationship of partnership between the woman and the professionals involved in her care, ensuring that she has continuity of care and carer from her lead professional.
▶ Keeping the woman well-informed about all aspects of her care and empowering her to make informed

choices in the knowledge that her autonomy is respected.

▶ The provision of appropriate support to promote psychological, emotional and social well-being in pregnancy.

▶ Health education to promote the maintenance and, where necessary, the improvement of health in pregnancy.

▶ Regular monitoring of the maternal and fetal conditions in pregnancy to ensure early detection of any deviations from the normal and the instigation of appropriate management.

▶ Preparation for labour and a safe, normal delivery that is a pleasurable, fulfilling experience for both the mother and her partner.

▶ The provision of education for parenthood.

▶ Preparation for successful breastfeeding, or artificial feeding if that is the mother's informed choice.

▶ Education for planned parenthood.

Provision of Antenatal Care

The traditional methods of delivering antenatal care which have been in existence since the 1940s are now under scrutiny. Increasing criticisms have been expressed during the 1980s and 1990s about large, impersonal hospital antenatal clinics where women are treated on a conveyor belt system, have long waiting times and are seen by a different midwife and doctor at each visit. In many clinics all women are seen by a doctor at every visit, irrespective of whether there were high risk factors, and the midwife's role was seriously eroded as she no longer performed antenatal examinations, or her examinations were duplicated by a doctor. *Shared care* between the general practitioner and midwife in the community and obstetricians and midwives in hospital has become the norm for most women and again there is often duplication of care and lack of communication between hospital and community staff. With these systems of care women experiencing uncomplicated pregnancies may receive the same care as those who are high risk or have developed complications. There is a tendency to ignore the woman's social circumstances and her psychological and emotional needs, and to focus on her as a 'case' and her pregnancy as a medical condition (Field, 1990). Only the few women booked for home confinement received continuity of care throughout pregnancy, labour and the postnatal period from their midwife and general practitioner, usually having been examined by an obstetrician early in pregnancy to ensure that they are suitable for home confinement.

Many changes have been made in the delivery of antenatal care in recent years to try and address these problems, but regretfully in some areas the process of change is slow and some of these problems still exist.

Changes in the delivery of antenatal care need to offer more effective care not only in terms of safety, but also in accessibility and acceptability to the women who use the service. Keirse (1994) says that it is not good enough for maternity services to be readily available to all women. They must also be accessible and not perceived as being alien, hostile or superfluous. Many of the changes which have taken place in the antenatal services offered to women in the last 20 years are due to increasing technology and the rising number of tests available for the diagnosis of fetal abnormality. It has been suggested that antenatal care has increasingly lost its '*care*' *component* and has become a package of other things – surveillance, monitoring and social control (Oakley, 1984). Yet to women the 'care' component, continuity of carer, being kept well-informed about the progress of their pregnancy and the options related to their care, and being able to make informed choices, thereby retaining their autonomy and control, are often the most important aspects of antenatal care (DOH, 1993). Midwives therefore need to develop a relationship of partnership with the women in their care and discuss their individual needs, wishes and expectations and ways in which they can be achieved. The move towards community-based care with midwifery teams and group practices and the implementation of the recommendations in the report, *Changing Childbirth* (1993) should help to achieve more individualized, women-centred care and revive the 'care' component which some consider has been lacking.

A special effort may be required to develop a partnership with women in the lower socio-economic groups and with young teenagers who tend to have more health problems associated with lifestyle, for example, anaemia due to poor diet and the many complications of smoking (McGreal, 1995; HEA, 1994a; Haglund and Chattingius, 1990; MacArthur *et al.*, 1987) (see Chapter 38). They are often ill-informed and inarticulate and the usual system of maternity care may fail to provide these women with appropriate care (Chadwick, 1994). This is an example of the Inverse Care Law, first described in 1971 by Tudor Hart, where those already at a disadvantage are further dis-advantaged by the system designed to help them. Increased social support during pregnancy has been shown to help overcome these problems and produce better outcomes for both mother and baby (Oakley, 1982; Oakley *et al.*, 1990). In some areas special ante-natal clinics for teenagers have improved the attendance rate for antenatal care and relationships with health professionals.

Some attempts have been made to redress these problems by the introduction of *community antenatal schemes* in deprived areas to offer care which is more accessible and in most cases acceptable to the local community. The Sighthill Clinic in Edinburgh was one of the first community schemes to be introduced where all mothers, apart from those who have diabetes or major cardiac problems, receive all their care in the local health centre (McKee, 1980). Each mother is carefully assessed for risk factors at the first visit to the clinic, using a checklist. If particular risk factors are elicited, then at subsequent visits a preplanned pro-gramme of management is followed which includes protocols for investigations and subsequent action. All staff involved in this scheme have regular group discussions about client care and work together as a team. The consultant obstetrician visits the health centre regularly and is available for consultation.

This scheme has greatly improved the quality of care and resulted in a significant reduction in the number of defaulters and in the perinatal mortality rate in an area with a high proportion of social class IV and V parents. The expectant mothers appreciate attending a local clinic and having continuity of care from their own midwife and general practitioner. Com-munity midwives and general practitioner obstetricians enjoy greater job satisfaction and there is close colla-boration between community and hospital personnel.

Since the introduction of the Sighthill scheme, many other community antenatal projects have been introduced which fully involve midwives in the deliv-ery of antenatal care (Reid *et al.*, 1983; Thomas *et al.*, 1987; Zander *et al.*, 1987; Davies, 1988).

Another scheme, this time in Glasgow, established a *satellite hospital clinic* about 6 miles from the city centre which made travelling easier and cheaper and reduced waiting times for those attending this clinic (Reid *et al.*, 1983). Attendance was no better than at the hospital clinic however and, although the women were more satisfied than those attending the hospital clinic, they perceived the attitude of the staff to be unfavourable

towards them. The clinic was staffed by a senior registrar, two hospital and two community midwives, plus a health visitor and a social worker. This high-lights the importance of appropriate attitudes of staff providing antenatal care and perhaps also the need for them to have a good understanding of the social con-text in which their clients live.

A project in deprived areas of Newcastle provides enhanced care by *community-based midwives* (Davies, 1988). Although attendance at the antenatal clinic has not improved, there are significant benefits of this scheme. These include improved attendance at the midwives' parentcraft classes, a decrease in smoking and improved maternal nutrition. This scheme also appears to be acceptable to the women in that they appreciate the enhanced care and refer themselves and their friends for care.

Another innovative scheme introduced by midwives was the '*Know Your Midwife Scheme*' (KYM) which was a randomized controlled trial whereby a small team of midwives gave total care to a group of women to test the feasibility of giving total care and the advantages of continuity of care (Flint *et al.*, 1987). The results showed greater client satisfaction with the care given to the KYM group and that it is feasible to provide total care by midwives in this way. Many other team and group practice midwifery schemes have been intro-duced in the 1980s and 1990s in efforts to give con-tinuity of care and carer and improve client satisfaction. The introduction of community-based group practices enables midwives to practise in a flexible manner, free from the constraints of an institution (Kroll, 1993), and to provide total care to a caseload of low-risk women (Ball, 1992; Page *et al.*, 1994). In 1993 the Institute of Manpower Studies published an evaluation of team midwifery and the report included recommendations that the team should have no more than six midwives and each team should have a defined caseload and provide total care.

The Winterton Report (DOH, 1992b) presented the case for woman-centred care which is planned to meet the individual physical, psychological, emotional, social and cultural needs and expectations of each woman (Magill-Cuerden, 1992). It was as a result of this report that the government set up an Expert Mater-nity Group to review the policy on NHS maternity care and to make recommendations. The report of the Expert Maternity Group, *Changing Childbirth*, was published in 1993 (DOH, 1993). It recommends fun-damental changes in the provision of maternity care in the UK. It is recognized that midwives have a key role in the provision of antenatal care that is flexible, sensitive and responsive to the needs of women and fully involves them as partners in care. To empower them to be partners, women must be well-informed, enabled to make choices and able to retain control throughout the process of pregnancy and childbirth. It also recommends continuity of carer for all women during pregnancy, labour and the postnatal period and this, together with other recommendations in the report, are now government policy for the maternity services.

In most hospital clinics now and in the community midwives give full antenatal care to *low-risk women*, sometimes after an initial examination by an obstetrician at the booking clinic, although this is not always considered necessary. More innovative schemes to try and improve continuity of care and carer have been introduced, such as different patterns of team midwifery, group practices and one-to-one practice (Page *et al.*, 1994), with midwives having a caseload of low-risk women to whom they give total care throughout the ante-, intra- and postnatal periods. Many of these schemes are community based, with continuity of care by midwives in community clinics or the woman's own home, rather than in a busy hospital clinic. The woman's named midwife also attends her in hospital if she is booked for a hospital delivery, and is responsible for her postnatal care which may start in hospital and then continues at home.

As more antenatal care is given in the community, obstetricians have more time to give to *high-risk women* in hospital antenatal clinics who need their specialist care. Formerly many of these women would have been admitted to an antenatal ward for assessment and rest, but this causes considerable family disruption and stress, and inpatient care is very expensive. Findings from studies concerning hospital admission for women in the antenatal period include the psychological and social stresses which they experience (MacDonald, 1990; Wilson-Barnett, 1976; White and Ritchie, 1984; Kemp and Page, 1984). In recent years many of these women with conditions such as non-proteinuric pregnancy-induced hypertension have been cared for at home by the community midwife. Several studies have shown that there are no adverse effects on pregnancy outcomes (Feeney, 1984; Hall *et al.*, 1985) and a randomized controlled trial carried out in Cardiff by Middlemass *et al.* (1989) showed that anxiety levels were considerably lower for the group cared for at home where they received a personal and informal approach to individualized care.

A recent development is the introduction of *hospital-based antenatal day units* where women can attend as outpatients for monitoring and a variety of other investigations and tests. Twaddle and Harper (1992) found that most women were prepared to attend an antenatal day unit five days a week to avoid hospital admission, although such frequent attendance is not usually necessary. Regular surveys and audit to assess the service offered by the antenatal day unit and consumer satisfaction with it are recommended by Haley (1995). Good liaison with the community enables easy access to the unit for expectant mothers who develop complications and are booked for care with their community-based midwife or general practitioner. In some areas self-referral is encouraged, usually to allay anxiety in women with a poor obstetric history, diminished fetal movements and multiple pregnancy (Morris de Lassalle, 1994). The development of antenatal day units has reduced antenatal hospital admissions, especially for non-proteinuric hypertensive women (Haley, 1995).

Booking for Confinement

The woman should be able to choose whether her first contact in pregnancy is with a midwife or her general practitioner (DOH, 1993). She should always be given clear, unbiased information and will choose whether she wishes to have a midwife, general practitioner or obstetrician as the lead professional to plan and give care during the ante-, intra- and postnatal periods. The choice of a lead professional does not prevent the woman from receiving care from other professionals if she wishes, or it becomes necessary. Certainly if complications arise she will be referred to an obstetrician. One of the objectives in the report *Changing Childbirth* is that all women should have the name of a midwife who practises locally whom she can contact for advice, even if she is not the lead professional.

It is important to encourage women to contact their midwife or family doctor when they first suspect pregnancy, which is usually after one or two missed periods. There are still women who seek medical supervision much later, when it is more difficult to assess uterine size accurately by clinical examination and consequently there may be confusion about the expected date of delivery until the gestational age is determined by ultrasound. After 28 weeks the assessment of gestational age by ultrasound is unreliable (Proud, 1994). Observations such as recording the blood pressure give an important baseline during the first trimester of pregnancy. After that time the blood pressure falls due to the physiological changes described later in this chapter and in Chapter 12. In the third trimester the blood pressure rises again and it is when this rise is greater than expected and cannot be compared with the baseline blood pressure recorded in the first trimester that problems in assessing the significance of the rise and subsequent management occur. Some investigations, such as the 'triple test', are only accurate if carried out at specific times, in this case between 15 and 18 weeks. The 'triple test' is for the detection of neural tube defects and Down's syndrome (see Chapter 21). Early detection of these conditions enables further investigations such as ultrasound scan or, in the case of Down's syndrome, amniocentesis, to be carried out at the optimum time, thus women who book late may lose this opportunity. Late booking also delays therapeutic treatment for conditions such as cervical incompetence. In some cases complications have already arisen by the time the mother books, which put both her and the fetus at risk, whereas such problems might have been avoided with early midwifery or medical supervision. During the early weeks of pregnancy many women feel exhausted, nauseated and anxious about many of the physiological changes that are occurring at that time. Early contact with their midwife or doctor gives them the opportunity to express their anxieties and receive the support, reassurance and advice which they may need during these early weeks.

The midwife or family doctor will examine the woman and perhaps arrange for a *pregnancy test* to be carried out to confirm pregnancy, although nowadays many women have already used a commercially available home testing pregnancy kit. Provided these tests are accurately carried out, they are 98% accurate and will be positive 8–14 days after the first missed period in pregnancy. They may also be positive with other conditions such as choriocarcinoma, however, therefore a false positive result should be investigated (Smith *et al.*, 1988). The midwife will then discuss the various options for care which are available locally for the woman. This will enable her to make an informed choice in her own time about her lead professional, arrangements for antenatal care, place of delivery and postnatal care. Although many women

choose their midwife or general practitioner as their lead professional, the report *Changing Childbirth* (DOH, 1993) recommends that all women should have the opportunity to meet an obstetrician at least once during pregnancy.

The number of hospital confinements in Engand and Wales has risen to nearly 99% as most professionals have considered it safer since the Peel Report of 1970 for women to be delivered in hospital rather than at home. In recent years, however, there has been increasing evidence to substantiate the view that home deliveries or Domino schemes for women with low-risk pregnancies are safe (Tew, 1990; Shearer, 1985; Lowe *et al.*, 1987; Klein *et al.*, 1983).

Domino scheme

In some areas of the country a domino scheme is available whereby a community-based midwife whom the mother knows accompanies her to hospital and cares for her throughout labour. After delivery she arranges to transfer the mother home when she is ready, usually within a few hours of delivery. Under this scheme the mother enjoys continuity of care from her known midwife, yet is delivered in hospital where specialist help and equipment are readily available should complications occur. In some cases the mother does not have to decide until she is in labour whether she wishes to remain at home or go into hospital for delivery. Many team and group midwifery practices offer a similar service now.

In some areas there is a midwife-led delivery suite for women who are considered to be low risk. A randomized controlled trial designed to examine whether intrapartum care and delivery in a midwife-managed unit differs from that in a consultant-led labour ward concluded that midwife-managed care results in more mobility and less intervention with no increase in neonatal morbidity. However, there was a high rate of transfer to the consultant unit, 34% antepartum and a further 16% intrapartum, mainly primigravidae (Hundley *et al.*, 1994).

Midwife/general practitioner unit or community hospital

Instead of booking in a consultant obstetric unit for hospital delivery the woman with a low-risk pregnancy may have her baby in a midwife-led or general practitioner-led community hospital. Again she enjoys continuity of care from her community-based midwife and her own doctor and usually appreciates the relaxed, friendly atmosphere of a small hospital.

The First Antenatal Visit

The expectant mother is given a friendly greeting and made welcome when she arrives at the clinic. Most women feel a little apprehensive at their first visit to the antenatal clinic, especially if they have not met the midwives or medical staff before. A warm, friendly greeting and a pleasant, comfortable environment can help to put the woman at ease. Young teenagers, women who do not speak English and those who are unhappy about their pregnancy feel especially vulnerable. Interpreters are required for non-English speaking clients and where possible they should be given written information in their own language. In many large cities where the number of teenage pregnancies is high, a special clinic or club may be held to meet the specific needs of young pregnant teenagers.

Whatever the background of the woman, or her reactions to her pregnancy, building a positive relationship with her is one of the midwife's most important aims during this first antenatal visit. It provides a foundation which will be built upon during the rest of pregnancy. The woman needs good communications with a midwife who is well-informed and committed to supporting her as an individual (Hutton, 1994). Mutual respect, trust and partnership then develop which gives satisfaction and pleasure to both mother and midwife. Garcia (1982) suggests that women are concerned with the uniqueness of their pregnancy while care-givers tend to aggregate pregnancies on the assumption that one is very much like another. Hutton (1994) investigated users' views of the maternity services and found that there were consistent messages about the importance of the quality of the women's relationship with their midwife and how this can make or mar their experience of pregnancy, labour and the early postnatal period. One of the best memories in pregnancy about midwives was being made to 'feel special'. Thoughtless remarks casting doubt on the outcome of the pregnancy was one of the worst memories.

HISTORY-TAKING

The history may be taken by the midwife in the mother's own home, or in a health centre, perhaps where her general practitioner is based, or at the first visit to a hospital antenatal clinic. When the history is taken at home or in a community clinic, the mother is likely to be more at ease and the midwife has the opportunity to make early contact with her and start building up a relationship in more relaxed surroundings. Often at this early stage in pregnancy the woman is suffering from nausea and fatigue and appreciates not having to travel to attend a busy clinic amongst strangers. Any problems can usually be discussed in private and the midwife may give information and offer advice, if appropriate, and also prepare the woman for her first visit to the antenatal clinic. On occasions there are other members of the family present during this initial assessment and this gives the midwife the opportunity to meet them, but she should also be sensitive to the fact that there may be information that the woman considers private or confidential and would prefer not to discuss in the presence of others. Later, when the mother makes her first visit to the antenatal clinic, she should be less anxious as she will have met her midwife and been prepared by her for the examinations and tests to be carried out. Also, it should be a shorter visit as her history has already been recorded and many of her questions answered. In a study conducted by Sikorski *et al.* (1995) it was surprising to find that general practitioners and obstetricians lacked enthusiasm for domiciliary booking visits conducted by midwives, despite a higher satisfaction rate for both women and midwives. If the history is taken in a hospital antenatal clinic, every effort should be made to put the woman at ease in a pleasant, non-clinical environment and privacy and sufficient time must be allowed.

The booking interview, whether it takes place at home, in a community clinic or a hospital antenatal clinic, should be a two-way process of interaction between the mother and midwife. It involves assessment of the woman's social, psychological, emotional and physical condition as well as obtaining information about the present and any previous pregnancies and the medical and family history. Care can then be planned in conjunction with the woman to meet her specific needs and wishes.

In her study, Methven (1982a,b) found that the antenatal booking interview merely recorded an obstetric history and that the promotion of a relationship between midwife and mother was not being achieved. This is an occasion when the midwife's ability to communicate well is of paramount importance. She needs to display warmth (Argyle, 1969) and friendliness which will help to put the woman at ease and establish a rapport with her. Other factors which promote a more relaxed atmosphere are an informal arrangement of the room without the barrier of a desk between the mother and midwife. Sitting side by side, preferably in easy chairs at an angle of approximately 90 degrees promotes easier conversation than a face-to-face position. A few minutes spent by the midwife in introducing herself and chatting informally enables the mother to settle down and relax before personal issues are discussed. Indeed, a skilled midwife can elicit most of the information required from the mother in a pleasant conversational manner without the mother realizing that she is being closely questioned at all. Open rather than closed questions should be employed because they encourage free responses and promote two-way interaction between the mother and midwife. Methven (1986, 1989) showed that the use of a *nursing/midwifery model* or framework for the booking interview significantly increases both the quality of the communication between mother and midwife and the relevance of the information obtained for planning subsequent care. Orem's self-care model was used by Methven but several models for midwifery have now been developed which are suitable for use at the booking interview (Mayes, 1987; Midgely, 1988; Hughes and Goldstone, 1989).

Some centres use *questionnaires* for obtaining the history, often sending them to mothers before they attend the booking clinic so that they can complete them in their own time at home and bring them to the clinic when they have their appointment. Other centres use computers which, according to Broadhurst (1988), are user friendly and midwifery orientated. Lilford *et al.* (1992) conducted a randomized controlled trial to compare the effectiveness of three methods of taking an antenatal history: an unstructured paper questionnaire, a structured paper questionnaire and an interactive computerized questionnaire. Structured questionnaires (paper or computer) were found to provide more and better information and their use improves clinical response to risk factors. However, the focus of the questions was medically orientated and there was limited information on the social, psychological and emotional state of the woman. Another study set out to discover if women themselves could complete part of the antenatal record at booking, instead of the midwife. The findings indicated that this method of collecting the necessary information is a useful alternative to the traditional way, but some women may prefer not to complete the form for a variety of reasons and their wishes should be respected (Galloway, 1994; Fawdry, 1994).

During the interview the midwife should be sensitive to the woman's attitude to her pregnancy and, if possible, to that of the father. Unusually adverse attitudes would be noted and counselling and support given, as required. Adverse attitudes often change as pregnancy advances, but occasionally an unwanted pregnancy results in a later case of non-accidental injury.

General particulars

The mother's full name, marital status, address, telephone number, age, date of birth, race, religion, occupation (and that of her partner) and number of years married are clearly recorded. Her age and duration of marriage or in a stable relationship may together be a guide to her fertility. A primigravida of 35 years may have been married only a year and be normally fertile, or she may have been married, or in a stable relationship, for 15 years and have almost given up hope of ever becoming pregnant. *Marital status* is established because some single mothers are unsupported and may need special help and understanding and referral to a social worker. Many single mothers today, however, are in a stable relationship or live an independent life and do not require any special help. In 1992, 31.7% of infants were born outside marriage in the UK, compared with 29.8% in 1991 (Central Statistical Office, 1994, 1993). *Race* is ascertained because some medical and obstetric conditions are more common in certain races and thus special diagnostic tests may be carried out, where appropriate. The *religion* of the woman is recorded because of the special requirements and rituals which may be practised and affect the mother and her baby. *Occupation* gives an indication of socio-economic status. Women in the socio-economic groups IV and V are more likely to have financial problems and substandard general health which may be associated with poor nutrition, smoking and inadequate housing. The outcome of pregnancy is adversely affected and the perinatal mortality rate is increased. Extra support and health education from the midwife and referral to a social worker, if the mother wishes, may be required. Unemployment adversely affects a family's standard of living and again special support from the midwife and referral to a social worker may be required.

Present pregnancy

Though not in correct chronological order, this is a convenient point at which to begin, since the present pregnancy is what is uppermost in the woman's mind.

The date of the first day of the *last menstrual period* (LMP) is ascertained, care being taken to check that this was the last *normal* menstrual period. Some women have a slight blood loss when the fertilized ovum embeds into the decidual lining of the uterus and many mistake this for the last period. By counting forwards nine months and adding seven days from the first day of the last normal menstrual period, it is possible to arrive at an *estimated date of delivery* (EDD); alternatively, count back three months and add seven days. This method of calculating the estimated date of delivery is known as *Naegele's rule*. It is important to explain to primigravidae that the actual day of delivery may be a week or so before or after this date and that it is quite normal.

Details of the mother's menstrual history must be sought: the age at which menstruation began, the duration of the periods and the number of days in the cycle. Conception occurs shortly after ovulation. With a regular cycle of about 28 days, the standard calculation is reasonably accurate to within a few days, provided the mother knows the date of her last normal menstrual period. In a 35-day cycle, however, ovulation would occur 21 days after the period; in a 21-day cycle, only seven days after. Adjustments may be made, therefore, when the woman has a regular long or short cycle. If the cycle is 33 days long the days in excess of 28 are added when calculating the EDD, e.g.

Cycle 33 days
LMP 12 August 1995
EDD 24 May 1996
i.e. 9 months + 7 days + 5 days = 24 May 1996

With a regular short cycle such as 23 days the number of days less than 28 are subtracted from the EDD, e.g.

Cycle 23 days
LMP 12 August 1995
EDD 14 May 1996
i.e. 9 months + 7 days − 5 days = 14 May 1996

The calculation is difficult or impossible, however, when the mother does not know the date of her last menstrual period or where there is a history of an irregular cycle, missed periods or no normal period since last taking the oral contraceptive pill. In some cases the mother may have a very good idea when conception occurred and then it is necessary to count forwards 38 weeks, or subtract seven days from nine months, to discover the expected date of delivery.

All mothers should be asked to make a note of the date when *fetal movements* are first felt. This is particularly helpful when there is doubt about the expected date of delivery, although nowadays with the widespread use of ultrasound in the UK, the correct gestational age is usually established during ultrasound examination, often between 16 and 18 weeks. Primigravidae normally become aware of fetal movements between 18 and 20 weeks, whereas multigravidae recognize the sensation a little earlier, between 16 and 18 weeks.

Although the use of ultrasound to estimate gestational age is very useful, it can cause distress to women if there are discrepancies in the date estimated by Naegele's rule, and that given following ultrasound examination, especially in those who are certain of the date of conception, or have a regular cycle and are certain of the date of the first day of their last menstrual period. In these cases open discussion between mother and her midwife or obstetrician is essential and in most cases it would be inappropriate to alter the expected date of delivery without the mother's agreement, especially when there is less than 10–14 days discrepancy with the previously given date (Proud, 1994).

Other pregnancy symptoms such as *breast changes*, *morning sickness* and increased *frequency of micturition* are noted. Morning sickness may mean anything from occasional slight nausea to quite serious vomiting with accompanying ketosis, when immediate medical treatment is necessary. Any history of *bleeding per vaginam* since the last normal menstrual period is recorded and the woman asked to seek medical attention immediately should further bleeding occur. In the first trimester of pregnancy a mother is quite likely to feel tired, perhaps nauseated and generally rather off-colour. A caring, approachable midwife who gives support, encourages the woman to express any worries and ask questions and gives clear information can be a great help to the woman at this time. Usually the woman can be reassured that soon she will feel very much better. Indeed, a mother in the second trimester often remarks that 'she never felt better in her life'. She is well adjusted to her pregnancy, her nausea is over, her appetite is good and she feels lively and full of energy.

Previous pregnancies

It is necessary to ask about all previous pregnancies, including miscarriages or terminations of pregnancy. If the woman has had a miscarriage she is asked at what stage in pregnancy it occurred, whether she knows of any possible cause, if she was transferred to hospital and, if so, whether she needed either an operation to remove retained products of conception, or a blood transfusion, or both.

She is asked similar questions about termination of pregnancy, including the reason for termination and how it was performed. Her previous notes should be available if treatment was carried out in the same district.

Details of all pregnancies, labours and puerperia are essential. Was the pregnancy normal or complicated, e.g. by vomiting, hypertension or haemorrhage? Was the labour at term and straightforward in all three stages? How long did it last? Was her baby born in hospital or at home? Was he born normally or did she require a forceps delivery, ventouse extraction or Caesarean section? If so, does she know why? Did she have a normal healthy baby and was he well at birth? And now? If she lost her baby she is asked if she knows why. Though it may distress her to have to recall this unhappy event, she will readily co-operate, realizing that this pregnancy and labour will be conducted with this misfortune in mind and that every effort will be made to achieve a happier outcome.

The *birthweight* of any previous baby is important, since it gives some indication of the capacity of the woman's pelvis. A woman who has, without difficulty, delivered herself of a healthy 3.5 kg (7½ lb) infant must have a roomy pelvis, while one who has had a forceps delivery of a 2.7 kg (6 lb) baby may have a small pelvis.

It is desirable to know, too, if the mother was *unwell after her baby's birth* or if she experienced excessive haemorrhage or any other complications. She is also asked how long she remained in hospital after baby's birth, since this may reflect the normal or complicated nature of the postnatal period. Finally, she is asked if she breastfed her baby and, if so, for how long. If not, she is asked the reason (unless, by now, it is obvious), since this may help in making arrangements for the feeding of the expected child, and she is asked how lactation was suppressed.

All pregnancies are dealt with thus, in chronological order. If the history reveals any obstetric or paediatric complications and previous notes are not accessible, the doctor will probably write to the appropriate hospital for further information.

Medical and surgical history

This includes inquiry about any *illness*, *operation* or *accident* which could complicate pregnancy. It is necessary to ask by name about rheumatic fever, chorea, cardiac, respiratory and renal diseases, thyrotoxicosis, diabetes, hypertension, thromboembolic disorders, tuberculosis and mental illness. A history of psychiatric disorders, especially postnatal depression or puerperal psychosis, is of significance because such conditions may recur following a subsequent pregnancy. The mother is asked about the infectious diseases of childhood and especially whether she has had rubella or been vaccinated against the disease. A blood test will confirm whether or not she is immune. The non-immune woman is warned to avoid contact with the disease because, if she develops rubella in pregnancy, the virus can cross the placenta and damage the developing fetus.

A woman who is thought to be at a high risk of acquiring the *human immunodeficiency virus* (HIV), perhaps because she is an intravenous drug abuser, will be counselled and offered a blood test which will detect the virus, if present. She is also counselled in a non-judgemental way about the risks of her lifestyle to her unborn child and offered referral for treatment of her drug addiction. If the HIV test is positive, the risks of transmission to her unborn child are discussed and referral for treatment is offered. Treatment with anti-retroviral drugs attempts to reduce the viral load in the mother and thereby reduce the risk of transmitting the virus to the fetus. The option of termination of the pregnancy is also discussed with the woman, but many women decide to continue with their pregnancy for a variety of reasons (Mandelbrot, 1993).

Operations on the uterus or the pelvic floor are significant. Following Caesarean section or myomectomy, there may be a weakened uterine scar, especially if the wound was infected, and there is a slight risk that it could rupture during a subsequent pregnancy or labour. Women of childbearing age sometimes have to undergo extensive pelvic floor repair operations. If a woman has had a successful operation for the relief of stress incontinence, both the mother and the obstetrician will be concerned about the mode of delivery; sometimes, another vaginal delivery is considered inadvisable and Caesarean section is planned.

Relevant *accidents* include those involving the spine and pelvis, particularly if a fracture has occurred and deformity resulted. Deformity of the spine or pelvis following poliomyelitis or congenital dislocation of the hip would cause similar concern, since in all these instances the bony pelvis may be asymmetrical and accordingly have a smaller capacity.

Details of any *blood transfusions* are important, including the reason and any adverse reaction.

It is important to ask the mother whether she is taking any *drugs*, because many which are quite safe for her may have a teratogenic (harmful) effect on the fetus. The mother should be informed about the risk of taking over-the-counter drugs without medical advice.

An increasing problem in pregnancy is drug addiction in women of child-bearing age and tactful enquiries about lifestyle and habits should elicit this information. It is essential that the approach and attitude of the midwife are caring, non-judgemental and constructively helpful, otherwise the woman may reject all the help which the health and other specialist services can offer. Medical illness and obstetric problems are common in these women and create a hostile intrauterine environment which places the fetus at risk.

Infections such as hepatitis B and HIV are also prevalent in those who are dependent on drugs and screening for these conditions is offered. Special arrangements may have to be made to try and ensure that these women receive regular antenatal care by the same professional who is acceptable to them. They are also offered referral to a drug dependency unit where help is available to help them to reduce their dependence on drugs and, if they are using opiates, methadone is prescribed as a substitute. Solvent abuse may be a problem for some women and again they will need special care and help in pregnancy.

Inquiry is also made about the woman's *eating*, *smoking* and *drinking habits*. A good mixed diet is advised (see Chapter 16). Women who smoke should be fully informed about the risks of smoking in pregnancy and offered constructive help to assist them to stop smoking. The Health Education Authority has produced some training materials for health professionals to help them to assist women stop smoking in pregnancy (HEA, 1994b). There is now a substantial body of evidence indicating that smoking causes intrauterine growth retardation, increases the perinatal and infant mortality and morbidity rates and has long-term detrimental effects on the growth and mental aptitude of the child and adolescent (Macleod Clark and Maclaine, 1992). Complications in pregnancy associated with smoking include a higher incidence of abortion and preterm labour. There are many problems associated with smoking in pregnancy which are discussed more fully in Chapters 15 and 25.

The alcohol consumption of the woman should also be ascertained. Women who drink excessively need help and support from the midwife as well as from alcohol dependency specialists and social services (Chadwick, 1993). A high level of alcohol consumption in pregnancy may lead to fetal alcohol syndrome (Plant, 1985). This condition has long-term detrimental effects on the child's mental and physical development (Streissguth *et al.*, 1985, 1991).

Unfortunately there are conflicting views about what constitutes a safe level of alcohol consumption in pregnancy, some considering that no more than two units a day should be consumed (Simms, 1989), while others suggest that this amount causes growth retardation, tremor and poor sucking in at least 10% of infants studied (Lewis, 1983). As the safe level is so uncertain, many suggest that it is wise to avoid alcohol altogether, except perhaps for an occasional small drink at a special occasion.

Family history

The mother's family medical history is important. *Familial diseases*, such as hypertension and diabetes, are sometimes discovered during routine antenatal examinations and it is useful to know the mother's medical background. It is essential to know if any near relative has pulmonary tuberculosis, since the newborn child is very vulnerable to the infection and must be protected. Arrangements are therefore made for the child to receive BCG vaccination before leaving hospital, as well as to be carefully segregated from the infected person.

There is a familial tendency to produce *twins*, especially dizygotic twins, thus it is important to ask if there are twins in the family and, if so, whether they are monozygotic (identical) or dizygotic (non-identical).

Finally, the mother should be asked if there is any history of *congenital defects* in the family. If so, a medical pedigree (Figure 1) should be obtained and the woman and her husband may be referred for genetic counselling (see Chapter 4). A number of diagnostic techniques are available for the diagnosis of congenital conditions in pregnancy and these may be discussed with the couple.

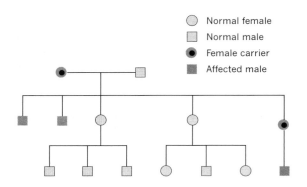

- ○ Normal female
- □ Normal male
- ◉ Female carrier
- ▩ Affected male

Figure 1 A medical pedigree showing three generations with X-linked haemophilia.

The midwife also carefully observes and enquires about the woman's reaction to her pregnancy, whether she is happy about it and coping with the initial minor disorders, or appears anxious, tense and unhappy. Guiding the conversation in a skilful, relaxed, unhurried manner and active listening and interpretation of both verbal and non-verbal communications helps to elicit the woman's feelings and concerns. Appropriate support and help can then be offered.

From this account it might appear that history-taking is a somewhat lengthy procedure. This is not usually so, however, since the majority of mothers are healthy young women who have never been seriously ill. This personal history provides a basis on which it is possible to assess the woman's physical, psychological and emotional health and well-being and, to some extent, to anticipate the outcome of her pregnancy. Another important aspect of this time spent taking the history is that the midwife and woman start getting to know one another and creating the relationship which has such a fundamental influence on the woman's experience of pregnancy and childbirth. On completion the midwife can assess the woman holistically and discuss her particular needs and wishes. She gives clear, accurate information about the services available to enable the woman to make informed choices and then the expectant mother and midwife together prepare a care plan for pregnancy tailored to meet individual needs.

EXAMINATION

At this first clinic visit a full medical examination of the woman is carried out. This includes:

- ▶ General appearance of the woman.
- ▶ General examination of mouth, mucous membranes, palpation of glands of neck.
- ▶ Height.
- ▶ Weight.
- ▶ Urinalysis.
- ▶ Blood pressure.
- ▶ Breast examination.
- ▶ Condition of heart and lungs.
- ▶ Abdominal examination.
- ▶ Cervical smear, if necessary.
- ▶ Legs for varicose veins and oedema.

General appearance

When taking particulars the observant midwife will notice the general appearance and demeanor of the woman she is questioning. Is she calm and happy or obviously worried and anxious? Does she look well or pale and tired? The midwife will also note any obvious physical defect, such as a limp which could be associated with a pelvic abnormality.

Height

The woman's height and sometimes the size of her shoes are ascertained, since stature and size of feet give some indication of pelvic size (Moore *et al.*, 1983). The petite woman, especially if under 1.52 m, may have a small pelvis, but it is worth bearing in mind that she may also have a small baby. Build is of interest. Tall, thin women tend to have easier labours than those who are short and heavily built. Moreover, women who are overweight have an increased tendency to develop hypertensive disorders.

Weight

Weight is usually ascertained at the first antenatal examination. When first recorded, usually at 10–12 weeks, it will differ little from before pregnancy and the subsequent gain is thus easy to assess. A survey conducted by the National Perinatal Epidemiology Unit in Oxford found there was little agreement between midwives and doctors about the usefulness of regular weighing in pregnancy, and how often it should be done, if at all. Consequently, the practice of routinely weighing women at each antenatal visit has been abandoned in many clinics because it is considered to be of limited value (Dawes and Grudzinskas, 1991). Although a higher than average weight gain is associated with the development of pre-eclampsia, there is considerable overlap between the weight gains of normotensive and pre-eclamptic women, and therefore the prediction of the occurrence of pre-eclampsia is unreliable (Green, 1989). When there is a particular indication the woman's weight may be monitored, preferably by the same person on the same scales and in similar attire each time, or the woman may be asked to record her weight at home on her own scales. Average total weight gain in pregnancy is 12–14 kg, usually 3–4 kg in the first 20 weeks and then approximately 0.5 kg a week until term, although the range of weight gain is very wide (Thomson and Billewicz, 1957; Hytten and Chamberlain, 1980). In developing countries weight gain in pregnancy is often well below this level in an apparently normal pregnancy. *Excessive weight gain* may be due to a wrong diet or to excessive retention of fluid; the latter may be associated with hypertensive disorders and should always be investigated. *Failure to gain sufficient weight* also requires investigation since it could be associated with poor diet, vomiting or placental insufficiency. The latter condition leads to retarded fetal growth and, in severe cases, to intrauterine fetal death.

Urine

At every clinic visit a specimen of urine is examined. At this first visit it is usual to obtain a mid-stream specimen, some of which is tested in the antenatal clinic. The colour, odour, specific gravity and reaction of the urine is noted. It is then tested for protein, sugar and ketone bodies. Protein may result from contamination, perhaps from a vaginal discharge or, more seriously, from a urinary tract infection or renal disease. Later in pregnancy, if associated with hypertension and oedema, it is a serious sign of pre-eclampsia, necessitating immediate admission to hospital. Glycosuria is not uncommon and may be related to a lowering of the renal threshold for sugar which occurs in pregnancy. Occasionally it is due to diabetes, however, and thus, if it occurs on two or more occasions, the doctor will usually request repeated random glucose estimates or a glucose tolerance test which will establish whether or not the woman has diabetes. Ketone bodies may be present if the woman is vomiting and may indicate that treatment is required.

The rest of the midstream specimen of urine is sent to the laboratory for bacteriological examination, as asymptomatic bacteriuria may be present and could lead to pyelonephritis later in pregnancy. Over 100 000 bacteria per ml of urine signifies infection. Treatment with the appropriate antibiotic is essential and it is followed by further bacteriological examination of a midstream specimen of urine to ensure that the infection has completely cleared. A reagent strip for testing urine specimens for infection has now been introduced and was tested in a study conducted by Etherington and James (1993) in an antenatal clinic. It was concluded that reagent strip testing of antenatal urine specimens for infection is a reliable and cheap alternative to culture of all urine specimens.

Blood pressure

The blood pressure is taken at this and every subsequent antenatal examination. The mother should be at rest and not breathless from recent exertion, otherwise the systolic reading may be higher than normal. Anxiety is also a cause of a raised systolic reading. The blood pressure reading in early pregnancy forms a baseline for subsequent readings. In a very anxious and nervous woman the blood pressure recording may need to be repeated when she is more relaxed. The blood pressure taken at home, or at a subsequent clinic visit may be a more reliable reading.

Correct recording of the blood pressure is essential to obtain an accurate reading. This includes using the correct size cuff for the woman, a well-maintained sphygmomanometer, palpating the brachial artery when first inflating the cuff to estimate the systolic pressure before auscultating with a stethoscope, and recording the diastolic pressure using the phase 4 Korotkoff sounds.

There is commonly a slight fall in blood pressure in the middle trimester of pregnancy due to the reduced viscosity of the blood and vasodilatation of peripheral vessels caused by the rising level of progesterone. In the third trimester, the blood pressure rises to its original level. A blood pressure of 140/90 mmHg or higher, or a diastolic rise of 20 mmHg or more above the level recorded in early pregnancy, is cause for concern in pregnancy and should be reported to the doctor.

Full medical examination

The woman then lies on the couch for a full medical examination, which is normally carried out by the doctor. The midwife assists the doctor, making sure that the mother is in the correct position and that only the necessary area is exposed at any one time. To the midwife, abdominal and vaginal examinations are commonplace, but to the mother they may be exceedingly embarrassing. Thoughtful preparation and reassurance will be appreciated by the mother and may encourage her to relax and so minimize the discomfort such examinations may cause. The doctor asks the mother how she feels and notes if she appears well. Then her *teeth* are inspected and she is advised to make an early appointment for a dental check-up, since any treatment required is best carried out in early pregnancy. Dental caries are septic foci and are potentially dangerous.

The *breasts* are examined to note the pregnancy changes, a useful aid in the diagnosis of pregnancy, and to note any features such as the presence of lumps or abnormal discharge from the nipples. Later the midwife will discuss breastfeeding with the mother.

Next the doctor auscultates the *heart and lungs*. A chest radiograph may be requested if there is any indication, such as a bad cough or a history of chest conditions, or if the woman is an immigrant, since in these cases tuberculosis is more common. When a chest X-ray is considered necessary it is deferred until about 20 weeks, when there is less risk of irradiation damaging the developing fetus.

The *abdomen* is examined to ascertain if there are any abdominal masses, if the uterus is palpable and, if so, if its size is compatible with the estimated period of gestation. Details of the abdominal examination are given later in this chapter.

A *vaginal examination* is only made in pregnancy if there is a specific indication, such as taking a Papanicolaou cervical smear for cytology to detect abnormal cells. Further investigations will be required if abnormal cells are found. If there is concern about the size and shape of the pelvis, a *pelvic examination* may be undertaken at 36–38 weeks if the fetal head is not engaged. At this stage in pregnancy the pelvic floor is relaxed and the examination causes less discomfort to the woman.

If the mother has a history of abortions, it is particularly important to avoid examination per vaginam in early pregnancy as the woman may associate the examination with the cause of abortion.

The *lower limbs* are examined for varicose veins and oedema. Varicosities are more likely in pregnancy because the veins become relaxed and dilated under the influence of progesterone.

Blood tests

Before the mother leaves the clinic on this first visit a specimen of blood is taken for investigations which are routinely carried out in pregnancy (see Chapter 21).

RISK FACTORS

At the end of the booking visit it should be possible to identify if there are any risk factors present which may adversely affect the outcome of pregnancy. James (1988) defines an at-risk pregnancy as follows: 'a pregnancy in which there is a risk of an adverse outcome in the mother and/or baby that is greater than the incidence of that outcome in the general population'.

Risk factors include poor general health, any significant medical conditions, a history of obstetric conditions which could recur, or complications which are already present in the current pregnancy, and significant social problems. Many risk-scoring systems have been devised, but have not proved sufficiently reliable to justify dependence on them (Lilford and Chard, 1983). Many of these scoring systems do not place sufficient emphasis on problems such as inability to speak English (Renfrew *et al.*, 1988) and social problems, although it is commonly accepted that these factors adversely affect the outcome of pregnancy. Individual assessment should be part of the antenatal care of every woman. In developing countries, where there are high maternal mortality rates and many women live a long distance from health care facilities, identification of risk is particularly important so that appropriate care can be arranged.

When risk factors are identified, the midwife will consult an obstetrician and, together with the mother, her care during pregnancy will be discussed and an initial care plan prepared in order to achieve the best possible outcome. Adaptations to the plan may need to be made as pregnancy advances.

ADVICE

Health in pregnancy is discussed with the woman and, if appropriate, advice is given and the woman is encouraged to ask questions and express any concerns she may have. Information is given about the maternity benefits for which she is eligible. Finally she is invited to attend a series of classes in preparation for parenthood, together with her partner.

Throughout the mother's time in the antenatal clinic, she is given clear information about all examinations and tests which are carried out and the opportunity to ask questions and discuss any problems.

Before she leaves, the date and time of her next appointment are arranged.

Antenatal Records

Contemporaneous, accurate and complete records must be made of all antenatal examinations and other relevant information and they are signed and dated by the midwife. It is now becoming normal practice for women to hold their own notes in pregnancy. Studies carried out on this practice indicate that women who are responsible for carrying their own records in pregnancy have a stronger sense of control (Hodnett, 1993), perhaps because they are better informed and can be more fully involved in discussions about their care (DOH, 1993). The fears of some professionals that women would lose or forget to bring their notes when they attend the antenatal clinic have proved to be ill-founded, although some find them difficult to read or worrying, but this has also been found to be the case with the co-operation card (Draper *et al.*, 1986). Pregnancy health records should be designed so that they can be effectively shared by all concerned in the woman's care and, as they should be held by the mother, language that is easily understood should be substituted for specialized terms (Fawdry, 1994). Before the woman leaves the clinic, the midwife should explain what she has written in the notes and encourage the woman to ask questions if there is anything which she does not fully understand. In some antenatal notes now there is an area for the mother to use if there is anything that she wishes to record.

Two of the objectives in the report *Changing Childbirth* are that providers should make the necessary arrangements to ensure that all women are able to carry their own case notes if they wish, and that they are fully informed on matters relating to their care and fully involved when decisions are to be made about their care.

Subsequent Care

FREQUENCY OF VISITS

The frequency of antenatal visits has come under scrutiny in recent years. They have followed the pattern of:

▶ every four weeks until the 28th week;
▶ every two weeks until the 36th week; and then
▶ every week until the onset of labour;

since the recommendations issued by the Ministry of Health in 1929 (Charles, 1992).

The main reason for the increasing frequency of visits in the third trimester is for the detection of pregnancy-induced hypertension which usually remains asymptomatic until the condition is serious. According to Hall *et al.* (1985), however, the prediction and detection of obstetric problems such as pregnancy-induced hypertension and intrauterine growth retardation is low. They suggest that normal multigravidae should have antenatal examinations at around 12, 22, 30, 36 and 40 weeks' gestation. Primigravidae should have extra blood pressure estimations and urinalysis, especially from 34 weeks' gestation because of the increased risk of pre-eclampsia during the latter weeks of pregnancy. Reactions to the reduced number of visits were varied. Some staff found it hard to form a relationship with a woman they saw so infrequently, whereas others were positive about the change. Mothers too had mixed reactions, some needing to attend for reassurance more than for the routine examinations (Laurent, 1992).

In 1982 the report of a Working Party set up by the Royal College of Obstetricians and Gynaecologists recommended a pattern of nine visits for primigravidae and six for multigravidae. The report of the Expert Maternity Group, *Changing Childbirth*, considers that these recommendations are still valid and recommends that providers should review the pattern of antenatal care in the light of current evidence (DOH, 1993). The time saved should be used to improve the quality and effectiveness of a reduced number of visits, including the provision of support and education (Thorley and Rouse, 1993).

Oakley (1982) poses many questions about the practice of antenatal care. These include whether the amount and type of antenatal care is either unequivocally beneficial or capable of overriding the effects of social deprivation. Increased social support during pregnancy has been shown to help overcome some of the problems associated with social deprivation and to produce better outcomes for both mother and baby (Oakley *et al.*, 1990). The provision of social and psychological support should nowadays be an integral part of antenatal care for all women.

With a reduction in the number of antenatal examinations it would be necessary to ensure that the woman knows she can telephone her midwife between visits if she has any worries or concerns which she wishes to discuss.

Defaulters

A few women fail to keep their antenatal clinic appointments and, in these cases, steps must be taken to follow them up. After a missed appointment it is usual to contact the mother, giving her another early appointment, or to visit her at home to make sure that she is well. The midwife usually examines the woman at home and will also, tactfully, try and find out why she has missed her appointments. Sometimes the care of young children is the problem and the midwife can then discuss what help may be available to enable the woman to attend the clinic, or arrange more home visits.

Most defaulters, like those who book after the 17th week, are in the lower socio-economic classes, under the age of 20 or of high parity (O'Brien and Smith, 1981). In the study conducted by Parsons and Perkins (1982) three types of non- or poor attenders were identified: the frightened teenagers, the competent childbearers, and those with social problems. The frightened teenagers were the largest group and all were single. Overall, the problem of non-attendance (includes poor attenders) in this study was small and, contrary to expectations, many appeared to have no major problems as a result. As already discussed, the way in which antenatal care is provided needs to be acceptable to and meet the needs of all women, especially those who are socially deprived in any way. Following the introduction of the Community Antenatal Care Scheme in Sighthill (McKee, 1980) there was a significant increase in the number of women booking early in pregnancy and a marked decrease in the defaulter rate. This is a good example of providing antenatal care which is acceptable and accessible to the local community.

Subsequent Antenatal Examinations

Subsequent antenatal examinations may be carried out by a midwife or doctor, depending on whether the woman is considered to be a low or high risk, and who she chooses to be her lead professional. The midwife is trained to practise normal midwifery, and thus can conduct and supervise the antenatal care of healthy women (UKCC, 1993, 1994).

Having greeted the woman in a friendly manner the midwife asks her how she feels and whether she has any problems. It is important to ask open rather than closed questions (see Chapter 14) and to give the woman time to answer fully and discuss any matters she wishes. The midwife exercises her listening skills, noting non-verbal as well as verbal communications.

She can give information and advice about minor disorders and do much to dispel fears when a mother's anxieties are brought to light. Extra support is often required by those with social problems and with obstetric or medical complications. This time should not be rushed as the woman needs time to discuss issues and assimilate information given by the midwife. Referral to a social worker for additional help and support may be offered, if appropriate.

The following examinations are carried out at each subsequent antenatal visit:

▶ In some clinics *weighing* is still carried out, but as discussed earlier in this chapter, many have abandoned it because it is considered of limited value. Many women weigh themselves at home regularly because they are concerned about putting on too much weight.

▶ *Blood pressure* is measured and compared with the last record, the overall trend being noted.

▶ *Abdominal examination* is performed to assess the height of the uterine fundus and, after the 28th week, to determine the lie, presentation and position of the fetus. From about 36 weeks engagement of the head is also determined. The fetal heart is auscultated.

Some mothers feel faint when they lie on their backs in the last trimester of pregnancy. This condition is called the *supine hypotensive syndrome* and is caused by the heavy uterus compressing the inferior vena cava, thereby impeding the return of the blood to the right side of the heart. The treatment is to turn the mother on her side immediately and she will rapidly recover.

▶ *Urine analysis* is undertaken to detect the presence of protein, glucose and ketones. Sometimes women are taught to test their own urine, as they are partners in care.

▶ Any *oedema* is noted.

The pretibial areas, ankles and fingers are examined for oedema. Some ankle oedema may occur in any pregnancy, since there is normally more tissue fluid in the body and it tends to gravitate towards the feet and ankles. In addition, the increased venous pressure in the legs predisposes to oedema. Moderate ankle oedema is normal and usually settles after a night in bed. Provided the blood pressure and urine are normal, it should not be a cause for concern because it occurs in 50–80% of healthy, normotensive women. Oedema may also occur in the hands, especially in the third trimester where it may be manifested by tightness of rings. Facial oedema is sometimes difficult to recognize, unless the midwife knows the woman well. She may say that a friend or relative has noticed the swelling and this information should be noted. Generalized oedema may occur and can be observed on the abdominal wall, when the fetal stethoscope leaves a depressed ring, or as vulval or sacral oedema.

Thomson and Hytten (1967) found that pregnant women with generalized oedema without hypertension have larger babies than those with little or no obvious oedema. Eighty-five per cent of women who develop pre-eclampsia also have oedema, and the outcome of pregnancy is improved when there is a combination of hypertension and oedema, rather than hypertension alone (Wallenburg, 1989).

At each antenatal examination the legs are examined for varicose veins. They may also occur in the vulva and the anal margin where they can give rise to considerable discomfort.

ABDOMINAL EXAMINATION

An abdominal examination is carried out at every visit to the antenatal clinic. At first, only the height of the fundus is ascertained to assess fetal growth, but as pregnancy advances more information is required.

The following terms are used in relation to the fetus *in utero* and must be understood when learning to make an abdominal examination:

Lie The lie (Figure 2) is the relationship of the long axis of the fetus to the long axis of the uterus. It may be

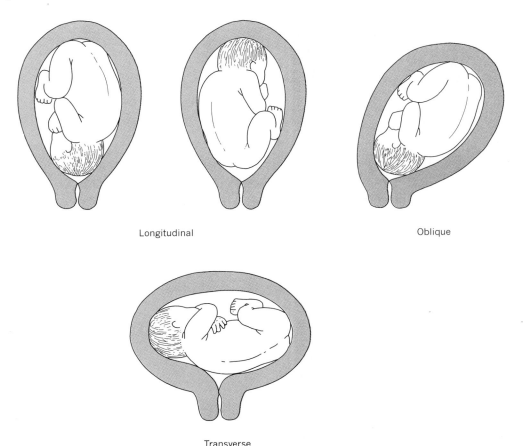

Longitudinal

Oblique

Transverse

Figure 2 The lie of the fetus.

longitudinal, *oblique* or *transverse*. In the latter weeks of pregnancy the lie should be longitudinal.

Attitude   The attitude (Figure 3) is the relationship of the fetal head and limbs to its body and may be *fully flexed*, *deflexed* or *partially or completely extended*. When fully flexed the head and spine are flexed, arms crossed over the chest, legs and thighs flexed. In this attitude the fetus forms a compact ovoid, fitting the uterus comfortably, though it can move freely.

Presentation   The presentation (Figure 4) is that part of the fetus lying in the lower pole of the uterus. A *cephalic* presentation is usual after about the 32nd week of pregnancy; other possible presentations are *breech*, *face*, *brow* and *shoulder*.

Denominator   The denominator is part of the presentation used to indicate the position:

▶ In a *cephalic* presentation, the denominator is the *occiput*.
▶ In a *breech* presentation, it is the *sacrum*.
▶ In a *face* presentation, it is the *mentum* (chin).

Position   The position (Figure 5) is the relationship of the denominator to six areas on the mother's pelvis. These areas are:

▶ Left and right anterior.
▶ Left and right lateral.
▶ Left and right posterior.

In a cephalic presentation the occiput is the denominator so the fetus is said to be in the:

▶ Left or right occipito-anterior position (LOA, ROA).
▶ Left or right occipitolateral position (LOL, ROL).
▶ Left or right occipitoposterior position (LOP, ROP).

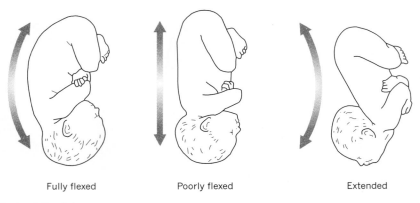

Fully flexed   Poorly flexed   Extended

Figure 3   The attitude of the fetus.

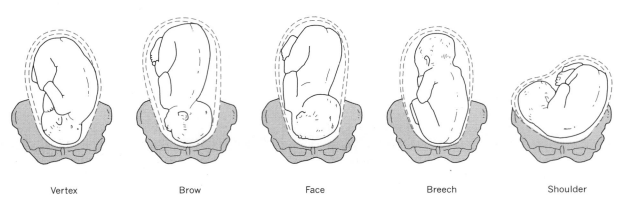

Vertex   Brow   Face   Breech   Shoulder

Figure 4   The presentation of the fetus.

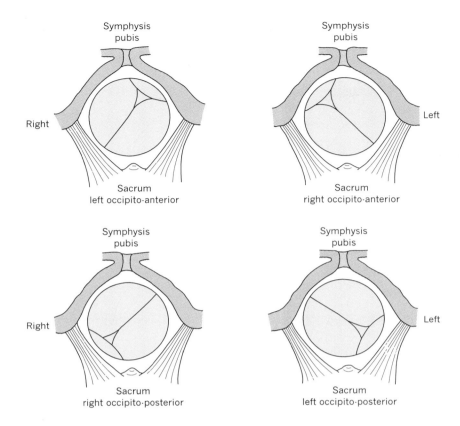

Figure 5 The positions of the fetal skull.

Anterior positions are more common than posterior positions and help to promote flexion of the fetus. This is because in an anterior position the fetal back is uppermost and can flex more easily against the mother's soft abdominal wall than when it lies against her spinal column, as occurs when the fetus adopts a posterior position. When the fetal head is well flexed, a smaller anteroposterior diameter presents to pass through the pelvis, and labour is therefore likely to be more straightforward.

Engagement Engagement of the fetal head (Figure 6) occurs when the transverse diameter (i.e. the biparietal diameter measuring 9.5 cm) has passed through the brim of the pelvis. Nowadays engagement of the fetal head is usually measured in fifths. The amount of fetal head palpable above the brim of the pelvis is assessed and described in fifths as follows (see Figure 7):

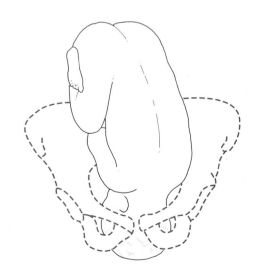

Figure 6 Engagement of the fetal head.

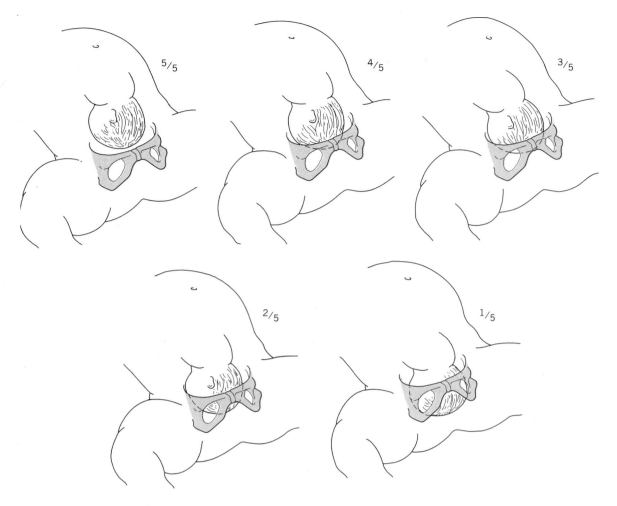

Figure 7 Examination per abdomen to determine the descent of the fetal head in fifths.

▶ **5/5**: The fetal head is *five-fifths* palpable on abdominal examination; that is, the whole head can be palpated above the brim of the pelvis.

▶ **4/5**: *Four-fifths* of the fetal head are palpable above the brim of the pelvis; one-fifth is therefore below the pelvic brim and cannot be palpated per abdomen.

▶ **3/5**: *Three-fifths* of the fetal head are palpable above the brim of the pelvis; two-fifths are below the brim of the pelvis.

▶ **2/5**: *Two-fifths* of the fetal head are palpable above the brim of the pelvis; three-fifths are below the brim of the pelvis. The widest transverse diameter of the fetal head has therefore passed through the brim of the pelvis and the head can be described as engaged.

▶ **1/5**: *One-fifth* of the fetal head is palpable above the brim of the pelvis, four-fifths are below the pelvic brim. The head can be described as being deeply engaged in the pelvis.

Method of abdominal examination

After emptying her bladder, the woman lies on a bed or couch where privacy can be assured. She lies flat on one pillow, unless she finds this very uncomfortable and requires a second pillow, and her knees may be flexed slightly if she wishes. Only her abdomen should be exposed. It is important that the mother should be relaxed and every effort must be made to put her at ease. Obesity, a thick, muscular abdominal wall, poly-hydramnios and twins make the examination difficult, but provided the woman is relaxed even these difficulties may be overcome.

Three ways are used to obtain the information required:

▶ Inspection.
▶ Palpation and measurement.
▶ Auscultation.

Normal findings in late pregnancy are summarized in Table 1.

Inspection   The most important features to be noted are the size and shape of the uterus. The *size* should correspond with the estimated period of gestation. If there is any discrepancy, the date of the last menstrual period should be rechecked. If the dates are correct and the uterus is too large, the main possibilities are:

▶ Large fetus.
▶ Multiple pregnancy.
▶ Polyhydramnios.
▶ Hydatidiform mole.

If the dates are correct and the uterus is small, the most likely causes are:

▶ Small fetus, probably due to placental insufficiency.
▶ Fetal death.
▶ Oligohydramnios.

If the midwife considers the girth to be excessive, she should measure it in centimetres: 95 cm at the umbilicus at 40 weeks is the average. Should a girth of 100 cm be reached or exceeded before that time, obesity may be the cause, but there may be polyhydramnios, twins or a transverse lie to account for it.

The normal *shape* is a longitudinal ovoid, usually very clear in the primigravida, but sometimes more

Table 1   Normal findings on abdominal examination in late pregnancy

Inspection	Uterus a longitudinal ovoid Uterine size consistent with supposed length of gestation
Palpation	Cephalic presentation Head engaged Position left occipito-anterior
Auscultation	Fetal heart sounds strong and regular Fetal heart rate 140 beats per minute

rounded in the multigravid woman. In late pregnancy, the unusual shape created by an oblique or transverse lie is usually unmistakable.

The dark line of pigmentation called the linea nigra, striae gravidarum, the quality of the muscle of the abdominal wall, obliquity of the uterus and fetal movements can also be observed. During this inspection any abdominal scars should be noted and the reason ascertained if not recorded in the notes.

Palpation   Palpation should be carried out gently with both hands. The hands should be clean and warm and the nails short to avoid causing the woman discomfort. They should be moved smoothly over the abdomen and the pads of the fingers used to palpate the fetal parts. A gentle, skilful touch conveys to the mother that she is being examined by a caring, competent midwife. Undue pressure produces pain and will tend to cause a tightening of the abdominal muscles, as well as the stimulation of uterine contractions, and so make palpation more difficult. First the midwife places the ulnar border of the left hand on the fundus and compares the height with the size expected for the period of gestation (Figure 8). In many clinics now the height of the fundus is measured from the symphysis pubis with a tape measure This may be plotted on a chart which gives average findings for gestational

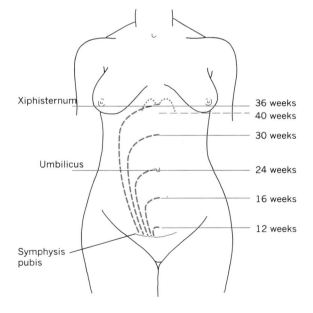

Figure 8   The height of the fundus at different stages of pregnancy.

age. Measurement of the symphyseal-fundal (SF) height is considered a useful guide in the detection of intrauterine growth retardation by many obstetricians, although a study in Denmark did not substantiate this (Lindhart *et al*. 1990).

The midwife then ascertains which part of the fetus is lying at the pelvic brim and confirms the diagnosis by palpating other points of the abdomen. Thus it should be possible to find out the lie, presentation and position and also the relationship of the fetal head to the mother's pelvis. This information is particularly important after the 32nd week of pregnancy.

There are three distinct manoeuvres (Figure 9) employed in abdominal palpation:

▶ Deep pelvic palpation.
▶ Lateral palpation.
▶ Fundal palpation.

Deep pelvic palpation This is the most important manoeuvre in abdominal palpation. The presentation is determined and from that the lie of the fetus is deduced. If the head is presenting, the degree of flexion can be ascertained. In the latter weeks of pregnancy it is most important to determine whether the fetal head is engaged or will engage. The amount of fetal head palpable above the brim of the pelvis is assessed and described in fifths. The midwife turns to face the woman's feet and places one hand on either side of the uterus near the pelvic brim. The fingertips are allowed to sink gently into the pelvis to feel the presentation. The fetal head feels hard and round and it may be possible to *ballotte* it if it is not engaged. This means that, when given a gentle tap on one side by the examining fingers, it floats away and is then felt to return against the examining fingers. When the fingertips can sink into the pelvis further on one side than they do on the other, it may be because the head is

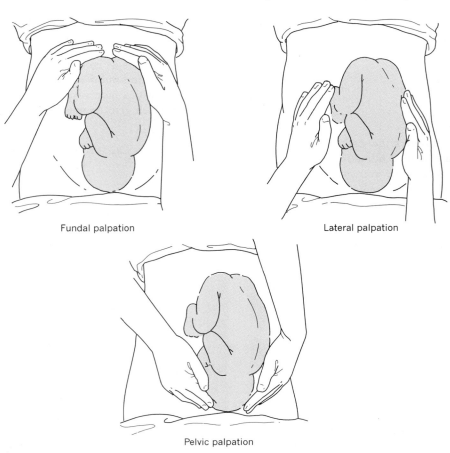

Fundal palpation

Lateral palpation

Pelvic palpation

Figure 9   Types of palpation per abdomen.

flexed and the occiput is lying on the side into which the fingers sink more deeply. The position of the occiput indicates the position of the fetus. Whilst carrying out this manoeuvre the midwife should turn her head to watch the mother's face for any sign of discomfort.

Lateral palpation This manoeuvre is carried out to locate the fetal back. The midwife turns to face the mother's face. One hand is placed flat on one side of the abdomen to steady it whilst the other hand gently palpates down the other side of the abdomen. The process is then reversed. The fetal back is felt as a continuous smooth resistant object, whereas the limbs are noted as small irregularities which are often felt to move. If the firm outline of the back cannot be easily palpated and fetal limbs are felt on both sides of the midline, the position is probably occipitoposterior. In this case the midwife may have observed a small depression on the abdomen just below the umbilicus.

Fundal palpation Still facing the mother's head, the midwife carries out this manoeuvre to determine which part of the fetus is lying in the fundus. In most cases it will be the breech. If the head is in the fundus it can be recognized as smooth, round, hard and ballotable, separated from the trunk by a groove, the neck. This is why it is more freely movable than the breech, which can only move from side to side, the back moving with it. The breech is also less hard, more irregular in outline, and the lower limbs may be palpated near it.

Auscultation   This is done with a stethoscope, either the Pinard monaural fetal stethoscope or the binaural stethoscope, or with an electronic fetal heart monitor. Having palpated the abdomen the midwife should know where to listen for the fetal heart sounds. They are heard at their maximum at a point over the fetal back. When the fetus is lying in an occipito-anterior or occipitolateral position the heart sounds are heard from the front and to the right or left according to the side on which the fetal back lies (Figure 10). The fetal heart sounds like the ticking of a watch under a pillow, the rate being about double that of the mother's heart beats observed at the wrist. The mother and her partner usually enjoy listening to their baby's heartbeat too.

A uterine *souffle* may be heard; this is a soft, blowing sound, the rate of which corresponds to the mother's pulse. It is caused by the flowing of blood through the uterine arteries.

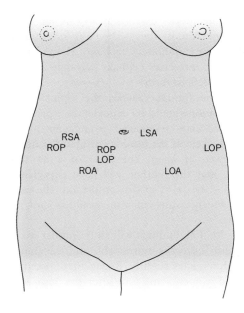

Figure 10   The approximate points of the fetal heart sounds in vertex and breech presentations.

Abdominal findings throughout pregnancy

▶ *At first* only the height of the fundus is ascertained.

▶ *Week 12* (or sometimes rather earlier): The fundus is just palpable above the symphysis.

▶ *Week 16*: The fundus is halfway to the umbilicus. At this stage a multigravida may have felt fetal movements.

▶ *Week 20*: The fundus reaches the lower border of the umbilicus and all mothers should be asked about movements. The fetal heart sounds may be audible.

▶ *Week 24*: The fundus reaches the upper border of the umbilicus, the fetus may just be palpable and the fetal heart sounds are heard.

▶ *Week 28*: The fundus of the uterus is one-third of the distance from the umbilicus to the xiphisternum. The fetus is now easily palpable, very mobile and may be found in any lie, presentation or position.

▶ *Week 32*: The uterus is two-thirds from the umbilicus to the xiphisternum. The fetus lies longitudinally and, usually, the head presents. If the midwife finds a breech presentation, she should refer the mother to a doctor. It may be decided to turn the fetus, though the doctor will probably want to wait to see whether it turns spontaneously.

▶ *Week 34*: The uterus extends nearly as far as the xiphisternum. Almost always the lie is longitudinal; usually the presentation is cephalic. If the breech presents then external cephalic version may be attempted or left to term.

▶ *Week 36*: The fundus reaches the xiphisternum. The presentation should be cephalic. In a primigravida the head may be engaged or engagement may occur a little later. If the head is engaged the fundus will be lower, at about the level of a 34 week pregnancy, and the mother will have experienced *'lightening'* – the relief of discomfort and the easier breathing which results when the head has sunk into the pelvis.

▶ *Weeks 37–40*: The findings will all be similar except that the fetus becomes more stable and the amount of liquor diminishes slightly. Engagement occurs in primigravid women some time after the 36th week. Usually it is later in multigravidae and it may not occur until labour is established.

The midwife must observe the woman carefully for signs of the *supine hypotensive syndrome* during abdominal examinations, especially as pregnancy advances and the weight of the uterus increases.

ENGAGEMENT OF THE FETAL HEAD

There is a popular myth that engagement of the head occurs at 36 weeks in a primigravida. In fact in about 50% of primigravidae engagement of the head occurs between 38 and 42 weeks (Weekes and Flynn, 1975). It has also been shown that in 80% of cases labour ensues within 14 days of the head engaging. In multigravidae, because of their lax uterine and abdominal muscles, engagement may not take place until labour is established. If the head is engaged the pelvic brim is certainly of adequate size and the probability is that the cavity and outlet are also adequate.

Engagement is often referred to as *lightening*, because the sense of lightness mothers feel as the pressure is lessened on the diaphragm.

Non-engagement of the fetal head

When, particularly in a first pregnancy, the head is not engaged at term, the cause should be sought. It may be something simple and easily remedied, such as a distended bladder or a full rectum. In occipitoposterior positions the head tends to be deflexed; the presenting diameter is then greater and the head has more diffi-

culty in becoming engaged. *Cephalopelvic disproportion* is an important, though not very common, cause of failure of engagement in the UK, but occurs more frequently in developing countries. In *polyhydramnios* non-engagement is expected because the fetus has plenty of room in which to move around. A persistently high head is sometimes a feature of *placenta praevia*, because the placenta occupies space in the lower segment of the uterus, thereby displacing the fetal head.

Occasionally a very small head fails to engage in an obviously large pelvis. This may indicate a *twin pregnancy*, the first with a deeply engaged head.

A *steep angle of inclination of the pelvic brim* tends to delay engagement until labour is well established. This is seen fairly commonly as a racial characteristic in West African and West Indian women (see Chapter 2).

Pelvic tumours and *gross malformations* are rare causes of a high head.

Head fitting   Various methods can be used to cause a non-engaged head to engage. The woman is invited to empty her bladder and then lies on the couch. Standing on the mother's right, the midwife or doctor defines the symphysis pubis with the fingers of the right hand. The thumb and fingers of the left hand are placed on either side of the fetal head. The woman is asked to breathe in deeply and as she breathes out the head is pushed downwards and backwards and the fingers of the right hand are used to estimate whether the greatest diameter of the head is passing through the pelvic brim. This is a simple and, with experience, accurate method of head fitting. Other methods with the woman either sitting or standing are available, but whatever method is used it is best learned by clinical demonstration and practice.

PELVIC ASSESSMENT

If there is doubt about the capacity of the pelvis the doctor may wish to make an examination per vaginam to assess the size and shape of the pelvis. This examination is easier during the latter weeks of pregnancy when the soft tissues are relaxed. Also, the fetal head is almost fully grown and can therefore be related to the size of the pelvis. This examination is particularly important for any woman in whom the head cannot be made to engage. An attempt is made to measure the diagonal conjugate since the obstetric conjugate cannot be reached (see Chapter 2). The size of the obstetric

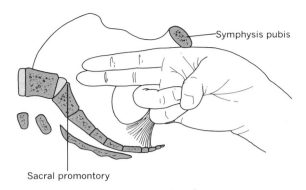

Symphysis pubis

Sacral promontory

Figure 11   Measurement of the diagonal conjugate.

conjugate can then be estimated (Figure 11). The obstetric conjugate is the actual space available for the fetal head to pass through at the brim of the pelvis. In order to assess the diagonal conjugate, the doctor measures with the fingers from the lower border of the symphysis pubis to the promontory of the sacrum. This is normally 12–13 cm. If the pelvis is a good size it is unlikely that the promontory of the sacrum will be reached. If it can be felt, however, the size of the obstetric conjugate can be estimated by subtracting 2 cm from the length of the diagonal conjugate to allow for the depth of the pubic bone.

The pelvic cavity is assessed by feeling the length and curve of the sacrum and by measuring the length of the sacrospinous ligament. It should comfortably accommodate two fingers.

Lastly, the size and shape of the pelvic outlet are assessed. The ischial spines are palpated. If they are prominent this could indicate a narrow transverse diameter of the pelvic outlet. The subpubic angle should be 90° or more and should accommodate two fingers in the apex of the arch. Finally, the distance between the ischial tuberosities is assessed by placing a closed fist on the perineum. A man-sized fist should fit between them.

Following this examination the findings and implications will be discussed with the woman. If there is any degree of cephalopelvic disproportion the mode of delivery will need to be considered (see Chapter 54).

BREAST CARE

There has been a general increase in breastfeeding in the UK since the 1970s when the decline in the number of women breastfeeding reached an all time low. At that time only 51% of women in England and Wales started breastfeeding (Martin, 1978), but after recommendations from the Department of Health and Social Security and a concerted effort by health care professionals and some voluntary groups, the incidence of breastfeeding rose to 67% within the next five years (Martin and Monk, 1982). However, only 26% of these mothers breastfed for the four months recommended by the Department of Health and Social Security (DHSS, 1980). Indeed, 19% of them had already discontinued by two weeks after delivery (Martin and Monk, 1982). The greatest increase in those who breastfed between 1975 and 1980 was amongst mothers having their second or subsequent baby (Silverton, 1985). These women are also most likely to be successful (Martin and Monk, 1982). Hytten (1976) suggests that this is because there is improved breast and nipple development with better lactation in multiparous women. Alexander (1991), however, reports that parity, of itself, does not influence nipple development in subsequent pregnancies, and women who have not breastfed before are almost two and a half times more likely to have inverted or non-protractile nipples.

In order to promote successful breastfeeding the midwife should have a knowledge of the factors which influence a mother's choice of feeding method and be competent to give appropriate information, advice and support during pregnancy and the postnatal period. In a study carried out by Hally *et al.* (1984) three-quarters of the mothers had already chosen their method of feeding before their hospital booking visit. Of these women one-third said they had made their choice before they were pregnant. This finding demonstrates the need to start education about breastfeeding early in schools, colleges and youth clubs since it is often too late when left until the woman is pregnant. In the majority of cases the women who had chosen their feeding method in early pregnancy did not change their decision (Hally *et al.* 1984; McIntosh, 1985). Hence the midwife is more likely to influence those women who are undecided about their choice of feeding method at the booking visit than those who have already decided to artificially feed.

Sociocultural influences have a major influence on the woman's choice of feeding method. Hally *et al.* (1984) found that those who lived in council-owned property or in overcrowded conditions, especially where there are children, are less likely to breastfeed. Similarly, fewer women breastfeed amongst the young, single, lower social classes, and poorly educated. Another interesting finding in this study is that mothers who have been breastfed themselves are more likely to breastfeed their own children. Also there is a greater incidence of breastfeeding in those who have seen a baby breastfed (Jeffs, 1977; Hally *et al.*, 1984). The partner's attitude to breastfeeding was found to have a significant influence on the method of feeding in a study carried out by Jeffs (1977). The influence of friends and young relatives was also found to be important since women seem to prefer the feeding method of their peer group (Jeffs, 1977; Hally *et al.*, 1984; Prince and Adams, 1987).

The main reasons given in support of a decision to bottle feed were that breastfeeding is inconvenient, embarrassing and the idea is distasteful. A survey of public attitudes to breastfeeding conducted by the Joint Breastfeeding Initiative in 1990 (an initiative established by the government) found that although 96% of the population supported the idea of breastfeeding, 60% disapproved of breastfeeding in public places, and 50% disagreed with feeding in restaurants.

By the time the woman attends the booking clinic she will have been exposed to a variety of social and cultural influences which influence her choice of feeding method.

Early in pregnancy the midwife takes the opportunity to explore the woman's attitudes to breastfeeding and discuss the advantages and disadvantages with her. It may be the first time the expectant mother has had the opportunity to discuss breastfeeding with a professional and the situation needs to be handled sensitively, particularly with women who appear uncomfortable or disinterested. Those who wish to breastfeed are encouraged, and the midwife will try to build up confidence in those who are uncertain about their ability to breastfeed successfully. Mothers need to believe that 'breast is not only best, but breast is possible' (Entwistle, 1991). Any mother who is unwilling to breastfeed is not coerced, but encouraged to reconsider her decision.

If a woman has successfully breastfed before, it is not necessary to carry out a routine antenatal examination of the nipples in a subsequent pregnancy (Alexander, 1991). For those who have not previously breastfed, it is recommended that the examination is deferred until the third trimester because spontaneous improvement in nipple contractibility occurs as pregnancy advances. A large, multicentre, randomized controlled trial of alternative treatments for inverted and non-protractile nipples in pregnancy was conducted between 1988 and 1993 (McCandlish *et al.*, 1992).

Women with inverted and non-contractile nipples who were treated with either breast shells or Hoffman's nipple stretching exercises and women with the same nipple problems who received no treatment were all breastfeeding at six weeks after delivery. As a result of these findings there appears to be no basis for recommending the use of breast shells or Hoffman's exercises for the treatment of inverted or non-protractile nipples in pregnancy.

Advice

Hygiene   It is advisable to wash the nipples with water only during pregnancy because soap has been found to remove the natural secretions of the sebaceous and sweat glands. These secretions increase in pregnancy and not only act as a natural lubricant, but also have bactericidal properties (Newton, 1952). The application of additional creams to lubricate the nipples in pregnancy should not therefore be required.

Support   There is no evidence that wearing a bra during the day and at night has any benefits, thus the woman should be advised to do what is most comfortable for her (Alexander, 1991). As the breasts enlarge during pregnancy, a larger size, well-fitting bra will be required.

Diet   A good, well-mixed diet is recommended for all women in pregnancy and is particularly important for women who intend to breastfeed so that their health is not compromised during lactation.

Antenatal education   The physiology of lactation and the management of breastfeeding is an important part of preparation during pregnancy. Perhaps most important of all, however, is to build up the woman's confidence in her ability to feed successfully.

WOMEN WITH SPECIAL NEEDS

Teenage pregnancies

Britain has the highest teenage birth rates in the European Union and the rates were rising annually until recently when there was a slight decrease. In 1992, 31.7% of all children were born outside marriage, compared with 29.8% in 1991 (Central Statistical Office, 1994, 1993). About 6% of all pregnancies of single women occur in teenagers under the age of 19 years (Lee, 1994). A number of young teenagers, about 8% of boys and 4% of girls, start sexual relationships before the age of 14 years. Women from higher social classes are more likely not to conceive at an early age, but if they do, often have a termination of pregnancy (Roberts, 1995). The government White Paper, *Health of the Nation*, aims to reduce the rate of conceptions in the under 16-year-olds by at least 50% by the year 2000 (DOH, 1992a).

There is particular concern about the high rate of teenage births, not only because of the increased risk of complications during pregnancy and childbirth, but also because of the social problems which ensue. Many of these young girls are already disadvantaged and the problems associated with poverty and poor education are often perpetuated into the next generation. Midwives have a particular role in offering emotional and social support to these young women, both on a one-to-one basis and increasingly in special clinics or clubs for pregnant teenagers (Minns, 1989). These groups not only offer peer and professional support during pregnancy, but also provide a forum for discussing many health education issues such as nutrition, smoking, drug abuse, alcohol consumption and unprotected sex. Good family planning advice is essential because many of these young teenagers will have a second baby by the age of 20. The problems of finance and accommodation are also discussed and appropriate information is given (Minns, 1994). Education for parenthood is included in the discussions which take place in these groups and many continue to meet as postnatal support groups.

In very young teenagers, their physical and psychological development is put at risk and their education severely disrupted. Complications in pregnancy are also more likely and these include pregnancy-induced hypertension, anaemia and preterm labour. Often too the infants are at risk after delivery due to poverty, neglect, malnutrition, abuse and infections (Akker, 1995). Maternal, perinatal and infant mortality and morbidity rates are increased with these young mothers. Continuity of carer, additional support, education and close surveillance in pregnancy are therefore particularly important for these young women so that problems can be identified and appropriate action taken. The co-operation of the teenager is essential if the best outcome is to be achieved for both mother and baby and therefore midwives need to tailor the care they offer to make it both acceptable and easily accessible to these young people. Drop-in antenatal clinics, where women can attend without an appointment, are often more acceptable, or special teenage clinics, as already described.

Midwives should have knowledge of national and local organizations which are available to support pregnant teenagers and young parents. The Teenage Parenthood Network is a national information and support system which publishes a quarterly newsletter giving useful information about resources, groups and study opportunities. Another source of help is *The Really Helpful Directory* which gives information about all the residential and non-residential services designed for young mothers in the UK. The addresses of both these organizations are given at the end of this chapter.

Ethnic minority groups

The perinatal mortality rates are increased in infants of women from many ethnic minority groups. For example, the perinatal mortality rate in the UK in 1987 was 8.6 per 1000 births, but for babies born to mothers whose country of origin was India it was 11.5, Bangladesh 12.5, and for Pakistan 14.9 (Narang and Murphy, 1994). The antenatal care for these women therefore needs to be tailored to meet their special needs and address their particular problems.

Communication is one of the major problems as many women from ethnic minority groups do not speak English, or their language is very limited. These women often bring an English-speaking relative to the clinic with them, often their husband or a child, but this is not always an ideal solution as sometimes the relative only interprets what they consider most important, or misunderstandings occur, and for the woman there is no confidentiality. A study conducted by Narang and Murphy (1994) concluded that the changes Asian women considered most necessary in antenatal care were the presence of an interpreter and the need for a female doctor. Health education and explanatory leaflets should be available in antenatal clinics for non-English-speaking women in appropriate languages.

Diet is a problem in some ethnic groups as certain foods which are of high nutritional value may be avoided in pregnancy. Many Asian women are vegetarians and, although a good vegetarian diet can be very nutritious, not all women are having the good mixed diet which they need in pregnancy. The midwife therefore needs to discuss diet carefully with women from ethnic minority groups and give dietary advice, if necessary, which is acceptable to women of different cultures.

Certain health problems are more prevalent in black, Asian or Mediterranean women and special investigations may be necessary in pregnancy. For example, sickle cell anaemia may be found in those who originate from Central and West Africa and parts of Asia, while thalassaemia may occur in those of Mediterranean origin. Anaemia due to hookworm infestation or malaria may be a problem in some women from the African continent and other parts of the world. Infectious conditions such as tuberculosis and HIV are also more prevalent in many overseas countries.

Attendance at parent education classes is poor for many women from ethnic minority groups, largely because of the language problem. Other women in the extended family tend to have a major influence on preparing younger members of the family for childbirth and parenthood. Some women from ethnic minority groups are very isolated, however, because most of their family are still in their country of origin. Midwives therefore need to offer support and parent education on a one-to-one basis or in small groups for women from ethnic minorities. Partners from some ethnic minority groups consider that support during pregnancy and childbirth is the role of women in the family and so tend not to become too involved. It may therefore be helpful for other female members of the family to be involved in preparation for childbirth and parenthood sessions too, so that they can support the pregnant woman appropriately during pregnancy, labour and the postnatal period.

Disabled women

Pregnant disabled women have special problems, not only because of their disability, but also due to the negative reactions of some professionals, as well as members of their families. Many people are concerned about how they are going to cope with a child and underestimate the parenting abilities and determination of women with disabilities.

Attendance at a busy antenatal clinic may be very difficult, if not impossible, for some women with major physical disabilities because of the problems of travel and access when they are there. Steps, small cubicles and having to move around from one area to another. climb on and off a couch and cope with a variety of different examinations and professionals may make the visit very difficult.

Those who are deaf or visually impaired also have problems and will need special help (Nolan, 1984a). Most deaf people lip read and so the midwife must ensure that her mouth is clearly visible to the woman at all times when she is speaking. A sign language interpreter should also be available at the clinic when the woman attends for her appointments (Kelsall, 1993). The midwife addresses her communications to the mother, however, and not to the interpreter. It is also important that the woman has her hands free for sign language and so the midwife should not expect a response from her when her hands are not free, for instance when her blood pressure is being taken. Written information and visual aids are particularly helpful to those who are deaf and should be used as much as possible to back up verbal explanations. The visually impaired will also need special help during the antenatal period, especially finding their way around a busy clinic and on and off an examination couch. Health education leaflets in Braille, audiocassettes and videos with a good commentary will be helpful for these women and some may be obtained from the Royal National Institute for the Blind.

One-to-one midwifery care from a very small group of midwives is most helpful for women with disabilities. This gives them the opportunity to build up a relationship of trust and become partners in care. They, too, have the right to be fully informed and make choices related to their care (Nolan, 1984b). The midwives need to find out the extent of the woman's disabilities and how she normally manages so that they can work out together the best way to cope in labour and with the care of the baby afterwards. The woman is the expert in her disability and the midwives can learn from her how to adapt their care to make it appropriate and as comfortable as possible for her. Antenatal care is often easier for the woman in her own home and this also gives the midwives the opportunity to see how the woman manages in her own surroundings and assess her ability to manage with a newborn baby. Help from social services may be required to provide support for the woman with the care of her baby and, if required, to make any necessary adaptations to her home.

Parent education needs to be adapted to make it suitable for the woman with disabilities and should involve partners wherever possible. The midwife needs to assess the woman carefully and devise effective ways of helping her to develop safe and appropriate parenting skills. For the visually handicapped learning by touch is effective and models to handle can be helpful (Nolan, 1994b). Audiocassettes can also be used to back up the spoken word. Those who are deaf appreciate visual aids, including demonstrations, videos, slides, films and also written information. It may be possible for some physically disabled women to attend the usual parent education classes with other women, but they may also need individual sessions to help them to adapt the skills they have observed to their special circumstances.

All women require individualized care and the midwives are striving to meet their needs and aspirations by working in partnership with them to achieve a safe, pleasurable and fulfilling experience of childbirth. Meeting the needs and aspirations of those who are disabled requires extra skill, insight and imagination but is especially rewarding when the outcome is successful for all concerned.

References

Akker, van den, O. (1995) Teenage pregnancy: a continued cause for concern. *Br. J. Midwifery*, 3(1): 6–7.

Alexander, J. (1991) The prevalence and management of inverted and non-protractile nipples in antenatal women who intend to breastfeed. Unpublished PhD thesis.

Argyle, M. (1969) *Social interaction*, 2nd edn. London: Tavistock/Methuen.

Ball, J. (1992) Who's Left Holding the Baby? An organisational framework for making the most of midwifery services. University of Leeds, The Nuffield Institute for Health Services Studies.

Broadhurst, M. (1988) Computers can improve the quality of care. News item. *Nursing Times* 84(48): 7.

Central Statistical Office (1993) *Social Trends*, no. 23. London: HMSO.

Central Statistical Office (1994) *Social Trends*, no. 24. London: HMSO.

Chadwick, J. (1993) Alcohol in pregnancy. *Modern Midwife* 3(2): 19–21.

Chadwick, J. (1994) Perinatal mortality and antenatal care. *Modern Midwife* 4(9): 18–20.

Charles, J. (1992) Pregnant pause. *Nursing Times* 88(34): 30–32.

Currell, R. (1990) The organisation of midwifery care. In Alexander, J., Levy, V. & Roch, S. (eds) *Antenatal Care*. Houndmills: Macmillan Educational.

Davies, J. (1988) Cowgate Neighbourhood Centre – a preventative health care venture shared by midwives and social workers. *Midwives Chronicle* 101(1200): 4–7.

Dawes, M.G. & Grudzinskas, J.G. (1991) Repeated measurement of maternal weight during pregnancy. Is this a useful practice? *Br. J. Obstet. Gynaecol.* 98: 189–194.

DHSS (Department of Health and Social Security) (1970) Domiciliary midwifery and maternity bed needs (Peel Report). London: HMSO.

DHSS (1980) *Present Day Practice in Infant Feeding*. London: HMSO.

DOH (Department of Health) (1992a) *The Health of the Nation. A Strategy for Health in England*. London: HMSO.

DOH (1992b) *Second Report of Maternity Services*, Vol. 1 (Winterton Report). London: HMSO.

DOH (1993) *Changing Childbirth*, Part 1. Report of the Expert Maternity Group. London: HMSO.

Draper, J., Field, S., Thomas, H. & Hare, M.J. (1986) Should women carry their own notes? *Br. Med. J.* 292: 603.

Entwistle, F. (1991) Breastfeeding: the most natural function. *Nursing Times* 87(18): 24–26.

Etherington, I.J. & James, D.K. (1993) Reagent strip testing of antenatal urine for infection. *Br J. Obstet. Gynaecol.* 100: 806–808.

Fawdry, R. (1994) Antenatal casenotes 1: comments on design. *Br. J. Mid.* 2(7): 320–327.

Feeney, J. G. (1984) Hypertension in pregnancy managed at home by community midwives. *Br. Med. J.* 288: 1046–1047.

Field, P.A. (1990) Effectiveness and efficacy of antenatal care. *Midwifery* 6(4): 215–223.

Flint, C., Poulengeris, P. & Grant, A.M. (1987) The 'Know Your Midwife' scheme: a randomised trial of continuity of care by a team of midwives. *Midwifery* 5: 11–16.

Galloway, L. (1994) Knowing the form. *Modern Midwife* 4(9): 24–26.

Garcia, J. (1982) Women's views of antenatal care. In Enkin, M. & Chalmers, I. (eds) *Effectiveness and Satisfaction in Antenatal Care*. London: Heinemann Medical Books.

Green, J. (1989) Diet and the prevention of pre-eclampsia. In Chalmers, I., Enkin, M. & Keirse, M.J.N.C. (eds) *Effective Care in Pregnancy and Childbirth*. Oxford: Oxford University Press.

Haglund, B.C. & Cnattingius, S. (1990) Cigarette smoking as a risk factor for sudden infant death sydrome: a population based study. *Am. J. Pub. Health* 80(1): 29–32.

Haley, J. (1995) Welcome to the antenatal day unit. *Modern Midwife* 5(6): 27–30.

Hall, M.H., Ching, P.K. & MacGillivray, I. (1980) Is routine antenatal care worthwhile? *Lancet* ii: 78–80.

Hall, M., MacIntyre, S. & Porter, M. (1985) *Antenatal Care Assessed*: A case study of an innovation in Aberdeen. Aberdeen University Press.

Hally, R., Bond, J., Crawley, J., Gregson, B., Phillips, P. & Russell, I. (1984) What influences a mother's choice of infant feeding method? *Nursing Times*, 80(4): 65–68.

HEA (Health Education Authority) (1994a) Smoking and pregnancy survey. *Midwives Chronicle* February: 53; *J. Obstet. Gynecol.*, 117: 1–9.

HEA (1994b) *Helping Pregnant Smokers Quit: Training for Health Professionals*. London: HEA.

Hodnett, E.D. (1993) Women carrying their own casenotes during pregnancy. In *Pregnancy and Childbirth Module. Database of Systematic Reviews*: review no. 03776. Oxford: Cochrane Updates.

Hughes, D.F.J. & Goldstone, L.A. (1989) Frameworks for midwifery care in Great Britain: an exploration into quality assurance. *Midwifery* 5(4): 163–172.

Hundley, V.A., Cruickshank, F.M., Lang, G.D. *et al.* (1994) Midwife managed delivery unit: a randomised controlled comparison with consultant led care. *Br. Med. J.* 309(6966): 1400–1403.

Hutton, E. (1994) What women want from midwives. *Br. J. Midwifery* 2(12): 608–611.

Hytten, F.E. (1976) The physiology of lactation. *J. Human Nutr.* 30: 225–232.

Hytten, F.E. & Chamberlain, G. (1980) *Clinical Physiology in Obstetrics*, Part 2, *Nutrition and Metabolism*. Oxford: Blackwell Scientific.

James, D.K. (1988) Risk at the booking visit. Chapter 4 in James, D.K. & Stirrat, G.M. (eds) *Pregnancy and Risk: the Basis of Rational Management*. Chichester: John Wiley & Sons.

Jeffs, J. (1977) Why do mothers breast feed? *Nursing Times* June 16: 911–914.

Joing Breastfeeding Initiative (1990) Survey of public attitudes towards breastfeeding. *Joint Breastfeeding Initiative Newsletter* 1: 6.

Keirse, M.J.N.C. (1994) Maternal mortality: stalemate or stagnant? *Br. Med. J.* 308: 344–345.

Kelsall, J. (1993) Giving midwifery care for the deaf in the 1990s. *Midwives Chronicle* 106(1262): 80–83.

Kemp, V.H. & Page, C.K. (1984) The psychological impact of a high risk pregnancy on the family. *J. Obstet. Gynecol. Neonatal Nursing* 13: 232–236.

Klein, M., Lloyd, I., Redman, C., Bull, M. & Turnbull, A.C. (1983) A comparison of low risk pregnant women booked for delivery in two systems of care. *Br. J. Obstet Gynaecol.* 90: 118–120.

Kroll, D. (1993) The name of the game – team midwifery now. *Modern Midwife* 3(3): 26–28.

Laurent, C. (1992) Pointless routine? *Nursing Times* 88(919): 22–23.

Lee, B. (1994) Teenage pregnancy. *J. Roy. Soc. Med.* 87: 485–486.

Lewis, D. (1983) Alcohol and pregnancy outcome. *Midwives Chronicle* December: 420–422.

Lindhart, A., Nielsen, L.A., Mouritsen, L.A. *et al.* (1990) The implications of introducing the symphyseal-fundal height measurement: a prospective randomized controlled trial. *Br. J. Obstet. Gynaecol.* 97(8): 675–680.

Lilford, R.J. & Chard, T. (1983) Problems and pitfalls of risk assessment in antenatal care. *Br. J. Obstet. Gynaecol.* 90: 507–510.

Lilford, R.J., Kelly, M., Baines, A. *et al.* (1992) Effect of using protocols on medical care: randomised trial of three methods of taking an antenatal history. *Br. Med. J.* 305: 1181–1184.

Lowe, S. W., House, W. & Garrett, T. (1987) A comparison of outcome of low risk labour in an isolated general practitioner maternity unit and a specialist maternity hospital. *R. Coll. Gen. Pract.* 37: 484–487.

MacArthur, C., Newton, J.R. & Knox, E.G. (1987) Effect of anti-smoking health education on infant size: a randomised controlled trial. *Br. J. Obstet. Gynaecol.* 94: 295–300.

Macleod Clark, J. & Maclaine, K. (1992) The effects of smoking in pregnancy: a review of approaches to behavioural change. *Midwifery* 8(1): 19–30.

MacDonald, S.J. (1990) Antenatal admissions: Women's perceptions of the experience. *Research and the Midwife*, Conference Proceedings, Manchester, pp. 72–82.

Magill-Cuerden, J. (1992) A question of communication. *Modern Midwife* 2(6): 4–5.

Mandelbrot, L. (1993) What determines seropositive women's choice to terminate or continue pregnancy? Paper presented at the Conference on HIV in Children and Mothers, Edinburgh, Abstracts, p. 301.

Martin, J. (1978) *Infant Feeding 1975: Attitudes and Practice in England and Wales* London: HMSO.

Martin, J. & Monk, J. (1982) *Infant Feeding*. London: Office of Population Censuses and Surveys.

Mayes, G.E. (1987) Developing a model of care in Waltham Forest. *Midwives Chronicle* 100 (1198): v–ix.

McCandlish, R., Renfrew, M.J., Ashurst, H. & Bowler, U. (1992) Getting results: the processes involved in organising and analysing data from the MAIN trial. *Research and the Midwife*, Conference Proceedings, pp. 17–25.

McGreal, I.E. (1995) Smoking and the pregnant woman. *Midwives Chronicle* 108(1290): 218–221.

McIntosh, J. (1985) Decisions on breast feeding in a group of first-time mothers. *Research and the Midwife*, Conference Proceedings, 46–64.

McKee, I. (1980) Community Antenatal Care: The Sighthill Community Antenatal Scheme. In Zander, L.I. & Chamberlain, G. (eds) *Pregnancy Care for the 1980s*. London: Royal Society of Medicine/Macmillan Press.

Methven, R.C. (1982a) The antenatal booking interview: recording an obstetric history or relating with a mother-to-be? *Research and the Midwife*, Conference Proceedings, Glasgow, pp. 63–76.

Methven, R.C. (1982b) The antenatal booking interview: recording an obstetric history or relating with a mother-to-be? *Research and the Midwife*, Conference Proceedings, Glasgow, pp. 77–86.

Methven, R.C. (1986) Care plan for a woman having antenatal care based on Orem's Self Care Model. In Webb, C. (ed.) *Woman's Health: Midwifery & Gynaecology*. Sevenoaks: Hodder & Stoughton.

Methven, R.C. (1989) Recording an obstetric history or relating to a pregnant woman? A study of the antenatal booking interview. In Robinson, S. & Thomson, A. (eds) *Midwives, Research and Childbirth*, Vol. 1. London: Chapman & Hall.

Middlemass, C., Dawson, A.J., Gauthe, N., Jones, N.E. & Coles, E.C. (1989) A randomised study of a domiciliary antenatal care scheme: maternal psychological effects. *Midwifery* **5**: 69–74.

Midgely, C. (1988) Survey of use of models for nursing in midwifery. Unpublished BEd. dissertation, Huddersfield Polytechnic.

Minns, H.R. (1989) Young Mum's Club. *Nursing Times* **85**: 53.

Minns, H. (1994) Teenage pregnancy. *Modern Midwife* **4**(7): 12–14.

Moore, J., Peters, A. & Frame, S. (1983) The relevance of shoe size to obstetric outcome. *Research and the Midwife*, Conference Proceedings, pp. 53–68.

Morris de Lassalle, S.H. (1994) The organization and work of a fetal assessment day unit. *Br. J. Midwifery* **2**(1): 20–25.

Narang, I. & Murphy, S. (1994) Assessment of the antenatal care for Asian women *Br. J. Midwifery* **22**(4): 169–173.

Newton, M. (1952) Nipple pain and nipple damage; problems in the management of breast feeding. *J. Pediat.* **41**: 411–423.

Nolan, M. (1994a) Care for the deaf mother. *Modern Midwife* **4**(7): 15–16.

Nolan, M. (1994b) Choice and control for the disabled mother. *Modern Midwife* April: 10–12.

Oakley, A. (1982) The relevance of the history of medicine to an understanding of current change: some comments from the domain of antenatal care. *Soc. Sci. Med.* **16**: 667–674.

Oakley, A. (1983) The development of antenatal care in the last eighty years. *Maternal and Child Health* **8**(2): 66–71.

Oakley, A. (1984) *The Captured Womb: a History of the Medical Care of Pregnant Woman*. Oxford: Blackwell.

Oakley, A., Rajan, L. & Grant, A. (1990) Social support and pregnancy outcome. *Br. J. Obstet. Gynaecol.* **97**(2): 152–162.

O'Brien, M. & Smith, C. (1981) Women's views and experiences of antenatal care. *Practitioner*, **225**: 123–125.

Orem, D. (1980) *Nursing: Concepts of Practice*. New York: McGraw-Hill.

Page, L. Jones, B. Bentley, R. *et al.* (1994) One-to-one midwifery practice. *Br. J. Midwifery* **2**(9): 444–447.

Parsons, W.D. & Perkins, E.R. (1982) *Why Don't Women Attend for Antenatal Care?* Leverhulme Health Education Project, Occasional paper no. 23, University of Nottingham.

Plant, M. (1985) *Women, Drinking and Pregnancy*. London: Tavistock.

Proud, J. (1994) *Understanding Obstetric Ultrasound*. Hale: Books for Midwives Press.

Prince, J. & Adams, M.E. (1987) *The Psychology of Childbirth*. Edinburgh: Churchill Livingstone.

Reid, M.E., Gutteridge, S. & McIlwaine, G.M. (1983) A comparison of the delivery of antenatal care between a hospital and a peripheral clinic. Social Paed. & Obstet. Research Unit, University of Glasgow.

Renfrew, M., Rosser, J., Kitzinger, S., Burns, E. & McKinney, T. (1988) Risk in childbirth: extracts from a discussion held in Oxford on 19 May 1988 MIDIRS Information Pack no. 9, November 1988.

Roberts, C. (1995) Families in Britain. *Midwives* **108**(1286): 71–74.

Royal College of Obstetricians and Gynaecologists (1982) Report of the RCOG Working Party on Antenatal and Intrapartum Care. Appendix 2.

Shearer, J.M.L. (1985) A five-year prospective survey on risk of booking for a home birth. *Br. Med. J.* **291**: 1478–1480.

Sikorski, J., Clement, S., Wilson, J. Das, S. & Smeeton, N. (1995) A survey of health professionals' views on the possible changes in the provision and organisation of antenatal care. *Midwifery* **11**(2): 61–68.

Silverton, L. (1985) Breast feeding yesterday and today. *Midwifery*, **1**(3): 162–166.

Simms, M. (1989) Misuse of drugs – who is to blame? *Midwife, Health Visitor & Community Nurse* **25**(4): 124–128.

Smith, D.B., Rustin, G.J.S. & Bagshawe, K.D. (1988) Don't ignore a positive pregnancy test. *Br. Med. J.* **297**: 1119–1120.

Streissguth, A., Clarren, S.K. & Jones, K. (1985) Natural history of the fetal alcohol syndrome. A ten year follow-up of 11 patients. *Lancet* ii: 85.

Streissguth, A., Aase, J., Clarren, S.K. *et al.* (1991) Reported social alcohol consumption during pregnancy and infants' development at 18 months. *Br. Med. J.* **303**(6793): 22–26.

Tew, M. (1990) *Safer Childbirth? A Critical Review of Maternity Care*. London: Chapman & Hall.

Thomas, H. Draper, J. Field, S. & Hare, M. (1987) Evaluation of an intregrated antenatal clinic. *J. R. Coll. Gen. Pract.* **37**: 544–547.

Thomson, A.M., Billewicz, W.Z. (1957) Clinical significance of weight trends during pregnancy. *Br. Med. J.* i: 243–247.

Thomson, A.M. & Hytten, R.E. (1967) The epidemiology of oedema during pregnancy. *J. Obstet. Gynaecol. Br. Commwealth.* **74**: 1–10

Thorley, K. Rouse, T. (1993) Seeing mothers as partners in antenatal care. *Br. J. Midwifery* **1**(5): 216–219.

Tudor Hart, J. (1971) The Inverse Care Law. *Lancet* **VI**: 405.

Twaddle, S. & Harper, V. (1992) An economic evaluation of day care in the management of hypertension in pregnancy. *Br. J. Obstet. Gynaecol.* **99**: 459–461.

UKCC (United Kingdom Central Council for Nursing, Midwifery and Health Visiting) (1993) *Midwives' Rules*. London: UKCC.

UKCC (1994) *The Midwife's Code of Practice*, pp. 3–4. London: UKCC.

Wallenburg, H.C.S. (1989) Detecting hypertensive disorders of pregnancy. In Chalmers, I., Enkin, M. & Keirse, M.J.N.C. (eds) *Effective Care in Pregnancy and Childbirth*. Oxford: Oxford University Press.

Weekes, A.R.L. & Flynn, M.J. (1975) Engagement of the fetal head in primigravidae and its relationship to the duration of gestation and time of onset of labour. *Br. J. Obstet. Gynaecol.* **82**: 7–11.

White, M. & Ritchie, J. (1984) Psychological stressors in

antepartum hospitalisation: Reports of pregnant women. *Matern. Child Nurs. J.* **13**: 47–56.

Wilson-Barnett, J. (1976) Patient's emotional reactions to hospitalisation, cited in *Research and the Midwife*, Conference Proceedings 1990, p. 82.

Zander, L., Lee-Jones, M. & Fisher, C. (1987) The role of the primary health care team in the management of pregnancy. In Kitzinger, S. & Davis, J. (eds) *The Place of Birth*. Oxford: Oxford Medical Publications.

Useful Addresses

Teenage Parenthood Network c/o Govanhill Action for Parents, 168 Butterbiggins Road, Glasgow G42 7AZ Tel. (0141) 424 0448.

The Really Helpful Directory TSA Publishing Ltd, 23 New Road, Brighton, East Sussex BN1 1WZ Tel. (01273) 693311.

20

Helping Women to Cope with Pregnancy Changes

Most women experience some of the so-called 'minor disorders' of pregnancy. These may be 'minor' in that they are not life-threatening, but they may be a major source of discomfort and anxiety. The expectant mother may need to cope with these disorders while continuing to work and care for her family, often having to look after other siblings while experiencing the fatigue and discomforts of pregnancy. Advice on how to relieve these disorders may be sought from the midwife or doctor, and occasionally serious conditions may develop from minor disorders. The midwife needs to refer to medical aid where complications arise (Rule 40, *Midwives Rules*, UKCC, 1993).

Problems Associated with the Gastrointestinal Tract

THE MOUTH

The gums, like all tissues with a large connective tissue component, swell in pregnancy and become spongy. Gingival oedema is not harmful but may lead to gingivitis (Hytten, 1990). As the gums may bleed, the use of a soft toothbrush is advised and the midwife should recommend regular dental check-ups during pregnancy. Dental care and treatment is free during pregnancy and for the year following childbirth.

NAUSEA AND VOMITING

Nausea and vomiting is a common disorder affecting up to 70% of the pregnant population (Weigel and Weigel, 1989) between the 4th and 14th week of pregnancy. Various remedies are available for the relief of nausea and vomiting. These are described fully in Chapters 22 and 29.

HEARTBURN

Heartburn – a painful retrosternal burning sensation – commonly occurs in pregnancy. If persistent, it may be a symptom of reflux oesophagitis, resulting from the regurgitation of acidic stomach contents. This may be due to the effects of progesterone relaxing the lower oesophageal (cardiac) sphincter. Hytten (1990) suggests the decreased response to raised intra-abdominal pressure may allow the sphincter to become incompetent and displace into the thorax, resulting in hiatus hernia. Dodds *et al.* (1978) discount the theory that heartburn is caused by upward pressure from the uterus.

The expectant mother should be advised to eat small, frequent meals, avoid spicy or fatty foods and very cold liquids. Smoking, alcohol, coffee and chocolate may potentiate gastrointestinal irritation (Brucker, 1988) and should be limited. An upright posture and avoiding lying down after meals may be helpful. Nocturnal heartburn may be alleviated by sleeping propped up with extra pillows.

Where simple measures do not relieve the heartburn, the midwife should refer the woman to a doctor (Rule 40, Midwives Rules, UKCC, 1993). Jewell (1993), reviewing *antacid therapy* for heartburn, cites that simple antacids can relieve heartburn, however 20–50% of the women studied by Shaw (1978) failed to gain substantial benefit from antacids. The use of antacids containing local anaesthetics may be more effective but their use requires further research. As Jewell (1993) states, the single trial of Atlay *et al.* (1978) that suggests there may be benefit in treating heartburn with dilute acid therapy needs verifying. With the increased interest in alternative health therapies the expectant mother may wish to use Shiatsu or homeopathic remedies for heartburn. These are discussed in Chapter 22.

CONSTIPATION

Constipation during pregnancy is caused by the general sluggishness and decreased peristalsis of the colon due to the relaxation of plain muscle by progesterone. The problem may be compounded by increased water absorption from the colon, probably due to the increased levels of aldosterone and angiotensin (Hytten, 1990).

Constipation can be overcome by adjusting the diet, adding extra fluid, fruit, vegetables and bran cereal. Iron supplements may aggravate the problem and the supplement may need to be changed to an alternative.

If constipation persists, *fibre supplements* or *vegetable laxatives* may be taken. These absorb water and swell in the gastrointestinal tract, giving bulk to the stool. They should be taken with extra fluids and may take some days to cause a bowel action. *Liquid paraffin* may interfere with the absorption of fat-soluble vitamins A and D and is rarely used, if at all. *Senna preparations* stimulate peristalsis and act in 8–12 hours. They may cause abdominal pain and discomfort and may not be well tolerated by the expectant mother. *Lactulose* is a hyperosmotic, causing an increase in fluid accumulation in the stool, distension, peristalsis and evacuation. It may take up to 48 hours to act. Laxatives should be a short-term treatment and used with information and education of dietary measures to prevent re-occurrence of constipation. The use of Shiatsu and abdominal massage for the treatment of constipation is discussed in Chapter 22.

Skin Changes in Pregnancy

SKIN PIGMENTATION

Increased pigmentation of the skin is very common in pregnancy, occurring in up to 90% of expectant women (Fitzpatrick *et al.*, 1979). The cause of skin changes is uncertain. They may be due to increased oestrogen, progesterone, adrenal hormones or an increase in melanocyte-stimulating hormone (Lewis and Chamberlain, 1990). The face, nipples, areola, vulva, perineum and perianal region commonly darken. The linea alba on the anterior abdominal wall frequently pigments to become the *linea nigra*. This may be more noticeable in dark-haired, dark-complexioned women. Scars on the abdomen may also pigment. The linea nigra fades after childbirth but may never completely disappear.

STRETCH MARKS

Stretch marks (striae gravidarum) may appear on the breasts, abdomen, thighs and buttocks. The purple-red striae fade to silver after pregnancy. Young (1993a) reviewed a cream to prevent striae gravidarum and records that the trial of Mallol *et al.* (1991) showed that Trofolastin cream (a topical cream containing extract of *Centella asiatica*, α-tocopherol and collagen hydrolysates) may protect against stretch marks developing in nulliparous women. No significant benefit was found for multiparous women. Further research is needed to identify the active ingredient(s) and to compare this with traditional remedies (Young, 1993a).

PRURITUS GRAVIDARUM

Pruritus gravidarum is intense itching that occurs without a rash or jaundice in late pregnancy. Itching occurs in about 17% of pregnant women (Fitzpatrick *et al.*, 1979). It may be caused by scabies, pediculosis, urticaria, atopic eczema, thrush, trichomonal infections or related to drug therapy (Black and Mayou, 1984). When these causes have been excluded a small group of women, 0.02–2.4%, continue to suffer from intense itching. Pruritus gravidarum may be generalized or localized to the abdomen. Calamine lotion may give relief of itching and antihistamine tablets may be prescribed by the doctor. The condition will spontaneously resolve after childbirth. The midwife should be aware of disorders that may occur and should refer to the doctor for treatment and management (Rule 40, *Midwives Rules*, UKCC, 1993).

The Musculoskeletal System

The physiological changes of pregnancy affect the musculoskeletal system, frequently causing pain and discomfort.

LOW BACK PAIN

Low back pain occurs frequently in pregnancy as progesterone and relaxin cause softening and relaxation of the ligaments of the pelvis. The weight of the pregnant uterus and the altered posture (*compensatory lordosis*) are likely to increase back strain, leading to pain. Sacro-iliac joint relaxation may cause pain in the back, lower abdomen or radiating down the legs (Heckmann and Sassard, 1994).

Back pain may be reduced by limiting physical activity, alteration of posture, wearing low-heeled shoes and adequate rest in bed. Supportive pillows beneath the knees and abdomen and the application of heat may relieve pain. Lying on the back with the feet elevated and supported approximately 60 cm above the hips for 20 minutes four times a day may relieve muscle spasm, decrease lumbar lordosis and reduce pain (Heckmann and Sassard, 1994).

Expectant mothers commonly attempt to get up from a lying position by raising themselves from their back without using their arms for support. Back strain may be reduced by the midwife advising the mother to turn on to her side and raising herself gradually, using her arms for support from a lying position. A physiotherapist may teach the expectant mother back and abdominal muscle exercises to strengthen these muscles, or apply a sacro-iliac or trochanteric support (see Chapter 25). The doctor may prescribe oral analgesia having considered the suitability of the different drugs and their effect upon the fetus. Alternative therapies to relieve back pain are discussed in Chapter 22.

CRAMP

Cramp, usually occurring at night in the legs, is reported in 50% of pregnant women (Hibbard, 1988). The cause is unclear. Massage and extension of the limb may be beneficial in relieving the pain. Young (1993b), in a review of the role of calcium in alleviating leg cramps in pregnancy, could find no conclusive benefit in treating leg cramps with calcium. A single trial conducted in 1947 suggesting that sodium chloride is an effective treatment needs replication to assess whether this should be recommended (Young, 1993b). Night cramp may be reduced by massage of the leg before going to bed and by raising the foot of the bed 20–25 cm.

Carpal Tunnel Syndrome

Compression of the median nerve in the wrist may lead to numbness, tingling and pain in the fingers, usually at night (Heckmann and Sassard, 1994). This usually occurs in the second and third trimesters of pregnancy. The physiotherapist may apply a lightweight splint to support the wrist, particularly at night. Heckmann and Sassard (1994), citing Wand (1990), state that the symptoms resolve completely and dramatically, often within days of delivery. Carpal tunnel syndrome may recur in subsequent pregnancies and women who experience this may be more at risk of developing the syndrome in later life.

Symphysis Pubis Pain

Pain in the symphysis pubis due to swelling within the joint, separation of the symphysis pubis or other unidentified factors, is a painful and disabling obstetric disorder, which may occur in pregnancy, during labour or after delivery. The true incidence of the condition is unknown. Lindsey *et al.* (1988) in a literature review cites incidences from one case in 521 deliveries (Boland, 1933) to one in 20 000 (Eastman and Hellman, 1966). Fry (1992), an obstetric physiotherapist at the Royal Berkshire Hospital (RBH), Reading, has noticed an increase in cases recently from the usual 1–2 per year to 15 cases in 18 months in a maternity unit of 5000 deliveries per year. Scriven *et al.* (1991) identified 9 cases in 21 months in a unit delivering 4200 women annually. Fry (1992), Scriven *et al.* (1991) and Taylor and Sonson (1986) suggest this is probably an underdiagnosed condition. The consequences for the expectant or newly delivered mother may be underestimated and the pain may persist for weeks, months or possibly years in extreme cases.

Causes

Pain in the symphysis pubis is thought to be caused by separation of the symphysis pubis joint (*diastasis symphysis pubis* or *symphysiolysis*), although a single review by Driessen (1987) suggests that it may be due to swelling within the joint. The hormones of pregnancy are commonly believed to cause an increase in the width of the symphysis pubis. Grieve (1976) noted that the normal 4 mm width increases to 9 mm in pregnancy. A separation of more than 10 mm is usually symptomatic. This may be due to partial or complete rupture of the joint.

Fry (1992) notes that symphyseal pain sometimes occurs in women who have had normal vaginal deliveries of 2.7–3.2 kg babies without obstetric trauma. This contrasts with the historical, traumatic reasons for separation of the symphysis pubis. Lindsey's literature review from 1927 to 1976 suggests that abnormal factors in labour compound the physiological effects of pregnancy. The forceful descent of the fetal head in a complicated labour exerts pressure on the pelvic bones.

Precipitous labour, difficult forceps delivery, cephalopelvic disproportion, abnormal presentation, multiparity, trauma caused by excessive or forced abduction of the maternal thighs during delivery are all suggested as possible causes. However, obstetric practice has changed during this time, Caesarean section is much more likely to be performed for cephalopelvic disproportion, delay in labour and abnormal presentation. Therefore it would be expected that the incidence would be decreasing. Instead the incidence of the condition occurring antenatally is being recognized more commonly.

Diagnosis

Diagnosis may be made by X-ray, where widening of the joint or vertical mobility of the joint may be apparent. However, X-ray examination does not always confirm separation or correlate with the severity of symptoms (Schwartz *et al.*, 1985) and is unlikely to be performed in pregnancy, although it is sometimes undertaken if the condition occurs postnatally. Diagnosis may be confirmed by ultrasound scan if the appropriate ultrasound transducer is available (Scriven *et al.*, 1991).

Driessen (1987) speculates from his study of 11 women in Malawi that the pain may not be caused by hormonal softening or rupture of the symphysis, but by swelling inside the fibrous confines of the joint. His hypothesis is based on the X-ray examination and clinical evidence that he was not able to demonstrate a separation of greater than 10 mm in all his subjects. Further research is required to support this theory. Realistically, cases will be treated symptomatically, with or without confirmation of joint separation.

Symptoms

The condition usually occurs in the second or third trimester of pregnancy. The onset of symptoms may be of insidious nature or follow a particular activity such as exercise in water, overenthusiastic housework or squatting while gardening (Fry, 1992). The woman may experience pain in the symphysis pubis and groins, which often radiates to the lower back or inner thighs. Increasing difficulty may be experienced with walking and weight bearing, a waddling gait becoming apparent. Moving in and out of bed and climbing the stairs becomes very difficult or may become impossible. Initially the back pain is sometimes mistaken for a urinary tract infection. However, there will be no other signs of this.

Management

The management of pain in the symphysis pubis is based upon the symptoms and severity of the pain and the physical limitation of movement. The midwife may help to reduce the longer term morbidity associated with the condition by early recognition and management antenatally and in labour. In some cases the pain may be so acute that hospital admission may be needed so that the expectant mother can have bedrest. She will need to be made as comfortable as possible with the hips adducted. A side-lying position may help to reduce the separation if the woman can be made comfortable with supportive pillows.

A pelvic binder or trochanteric belt may give relief if the woman is able to wear it. McIntosh (1995) has found a simple, effective support may be made from an elasticated tubular support bandage (size K or L Tubigrip) tripled and worn around the ilium and symphysis pubis (Figure 1), or the lower portion tripled and the upper portion doubled as in Figure 2. This offers an acceptable support either antenatally or postnatally. Analgesia should be prescribed by the doctor and given regularly. Ice and ultrasound therapy are suggested by Polden and Mantle (1990) to relieve pain. However, this may or may not prove to be beneficial.

If the mother is having bedrest, ankle and calf exercises should be actively promoted to avoid the formation of deep vein thrombosis. When the pain subsides, very gradual mobilization may be undertaken. The woman will be able to go to the toilet in a wheelchair, and elbow crutches or a walking frame can be used to promote minimal weight-bearing. Showering rather than bathing will be easier, and if the woman wishes to use the bidet she should avoid sitting astride it as this will abduct the hips, placing strain on the symphysis pubis.

Care during labour

A plan of management needs to be formulated for the care during labour of the expectant mother with symphysis pubis pain. A multidisciplinary approach will be needed. The expectant mother and her labour partner will need to be involved in planning her care so that they are aware of the positions that are most likely to be comfortable during the different stages of labour. Involvement and clear information about the forthcoming labour may help to reduce the anxiety that the expectant mother may experience.

The range of hip abduction should be assessed prior to labour (Fry, 1992) by an obstetric physiotherapist and advice on suitable positions for labour given. Attempts should be made to ensure that the woman is not placed in any position that is outside her range of hip movement. Finding a position of comfort for the labouring mother may be difficult as her mobility may be severely limited and lying down may cause pain. The midwife needs to be aware that epidural anaesthesia, although offering valuable pain relief, could mask the symptoms of symphysis pubis pain and allow excessive mobilization of the joint. For the second stage of labour the left lateral position or a supported 'all fours' position will reduce strain on the symphysis pubis.

If the lithotomy position is needed for a forceps delivery or ventouse extraction, the hips should be abducted for as short a time as possible. Extreme pain is likely throughout the procedure. The midwife

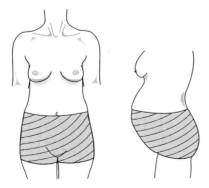

Figure 1 Elasticated tubular support bandage tripled around ilium (redrawn with permission from McIntosh, 1995).

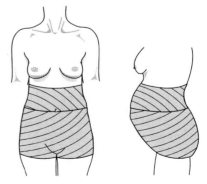

Figure 2 Elasticated tubular support bandage doubled around upper abdomen and tripled around symphysis pubis (redrawn with permission from McIntosh, 1995).

should be aware that symphysis pubis pain experienced by a woman while in the lithotomy position could signify the onset of symphysis pubis separation.

Labour care should be undertaken as is usual for any client in labour, with emotional support, pain relief, observation of the maternal and fetal condition, recognition of normal labour progress and record keeping. Giving individualized physical care and meeting the emotional needs of a mother who may be very anxious represents a challenge for the midwife.

Following delivery, the midwife will need to assist the mother in finding a comfortable position to breastfeed her new baby. If she can be made comfortable with supportive pillows in a side-lying position this may be suitable for mother and baby at this time.

Postnatal management of the condition is very similar to antenatal management and is discussed in Chapter 37. The mother will require complete bedrest and all physical care from the midwife for the first 48 hours following delivery. Assistance will be needed with personal hygiene. Ankle and calf exercises are important to prevent deep vein thrombosis. The midwife will need to hand the baby to the mother for cuddles and give help with feeding the baby. A comfortable position will need to be found for breastfeeding and assistance given with correct positioning. Pelvic floor exercises, pelvic tilting and abdominal exercises should be encouraged as the symphysis pubis pain subsides.

Transfer home

Whether transfer home occurs antenatally or postnatally the home circumstances need careful review. The proximity of the bathroom, number of stairs, help available from the partner, family and friends will be required prior to transfer. The multiparous mother may require substantial help in caring for other children. Driving may be impossible for a period of time, thus increasing the mother's dependence upon family or friends for social activities, shopping and taking siblings to playgroup or school.

Recovery

Whether the condition occurs antenatally, during labour or postnatally, a very clear explanation of the condition, treatment and prognosis will be needed by the woman and her partner. The recovery period varies from weeks to months (Lindsey et al., 1988), or even years in extreme cases (Scriven et al., 1995). Pain may continue during this time, and may be worse during the secretory phase of the menstrual cycle. In chronic cases surgical fixation may be required to stabilize the joint. Further research is required to determine if the condition re-occurs in subsequent pregnancies, and if so which mode of delivery is advisable.

The lack of awareness of health professionals and limited information available about the long-term effects of symphysis pubis pain can make the sufferer feel very isolated. Sometimes health professionals fail to appreciate the severity of the symptoms. A lack of sympathy and little information about this 'rare' condition, especially if the pain persists over a period of months, is common. The early recognition and management of the condition by the midwife may help to reduce morbidity in the longer term.

References

Atlay, R.D., Weeks, A.R.L., Entwistle, G.D. & Parkinson, D.J. (1978) Treating heartburn in pregnancy. *Br. Med. J.* **2**: 919–920.

Boland, B.F. (1933) Rupture of the symphysis pubis. Articulation during delivery. *Surg. Gynecol. Obstet.* **57**: 517–522.

Black, M. & Mayou, C. (1984) Skin diseases in pregnancy. In De Swiet, M. (ed.) *Medical Disorders in Obstetric Practice*, 2nd edn. Oxford: Blackwell Scientific.

Brucker, M.C. (1988) Management of common minor disorders in pregnancy. Part 3, Managing gastro-intestinal problems in pregnancy. *J. Nurse Midwifery* **33**(2) March/April: 67–73.

Dodds, W.J., Dent, J. & Hogan, W. (1978) Pregnancy and the lower oesophageal sphincter. *Gastro-enterology* **74**: 1334–1336.

Driessen, F. (1987) Postpartum arthropathy with unusual features. *Br. J. Obstet. Gynaecol.* **94**: 870–872.

Eastman, N.J. & Hellman, L.M. (1966) *Obstetrics*, 13th edn. New York: Appleton Century Crofts.

Fitzpatrick, T.B., Eisen, A.Z. & Wolff, K. (1979) *Dermatology in General Medicine*. New York: McGraw-Hill.

Fry, D. (1992) Diastasis symphysis pubis. *J. Assoc. Chartered Physiother. Obstet. Gynaecol.* **71**: 10–13.

Grieve, F. (1976) The sacro iliac joint. *Physiotherapy* **62**: 386–399.

Heckmann, J. & Sassard, R. (1994) Muskuloskeletal considerations in pregnancy. *J. Bone Joint Surg.* **76A**(11): 1720–1730.

Hibbard, B.M. (1988) *Principles of Obstetrics*. London: Butterworth.

Hytten, F. (1990) The alimentary system in pregnancy. *Midwifery* **6**: 201–204.

Jewell, M. (1993) Antacid therapy for heartburn in pregnancy. In Enkin, M.W., Keirse, M.J.N., Renfrew, M. &

Neilson, J.P. (eds) *Pregnancy and Childbirth Module Cochrane Database of Systematic Reviews*, No. 06885. Cochrane updates on disk, Disk issue 1. Oxford: Cochrane.

Lewis, T.L. & Chamberlain, G. (eds) (1990) *Obstetrics by Ten Teachers*, 15th edn. London: Edward Arnold.

Lindsey, M.D., Leggon, R., Wright, D. & Nolasco, D. (1988) Separation of the symphysis pubis in association with childbearing. *J. Bone Joint Surg.* **70-A**(2): 289–292.

McIntosh, J. (1995) Treatment note: an alternative pelvic support. *J. Assoc. Chartered Physiother. Womens Health* **76**: 28.

Mallol, J., Belda, M.A., Costa, D., Noval, A. & Sola, M. (1991) Prophylaxis of striae gravidarum with a topical formulation. A double blind trial. *Int. J. Cosmetic Sci.* **13**: 51–57.

Polden, M. & Mantle, J. (1990) *Physiotherapy in Obstetrics and Gynaecology*. London: Butterworth Heinemann.

Schwartz, Z., Katz, Z. & Lancet, M. (1985) Management of puerperal separation of the symphysis pubis in association with childbearing. *Int. J. Gynaecol. Obstet.* **23**: 125–128.

Scriven, M., McKnight, L. & Jones, D. (1991) Diastasis of the symphysis pubis in pregnancy. *Br. Med. J.* **303**:56.

Scriven, M., McKnight, L. & Jones, D. (1995) The importance of pubic pain following childbirth: a clinical and ultrasonographic study of diastasis of the symphysis pubis. *J. R. Soc. Med.* **88**: 28–30.

Shaw, R.W. (1978) Randomized controlled trial of Syn-Ergel and an active placebo in the treatment of heartburn in pregnancy. *J. Int. Med. Res.* **6**: 147–151.

Taylor, R.N. & Sonson, R.D. (1986) Separation of the symphysis pubis: an under recognised peripartum complication. *J. Reprod. Med.* **31**: 203–206.

UKCC (United Kingdom Central Council) (1993) *Midwives Rules*. London: UKCC.

Wand, J. (1990) Carpal tunnel syndrome in pregnancy and lactation. *J. Hand. Surg.* **15-B**: 93–95.

Weigel, M. & Weigel, R. (1989) Nausea and vomiting of early pregnancy and pregnancy outcome. An epidemiological study. *Br. J. Obstet. Gynaecol.* **96**: 1304–1311.

Young, G.L. (1993a) A cream to prevent striae gravidarum. *Pregnancy and Childbirth Module Cochrane Database of Systematic Reviews*, No. 06519. Cochrane updates on disk, Disk issue 1. Oxford: Cochrane.

Young, G.L. (1993b) Calcium for leg cramps in pregnancy. In Enkin, M.W., Keirse, M.J.N., Renfrew, M. & Neilson, J.P. (eds) *Pregnancy and Childbirth Module Cochrane Database of Systematic Reviews*, No. 04385. Cochrane updates on disk, Disk issue 1. Oxford: Cochrane.

21

Antenatal Investigations of Maternal and Fetal Well-being

Continuing advances in medical knowledge and technology make available increasingly effective techniques for investigating maternal and fetal well-being. Many of these techniques are applied as screening tests to all pregnant women; others are only used for those who are particularly at risk and give reassurance of normality, or early indication of problems so that action can be taken, where appropriate.

The obverse of the benefits is that many of the tests require invasive procedures, some of which involve a small element of hazard. The proliferation of tests may place an additional burden on pregnant women and their partners, causing them anxiety and involving them in taking difficult decisions. Midwives have an important part to play in providing information, counselling, facilitating decision-making and relieving anxiety.

Cervical Cytology

Cervical cytology is a diagnostic investigation which may be carried out in pregnancy. It involves the removal of a sample of cervical cells for cytological investigation (study of cells) to detect cervical intra-epithelial neoplasia (CIN), a precursor of invasive carcinoma. The cells are removed by means of a Papanicolaou (Pap) cervical smear (Wilkinson, 1990). Carcinoma of the cervix, the eighth most common cancer in women in the UK, is a significant condition responsible for mortalities (CRC, 1990). Globally, it is the second most common cancer, 77% of cases occurring in the developing countries. It is recommended that all women aged 20–64 years or who are sexually active should have cervical screening every five years. In practice there is considerable local variation in the arrangements and the time of recall may be 3–5 years; the optimum interval for screening is debatable and further research is recommended. Setting up a systematic national call and recall system in 1988 has facilitated the screening programme. Sexual activity is thought to be a primary factor in the incidence of cervical cancer and the disease has increased in the age group 24–34 (Austoker and McPherson, 1992).

Risk factors for cervical cancer

Although the cause of cervical carcinoma is unknown, current evidence suggests that it is a multifactorial process associated with a number of clinical epidemiological factors (Wilkinson, 1990). These factors may be directly or indirectly implicated and include the following (Austoker and McPherson, 1992):

▶ Sexual behaviour (early onset of sexual intercourse, multiple partners).
▶ Sexual transmission.
▶ Parity (virgin women low risk).
▶ Age at first pregnancy (late first pregnancy, low risk).
▶ Methods of contraception (barrier offers more protection).
▶ Long-term use of oral contraceptive increases risk.
▶ Occupation (less common in professional groups).
▶ Social class (commoner in lower social groups).
▶ Heavy smoking.
▶ History of papilloma or wart virus.
▶ History of dyskaryosis.
▶ Sexual partners with penile warts (unless a sheath is used).

Method

A sample of superficial cells is taken from the squamo-columnar junction between the endocervix (columnar epithelium) and the ectocervix (squamous epithelium) in the transformation zone. The position of this zone varies during a woman's lifetime. It is the area where the initial cellular changes occur. The smear is obtained by using either a wooden spatula (Aylesbury or Ayre's spatula), or a plastic multi-spatula, and by rotating it through 360° with the spatula firmly applied to the cervix (Wolfendale, 1989). The quality of the smear and the expertise of the cytologist in microscopic examination are important factors in interpretation of the results. The smear is repeated if abnormal cells are found and further investigations are required following a second abnormal smear (Austoker and McPherson, 1992). In addition to the diagnosis of cervical intra-

epithelial neoplasia, other conditions may be discovered such as herpes simplex virus infection, *Trichomonas* infection, *Candida albicans* (monilia), threadworm ova. Appropriate treatment for such conditions is instituted.

Management of abnormal cervical cytology in pregnancy

Management of abnormal cervical cytology depends upon the severity of the condition. A positive result causes anxiety in a woman and her partner, requiring sensitive and effective counselling. Abnormal cervical cytology requires an evaluation of the cervical condition by *colposcopy* (microscopic examination of the cervix), when cervical biopsies may be taken. This technique is available in many large medical centres but in areas where colposcopy is not available, a *cone biopsy* is taken. This may be delayed until after pregnancy, however, because of the risks of inducing abortion and of haemorrhage from the cervix which is very vascular. The accepted treatment following colposcopy is usually by *laser* or *cryotherapy* (Hannigan, 1990).

In advanced disease, which is uncommon in pregnancy, a decision may have to be taken on the methodology of treatment. This may be termination of pregnancy or maintenance of the pregnancy until the fetus is viable. The decision will depend on a number of factors such as the stage of the disease, maternal condition, and stage of pregnancy, each case being considered individually together with the woman and her partner. There is no evidence to suggest that the progression of the disease is affected by the pregnancy.

Cervical intraepithelial neoplasia (CIN)

CIN is classified into three groups as follows (Draper Report, 1980):

▶ *CIN I* Lesions of mild dysplasia in which the epithelium has lost some form of order and differentiation and cells are of variable size with an increased nucleocytoplasmic ratio. This is a reversible condition.
▶ *CIN II* Moderate dysplasia with further loss of differentiation in cell structure. This is also reversible.
▶ *CIN III* Severe dysplasia and carcinoma *in situ* extending to a depth of 3 mm or more with invasion of malignant cells into the underlying stroma. This condition is irreversible and surgery is usually

required to prevent the development of invasive carcinoma.

Blood Tests in Pregnancy

At the first visit to an antenatal clinic a venous sample of blood is taken from the woman for a number of laboratory investigations. Full explanation as to the nature, purpose and implications of the investigations should be given to the woman by the midwife. This enables the woman to make informed decisions on the information given and to give her consent to the procedure (NHSME, 1992). Evidence suggests that many women are unaware of the nature of such tests in pregnancy (Marteau et al., 1992). At subsequent visits to the antenatal clinic further venous blood samples may be taken for specific laboratory investigations, including the estimation of serum alpha-fetoprotein, antibodies and other investigations which may be required.

ABO and rhesus blood group system

Identification of the maternal ABO and rhesus blood group systems have clinical significance in pregnancy and childbirth (Campbell, 1993). This is essential for the purpose of accurate cross-matching without delay, safety in blood transfusion in cases of severe haemorrhage or anaemia and in cases of rhesus and ABO incompatibility. The rhesus blood group system is important for the detection and management of rhesus iso-immunization (Bowell et al., 1986).

Antibodies

Maternal blood serum is examined for the presence of antibodies, especially rhesus antibodies if the mother is rhesus-negative. Other uncommon antibodies may be significant in pregnancy such as anti-Kell and anti-c, and these antibody levels, if detected, need monitoring (Mackenzie et al., 1991). In rhesus-negative women repeat antibody tests are carried out in the last trimester of pregnancy as the presence of antibodies may not be detected in the first specimen (Bowell et al., 1986). Antibodies may be stimulated by the occurrence of a feto-maternal haemorrhage when 'leaks' occur and some fetal rhesus-positive cells pass into the maternal circulation as pregnancy advances. This may also follow invasive interventions such as amniocentesis, chorionic villus biopsy or cordocentesis, external cephalic version or in abnormal conditions such as antepartum haemorrhage. The rhesus-negative mother responds by producing antibodies which may cross the placenta to the fetal circulation and cause haemolysis of fetal red cells. The administration of anti-D immunoglobulin is effective in preventing the production of antibodies (Mackenzie et al., 1991).

Serology

A serological test is carried out to detect the presence of specific sexually transmitted diseases, e.g. syphilis (causative organism *Treponema pallidum*). The usual investigation is the *venereal disease research laboratory test* (VDRL), a non-treponemal test. Occasionally the findings are doubtful or positive and further confirmatory tests such as the *fluorescent treponemal antibody absorption test* (FTA-ABS) and the *microhaemagglutination test* (MHA.TP) are used. A minority of women will have the disease and prompt curative treatment with penicillin is necessary. If started before the 20th week of pregnancy, this may prevent the infant being born with congenital syphilis. In addition, contact tracing should be instituted and sexual partners should be treated, if positive (Wang and Smaill, 1989).

Surveillance studies to assess the current incidence of syphilis in pregnancy and congenital syphilis in the UK are being conducted (Nicoll and Moisley, 1994).

Haemoglobin estimation

Haemoglobin, a protein, has a significant part to play in pregnancy. The haemoglobin level is used to indicate the presence of anaemia, 11.0 g/dl being considered the lower limit of the normal range (WHO, 1972). Occasionally other arbitrary figures may be used (Mahomed and Hytten, 1989). If the haemoglobin is below this level, the woman is said to be anaemic. Haemoglobin is checked at the first antenatal visit and repeated according to individual need. If the level is below 9.0 g/dl, further investigations such as folate levels and serum ferritin may be necessary. The haemoglobin is likely to fall because of the haematological changes in pregnancy, including an increase in plasma volume (Mahomed and Hytten, 1989), and this may be more marked in multiple pregnancy (Chamberlain, 1992).

Anaemia is a common medical disorder in pregnancy, usually because of *iron deficiency*. It may also be due to folate deficiency which is diagnosed by low haemoglobin levels, often below 8.0 g/dl, high serum iron, low erythrocyte folic acid, and megaloblastosis (Chamberlain, 1992). *Folic acid deficiency* is more common in women with multiple pregnancy, haemoglobinopathies, and those taking anticonvulsive drugs, when daily supplements are recommended. A directive from the Department of Health (DOH, 1992) on the prevention of first occurrence neural tube defects recommends that all women take daily supplements of 0.4 mg (400 µg) of folic acid, if planning a pregnancy and for the first 12 weeks following conception. To prevent recurrence of neural tube defect, the recommended dosage of folic acid is 4 mg (4000 µg) taken for a minimum of four weeks prior to conception and until at least eight weeks' gestation (RCOG, 1993).

Epileptic women require individual counselling as folic acid may interfere with the efficacy of anticonvulsive drugs (DOH, 1992). The recommended daily dosage of folic acid for epileptic women is 5 mg (5000 µg) (O'Brien and Gilmour-White, 1993).

Recent evidence suggests that daily treatment of all women in pregnancy with iron is not necessary and it should be reserved for those with genuine evidence of iron deficiency (Mahomed and Hytten, 1989). Steer (1995) found that a fall in haemoglobin during pregnancy is associated with positive outcomes in terms of birth weight and gestation at birth. He confirms that the routine administration of iron during pregnancy is therefore not usually required. Iron tends to cause digestive upsets and is better started after morning sickness has settled. The colour of the stools changes to black and women should be advised of this. If severe anaemia develops, further laboratory investigations such as *ferritin levels* (normal 10–200 µg/l) and total *iron-binding capacity* (TIBC) (normal 40–70 µmol/l) may be conducted and appropriate treatment will be necessary (see Chapter 42).

Serum ferritin

Ferritin is the body's major iron-storage protein, ensuring that iron is readily available when demand is high, and is found in the liver, marrow and spleen. Serum ferritin falls in proportion to a decrease in iron store and is a more reliable test of iron status than haemoglobin level (Montgomery, 1990).

Haemoglobinopathies

Haemoglobinopathies are a diverse group of inherited single-gene disorders involving abnormal haemoglobin patterns which constitute two major conditions: *thalas-*saemia (HbS-Thal) and *sickle-cell trait* (SCT or HbS) or sickle cell disease (SCD or HbS-S) (Old, 1992). These conditions affect women of African, Asian, Middle Eastern or Mediterranean origin and women from these groups should have haemoglobin electrophoresis investigations.

If thalassaemia or sickle cell trait are detected, meticulous management of the pregnancy will be required, including screening of the partner and frequent antenatal visits, usually every two weeks. Rigorous assessment is required of the degree of anaemia, reticulocyte counts, bilirubin levels, degree of sickling and presence of infection, detection of pregnancy-induced hypertension and intrauterine growth retardation, so that prompt and appropriate treatment may be given. Appropriate counselling and health education is also given to prevent maternal and neonatal morbidity and mortality which is higher in this group (Blake *et al.*, 1993). The midwife has a key role to play in these conditions.

Rubella

This common virus infection is a significant condition in pregnancy due to the teratogenic effect on the developing fetus caused by transplacental transmission of the virus (Sidle, 1985). Detection of rubella antibodies is carried out by serological testing to detect immunity (IgM and IgG antibodies) (Dawson, 1988).

The majority of women in the UK (85%) are immune as a result of vaccination against rubella at 11–14 years of age (Wang and Smaill, 1989). Vaccination is now by measles, mumps and rubella (MMR) vaccine (introduced in 1988) administered usually before 15 months to male and female infants (HEA, 1992). It is reported that the incidence of rubella infection in pregnancy has decreased substantially (Miller *et al.*, 1993) and it is hoped that with over 95% take-up, rubella will be eradicated altogether (Sense, 1990).

If a woman is non-immune and comes into contact with rubella she may develop the disease. The extent of the damage to the developing fetus varies with the period of gestation, but is particularly high in the first trimester of pregnancy (Sidle, 1985). Termination of the pregnancy is offered and may be carried out under the Abortion Act 1967 as amended 1990 (FPA, 1992). Women who have been in contact with, or develop a rubella-type illness in pregnancy will have additional testing to detect antibody levels, high levels of IgM indicating recent infection. Detailed information is required by the laboratory to aid the diagnosis which may need expert consultation (Wang and Smaill, 1989). Immune serum globulin may be administered if maternal rubella occurs. To avoid the danger of rubella in future pregnancies the non-immune woman is offered vaccination in the puerperium, together with contraceptive advice for a period of three months. Factors contributing to the continuing occurrence of congenital rubella include missed opportunities for immunization at school or postpartum, maternal reinfection and recent immigration into the UK, especially amongst Asian and Oriental women (Miller *et al.*, 1993).

Serum alpha-fetoprotein (SAFP)

Maternal serum is tested at 16–18 weeks' gestation to measure the level of alpha-fetoprotein. This protein was first discovered in 1956 (Bergstrand and Czar, 1956). It is excreted first by the yolk sac and then by the fetal liver and may be detected in maternal serum or the amniotic fluid during pregnancy. Elevated levels may be associated with open neural tube defects.

The levels vary according to the duration of pregnancy, hence the need for accurate assessment of gestation period. They are measured in terms of multiples of the median (MoM) level for unaffected pregnancies for the gestation period in question (Green and Statham, 1993). For a reliable result this test must be carried out on maternal serum between the 16th and 18th week of pregnancy (Brock, 1992).

A raised maternal serum alpha-fetoprotein (MSAFP) may be associated with:

▶ Incorrect dates (underestimation of gestational age).
▶ Multiple pregnancy.
▶ Intrauterine fetal death.
▶ Neural tube defect or other fetal abnormality, such as exomphalos, gastroschisis.
▶ Rhesus disease, cystic hygroma and other conditions associated with fetal oedema (raised levels due to alpha-fetoprotein transudation).
▶ Fetal growth deficiency.
▶ Congenital nephrosis.
▶ Certain skin disorders.
▶ Upper fetal bowel obstruction.
▶ Maternal liver disease.

A raised level in the second trimester may be associated with complications of pregnancy such as *hypertension* (Simpson and Elias, 1994).

Levels of serum alpha-fetoprotein are reported to vary with maternal age, maternal weight, insulin-dependent diabetes mellitus (IDDM), cigarette smoking and race. Measured levels should therefore be adjusted accordingly (Cuckle and Wald, 1990; Wald and Cuckle, 1992). Evidence suggests that there is an increased risk of adverse pregnancy outcome after an unexplained high maternal level of alpha-fetoprotein (Crandall *et al.*, 1991).

After discussing the implications of raised serum alpha-fetoprotein levels with the woman and her partner, the doctor may, with her agreement, proceed with further investigations such as amniotic fluid alpha-fetoprotein and ultrasound scan. A detailed ultrasound scan is necessary to determine the period of gestation and to detect other possible causes such as multiple pregnancy and intrauterine fetal death.

If these conditions are excluded an attempt is made to visualize a neural tube defect by high-resolution ultrasound examination (Campbell and Pearce, 1983). This technique is well-established in some centres for the diagnosis of neural tube and other craniospinal defects. The accuracy of the diagnosis, however, depends very much on the expertise and experience of the operators and clinicians and on the quality of the ultrasound equipment used.

Where high-resolution ultrasound equipment is not available or further confirmation of the diagnosis is required, an amniocentesis is carried out to estimate the amniotic fluid alpha-fetoprotein, as this is a more accurate test than serum. Chromosomal studies may also be carried out on the fetal cells in the liquor to detect other congenital abnormalities. A raised liquor alpha-fetoprotein level suggests that the fetus has a neural tube defect.

Once the diagnosis has been made, termination of pregnancy usually follows if this is the parents' wish. Careful counselling is required prior to the test to inform the woman and her partner of the implications of a positive test; understandably, many couples still suffer from anxiety (Green, 1990).

A low serum alpha-fetoprotein in the second trimester has been associated with fetal trisomies 18 (Edward's syndrome) and 21 (Down's syndrome) (Merkatz *et al.*, 1984). Some doctors recommend that amniocentesis for chromosomal studies should be offered to women with low serum alpha-fetoprotein values to increase the detection of Down's syndrome.

Down's syndrome testing (Bart's or triple test)

The blood test for Down's syndrome is available to most women and identifies an individual woman's risk of having an affected pregnancy. It is performed between 16 and 18 weeks' gestation. Three principal markers are used:

▶ MSAFP (low in Down's syndrome);
▶ maternal serum human chorionic gonadotrophin (MShCG) (raised in Down's syndrome); and
▶ maternal serum unconjugated oestriols (MSuE₃) (low in Down's syndrome).

Maternal age is also taken into consideration because of the association between advanced maternal age (over 35) and Down's syndrome. The individual risk factor is calculated on these markers. Risks higher than 1:250 are 'high' or 'screen positive'; those below 1:250 'low' or 'screen negative' (Cuckle and Wald, 1990; Green and Statham, 1993).

This test was developed from work done by Wald *et al.* (1988) at St Bartholomew's Hospital, hence the name, and has been found to be effective in practice in detecting 58% of Down's syndrome babies (Wald *et al.*, 1992). Pre-test counselling is essential to allow women and their partners to understand the rationale and implications of the test.

Hepatitis B (Australian antigen; AA)

Hepatitis B (HBsAg) surface antigen is found in the serum of a person who has acute or chronic serum hepatitis or is a carrier for that virus. An investigation may be carried out to detect the presence of HBsAg in women considered to be at risk of the condition, for example those from tropical countries, drug abusers and those who have been tattooed. Adequate precautions must be taken to prevent autoinoculation of all health care workers involved, and biohazard identification of samples is mandatory (Goodlad, 1989).

Toxoplasmosis

Toxoplasmosis is a protozoan parasitic infection caused by the protozoan *Toxoplasmosis gondii* which is endemic in Europe, especially France (Pope, 1992). It causes a number of abnormalities of the developing fetus by transplacental infection (RCOG, 1992). The domestic cat is a host for the oocytes, which are excreted in cat faeces, but cat ownership is not an indication for testing (Hall, 1993). The true incidence in the UK is unknown but is reported to be 2:1000. Routine prenatal screening was not advised by the RCOG in 1992, but this is under review. The test may be carried out on women at risk, for example immunocompromised women such as those with AIDS (due to reactivation of latent infection) or following organ transplantation (Pope, 1992). It may be carried out on maternal request to allay anxiety. Maternal awareness has been raised due to the publicity generated by the Toxoplasmosis Trust founded in 1989.

The test, which examines the immunity status of the woman by looking at IgG and IgM antibodies, should be performed in a Toxoplasmosis Reference Laboratory (RCOG, 1992), as diagnosis is not straightforward (Hall, 1993). Pre-test counselling is recommended as a positive result will require decisions regarding termination of pregnancy or tests for diagnosis of fetal abnormalities. Berrebi *et al.* (1994) report that pregnancy need not be terminated if repeated fetal ultrasound is normal and antiparasitic treatment is given. Primary prevention by health education is recommended and the Department of Health has published a leaflet (DOH, 1991) to facilitate this.

Phenylketonuria (PKU)

Phenylketonuria is an inherited inborn error of metabolism whereby there is a deficiency of the enzyme *phenylalanine hydroxylase*. The condition causes irreversible brain damage if untreated, due to a build-up of phenylalanine in the body, but can be managed by following a low-phenylalanine diet. Serum phenylalanine testing may be carried out on women with phenylketonuria to establish their serum phenylalanine levels as there is a high risk (80%) of transplacental fetal brain damage. It is recommended that these women revert to a low-phenylalanine diet to reduce serum phenylalanine before conception to improve the outcome of pregnancy (MRC, 1993).

Human immunodeficiency virus infection (HIV) or acquired immune deficiency virus (AIDS)

A test for HIV may be carried out on women at risk, including drug abusers and prostitutes, and on request. Confidentiality is of paramount importance. Blood samples must be obtained with the consent of the woman based on appropriate information (UKCC, 1993). Unlinked anonymous testing, whereby unidentified specimens are tested, is carried out on blood submitted for other antenatal investigations from selected geographical areas to establish the prevalence of HIV. This commenced in 1990 after being sanctioned by the Secretary of State for Health and is coordinated by the Public Health Laboratory Service (DOH, 1989). In some centres voluntary, named testing for HIV is now offered to all women in pregnancy to detect the prevalence of the condition and attempt to prevent transmission to the fetus (Chrystie *et al.*, 1995; Lindgren *et al.*, 1993; Banatvala and Chrystie, 1994). The UKCC (1993) sets out its position and advice to practitioners in a set of principles on which agreement to participate should be based. Midwives need to keep abreast of current knowledge of HIV/AIDS so as to be able to inform pregnant women appropriately (Cohn, 1993).

Urea-resistant neutrophil alkaline phosphatase (UR-NAP)

Research indicates that in the presence of a Down's syndrome fetus, the levels of urea-resistant neutrophil alkaline phosphatase in the maternal blood are raised (Cuckle *et al.*, 1990). This is thought to be the single most effective marker for Down's syndrome. The test is not routine at the present time as more information is needed, but research work continues.

Ethical issues of prenatal screening

Prenatal diagnostic and risk factor tests bring complex ethical problems for health care professionals, women and their partners and for society. Women and partners are faced with difficult decisions on complex issues. Fletcher and Wertz (1992) summarize the problems involved in prenatal diagnosis:

▶ Access to services.
▶ Increasing demands for genetic services.
▶ Abortion choices.
▶ Dilemmas regarding disclosure.
▶ Directive versus non-directive counselling.
▶ Protection of confidentiality and privacy.
▶ Controversial indications for prenatal diagnosis.
▶ Fetal abnormality in multiple pregnancy.
▶ Multifetal pregnancies.
▶ Third trimester dilemmas.
▶ Research issues.

Midwives need to consider their ethical and moral stance in relation to these issues.

Invasive Tests

AMNIOCENTESIS

Amniocentesis is a well-established, relatively safe prenatal diagnostic invasive intervention performed under ultrasound imaging which involves the removal of liquor amnii from the gestational sac through the abdominal wall. It is performed for a range of biochemical, cytogenetic and other investigations (MacLachlan, 1992). The technique is one of the commonest prenatal diagnostic tests for the diagnosis of chromosome abnormalities and may be performed at various times during pregnancy, usually at 15–16 weeks' gestation (mid-trimester amniocentesis) or later (late trimester amniocentesis), but increasingly between 9 and 13 weeks (first trimester amniocentesis) (Hanson *et al.*, 1992).

Introduced in the late nineteenth century, the technique is now successfully performed under ultrasound imaging which reduces bloody and dry taps and fetal loss rates (MacLachan, 1992). Great care must be taken to avoid the introduction of infection into the amniotic sac. There is a slightly increased risk of abortion (1%) following amniocentesis (Tabor *et al.*, 1986), so mothers and partners should be counselled prior to the intervention.

Apart from cytogenic and biochemical information available from cultured amniotic fluid cells or supernatant, amniotic fluid may also be assayed for other fetal products which are used for prenatal diagnosis, e.g. alpha-fetoprotein, bilirubin and pulmonary phospholipids. Amniocentesis may also be used to regulate the intra-amniotic fluid volume, in cases of oligohydramnios by amnioinfusion, and intra-abdominal fluid pressure in polyhydramnios by decompression amniocentesis.

Early (first trimester) amniocentesis

This is reported to be a safe, simple, accurate method of prenatal diagnosis of numerical and structural chromosome aberrations if carried out between 9 and 13 completed weeks of pregnancy (Fogarty and Dorman, 1992). Amniotic cell culture time may be increased relative to mid-trimester amniocentesis (Djlali *et al.*, 1992). Due to the presence of two sacs (amniotic and extra-embryonic coelom) in the first trimester it is important to identify the site of the fluid sampled as concentrations of human chorionic gonadotrophin and alpha-fetoprotein levels vary, and biochemical results will be affected. At the present time the value of alpha-fetoprotein levels in the first trimester diagnosis of neural tube defects is unknown; if found to be important, the type of fluid sampled will be important (Neilson and Godsen, 1991).

The intervention is not without risks, it may increase the incidence of fetal loss, compared with mid-trimester amniocentesis (Assel et al., 1992) and there is an associated risk of antenatal impaired lung growth thought to be due to the reduction in amniotic fluid volume (Thompson et al., 1992). Jorgenson et al. (1992) advise caution before the intervention is adopted as a routine, and recommend further research.

Indications

Improvements in biochemical diagnostic techniques, for example enzyme activity or protein deficiencies, have increased the indications for amniocentesis (MacLachlan, 1992). Today, the technique may be indicated for:

▶ Detection of chromosomal abnormalities.
▶ Determination of the sex of the fetus.
▶ Assessment of alpha-fetoprotein level.
▶ Assessment of lecithin–sphingomyelin ratio.
▶ Measurement of creatinine level.
▶ DNA analysis.
▶ Detection of rhesus incompatibility.
▶ Treatment of polyhydramnios.
▶ Augmentation of amniotic fluid volume.
▶ Enzyme assay.

Chromosomal studies   Chromosomal abnormality associated with maternal age of more than 35 years is the commonest indication for amniocentesis, accounting for more than 5% of cases (MacLachlan, 1992). Down's syndrome (trisomy 21) is the main indication, with 30% of Down's syndrome fetuses being detected in this age-group from amniotic fluid cell culture (Mikkelson and Neilson, 1992).

A previous child with a chromosomal aberration is the second most common indication. However, with the increased use of the 'triple test' amniocentesis is likely to be made available to younger women who may be shown to be at risk by this test. Other trisomies such as Patau's syndrome (trisomy 13), Edwards' syndrome (trisomy 18), Turner's syndrome and Klinefelter's syndrome and other chromosome abnormalities can

also be detected by amniocentesis (Mikkelson and Neilson, 1992).

Amniocentesis may be performed following the detection of choroid plexus cysts on ultrasound imaging as this may be associated with chromosomal abnormality, e.g. trisomy 18 (Howard et al., 1992; Gupta et al., 1995).

Sex of the fetus   Certain X-linked recessive disorders such as Duchenne muscular dystrophy and haemophilia generally affect males and are transmitted from the carrier mother, the risk being 1:2 that a son will be affected, or that a daughter will be a carrier (Young, 1990). The woman may have an amniocentesis to determine the sex of the fetus, followed by a termination of pregnancy if the fetus is a male.

Alpha-fetoprotein   The connection between raised amniotic alpha-fetoprotein levels, open neural tube defects and other fetal abnormalities such as exomphalos, gastroschisis and congenital nephrosis is well-documented (MacLachlan, 1992; Brock, 1992). Although the discovery of reduced levels of amniotic fluid alpha-fetoprotein in Down's syndrome fetuses is significant, the wide range of variation militates against the use of this as a practical method for diagnostic purposes (Brock, 1992).

Lecithin–sphingomyelin ratio (L/S ratio)   Surfactant is a phospholipid secreted by the fetal lungs into the amniotic fluid. Its function is to reduce surface tension where gas meets tissue and to facilitate lung expansion. Surfactant contains two phospholipids: lecithin and sphingomyelin. Before 34 weeks they are found in equal amounts, that is a ratio of 1:1. After this the lecithin level rises sharply to a ratio of 2:1. This increased lecithin indicates the presence of adequate surfactant in the fetal lungs and the test is used for the prenatal diagnosis of lung maturity. Concentration of lecithin above 3.5 mg/100 ml indicates maturity of the fetal lungs. In conditions such as insulin-dependent diabetes mellitus and drug addiction, fetal lung maturity may be delayed (Hollingsworth, 1992; Finnegan and Wapner, 1988).

Creatinine   As pregnancy advances, the concentration of creatinine in the liquor increases. At 36 weeks it is 150 μmol/l. This is a useful indication of fetal maturity.

Rhesus incompatibility Since the pioneering work of Liley (1961), amniocentesis remains an important method for assessing the degree of fetal haemolysis after 28 weeks' gestation in cases of Rhesus incompatibility. The liquor bilirubin level is usually estimated in rhesus iso-immunized women. The fetus passes urine into the liquor and where there is excessive breakdown of fetal red blood cells, as occurs in rhesus incompatibility, the amount of bilirubin excreted into the liquor from the fetal urine is increased.

This can be assessed by measuring the increment in optical density of the liquor due to bilirubin at 450 nm and plotting against gestational age on the Liley curve. If serial readings fall into the upper 80–85% level of zone 2 before 30 weeks' gestation, into level 3 after 30 weeks, or there is a single reading well into zone 3 at any gestation, then intrauterine transfusion is indicated. Induction or delivery of the infant would be carried out according to fetal lung maturity which is estimated by lecithin–sphingomyelin ratio, and placental location if anterior or posterior (Bowman, 1994).

Polyhydramnios Amniocentesis is sometimes used for women with polyhydramnios to relieve extreme maternal discomfort by reducing the intra-abdominal pressure (decompression amniocentesis), giving some relief of symptoms and attempting to prolong gestation. This treatment only gives temporary relief as the amniotic fluid quickly increases again. In some cases the woman goes into labour following decompression amniocentesis, especially when a considerable amount of liquor has been withdrawn. It may also be performed for fetal karyotyping. Evidence indicates a 5% chance of fetal chromosome abnormality in moderate to severe polyhydramnios associated with structural abnormality of the fetus (Carlson *et al.*, 1990).

Amnioinfusion This invasive procedure is the infusion of a saline solution into the amniotic cavity transabdominally, or by means of a transcervical catheter, with the objective of augmenting amniotic fluid volume or diluting meconium (Hofmeyer, 1992). It may be performed in the antenatal or intranatal period to:

▶ improve ultrasound imaging in cases of oligohydramnios associated with fetal abnormality;
▶ facilitate rapid fetal karyotyping;
▶ provide conservative treatment of preterm premature rupture of the membranes;
▶ attempt to prevent fetal lung hypoplasia in pregnancies complicated by oligohydramnios (Hofmeyer, 1992);
▶ prevent fetal distress in the intrapartum period by decreasing cord compression in cases of oligohydramnios, thereby reducing fetal hypoxia with associated release of meconium;
▶ reduce recurrent variable decelerations; or
▶ dilute meconium and improve fetal outcome (Snell, 1993).

The number of Caesarean section births for fetal distress is reported to be reduced with amnioinfusion. The procedure, which is time-consuming to complete, restricts the woman to bed and may cause umbilical cord prolapse. It is still in the experimental stage. It is contraindicated in a number of cases, e.g. breech presentation, antepartum haemorrhage, fever, vaginal birth after Caesarean section, fetal distress, and elective lower segment Caesarean section, and it is not recommended in cases where late deceleration patterns are recorded (Snell, 1993). Further research work is needed to confirm or refute the possible benefits suggested by the earlier research (Hofmeyer, 1992).

DNA analysis Referred to as molecular genetics, this has developed from the Southern blot or DNA transfer technique, in which DNA extracted from cells is fragmented by means of a restriction enzyme and the fragments separated by size using electrophoresis on an agarose gel. The fragments are denatured with alkali to form single strands and a permanent copy of the single-stranded fragments is made by transferring them on to a nitrocellulose filter (the Southern blot). A particular DNA fragment can then be localized using a radioactively labelled DNA probe which facilitates visualization by autoradiography (Mueller, 1990).

Currently the *polymerase chain reaction (PCR)* or *DNA amplification* is used. Small amounts of DNA are amplified by enzyme synthesis then visualized by special staining of an agarose gel. This is a more effective technique in the detailed analysis of specific genes (Malcolm, 1992). Continuing progress has led to the isolation and characterization of the most important genes.

Fetal DNA can be obtained from fetal cell cultures obtained from amniocentesis or, more recently, from chorionic villus biopsy or by cordocentesis. DNA analysis for haemoglobinopathies (Old, 1992) and for fetal sexing (Gosden, 1990) can now be carried out.

As more gene probes are developed, the scope of this analysis will expand rapidly. Early work suggests that amniocentesis may be useful in the prenatal diagnosis of cytomegalovirus infection (Hogge *et al.*, 1993).

Enzyme assay Prenatal diagnosis is possible for over half the inborn errors of metabolism in which the enzyme defect is known by measuring the enzyme in question in amniotic fluid cells following culture.

Method

Detailed explanation of amniocentesis should be given to minimize parental anxiety and informed consent is obtained following non-directive counselling to advise of the risks and benefits. The woman and her partner may then make informed decisions based on up-to-date information (Donnai, 1992).

The pregnant woman is asked to empty her bladder before the procedure is performed. Depending on the period of gestation, abdominal examination and auscultation is performed to determine lie, presentation and position of the fetus. Ultrasound imaging is used to confirm viability, singleton pregnancy or not, placental site, to date the pregnancy and locate a suitable site for insertion of the needle. The skin is cleansed and may be infiltrated with a local anaesthetic, if deemed necessary. A long needle 20 gauge or smaller is attached to a syringe and inserted through the abdominal and uterine walls into the amniotic sac; 20 ml of amniotic fluid is aspirated. The first few millilitres are discarded to minimize the risk of maternal cell contamination (MacLachlan, 1992). The sample is placed in the bottle, labelled and sent to the cytogenetics department with the completed request form. The puncture hole is sealed with a plastic dressing spray. The fetal heart is checked and recorded both before and after the procedure. Rhesus-negative mothers are given anti-D immunoglobulin as prophylaxis against possible antibody production arising from feto-maternal haemorrhage.

Risks

The risks to the mother are low but may include maternal infection, rhesus iso-immunization and anxiety. These may be reduced by attention to good technique, information and counselling. The risks to the fetus may be direct, leading to fetal death, or indirect, that is secondary to removal of liquor. They are reduced by operator expertise and meticulous

technique (MacLachlan, 1992). It has been found retrospectively that fetal loss is higher if the serum alpha-fetoprotein is raised in the second trimester; this is due to pregnancy complications (Simpson and Elias, 1994).

Causes of fetal loss include:

▶ Spontaneous abortion.
▶ Infection.
▶ Haematoma.
▶ Haemorrhage.
▶ Leakage of amniotic fluid.
▶ Preterm labour.

Reports of respiratory problems at birth have not been supported by recent research and there is no evidence that amniocentesis causes orthopaedic postural abnormalities (MacLachlan, 1992). A specimen of amniotic fluid contaminated with fetal blood will falsely raise the alpha-fetoprotein level. Contamination with maternal blood makes it difficult to distinguish female fetal cells from the mother's. A Kleihauer test would therefore be necessary.

Psychological effects

Amniocentesis is commonly carried out at 15–16 weeks' gestation if there is thought to be a high risk of fetal abnormality. This causes the parents considerable anxiety, especially as they have to wait 3–4 weeks for the result. Further stress ensues if a late termination of pregnancy is then considered (Green, 1990). The introduction of chorionic villus sampling has the advantage that it can be carried out as early as eight weeks' gestation and the results are available quickly. It has a number of risks, however, including increased risk of abortion and limb abnormalities. These risks have restricted its use in some centres.

CORDOCENTESIS

Cordocentesis percutaneous umbilical blood sampling (PUBS) is an invasive intervention performed using ultrasound imaging whereby a sample of fetal blood is obtained from the umbilical cord or intrahepatic vein, usually in the second and third trimester of pregnancy. The site of sampling is selected on consideration of accessibility, quality of visualization, gestational age and safety. It was developed from a number of earlier interventions, including fetoscopy, for the purpose of prenatal diagnosis of the following conditions (Lilford, 1990; Nicolini and Rodeck, 1992):

▶ Genetic disorders, e.g. haemoglobinopathies, coagulopathies including haemophilia, inherited immunodeficiency disorders.

▶ Fetal karyotyping in structural anomaly, e.g. exomphalos, cardiac, duodenal atresia.

▶ Fetal infections, e.g. toxoplasmosis, rubella, cytomegalovirus, human parvovirus.

▶ Fetal haematological status in rhesus iso-immunization (feto-maternal allo-immunization).

▶ Fetal platelet counts in autoimmune thrombocytopaenia.

▶ Rapid fetal karyotyping in intrauterine growth retardation.

▶ Biochemical status in cases of intrauterine growth retardation.

▶ Clarification of ambiguous amniocentesis or chorionic villus biopsy chromosome results.

▶ Diagnosis of fragile X.

Real-time ultrasound imaging is essential prior to and independent of the procedure to establish fetal number, viability and size, presence or absence of structural abnormalities, placental implantation and amniotic fluid volume. In intrauterine growth retardation preliminary measurement of blood flow waveforms by Doppler ultrasound is essential (see later in this chapter). To ensure accuracy of diagnostic results, it is essential to confirm that the blood sample is uncontaminated fetal blood (Nicolini *et al.*, 1992).

Complications

No maternal complications are reported. Incidence of fetal loss (within two weeks of the procedure) is small, 57% of these being due to chorioamnionitis or prelabour rupture of the membranes. The remainder were due to bleeding, persistent bradycardia or thrombosis. Factors which influence the success of the intervention are reported to be the expertise of the operator and gestational age; fewer losses occurring in the second trimester (Nicolini *et al.*, 1992).

FETAL SKIN SAMPLING

This is a prenatal diagnostic intervention performed under ultrasound imaging for the diagnosis of fetal congenital skin disorders, e.g. epidermolysis bullosa or albinism. The site of fetal biopsy varies; for example, for epidermolysis bullosa the sample is taken from the buttock or leg, for albinism from the eyebrow or scalp.

Skin biopsies may be obtained by direct fetoscopy using a fetoscope with an operating side arm which allows for direct vision; by blind or ultrasound-directed fetoscopy, in which the fetoscope is removed and the sample obtained via the cannula; or by ultrasound-guided transabdominal skin biopsy, in which an 18 gauge trocar and cannula with biopsy forceps is used (Nicolini and Rodeck, 1992). The indications are epidermolysis bullosa letalis and epidermolysis bullosa dystrophica.

CHORIONIC VILLUS SAMPLING

Chorionic villus sampling (CVS) is a relatively new prenatal diagnostic invasive intervention carried out at 8–11 weeks of completed pregnancy. Guided by ultrasound imaging, chorionic villi are aspirated from placental tissue (chorion frondosum) and investigated for a number of disorders in the fetus.

CVS can be used to diagnose a number of conditions such as cytogenetic disorders, inborn errors of metabolism and other genetic disorders using recombinant DNA analysis, biochemical investigation and chromosome analysis (Lilford, 1990). It may be performed by a transvaginal or transabdominal route, and both are reported to be equally safe at 9–12 weeks. The transvaginal route is absolutely contraindicated in the presence of active herpes, gonorrhoea or chlamydial infection (Simpson and Elias, 1994).

Chorionic villus biopsy is reserved for women at high risk of cytogenetic conditions and is only available in a number of large centres. The test is now widely used in European countries and the USA where a register, commenced in 1984, is kept of all cases (Silverman and Wapner, 1992).

The expertise of the operator plays a significant role in both sampling routes in the safety and efficacy of the test. It is suggested that for overall safety, accuracy and improved pregnancy outcome a centre should adopt both methods of sampling (Silverman and Wapner, 1992). Expertise in the technique was gained by using cases where a decision has been taken to terminate the pregnancy (Blakemore, 1988).

One of the advantages of this test is that it can be carried out in the first trimester of pregnancy, usually between 8 and 10 weeks' gestation (Silverman and Wapner, 1992). This makes the test more acceptable to parents since there is less psychological stress at this early stage in pregnancy (Richards, 1989; Green 1990). It allows the couple 'privacy' as the pregnancy is not yet obvious, and permits earlier and therefore safer therapeutic abortion should it be considered. These two factors in particular made an earlier diagnostic test desirable (Silvermann and Wapner, 1992).

A number of cases have been reported in the literature of fetal structural abnormalities such as limb deformities attributed to this technique (Firth, 1991; Burton *et al.*, 1992). This occurred more frequently when the transabdominal route was employed and the procedure was performed at less than nine weeks' pregnancy. A number of hypotheses have been postulated, including hypoperfusion due to feto-maternal haemorrhage or pressor substances, vascular aetiology, possible thrombosis with subsequent embolization, amniotic puncture and limb entrapment. The substantive risk of congenital abnormality is reduced if chorionic villus biopsy is performed after eight completed weeks of pregnancy. It is recommended that prospective parents are informed of this risk prior to having the procedure performed (Simpson and Elias, 1994).

Technique

Chorionic villi may be obtained by aspiration transcervically or transabdominally (Silverman and Wapner, 1992). *Transcervical aspiration* is a simple technique whereby a needle or a plastic tube with a metal guide is placed through the cervix with the use of ultrasound imaging until it reaches the edge of the chorion frondosum. Chorionic villi are aspirated into the tube with the aid of a syringe attached to the tube. Great care is exercised to exclude the aspiration of maternal rather than chorionic tissue. The amount of aspirate required depends on the tests to be performed: approximately 10–20 mg are required for direct chromosomal analysis, only 1–2 mg for biochemical analysis and as much as 30–60 mg for the diagnosis of beta-thalassaemia.

Transabdominal aspiration is carried out by inserting a needle through the abdominal and uterine walls, using ultrasound imaging for guidance.

Risks of CVS

Infection This is a potential risk, especially with the transvaginal route, but evidence suggests that it is minimal, especially when a catheter is used once only, then discarded. Chorionamnionitis has been reported in the literature, but the incidence is low (Silvermann and Wapner, 1992).

Rupture of the membranes This is a rare complication which has a low incidence of occurrence (Hogge *et al.*, 1986). It is due to trauma to the chorion which allows subsequent exposure and damage to, or a low-grade infection of, the chorion.

Rhesus iso-immunization A transient increase in the levels of serum alpha-fetoprotein may occur, implying a degree of feto-maternal bleeding (Blakemore, 1988). It is recommended that rhesus-negative women undergoing CVS receive anti-D immunoglobulin subsequent to the procedure. In women already sensitized, CVS may be contraindicated, the exceptions being evaluation of fetal blood type in red cell antigen incompatibility and when termination of an antigen-positive pregnancy has been discussed and planned (Silvermann and Wapner, 1992).

Accuracy of CVS

It is reported that there is a risk of maternal cell contamination which leads to subsequent errors of diagnosis. This risk has been reduced with the improved expertise of operators and laboratory personnel.

Fetal damage

The risks to the fetus have already been discussed.

Indications

DNA analysis This involves DNA transfer or Southern blot technique or polymerase chain reaction (PCR) (see earlier in this chapter) (Malcolm, 1992). The technique enables the use of gene probe diagnosis to determine a number of inherited disorders including the haemoglobinopathies (Old, 1992). Sickle cell disease can now be diagnosed but not all beta-thalassaemias.

Fetal sex selection Fetal sex can be determined using CVS. This allows carriers of severe X-linked diseases, such as Duchenne muscular dystrophy (DMD), to opt for a first trimester abortion if it is found that the fetus is male (Bakker and van Ommen, 1992).

Chromosome analysis Chromosomal analysis is possible but is not yet as reliable as the diagnosis of sickle cell disease or the sex of the fetus.

Inborn errors of metabolism Metabolic diseases such as Tay–Sachs disease may be diagnosed from chorionic villi. In due course it is hoped that many more metabolic diseases will be diagnosed in this way, once the normal enzyme activities in the villi have been established.

Preparation of the woman and partner

Appropriate and adequate information in the form of non-directive counselling should be given to the woman and her partner prior to the procedure and at the time of testing to enable them to make informed decisions as to the risks and benefits, and to prepare them for the difficult decisions which may arise from the results of the tests performed (Donnai, 1992). Couples should be aware that chorionic villus biopsy is a diagnostic test, treatment of the fetus is not an option and the only course open is to proceed with the pregnancy, or termination. Rothman (1988) has explored these hard options in relation to amniocentesis.

Fetal therapy, which is in its infancy at the present time, may be a reality for more conditions in the future (Kuller and Golbus, 1992). However, the work on this area is still at the experimental stage and there are associated problems which require to be resolved before fetal therapy is offered generally to the pregnant woman.

Post-termination support and counselling is essential to alleviate the adverse psychological sequelae which may occur following detection of fetal abnormalities and subsequent termination. Midwives may refer women to voluntary groups, such as Support After Termination for Fetal Abnormality (SATFA), which are active nationally in providing support for such women and their partners.

The need for continued support in relation to the next pregnancy is recommended. For accurate genetic counselling of families, pathological, cytogenetic and clinical geneticist expertise is essential (Donnai, 1992).

Social and psychological aspects

The social and psychological aspects of CVS have been explored by a number of authors including Richards (1989) and Green (1990). The anxiety engendered by the tests, the waiting times, the results and the termination of pregnancy, if decided upon, place great stresses on the woman and her partner. It is documented that couples experience less anxiety with CVS and have a greater attachment

to the fetus in the second trimester (Spencer and Cox, 1988).

Non-invasive Tests

ASSESSMENT OF FETAL WELL-BEING

Biophysical monitoring of high- and low-risk pregnancies to provide indirect information about the integrity and functional state of neurological, neuromuscular and excretory function has largely replaced biochemical tests of endocrine function of the fetoplacental unit (e.g. oestriol estimation). It is thought that antenatal biophysical monitoring, as described at the end of the chapter, may detect or predict adverse perinatal events and, when combined with appropriate obstetrical intervention, reduce the severity or frequency of these events, e.g. antepartum stillbirth (Mohide and Kierse, 1989).

Fetal movements

Monitoring fetal movements is a simple, inexpensive, daily test of fetal well-being developed from early work by Sadovsky in the 1970s. He showed that decrease or cessation of fetal movements precedes fetal death by one day or more.

The risk of fetal death from known and unexplained causes varies with gestation period, being greatest at 28 weeks, reducing to term and rising post-term. Ultrasound evidence shows that the fetus moves *in utero* in two distinct patterns: *active* (40 minutes average) and *quiet* phases (23 minutes average). An extended length of the quiet phase (greater than 60 minutes) is abnormal (Grant and Elbourne, 1989). Estimation of fetal movement patterns using fixed time/number counting has been explored by a number of authors, including Pearson (1979), who developed a fetal activity chart – the Cardiff 'Count to Ten Kick Chart'.

Women in high-risk groups may be asked to count and chart fetal movements daily during the latter weeks of pregnancy. Ten movements in a 12-hour period is considered the minimum safe number. Less than ten movements in 48 hours or no fetal movements for more than 12 hours are indicative of serious intrauterine hypoxia. Delivery may then be expedited, after consideration of the possibility of congenital malformation. A number of factors may alter the activity of a fetus (e.g. fetal malformations), and evidence suggests that fetuses have inherent individual rates of activity. Sedatives taken by the mother may be a cause of diminished fetal movements. It is recommended that fetal movement counts should be used for all women as a screening test which prompts the use of other diagnostic tests, e.g. biophysical assessment, rather than more definitive obstetric intervention such as expediting delivery, and for diagnosing late antepartum deaths (Grant and Elbourne, 1989).

In a large study covering a five-year period it was found that maternal monitoring of fetal movements did not reduce the risk of intrauterine fetal death (Lobb *et al.*, 1985). Problems associated with this method of fetal assessment include non-compliance, maternal anxiety, false reports of the cessation of fetal movements and the wide range of variations between individuals due to individual fetal activity, individual perception of movements by mothers and variation in activity between fetuses.

Draper *et al.* (1986) report that filling in the charts worries one-quarter of women and most do not have the aims fully explained to them. Many women have difficulty in deciding which movements to record. It is important that mothers are given clear instructions on how to count fetal movements and have a good understanding of the reasons for doing so. Research is ongoing in an attempt to elicit the effectiveness of fetal movement counting in relation to teaching the technique, encouraging compliance and response to reported reduction in fetal movements (Grant and Elbourne, 1989).

Pathophysiology

Research has indicated that, in the presence of hypoxia, a fetus undergoes changes in biophysical activities, one of which is fetal movements. This is thought to be due to cellular dysfunction of the central nervous system which is very sensitive to oxygen supply (Tsang and Manning, 1992). Fetal biophysical activities reflect CNS activity and response to oxygen depletion and may provide evidence of fetal oxygenation.

Fetal heart sounds in pregnancy

The fetal heart rate gradually falls after 28 weeks, the normal range being between 110 and 150 beats per minute (bpm) (FIGO, 1987), and two patterns of variability emerge. These are *saltatory episodes* produced by frequent accelerations above the baseline due to fetal activity and *undulatory episodes*, which are associated with a stable baseline and variability usually between 5 and 15 bpm lasting 10–40 seconds. The fetal heart may be monitored by means of a Pinard's stethoscope, Doppler ultrasound or cardiotocograph monitor. In high-risk mothers it may be continuously monitored in pregnancy, for periods varying from half an hour to about two hours, with or without monitoring uterine contractions or recording fetal movements. Abnormal fetal heart patterns (see Chapter 29), such as decelerations or loss of beat-to-beat variation, may be detected on the trace and indicate the need to expedite delivery.

Cardiotocography is a correlation of fetal heart rate patterns with fetal movements or uterine contractions. It is a useful method of assessing fetal well-being. The fetal heart should accelerate by up to 20 bpm when the fetus moves. Failure of the fetal heart rate to rise indicates that the fetus is at risk because of placental dysfunction.

Fetal breathing movements

Fetal breathing movements, which are episodic separated by periods of apnoea, may be detected by ultrasound scanning and individual fetal breaths are recognized by paradoxical inward movement of the anterior chest wall and outward movement in the opposite direction of the anterior abdominal wall (Richardson and Gagnon, 1994). In a healthy fetus breathing is rapid, intermittent and irregular. Fetal breathing varies with gestation period. In the last trimester of pregnancy fetal breathing occurs approximately 30% of the observed time and is clustered; earlier in pregnancy at 24–28 weeks, it is reduced with shorter period of apnoea. Factors which affect breathing movements are behavioural state, physiological characteristics (e.g. eye and somatic movements and fetal heart rate), gestational age, time of day and maternal alcohol ingestion, cigarette smoking and drug ingestion (e.g. methadone, diazepam, caffeine) (Richardson and Gagnon, 1994). Fetal breathing is seen as a reliable index of fetal health and is used as a variable in the biophysical profile in conjunction with body movement, but false results may occur. Decreased fetal breathing may be indicative of fetal compromise due to hypoxia and or acidaemia. Long periods of apnoea suggest that the fetus is seriously at risk.

ULTRASONOGRAPHY

Ultrasound imaging is a non-invasive diagnostic technique using sound waves with a frequency well above the range of human hearing, that is over 20 000 cycles/second or hertz (Hz) (Gegor, 1993). It was introduced into obstetrics by Donald in the 1950s (RCOG, 1984) and, although there is little or no evidence at the present time that it is harmful to mother or fetus (Green, 1990; Proud, 1991; Gegor, 1993), the issue of safety is still of concern as the use of ultrasound in pregnancy has never been fully evaluated (Robinson and Lawrence Beech, 1993).

Reasons given to support the use of ultrasound for all women at 18 weeks' gestation include measurement and imaging of the fetus and associated maternal structures as an aid to the diagnosis of abnormalities and deviations from normal development (Pearce, 1987; Chitty et al., 1991; Gegor, 1993).

Technical aspects of ultrasonography

The use of ultrasound for medical purposes was developed from SONAR (sound navigation and ranging), a system used to detect submarines by emitting pulses of sound and evaluating echoes (Chudleigh and Pearce, 1992). The pulses can be generated by passing a high voltage through a crystal and causing it to vibrate at a high frequency. Sound waves are emitted, formed into a beam and directed on to the abdomen. Whenever the beam crosses a boundary (interface) between two tissues of differing properties it is partially reflected back to the crystal. The crystal (or transducer) converts the sounds into electrical energy which can be displayed on a cathode ray screen, either as a vertical deflection of a horizontal line (an A–scan) or as a bright spot (a B–scan).

Information can be displayed on the monitor screen in several ways as follows:

▶ *Amplitude (A) mode*: This gives a measure of the distance between features as shown in Figure 1.
▶ *Brightness (B) mode*: In this case an echo is displayed as a bright spot varying in intensity with the strength of the echo. The combination of many thousands of such spots produces a two–dimensional image of a selected plane orthogonal to the direction of the ultrasound beam. This may be a static image or a real–time image in which movement is simulated by a rapid series of static images (greater than 20 per second) to avoid flicker. The probe is moved manually to scan the target area.
▶ *Time–motion (T–M) mode*: This is a means of imaging fast-moving structures such as heart valves in such a way as to indicate their operation against a base of time.

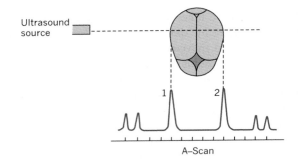

Figure 1 An A-scan sonogram; 1 and 2 indicate the parietal eminences.

▶ *Doppler ultrasound*: This is a means of imaging blood flow in vessels based on the Doppler effect, where the frequency shift in the echo from flowing blood indicates the nature of the flow.

Introduction of linear array real-time scanners in the 1970s made the equipment cheaper, smaller and easier to use. The time required to produce an image with this equipment is only a fraction of a second, whereas it takes 20–30 seconds for hand-held mechanical B-scans. When the entire image of many B-mode lines can be constructed faster than the flicker fusion rate of the eye, the image appears to be in real time.In obstetrics two types of transducers are commonly used, the *transabdominal* 3.5–5.0 MHz and the *transvaginal*, which may be brought closer to the structures of interest, 5.0–7.5 MHz (Chudleigh and Pearce, 1992).

Preparation of the woman and partner

Ultrasound scanning is routine practice in most midwifery units and women and partners usually expect this (Proud, 1991). It is recommended that informed consent is obtained and women and partners should be informed of the choices, risks, benefits and options so that they may make a decision (Gegor, 1993). The preparation should also include attention to the anxiety of mothers and partners relating to ultrasound scanning and sensitive handling in the event of an abnormality being detected (Proud, 1991).

Method

Ultrasound scanning may be performed by an ultrasonographer or a midwife trained in the technique. The ability of the operator to give individualized attention is important (Green, 1990).

A water-soluble gel is smeared over the mother's

abdomen to ensure proper contact of the ultrasound probe. If performed in early pregnancy the only discomfort experienced by the mother is that of a full bladder. This is necessary to raise the uterus out of the pelvis, displace the intestine, and serves as a useful landmark as it is seen as a well-defined black area on the monitor screen. An A-scan facilitates very accurate measurements (Figure 1). A B-scan gives a composite two-dimensional picture (Figure 2). The bright spots indicating the position of the echoes as the probe moves across the abdomen coalesce to give an anatomical outline which appears to be in real time. The screen should be positioned so as to be visible to the mother.

An ultrasound scan is usually performed between 16 and 18 weeks' gestation, and may be repeated later in pregnancy if indicated, e.g. for intrauterine growth retardation. The objectives are:

1   to establish the correct gestational age by measurements, e.g. biparietal diameter, head circumference, femoral length, crown rump length;
2   to diagnose multiple pregnancy;
3   to identify fetal abnormalities by looking at brain, spine, chest, abdomen, cord, heart, kidneys, diaphragm;
4   to locate the placenta and estimate liquor volume;
5   to assess fetal growth (eg. by measuring abdominal circumference);
6   to detect any abnormality in early pregnancy, e.g. hydatidiform mole, missed abortion; and
7   to diagnose uterine abnormality, e.g. bicornuate uterus.

Indications for diagnostic ultrasonography

Diagnosis of pregnancy   The embryonic sac may be identified as early as five weeks' gestation using a transabdominal probe and at four weeks with a transvaginal probe. Fetal heart movements can be visualized

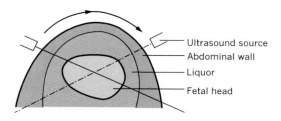

Figure 2   A diagram showing the abdominal wall and the fetal head.

at 6–7 weeks' gestation. Lack of fetal heart movement is a reliable method of diagnosing fetal death. Actual movements of the fetus can be observed from 8–9 weeks. Doppler ultrasound machines may be used to hear the fetal heart after 10–12 weeks' gestation, but failure to hear the fetal heart does not always indicate fetal death.

Ectopic pregnancy   This may be detected by ultrasound scan, the transvaginal route being more accurate than the transabdominal route (Chudleigh and Pearce, 1992). Diagnosis is difficult, but identification of high-risk groups, clinical examination and biochemical tests usually assist the diagnosis.

Missed abortion   This will be suspected if the fetal sac fails to grow, a fetal pole is visible but no fetal heart beat is seen.

Hydatidiform mole   This can be accurately diagnosed by seeing a classic white mottled area 'snowstorm' appearance on B mode scanning and by the lack of any recognizable structures. Ultrasound scan confirms the diagnosis following painless bleeding per vaginam, a large-for-dates uterus, hyperemesis gravidarum and absence of fetal heart sounds by 14 weeks' gestation using Doppler ultrasound.

Cervical incompetence   Serial ultrasound from 16 weeks reveals cervical funnelling of the amniotic membranes and shortening of the cervix (Jackson and Garity, 1992).

Multiple pregnancy   Multiple pregnancy can be identified from four weeks transvaginally, and five weeks abdominally (Chudleigh and Pearce, 1992). Initially it is diagnosed by seeing more than one fetal sac; the presence of two viable fetuses confirms the diagnosis. Serial ultrasound to estimate fetal growth and development may be carried out throughout pregnancy as complications are more likely to arise in a multiple pregnancy.

Estimation of gestational age   This can be accurately determined by ultrasound scan and the commonest parameters used are gestation sac volume, crown–rump length, biparietal diameter, femoral length, head circumference and abdominal circumference (Chudleigh and Pearce, 1992). The most accurate time to measure the gestational sac is between the fifth and sixth week of pregnancy (transabdominal) or earlier if a transvaginal probe is used. This examination confirms an intrauterine pregnancy, enables calculation of gestational age before the fetus is visible and diagnosis of anembryonic pregnancy (no embryonic tissue).

The *crown–rump length* is considered to be the most reliable means of determining gestational age from 7–14 weeks' gestation. From 14 weeks until term, gestational age may be estimated by measuring the *biparietal diameter, head circumference, abdominal circumference* or *length of the femur.* The biparietal diameter is the most widely used, easily obtained, and most accurate ultrasound parameter for estimation of gestational age. Standard sections for the measurement of biparietal diameter in conjunction with head circumference and occipitofrontal diameter are laid down by the British Medical Ultrasound Society (BMUS). A biparietal measurement between 13 and 20 weeks is as accurate as a crown–rump length measurement in the first trimester of pregnancy (Chudleigh and Pearce, 1992). Femur length is as accurate as the biparietal diameter in predicting gestational age. It can be measured from 12 weeks' gestation to term and may be used to confirm age estimated from the biparietal diameter. For accuracy the measurements to assess gestational age should be done between 16 and 20 weeks' gestation as prediction of gestational age by ultrasound scan cannot be accurately made after 24 weeks (Chudleigh and Pearce, 1992).

Assessment of fetal growth　To assess fetal growth, the age of the fetus must be accurately established before 24 weeks' gestation. Fetal growth may be monitored by serial measurements, usually the head and abdominal circumferences every four weeks, but any of the parameters, namely biparietal diameter, head and abdominal circumference, femoral length may be used. Measurement of head and abdominal circumference are used to estimate the growth in small-for-gestational-age fetuses, both asymmetrical and symmetrical, and large-for-gestational-age fetuses. In the symmetrical small-for-gestational-age fetus the normal growth shows deviation in later pregnancy below the 5th centile. In the asymmetrical condition, the abdominal circumference growth is slow and may stop, and eventually the head circumference stops growing. As a rule of thumb the abdominal circumference slows 2–3 weeks before the head circumference (Chudleigh and Pearce, 1992). Growth acceleration (large abdominal circumference) above the 90th cen-

tile may be due to maternal diabetes mellitus, especially if associated with polyhydramnios and a large thick placenta.

Estimation of fetal weight　This may be carried out in a number of situations, e.g. preterm labour, fetal macrosomia, e.g. diabetic babies, but is subject to errors of 160 g per kg of fetal weight. It may involve measurement of the biparietal diameter and abdominal circumference or, if this is not possible, abdominal circumference and femoral length.

Placental location　This is important for success prior to invasive procedures, e.g. amniocentesis, chorionic villus biopsy. It can be determined by ultrasound at 16–20 weeks and is considered to be worthwhile as 95% will be a fundal implantation. Approximately 5% of placentae will be defined as low lying on ultrasound examination early in the second trimester of pregnancy. A repeat ultrasound scan at 32 weeks, or earlier should bleeding occur, would be performed on those women with a low-lying placenta in the second trimester. However, most will no longer exhibit this by term unless the placenta is central (type IV). The umbilical cord and placenta, including any deviations from normal, e.g. circumvallata, chorioangioma, can all be visualized during ultrasound scanning (Chudleigh and Pearce, 1992).

Ultrasound in late pregnancy

This is usually reserved for high-risk cases, such as a suspected small-for-gestational-age fetus, low-lying placenta diagnosed at early scan, suspected placenta praevia on clinical findings, fetal presentation, e.g. confirmation of breech, fetal anomaly, fetal weight estimation, confirmation of fetal death *in utero*, as an aid to external cephalic version and for 'women who book late for ante-natal care' (Chudleigh and Pearce, 1992). Occasionally a previously undetected fetal malformation will also be found at this time.

Congenital abnormalities

A detailed scan is performed by an expert looking specifically at fetal anatomy for any structural abnormalities. Information gained is used for decisions regarding termination of pregnancy, appropriate timing and mode of delivery, facilities for neonatal surgery, fetal therapy and psychological preparation of the parents

(Neilson and Grant, 1989). Fetal abnormalities which may be detected include the following:

▶ *Craniospinal defects*, e.g. anencephaly, spina bifida, choroid plexus cysts.
▶ *Cardiac defects*, such as ventricular septal defect, Fallot's tetralogy, mitral or tricuspid atresia.
▶ *Gastrointestinal defects*, e.g. gastroschisis, diaphragmatic hernia, oesophageal and duodenal atresia.
▶ *Renal defects*, e.g. renal agenesis (Potter's syndrome), polycystic disease, hydronephrosis.
▶ *Skeletal abnormalities*, e.g. dwarfism.
▶ *Miscellaneous conditions* include chromosome abnormalities, e.g. trisomy 21 (Down's syndrome), trisomy 18 (Edwards' syndrome), trisomy 13 (Pattau's syndrome), non-immune hydrops, cleft lip and palate and fetal tumours, e.g. cystic hygroma, and teratomas (Chitty and Campbell, 1992).

It is recommended that ultrasound scanning is performed when the serum alpha-fetoprotein is found to be raised, to elicit possible causes.

Down's syndrome   A number of ultrasound markers (i.e. signs) have been reported for Down's syndrome, the most significant being duodenal atresia, and cardiac defects, e.g. atrioventricular canal defects, ventricular septal defects, atrial septal defects, and patent ductus arteriosis. A number of other markers have been reported, e.g. cystic hygroma (5%), hydrops, hydrothorax, omphalocele, shortened femoral length, pyelectasis (mild dilation of the renal pelvis), and thicker nuchal fold, but current evidence suggests these are unsuitable for use as a reliable marker of Down's syndrome (Lockwood *et al.*, 1991).

Other uses for ultrasonography

Fetal therapy   Ultrasound may be used in conjunction with karyotyping and echocardiogram to establish accurate diagnosis of the fetal condition prior to selection of fetuses for possible therapy. Kuller and Golbus (1992) stress the need for strict criteria to be met before fetal therapy is embarked upon. *In utero* fetal therapy is still in the experimental stage, but has been successfully used in the treatment of bilateral urinary tract obstruction. Ultrasound scanning may be used to monitor the degree of ventriculomegaly in fetal hydronephrosis to aid decision making regarding treatment. Ultrasound scanning is used also after birth to aid in the management of certain conditions.

Ultrasound guidance for special procedures   Ultrasound guidance for procedures such as amniocentesis, intrauterine transfusions, fetoscopy, cordocentesis and chorionic villus sampling has added to the safety and accuracy of these investigations and treatments.

Tumours   Some tumours, such as maternal ovarian cysts and uterine tumours, may be detected by ultrasound scanning.

Infertility   Ovarian follicular development is monitored and measured by transvaginal ultrasound scanning in cases of infertility as an aid to establish ovulation and for the management of individual cases, usually in conjunction with pharmacological treatment.

Retained products of conception   Ultrasound is used to confirm the diagnosis in suspected cases of retained products in the puerperium when clinical findings are suggestive of this, e.g. excessive lochia and subinvolution of the uterus.

Congenital dislocation of the hips   Ultrasound has been used to diagnose this condition when suspected in the neonate.

Effect of ultrasound on mothers and partners

Most mothers and partners find the ultrasound scan a positive experience; however, the psychological effect of the experience depends on the quality of the communication that accompanies it (Proud, 1994). The experience is thought to enhance maternal–fetal bonding (Green, 1990). Problems can arise, however, when abnormalities are detected, and this can be a devastating experience because of anxiety (Proud, 1991). Arrangements should always be made for the obstetrician to see the parents at the earliest opportunity so that the findings can be fully discussed with them.

Doppler ultrasound

This technique is used to measure blood flow in the umbilical artery and uteroplacental vessels from a waveform recording on a monitor screen. The waveform is measured crudely using three indices: the *systolic/diastolic* (S/D or A/B) *ratios, resistance index* (RI) and the *pulsatility index* (PI). Current indications for umbilical artery waveforms are mainly intrauterine growth retardation, fetal assessment in maternal systemic lupus erythematosus, differing growth patterns in twin pregnancy and in conjunction with uteroplacental waveforms in oligohydramnios. They are not of value in screening the small-for-gestational-age fetus, and do not predict fetal death or placental abruption (Chudleigh and Pearce, 1992).

Uteroplacental waveforms are used mostly in cases of hypertensive disorders of pregnancy (Chudleigh and Pearce, 1992). The use of Doppler is still in its infancy, and its potential in obstetrics is as yet undetermined. Further research work is needed to evaluate it.

RADIOLOGICAL AND MAGNETIC VISUALIZATION TECHNIQUES

Ultrasound has replaced radiology as a means of imaging in obstetrics since the latter is considered to be harmful to the fetus (Johnson, 1992). In a small number of cases X-ray pelvimetry may be performed, for example, when considering vaginal breech delivery. Radiology should be delayed until 30–32 weeks when it is less harmful to the fetus.

Magnetic resonance imaging (MRI) in pregnancy

MRI is used as a diagnostic tool in medicine but research in obstetrics has shown that it is unsuitable as a means of imaging the fetus due to fetal movement and difficulties in selecting the plane of imaging. However, it has been found to be satisfactory for imaging maternal structures (Johnson, 1992). It may be useful in a few cases, e.g. oligohydramnios, but at present ultrasound scanning is considered to be superior in prenatal diagnosis.

BIOPHYSICAL PROFILE

This is a non-invasive accurate test of fetal well-being which was first described in 1980 using ultrasound imaging to measure five biophysical variables:

- Fetal heart rate.
- Fetal tone.
- Somatic movements.
- Breathing movements.
- Amniotic fluid volume (James, 1993).

The variables are scored individually and totalled to give a biophysical score. Biophysical profile is an accurate predictor of fetal death in a large number of high-risk pregnancies, where the fetus is at risk from diverse pathologies. It may be influenced by a number of factors, most of which are linked to gestation period. These include:

Physiological factors:

- Fetal heart rate.
- Fetal activity organized into periods of rest and activity.
- Fetal breathing and liquor volume (Pillai and James, 1990).

Pathological factors:

- Chronic asphyxia, e.g. pre-eclampsia, recurrent placental bleeding.
- Endocrine conditions: maternal diabetes.
- Cardiovascular problems: fetal cardiac problems, structural problems.
- Neurological problems: anencephaly (James, 1993).

Other problems which may affect the biophysical profile are maternal drug abuse or therapeutic medication or fetal chromosome abnormalities.

References

Assel, B.G., Lewis, S.M., Dickerman, L.H., Murtif Park, V. & Jasani M.N. (1992) Single-operator comparison of early and mid-second-trimester amniocentesis. *Obstet. Gynecol.* 79(6): 940–944.

Austoker, J. & McPherson, A. (1992) *Cervical Screening.* Oxford: Oxford University Press.

Bakker, E. & van Ommen, G.J.B. (1992) Muscular dystrophies. In Brock, D.J.H., Rodeck, C.H. & Ferguson-Smith, M.A. (eds) *Prenatal Diagnosis and Screening.* Edinburgh: Churchill Livingstone.

Banatvala, J.E. & Chrystie, I.L. (1994) HIV screening in pregnancy: UK lags. *Lancet* 343: 113.

Bergstrand, C.G. & Czar, B. (1956) Demonstration of a new protein fraction in serum from the human fetus. *Scand. J. Clin. Lab. Invest.* 8: 174.

Berrebi, A., Kobuch, W.E., Bessieres, M.H. *et al.* (1994) Termination of pregnancy for maternal toxoplasmosis. *Lancet* 344: 36–39.

Blake, P.G., Martin, J.N. & Perry, K.G. (1993) Haemoglobinopathies. In Knuppel, R.A. & Drukker, J.E. (eds) *High Risk Pregnancy: A Team Approach.* Philadelphia: W.B. Saunders.

Blakemore, K.J. (1988) Prenatal diagnosis by chorionic villus sampling. *Obstet. Gynecol. Clin. North Am.* 15(2): 179–213.

Bowell, P.J., Allen, D.L. & Entwistle, C.C. (1986) Blood group antibody screening tests during pregnancy. *Br. J. Obstet. Gynaecol.* 93: 1038–1043.

Bowman, J.M. (1994) Haemolytic disease (Erythroblastosis fetalis). In Creasy, R.K. & Resnik, R. (eds) *Maternal, Fetal Medicine, Principles and Practice*. Philadelphia: W.B. Saunders.

Brambati, B., Simoni, G. & Travi, M. (1992) Genetic diagnosis before 8 gestational weeks: efficiency, reliability and risks on 317 completed pregnancies. *Prenatal Diagnosis* 12(10): 789–799.

Brock, D.J.H. (1992) Alphafetoprotein and acetylcholinesterase. In Brock D.J.H., Rodeck, C.H. & Ferguson-Smith, M.A. (eds) *Prenatal Diagnosis and Screening*. Edinburgh: Churchill Livingstone.

Burton, B.K., Schulz, M.S. & Burd, L.I. (1992) Limb anomalies associated with chorionic villus sampling. *Obstet. Gynecol.* 79(5): 730–736.

Campbell, J. (1993) Making sense of blood groups. *Nursing Times* 89(22): 36–38.

Campbell, S. & Pearce, J.M. (1983) Ultrasound visualisation of structural anomalies. *Br. Med. Bull.* 39: 322.

Carlson, D.E., Platt, L.D., Medearis, A.L. & Horenstein, J. (1990) Quantifiable polyhydramnios: diagnosis and management. *Obstet. Gynecol.* 75: 989–993.

Chamberlain, G. (1992) *ABC of Antenatal Care*. London: BMA.

Chitty, L. & Campbell, S. (1992) Ultrasound screening for fetal abnormalities. In Brock D.J.H., Rodeck, C.H. & Ferguson-Smith, M.A. (eds) *Prenatal Diagnosis and Screening*. Edinburgh: Churchill Livingstone.

Chitty, L.S., Hunt, G.H., Moore, J. & Lobb, M.O. (1991) Effectiveness of routine ultrasonography in detecting fetal structural abnormalities in a low risk population. *Br. Med. J.* 303: 1165–1169.

Chrystie, I.L., Wolfe, C.D.A., Kennedy, J. *et al.* (1995) Voluntary named testing for HIV in a community based antenatal clinic: a pilot study. *Br. Med. J.* 311: 928–931.

Chudleigh, P. & Pearce, M.L. (1992) *Obstetric Ultrasound, How, Why and When*. Edinburgh: Churchill Livingstone.

Cohn, J.A. (1993) Human immunodeficiency virus and AIDS, 1993 update. *J. Nurse-Midwifery* 38(2): 65–85.

Crandall, B.F., Robinson, L. & Grau, P. (1991) Risks associated with an elevated maternal serum alpha-fetoprotein level. *Am. J. Obstet. Gynecol.* 165(3): 581–585.

CRC (Cancer Research Campaign) (1990) *Cervical Cancer, Factsheet 12*. London: CRC.

Cuckle, H.S. & Wald, N.J. (1990) Screening for Down's syndrome. In Lilford, R. (ed.) *Prenatal Diagnosis and Prognosis*. London: Butterworth.

Cuckle, H.S., Wald, N.J., Goodburn, S.F. *et al.* (1990) Measurement of urea resistant neutrophil phosphatase as an antenatal screening test for Down's syndrome. *Br. Med. J.* 301: 1024–1026.

Dawson, M. (1988) Immunology, specific immunity 1 and 2. *Nursing Times* 84(17, 18, 19): 75–78; 73–76; 69–71.

Djlali, M., Barbi, G., Kennerknecht, L. & Terinde, R. (1992) Introduction of early amniocentesis to routine prenatal diagnosis. *Prenatal Diagnosis* 12(8): 661–669.

DOH (Department of Health) (1989) *Unlinked Anonymous HIV Surveys, guidance for health service staff* (leaflet AHT4). London: HMSO.

DOH (1991) *While you are Pregnant: Safe Eating and Safe Contact with Pets*. London: HMSO.

DOH (1992) *Folic Acid and the Prevention of Neural Tube Defect*. London: DOH.

Donnai, D. (1992) Genetic counselling and the pre-pregnancy clinic. In Brock D.J.H., Rodeck, C.H. & Ferguson-Smith, M.A. (eds) *Prenatal Diagnosis and Screening*. Edinburgh: Churchill Livingstone.

Draper, J., Field, S., Thomas, H. & Hare, M.J. (1986) Women's views on keeping fetal movement charts. *Br. J. Obstet. Gynaecol.* 94: 334–338.

Draper Report (1980) *Screening for Cervical Cancer*. London: HMSO.

FIGO (International Federation for Gynaecology and Obstetrics) (1987) Guidelines for the use of fetal monitoring. *Int. J. Gynaecol. Obstet.* 25: 1159–1167.

Finnegan, L.P. & Wapner, R.J. (1988) Narcotic addiction in Pregnancy. In Niebyl, J.R. (ed.) *Drug Use in Pregnancy*. Philadelphia: Lea & Febiger.

Firth, H.V., Boyd, P.A., Chamberlain, P., Mackenzie, I.Z., Lindenbaum, R.H. & Huson, S.M. (1991) Severe limb abnormalities after chorion villus sampling at 56–66 days gestation. *Lancet* 337: 762–763.

Fletcher, J.C. & Wertz, D.C. (1992) Ethics and prenatal diagnosis. In Brock D.J.H., Rodeck, C.H. & Ferguson-Smith, M.A. (eds) *Prenatal Diagnosis and Screening*. Edinburgh: Churchill Livingstone.

Fogarty, P. & Dorman, J.C. (1992) Early amniocentesis. *Contemp. Rev. Obstet. Gynaecol.* 4(2): 66–70.

FPA (Family Planning Association) (1992) *Factsheet 6B, Abortion: Legal and Ethical Issues*. London: FPA.

Gegor, C.L. (1993) Third trimester ultrasound for nurse midwives. *J. Nurse-Midwifery* 38(2) (Suppl.): 49S–61S.

Goodlad, J. (1989) Understanding Hepatitis B. *Nursing Times* 85(24): 69–71.

Gosden, C. (1990) Prenatal diagnosis of chromosome abnormalities. In Lilford, R. (ed.) *Prenatal Diagnosis and Prognosis*. London: Butterworth.

Grant, A. & Elbourne, D. (1989) Fetal movement counting to assess fetal well-being. In Chambers, I., Enkin, M. & Keirse, M.J.N. (eds) *Effective Care in Pregnancy and Childbirth*, Vol. 1. Oxford: Oxford University Press.

Green, J. (1990) Calming or harming? A critical review of psychological effects of fetal diagnosis on pregnant women. Occasional Paper No. 2. London: Galton Institute.

Green, J. & Statham, H. (1993) Testing for fetal abnormality in routine antenatal care. *Midwifery* 9: 124–135.

Gupta, J.K., Care, M., Lilford, R. *et al.* (1995) Clinical significance of fetal choroid plexus cysts. *Lancet* 8977: 724–726.

Hall, S.M. (1993) How common is congenital toxoplasmosis and what are its clinical manifestations? *Maternal and Child Health* July: 204–209.

Hannigan, E.V. (1990) Cervical cytology in pregnancy. *Clin. Obstet. Gynecol.* 33(4): 837–845.

Hanson, F.W., Tennant, F., Stacy Hune, M.S. & Brookhyser, K. (1992) Early amniocentesis: outcome, risks, and technical problems at <12.8 weeks. *Am. J. Obstet. Gynaecol.* **166**(6, Pt 1): 1707–1711.

HEA (Health Education Authority) (1992) *Vaccination Leaflet MMR Vaccination*. London: HEA.

HMSO (1967) The Abortion Act of 1967 and as amended 1991 (Human Fertilisation and Embryology Act, 1990). London: HMSO.

HMSO (1990) Human Fertilisation and Embryology Act, 1990, London: HMSO.

Hofmeyer, G.J. (1992) Amnioinfusion: a question of benefits and risks. *Br. J. Obstet. Gynaecol.* **99**: 449–451.

Hogge, J.S., Hogge, W.A. & Golbus, M.S. (1986) Chorionic villus sampling. *J. Obstet. Gynecol. Neonatal Nurs.* January/February: 24–28.

Hogge, W.A., Bufone, G.J. & Hogge, J.S. (1993) Prenatal diagnosis of cytomegalovirus (CMV) infection: a preliminary report. *Prenatal Diagnosis* **13**: 131–136.

Hollingsworth, D.R. (1992) *Pregnancy, Diabetes and Birth*. Baltimore: Williams & Wilkins.

Howard, R.J., Tuck, S.M., Long, J. & Thomas, V.A. (1992) The significance of choroid plexus cysts in fetuses at 18–20 weeks. An indication for amniocentesis? *Prenatal Diagnosis* **12**: 689–693.

Jackson, D.J. & Garity, T.J. (1992) Surgical correction of uterine abnormalities. In Plauche, W.C., Morrison, J.C. & O'Sullivan, J. (eds) *Surgical Obstetrics*. Philadelphia: W.B. Saunders.

James, D. (1993) Monitoring the biophysical profile. *Br. J. Hospital Med.* **49**(8): 561–563.

Johnson, I.R. (1992) Radiological and magnetic visualisation techniques. In Brock D.J.H., Rodeck, C.H. & Ferguson-Smith, M.A. (eds) *Prenatal Diagnosis and Screening*. Edinburgh: Churchill Livingstone.

Jorgenson, F.S., Bang, J. & Lind, A.M. (1992) Genetic amniocentesis at 7–14 weeks of gestation. *Prenatal Diagnosis* **12**(4): 277–283.

Kuller, J.A. & Golbus, M.S. (1992) Fetal therapy. In Brock D.J.H., Rodeck, C.H. & Ferguson-Smith, M.A. (eds) *Prenatal Diagnosis and Screening*. Edinburgh: Churchill Livingstone.

Liley, A.W. (1961) Liquor amnii analysis in the management of the pregnancy complicated by rhesus sensitisation. *Am. J. Obstet. Gynecol.* **82**: 1359–1370.

Lilford, R. (1990) *Prenatal Diagnosis and Prognosis*. London: Butterworth.

Lindgren, S., Bohlin, A.B., Forsgren, M. *et al.* (1993) Screening for HIV-1 antibodies in pregnancy: results from Swedish national programme. *Br. Med. J.* **307**: 1447–1451.

Lobb, M.O., Beazley, J.M. & Haddad, N.G. (1985) A controlled study of daily fetal movement counts in the prevention of stillbirths. *J. Obstet. Gynaecol.* **60**: 87–91.

Lockwood, C.J., Lynch, L. & Berkowitz, R.L. (1991) Ultrasonographic screening for the Down's syndrome fetus. *Am. J. Obstet. Gynecol.* **165**(2): 349–352.

MacKenzie, I.Z., Selinger, M. & Bowell, P.J. (1991) Management of red cell isoimmunisation in the 1990s. In Studd, J. (ed.) *Progress in Obstetrics and Gynaecology*, Vol. 9: Edinburgh: Churchill Livingstone.

MacLachlan, N.A. (1992) Amniocentesis. In Brock D.J.H.,

Rodeck, C.H. & Ferguson-Smith, M.A. (eds) *Prenatal Diagnosis and Screening*. Edinburgh: Churchill Livingstone.

Mahomed, K. & Hytten, F. (1989) Iron and folate supplementation in pregnancy. In Chalmers, I., Enkin, M. & Keirse, M.J.N. (eds) *Effective Care in Pregnancy and Childbirth*. Oxford: Oxford University Press.

Malcolm, S. (1992) Molecular genetics. In Brock D.J.H., Rodeck, C.H. & Ferguson-Smith, M.A. (eds) *Prenatal Screening and Diagnosis*. Edinburgh: Churchill Livingstone.

Marteau, T.M., Slack, J., Kidd, J. & Shaw, R. (1992) Presenting a routine screening test in antenatal care: practice observed. *Public Health* **106**(2): 131–141.

Merkatz, I.R., Nitowsky, H.M., Macri, J.N. & Johnson, W.E. (1984) An association between low maternal serum alpha-fetoprotein and fetal chromosome abnormality. *Am. J. Obstet. Gynecol.* **148**: 886–894.

Mikkelson, M. & Neilson, K.B. (1992) Karyotype analysis and chromosome disorders. In Brock D.J.H., Rodeck, C.H. & Ferguson-Smith, M.A. (eds) *Prenatal Diagnosis and Screening*. Edinburgh: Churchill Livingstone.

Miller, E., Wraight, P.A. & Vurdien, J.E. (1993) *Communicable Disease Report Review* **3**(3): 35–40.

Mohide, P. & Kierse, M.J.N.C. (1989) Assessment of fetal wellbeing. In Chambers, I., Enkin, M. & Keirse, M.J.N. (eds) *Effective Care in Pregnancy and Childbirth*. Oxford: Oxford University Press.

Montgomery, E. (1990) Iron levels in pregnancy, physiology or pathology? Assessing the need for supplements. *Midwifery* **6**: 205–214.

MRC (Medical Research Council) (1991) Medical Research Council European Trial of chorion villus sampling. *Lancet* **337**(8756): 1491–1499.

MRC (1993) Phenylketonuria due to phenylalanine hydroxalase deficiency: an unfolding story. *Br. Med. J.* **306**: 115–119.

Mueller, R. (1990) Technology for DNA diagnosis. In Lilford, R. (ed.) *Prenatal Diagnosis and Prognosis*. London: Butterworths.

Neilson, J.P. & Gosden, C. (1991) First trimester prenatal diagnosis. *Br. J. Obstet. Gynaecol.* **98**: 849–852.

Neilson, J. & Grant, A. (1989) Ultrasound in pregnancy. In Chalmers, I., Enkin, M. & Keirse, M.J.N. (eds) *Effective Care in Pregnancy and Childbirth*. Oxford: Oxford University Press.

NHSME (National Health Service Management Executive) Department of Health (DOH) (1992) *A Guide to Consent for Examination*. London: DOH.

Nicolini, U. & Rodeck, C.H. (1992) Fetal blood and tissue sampling. In Brock D.J.H., Rodeck, C.H. & Ferguson-Smith, M.A. (eds) *Prenatal Diagnosis and Screening*. Edinburgh: Churchill Livingstone.

Nicoll, A. & Moisley, C. (1994) Antenatal screening for syphilis. *Br. Med. J.* **308**: 1253–1254.

O'Brien, M.D. & Gilmour White, S. (1993) Epilepsy and pregnancy. *Br. Med. J.* **307**: 492–495.

Old, J.M. (1992) Haemoglobinopathies. In Brock D.J.H., Rodeck, C.H. & Ferguson-Smith, M.A. (eds) *Prenatal Diagnosis and Screening*. Edinburgh: Churchill Livingstone.

Pearce, J.M. (1987) Making waves: current controversies in obstetric ultrasound. *Midwifery* **3**: 25–38.

Pearson, J.F. (1979) Fetal movement recording: a guide to fetal well-being. *Nursing Times* 75: 1639–1641.

Pillai, M. & James, D. (1990) The development of fetal heart rate patterns during normal pregnancy. *Obstet. Gynecol.* 76: 812–816.

Pope, E. (1992) Toxoplasmosis. *Midwives Chronicle and Nursing Notes* October: 300–303.

Proud, J. (1991) The ultrasound scan – is it really necessary? *Modern Midwife* September/October: 6–8.

Proud, J. (1994) *Understanding Obstetric Ultrasound*, p. 19. Hale: Books for Midwives Press.

RCOG (Royal College of Obstetricians and Gynaecologists) (1984) *Report of the Working Party on Routine Ultrasound Examination in Pregnancy*. London: RCOG.

RCOG (1992) *Prenatal Screening for Toxoplasmosis in the UK*. London: RCOG.

RCOG (1993) *Effective Procedures in Obstetrics*. Manchester: RCOG, Medical Audit Unit.

Richards, M. (1989) Social and ethical problems of fetal diagnosis and screening. *J. Reprod. Infant Psychol.* 7(3): 171–185.

Richardson, B.S. & Gagnon, R. (1994) Fetal breathing and body movements. In Creasy, R.K. & Resnik, R. (eds) *Maternal, Fetal Medicine*. Philadelphia, W.B. Saunders.

Robinson, J. & Lawrence Beech, B. (1993) Ultrasound??? unsound, editorial. *Assoc. Improv. Maternity Serv.* 5(1).

Rothman, B.K. (1988) *The Tentative Pregnancy, Prenatal Diagnosis and the Future of Motherhood*. London: Pandora.

Sadovsky, E. & Polishuk, W.Z. (1977) Fetal movements in utero, Nature assessment, prognostic value, timing of delivery. *Obstet. Gynecol.* 50: 49.

Sense (1990) *Rubella in pregnancy: what does it do?* London: Sense (National Deaf–Blind and Rubella Association).

Sidle, N. (1985) *Rubella in Pregnancy*. London: Sense.

Silverman, N.S. & Wapner, R.J. (1992) Chorionic villus sampling. In Brock D.J.H., Rodeck, C.H. & Ferguson-Smith, M.A. (eds) *Prenatal Diagnosis and Screening*. Edinburgh: Churchill Livingstone.

Simpson, J.L. & Elias, S. (1994) Prenatal diagnosis of genetic disorders. In Creasy, R.K. & Resnik, R. (eds) *Maternal, Fetal Medicine*. Philadelphia, W.B. Saunders.

Snell, B.J. (1993) The use of amnioinfusion in nurse-midwifery practice. *J. Nurse-Midwifery* 38 (Suppl.): 62S–71S.

Spencer, J.W. & Cox, D.N. (1988) A comparison of chorionic villi sampling and amniocentesis: acceptability of procedure and maternal attachment to pregnancy. *Obstet. Gynaecol.* 72: 714–718.

Steer, P. (1995) Maternal haemoglobin and birthweight. What is the relationship? *Maternity Action* 69: 3.

Tabor, A., Madsen, M., Obel, E.B., Philip, J., Bang, J. & Noorgaard-Pederson, B. (1986) Randomised controlled trial of genetic amniocentesis in 4606 low risk women. *Lancet* 1: 1287–1289.

Thompson, P.J., Greenhough, A. & Nicolaides, K.H. (1992) Lung volume measured by functional residual capacity in infants following first trimester amniocentesis or chorionic villus sampling. *Br. J. Obstet. Gynaecol.* 99: 479–482.

Tsang, H.H. & Manning, F.A. (1992) Fetal biophysical profile scoring. In Druzin, M.L. (ed.) *Antepartum Fetal Assessment*. London: Blackwell Scientific.

UKCC (United Kingdom Central Council) (1992) Registrar's letter, 8/1992, replacing circular PC/89/02. London: UKCC.

UKCC (1993) *HIV/AIDS Guidelines for Staff*. London: UKCC.

Wald, N.J. & Cuckle, H.S. (1992) Biochemical screening. In Brock D.J.H., Rodeck, C.H. & Ferguson-Smith, M.A. (eds) *Prenatal Diagnosis and Screening*. Edinburgh: Churchill Livingstone.

Wald, N.J., Cuckle, H.S., Demson, J.W. *et al.* (1988) Maternal serum screening for Down's syndrome in early pregnancy. *Br. Med. J.* 297: 883–887.

Wald, N.J., Kennard, A., Demson, J.W., Cuckle, H.S., Chard, T. & Butler, L. (1992) Antenatal maternal serum screening for Down's syndrome: results of a demonstration project. *Br. Med. J.* 305: 391–394.

Wang, E. & Smaill, F. (1989) Infection in pregnancy. In Chalmers, I., Enkin, M. & Keirse, M.J.N. (eds) *Effective Care in Pregnancy and Childbirth*, Vol. 1, pp. 534–564. Oxford: Oxford University Press.

WHO (World Health Organisation) (1972) *Nutritional Anaemias, Report of a Group of Experts*. WHO Technical Report Series No. 503, p. 29.

Wilkinson, E.J. (1990) Pap smears and screening for cervical neoplasia. *Clin. Obstet. Gynecol.* 33(4): 817–825.

Wolfendale, M.R. (1989) *Taking Cervical Smears*. London: British Society Clinical Cytology (BSCC).

Young, I.D. (1990) DNA Diagnosis: calculation of genetic risk. In Lilford, R. (ed.) *Prenatal Diagnosis and Prognosis*. London: Butterworth.

Further Reading

Daker, M. & Bobrow, M. (1989) Screening for genetic disease and fetal anomaly during pregnancy. In Chalmers, I., Enkin, M. & Keirse, M.J.N. (eds) *Effective Care in Pregnancy and Childbirth*. Oxford: Oxford University Press.

Canadian Collaborative CVS–Amniocentesis Clinical Trial Group (1989) Multicentre randomised controlled trial of chorion villus sampling and amniocentesis. *Lancet* i: 1–6.

Neilson, J.P. & Gosden, C.M. (1991) First trimester prenatal diagnosis: chorion villus sampling or amniocentesis: *Br. J. Obstet. Gynaecol.* 98: 849–852.

RCOG (Royal College of Obstetricians and Gynaecologists) (1987) *Report of the Intercollegiate Working Party on Cervical Cytology Screening*. London: RCOG.

Simpson, D. (1989) Phenylketonuria. *Midwives Chronicle and Nursing Notes* February 37–41.

Smidt-Jenson, S., Permin, M., Philip, J. *et al.* (1992) Randomised comparison of amniocentesis and transabdominal and transcervical chorionic villus sampling. *Lancet* 340(8830): 1237–1244.

22

Complementary Therapies and Childbearing

There is increasing interest in the use of complementary or alternative therapies amongst both consumers and health professionals. The British Medical Association's report on 'non-conventional' medicine (BMA, 1993) recognized the potential value of many aspects of complementary therapies, and made recommendations for education and practice. General practitioners are able to employ therapists in their surgeries, and many health authorities and trusts are considering purchasing these services.

Childbearing women in particular are keen to use natural remedies because they do not wish to expose their unborn children to the potential dangers of drugs: they also wish to remain in control of their own bodies during a period when they can feel very vulnerable. They want more choices available for relieving physiological symptoms of pregnancy and the puerperium, and for pain relief in labour; and there has been a growing dissatisfaction with the dependence of obstetricians on technology. This trend, apparent in all aspects of maternity care, contributed to the *Changing Childbirth* report (DOH, 1993) which advocates more 'choice, control and continuity' for women. In essence, the use of complementary therapies provides more choice and they should be viewed as additional tools to enhance care, rather than as a threat to conventional treatments.

Professional Accountability

The professional autonomy of the midwife places her in an excellent position to offer women advice about and treatment with complementary therapies, but she must take care not to jeopardize either the health of clients or her own integrity by injudicious use or inadvertent misuse (Cresswell, 1993). Expectant parents put their trust in the professional skills of the midwife, who would be liable to destroy that trust if she made suggestions, perhaps through lack of knowledge, about using complementary therapies which were harmful to the pregnant woman or the fetus (Tiran, 1994).

Rule 40(2) in the *Midwives Rules* (UKCC, 1993) states that midwives should not undertake any practices for which they have not previously received training. Well-meaning midwives wanting to recommend homeopathic remedies or utilize aromatherapy oils for their clients must have adequate knowledge about the substances to provide safe care for mothers and their babies, and to enable them to facilitate the mother's informed choice. Therefore it is essential that any midwife using complementary therapies should be adequately and appropriately qualified in the relevant therapy. Many midwives attempt to 'dabble' in a variety of complementary or alternative strategies, without considering the implications of doing so when not properly trained. The United Kingdom Central Council for Nursing, Midwifery and Health Visiting does not seek to restrict the practice of midwives, but rather to facilitate the expansion of their role, within the parameters of the *Scope of Professional Practice* (UKCC, 1992), whilst acknowledging its own responsibilities in regulating practice to protect the public.

The *Midwife's Code of Practice* (UKCC, 1994) mentions specifically the use of homeopathic or herbal substances (paragraphs 34/35) and other complementary or alternative therapies (paragraph 56) and stresses the right of individuals to administer substances to themselves or to consult an alternative practitioner. The midwife is urged to act as an advocate for mothers, to gain consent to treatment, and to base the use of complementary therapies on all available knowledge and skill.

It is vital that midwives and their managers and supervisors develop local policies or protocols regarding the use of complementary therapies, to protect their clients and themselves (Tiran, 1995a). A working group could be established to consider several policies, including the use of therapies by midwives in the unit, issues pertinent to the care of women who are accompanied by visiting therapists, and specific procedures on therapies such as aromatherapy or reflexology. Even when a midwife is qualified in a therapy she should work within the local guidelines, and needs to differentiate between her role as a midwife and as a complementary therapist.

Implementation of Complementary Therapies

The availability of a complementary therapy service as part of maternity care may be dependent on local interest and demand from mothers and midwives, support from medical colleagues and on relevant expertise. Most often midwives who have trained in areas such as aromatherapy or reflexology (usually at their own expense and in their own time) incorporate the therapy into their personal practice. Some units have established a more formal service, with managers being willing to send staff on courses, or to appoint midwives with specific responsibility for a particular therapy, for example acupuncture (Yelland, 1995). Where obstetricians have seen the benefits to mothers – in increased satisfaction and physical comfort, and the benefits to the unit – in reduced costs of inpatient admissions or iatrogenic complications, they do not view the use of such therapies as a threat to their own position, and can often be extremely supportive.

The Therapies

There is a confusing plethora of complementary therapies from which to choose but the fundamental feature common to all therapies is that they attempt to treat the whole person rather than a disease process, believing that a person's mind, body and spirit are interlinked and that one aspect cannot be treated in isolation from the others. However, certain therapies may be more appropriate for some conditions than for others; as with conventional medicine a decision is made to determine the best treatment for an individual. Client co-operation is important as much of the advice or treatment given depends on lifestyle changes; often, too, there is an initial worsening of the client's condition as the body responds to treatment with a healing crisis. Many of the therapies are used symbiotically, or therapists will refer clients to practitioners of other therapies.

The NAHAT Report (1993) identified the five main therapies as: *homeopathy, acupuncture, osteopathy, chiropractic* and *herbalism*, which are all complete systems of care in their own right and may sometimes be used as an alternative to conventional treatment. The therapies which are most often used by midwives, nurses and health visitors, and which may be termed complementary or supportive, include *aromatherapy, shiatsu, reflexology, massage, hypnotherapy*, and a variety of *relaxation techniques* such as art, music or drama therapy, visualization or yoga. There are also many more obscure therapies not currently accepted in conventional medical circles, and which are not founded on any known scientific fact.

MASSAGE

Massage, or healing touch, is already used spontaneously by many midwives in the labour ward. Massage is an excellent means of relieving stress, aiding relaxation and inducing sleep, and because touch impulses reach the brain faster than pain impulses, it can be used to alleviate pain in labour.

There are few contraindications to the use of massage in pregnancy, although lower abdominal and sacral massage should be avoided during the first trimester. No research has been undertaken that proves that massage at this time can actually cause miscarriage, but neither is it disproved.

Massage should not be applied directly to varicosed areas to avoid the risk of dislodging clots into the bloodstream, but can be substituted by simple stroking down the legs.

Massage has a warming effect as a result of circulatory stimulation so it should not be used in cases of pyrexia, but it is an excellent (and cost-effective) method of lowering the blood pressure. This effect can also be put to good use in reducing oedematous legs, especially in the puerperium.

Massage of the neonate has become increasingly popular and has been found to be of particular benefit for preterm babies (Adamson-Macedo and Attree, 1994; Isherwood, 1994; Acolet *et al.*, 1993; Roiste and Bushnell, 1993; Kuhn *et al.*, 1991; Harrison *et al.*, 1990).

AROMATHERAPY

Aromatherapy involves the use of highly concentrated essential oils distilled from plants, whose chemical constituents produce a variety of therapeutic properties. Essential oils may be used in massage, in the bath or for inhalation, but must never be taken internally, nor, with very few exceptions, should they be applied to the skin undiluted. The essential oils should be treated with the respect given to drugs, and indeed it is possible to overdose someone by using too high a concentration. For example, some essential oils will raise or lower the blood pressure, some may initiate epileptic fits, others potentiate the effects of alcohol or should be avoided when driving. There are many oils which should not be used in pregnancy, either because they may be teratogenic, emmenagogic (i.e. they induce uterine bleeding) or may have an undesirable systemic effect, such as hypertension.

Contraindicated essential oils include lavender, marjoram, rosemary, sage, jasmine, camomile. The safest and most versatile oils are the citrus ones – mandarin, lemon, grapefruit, lime, bergamot and neroli. On no account should midwives attempt to use essential oils in their practice unless they have been trained to do so (see Tiran, 1996, for a more comprehensive discussion on the safety of essential oils in pregnancy).

Essential oils should be diluted in a base oil such as sweet almond or grapeseed, usually to a maximum dose in pregnancy of 2%, i.e. two drops of essential oil to 5 ml of base oil. This is suitable for massage or baths, although a 4% mix can be used in the bath.

REFLEXOLOGY

Reflexology, or reflex zone therapy, works on the principle that the feet are a map of the rest of the body and that, by performing a sophisticated massage and manipulation of the feet, other parts of the body can be treated. However, it is a skill underpinned by a thorough knowledge of anatomy, physiology, health and disease and should not be used by unqualified personnel. It is possible to do more damage than good either by overdosing the recipient or by using incorrect techniques to achieve the desired results.

Reflexology is *not* simply foot massage. It is important to point out that vigorous massage of the heel should be avoided throughout pregnancy, as the reflex zone for the pelvic area is in the heels and the pregnancy could potentially be disrupted by such massage.

Reflex zones are also found on the hands but as they are less sensitive than the feet it is more usual to work on the latter.

OSTEOPATHY AND CHIROPRACTIC

Osteopathy and chiropractic are related therapies in which manipulation of the musculoskeletal system can affect the rest of the body by realignment of the spine and its appendages. It is especially useful for spinal conditions but may be beneficial for other problems. For example, menstrual problems of pituitary aetiology may be relieved by correction of the position of the cervical vertebrae. The British School of Osteopathy runs an Expectant Mothers' clinic to which women can refer themselves or be referred by their midwife or doctor (see Useful Addresses). Osteopathy is generally a gentler technique, relying on massage to relax muscles before commencing manipulative work; chiropractic is more specific and uses X-rays as a means of diagnosis.

Cranial osteopaths work only on the head by finely manipulating the skull bones to alleviate symptoms. Some cranial osteopaths advocate their therapy for babies delivered by forceps to relieve pressure on the brain from the forceps blades (Bullen, 1989) or for neonatal colic (Searle, 1988) and research is ongoing into its use for hyperactive children.

The Osteopathy Act of 1993 and a similar Act for chiropractic in 1994 have enabled the therapies to become part of mainstream medicine.

ACUPUNCTURE AND SHIATSU

Acupuncture is an ancient Chinese technique based on the belief that one's life force flows round the body along energy lines called meridians which link major organs and that the flow is uninterrupted when one is in good health. An imbalance of the energy flow will cause symptoms to appear. Introducing needles, applying heat or electromagnetism at certain points along the meridians will rebalance the energy and improve the condition. A similar principle is used in *Shiatsu* (originally a Japanese therapy but now virtually indistinguishable from acupressure) in which finger and thumb pressure is appied to the points on the meridians to improve the flow of energy. *Auricular acupuncture* is a variation of acupuncture, in which the ear, which has a complete set of acupuncture points, is used to restore the balance of energy within the body. Many people worry that acupuncture is painful but the needles are so fine that this is not so. There has also been concern about the transmission of HIV via the needles, but many practitioners use disposable needles while others autoclave them.

HOMEOPATHY

In homeopathy, minute doses of various substances are used which, if given in much larger doses, would actually cause the symptom they are intended to treat. Homeopaths need to discover the client's personality and the precise nature of the symptoms in order to select the correct remedy. For example, if a woman complained of insomnia, characterized by headaches, irritability, being jittery and needing to urinate frequently, the most appropriate homeopathic remedy would be coffea, derived from coffee – an excess of which would produce exactly the same symptom picture. Although many remedies are available in health stores, it is advisable to seek professional help. It is often thought that no harm can be done by taking the wrong remedy but this may not be so. Many homeopaths are also medically qualified and it is one of the few therapies which is already available on the National Health Service, there being five homeopathic hospitals in the UK.

If a woman decides to treat herself with homeopathy it is important to know how to administer the remedies correctly. The mouth should be clean from all food, drink, tobacco and toothpaste for an hour before administration and tablets should be placed directly in the mouth, avoiding overhandling. The remedies should be stored away from any strong smelling substances (including essential oils) and with some of the remedies, other odorous substances such as peppermint toothpaste and coffee should be avoided for the duration of the treatment. Proof that homeopathy works has been documented in the *British Medical Journal* (Kleijnen *et al.*, 1991) and its use in veterinary work disproves the theory that belief in the therapy will make it work (Richards-Williams, 1991).

Midwives and doctors may be concerned about possible interaction with prescribed pharmaceutical preparations but the dose of homeopathic remedies is negligible and will not affect other drugs. It is far more likely that the drugs will interfere with the homeopathic treatment and, in particular, steroids and strong antibiotics may antidote them (Castro, 1992).

A branch of homepathy involves the use of *Bach*

flower remedies which are used to treat emotional disorders rather than physical complaints, and includes Rescue Remedy, a combination of five of the flower remedies, which is excellent for stress.

HERBALISM

Herbalism (phytotherapy) makes use of the same or similar chemical constituents in plants as aromatherapy, although they are extracted and prepared in different ways. Due to the persecution of many people as witches in the Middle Ages much of the knowledge and most of the skills of herbalism were lost and its reputation declined and is only now being rediscovered. Many herbal remedies are available over the counter in health food stores but it is best to seek help from a qualified practitioner, especially during pregnancy. As with essential oils there are many herbs which should not be used in pregnancy, especially broom, Devil's claw and pennyroyal which are abortifacient.

However, plants produce no side-effects when used in the context of the whole plant, unlike modern drugs in which the therapeutic substances have been isolated or synthetically produced.

HYPNOTHERAPY

Hypnosis is a means of altering a person's level of consciousness, inducing relaxation and enhancing concentration and awareness. It is useful for treating many stress-related problems as well as certain physical ailments and is particularly valuable as a method of pain relief in labour.

NUTRITIONAL MEDICINE

This is a relatively new therapy, often practised by qualified doctors. It relies on identifying vitamin and mineral deficiency, due to inadequate intake, absorption or utilization of nutrients from food, and which may result in a variety of symptoms and non-specific conditions. Along with suggestions for dietary adaptations, supplements of the deficient elements are prescribed.

The Use of Complementary Therapies During Pregnancy

Complementary therapies lend themselves admirably to helping women with the various physiological disorders of pregnancy, which midwives and medical practitioners are naturally averse to treating with drugs unless absolutely necessary. It is precisely because these discomforts are physiological that they are often called 'minor disorders', but for the women who suffer them they may be anything but minor. In order to provide optimum care for all expectant women it is useful to have additional tools at our disposal and it is with this objective that midwives can learn to utilize some of the therapies.

Vomiting

Sickness is perhaps one of the commonest and most distressing of the early effects of pregnancy, and conventional suggestions such as tea and dry toast on waking will be effective for only a small percentage of women. Nutritional therapists suggest that dairy produce exacerbates the condition and because prolonged vomiting may lead to vitamin B deficiency, supplements of vitamin B_6 50–100 mg once a day may help, accompanied by magnesium 200–500 mg daily (Davies and Stewart, 1987). Butler (1985) found that yoghurt may be of use in some cases.

Phytotherapeutic ginger capsules or ginger tea can be very effective (Roach, 1985; Stewart, 1987; McIntyre, 1988), as well as chewing on crystallized ginger. Lemon balm, red raspberry leaf, chamomile or lavender flowers and black horehound have also been found to be effective. Acupressure/shiatsu techniques may be of use and one popular, commercialized version is now available as bands worn on the wrist, which apply pressure to the appropriate point on the affected meridian. Indeed the use of acupuncture and acupressure has been well researched, not only in relation to pregnancy sickness but also for vomiting induced by chemotherapy (Dundee *et al.*, 1988; Hyde, 1989; Stannard, 1989; Barsoum *et al.*, 1990; Price *et al.*, 1991; Evans *et al.*, 1993; Belluomini *et al.*, 1994) (Figure 1).

A homeopath would need to determine the exact nature of the symptoms, but remedies which may be used include nux vomica or sepia (Castro, 1992). Treatment from a qualified reflex zone therapist may alleviate the symptoms and reduce anxiety, but should not be used for those women whose pregnancies are at risk (Wagner, 1987).

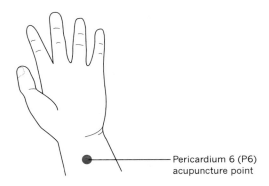

Pericardium 6 (P6)
acupuncture point

Figure 1   Acupressure point P6 for relief of nausea and vomiting. The point is 2–3 finger widths below the wrist crease on the inner aspect of the arm.

Heartburn

Heartburn responds well to phytotherapy in the form of garlic capsules to reduce the severity but clients should be careful when purchasing the capsules. The active ingredient is in the allicin and various sulphur-containing compounds which also give garlic its characteristic odour. This means that they are 'slow release' capsules, odour-free ones may be ineffective. Stapleton (1995) recommends various herbal remedies such as slippery elm, dandelion root, peppermint, chamomile and ginger.

Nutrition therapists would advise avoiding E additives in the range E200–E276 as well as eliminating milk products from the diet (contrary to popular belief) (Davies and Stewart, 1987).

A simple self-administered shiatsu remedy for heartburn involves finding the point four fingers above the umbilicus and pressing with two fingers intermittently for 10 seconds at a time for about 10 minutes (Figure 2).

As always, depending on the symptoms, homeopathic remedies may include capsicum, lycopodium or phosphorus.

Osteopathy is effective not only for direct musculoskeletal problems but can also be good for heartburn, for the principle of osteopathy is that all organs in the body are related to the spine and thus spinal manipulation will release tensions which either cause, or are an effect of heartburn (Conway, 1995).

Constipation

Nutrition therapists recommend that tea intake should be reduced as the tannin has been found to exacerbate

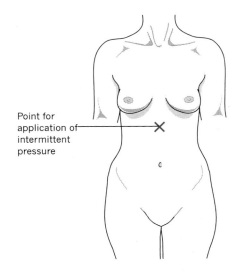

Point for application of intermittent pressure

Figure 2   Shiatsu remedy for heartburn. Intermittent pressure is applied at a point four fingers above the umbilicus.

constipation (Sharon, 1989), although Davies and Stewart (1987) state that it may cause either constipation or diarrhoea depending on the woman's constitution.

In phytotherapy artichoke capsules, or the vegetable itself, used in cooking, provides a high quality of fibre and acts as a non-purgative laxative.

Firm abdominal massage in a clockwise direction can stimulate peristalsis and promote movement of faecal matter towards the rectum. Essential oils such as mandarin or orange enhance the effects of the massage (Figure 3). Alternatively, clockwise massage of the arches of the feet will work on the reflex zones for the abdomen.

Shiatsu, possibly after abdominal massage, involves intermittent pressure for about 10 seconds being applied at the point midway between the symphysis pubis and the umbilicus over a period of about five minutes (Figure 4).

Varicosities

Essential oil of cypress with its astringent properties and geranium to balance the circulation can be added to the bath (in a carrier oil), as massage of varicosed areas of the legs is contraindicated. For anal varicosities Worwood (1990) suggests adding geranium oil to a proprietary lubricating gel and applying this, especially when there are protruding haemorrhoids.

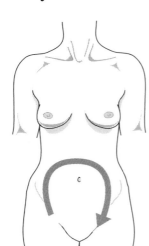

Figure 3 Constipation can be treated using abdominal massage in a clockwise direction.

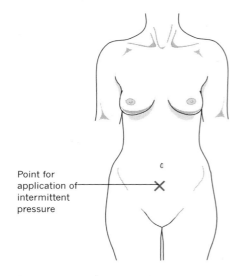

Point for application of intermittent pressure

Figure 4 Shiatsu technique for treatment of constipation. Intermittent pressure is applied at a point midway between the symphysis pubis and the umbilicus.

Once again garlic, either in capsule form or eaten in food, is noted for its beneficial effects on the circulatory system. Other herbal remedies such as golden seal, horse chestnut, lime blossom, and, externally, marigold may also be used.

A homeopathic dose of *Hamamelis virginica* may alleviate the discomfort of varicosities, and indeed, hamamelis water (witch hazel) can be applied directly to the varicosed area. In certain circumstances pulsatilla tablets may be used.

Oedema

Ankle and lower leg oedema responds well to bimanual massage, moving upwards from ankles to knee. The massage can be enhanced by adding one drop of lemon (detoxifying) and one drop of geranium (balancing) to 5 ml of base oil (Figure 5).

It is also possible for the mother to learn various yoga positions which will help to alleviate the discomfort of severe oedema. One of the most effective remedies for ankle oedema (and for early postnatal breast engorgement), is to apply dark green cabbage leaves over the affected area. Rhubarb or olive tree leaves work equally well (McIntyre, 1988). The leaves should be wiped clean, and either cooled in the refrigerator or ironed to warm them. They are then applied to the legs (or breasts) and replaced when wet, until relief is obtained. Community midwives in one health authority have used this method for breast engorgement for many years, and research is beginning to attempt to elicit why it should be so effective. It is thought that it may be related to the amount of chlorophyll in the leaves.

Backache

Many women will spontaneously massage their backs when aching, especially the sacral area, and midwives can suggest that a partner performs this as well. Firm pressure with the heel of the hand over the area of the

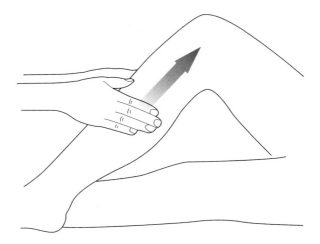

Figure 5 Direction of bimanual leg massage for the reduction of ankle oedema.

sacral alae is often the most effective, although massage using small circular movements may also be helpful. Certain essential oils can be used to alleviate backache in late pregnancy or during labour, but most of those traditionally used for muscular backaches, such as lavender and camomile, are contraindicated in early pregnancy.

It is possible to treat backache with reflex zone therapy, working on the inner edge of each foot on the zone related to the back, but it would not necessarily be the treatment of choice, as it may only relieve the symptoms rather than treat the cause.

Osteopathy and/or chiropractic are probably the most effective treatments for women with chronic backache. Many of these mothers continue to have problems in the early postnatal period as hormonal levels readjust, and the practitioner would be able to complete the course of treatment appropriately.

Treatment to the relevant acupuncture points will re-balance the meridians to relieve the backache. This can also be done with shiatsu (acupressure).

Headache

Headache in the first trimester of pregnancy is often a result of dilatation of the cerebral blood vessels under the influence of progesterone, and may be eased by a variety of massage techniques. Simple application of one drop of neat lavender essential oil to the temples can be effective on isolated occasions, but excess administration of lavender oil is inadvisable in early pregnancy. For a more diversified ache, firm scalp massage in a 'hairwashing' action can bring relief. This massage does not require the application of any oils and can be done by the woman herself or by a partner. Pressure of two fingers directly under the occiput will rebalance the meridians as there is an acupressure point there. Firm massage of the big toes, particularly if they feel painful to touch, will act on the reflex zone for the head and may be effective. More chronic headache for which no pathological cause has been found will benefit from osteopathy. Alternatively the postural realignment of the Alexander technique may be of help.

Nutrition therapists suggest the elimination of stimulants such as tea, coffee, cola and chocolate from the diet as well as avoiding the food additives in the E200–E274 range.

Insomnia

Many women have difficulty sleeping, especially in later pregnancy, and in addition to advice about positioning they may find a cup of camomile tea of use, or alternatively a few drops of camomile and lavender essential oil (in a base oil) in the bath water. Phytotherapists advocate taking valerian capsules or the use of a herb or hop-filled pillow on which to rest the head.

Midwives can remind mothers about relaxation exercises, or a hypnotherapist may provide an audiocassette for more chronic problems with sleeplessness. A variety of homeopathic remedies is also available but the relevant remedy needs to be selected according to the precise nature of the complaint.

Labile emotional state

The many mood swings through which expectant mothers pass as a result of hormonal fluctuations can be alarming to the whole family. Using a room spray to which have been added the essential oils of orange, lavender, rose, geranium, in any combination, will not only help the mother but also ease the atmosphere for the rest of the family.

For those women who are anxious about their impending labours and the advent of parenthood, several stress-relieving remedies may be used. A visit to a reflexologist, or aromatherapist may restore the woman's sense of self-esteem and confidence in herself. She may wish to attend yoga classes which will produce the additional benefit of relieving some of the physical discomforts of pregnancy as well as being relaxing. For any woman who suffers panic attacks a few drops of the Bach flower remedy Rescue Remedy can be helpful. This is also a valuable substance for the woman to have in the labour room for episodes of panic and for transition from first to second stage. As this is a homeopathic remedy, the dose of active ingredients is negligible so can do no harm to the mother or fetus. It is, however, preserved in brandy and this needs to be explained to the mother in case she objects to alcohol. The mother can take Rescue Remedy orally, either neat direct onto the tongue (four to five drops) or the same amount in a small glass of water to sip at intervals.

Several more serious complications can be helped by the use of complementary therapies, even if only as an adjunct to conventional care. For example the de-stressing and relaxing effects of massage, with or without essential oils, or of reflex zone therapy, could assist in reducing hypertension, or calming mothers awaiting procedures such as chorionic villus biopsy or prior to Caesarean section. Candidal infections respond well to acidophilus, and proprietary pessaries containing the active ingredients from the Australian ti tree are now available.

Persistent breech presentation after 34 weeks' gestation can be corrected in almost 80% of cases using an acupuncture technique called moxibustion. This involves the application of a moxa stick containing the herb mugwort to the B67 acupuncture point at the base of the little toenails, twice daily for five days (Budd, 1992).

The Use of Complementary Therapies During Labour

ONSET OF LABOUR

Labour may be induced (with medical permission) or accelerated, using a variety of complementary methods. Many midwives have long advocated sexual activity as an aid to ripening the cervix, in the belief that prostaglandins in semen, local cervical stimulation and uterine contraction from orgasm will initiate labour. Nipple stimulation can also be used, both as a way of cervical ripening from about the 37th week (although only one breast should be massaged at a time to avoid overstimulation) and to increase the length, strength and frequency of contractions in labour. This obviously increases pituitary output of oxytocin and can be very useful during the transition phase at the end of the first stage of labour, when contractions may slow down, or if there is delay in separation of the placenta during the third stage.

Phytotherapists recommend taking raspberry leaf in the form of a tea or tablets. This has a toning effect on the uterus and can be drunk from mid-pregnancy to prepare for labour, as well as during labour to assist with contractions, and postnatally to aid involution of the uterus.

Homeopaths also have many remedies at their disposal, but as with any other situation the remedy must be appropriate for the individual. For example caulophyllum (blue cohosh) which stimulates uterine muscle, can be useful if the cervix is slow to dilate, contractions are weak or the mother is exhausted. Care should be taken with this remedy however for if it is inappropriately administered it may be so powerful that labour is short and violent, or it may work in reverse and, instead of accelerating labour, it could cause it to become protracted (Castro, 1992).

Aromatherapists may choose to massage the suprapubic and sacral areas with a blend of jasmine and lavender for a few days before labour as this will aid in strengthening the uterus, and its use can be continued into labour. Stimulation (by either acupuncture or acupressure) of the B67 point at the base of the little toenail can, in addition to turning a breech presentation to cephalic, enhance and co-ordinate uterine action during labour.

PAIN AND DISCOMFORT IN LABOUR

The relief of pain and discomfort in labour is one of the main areas of midwifery in which alternative treatments can truly act as a complement to any other conventional care, and is also the time when midwives may feel deficient in what they have to offer women. The range of analgesia is limited in conventional terms, and many women find them ineffective or unpleasant.

Mothers may wish to be accompanied in labour by a professional therapist and midwifery management and medical attendants should facilitate this. It may require a change in attitude for many doctors and midwives to accept that a different professional can be of help. Our aim in caring for childbearing women should be to relinquish control, and to provide choices and optimum care for each individual woman. Those midwives who feel unable to cope with a situation in which there is a complementary therapist in attendance should defer to another midwife to care for that mother. However it is also encumbent upon us to increase our awareness and understanding of the various therapies in order to provide good quality care.

Appropriately trained midwives may use essential oils of clary sage, lavender and jasmine, which not only strengthen the uterus but also alleviate pain, discomfort and anxiety. These can be massaged into the abdomen, put into a warm bath or used as a room spray, although the concentration of jasmine should not be too high as some women find its strong aroma rather cloying. Other oils which can be useful in relaxing both mother and father (and carers!) include rose, orange and geranium and the oils selected should depend on the mother's preference (Reed and Norfolk, 1993; Burns and Blamey, 1994). Simple massage of the abdomen without essential oils can also be effective in reducing the mother's perception of pain.

Reflex zone therapy is relaxing and will increase uterine efficiency (Feder *et al.*, 1993). Alternatively, either the midwife or the father could perform simple foot massage without reflexology which will redirect the mother's attention away from her contractions. It will also warm the mother's feet, for many women in labour literally have cold feet, and if done by the father, will make him feel useful.

Hypnotherapy can be taught to the mother during pregnancy and self-induced during labour, or she may choose to have her hypnotherapist with her. Trials have shown that hypnotherapy can be particularly valuable in labour without the danger of side-effects (Gartside, 1982; Guthrie *et al.*, 1984; Brann and Guzvica, 1987; Woods, 1989; Jenkins and Pritchard, 1993).

Acupuncture has also been well-documented for its use in labour in Western cultures although it is interesting to note that it is not used in China as a means of relieving pain in labour because contractions produce physiological rather than pathological discomfort (Budd, 1992; Skelton and Flowerdew, 1985, 1986; Meiyu, 1985; Ledergerber, 1976).

A simple shiatsu technique to ease the pain of labour contractions, or of dysmenorrhoea, can be performed by midwives or taught to partners, and is as follows: standing or kneeling behind the mother, the thumbs are pressed into the 'dimples' visible on either side of the spine, starting at the coccyx and working up intermittently to the lumbo-sacral area (i.e. from the coccyx to the waist). This should be done with a rocking motion with the fingers resting over the areas of the sacroiliac joints and performed throughout each contraction (for dysmenorrhoea the procedure is carried out for about 5–10 minutes until relief is obtained and repeated as necessary) (Figure 6).

Again, there are many homeopathic remedies which can be of use, but because of the changing nature of the process of parturition it is vital to have knowledge and experience of using them.

As mentioned previously the Bach flower remedy Rescue Remedy is excellent for relieving panic, anxiety and hysteria and lends itself very well to use in labour, particularly during transition from the first to second stage. Many mothers have their own bottle but midwives may wish to consider stocking it for professional use. Although it is used by some midwives further trials need to be carried out and published in accepted journals to promote more widespread use.

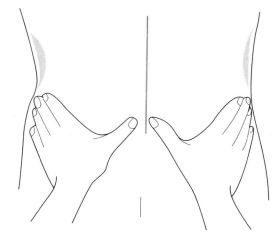

Figure 6   Shiatsu technique for relief of pain in labour.

There are many herbal substances which can be suitable for women in labour, including squaw vine and birth root, but qualified assistance is required to select the most appropriate one. However the ubiquitous raspberry leaf tea is safe and can be drunk throughout labour, either hot or iced to strengthen contractions and relieve the intensity of pain.

Other natural means of relieving pain and discomfort in labour include the use of warm water for bathing during the first stage (some mothers wish to remain in the water for the delivery) (Garland, 1995) and a range of relaxation techniques including visualization, meditation, music, yoga postures and breathing exercises. The midwife should consider the whole range at her disposal in order to offer a comprehensive choice to women. However, at present it is unlikely that any one midwife or maternity service will be able to provide the entire selection as many depend on having appropriately trained practitioners within the area.

It would be preferable for each maternity services manager to identify the skills and knowledge available amongst the staff and to build on them in order to expand the facilities for the local clientele, focusing on a limited number of therapies. The unit to which this author is attached maintains a register of those midwives qualified in massage, aromatherapy and reflex zone therapy/reflexology and, within the restrictions laid down in the unit policy, allows those midwives to apply their skills to their normal midwifery practice. In this way, managers/supervisors are aware of which midwives can practise alternative therapies, and the service can be offered to mothers as there are enough midwives using each of the therapies for one of them to be available most of the time.

There are other situations which occur during labour that can be adequately treated with various complementary therapies. Where there is *mild cephalopelvic disproportion*, reflex zone therapy can be effective in enlarging the pelvic outlet by working on the part of the feet relating to the sacroiliac joints and the symphysis pubis. This may have the effect of loosening the pelvic joints sufficiently to facilitate a normal rather than a forceps delivery, or perhaps a forceps rather than a Caesarean delivery.

Reflex zone therapy can also be used to separate a *retained placenta*, saving time and money by avoiding the need for removal of placenta under anaesthetic. (This is effective in cases where the placenta has not yet separated, by stimulating uterine contraction, but will not deal with a morbidly adherent placenta.) Acupuncture can also be effective in promoting placental separation (Skelton and Flowerdew, 1986) as can homeopathic remedies such as pulsatilla (Holt, 1988), while phytotherapists might use myrrh, feverfew or raspberry leaf. Nipple stimulation can be advised and discreetly practised to increase the pituitary output of oxytocin, or of course the baby could be put to the breast. Jasmine essential oil has been found to be of use when massaged into the abdomen, and could be combined with massage over the area of the fundus to stimulate the uterus to contract (Davis, 1988).

The Use of Complementary Therapies in the Postnatal Period

Much of our care in the puerperium revolves around helping the mother to return to her non-pregnant state both physically and mentally, as well as facilitating the establishment of a suitable feeding method for the baby. Complementary therapies have much to offer the mother at this time, especially for enhancing her confidence and self-esteem.

Postnatal depression

Those women who are susceptible to postnatal depression, either because of a previous personal or a family history, may benefit from the use of essential oils of jasmine, with its anti-depressant properties, and rose, which has a particular affinity for the reproductive tract and can help to cleanse, tone and purify the

uterus. Both of these oils are extremely expensive but only a few drops would be used and the effects are profound in some cases. The oils could be massaged into the back, abdomen and legs, added to bath water or sprayed around the room.

Agnus-castus or squaw vine may be advocated by herbalists for depression, and cups of camomile tea will calm the mother, help her to sleep and also act as a diuretic to cleanse the urinary tract (McIntyre, 1988).

The elimination of all sugars from the diet will enable the hormones to rebalance themselves and nutrition therapists also suggest taking supplements of vitamin B_6 and zinc (Davies and Stewart, 1987).

Inadequate lactation

Where the mother has poor lactation, reflex zone therapy can be of enormous help. The part of the foot which, in reflex zone therapy, relates to the breast is an area on the dorsum situated above the point where the toes join the foot. If this principle is related to the hand, the place in which an intravenous cannula may be sited lies directly over the zone for the breast, and the theory that women who receive intravenous fluids in labour may have impaired lactation would certainly be worth investigating. This then is the area which midwives could massage firmly on the hands and the feet in order to increase lactation. The mother could also be shown how to perform this for herself (Figure 7).

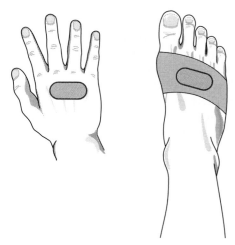

Figure 7   Reflex zones to breasts on dorsum of foot and back of hand. These areas can be massaged to stimulate lactation.

Fennel and dill teas have been found to aid lactation and are now available as proprietary teas, although they can be high in sugar content.

Breast engorgement

Early breast engorgement responds well to the application of either dark green cabbage or rhubarb leaves. The cabbage leaves are wiped clean and cooled in the refrigerator, then applied to the engorged breasts. Within minutes the leaves become soaking wet, after which time they are replaced with dry ones. This process is repeated until relief is obtained. The technique may also be of use when mothers wish to suppress lactation, and research by Shrivastav *et al.* (1988) demonstrated that jasmine flowers are also effective for this purpose. Homeopaths may recommend belladonna, particularly where the breasts have red streaks on them, or bryonia in cases where the discomfort is greater with movement. However Castro (1992) advises that arnica tablets should be discontinued while the remedy for engorgement is used.

Nipple soreness may respond to Bach Rescue Remedy cream, calendula or camomile creams (now used in a proprietary form in many units) or phytolacca tincture.

Perineal problems

One of the commonest discomforts in the early postnatal period is that of the perineum while healing from lacerations, bruising or episiotomy. Dale and Cornwell's trial (1994) found that using lavender essential oil in the bath water did not significantly accelerate healing of the perineum, as anticipated. However, it was found to ease discomfort and relax the mothers, particularly between the third and fifth postnatal days.

If there is bruising of the buttocks and surrounding area, arnica homeopathic tables can be taken or arnica cream applied direct (although this should not be used on open wounds). Arnica is one of the few homeopathic remedies which can be universally used in cases of trauma, shock or bruising. Other homeopathic remedies suitable for perineal discomfort include hypericum, bellis perennis or nux vomica, but as with all other situations it is important to find the correct remedy for the individual. Phytotherapeutic marigold tincture may also be of use.

Various complementary strategies can also be utilized for other postnatal problems. For example, *retention of urine* in the early puerperium can be relieved with reflex zone therapy. This is useful also for easing the *stiff neck* and *headache* which occasionally follow epidural anaesthesia.

The Future of Complementary Therapies in Pregnancy and Childbirth

The future for the use of complementary medicine in Britain appears promising if rather uncertain. Many more changes in legislation and regulation are on the horizon for the various therapies available. Pressure from consumers who express a general dissatisfaction with conventional medical care may force the government to reconsider the position of 'alternative' therapies, and to accept some of them as deserving of equal status alongside orthodox methods. Tighter regulation of the different therapies with standardization of training and practice requirements should prove beneficial to clients by eliminating underqualified therapists, and to practitioners by enhancing their public image. The move towards the use of the National Vocational Qualifications should assist in this process.

Within maternity care, complementary therapies can be extremely valuable in alleviating many of the physiological disorders of the childbearing period, and can be incorporated into midwifery practice relatively easily. The suggestion that all student midwives should receive an introduction to the subject during their initial education programmes, and proposals for the development of a new complementary therapy speciality within the midwifery profession, have been made (Tiran, 1995b).

The explosion of interest amongst doctors, midwives and nurses will stimulate research projects which will give further credibility to the practice of alternative therapies. Only in this way can there be any hope of those therapies which are currently 'alternative' becoming truly 'complementary' to the care on offer.

References

Acolet, D., Modi, N. Giannakoulopoulos, X. *et al.* (1993) Changes in plasma cortisol and catecholamine concentrations in responses to massage in preterm infants. *Arch. Dis. Childh.* **68**(1): 29–31.

Adamson-Macedo, E.N. & Attree, J.L.A. (1994) TIC TAC therapy: the importance of systematic stroking. *Br. J. Midwifery* **2**(6): 264–269.

Barsoum, G., Perry, E.P. & Fraser, I.A. (1990) Postoperative nausea is relieved by acupressure. *J. R. Soc. Med.* **83**(2): 86–89.

Belluomini, J., Litt, R.C., Lee, K.A. *et al.* (1994) Acupressure for nausea and vomiting of pregnancy: a randomized, blinded study. *Obstet. Gynaecol.* **84**(2): 245–248.

BMA (British Medical Association) (1993) *Complementary Medicine – New Approaches to Good Practice.* Oxford: Oxford University Press.

Brann, L.R. & Guzvica, S.A. (1987) Comparison of hypnosis with conventional relaxation for antenatal and intrapartum use: a feasibility study in general practice. *J. R. Coll. Gen. Pract.* **37**(303): 437–440.

Budd, S. (1992) Traditional Chinese medicine in obstetrics. *Midwives' Chronicle* **105**(June): 140–143.

Bullen, J. (1989) Cranial osteopathy: an experience *Cry-sis* **12**(Spring): 4.

Burns, E. & Blamey, C. (1994) Using aromatherapy in childbirth. *Nursing Times* **9**(9): 54–60.

Butler, K. (1985) Nausea in pregnancy. *Women Wise* **8**(1): 3–4.

Castro, M. (1992) *Homeopathy for Mother and Baby.* London: Macmillan.

Conway, P. (1995) Osteopathy during pregnancy. In Tiran, D. & Mack, S. (eds) *Complementary therapies for pregnancy and childbirth.* London: Baillière Tindall.

Cresswell, J. (1993) Handle with care. *Nursing Times* **89**(1): 18–19.

Dale, A. & Cornwell, S. (1994) The role of lavender oil in relieving perineal discomfort following childbirth: a blind randomised clinical trial. *J. Adv. Nursing* **19**(1): 89–96.

Davies, S. & Stewart, A. (1987) *Nutritional Medicine.* London: Pan.

Davis, P. (1988) *Aromatherapy An A–Z.* London: C. W. Daniel.

DOH (Department of Health) (1993) *Changing Childbirth.* Report of the Expert Maternity Group. London: HMSO.

Dundee, J. W., Sourial, F.B.R. & Ghaly R.G. (1988) P6 acupuncture reduces morning sickness. *J. R. Soc. Med.* **81**(8): 456–457.

Evans, A.T., Samuels, S.N., Marshall, C. *et al.* (1993) Suppression of pregnancy-induced nausea and vomiting with sensory afferent stimulation. *J. Reprod. Med.* **38**(8): 603–606.

Feder, E., Liisberg, G.B., Lenstrup, C. *et al.* (1993) Zone therapy in relation to birth. In *Midwives: hear the heartbeat of the future. Proceedings of the International Confederation of Midwives 23rd International Congress*, Vol. 2, pp. 651–656. International Confederation of Midwives.

Garland, D. (1995) The uses of hydrotherapy in today's

midwifery practice. In Tiran, D. & Mack, S. (eds) *Complementary Therapies for Pregnancy and Childbearing.* London: Baillière Tindall.

Gartside, G. (1982) Easy labour – personal experience of childbirth under hypnosis. *Nursing Times* **51**(78): 2187.

Guthrie, K., Taylor, D.J. & DeFriend, D. (1984) Maternal hypnosis induced by husbands during childbirth. *J. Obstet. Gynaecol.* **4**(5): 93–95.

Harrison, L.L., Leeper, J.D., Yoon, M. (1990) Effects of early parent touch on preterm infants' heart rates and arterial oxygen saturation levels. *J. Adv. Nursing* **15**(8): 877–885.

Holt, M. (1988) Homeopathy in childbearing. *Midwives' Chronicle* **1206**(101): 225–226.

Hyde, E. (1989) Acupressure therapy for morning sickness – a controlled clinical trial. *J. Nurse-Midwifery* **43**(4): 171–178.

Isherwood, D. (1994) Baby massage groups. *Modern Midwife* **4**(2): 21–23.

Jenkins, M.W. & Pritchard, M. (1993) Practical applications and theoretical considerations of hypnosis in normal labour. *Br. J. Obstet. Gynaecol.* **100**: 221–226.

Kleijnen, J. Knipschild, P. and Gerben, T.R. (1991) Clinical trials of homeopathy. *Br. Med. J.* **302**: 316–321.

Kuhn, C.M., Schanberg, S.M., Field, T. *et al.* (1991) Tactile-kinesthetic stimulation effects on sympathetic and adrenocorticol function in preterm infants. *J. Pediat.* **119**(3): 434–440.

Ledergerber, C. (1976) Electroacupuncture in Obstetrics. *Acupuncture Electrother. Res. Int. J.* **2**: 105–118.

McIntyre, A. (1988) *Herbs for Pregnancy and Childbirth.* London: Sheldon.

Meiyu, C. (1985) Acupuncture anaesthesia for Caesarian section. *Midwives' Chronicle* **1168**(98): 107.

NAHAT (1993) *Complementary therapies in the NHS.* London: National Association of Health Authorities and Trusts.

Price, H., Lewith, G. & Williams, C. (1991) Acupressure as an anti-emetic in cancer chemotherapy. *Complementary Med. Res.* **5**(2): 93–94.

Reed, L. & Norfolk, L. (1993) Aromatherapy in midwifery. *Aromatherapy World* **10**: 12–15.

Richards-Williams, J. (1991) It works for animals too. *Here's Health* April: 51.

Roach, B. (1985) Ginger root (*Zingibar officinale*). *California Assoc. Midwives Newsl.* **1**: 2.

Roiste, A.D. & Bushnell, I.W.R. (1993) Tactile stimulation and preterm infant performance on an instrumental conditioning task. *J. Reprod. Infant Psychol.* **11**(3): 155–163.

Searle, L. (1988) A case of colic? *New Generation* **1**(7): 35.

Sharon, M. (1989) *Optimum Nutrition.* London: Prion.

Shrivastav, P., George, K. Balasubramaniam, N. *et al.* (1988) Suppression of puerperal lactation using jasmine flowers. *Aust. NZ J. Obstet. Gynaecol.* **1**(28): 68–71.

Skelton, I. & Flowerdew, M. (1985) Midwifery and acupuncture. *Midwives' Chronicle* **1168**(98): 125–129.

Skelton, I. & Flowerdew, M. (1986) Is there a place for

acupuncture on labour wards? *Midwife, Health Visitor and Community Nurse* 12(22): 423–426.

Stannard, D. (1989) Pressure prevents nausea. *Nursing Times* 4(85): 33–34.

Stapleton, H. (1995) Women as herbalists and midwives. In Tiran, D. & Mack, S. (eds) *Complementary Therapies for Pregnancy and Childbirth*. London: Baillière Tindall.

Stewart, N. (1987) New ways to beat sickness. *Mother* May.

Tiran, D. (1994) Complementary therapies and midwifery practice. *Modern Midwife* 4(9): 8–10.

Tiran, D. (1995a) Introduction. In Tiran, D. & Mack, S. (eds) *Complementary Therapies for Pregnancy and Childbirth*. London: Baillière Tindall.

Tiran, D. (1995b) Complementary therapies education in midwifery. *Complementary Ther. Nursing Midwifery* 1(2): 41–43.

Tiran, D. (1996) *Aromatherapy in Midwifery Practice*. London: Baillière Tindall.

UKCC (United Kingdom Central Council) (1992) *Scope of Professional Practice*, London, UKCC.

UKCC (1993) *Midwives Rules* 40(2), London, UKCC.

UKCC (1994) *The Midwife's Code of Practice*, London, UKCC.

Wagner, F. (1987) *Reflex Zone Massage*. London: Thorsons.

Woods, M. (1989) Pain control and hypnosis. *Nursing Times* 7(85): 38–40.

Worwood, V. (1990) *The Fragrant Pharmacy*. London: Bantam.

Yelland, S. (1995) Using acupuncture in midwifery care. *Modern Midwife* 5(1): 8–11.

Further Reading

Trevelyan, J. & Booth, B. (1995) *Complementary Medicine for Nurses, Midwives and Health Visitors*. London: Churchill Livingstone.

Wells, R. with Tschudin, V. (1995) *Wells' Supportive Therapies in Health Care*. London: Baillière Tindall.

Useful Addresses

British Complementary Medicine Association Harold Gillies Ward, St Charles' Hospital, Exmoor Street, London W10 Tel. 0181 964 1205

An organization which acts as a resource on all matters related to complementary therapies, the BCMA is also attempting to set up registers of practitioners of their member organizations and to press for greater recognition of the therapies within mainstream healthcare.

British Homeopathic Association 27a Devonshire Street, London W1N 1RJ Tel. 0171 935 2163

Maintains registers of homeopathic doctors, dentists and veterinary surgeons.

British School of Osteopathy 1–4 Suffolk Street, London SW1Y 4HG Tel. 0171 930 9254/8

Offers four-year course in osteopathy. Runs an expectant mothers' clinic at which students under the supervision of senior tutors provide appropriate treatment for women during pregnancy. Women may refer themselves or be referred by their midwife or doctor.

British School of Reflex Zone Therapy Department of Continuing Education, Royal Masonic Hospital, London W6 0TN Tel. 0181 846 8066

Offers courses only to those who are already registered in some form of medically related profession, e.g. doctors, nurses, midwives, health visitors, physiotherapists, osteopaths, chiropodists. Maintains register of those who have completed the School's full training course.

Institute for Complementary Medicine PO Box 194, London SE16 1QZ Tel. 0171 237 5165

A resource centre on issues related to all complementary therapies, the ICM also has a regiser of complementary practitioners and is working towards the development of a college of complementary medicine offering courses at certificate, diploma and degree level.

International Federation of Aromatherapists Department of Continuing Education, Royal Masonic Hospital, London W6 0TN Tel. 0181 846 8066

The IFA maintains a register of members who have successfully completed their examinations; as well as training centres for the IFA courses.

National Institute of Medical Herbalists Department H, 9 Palace Gate, Exeter EX1 1JA Tel. 01392 426022

Maintains register of practitioners and lists of

phytotherapy courses. Members use MNIMH or FNIMH after their name.

Research Council for Complementary Medicine
60 Great Ormond Street, London WC1N 3JF Tel. 0171 833 8897

Centre with access to several international databases; staff will discuss, over the telephone, the requirements of the enquirer and conduct literature searches for a moderate fee; off-prints of articles can be purchased following the literature search.

Part Seven

Education in Preparation for Childbirth and Parenthood

23

Health Promotion and Education

Health is a state of being to which most people aspire. Yet it is difficult to define what is understood by the term, as it can be interpreted differently by individuals and communities depending on their surroundings and circumstances. In 1946, the World Health Organization described health as 'a state of complete physical, mental and social well-being and not merely the absence of disease or infirmity' (Aggleton, 1990). Health is thus seen as an ideal state of being which may be impossible to achieve. A sociological definition of health from a functionalist perspective could be 'the state of optimum capacity of an individual for the effective performance of the roles and tasks for which he has been socialized' as defined by Talcott Parsons in 1951 (Morgan *et al.*, 1985). This definition emphasizes the functional importance of health for society rather than for the individual. A more modern view of health could

be that it is a commodity which can be supplied by others (Seedhouse, 1986). Health has become a growing business in the marketplace with the increase in private health and purchaser/provider contracts.

In the UK in the 1990s the emphasis tends to be on personal prevention and responsibility for health (DOH, 1991), though it must be recognized that social and environmental factors are important influences which also need to be addressed. People are becoming more aware of their own contribution to physical health as evidenced by the growth in numbers of leisure centres and health clubs. There seems to be also an increased awareness of psychological health needs, if we consider how the numbers of counsellors, self-help and support groups have increased over the last decade or so. The humanist approach to health recognizes that there is a latent ability for self-development in all human beings who have the actual or potential ability to understand the implications of their actions; there are interconnections between the physical, the spiritual and the intellectual (Seedhouse, 1986).

The lifestyle behaviours and personal habits of individuals are major contributors to health and illness. A person's attitudes and beliefs affect his or her behaviour and can influence health as a result. This means therefore, that with regard to health education, health professionals must take account of individual differences in attitudes and beliefs and try to effect change in those which are unhealthy. They need also to be aware of their own health-related behaviour and their potential influence as role models.

Health Models

Over the last decade or so health psychology has developed as a new discipline. Health models have been developed by psychologists in this field which try to explain why some individuals indulge in healthy behaviour and others do not. Some of the most well-known models will be briefly examined in the following paragraphs.

The Health Belief Model

The Health Belief Model, originally formulated by Rosenstock in the 1960s and further developed by Becker in the 1970s (Becker *et al.*, 1977), was developed specifically to explain and predict preventive health behaviours (Rosenstock, 1974). Readiness to take action and engage in health-related behaviour depends on a number of factors according to this model. These are the individual's perception of:

1 susceptibility to the illness;
2 seriousness of the illness;
3 potential benefits of taking action to prevent or reduce the threat of illness; and
4 the potential barriers or negative consequences of taking that action (e.g. inconvenience, financial cost, etc.).

The first two components combined mobilize the person to act and the preferred course of action is determined by the person's assessment of perceived benefits minus negative consequences. Other factors, in addition to beliefs which influence health behaviour, are cues to action and client motivation. An individual

may have a high degree of perceived susceptibility, perceived severity and perceived benefits of action and still not engage in health behaviour. Cues to action may be required. These may be internal (e.g. the perception of symptoms), or external (e.g. health education message). As regards client motivation, the person who values their health will engage in health activity more readily than the person who does not. Some may put recreation or work, etc. before health, whilst others with low self-esteem may not view their health status as of any importance to themselves or others (Dummer Clark, 1984).

The Health Belief Model has been used in studies of the uptake of numerous health-promoting behaviours, such as stopping smoking, reducing alcohol consumption and diet alterations. The strongest predictors of preventive health behaviours are perceived barriers to the behaviour and perceived susceptibility to the illness in question (Marteau, 1989a).

In utilizing the Health Belief Model, the midwife must first identify the individual's beliefs and their influence on behaviour, as well as the presence of any cues to action and any motivational factors which may influence behaviour. She should reinforce positive attitudes to health and counter myths and negative attitudes (e.g. it is better to smoke during pregnancy as the delivery of a smaller baby will be easier). When behaviours conducive to ill-health are found to be the result of erroneous or unrealistic beliefs, cues or motivators, the midwife intervenes to change these factors and thereby change unhealthy behaviour (e.g. as regards smoking in pregnancy, she explains that it causes reduced blood supply to the fetus which affects other aspects besides growth etc.).

Health Locus of Control

Locus of control was proposed by Rotter (1966) as a concept of his social learning theory put forward in 1954. It refers to the amount of personal control over events that people believe they possess. Individuals who believe that they have personal control are said to have an *internal locus of control*, whereas those who believe that events are under the control of external forces, such as other people, luck, or fate, are said to have an *external locus of control*. These beliefs are thought to develop from specific experiences and past reinforcement. If a person's attempts at personal control were successful in the past, an internal locus of control develops. However, if attempts were unsuccessful an external locus of control develops (Niven, 1989).

Rotter's theory has been applied in the Health Locus of Control model which seeks to examine the relationship between locus of control and health-related behaviour. It has been linked to various health-related behaviours such as ability to stop smoking, lose weight and use birth control effectively. In studies using this model it has been found that people with an internal locus of control combined with a high value placed on health were more likely to perform a variety of health-promoting behaviours (Lau, 1982). They are more sensitive to health messages, more likely to take preventive measures and perhaps are less susceptible to physical and psychological ill-health than those with an external locus of control. On the other hand, those who are predominantly 'internal' may feel guilty if they become ill, whereas those who think they have no control over events and expect negative events to happen to them can suffer a condition called 'learned helplessness' and become depressed (Abramson et al., 1978).

There are various strategies which the midwife can employ to modify a woman's locus of control, particularly if it is an external one. She should try to persuade her that her health and well-being can be affected by her behaviour and lifestyle and that she has some control over health events (e.g. breastfeeding helps to reduce the risk of breast cancer). The midwife can encourage the woman with internal locus of control by reinforcing health-promoting behaviours.

Salience of Lifestyle

This model was developed by Pill and Stott in the early 1980s as a concept to predict preventive health behaviour (Pill and Stott, 1982). They developed an index to assess the importance that individuals attach to their lifestyle and the extent to which they recognize that individual choices can affect future health status (Pill and Stott, 1987). Those who score high on this measure are called 'lifestylists'. They are more likely to take positive action to improve their health such as eating a healthy diet, not smoking, taking regular exercise and avoiding stress. Health is viewed as a dynamic relationship between the individual and the environment and therefore susceptible to a variety of influences, some of which are under individual control. Although 'lifestylists' have positive attitudes to preventive health behaviour, they do not necessarily

use professional screening facilities as they tend to reject the idea of others controlling their health.

The Salience of Lifestyle index has been shown to discriminate effectively for personal health practices, e.g. smoking and drinking, but not for health procedures which rely on health professionals, e.g. immunizations and routine health checks.

Pill and Stott's research is highly relevant for primary care workers, including midwives. It emphasizes the importance of using simple techniques to elicit an individual's own beliefs about lifestyle and health and of having a patient-centred approach rather than applying stereotypes, e.g. 'working class fatalism'. They also advocate a 'practise what you preach' approach for health professionals, who should themselves demonstrate a healthy lifestyle by not smoking, eating a healthy diet and taking regular exercise (Stott and Pill, 1990).

Sociocultural and Gender Influences on Health

In health promotion and education it is important to consider health and illness in a social context, as it is influenced by many important factors in society. Social class, employment status, gender and ethnic differences are particularly significant.

It has long been recognized that *poverty* has an adverse effect on health. In the UK the National Health Service was set up in 1948 to provide a range of free medical care to the whole population and thereby achieve equality of access to health services for those in need. It was hoped that this would eliminate or greatly reduce inequalities in health but this has not proven to be the case. Many studies have shown that the higher income groups make better use of health services than the lower income groups and that social classes IV and V make less use of preventive services, such as cervical cytology, infant welfare, dentistry, antenatal and family planning clinics (McMahon, 1993). The Black Report in 1980 demonstrated substantial differences in mortality and morbidity rates of social class groups (Townsend and Davidson, 1992). In a further report 'The Health Divide', which was commissioned by the Health Education Council in 1986, Margaret Whitehead, its author, concluded that there was a widening of health inequalities as 'in some respects the health of the lower occupational classes had actually deteriorated against the background of a general improvement in the population as a whole' (Whitehead, 1992: 275). Although overall death rates fell in Britain between 1974 and 1984, non-manual groups experienced a much greater decline than manual groups and there was a widening gap between the two as regards chronic sickness. Coronary heart disease, lung cancer, stroke, peptic ulcer and a wide range of other diseases are more common in the manual classes. Perinatal and infant deaths are higher in the lower socio-economic groups, as is low birthweight.

Housing tenure and *employment* are other measures which have been used to investigate the association between poverty and ill-health. There are marked and consistent differences in mortality and morbidity between those in owner-occupied and local authority accommodation. Homelessness has risen considerably in recent years and has many implications for health, including stress and poor nutrition. Those who are unemployed experience worse physical and mental health than those in work and higher death rates, particularly from lung cancer, suicide, accidents and heart disease (McMahon, 1993). Poorer health and development have been found in the children of the unemployed (Whitehead, 1992).

Single-parent families are another group who can experience financial hardship and stress. These families are dependent on solitary breadwinners, the vast majority of whom are women. Childcare responsibilities can restrict their job opportunities and the cost of childcare can be prohibitive, resulting in unemployment and low income for many. Babies born to unsupported mothers are most vulnerable to perinatal death (Graham, 1984) and infant death (Judge and Benzeval, 1993).

Cultural background is another important influence on health. There are wide variations in lifestyle and perceptions of health and illness between cultures. There are also a number of specific conditions which are much more common in certain ethnic groups. For example, people from northern and central Europe are more prone to cystic fibrosis; sickle cell disease and hypertension occur mainly in people of African and Afro-Caribbean descent; spina bifida in people of Celtic origin; and rickets and osteomalacia particularly affect people of Asian origin. The perinatal and infant mortality rates are higher in babies of Asian-born women and in particular of those born in Pakistan (Whitehead, 1988).

As regards *gender* and health, women have a longer life expectancy than men but are more likely to suffer chronic and acute disorders. This may reflect the differences in working conditions, lifestyle and behaviour of women and men. Poor housing and living conditions have a more marked effect on the health of women and pre-school children, than on other members of the family, as they tend to spend more of their time at home (Graham, 1984). The numbers of married women in paid employment in the UK has increased considerably since the Second World War but housework and childcare are still largely women's responsibility rather than being equally shared between both partners. Domestic violence is a serious threat to women's health and there is increasing awareness of this problem by government departments, police, etc., though it is believed that it is significantly under-reported.

Advice Given in Pregnancy

THE IMPORTANCE OF ANTENATAL CARE

Ideally, schoolchildren should be taught the importance of antenatal care in an effort to improve their understanding of the value of early booking and regular antenatal clinic attendance. At the expectant mother's first visit to the antenatal clinic, the midwife should explain how normal progress of pregnancy can be monitored with regular examinations and tests. Questions should be encouraged and answered with skill and understanding. Although this is time-consuming, it is essential that the woman and her family understand and accept the care offered. The health of pregnant women influences that of their babies and fetal and infant health are major determinants of health in childhood and later life. It follows that antenatal care should be as accessible as possible to all cultures and social classes. If women feel ill-at-ease or have difficulty communicating with carers, they will be less inclined to seek antenatal care. The women's perception of care during pregnancy should be that it takes account of social and psychological as well as physical needs, so that uptake of antenatal services is optimal.

THE ROLE OF THE MIDWIFE IN HEALTH PROMOTION AND EDUCATION

Health promotion and education are important aspects of the midwife's role. She has many opportunities to teach, either on a one-to-one basis in the antenatal clinic and in the mother's home or in groups when prospective parents attend parent education classes. Most women are very receptive to teaching in pregnancy and are keen to learn how to maintain their own health and that of their baby. The midwife needs to be aware of this fact and give advice sensitively and accurately. She should be careful not to instil guilt in a woman who is unable to comply with advice. The pregnant woman may have other priorities and valid reasons for not following advice. For example, she may not be able to follow dietary advice, because it has cost implications or does not fit in with cultural or family customs.

The midwife must ensure that advice is appropriate and acceptable with consideration of the individual's circumstances and lifestyle. She must also be aware of her own feelings when well-meaning advice given by her is not taken and acted upon and not react negatively. In particular, she needs to be aware of any tendency to stereotype. This occurs when people of a particular social class or ethnic group are attributed certain characteristics because they are members of that group (Gross, 1992). The dangers of stereotyping are that these characteristics are not necessarily accurate and are often negative or derogatory (Green *et al.*, 1990; Bowler, 1993). It does not take account of individual differences and needs and overestimates the differences between groups. The midwife can overcome this problem by being open to learning about and increasing her awareness of individual needs.

DIET

The importance of nutrition and nutritional advice in pregnancy is covered in Chapter 16.

EXERCISE AND SPORT

Most people are well aware of the benefits of exercise and sport and many women nowadays are fitness conscious. Exercise has many positive effects for the pregnant woman such as improving stamina and posture and maintaining muscle tone. Healthy women may undertake exercise to which they are accustomed, such as cycling, swimming and riding as well as walking, light gardening and ordinary housework. The woman with a sedentary lifestyle before pregnancy should be encouraged to increase her activity level during pregnancy. A half-hour walk each day is a

good introduction to regular exercise (Edelman and Mandle, 1990).

Water is an attractive medium for the pregnant woman as it gives buoyancy, increases mobility, puts less strain on the joints and may relieve backache. Aquanatal classes are becoming more common in recent years though not all with qualified teachers in attendance (Baddeley, 1993). The physiology of pregnancy must be understood and appreciated by teachers so that exercises are appropriate for pregnant women and their response to exercise monitored. This principle applies to all types of exercise both in and out of water. The ligaments which support joints are relaxed by the hormone relaxin in pregnancy and the pregnant woman should be instructed to employ minimum muscle tension during exercise so as not to overstretch the ligaments permanently. The abdominal muscles are already stretched over the growing uterus and women should not do exercises, such as sit-ups, which put further strain on these. Pelvic tilting exercises and abdominal retraction are advised in pregnancy (see Chapter 25) (Baddeley and Green, 1992).

Most physically active sports become more difficult as weight increases and the breasts and abdomen enlarge. Balance is affected with lowered centre of gravity. More stress is placed on weight-bearing joints and musculoskeletal injury becomes more common (Thistlethwaite, 1989). Other physiological changes in pregnancy, such as raised cardiac output, reduced lung capacity and decreased agility, mean that the pregnant woman may want to choose less active sports than those pursued when not pregnant. Any sport which causes undue fatigue, muscle cramps, or joint pain should obviously be modified or discontinued and women should avoid becoming overheated and dehydrated. Strenuous unaccustomed exercise and heavy lifting should be avoided in pregnancy.

Contraindications to exercise in pregnancy include hypertension, diabetes, cardiac and thyroid disease, as well as obstetric complications such as intrauterine growth retardation, incompetent cervix and uterine bleeding (Carbon, 1994).

HYGIENE AND DENTAL CARE

A daily shower or bath is particularly necessary in pregnancy because the sweat and sebaceous glands are more active, there is increased leucorrhoea and colostrum may leak from the nipples. The use of bubble bath is contraindicated for women who are inclined to cystitis and urinary tract infection. The teeth and gums should be brushed with a fluoride toothpaste at least twice daily and ideally after every meal. This reduces the build-up of plaque which can cause gum disease and tooth decay. Many dentists recommend the use of dental floss after meals also for this purpose. Unhealthy gums look red and swollen and bleed easily. With the hormonal changes in pregnancy, plaque can cause increased inflammation of the gums. Dental caries are septic foci and therefore require attention as they are potentially dangerous. The woman is advised to avoid sugary snacks and drinks and to visit the dentist for a check-up early in pregnancy. Dental care in the UK is free during pregnancy and for one year after the birth of the baby.

CLOTHING

Clothing generally should be loose, light, comfortable and easily laundered. A properly fitting brassière is usually comfortable in early pregnancy when the breasts enlarge and need support. It will need to be one or two sizes larger than usual; it should have wide straps that do not cut into the shoulders; the cups should be deep so as not to flatten the nipples. Some types may be used during lactation, the most useful being the front-opening type. As pregnancy advances the woman has to lean backwards to counterbalance the weight of the uterus. High-heeled shoes aggravate this tendency to tilt forward and the strain on the spine and sacro-iliac ligaments may cause backache. The woman is therefore advised to wear lower heeled shoes.

SEXUAL HEALTH

Sexuality in pregnancy is an important aspect of health which is not always adequately addressed. Some women may feel embarrassed broaching the topic and some midwives, fearing intrusion of privacy, may also be reticent about discussing the issue. There may be religious, cultural and social taboos about having sexual intercourse during pregnancy. However, some couples may have anxieties which could be relieved through frank discussion. There is little evidence that sexual intercourse during normal pregnancy is harmful and couples can be reassured of this. Sexual desire can vary during pregnancy and from one individual to another. In the first trimester loss of sexual interest is very common, as the woman may feel sick and/or tired due to physical and hormonal changes. If the pregnancy is unplanned she may also be in an emotional dilemma about whether to continue the pregnancy or not. By the second trimester these problems will have usually been resolved and the woman's interest in sex returns. As pregnancy advances the woman will find intercourse more comfortable if positions are used which do not put undue pressure on her enlarging abdomen, such as lying side by side with her legs across her partner or the female superior position (see Chapter 59).

In the last weeks of pregnancy sexual intercourse and orgasm may stimulate strong uterine contractions which can make the woman feel uncomfortable. Seminal fluid contains a large amount of prostaglandins and intercourse may help to ripen the cervix or induce labour. Oxytocin is thought to be released during female orgasm and some women experience painful contractions. This experience may have a negative effect on the frequency of intercourse, though no significant fetal effects, such as fetal distress or reduced Apgar scores, have been shown (Savage and Reader, 1984).

Penetration may also cause the woman discomfort if the fetal head is deeply engaged. Couples may then wish to consider other ways to feel close and show love and affection to one another. This is especially important if the woman is feeling tired, unwell or unattractive and for couples who have been advised against having intercourse during pregnancy.

For women with a history of recurrent abortion, intercourse should be avoided in the early months of pregnancy, especially at the time when menstruation would normally occur and around the time of previous abortions. Similarly when bleeding occurs in pregnancy, intercourse should be avoided. In the last month of pregnancy, there is an increased risk of introducing infection into the uterus during intercourse because the cervix is beginning to efface and slightly dilate. The midwife should advise about the importance of good hygiene for the couple. She can also show understanding and support to couples with sexual problems and advise them about how to get sexual counselling if required. Couples can seek referral to a counsellor through their general practitioner, or apply to a counselling service such as Relate for an appointment. As pregnancy affects sexual interest, couples are advised to wait for a few months after delivery before starting therapy.

EMPLOYMENT

Most women in paid employment continue working until maternity leave, so long as they are fit and healthy. Since maternity benefit payment in the UK has become more flexible, women are increasingly more likely to work into the third trimester. They may wish to have maximum income for as long as possible to meet outgoings like mortgage repayments etc. or they may not want to interrupt progress in career prospects for any longer than necessary. They may also prefer to prolong contact with working colleagues to enjoy their support and encouragement rather than to be isolated at home.

For the majority of women, work during pregnancy does not pose a threat to their health or that of their babies. For some it may be necessary to modify working practices to promote safety and comfort. The pregnant woman should avoid heavy lifting. Seating for sedentary workers should be supportive to the back because of increased lordosis. Standing for long periods should be avoided and more rest periods instituted, because of reduced venous return and risk of varicosity development. Smoky environments should be avoided because of the risks of passive smoking.

Some occupations may actually be hazardous to the health of fetus and expectant mother, such as work exposure to toxic chemicals (e.g. lead and pesticides), anaesthetic gases and radiation (Keleher, 1991). Women who do work that is dangerous, or who cannot do their work adequately because of pregnancy may have the right to move to another job in the same firm, if one is available. In the UK under the Trade Union Reform and Employment Rights Act 1993, all women are entitled to this right, regardless of how long employed or how many hours worked. If there is no suitable alternative work, the employer can fairly dismiss the pregnant woman. Ideally the woman should seek advice before pregnancy or as soon as possible after conception if she is concerned.

The midwife should be aware of potential hazards in the workplace so that she can advise women when required. She should also be able to give advice regarding maternity benefits and employment rights. It is particularly important that pregnant women are aware of their legal right to have paid time off work for antenatal care and that this should not be unreasonably refused, whether in part-time or full-time employment. UK law does not make it clear whether or not antenatal classes are included in antenatal care. An industrial tribunal has ruled that it can, so women should get paid for time off to attend classes (Maternity Alliance, 1991). The employer may require a letter from the midwife or doctor saying that the classes are part of antenatal care.

Occasionally, it may be necessary to advise a woman against continuing to work during pregnancy, if she develops complications like uncontrolled diabetes, hypertension or threatened preterm labour. A certificate from the doctor would be required so she can claim sickness benefit until such time as maternity benefit payment is possible.

TRAVEL

Women with a history of recurrent abortions or preterm labour would be advised to avoid long journeys in pregnancy. Preterm labour is more likely after 32 weeks, thus special care should be taken after this time. When long journeys are necessary, frequent breaks help to relieve fatigue and discomfort. When travelling by car, pregnant women should wear shoulder harness seatbelts if possible as in the event of an accident, there is less abdominal trauma than with the single lap-type belt (Markos, 1990). The diagonal strap should be worn across the body between the breasts and the lap belt across the upper thighs.

Airlines may require a doctor's certificate stating that a pregnant woman is fit to travel. It may be inadvisable for her to fly in the early weeks of pregnancy if sickness is a problem. Most airlines will not carry pregnant women after 32 weeks.

STRESS IN PREGNANCY

Stress is something which all people experience occasionally. It is usually seen in a negative light because of its potential for physical and psychological harm though it does have positive effects also. There is an optimal level of stress for each individual. If it is too little, the person does not feel challenged and stimulated. With too much stress, the person can develop physical disorders such as heart disease, peptic ulcer, migraine and infections, or have psychological effects such as anxiety, anger, depression and burn-out. Stress arises from an interaction between people and their environment. When a person's perception is that there is an imbalance between a demand and their ability to meet that demand they are subject to stress (Gross, 1992). Perception varies from one individual to another and this is why there are differences in stress reactions, sources and degree of stress experienced. Controllability is an important factor to consider in relation to stress. The more uncontrollable an event seems, the more likely it is perceived as stressful. Pregnancy and the addition of a new family member are recognized as stressful life events (Atkinson *et al.*, 1993).

In pregnancy, the woman has to deal with the effects of major physiological changes in her body as well as changes in her role, self-image, body-image, and other aspects. She may already have ongoing stresses in her life, such as poverty, difficult relationships or unsatisfactory living or working conditions. How she handles these stresses, including the changes that pregnancy brings, is influenced by her individual personality, physical state, spiritual beliefs and sociocultural background. Whether or not the pregnancy was desired and how supportive the woman's family is, especially her partner, are other aspects which may influence how the woman will cope with her pregnancy and future role (Edelman and Mandle, 1990).

The pregnant woman tends to become more introverted and passive, which allows her to centre her attention on the growing child and on her own growth and development as a person. The woman who is expecting her first baby has to adjust to becoming a mother. To do this, she will draw on past experiences including her own mothering as a child. If this was a positive experience for her, she is likely to be optimistic. Conversely, if her relationship with her mother was poor, she may have anxieties about her relationship with her baby (Prince and Adams, 1978). A pregnant teenager who is still in adolescence may be searching for her own identity and have difficulty adjusting to her pregnant body and role of mother all at the same time.

The woman with other children may have different concerns. She may worry about whether she will be able to love and care for the new baby and the older children as much as needed. She may be much more aware of the problems involved with caring for a new infant than the woman who has not had this experience and be less excited about it. There may be anxieties about fetal well-being, especially for the older mother or the woman who has a poor reproductive history. Fetal screening may bring reassurance to some women who are tested, for others it may give rise to anxiety by raising the question of abnormality (Marteau, 1989b). Some test results can take weeks which adds to the stress the woman and her partner may feel. The woman's perceived lack of control over her care in

pregnancy may be another stressor. This will depend on how involved she is in decision-making about aspects of her care and the attitudes of carers (Reid and Garcia, 1989). Perhaps she is referred to and treated as a 'patient' even though she is a healthy woman with an uncomplicated pregnancy.

Anxiety tends to be high in the first trimester as the woman makes her initial adaptations to pregnancy and anticipated life changes. These feelings tend to decrease in the second trimester and then increase during the final weeks as labour and delivery become imminent. They may be expressed as dreams and fantasies, with the woman dreaming that her baby is born deformed or dead, or that she herself dies. Some women manifest their anxieties by smoking or drinking more, or through psychosomatic complaints, such as nausea and vomiting after the first trimester, excessive eating and sleeplessness. The fetus can be affected by the mother's reaction to stress, e.g. if she drinks or smokes excessively. It may be that stress affects the fetus. In a large Danish study, psychological distress later in pregnancy was associated with an increased risk of preterm delivery (Hedegaard *et al.*, 1993).

The pregnant woman may perceive a decrease in her ability to cope with the stresses specific to pregnancy but also the everyday stresses that she managed in the past (Edelman and Mandle, 1990). The midwife should encourage her to express her feelings and air her problems. Some women have their own ways of dealing with stress which are not harmful to them or the fetus and the midwife should encourage the use of those they have found effective. These may include talking to a friend, listening to soft music, exercising or sleeping. Antenatal classes may help also. Relaxation techniques can be used in times of stress. Information gained about pregnancy, labour and parenting may help to dispel anxieties. As already stated, perception of control is important and the woman's individual needs and her right to choose must always be acknowledged if stress is to be reduced.

SMOKING IN PREGNANCY

Smoking is the largest single preventable cause of mortality and it accounts for a third of all deaths in middle age. Ninety per cent of lung cancers are smoking related and it is a contributory cause of cancers of the larynx, oesophagus, pancreas, bladder, cervix and other organs (DOH, 1991). It is a major cause of coronary heart disease, stroke and chronic bronchitis and is also associated with reduced fertility and early menopause in women (Rosevear *et al.*, 1992). In pregnancy, smoking is related to spontaneous abortion, placenta praevia, placental abruption, preterm labour and low birthweight (Plant, 1990). Women from lower socio-economic groups are more likely to smoke in pregnancy and it significantly increases the risk of perinatal and infant mortality. Children who are exposed in the home to cigarette smoke are more likely to develop otitis media and asthma and have higher hospitalization rates for severe respiratory illness (Walsh and Redman, 1993). Passive smoking is also associated with sudden infant death syndrome (Gilbert *et al.*, 1995).

The Department of Health paper *The Health of the Nation* (DOH, 1991) sets out an objective to reduce significantly the numbers of people starting to smoke and increase the numbers who stop smoking. According to the document, 33% of men, 30% of women and 8% of children aged 11–15 smoke cigarettes. Teenage smoking is a difficult problem as there can be powerful pressures on teenagers to smoke, even when they are aware of the dangers. Peer pressure, the need to experiment, cigarette advertising, imitation of parents and self-image can influence them to smoke.

At the first antenatal visit, the midwife should enquire of all women as to whether they smoke or not and if they do, how many cigarettes are smoked daily. If she smokes, the woman's knowledge as to the risks to her own health and that of her baby should be assessed and information given as appropriate. The midwife should acknowledge the physical and psychological addiction to tobacco experienced by smokers and not expect cessation to be simply a matter of advising them to cut down or stop. Women who are highly dependent on tobacco may feel guilty and inadequate at not being able to give it up. This may affect the relationship with the baby as well as causing stress, the effects of which have already been discussed. More than half of smoking women worry about smoking in pregnancy and 10% smoke more heavily during this time (Enkin *et al.*, 1989). The midwife should be encouraging and supportive and ready to offer help to women who express the desire to stop smoking. Smoking cessation programmes which involve education and behavioural modification are thought to be effective in reducing smoking during pregnancy (Walsh and Redman, 1993). Midwives are well-placed to provide such programmes because of their regular contact with women. The benefits to the mother as well as the baby should be emphasized. The risks of developing smoking-related diseases start to fall rapidly when the person stops and this information can be encouraging. Strategies for women wanting to stop or reduce smoking include the following:

1 Set a date to stop and stick to it.
2 Get someone else to give up with you for the moral support (e.g. your partner).
3 Choose a time to give up when there are fewer triggers to smoke (e.g. stress).
4 Avoid other smokers and look for no-smoking areas in public places.
5 Identify times and situations when you are most likely to want to smoke and consider how to avoid or deal with them.
6 When faced with the urge to smoke, try an alternative activity (e.g. exercising, phoning a friend, pursuing a hobby).
7 When trying to reduce the number smoked, smoke cigarettes only halfway down.
8 Delay having the first cigarette of the day.
9 Never keep your cigarette in your hand – put it down after each puff.

Carbon monoxide monitors can be used in antenatal clinics to help women check their own progress in cutting down or stopping smoking. Health education leaflets and self-help groups may also be offered. Nicotine gum and patches are contraindicated in pregnancy.

ALCOHOL IN PREGNANCY

Many women in Western society drink alcohol and over the past 30 years the number of women drinkers has increased much more than that of men. There has been a corresponding increase in alcohol-related problems among women, such as illness, hospital admissions, deaths and drunken driving prosecutions (Chadwick, 1993). There has also been a large increase in female adolescent drinking. Women who are single and under 25 are considered most at risk of excessive drinking in the UK and especially those who are career-orientated. Divorced and separated women are another high-risk group (Clemenger, 1993).

The vast majority of people who drink do so sensibly without harming either themselves or others. Nevertheless, individuals should be aware of the amount and pattern of their consumption. Excessive alcohol intake is potentially lethal, affecting virtually every organ system in the body, including the liver, gastrointestinal tract, cardiovascular and neurological systems. It affects nutrition by altering the metabolism, mobilization and storage of nutrients and by its effect on appetite. Excessive or chronic alcohol abuse is associated with several vitamin and mineral deficiencies, including folic acid, vitamin B, magnesium and iron. Learning difficulties, loss of memory and other mental process problems are associated with alcoholism (Edelman and Mandle, 1990). Women cannot tolerate as much alcohol as men because of differences in body size, absorption and metabolism. They have a higher proportion of fat to water, so that alcohol becomes more concentrated in the body fluids. Damaging effects are therefore more likely to develop and women take longer to recover from them. Women who abuse alcohol are particularly at risk of breast cancer and liver disease (Anderson *et al.*, 1993), as well as other conditions such as gastritis, pancreatitis, peptic ulcers and malnutrition.

There is much speculation about the causes of alcohol abuse. It is known that the children of alcoholic parents have a greater risk of becoming alcoholics themselves. This tendency may be hereditary, as a gene for alcoholism has been identified. It may be environmental, as a consequence of a dysfunctional family background (Bradshaw, 1988). Perhaps it is a combination of both. Psychological factors often lead to excessive drinking, such as anxiety, anger, guilt, shame and grief (Long and Mullen, 1994). Stress and depression are other contributory causes, as is the experience of sexual abuse (Bullows and Penfold, 1993). Alcohol problems are evident in all occupations and at all levels of seniority, from shop floor to boardroom (Hartz *et al.*, 1990).

Though female drinking has become more publicly acceptable, a woman's excessive drinking is still regarded differently from that of her male counterpart. As a result, women are more inclined to hide their drinking and receive less help (Clemenger, 1993). Denial of the problem is a well-recognized feature of alcoholism generally. The alcoholic has to acknowledge the problem and be prepared to do something about it, before she or he can begin recovery. The family of the alcoholic often needs help to recover also, as alcoholism can affect the whole family. They may be suffering from the effects of both physical and mental abuse. Some people who are involved in relationships with addicts, such as alcoholics, can exhibit what is known as co-dependent behaviour. The co-dependent feels responsible and overcommits to caring for the

addict, with the result that the addiction is unwittingly supported rather than discouraged (Barker, 1991). Self-help groups like Al-anon and Alateen (for teenage children of alcoholics) are useful reference points for those who are friends and relatives of alcoholics.

Drinking excessively in pregnancy can adversely affect the pregnancy and fetal development (see Chapter 15) and the babies of alcoholics may be more at risk of child abuse and neglect. The pregnancy may have been conceived when the woman was under the influence of alcohol and be unplanned and unwanted. She may also have an increased risk of sexually transmitted disease for the same reason. General advice as regards sensible drinking for women who are not pregnant is to drink up to 14–21 units of alcohol per week with two or three drink-free days. One unit is half a pint of beer, a glass of wine or a measure of spirits. In pregnancy, it is still not known what constitutes a safe limit. The midwife is thus faced with the dilemma of whether to encourage abstinence or not. The evidence suggests that one or two units once or twice a week will not cause adverse effects (Plant, 1990).

At the first antenatal visit, the midwife should enquire about the woman's alcohol consumption in a tactful and professional manner. A useful way of taking a drinking history is to ask specifically about the preceding seven days. If she has taken alcohol, the amount in units should be recorded. If she is drinking more than the recommended amount for pregnancy, the midwife should try to explore the reasons for this with her and counsel her about how she may reduce her consumption. Any intervention should seek to maximize the individual's sense of responsibility for their own drinking behaviour (Royal College of Psychiatrists, 1986). The following advice may be useful for women wanting to reduce their alcohol consumption:

1   Do not drink daily, make five or six days a week drink-free.
2   Do not have more than one or two units of alcohol on the same day.
3   Quench your thirst first with a non-alcoholic drink.
4   Dilute spirits with at least as much water or something non-fizzy to slow absorption.
5   Make every second drink alcohol-free or low alcohol.
6   Sip your drink, do not gulp.
7   Always put your glass down between sips.

8 Be firm and do not give in to people who try to press you to drink more.

9 Do not use alcohol to try to solve emotional problems.

10 Avoid drinking as a means of unwinding, use effective alternatives: music, reading, warm bath.

If it appears that a woman is dependent on alcohol, a referral to a specialist may be required. It may also be appropriate to refer her to Alcoholics Anonymous (AA) or any other self-help group available. The proportion of women in AA has risen considerably in recent years as there is less stigma about women's drinking than in the past. Many find the help and understanding they require from those who can identify with the alcoholic's feelings and needs. The philosophy of AA may also offer them a new way to deal with the problems of life (Royal College of Psychiatrists, 1986).

DRUGS IN PREGNANCY

All drugs taken by the pregnant woman and achieving a plasma concentration cross the placenta to the fetus, except for insulin and heparin. This usually occurs by the process of simple diffusion from a high to a low concentration (Ledward *et al.*, 1991). Some drugs which are normally considered safe may have a teratogenic effect on the developing fetus, especially in the first trimester. This may occur because:

▶ fetal tissues are more sensitive to the effects of drugs;
▶ the fetal plasma has a lower protein-binding ability which affects the level of free drug;
▶ the fetal liver is less able to detoxify and deal with them.

Some drugs accumulate in the placenta and may affect placental perfusion.

Pregnant women should be advised to take only those drugs which are prescribed by a doctor. If already taking prescribed medication prior to pregnancy, they should discuss with their doctor as to whether an alternative needs to be considered for pregnancy. Major teratogenic drugs include tetracycline, thalidomide, radioactive iodine and local anaesthetic prilocaine. There are many others which are known or suspected to carry a teratogenic risk. Over-the-counter drugs may also have the potential to harm the fetus and should be avoided.

Drug and volatile substance abuse

Drug abuse, including narcotics, tranquillizers, cocaine and amphetamines, is a serious health problem for the mother and the fetus. Male drug abusers have always outnumbered female drug abusers, but the gap is closing with a steadily increasing proportion of young females abusing a wide range of drugs. Women are twice as likely as men to use sedatives and tranquillizers and these drugs can provoke misuse and dependence. Women who are restricted to the traditional role of housewife are more at risk of becoming dependent on these drugs, than those fulfilling numerous roles (Das Gupta, 1990).

The causes of drug addiction are multifactorial. Many theories have been expounded, including personality disorder, disrupted parenting, socio-economic deprivation, cultural and peer influence (Johns, 1990). It has also been suggested that a propensity for opiate addiction may be the result of imprinting on the fetus when these drugs are used as pain relief for the mother in labour (Jacobson *et al.*, 1990).

Drug addiction is usually compounded with poor nutrition, abnormal behaviour and especially when used intravenously, the risk of viral, bacterial and occasionally fungal infection. The most serious infections include hepatitis, infective endocarditis and HIV. The severely dependent addict may be constantly pre-occupied with the need to obtain drugs. Some may turn to prostitution to get money to finance their habit which gives them the additional risk of contracting sexually transmitted diseases. This is also a risk for those who engage in casual sexual relationships when under the influence of drugs. Young and immature people who experiment with drugs are at particular risk. Violent injury is another risk for those who engage in illegal activity and who associate with criminals in order to procure or sell drugs. Drug abusers are also at increased risk of accidental injury when intoxicated or withdrawing from drugs. Drug overdose is the most common cause of death in drug abusers. This can occur accidentally due to loss of tolerance to the drug following a period of abstinence or due to impaired judgement. Pulmonary embolism can occur following the development of deep vein thrombosis in intravenous drug abusers. Inhalation of heroin can precipitate asthma or acute bronchitis and the snorting of cocaine can cause rhinitis and, if prolonged, nasal damage.

Cocaine is becoming recognized as one of the most

dangerous illicit drugs in common use today. It can produce profound dependence, psychological disturbance and various medical disorders including cardiovascular, neurological and gastrointestinal complications. Preparations can be swallowed, injected, sniffed or smoked. Rock cocaine, or 'crack' as it has come to be known, is the form that is smoked and its effects are felt some 8 seconds after inhalation. For this reason it has become the most favoured route and has led to an increase in the rate of acute fatalities. Most deaths after cocaine use are attributed to generalized convulsions, respiratory failure or cardiac arrhythmias. These risks depend on the dose taken but also on the purity of the drug, which can vary enormously when purchased on the street (Maxwell, 1990).

Since the late 1980s the drug methylenedioxymethamphetamine (MDMA) commonly known as 'ecstasy' or 'E' has gained popularity in conjunction with the acid house/rave explosion. It is one of the most widely used illicit substances in the UK (McGuire *et al.*, 1994). MDMA is a synthetic hallucinogenic amphetamine and comes in a variety of tablets and capsules for oral or rectal administration. Users often refer to them by 'brand-names' such as 'white diamonds', 'burgers', 'banana splits', 'love doves', 'rhubarb and custards', and 'Dennis the Menace' (Cook, 1995). MDMA is complex and expensive to produce and drugs purported to be 'ecstasy' contain various concentrations in the range 2–200 mg. The tablets or capsules may also contain other substances such as MDEA and MDA (precursors to MDMA), caffeine, paracetamol or ketamine (an anaesthetic drug) and thus users are vulnerable to various effects (Wolff *et al.*, 1995). In Holland the Amsterdam drug advice bureau offers the service of checking ecstasy tablet content for a small fee. Users can then be advised if tablets are of high MDMA content or are adulterated with other substances, so that the user can decide not to take it or reduce the dose (Sheldon, 1995).

MDMA inhibits the reabsorption of the neurotransmitter serotonin, thus reducing brain reserves and effecting psychedelic mood changes. It appeals to users because they experience increased sensuality, euphoria and a strong desire to bond with others. They also have the energy to dance continuously for hours. However, these effects decrease with frequent use and unwanted side-effects increase with both dose and frequency. Loss of appetite, sweating, palpitations, jaw stiffness, insomnia, grinding of teeth and the desire to urinate are lesser side-effects. More serious effects have also been shown such as cardiac arrhythmias, hepatotoxicity, neurological and psychiatric conditions. It can also affect thermoregulation. Hyperpyrexia, the most lethal effect, can occur when the user subjects him/herself to intense physical exertion, such as rave dancing in a hot environment and with inadequate hydration. Disseminated intravascular coagulation, severe metabolic acidosis, hyperkalaemia, rhabdomyolysis and acute renal failure are associated with hyperpyrexia and the user convulses or collapses unconscious. Treatment of hyperthermic syndrome is a medical emergency. There is an urgent need to control body temperature as the severity and duration of hyperthermia are important prognostic indicators for survival or death (O'Connor, 1994).

Inhalation of volatile substances usually takes place as a group pastime among young people in their early or middle teens. It is usually experimental and of short duration. The main volatile substances inhaled include gas fuels such as butane; glue solvents such as toluene; and others such as cleaning agents, correcting fluid thinners and aerosol sprays. There is uncertainty about organ damage following solvent abuse but it is thought that toluene causes cerebral atrophy and brain dysfunction. Epilepsy, liver and kidney damage are other rare attributed complications. A minority of inhalers go on to develop a psychological dependence. About a third of UK deaths occur in persons aged 20 years or more and most take place during solitary rather than group inhalation. Death can result mainly from the toxic effects of the substances, such as cardiac arrhythmias; or due to asphyxiation from the use of a plastic bag placed over the head to inhale solvents; or from vomiting and aspiration (Madden, 1990).

Pregnancy may be the first time that drug addictions come to light as the mother may be concerned for the welfare of her baby. Some may be afraid to admit their dependence and stay away from health professionals. The drug abuser may not even realize for some time that she is pregnant. Amenorrhoea and abnormal menstrual cycles can occur as a result of opiate abuse or because of the effects of her lifestyle. For this reason it may be difficult to estimate gestation of pregnancy. It is most important that midwives and other health professionals are tactful and sensitive in their encounters with pregnant addicts so that they are not discouraged from seeking help and treatment. The individual should be considered rather than the stereotype, with the ultimate goal being that she can regain responsibility for the areas of her life over which she has lost control. She may be feeling very anxious and vulnerable as well as guilty about the possible effects of her addiction on the baby. The social isolation experienced by some drug addicts can mean few role models as regards childbearing and motherhood. The midwife will need to give special care and support to the addict so that her health and that of the fetus is promoted and she learns how to parent her child.

Ideally, she should be helped to come off drugs as early in pregnancy as possible or at least two months before expected delivery to ensure a non-addicted infant. The opiate-dependent woman may need to be stabilized on methadone which should then be withdrawn gradually so as not to cause fetal distress or preterm labour. If lacking in experience of treating drug dependency the doctor may need to refer her to the local drug dependency unit. There should be close liaison between those treating her drug problem and the maternity and paediatric teams. The woman who is withdrawing from drugs can experience feelings of bereavement. Counselling by a professional experienced in drug addiction may be indicated. Narcotics Anonymous may also be useful as a self-help group. This is a 12-step programme similar to AA, which offers mutual support in a non-judgemental manner through the sharing of 'experience, strength and hope' (Wells, 1990). Marital and family therapy may also be necessary to help families change patterns of interaction that have developed to deal with the problem and which are counterproductive when the addict is in recovery.

DOMESTIC VIOLENCE

Violence in the home poses a serious threat to women's health. It includes emotional, sexual and physical abuse and is usually by the male partner or ex-partner. Abused women and abusers come from all cultural, educational, racial, religious and socio-economic backgrounds. Research indicates that domestic violence is widespread in the UK but it is difficult to obtain reliable statistics, as it is generally accepted to be under-reported. A study of women living in Islington, London, showed that one in four women were assaulted by their partners in the course of their relationship (Andrews and Brown, 1988). An American study revealed that the incidence of abuse during pregnancy was between one in 11 and one in 50 women

from the general population (Bohn, 1990). Physical assault can cause injuries such as cuts, bruises, serious disfigurement, broken bones, and internal injuries. Women also die as a result of domestic violence. The latest Home Office figures for England and Wales for 1990 suggest that 43% of female homicides were killed by their partners and 19% were killed by another family member (cited by Friend, 1993).

The psychological trauma experienced by women who are abused by their partner is considerable. Children who witness the abuse may also be traumatized and short- and long-term emotional and behavioural effects can result. A cycle of violence has been described by Walker (1984), which consists of three phases:

1 *Phase one* can last from minutes to months, during which there is a gradual increase in tension. It is characterized by minor battering incidents, such as throwing objects and pushing, as well as psychological abuse and humiliation, which occur with increasing frequency.
2 *Phase two* is the acute battering incident which is a discharge of tension and may last for 24 hours.
3 *Phase three* is the loving contrition phase, in which the abuser expresses remorse, reaffirms his love for her and promises that it will never happen again.

Over time as the cycle is repeated, the tension-building phase lasts longer, the violent episodes are more frequent and severe and the loving contrition phase may decrease or disappear. At first, the woman may disbelieve or deny what has happened. Following further violence, she may experience fear, hatred or rage and her sense of betrayal, humiliation, powerlessness, and low self-esteem intensifies. This may lead to substance abuse, depression or suicide. Some women blame themselves for provoking the attack, an attitude which is encouraged by the abuser who seeks to justify his actions by blaming the victim.

Domestic violence is thought to reflect patriarchal attitudes towards women. The woman is seen as property, having a subservient role in the household and deserving to be abused (Chez, 1988). The woman with low self-esteem and self-confidence can feel trapped in a violent relationship. She may be economically or emotionally dependent on the abuser, fear reprisals if she leaves him, or wish to maintain society's ideal of the family staying together. There is evidence that violence begins or escalates during pregnancy (Bohn, 1990; Andrews and Brown, 1988). Attacks to the abdomen, breasts and genitals are more common at this time and may result in miscarriage, placental abruption, preterm labour and stillbirth. The abuser may be consciously or subconsciously trying to terminate the pregnancy. He may feel jealous of the woman's ability to carry a pregnancy, or see the fetus as an intruder. He may also become violent because of strained finances or because the woman is not fulfilling his expectations of her. Characteristics of such violent men are likely to include jealousy, possessiveness and emotional dependence on their partner. Women are more likely to become involved in a violent relationship if they experienced lack of care in childhood, premarital pregnancy and teenage marriage (Andrews and Brown, 1988).

The midwife has a role in prevention and detection of domestic violence. She may need to examine her own attitude to this issue to ascertain if she sees violence as the responsibility of the victim or the perpetrator. She may see it as a private matter for the couple or feel unsure about getting involved. In recognizing that domestic violence is a public health issue and a possible complication of pregnancy, it is appropriate that guidelines for dealing with the problem should be developed in maternity units. Sexual inequality and acceptibility of male aggression should be challenged by individuals, professionals and professional organizations, at social and political level. Antenatal classes could provide a forum for discussion and education of parents about domestic violence.

The midwife is ideally placed to detect cases of domestic violence and it is important that she responds appropriately. The woman may try to keep the abuse secret because she feels ashamed or afraid. She may give a history of being accident prone or bruising easily. The nature of the injuries may not match the description of how they were caused and they may be at several sites and in different phases of healing. The woman may display low self-esteem or signs of anxiety and depression. Her partner may make adverse or belittling comments about her in front of others or appear overly solicitous. The midwife should ensure privacy and be non-judgemental and encouraging to the woman so that she can express herself without fear. It is suggested that when abuse is suspected, the best way to confirm suspicions is by direct questioning, such as: 'Did somebody cause these injuries?' or 'Has somebody been hurting you?' (Chez, 1988; Bohn 1990; Bewley and Gibbs, 1991). She

may choose to deny it, but at least she can be made aware that help is available.

When the woman acknowledges that she has been abused, the midwife should emphasize that violent behaviour is the responsibility of the aggressor and not the victim, that no-one deserves to be abused and that it must cease. The woman may not be aware of the resources available to help her, such as the police, social services or primary health care team. The police are now more willing to intervene in such cases and have set up domestic violence units in some areas. In the UK, the Women's Aid Federation also offers help and advice to women and children who are abused and they can be contacted through a national helpline number. They can provide a safe refuge for those who have to leave home and have nowhere else to go. The Samaritans, Relate and Victim Support are other agencies which can offer counselling and support. The midwife should be able to supply the woman with relevant local telephone numbers and addresses. It may also be useful to post these on noticeboards in the maternity unit or health centre.

Needs of Special Groups

TRAVELLERS

The term travellers includes Gypsies, New Age travellers and others who lead a nomadic way of life but excludes travelling showmen and circus personnel. In the UK local authorities used to be obliged to provide adequate permanent legal caravan sites for such travellers, though many areas were underprovided for, especially in London boroughs and metropolitan districts. However, under the 1995 Criminal Justice Act, this requirement is removed from statute and local authorites have discretion to decide on site provision and expenditure. The Act also gives greater powers of eviction from unauthorized sites and harsher penalties can be levied (Lloyd, 1994).

Travellers face particular problems when it comes to health as a consequence of either living on unsuitable sites or because of reduced access to health services through enforced or voluntary mobility. Some travellers may be parked on sites which are close to motorways or railways, have unclean water or are in the vicinity of dangerous waste or chemicals. Even official sites may lack basic facilities and provide unhealthy environments in which to live. Research by the Association of Metropolitan Authorities and the Maternity Alliance has shown that many local authorities evict traveller women from unofficial sites when they are close to delivery or have just given birth (Durward, 1990). Pregnant women are thus subjected to additional stress with the threat of enforced mobility.

Continuity of care and the transfer of health records are particularly difficult when traveller families move on to other areas. To obtain health care, the local general practitioner, midwife or health visitor must be sought out after every move. Pregnant women or mothers are faced with health professionals who do not know them or their children and who may have no access to their health records. They may also face prejudice or lack of respect from health care personnel and be exploited. Fundholder general practitioners may be unwilling to accept them on their lists because they need to meet their targets for immunization and cytology and do not want temporary residents (Reid, 1993). For these reasons, traveller women may not avail themselves of health services such as antenatal care, six-week postnatal checks and family planning. Their children may not have routine developmental checks and immunizations.

Communication of health information is a problem for travellers because of high levels of illiteracy and because they have no regular postal address or telephone. Discrimination, hostile attitudes and lack of understanding of their cultural differences may also be barriers to communication. Health promotion and education are important for travellers and problems of communication need to be overcome. Their lifestyle can be stressful as they are self-employed. Smoking is common among travellers and their diet tends to consist mainly of convenience foods which are high in cholesterol. There is a high incidence of hypertension, coronary artery disease and gallstones and many are overweight (Rose, 1993).

Midwives and other health professionals need to be aware of the difficulties and problems faced by travellers and avail themselves of opportunities for health promotion when they arise. Visual aids and health promotional materials have been produced by Save the Children Fund, Maternity Alliance and traveller groups which could be useful. Gypsies have traditional attitudes towards health, hygiene and healing and there needs to be increased awareness and consideration of these by health professionals (Rose, 1993). A record of the care given should be made available to travellers so they can achieve some continuity if they move on to another area. Midwives and health visitors should liaise with local authorities if there is a threat of eviction for pregnant women or those who have young babies. A compromise solution may be negotiated. The Maternity Alliance recommends that health authorities identify a named person to co-ordinate information relating to travellers and to be responsible for liaison with other agencies (Durward, 1990).

IMMIGRANT FAMILIES

Immigrants to Britain come from various racial, cultural and social backgrounds. The majority come from Asian, European and African countries, with smaller numbers coming from the Caribbean, America and Commonwealth countries (OPCS, 1991). Some may not be able to speak English and for many it is a second language, which can present major barriers to communication. Adjusting to a new culture and totally different environment can be very stressful, particularly for those who have moved from a developing country or for those who lack the support of their extended family. Some immigrant families may choose to live in an area where their community is already well established with its own religious centres, shops, newspapers and support groups. Adaptation to the new country is easier if at least one adult member of the family can speak and write English and has a profession or skill appropriate to life in Britain (Black, 1987).

In some Asian cultures the man is seen as the breadwinner and the woman is expected to stay at home or not go out without a male escort. The immigrant woman has thus little opportunity to experience the culture of the adopted country and it may be difficult for her to attend classes to learn English. Some women of Muslim and Hindu religious backgrounds may come to Britain following an arranged marriage, so they have also to adjust to marriage and a new family. Racial harassment and discrimination contribute to the stress experienced by some immigrants to the UK. Health care providers do not always consider the needs of ethnic minorities (Mares *et al.*, 1985; Bowler, 1993).

There are various health risks for immigrants depending on their race, religion, culture and country of origin. They may suffer from dietary deficiencies such as vitamin D, calcium and iron. These may arise because of the restrictions of a vegetarian diet as with Hindu and Rastafarian religions. When the mother is vitamin D deficient, her infant is also at risk if fed with unfortified milk or breastfed without vitamin supplementation. Vitamin D deficiency can also be the result of inadequate exposure of the skin to sunshine. People who emigrate from countries with a hot climate may find Britain too cold and as a result wrap themselves up and stay indoors. Muslim tradition requires women and girls to cover their limbs and heads which further prevents synthesis of vitamin D by the available sunshine in Britain.

A deficiency of vitamin D can cause hypocalcaemia and rickets. Symptoms of this condition include limb pain and backache, bending of weight-bearing bones and other bony malformations. It may affect the female pelvis and result in cephalo-pelvic disproportion. Iron-deficiency anaemia can also occur when immigrant families in poor socio-economic circumstances cannot afford to buy iron-rich foods. It may also be as a consequence of parasitic disease, such as hookworm infestation, acquired before emigration or on return visits to tropical countries. Other acquired tropical infections may include *Giardia lamblia, Entamoeba histolytica,* filaria, tuberculosis, malaria, typhoid and dysentery. Many may be asymptomatic and specific blood tests and stool microscopy may be indicated for those whose history suggests a risk (Carroll *et al.,* 1993).

Thalassaemia and sickle cell disease are major haemoglobin abnormalities which may affect immigrant communities. Those mainly affected by thalassaemia are Greeks, Greek Cypriots, Southern Italians and Asians. Sickle cell disease affects mainly black people who originate from Central and West Africa (including Afro-Caribbean) and parts of Asia. The midwife should be able to discuss the implications of these diseases with pregnant women who may be affected and preferably before conception. She should encourage them to have haemoglobinopathy screening and, if positive, their partners also. If both partners are found to be carriers or if the partner is not available for screening, the potential parents need to be counselled and offered fetal screening.

The midwife needs to be aware of the potential health problems experienced by immigrant women and their families, so that effective counselling, screening and treatment can be offered. The diversity of women's lifestyles needs to be recognized. It cannot be presumed that women from particular religious or cultural backgrounds all behave the same or have the same beliefs (Phoenix, 1991). Good communication is essential for assessment of individual needs as regards health education and promotion. Language support and advocacy need to be available to women who do not speak English. Some health authorities provide this service in the form of linkworkers and translators who are able to interpret and communicate for women. Health education and information about pregnancy and childbirth leaflets have been interpreted into a variety of different languages by the Health Education Authority. Some Community Health Councils also provide translators.

FORCES FAMILIES

Women who are married to men in the army, navy and airforce face life experiences which are very different from those of other married women. Many are subject to frequent residential mobility over which they have little or no control. The needs of the respective force take precedence over personal and family needs. Frequent mobility inhibits the maintenance of stable social networks and moves wives away from their family of origin. Their career development is jeopardized as they have to leave and enter the labour market with each move and are more likely to be full-time housewives. They may also lack support from their husbands due to frequent and sometimes unplanned separation. This 'intermittent husband syndrome' can result in acute psychological strain and lead to symptoms of depression and anxiety as well as sexual problems. When husbands are on active service, wives may have additional worries for their safety. All of these factors can contribute to the stress experienced by forces families. The lack of support networks may affect the general coping ability of wives dealing with marital and military life stress. However, the evidence suggests that in the armed forces the wives learn to cope with these stresses (Anson *et al.,* 1993; Martin and Ickovics, 1987).

There is evidence that children born to army families may be affected by the stresses mentioned above, as visits to the family doctor have been found to be significantly more frequent than controls (Anson *et al.,* 1993). The infant mortality rate has been found to be higher in children of army families than in the general population. In one study, a higher rate of sudden infant death syndrome was found in babies whose fathers were in the army (Rao and Hoinville, 1988). In another study, the infant death rate was found to be three times higher in army families than in controls, yet there were no cases of sudden infant death syndrome (Kimmance and Waters, 1992). It may be that isolation and lack of family support for their mothers contribute to the higher mortality rate in these babies, but more research into the reasons is needed.

YOUNG TEENAGERS

Teenage pregnancy is generally seen as a major problem in the Western world. In England and Wales, the rate of conceptions for teenagers under the age of 16 has risen steadily from the late 1950s and more steeply following the Abortion Act of 1967. By 1991 the rate had reached 9.3 per 1000 girls of this age-group, with total conceptions amounting to 7829, according to OPCS figures. One of the targets in the *Health of the Nation* report is to halve the conception rate in girls under 16 by the year 2000 (DOH, 1991).

Various factors contribute to teenage pregnancy. Society's attitude towards premarital sex and illegitimate birth has changed considerably since the 1950s and many couples nowadays co-habit outside of marriage. There is an emphasis on sexuality in the media and in pop music. Peer pressure can be a powerful influence and some girls may wish to appear more grown-up by having a sexual relationship. Teenagers' knowledge about contraception varies. They may not understand the need for contraception, not like the idea of using contraceptives or not wish to acknowledge openly that they are sexually active. When contraceptives are used they may not be used correctly. Pregnancy may be planned by some girls who have an unhappy home life when it is seen as a means of escape (Mills, 1990). It may provide a boost to self-esteem to be pregnant with the image of motherhood seen as more romantic than realistic. The young mother is in many ways still a child herself and very needy emotionally if deprived of love in her own childhood. She would therefore be unable to meet her baby's emotional needs (Birch, 1992).

Early sexual activity places the teenager at increased risk of contracting sexually transmitted diseases and pelvic infection with resultant infertility. It also increases the risk of developing cervical carcinoma in later years, especially if it is with more than one partner (Barron, 1986). Pregnancy can have implications for the health of the young teenager and may be associated with social, psychological, educational and legal problems. It has much less impact on the older teenager, who has reached the age of consent, completed her basic education and is more physically and emotionally mature.

The young teenager is more likely to present later in pregnancy. She may not know the signs of pregnancy or have not yet established a regular menstrual cycle. She may also be afraid that her boyfriend will be prosecuted for having intercourse with a girl below the age of 16. Her pregnancy may even be the result of an incestuous relationship with a close male relative and she may be afraid to acknowledge the fact for fear of the consequences. More than 50% of young teenagers opt for abortion. Many of these are in the second trimester because such pregnancies go unrecognized for a time. The immature cervix resists dilatation and as a result, therapeutic abortion carries more risk of cervical laceration. This in turn leads to a greater risk of spontaneous abortion in subsequent pregnancy (Russell, 1988).

There are increased risks also when pregnancy is continued though they are diminished greatly with good antenatal care. Pregnancy-induced hypertension and iron-deficiency anaemia are slightly increased. The baby is at increased risk of low birthweight, congenital malformation and perinatal death. This may be as a consequence of low socio-economic status, smoking and alcohol or drug abuse. Poor dietary habits in adolescents may be the cause of anaemia, especially in those from a socially deprived background (Mills, 1990) (see Chapter 19).

Teenage pregnancy is more common in lower socio-economic groups and the whole family can be affected by the arrival of a new baby. Family relationships can be placed under great strain because of extra demands on space and finances. In the UK a family are expected to support a girl under 16. They will be receiving child benefit for her and can claim for the new baby when it is born. The girl herself will not be able to claim any benefits. Under the 1993 Child Support Act, the baby's father would be required to contribute financially. If he himself is a teenager, the prospects of his being able to do this are small. The girl's parents may decide to accept her baby into the family and raise the child as their own. This can sometimes lead to difficulties. The girl may resent their control over her baby and the child may become confused about who is the natural mother. Sometimes parents reject their daughter and she may have to leave home and go into residential care. Adoption may be considered as in the best interests of the baby or as a way of providing a fresh start for the young teenager though it can mean emotional difficulties such as grief and guilt. Future employment prospects can be seriously affected by pregnancy at an early age. Many leave school during pregnancy and do not return to complete their education (Russell, 1988).

Prevention of teenage pregnancy is an important aspect of health education in schools. The aim should be to enable teenagers to make informed, responsible decisions about their sexual behaviour. Boys and girls should have opportunities to discuss and learn about relevant issues, such as sex and reproduction, sexually transmitted diseases, contraception and human relationships including parenthood. Teachers should be appropriately experienced in the field of health education, such as health visitors, midwives and nurses.

The midwife should be sensitive to the needs and feelings of the pregnant teenager. It may be embarrassing and intimidating for the young girl to attend the antenatal clinic alongside more mature women. In some areas, midwives have set up teenage antenatal clinics and parent education classes which help to overcome this problem. A social worker, health visitor and dietician may be involved to give advice as required. The atmosphere should be kept as informal as possible so as to encourage attendance for antenatal care. Peer support should be fostered so the girls can get to know one another and develop friendships. They are often in great need of parent education, yet are reluctant to attend. When classes are specifically geared towards

teenagers, attendance and motivation to learn can be improved. Continuity of care for pregnancy, labour and postnatal period is particularly important for the young teenager so that she is familiar with her carers and trusts them. It is important that the girl continues her education if possible and she should be encouraged and supported to do so, especially by her family. Educational provision for pregnant schoolgirls varies from one authority to another. Some authorites provide special tuition, others are wary of being seen to be accepting of teenage pregnancy and its effect on their reputation. The cost of crèche facilities is another consideration which may be prohibitive (Mills, 1990).

There are various agencies and charities which exist to provide help and support for pregnant teenagers. In the UK, Youth Support, a self-funding charity, is working to overcome the problems of inadequate education and support of pregnant schoolgirls and other teenagers. Its membership is drawn from various professions including medical, social work, teaching, nursing and midwifery. It provides a forum for professionals to discuss adolescent health and welfare as well as education for professionals involved in working with teenagers. Youth Support House in south-east London offers residential care for pregnant girls and school-age mothers. There, they receive education, support and psychotherapy. The aim is that they are equipped to survive and succeed in the world.

References

Abramson, L.Y., Seligman, M.E.P. & Teasdale, J.D. (1978) Learned helplessness in humans: critique and reformulation. *J. Abnormal Psychol.* 87: 49–74.

Aggleton, P. (1990) *Society Now Health.* London: Routledge.

Anderson, P., Cremona, A., Paton, A., Turner, C. & Wallace, P. (1993) The risk of alcohol. *Addiction* 88: 1493–1508.

Andrews, B. & Brown, G.W. (1988) Marital violence in the community. *Br. J. Psychiatry* 153: 305–312.

Anson, O., Rosenzweig, A. & Shwarzmann, P. (1993) The health of women married to men in regular army service: women who cannot afford to be ill. *Women & Health* 20: 33–45.

Atkinson, R.L., Atkinson, R.G., Smith, E.E. & Bem, D.J. (1993) *Introduction to Psychology,* 11th edn. Fort Worth, Texas: Harcourt Brace Jovanovich.

Baddeley, S. (1993) Aquanatal advantages. *Modern Midwife* July/August: 16.

Baddeley, S. & Green, S. (1992) Physical education and the pregnant woman: the way forward. *Midwives Chronicle & Nursing Notes* 105(1253): 144–145.

Barker, P. (1991) Co-dependency caring chameleons. *Nursing Times* 87: 51, 55–57.

Barron, S.L. (1986) Sexual activity in girls under 16 years of age. *Br. J. Obstet. Gynaecol.* 93: 787–792.

Becker, M.H., Haefner, D.P., Kasl, S.V., Kirscht, J.P., Maiman, L.A. & Rosenstock I.M. (1977) Selected psychological models and correlates of individual heath-related behaviours. *Medical Care* 15: 27–46.

Bewley, C.A. & Gibbs, A. (1991) Violence in pregnancy. *Midwifery* 7: 107–112.

Birch, D. (1992) Teenage pregnancy a problem for the nineties. *Novum* 50: 8.

Bohn, D.K. (1990) Domestic violence and pregnancy implications for practice. *J. Nurse-Midwifery* 35(2): 86–98.

Bowler, I. (1993) Stereotypes of women of Asian descent in midwifery: some evidence. *Midwifery* 9: 7–16.

Black, J.A. (1987) Paediatric problems in the Asian community. *Update* 15 December: 1300.

Bradshaw, J. (1988) *Bradshaw on the Family.* Deerfield Beach. Florida: Health Communications Inc.

Bullows, J. & Penfold, A. (1993) Tackling dependency women and alcohol. *Nursing Times* 89(2): 27–29.

Carbon, R. (1994) Female athletes. *Br. Med. J.* 309: 254–258.

Carroll, B., Dow, C., Snashall, D., Marshall, T. & Chiodini, P.L. (1993) Post-tropical screening: how useful is it? *Br. Med. J.* 307: 541.

Chadwick, J. (1993) Alcohol in pregnancy. *Modern Midwife* March/April: 19–21.

Chez, R.A. (1988) Woman battering. *Am. J. Obstet. Gynecol.* 158(1): 1–4.

Clemenger, M. (1993) Under the influence: women and alcohol. *Nursing Times* 89(2): 24–26.

Cook, A. (1995) Ecstasy (MDMA): alerting users to the dangers. *Nursing Times* 91(16): 32–33.

Das Gupta, S. (1990) Extent and pattern of drug abuse and dependence. In Ghodse, H. & Maxwell, D. (eds) *Substance Abuse and Dependence – an Introduction for the Caring Professions.* London: Macmillan.

DOH (Department of Health) (1991) *The Health of the Nation: A Consultative Document for Health in England.* London: HMSO.

Dummer Clark, M.J. (1984) *Community Nursing Health Care for Today and Tomorrow.* Virginia, USA: Reston Publishing.

Durward, L. (ed.) (1990) *Traveller Mothers and Babies.* London: Maternity Alliance.

Edelman, C.L. & Mandle, C.L. (1990) *Health Promotion throughout the Lifespan*, 2nd edn. St Louis, Missouri: C.V. Mosby.

Enkin, M., Keirse, M.J.N.C. & Chalmers, I. (1989) *A Guide to Effective Care in Pregnancy and Childbirth.* Oxford: Oxford University Press.

Friend, B. (1993) The enemy within. *Nursing Times* 89(23): 16.

Gilbert, R.E., Wigfield, P.J., Fleming, P.J. *et al.* (1995) Bottle feeding and the sudden infant death syndrome. *Br. Med. J.* 310: 88.

Graham, H. (1984) *Women Health and the Family.* Herts: Wheatsheaf Books.

Green, J.M., Kitzinger, J.V. & Coupland, V.A. (1990) Stereotypes of childbearing women: a look at some evidence. *Midwifery* 6: 125–132.

Gross, R.D. (1992) *Psychology The Science of Mind and Behaviour*, 2nd edn. London: Hodder & Stoughton.

Hartz, C., Plant, M. & Watts, M. (1990) *Alcohol and Health: A Handbook for Nurses, Midwives and Health Visitors.* London: The Medical Council on Alcoholism.

Hedegaard, M., Henriksen, T.B., Sabroe, S. & Secher, N.J. (1993) Psychological distress in pregnancy and preterm delivery. *Br. Med. J.* 307: 234–239.

Jacobson, B., Nyberg, K., Grondbladh, L., Eklund, G., Bygdeman, M. & Rydberg, U. (1990) Opiate addiction in adult offspring through possible imprinting after obstetric treatment. *Br. Med. J.* 301: 1067–1070.

Johns, A. (1990) What is dependence? In Ghodse, H. & Maxwell, D. (eds) *Substance Abuse and Dependence – an Introduction for the Caring Professions.* London: Macmillan.

Judge, K. & Benzeval, M. (1993) Health inequalities: new concerns about the children of single mothers. *Br. Med. J.* 306: 677–680.

Keleher, K.C. (1991) Occupational health: how work environments can affect reproductive capacity and outcome. *Nurse Practitioner* January: 23–37.

Kimmance, K.J. & Waters, W.E. (1992) Infant mortality and army families: a case-control study. *Br. Med. J.* 305(6863): 1197.

Lau, R.R. (1982) Origins of health locus of control beliefs. *J. Pers. Soc. Psychol.* 42(2): 322–334.

Ledward, R.S., Hawkins, D.F. & Stern, L. (1991) *Drug Treatment in Obstetrics*, 2nd edn. London: Chapman & Hall Medical.

Lloyd, L. (1994) The Criminal Justice Bill: Implications for midwifery practice. *Br. J. Midwifery* 2(11): 559–561.

Long, A. & Mullen, B. (1994) Exploration of women's perception of major factors that contributed to their alcohol abuse. *J. Adv. Nursing* 19: 623–639.

Madden, S. (1990) Effects of drugs of dependence. In Ghodse, H. & Maxwell, D. (eds) *Substance Abuse and Dependence – an Introduction for the Caring Professions.* London: Macmillan.

Mares, P., Henley, A. & Baxter, C. (1985) *Healthcare in Multiracial Britain.* Cambridge: Health Education Council and National Extension College Trust Ltd.

Markos, A.R. (1990) Use of conventional seat-belts in pregnancy. *Midwife Health Visitor & Community Nurse* 26(7&8): 256.

Marteau, T.M. (1989a) Health beliefs and attributions. In Broome, A.K. (ed.) *Health Psychology Processes and Applications.* London: Chapman & Hall.

Marteau, T.M. (1989b) Psychological costs of screening. *Br. Med. J.* 299: 527.

Martin, J.A. & Ickovics, J.R. (1987) The effects of stress on the psychological well-being of army wives: initial findings from a longitudinal study. *J. Human Stress* 13: 108.

Maternity Alliance (1991) *Know your Rights 3: Pregnant at Work.* London: Maternity Alliance.

Maxwell, D. (1990) Medical complications of substance abuse. In Ghodse, H. & Maxwell, D. (eds) *Substance Abuse and Dependence – an Introduction for the Caring Professions.* London: Macmillan.

McGuire, P.K., Cope, H. & Fahy, T.A. (1994) Diversity of psychopathy associated with use of 3,4-methylenedioxymethamphetamine ('Ecstasy'). *Br. J. Psychiat.* 165(3): 391–395.

McMahon, B. (1993) Time for a change in direction: effects of poverty on ill health and service provision. *Professional Nurse* June: 610–613.

Mills, M. (1990) Teenage Mothers. In Alexander, J., Levy, V. & Roch, S. (eds) *Postnatal Care A Research-based Approach.* London: Macmillan.

Morgan, M., Calnan, M. & Manning, N. (1985) *Sociological Approaches to Health and Medicine.* Beckenham Kent: Croom Helm.

Niven, N. (1989) *Health Psychology – an Introduction for Nurses and other Health Care Professionals.* Edinburgh: Churchill Livingstone.

O'Connor, B. (1994) Hazards associated with the recreational drug 'Ecstasy'. *Br. J. Hosp. Med.* 52(10): 507–514.

OPCS (Office of Population Censuses and Surveys) (1991) *1991 Census GB Report Part 1.* London: OPCS.

Phoenix, A. (1991) Black women and the maternity services.

In Garcia, J., Kilpatrick, R. & Richards, M. (eds) *The Politics of Maternity Care*. London: Clarendon Press.

Pill, R. & Stott, N.C.H. (1982) Concepts of illness causation and responsibility: some preliminary data from a sample of working class mothers. *Soc. Sci. Med.* **16**: 43–52.

Pill, R. & Stott, N. (1987) Development of a measure of potential health behaviour, a salience of lifestyle index. *Soc. Sci. Med.* **24**(2): 125–134.

Plant, M. (1990) Maternal alcohol and tobacco use during pregnancy. In Alexander, J., Levy, V. & Roch, S. (eds) *Antenatal Care A Research-based Approach*. London: Macmillan.

Prince, J. & Adams, M.E. (1978) *Minds, Mothers and Midwives. The Psychology of Childbirth*. Edinburgh: Churchill Livingstone.

Rao, M. & Hoinville, E. (1988) Review of postperinatal mortality in a health district with a garrison town. *Br. Med. J.* **297**: 662.

Reid, T. (1993) Partners in care. *Nursing Times* **89**(33): 28–31.

Reid, M. & Garcia, J. (1989) Women's views of care during pregnancy and childbirth. In Chalmers, I., Keirse, M. & Enkin, M. (eds) *Effective Care in Pregnancy and Childbirth*. Oxford: Oxford University Press.

Rose, V. (1993) On the road. *Nursing Times* **89**(33): 31.

Rosenstock, I.M. (1974) Historical origins of the health belief model. In Becker, M.H. (ed.) *The Health Belief Model and Personal Health Behaviour*. Thorofare, New Jersey: Charles B. Slack.

Rosevear, S.K., Holt, D.W., Lee, T.D., Ford, C.L., Wardle, P.G. & Hull, M.G.R. (1992) Smoking and decreased fertilisation rates in vitro. *Lancet* **340**: 1195–1196.

Rotter, J.B. (1966) Generalized expectancies for internal versus external control of re-inforcement. *Psychological Monographs* **80**: 1.

Royal College of Psychiatrists (1986) *Alcohol Our Favourite Drug*. London: Tavistock Publications.

Russell, J.K. (1988) Early teenage pregnancy. *Maternal and Child Health* February: 43–46.

Savage, W. & Reader, F. (1984) Sexual activity during pregnancy. *Midwife, Health Visitor and Community Nurse* **20**(11): 398.

Seedhouse, D. (1986) *Health: The Foundations for Achievement*. Chichester: J Wiley & Sons.

Sheldon, T. (1995) Agony and ecstasy. *Nursing Times* **91**(44): 14–15.

Stott, N.C.H. & Pill, R.M. (1990) *Making Changes – a Study of Working Class Mothers and the Changes Made in their Health-related Behaviour over 5 Years*. Cardiff: University of Wales College of Medicine.

Thistlethwaite, J. (1989) Exercise in pregnancy: what advice should we give? *Maternal and Child Health* November: 368–370.

Townsend, P. & Davidson, N. (1992) The Black Report. In *Inequalities in Health* (Townsend, P. & Davidson, N. eds.), New Edition Revised and Updated. London: Penguin.

Walker, L. (1984) *The Battered Woman Syndrome*. New York: Springer Publishing.

Walsh, R. & Redman, S. (1993) Smoking cessation in pregnancy: do effective programmes exist? *Health Promotion International* **8**(2): 111.

Wells, B. (1990) Psychological interventions. In Ghodse, H. & Maxwell, D. (eds) *Substance Abuse and Dependence – An Introduction for the Caring Professions*. London: Macmillan.

Whitehead, M. (1992) The Health Divide. In (Townsend, P. & Davidson, N. eds.) *Inequalities in Health*, New Edition Revised and Updated. London: Penguin.

Wolff, K., Hay, A.W.M., Sherlock, K. & Conner M. (1995) Contents of 'Ecstasy'. *Lancet* **346**: 1100–1101.

24

Education for Parenthood

> In the demands they make upon your body and soul, few careers are more exacting than that of a parent.
> (Spiers, 1950)

As any parent will agree, parenting skills are as complex as life itself. They involve providing for the holistic needs of the child into adulthood and few people are fully prepared for the task at the arrival of their first child. Parents require guidance, advice and teaching that is directed towards their needs to help them cope with the demands of parenthood.

Historical Background

The provision of formal education for parenthood in the UK emerged from a concern for public health during the second half of the nineteenth century (Coombes and Schonveld, 1992). In the 1950s various books were written which attempted to provide complete and comprehensive guides for mothers. These authoritative works presented advice from experts in every branch of maternal care and childcare and they were welcomed as it was recognized that something was needed to fill the gap left by the decline of the extended family due to social and demographic changes. New mothers at this time were considered to be isolated, ignorant and unsupported and education for women was seen as important for the nation. At the same time, teaching about the body and its functions became acceptable.

The National Health Service began to provide mothercraft classes in the 1950s. Later it was recognized that in the absence of traditional support networks, the father was the primary source of social support. This led to the inclusion of fathers in 'preparation for baby' groups and eventually the arrival of 'parentcraft classes'.

As childbirth became increasingly medicalized in the decades that followed, parentcraft started to encompass information designed to promote compliance with hospital routines and procedures, and tended to encourage parents to depend on the 'experts' (Priest and Schott, 1991; Coombes and Schonveld, 1992). The Report of the Expert Maternity Group, *Changing Childbirth* (DOH, 1993), however, promoted the move towards a flexible approach. It emphasized the partnership between parents and professionals, underlining the need for a more negotiated and parent-led approach to care. This changes the emphasis from a teacher-led instruction (didactic) to a more facilitative, flexible approach, giving choice and widening the scope to target those who would otherwise be unlikely to attend parent education, such as teenagers and parents from lower socio-economic groups.

Increasingly it has been recognized that emotional as well as physical needs should be addressed during sessions. The trend in classes is now to concentrate less on the 'craft' and more on sharing feelings, emotions and experiences, and 'parenthood education' has become the preferred term.

It is valuable to reflect upon the historical basis of the aims and delivery of classes as approaches and issues remain in practice that are questionable in meeting the needs of today's parents. Many historical practices which continue have an adverse effect on the quality of preparation for parenthood.

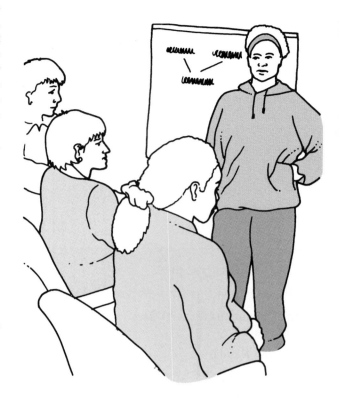

Figure 1   Educational quality poor; less didactic methods of teaching required.

Critique of the Quality of Parent Education

The 'expert' authoritarian advice-giver is still found in practice today. As O'Mearea (1993) points out, 'Childbirth educators tend to be action-centred practitioners who concentrate their efforts on teaching and instruction.' In their report *Life will Never be the Same Again*, Coombes and Schonveld (1992) found that in general the educational quality of parenthood classes in England left much to be desired. In particular, they reported that:

▶ Educational quality is poor.
▶ Midwives underestimate the educational opportunities in care settings.
▶ Health professionals tend to ignore or skim over social, emotional and psychological needs of parents.
▶ Certain groups are missing out, in particular young,

single, lower socioeconomic classes, ethnic minority groups, and men.
▶ There is a lack of information and advice in early pregnancy
▶ There is tribalism evident between professionals involved in education for parenthood
▶ Management support is lacking in key areas of training development and resources.

On the other hand, Coombes and Schonveld also found that change had occurred in isolated areas and that there were many examples of exciting innovation and effective use of participative group methods. Nevertheless, classes remain poorly attended and the same old critique by professional carers was expressed that 'those who need it' – i.e. lower socio-economic, single, young, ethnic minority clients – do not attend.

One of the main reasons that these parents miss out may be that they experience inappropriate interactions with professionals. Kirkham (1993: 3) looked at how midwives disable the client from asking questions by using unconscious behaviour patterns that suppress interaction. The non-verbal communications we send during care are often 'do not disturb' messages. Clients often say that practitioners appear to be pressed for time. Thus the way in which professionals interact during delivery of care is the likely cause of lack of parent education on a one-to-one basis. It is not that the midwife is unwilling or that the woman is uninterested.

Midwives tend to underestimate the educational opportunities in care settings. In their report, Coombes and Schonveld (1992) found lack of information and advice in early pregnancy. Anxieties and worries of parents, particularly about test results, were not addressed. Care is focused on medical and physical health, and our emphasis is still on the body and its functions. These are subjects which are taught in school, portrayed on television and readily found in books. Yet the social and emotional needs of parents are unmet.

Perkins (1980) and Coombes and Schonveld (1992) found that parents are keen to address feelings, they want to explore negative as well as positive experiences and yet health professionals tend to ignore or skim over social, emotional and psychological aspects in classes. There is 'notable lack of knowledge concerning psychological factors involved in the transition to parenthood . . . [physiotherapists and midwives are] relatively untrained in teaching methods of value in childbirth education' (Chalmers *et al.*, 1987). Indeed, there seems

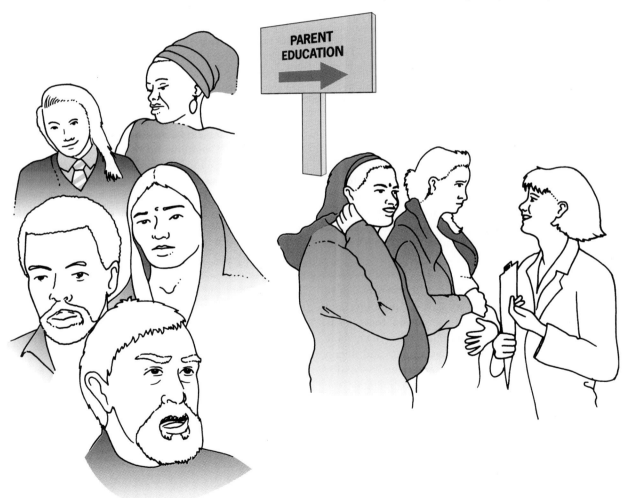

Figure 2   Certain parents are missing out.

to be an undercurrent of interprofessional rivalry with the three main groups – midwives, health visitors and physiotherapists – as to which is best suited to take the role of parenthood educator. This tribalism can result in disagreements and is wholly counterproductive.

Another group of parents who are missing out on education for parenthood are men. In general, women are seen as the target group for parenthood classes and such education is less accessible to men (Coombes and Schonveld, 1992). The social support required by new mothers – physical and emotional support from family, friends and professionals – and the need to involve partners/fathers in parenthood education was recognized in the middle of this century. Social support has been shown to be important in promoting better physical and emotional adjustment to parenthood (Nichols and Smith-Humenick, 1988).

Coombes and Schonveld (1992) criticized the managers of parenthood educators. Support was found to be lacking in key areas of training, development and resources. To help managers to improve access to quality parent education, a separate publication for managers is available from the Health Education Authority (Rowe and Mahoney, 1993).

In his book *Antenatal Illustrated*, published in 1955, Dick Read put forward recommended principles for preparation for parenthood. Although now outdated in many respects, in particular in its use of imagery, in other ways Dick Read's book was way ahead of its time, suggesting making use of care settings, using small groups for discussion, and encouraging women to air their problems.

Do keep these classes friendly, informal and give plenty of time for women to ask questions and ventilate their problems. It is during these chats whilst patients are being weighed and shown some of the illustrations that they learn most and obtain confidence in the replies they are given. Secondly, do keep the classes small in order to maintain the personal touch. Eight or ten in a class is the maximum number that one instructress can handle adequately, and is ideal from the patients' point of view.

(Dick Read, 1955)

With a more humanized care setting, the opportunities for parenthood education can be more effectively utilized.

The Role of Midwives in Providing Education

During initial midwifery education, one of the duties student midwives are prepared for is to undertake parenthood education (UKCC, 1994). The midwives' responsibility and ability to educate is often said to be good on a one-to-one basis, but when asked to take up this role with groups, they feel ill-prepared and seek support. Perhaps as midwifery education programmes incorporate more facilitative teaching methods, including seminar and peer presentations, they will prepare future midwives more effectively for their role as educators. The current changes in the provision of care will also help midwives who will know and better understand their clients.

The use of small teams of midwives and provision of continuity of care for clients recommended in *Changing Childbirth* (DOH, 1993) will give greater opportunity for personal contact between midwives and their clients. Perhaps parents will then find it easier to express their fears and anxieties freely to their named midwife. Some concern has been expressed that the recommendations by the Expert Committee to re-examine antenatal care and to rationalize the provision of this service may lead to less investment in education and support antenatally (Warren, 1993).

With the implementation of choices in childbirth, a social model of care which is client orientated and client centred will render the teaching of compliance to hospital rules irrelevant. For example, there is no longer any need to teach rules such as who can be present at birth, or the position to be adopted in labour. In the past, it was not uncommon for women to leave parentcraft sessions believing that procedures such as an enema and shave were necessary prior to delivery.

The market economy created as a result of recommendations from the White Paper *Working for Patients* (DOH, 1989) has resulted in a variety of changes in the provision of the maternity services. NHS classes now may consist of only three or four two-hour sessions instead of six to eight classes. In contrast, in other areas innovations such as weekend courses have been introduced to meet the needs of parents. Another innovation is the teaching of aqua-natal classes by midwives. Some progressive practitioners have chosen to teach all aspects of parenthood education – the physical, theoretical and emotional aspects – within one course. Recognizing that parent-led groups may not need the different experts to come and do 'their' session, one knowledgeable facilitator can provide the information parents seek.

These innovations demonstrate how midwives are adjusting to the needs of parents, working women and their partners. It is appreciated that the parent-led approach may need only one facilitator who has good communications and liaison with the related disciplines.

As a partner in care, a midwife may discuss the wide variety of preparation-for-parenthood sessions available, matching the client to the class. The consumer has a rich selection from which to choose (Figure 3). In addressing the needs of parents, each class provided may target a small, specialized group and/or a normative group for the geographical area. Parent education for special groups may be needed in areas where there is a large ethnic minority population, for example. In an ideal world, all would be catered for, but realistically, limited resources mean that some people will miss out.

However, particular problems and aspects can be discussed on an individual basis and information can also be supplied about other resources available, such as video loan, or referral to specialist classes such as the multiple birth monthly lecture at Queen Charlotte's Hospital in London.

Meeting Needs

Midwives and other health care professionals inevitably enter their parenthood education role with their own agenda. They may feel that it is important to cover a certain topic because of their knowledge and experience, but it is important to remember that this may or may not be useful to the parents attending – they may have other issues uppermost in their minds.

In the report *Life will Never be the Same Again*, Coombes and Schonveld (1992: 17) outlined the experiences, feelings and concerns of parents during the infant's first year. How can professionals best

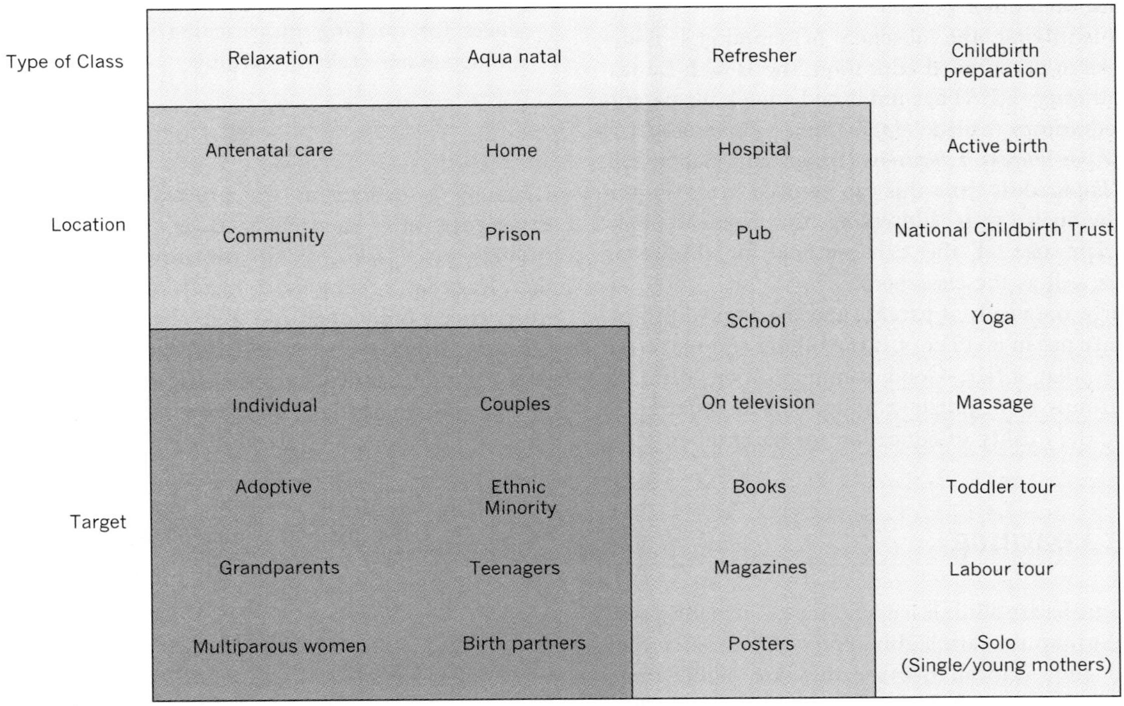

	Relaxation	Aqua natal	Refresher	Childbirth preparation
Type of Class	Relaxation	Aqua natal	Refresher	Childbirth preparation
Location	Antenatal care	Home	Hospital	Active birth
	Community	Prison	Pub	National Childbirth Trust
			School	Yoga
Target	Individual	Couples	On television	Massage
	Adoptive	Ethnic Minority	Books	Toddler tour
	Grandparents	Teenagers	Magazines	Labour tour
	Multiparous women	Birth partners	Posters	Solo (Single/young mothers)

Figure 3 A wide variety of preparation-for-parenthood resources and classes are available in different settings from which the client can choose.

provide for those needs? The broad aims of parenthood education are:

- ▶ To improve health.
- ▶ To give information and support.
- ▶ To enable preparation for labour.
- ▶ To develop confidence and parenting skills.
- ▶ To provide emotional and psychological preparation/support for the new role as parents.
- ▶ To encourage peer support.

Coombes and Schonveld suggest that these aims are too wide and that educators need to examine closely whether the needs of parents are being met. In addressing this difficulty, Parr (1996) concentrated on the area of psychological and group support to produce a programme – the Pippin programme – that aims to supplement traditional parenthood education. Pippin begins in the antenatal period and continues postnatally and the results are encouraging. 'Pippin parents develop significantly more realistic perceptions and expectations of the challenges of new parenthood' (Parr, 1996). The research also suggests that 'Pippin parents' have more positive relationships with their child and each other.

In identifying the absence of emotional issues addressed in parenthood education, the Health Education Authority (HEA) has published a book for parenthood educators called *Approaching Parenthood: A Resource for Parent Education* (Braun and Schonveld, 1993). Topic ideas from this can be used in a group or for individuals, thus addressing the need to make appropriate use of the care setting for discussing issues as well as the classroom.

Clearly, the needs of parents and the aims of professionals are not in conflict, it is the timing and perceived priorities that differ. Good communication with the client groups to negotiate a united aim is required to improve the quality of education for parenthood.

Adult Learning

Parents-to-be are adult learners; they are usually a self-selected group that are highly motivated. As such they are also quite critical. Because they are highly motivated they are more likely to be receptive to any lifestyle changes, both physical and psychological, that are advocated to improve health in pregnancy. It is helpful to bear the characteristics of the adult learner in mind.

Knowles (1984: 56) suggests that adult learners increase in self-directedness as they mature and move away from dependency as their self-concept grows. For the facilitator, Knowles' underlying assumptions about adult learners leads to the following principles in parenthood education which have been adapted from his theories.

PRINCIPLES FOR ADULT LEARNING

- ▶ It is essential that the physical and psychological climate is comfortable for parents. This will aid confidence and promote a feeling of acceptance and lack of threat, thereby encouraging participation whether they know the answer or not.
- ▶ The parents' need for self-direction is nurtured by enabling them to be in control of their learning by joint negotiation of learning goals and a parent-centred approach.
- ▶ The teaching–learning process needs to be seen as a mutual responsibility. The leader or facilitator of the group is more of a catalyst, guide and resource person.
- ▶ The facilitator needs awareness of her own preferences for teaching and learning styles as this will influence her style of teaching.

Learning

Learning is defined as the process of transforming experience into knowledge, skills, attitudes, values, feelings, etc. (Jarvis, 1995). Mezirow (1990) suggests that learning occurs as a result of *reflecting* upon experience. Individuals do not always reflect upon and learn from their experiences, however, and when this does not happen, non-learning can occur. It may be due to *presumption*, that is, a typical response to a familiar situation, *non-consideration* or *rejection*. Very simple skills learning may be non-reflective, for instance when acquired by imitation or role-modelling, but most skills learning is more complex and reflection upon the experience is a necessary part of the process.

Learning styles

The way people learn best is different for each individual. Consider experiences of formal and informal learning; the styles adopted may have a common mode despite the different setting. The example below illustrates the differences between individuals in learning styles:

> I was given written directions which were linear words. Turn left out of the drive, go over three traffic lights, at the roundabout take the first exit . . . I thanked my host and got out a map as the words had no meaning for me, I had to see the picture first.

Honey (1986) describes four learning styles:

- ► *Activists* are people who thrive on new experiences and active learning.
- ► *Reflectors* are people who prefer time for thorough exploration and review.
- ► *Pragmatists* are people who like to apply ideas to see if they work.
- ► *Theorists* are people who enjoy logical integrated information within a rational theory.

These are extreme characterizations and it is possible to enjoy all styles, but most people find they have a tendency to use one or two styles. For example, in a learning experience in parent education:

- ► the activists would like to do the baby bath themselves;
- ► the reflectors would probably like to observe a bath demonstration;
- ► the pragmatists probably would like a problem sheet whereby they would have to find out and think about how to bath a baby in different circumstances; and
- ► the theorists would probably view the baby bath like a surgical procedure and would like to know how to place the cotton balls, the temperature of the water (with thermometer), what type of towels, etc.

The parent educator needs to approach teaching with an awareness of all these differences and needs to avoid teaching only in their preferred style of learning. Group work lends itself well to meeting all these learning types. These four groups if asked to discuss and try out baby equipment together will naturally learn in their preferred style and share information with each other.

Appropriate Teaching Methods

More extensive use of group work for parent education has been widely advocated in recent years, but it seems the most common method of teaching is still the lecture. Most antenatal educationalists do a bit of chat, followed by a video and/or a discussion. This is not necessarily wrong, provided the needs of the group are met. Unfortunately, however, it is hard to promote interaction on emotional and social issues using this method. Nor will the variety of learning styles be catered for. A brief guide to some of the alternative teaching methods possible and their application are described next.

Brainstorming

This is when parents are asked to consider a topic and say or write what immediately comes to mind about it. Their thoughts are briefly recorded without comment or criticism by the facilitator on a board or paper that everyone can see. Brainstorming can also be conducted in pairs, and then fed back to the whole group. This can be a useful way of beginning negotiation of the programme for parent education or a preliminary to ascertain the main issues about pain in labour and other topics.

Buzz groups

Parents are asked to discuss a topic/issue in small groups of about three and then feed back to the whole group. This can also be used for negotiating the course content. In this way even the less confident members of the group will contribute.

Quizzes

A fun set of questions can act as an icebreaker. Stock-taking worksheets can provide a starter for discussion. For example, to begin an infant feeding discussion, a list of questions on the facts, feelings and myths of breastfeeding can be posed, then responses shared with other members of the group.

Birth stories

These are used as case studies, fictitious ones being built up. Parts of the story are distributed and the parents are asked to discuss the circumstances. When they have discussed the situation fully the next part of the story is given. This helps parents to consider realistic situations, test out ideas and explore attitudes.

Problem-solving

Realistic problems are posed for small groups of parents to solve. Such topics as 'Your waters break in the supermarket. What do you do?' 'Your baby only sleeps two hours at a time and is now six weeks old. What do you do?' This approach encourages self-direction and self-investigation of resources available.

Snowballing

This is begun by allowing time for thought on a topic individually, followed by sharing in pairs, then fours, eight and perhaps 16. Each stage has a task which builds on the one before. An example might be a discussion about pain and coping in labour. Individually, the parents are asked to consider their most painful experience. Then they share it with the person next to them and discuss their reactions to pain and physiological response. In groups of four the parents then discuss labour and how they intend to cope with pain.

Games

Games that are successful often use the rules of well-known games such as Trivial Pursuit or Snakes and Ladders (Aikman and Murphy-Black, 1993). For parenthood education a variety of games has been developed to explore many topics. A popular variation is the 'grab bag', in which a selection of items of equipment used in labour (either real or cardboard cut-outs) are placed in a bag. Participants dip in the bag, pull out a piece of equipment, an amnihook, for example, identify it and then discuss their feelings.

Learning in Groups

It is important for the parent educator to understand the group process as it has a strong influence on learning, affecting motivation, providing mutual support and friendship.

There are many advantages of learning in groups. Group discussion helps to explore and clarify issues, clear up misunderstandings and resolve problems. There are also the social benefits; as group cohesion is established, mutual support is nurtured and group members are able to support each other rather than relying on the leader. Skilful, democratic leadership can promote a heightened sense of sensitivity to others within the group and a greater tolerance of other viewpoints. Motivation to learn is increased and parents develop insights into their own feelings and

behaviours and those of others. All these factors help to promote effective learning in groups.

Problems may arise in groups, however, and a skilful group leader should be perceptive to feelings and situations, and thus be both participant and observer. Occasionally there are one or two people who monopolize or dominate the group and this can give rise to feelings of frustration in other group members, especially if the facilitator does not intervene. Intervention may take the form of thanking the vocal parent for her or his contributions and then making it clear that you would like to give others the opportunity to express their views.

Another problem which may occur is a low level of participation from the group as a whole. This could be in response to a rather autocratic style of leadership, in which case the midwife needs to review her approach as a facilitator. Other reasons include talking about issues which are frightening, or seem irrelevant and unimportant to the group, or perhaps there is some conflict amongst members which has not been resolved. There are often one or two quiet or inarticulate members of a group who feel uncomfortable if pushed to contribute to discussion before they feel ready, although they usually participate in work in pairs, buzz groups or other small group sessions.

GROUP PROCESS

There are several models of the group process (Satow and Evans, 1983). The most often quoted is Tuckman's model of 'Forming, Storming, Norming and Performing' (Satow and Evans, 1983; Nichols and Smith-Humenick, 1988). In any group the members who come to meet for the first time begin by being polite to each other when their relationships are *forming*. By the end of six sessions, the group process has usually just become comfortable. Parents know each other well enough to chat spontaneously and have reached the *norming* stage. Few parenthood education groups will go through a *storming* stage, when they challenge and confront each other and the leader. Those groups that reach the *performing* stage are often groups that continue to meet for months or years. This stage may occur with those who continue to meet once the main group has disbanded. Sometimes good friendships develop between the parents and often between the children as well which may continue for years.

In the first session of a parent education programme it is useful to avoid sensitive topics until the parents know each other better. The better people know one another, the more comfortable the group. The way in which the leader accepts them and treats self-disclosure will influence how trusting and safe the group becomes. Creating a trusting environment is not easy, but some suggested factors that indicate success are listed here. A trusting environment is usually one in which:

▶ the members feel their values, beliefs, rights and practices are respected;
▶ confidentiality is maintained;
▶ feelings of acceptance are promoted;
▶ communication is open; and
▶ assumptions about others are avoided.

Other factors for consideration are the mix of social class, race and religion. A trusting, supportive group will minimize any misunderstandings that may arise. Small group interaction will vary because of the factors which influence group interaction. All these need to be kept in mind by the parent educator. If resources allow, it may be beneficial to create a new special group to allow, for example, single parents to be more comfortable discussing their different needs.

Parenthood education may be facilitated in closed or open groups. Priest and Schott (1991) outline the advantages and disadvantages of these groups. An *open group* is one in which the group members have an open invitation to attend and often the individuals and total number of parents which arrive are unknown to the leader. An example of this is an early pregnancy group, or a fathers' evening. A *closed group* is a regular, small group of known parents expected to attend over a defined period of time. The group dynamics will be different for these two types of group and the parenthood educator needs to approach them differently.

Closed groups

The first step in promoting the group process is to plan the first session. One suggestion is described here.

Planning the first session   The first thing to do is to reflect on the philosophy for the course (Deane-Gray and Nunnerley, 1988) and make a list of the objectives. For the first session, the following may be on your list (Batchelor and Napper, 1989):

1   The parents will begin to know each other and the leader.

2   The parents will state their expectations of the course and content of the programme.
3   The parents will receive answers to their most urgent questions.
4   The leader will give important health information perceived as essential if the parents have not raised the issue.

Many people are reluctant to talk to strangers. The facilitator's role is to help parents overcome this barrier and to encourage more active participation by individuals within the group as they become more comfortable with each other. Ideas on icebreakers can be found in *The Gamester's Handbook* (Brands, 1982), *Antenatal Skills Training* (Murphy-Black and Faulkner, 1988) and *Leading Antenatal Classes* (Priest and Schott, 1991).

The facilitator needs to consider how warm-up exercises will be received by the group members. This will depend on the type of clientele. If there is an odd number and a pairs exercise is chosen then a threesome may be used, or the facilitator may join in. In couples groups separating the men and women may produce better interaction, as like sexes may have more in common.

Some tips for success are as follows:

▶ *Make everyone feel comfortable*: An uncomfortable silence while waiting for parents to arrive can be filled by some quiet music. This will make it feel less awkward. Begin by introducing yourself, explaining the location of the toilets, availability of refreshment, timing of breaks and the length of the course. This gives people time to settle down and get used to the environment.
▶ *Explain why it would be beneficial for them to get to know each other*: The parents are a group and conversation is easier amongst friends. They will be sharing similar experiences and have much in common. They may find themselves sitting next to a neighbour.
▶ *Explain and give clear instructions on each exercise*: Introduce the icebreaker, explaining the method you have chosen. You might underline the value of participating in the exercise by pointing out the silence that reigned while you were all waiting for everyone to arrive. *Repeat the instructions again.* This helps people to internalize what is being asked of them. Organize the parents as required for the exercise chosen. *Check understanding one more time.* Before moving on, check individually that they have

completed the exercise to their satisfaction. Then obtain feedback or build on the exercise.

Open groups

In a lecture environment or an open group, interaction can be improved by encouraging the group members to talk to each other. This is done by suggesting that they lean over or turn around and tell the person near them how they feel about being pregnant/expecting a baby, or perhaps how they met their partner. Breaking the 'ice' is the first step in the process of creating a cohesive group.

Facilitating and Structuring Learning

To facilitate learning the parent educator embraces concepts of adult learning already discussed. As a conductor of learning, the job of the facilitator is to structure the topics that parents want and have negotiated. It is helpful to state what is planned for a class and check that other items have not taken precedence since the last class.

In planning the session, consider the needs of the parents.

The aims of the learning will affect the learning methods selected. The facilitator can try to put herself in the shoes of the client. This will help her to make the learning more realistic and meaningful to the parents. Information is presented by building on the known and progressing to the unfamiliar.

The learning methods should be appropriate to the group topic and length of the session. If the group consists of just three parents then a snowball technique is inappropriate. However, unlike a large group, a group of three is entirely suitable for a board game.

Consider the amount of time for information-giving and activities. A useful structure to use is a warm-up exercise followed by a short introduction/information, then an activity which involves pairs or small groups, then sharing in the whole group. To divide up the time available, a suggested balance is to have one third information-giving, one third parents discussing and one third physical preparation. The parents, as members of the orchestra, must play the tune themselves, the facilitator cannot do it for them.

Organize resources such as books, leaflets, flipchart, posters, slides and video. As has been said many times,

a picture is worth a thousand words. The majority of information stored in the memory is received visually. Confucius pointed out:

I hear and I forget
I see and I remember
I do and I understand.

However, take care to ensure that the visual aid is appropriate to the objective of the class. Does its use help the audience or the facilitator? One midwife was asked why she used such a long and out-of-date film in her classes. Her reply was that it gave her a rest!

Back-up activities should be planned to allow flexibility. Any number of unexpected problems may come up, such as the following:

▶ The planned session does not seem to be going well.
▶ The visual aid equipment has broken down.
▶ The knowledge of the parents is greater than anticipated.
▶ The topic is finished earlier than planned.

A flexible approach allows activities to be added or subtracted as needed. One of the dangers to be avoided is to end up adhering to a rigid plan that must be completed and yet is taking far longer than the agreed length of the session.

Principles for enabling the learning of parenting skills   In summary:

▶ Find out what the parents already know and what they want to learn.
▶ Give them the information on the topic and let them explore the information themselves.
▶ Do not do it for them, but be there if they ask for help.
▶ Let the parents, with help, realize that they can use resources to make choices. Try not to be the expert; the parents need to feel that they are the experts based on their experience.
▶ Be clear in giving instructions on the forthcoming activity, repeat instructions a few times, and check for understanding.
▶ Allow parents to come to answers that are different to the ones you expected (provided they are not harmful).

Keeping the group going

The parent educator is balancing the management of the group process as well as facilitating learning. The qualities you will need as a group facilitator to achieve success in this balancing act include the following (Rogers, 1983):

▶ Respect: believe that each course member will make constructive use of the course.
▶ Be honest and act according to your own feelings.
▶ Understand the feelings a group member is experiencing. Use specific examples rather than theory.
▶ Use a range of teaching/learning methods to utilize the skills and experience of the group.
▶ Help them relate theory to practice.
▶ Listen, reflect, clarify and draw relevant points together.
▶ Be supportive and non-judgemental.

As Bedford and Pepper (1992: 107) point out 'Perhaps good working practice involves the tutor taking responsibility for structuring events, and the group also taking a share of the responsibility for the learning that takes place.' For the group process to evolve successfully, the leader must portray what Rogers (1983) called 'genuine positive regard'. Common factors that inhibit successful group process are lack of confidence in the facilitator and large numbers in the group. Twenty or more people are unable to function effectively as a group (Nichols and Smith-Humenick, 1988: 401). If a large number is unavoidable, it is helpful to split large groups into smaller ones. If a safe group is achieved the advantages are that it allows extra freedoms as parents share ideas, trigger hidden fears and give each other the support and strength to cope with them.

As the course progresses, facilitation involves keeping the group united, focusing them on the issues under discussion and mobilizing the group. Help them move from dependence to independence. The stages of structure and control as described below are adapted from the film *Meetings Bloody Meetings* (Video Arts, 1993).

Structure and Control

Unite the group

Get group members to share common experiences, let them express their anger or fears, do not take sides, remain neutral as far as possible and bring in the other group members, inviting them to comment. Meet the challenges not by defence but by clarification and acceptance. Stick to facts if the interaction becomes steamy!

Focus the group

Parents needs come first and they should have an opportunity to do more than exchange facts; therefore help them to express their feelings also. Avoid personal hobby horses, listen and help them discover what they want to do and learn. Help them face reality and do not endorse fantasies. The facilitator is part of a group, not a performer with an audience. Stay alert; if they stray off the point guide them back. This can be done by testing understanding, paraphrasing the discussion so far and checking back with the group. This can also raise personal awareness of group members by reflecting what has been heard and understood.

Mobilize the group

Try to build the self-esteem of the parents by thanking them for their contribution and perhaps comment on any new awareness which the facilitator has gained from the session. Protect the weak and check around the group for any problems or issues that are unresolved. Record items that would be best discussed later because they are off the point. Give the group problems and the opportunity to share ideas, but also be prepared to supply possible solutions. Try not to be too ambitious and aim to cover three main points only during each class.

Keeping a group discussion going

Verbal prompts can be employed by the facilitator to promote discussion, for example short phrases such as 'go on', 'I see', or 'has anyone else an opinion on that?'.

The facilitator can repeat key words, confirming that the parent has been heard. This is a playback technique. For example, a woman may say 'I am really scared' and the facilitator says 'scared?'

Rather than supplying an immediate answer to a question the question can be clarified by posing another question. For example, 'How do you feel about it?' or 'Can you give an example?'

Evaluation

To improve the quality of parenthood education it is helpful to find out if the facilitation was of value to the clients. The feedback will give a measure of the effectiveness of the teaching/learning process. This will help the facilitator to reflect on the experience and promote personal growth. Evaluation is used to aid effective changes in the programme where required, and also affirms the positive and valuable aspects of the teaching/learning process.

Evaluation is a continuous process because, as the facilitator moves to a new point, relevance and understanding is checked. The pace and level of the content is immediately fed back. Continuous comments and feedback are asked for during a session.

Self-evaluation involves reflection on the educator's style and effectiveness as a facilitator. What was done well? Is there anything that was unsatisfactory and could be done differently? Did discussion flow and were the silences comfortable? What could be done to improve the situation if it occurred again?

Client behaviour can give specific clues to achievement by observation of change in their attitude, knowledge and skills. Note what parents say and do as a result of their learning. After reflection, note what has been learned about facilitation from the experience.

Formal evaluation by written questionnaire is the most common form of seeking information from parents about the positive and negative aspects of the course. Formulating questionnaires is not a simple exercise and expert advice may be advisable, although the midwife responsible for facilitating the classes will know the particular areas where feedback would be helpful. Open questions will give more information than closed questions. For example, parents could be asked:

▶ What do you think you have achieved?
▶ If a friend of yours was to attend the classes, what information would you give to her about the class?

Verbal feedback is often obtained at the reunion held postnatally. Peers can be asked to sit in on a class and give constructive criticism. The person who is usually the most critical is the facilitator. Although parents and peers are usually very kind with their comments, some feedback can be painful to hear. Evaluation data, good or bad, should be used in making decisions about future classes, but many childbirth educators collect data which has no relevance to them (Nichols and Smith-Humenick, 1988: 473). Sadly, some information is ignored because the evaluator does not know what to do about it or is unwilling to do anything about it. A forum for discussion with other facilitators would be beneficial in that problems can be shared and possible solutions discussed with peers in a supportive environment.

> Childbirth educators should seek to communicate more among themselves and with other health professionals to increase awareness of their role and enlist more co-operation and support for their efforts.
>
> (O'Mearea, 1993)

To prevent the isolation often expressed by those facilitating parenthood education the midwife can utilize the support networks that have grown up to overcome this problem. The midwife, as a provider of parenthood education has a wealth of information to share with other colleagues. In recent years, several support groups for those facilitating parenthood education have developed. The Parent Educators Group Support (PEGS) which started in London has now merged with the Professional Association of Childbirth Educators (PACE). However, many local areas have created PEGS networks. Another similar group has emerged from a group of health visitors, the Progressive and Innovative Parentcraft Teachers Support and Interest Group (PIPSI).

It is hoped that these developments will not only give support to those facilitating parenthood education but also lead to research and thereby to a higher quality of education which meets the needs of parents of today and in the foreseeable future.

References

Aikman, N. & Murphy-Black, T. (1993) Playing and learning in the antenatal class. *Modern Midwife* 3(6): 41–42.

Batchelor, D. & Napper, R. (1989) *Tutor's Toolkit: An Open Learning Resource for First Time Tutors*. National Extension College Trust Ltd.

Bedford, J. & Pepper, L. (1992) *Women Together: A Health Education Training Handbook for Ourselves and Others*. London: Health Education Authority.

Brands, D. (1982) *The Gamesters Handbook*. London: Hutchinson.

Braun, D. & Schonveld, A. (1993) *Approaching Parenthood: A Resource for Parent Education*. London: Health Education Authority.

Chalmers, B., Meyer, D. & Werner, S. (1987) Training childbirth educators: assessing changes in intent following an educational intervention. *J. Psychometric Obstet. Gynaecol.* **6**: 233–255.

Coombes, G. & Schonveld, D. (1992) *Life Will Never be the Same Again: A Review of Antenatal and Postnatal Education*. London: Health Education Authority.

Deane-Gray, T. & Nunnerley, R. (1988) Parent education. *Nursing Times* **84**(29).

Dick Read, G. (1955) *Antenatal Illustrated*. Oxford: William Heinemann Medical.

DOH (Department of Health) (1989) *Working for Patients: a Review of the NHS*. London: HMSO.

DOH (1993) *Changing Childbirth*. The Report of the Expert Maternity Group. London: HMSO.

Honey, P. (1986) *The Manual of Learning Styles*. P. Honey, 10 Linden Avenue, Maidenhead SL6 6HB.

Jarvis, P. (1995) *Adult and Continuing Education*, 2nd edn. London: Routledge.

Kirkham, M. (1993) Communication in midwifery. In Alexander, J., Levy, V. & Roch, S. (eds) *Midwifery Practice: A Research Based Approach*, London: Macmillan.

Knowles, M. (1984) *The Adult Learner: A Neglected Species*, 3rd edn. Houston, USA: Gulf Publishing.

Mezirow, J. & Associates (1990) *Fostering Critical Reflection in Adulthood*. San Francisco: Jossey Bass.

Murphy-Black, T. & Faulkner, A. (1988) *Antenatal Skills in Training*. Chichester: John Wiley and Sons.

Nichols, F. & Smith-Humenick, S. (1988) *Childbirth Education: Practice, Research, and Theory*. Philadelphia: W.B. Saunders.

O'Mearea, C. (1993) Childbirth and parenting education – the providers' viewpoint. *Midwifery* **9**: 76–84.

Parr, M. (1996) *PIPPIN: Support for Couples in the Transition to Parenthood*, PhD dissertation. University of East London: Department of Psychology.

Perkins, E. (1980) *Education for Childbirth and Parenthood*. London: Croom Helm.

Priest, J. (1992) Comparative approaches to childbirth education, Keynote address Professional Association of Childbirth Educators Study Day. *Pacenews* 4.

Priest, J. & Schott, J. (1991) *Leading Antenatal Classes: A Practical Guide*. Oxford: Butterworth Heinemann.

Rogers, A. (1992) *Teaching Adults*. Milton Keynes: Open University Press.

Rogers, C. (1983) *Freedom to Learn for the 80's*. Columbus, OH: C.E. Merrill.

Rowe, J. & Mahoney, P. (1993) *Parent Education: Guidance for Purchasers and Providers*. London: Health Education Authority.

Satow, A. & Evans, M. (1983) *Working with Groups*. London: Health Education Council & TECADE.

Spiers, B.G. (ed.) (1950) *The Complete Book of Mothercraft: A Collection of Expert Advice for Successful Parenthood*. London: Universal Textbooks.

UKCC (1994) *A Midwife's Code of Practice*. London: UKCC.

Video Arts Ltd (1993) *Meeting Bloody Meetings*. London: Video Arts Limited.

Warren, C. (1993) A.R.M.'s response to Changing Childbirth. *Midwifery Matters* **59**: 3–5.

25

Physical Preparation for the Ante-, Intra- and Postnatal Periods

Physical preparation for childbirth has been recommended for many years. Minnie Randall, a physiotherapist with a midwifery qualification, introduced bed exercises for postnatal mothers as early as 1912 to help prevent the numerous problems arising from prolonged postpartum immobility. Following their success, she encouraged mobilizing exercises for pregnant women. Then in the 1930s, Minnie Randall teamed with Dr Grantly Dick-Read and they introduced the principles of relaxation and deep breathing into antenatal preparation classes. These classes were continued by another well-known physiotherapist – Helen Heardman – who was one of the founder members of what is now known as the Association of Chartered Physiotherapists in Women's Health (ACPWH).

It has been acknowledged by the Royal College of Midwives (RCM) and the Health Visitors Association (HVA) that the obstetric physiotherapist is an invaluable member of the obstetric team and the ideal professional to help women to adjust to the physical changes which occur throughout pregnancy and the puerperium, to prepare them for labour using relaxation and breathing awareness, to teach postnatal exercises and to carry out specialized treatments where necessary.

However, as more and more women and couples are demanding antenatal education, there are insufficient numbers of obstetric physiotherapists and, in some areas, midwives may be asked to teach antenatal and postnatal exercises and coping skills for labour.

Anatomy and Functions

Before teaching exercises for specific muscle groups, their anatomy and functions must be fully understood. The anatomy of the pelvic floor is explained in Chapter 34, but little is mentioned of the abdominal wall anatomy in any midwifery textbook.

Anatomy of the abdominal muscles
(Figure 1)

The abdominal muscles form the anterior and lateral parts of the abdominal wall or corset and consist of three layers of muscle and fascia. The deepest muscle layer is formed by the *transversus abdominis* which runs in a horizontal direction from the thoracolumbar fascia, iliac crest and inguinal ligament at each side. It attaches to the inner surface of the lower six ribs and its aponeurosis inserts into the linea alba.

The next layer is composed of two sets of oblique muscles. The deeper are the *interal obliques* which run upwards and inwards from the thoracolumbar fascia, iliac crest and inguinal ligament and insert into the inferior borders of the lower three ribs and by an aponeurosis into the linea alba. Directly superficial and running at right angles to these muscles are the *external obliques*. Their origin is the outer surface of the lower eight ribs and they insert into the anterior half of the iliac crest, pubic crest and by an aponeurosis into the linea alba. The lower border of each external oblique muscle forms the *inguinal ligament*

The most superficial group of abdominal muscles are the *recti abdominis* which run in a vertical direction. They are narrow and anterior, being enclosed in the aponeuroses formed by the other abdominal muscles. This enclosure of the recti is known as the *rectus sheath*. The rectus muscles attach superiorly to the cartilages of the fifth, sixth and seventh ribs and to the xiphisternum. Inferiorly there are two tendons: one from the crest of the pubis at the same side, the other from that of the opposite side. The muscles are intersected by three fibrous bands known as *tendinous intersections*.

Functions of the abdominal muscles

The abdominal corset provides support for the abdominal organs and for the pelvis and spine. It helps to control the intra-abdominal and intrapelvic pressures and so aids in any expulsive actions such as defaecation, parturition and, together with the diaphragm, helps with breathing and coughing. The abdominal muscles perform the trunk movements of forward and side flexion and rotation. With the hip and back extensors, they control the tilt of the pelvis and splint the spine, thus making a large contribution to body posture.

Anatomy of the pelvic floor
See Chapter 34.

Functions of the pelvic floor muscles

The two most important functions of the pelvic floor are the control of the sphincters of the bladder and bowel and the support of the pelvic contents in their correct anatomical position. However, it must be remembered that the pelvic floor muscles also play a large part in the sexual satisfaction that both partners gain from intercourse. Muscles with good tone will stretch and recoil more effectively than weak muscles and therefore will relax more easily.

Physiological Effects of Pregnancy on the Musculoskeletal System

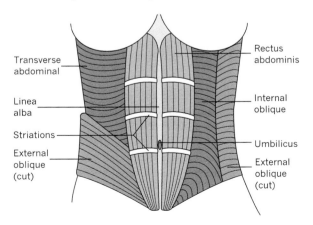

Figure 1 Anterior abdominal wall showing muscle layers and striations of the rectus muscle.

Transverse abdominal

Linea alba

Striations

External oblique (cut)

Rectus abdominis

Internal oblique

Umbilicus

External oblique (cut)

The physiological effects on the musculoskeletal system in pregnancy are mainly due to the hormonal influence of oestrogen, progesterone and relaxin. Oestrogen is thought to help the action of relaxin which is produced at two weeks and is at its highest level in the first trimester (Weiss, 1984). Relaxin alters the composition of collagen which is present in joint capsules, ligaments and fibrous tissue such as the linea alba. This collagen is remodelled, having a higher water content which leads to greater pliability and extensibility. This means, however, that joints do not receive the same protection from the ligaments as before and become lax. Muscles which are intersected with fibrous bands, e.g. the recti, or those interspersed with fascial layers, e.g. the pelvic floor, are weakened.

An increase in joint laxity leads to an increase in joint range. Calguneri et al. (1982) have shown that this increase is greater in second pregnancies than in first pregnancies. Increased range in the pelvic joints, coupled with the weight of the developing uterus may cause backache and referred 'sciatica-like' pain down the leg. Posture is altered. The pelvis tips forward and the pregnant woman adopts a typical stance, with exaggerated spinal curves and protruding abdomen which again can produce backache (Figure 2). The woman may also experience a dragging sensation in the lower abdomen as the weight of the uterus is transmitted through these muscles instead of through the thighs. The centre of gravity is shifted further forward, causing the mother to be unbalanced and more prone to falling.

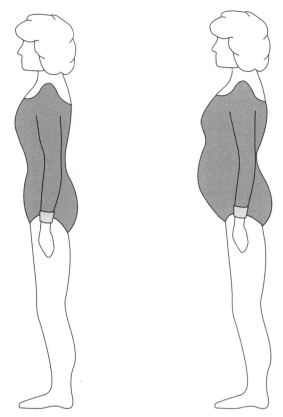

Figure 2 Normal posture (left) and posture in pregnancy (right).

Care of the Back During Pregnancy

During pregnancy the back is especially vulnerable. The stretching ligaments, increased joint range, extra weight and altered posture all mean that the woman should pay particular attention to back care in order to avoid long-term back problems. She should be taught correct lifting, keeping her back straight and holding the object close to her body (Figure 3). She should, however, be discouraged from lifting at all if it can be avoided, certainly anything heavy.

The midwife can make sure that the woman knows how to get up from the examination couch or bed and how to get up and down from the floor. Trying to sit up forwards from lying with the legs straight is the same as performing sit-ups and puts a great strain on the abdominals as well as the back. All women should be shown how to bend the knees up, keep them together,

roll over on to one side, and to push up on the upper hand and underneath elbow into a sitting position with the legs over the side of the bed before slowly standing. If on the floor, the woman will go over on to her hands and knees before slowly standing.

Antenatal Exercises

It is inadvisable to take up any new sporting activities in pregnancy (Sady and Carpenter, 1989) but it is usually considered safe to continue with familiar activities as long as they do not involve lifting or twisting. Swimming and walking are especially beneficial, but competitive or contact sports should be discontinued during pregnancy. If in doubt, an obstetric physiotherapist should be consulted.

The following exercises could lead to long-term back problems and should be avoided at all times, but especially during pregnancy and the postnatal period:

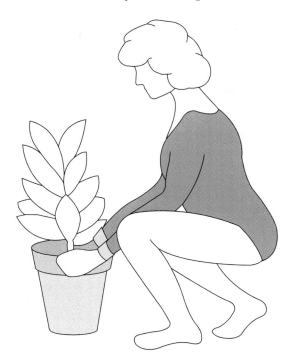

Figure 3 Correct lifting technique.

▶ *Double leg lifting*: Lying on the back with both legs straight, lifting both legs up into the air, then lowering them back down.
▶ *Sit-ups*: Lying on the back with both legs straight, sitting up to touch the toes, then lowering the head and shoulders back down to the floor (Figure 4).

The exercises described below *are* recommended during pregnancy and may be started in the first two or three months unless the woman has specific orders to rest, in which case, only the circulatory exercises are advised.

In the last two trimesters, women may suffer from supine hypotension so should never be asked to lie flat on their backs to exercise. Half-lying, i.e. lying with the back supported at an angle of 45 degrees, is a safe position.

CIRCULATORY EXERCISES

Because of the hormonal effects and the increasing size of the baby, the circulation – particularly the venous return – becomes more sluggish. This may lead to foot and ankle oedema, varicose veins and cramp. To stimulate the circulation and alleviate/prevent these

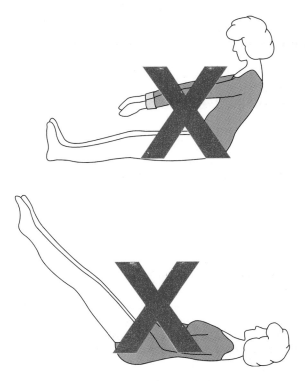

Figure 4 Exercises to avoid.

problems, the following exercises should be performed vigorously and regularly:

▶ *Ankle circling*: Sitting or half-lying with legs stretched out and supported, circle both ankles round in as large a circle as possible whilst keeping the knees still. This should be done at least 12 times before rotating the ankles in the opposite direction for the same number of repetitions.
▶ *Leg tightening*: Still in the same position as above, bend both feet upwards at the ankle joint and press the back of both knees down on to the underneath surface, tightening both the calf and the thigh muscles. Hold these muscles tight for a couple of seconds, breathing normally, before relaxing. Repeat 12 times.

Both these exercises should improve the distal circulation, particularly the venous return. They should be performed frequently throughout the day, especially first thing in the morning and last thing at night.

Prolonged standing should be avoided as this could compound circulatory stasis, and mothers will benefit from sitting with legs supported on a stool whenever possible. If there is oedema present, the mother may find it helpful to lie supported at an angle of about 45 degrees with the legs elevated just higher than the level of the groin to aid drainage by gravity. Great care must be taken to ensure as wide an angle as possible at the groin to prevent circulatory stasis in that region.

ABDOMINAL EXERCISES

As already mentioned, the pelvis will tilt further forwards as pregnancy advances, putting a strain on the ligaments and joints of the pelvis and on the abdominal and back muscles. Tilting the pelvis in the opposite direction will help to alleviate this strain. The action involves all the abdominal muscles and the hip extensors so will help to maintain their tone. These muscles will assist in supporting the pelvic joints as the ligaments stretch.

▶ *Pelvic tilting exercise*: In half-lying with both knees bent up and feet resting on the floor, tighten and pull in the abdomen, tighten the muscles of the buttocks and press the small of the back downwards on to the supporting surface. Hold the contraction for a couple of seconds whilst breathing normally, then relax. Repeat five times (Figure 5).

This exercise may be performed in a supported sitting position, prone kneeling or standing, but most pregnant women find it easier to learn the exercise in the half-lying position.

Because of the hormonal effects on the linea alba, exercises which cause contraction of the muscles inserting into this area should be avoided in later pregnancy to minimize the risk of diastasis of the recti. In the last trimester it is difficult to check for diastasis, so to avoid further strain it is wiser to omit rotation exercises and stronger abdominal exercises such as curl-ups.

PELVIC FLOOR EXERCISES

Pelvic floor exercises should be introduced during pregnancy to maintain muscle tone and promote understanding of the effects of pregnancy on the

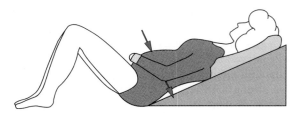

Figure 5   Pelvic tilting exercise in half-lying position.

functional ability of the pelvic floor postnatally. Few women will have performed pelvic floor exercises before coming to antenatal classes, so it is important to take time to explain in simple terms, the relevant anatomy and the importance of the muscles before embarking on the exercise itself.

Pelvic floor contractions can be performed in any position except with crossed legs. Probably the easiest position is in sitting, leaning forwards with the legs slightly apart.

▶ *Pelvic floor exercise*: Close the back passage as though preventing a bowel action, close the middle and front passages too as though preventing the flow of urine, then draw up all three passages inside. Hold as strongly as possible for as long as possible up to a count of 10, breathing normally throughout. Relax and rest for 5 seconds. Repeat the above *slowly* up to a maximum of 10 repetitions.

Tighten and relax more *quickly* up to 10 times without holding the contraction.

It is an excellent idea to relate the practice of this exercise to the performance of everyday activities, e.g. washing hands, *after* emptying the bladder, answering the telephone. This will establish a routine for postnatal practice.

Some women find the exercise difficult to comprehend at first and may need other suggestions to describe the sensation of tightening their pelvic floor. It may be helpful to try to stop the flow of urine midstream occasionally, but this is not advisable as a regular habit as it is not good bladder training and could possibly lead to urinary tract infection due to reflux of urine.

Stress and Relaxation

Most of us show some signs of stress at times when problems accumulate, workload increases and there are staff shortages. It is often a very insignificant factor which can be enough to break the 'camel's back'. Consider the pregnant woman who may have all the everyday stresses we undergo plus the added mental stresses which even a planned and longed-for pregnancy can bring, let alone an unplanned and unsupported one. Pregnancy also brings its own physical stresses – fatigue, aching joints, reduced mobility. The whole process increases the work of every system of the body, so acquiring the art of relaxation during pregnancy can only be greatly beneficial.

The automatic reaction of the body to stress is the 'fight or flight' response. We assume a tense position with hunched shoulders, elbows close to the body, hands clenched, legs crossed, feet pulled up and body leaning forward. The face assumes a worried look, jaw is tense with teeth touching and mouth dry. The heart beats faster, there may be sweating and the breathing is often shallow and rapid.

Adopting this position in itself increases tension and fatigue. Part of mastering relaxation techniques is gaining an awareness of the tense situation before it is too late and changing it to a position of ease. This position is the exact opposite of one of tension and allows all joints to assume a comfortable mid-position and the muscles around the joints to be as relaxed as possible.

Physiological relaxation, first taught by Laura Mitchell, works the joints into positions of ease which the brain can accept as a neutral position. With practice the method becomes easy and the brain will receive messages from receptors in the joints if there is any deviation from the position of ease.

The method works on the principle of reciprocal innervation of opposite muscle groups, e.g. if one muscle group shortens or contracts, the opposite muscle group lengthens or relaxes to allow that action to take place. For instance as the finger muscles flex to make a fist, the extensor muscles of the fingers are stretched or lengthened. Conversely, the flexors are stretched or lengthened as the fingers extend or straighten. This principle is applied to the tense muscles of each joint in the stressed position.

There are specific instructions for this method of relaxation:

1 Work the opposite muscle group to the tense ones strongly.
2 Stop the action of those muscle groups.
3 Pause to 'feel the difference' now the joint is in a position of ease.

The mothers need to be aware of the groups which exhibit tension, then work their way through the opposite ones. Relaxation can be practised in any comfortable and supported position but half-lying and side-lying are often preferred in pregnancy (Figure 6).

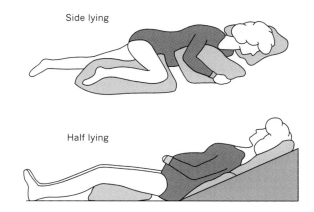

Side lying

Half lying

Figure 6   Relaxation in half-lying and side-lying positions (recovery position).

RELAXATION INSTRUCTIONS

▶ *Shoulders*: Pull your shoulders down towards your feet. *Stop* pulling your shoulders down. Your shoulders are now lower and your neck feels longer.

▶ *Elbows*: Move your elbows slightly away from your side. *Stop* moving your elbows. Be aware that your elbows are open and slightly away from your side.

▶ *Hands*: Stretch out and separate your fingers and thumbs. *Stop* stretching. Your fingers are fully supported. Feel the surface they are resting on.

▶ *Hips*: Roll your hips and knees outwards. *Stop* rolling outwards. Your legs are slightly apart and feel heavy.

▶ *Feet*: Push your feet away from your body. *Stop* pushing. Your feet feel loose and heavy.

▶ *Body*: Press your body into the support. *Stop* pressing. Feel your body resting on the surface.

▶ *Head*: Press your head into the pillow. *Stop* pressing. Your head is nestling comfortably in the hollow you have made in the pillow.

▶ *Jaw*: Pull down your lower jaw. *Stop* pulling down. Your teeth are no longer touching and your tongue is resting on your lower jaw.

▶ *Eyes*: Close your eyes if you want to.

▶ *Forehead*: Imagine someone smoothing away your frown lines from your eyebrows up over to the top and the back of your head.

▶ *Breathing*: Give a big sigh out. Breathe fairly low down in your chest at your own natural resting breathing rate. To prevent your brain being too active during your relaxation think about something pleasant which helps you to feel comfortable.

After complete relaxation, the circulation should be stimulated by stretching or performing foot and hand movements before sitting up slowly, then standing.

Women should be encouraged to practise the relaxation technique every day of their pregnancy, either sitting supported in an armchair whilst watching the television, or lying on the bed for an afternoon rest or in bed before going to sleep. Apart from allowing the body's systems to slow down, practice makes perfect for labour.

Coping Strategies for Labour

The answer to the question 'Why have you come to antenatal classes?' is almost invariably 'To learn what to do in labour' from the women, and 'To find out how I can help and share in the experience' from the fathers.

Each couple is different and every labour unique, but there are common coping skills that couples can learn during pregnancy and put into practice in labour. The main tools are relaxation, breathing awareness and positions of ease. All three are interrelated and all can be practised together at home.

The physiological method of relaxation lends itself very well to both stages of labour. If the mother can conserve her energy during the first stage she is preparing herself for the hard work to come, as well as ensuring that her baby and uterus both receive sufficient oxygen. Any position which she finds comfortable is acceptable, allowing for the possibility of drips or monitors being attached. Alteration of maternal position during the first stage encourages productive contractions (Roberts *et al.*, 1983), and suggestions for different positions appear in Chapter 29.

Breathing has been the subject of much debate and much criticism over the years. Levels of breathing and breathing patterns formed the basis of the *psychoprophylaxis teaching* in the 1960s. It has now been shown that these can cause hyperventilation which may be disadvantageous for both mother and baby. The emphasis nowadays is to encourage the mother to tune in to her own natural breathing rhythm and to recognize times in labour when she may have to adapt this if the situation arises. This '*breathing awareness*' is being accepted as non-interfering and is unlikely to lead to hyperventilation. It is the outward breath which is the relaxing phase of respiration, so mothers should be encouraged to concentrate on that when

tuning in to their breathing. They may also become aware of a slight pause at the end of the outward breath before the next inward breath follows. There is never any need to instruct anyone to breathe in as this happens automatically. It may be necessary, however, to encourage the breath out or to extend the expiratory phase.

Breathing is one of the first obvious signs of tension or panic. It becomes rapid and shallow involving only the upper part of the lungs and increasing tension in the shoulder muscles. If this type of breathing continues it may lead to hyperventilation or hyperoxygenation – a state where too much oxygen has been inhaled and too much carbon dioxide has been exhaled.

The symptoms of *hyperventilation* are pallor, dizziness, sweating and pins and needles in the face and extremities. The woman feels very unwell and the baby's blood gases may also be compromised. The immediate remedy is to breathe in carbon dioxide as soon as possible, the quickest way being for the mother to breathe in and out of her own cupped hands until the blood gas levels are stabilized. To prevent hyperventilation in the first place, *SOS breathing* can be practised during the contraction. This stands for 'sigh out slowly' and is a relaxed breathing exaggerating the outward breath by making a sighing noise. It will slow down 'panic breathing' and also leads to relaxation of the shoulder muscles. As SOS represents an emergency situation (as indeed hyperventilation would be) it is a useful phrase for couples to remember.

The end of first stage can be a difficult time for all mothers but particularly those who experience a premature urge to push. In addition to altering their position, these mothers can adapt their breathing to prevent themselves from pushing. The diaphragm should not be allowed to fix, so breath holding must be discouraged. Panting, as used at the crowning of the fetal head, would prevent pushing but it is not possible to sustain panting for any length of time without hyperventilation occurring. Instead, a *modified panting breathing* may be useful – breathing in threes with the emphasis on two short breaths out followed by a longer breath out. This method is known variously as pant–pant–blow or puff–puff–blow breathing and can be practised for the length of a contraction without hyperventilation occurring.

Midwives will have their own ideas and policies on the management of the second stage of labour and the question 'to push or not to push' initiates much discussion. It is now known that the continued practice of the Valsalva manoeuvre when pushing could lead to loss of maternal consciousness if the mother's cerebral blood flow is already compromised (Bush, 1992). It is also documented that holding the breath for more than 5 or 6 seconds alters the blood gases in the placenta and may compromise the fetal circulation (Caldeyro-Barcia, 1978). Certainly the mother is less exhausted when she has been allowed to push whenever and for however long she chooses.

The *position* she adopts for the second stage will also have an effect on the outcome (Russell, 1982). Chapter 30 discusses practical positions for delivery. **Note** that if a separation of the symphysis pubis has presented antenatally, side-lying or prone-kneeling may be the only safe positions (Fry, 1992). Between contractions, mothers may need to be reminded to relax quickly using the physiological method.

Postnatal Exercises

The overall aim of postnatal exercises is to restore the mother to her pre-pregnancy state as soon as possible.

CIRCULATORY EXERCISES

Exercises to improve the sluggish circulation can be started immediately following delivery. The *foot and leg exercises* described in the antenatal section should be practised as frequently as possible and continued until the mother is fully mobile and there is no oedema present. The advice given antenatally to avoid sitting or lying with legs crossed or prolonged standing still holds good, as does encouraging sitting with feet on a stool or even higher if oedema is present.

ABDOMINAL EXERCISES

The abdominal corset has stretched to approximately twice its length and two-thirds of its girth by the end of pregnancy. All its component muscles will need exercising to regain their former length and strength. However because of their insertion into the linea alba and rectus sheath (see earlier in this chapter) the oblique muscles should not be exercised before checking for any undue diastasis of the rectus muscles (Noble, 1988). Up to two fingers' width is considered normal 48 hours after delivery, but if the gap is more than that, rotation exercises should not be performed since they may cause further separation of the rectus muscles.

The midwife is the ideal person to measure diastasis when she is checking the fundus on the third day post-delivery. The mother should lie on her back with knees bent up and feet flat on the bed. With the midwife's fingers pressed into the midline of the abdomen either just above or just below the umbilicus, the mother is asked to lift her head and shoulders off the pillow and look towards her knees. If there is no undue diastasis, the rectus muscles will be felt taut either side of the fingers.

If the rectus muscles cannot be felt until two or more fingers are inserted, only pelvic tilting exercises with head lifting should be performed until the gap is reduced (Figure 7).

Pelvic tilting, as described earlier in this chapter, can be started on the first or second day postdelivery. As well as toning up the straight abdominal muscles, this exercise will help to relieve any postural backache which may be present after delivery. Pelvic tilting must be encouraged in sitting and standing as well as in lying positions and, as with the pelvic floor exercise, it can be related to activities with the baby to ensure frequent practice.

If there is no undue diastasis or when the gap has reduced, other exercises can be started:

▶ *Curl-ups*: Lying on the back with both knees bent up, tilt the pelvis backwards, then lift the head forwards reaching towards the knees with the hands (Figure 8). Hold the position for a couple of seconds before lowering the head back slowly, then relax the abdominal muscles. Repeat the exercise up to six times, building up to 12 times over the next six weeks. NB. This exercise must always be

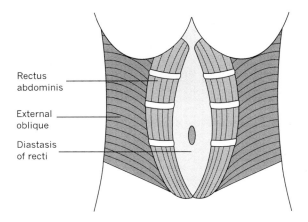

Rectus abdominis

External oblique

Diastasis of recti

Figure 7   Diastasis recti postpartum.

done with knees bent and never without pelvic tilting first.

▶ *Knee rolling*: Lying on the back with both knees bent up, tilt the pelvis backwards and roll both knees over to the left as far as possible, keeping shoulders flat (Figure 9). Return knees to the centre and relax the abdominals. Pelvic tilt again and repeat the exercise to the right side, before returning the knees to the centre and relaxing. Repeat the exercise six times, progressing up to 12 times over the following six weeks.

▶ *Hip updrawing*: Lying on the back with left knee bent and right knee straight, push the right heel downwards to lengthen the leg, pull in the abdominal muscles, then pull the right hip up towards the ribs at the same side to shorten the leg (Figure 10). Return the leg to its normal position and relax the abdominals. Repeat the exercise up to six times before bending up the right knee and exercising the muscles of the left side. Hip updrawing (or hitching) can be progressed up to 12 repetitions over the following six weeks. This exercise can also be done in the standing position whilst holding on to a firm support.

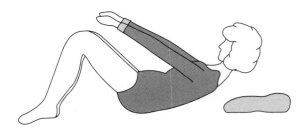

Figure 8   Curl-up exercise.

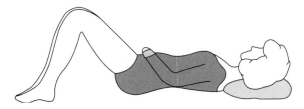

Figure 9   Knee rolling exercise.

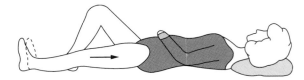

Figure 10   Hip updrawing exercise.

PELVIC FLOOR EXERCISES

(See earlier in this chapter)

These must be started as soon after delivery as possible to avoid disassociation by the brain (Shepherd, 1980). The mother should be warned that contracting the pelvic floor will be much more difficult postnatally because of the stretching that has taken place during delivery and possible discomfort from a bruised or sutured perineum. However, if she can persevere with the pelvic floor exercise as described in the antenatal section, then urinary problems and prolapse may well be avoided. Good tone in the pelvic floor is also necessary for the sexual satisfaction of both partners during intercourse.

Frequent performance of the pelvic floor exercise is vital in the postnatal period – every hour or so – and its performance can be linked to activities associated with the baby, e.g. feeding, bathing, washing and also *after* the mother has emptied her bladder. It is not a good idea to encourage a midstream stop during each bladder emptying as this is not promoting good bladder function, but the activity may be performed occasionally as a test. If a sore perineum makes the exercise difficult in sitting, then it could be done in prone or side-lying or standing.

Mothers can test the strength of their pelvic floor muscles 2–3 months postdelivery by stride jumping with a full bladder and coughing deeply twice whilst doing so. If any leakage occurs then the muscles have not regained their former strength and function and need further intensive exercising. The test can be repeated 4–6 weeks later and if there are still problems the mother should be referred to the gynaecologist or obstetric physiotherapist before embarking on any strenuous exercise or a subsequent pregnancy. Even when the muscles are functioning adequately, women are advised to continue regular pelvic floor contractions for the rest of their lives to prevent gynaecological problems in the future.

Care Following Caesarean Delivery

Circulatory exercises and *deep breathing* (no more than 3 or 4) are extremely important following Caesarean delivery and should be performed regularly whilst the mother is relatively immobile.

She should be taught how to *move up and down the*

bed by bending her knees, curling forwards and pushing on her hands and feet to move herself in a forwards or backwards direction. She should not attempt to sit up forwards from a lying position, but instead to roll over on to her side as described earlier in this chapter. This is also the easiest way of getting out of bed – pushing up into a sitting position on the edge of the bed.

If the mother needs to *cough*, she should bend her knees and support her wound with a pillow or her hands whilst leaning forwards. This will prevent undue strain on her sutures.

Pelvic tilting may be performed as soon as the mother feels able, as this exercise will relieve postural backache from the tilted position on the operating table, as well as helping to disperse wind. It is probably not possible to check for diastasis of the recti until about the fifth day postdelivery, so other abdominal exercises should be left until after this time, then progressed more gently than after a normal delivery.

Pelvic floor exercises should be performed regularly even though the muscles have not been stretched at birth as in a vaginal delivery. The hormonal influence during pregnancy causes most urinary problems (Francis, 1960) so the muscles will still need strengthening.

It must be remembered that a Caesarean birth has necessitated major surgery and these mothers will require more rest and more support at home. Many relatives do not appreciate this fact and the community midwife is the ideal professional to convey this message.

Care of the Back Postnatally

The early postpartum period is when the mother's joints, particularly those of the spine and pelvis, are at their least protected because the ligaments are at their most relaxed. Unfortunately this is the time when the mother has numerous objects to lift, e.g. baby bath, carrycot, and tasks which involve bending and stooping. It is important that the midwife explains the underlying physiology to the mother and reinforces good back care routines both in hospital and at home, now and for the future.

Positions for feeding, bathing and nappy changing must be discussed (Figure 11). To avoid a slouched position whilst feeding, the mother should sit well-supported with baby resting on pillows on her knee. Baby bathing and nappy changing can be done on a surface at waist height if standing, or at coffee table height if kneeling. Both these postures avoid stooping. Lifting should be kept to an absolute minimum and, if unavoidable, only light objects lifted and held as close to the body as possible. The correct lifting procedures as described earlier in this chapter must be followed to avoid back strain at this very vulnerable time.

Daily Activities

If possible, heavy housework, e.g. vacuuming, moving furniture, cleaning windows, should be avoided for several weeks after delivery to prevent back strain.

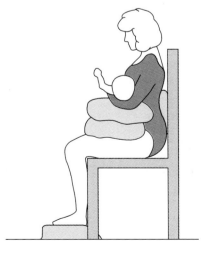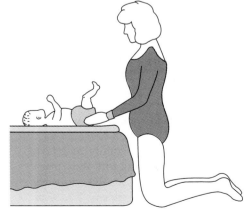

Figure 11   Positions for feeding and nappy changing.

Walking and swimming are good ways of supplementing the above postnatal exercises, but more strenuous keep-fit classes, aerobics or competitive sports should be left for 10–12 weeks or even longer if there are any joint or bladder problems. *Double leg lifting and sit-ups should never be performed.*

Postnatal Complications

The pain from a *bruised or oedematous perineum* can be eased by the application of ice (Knight, 1989), therapeutic ultrasound or pulsed electromagnetic energy by an obstetric physiotherapist (McIntosh, 1988).

Testing for *diastasis recti* has already been described. If a gap of more than two fingers' width is discovered, 'J' or 'K' size tubigrip applied from xiphisternum to below the buttocks will give some support in the early stages. Advice about posture, getting out of bed and special exercises for the rectus muscles are all important and an obstetric physiotherapist will advise.

Separated symphysis may require complete bedrest in the acute stage until the severe pain has subsided, then limited walking with the aid of a frame or crutches. Local pain relief will help (see Chapter 20).

Backache is usually postural and advice on positions, pelvic tilting and lifting plus some local heat should ease it considerably. Women with long-term back problems should be referred for individual assessment by a physiotherapist.

Coccydynia can be incapacitating, the mother finding it impossible to adopt a sitting position. Pain-relieving therapies such as ice, therapeutic ultrasound or pulsed electromagnetic energy may help.

Urinary problems, such as *stress incontinence, frequency* and *urgency*, which do not respond to postnatal exercise must be referred to a gynaecologist or obstetric physiotherapist before a subsequent pregnancy compounds the problem.

Dyspareunia can often be treated successfully by physiotherapy (McIntosh, 1988), though some women may require psychosexual counselling.

Most mothers welcome the opportunity to return with their babies and discuss progress with their peers at a reunion session. It may be in this informal atmosphere that urinary and back problems are mentioned and referrals made to the appropriate professionals.

Teaching Physical Skills

Before teaching physical skills, the tutor must be proficient in those skills herself. She should then memorize the appropriate instructions for each skill and practise teaching them to family members or a small group of colleagues. It will be more helpful if the 'guinea-pigs' are previously unaware of the skills and are willing to give constructive criticism of the instructions.

When teaching physical skills to groups, there are a number of points to consider:

▶ The room should be of adequate size with appropriate facilities for exercises, e.g. mats or carpeted floor, wedges and/or sufficient pillows.
▶ The group should be arranged so that each individual can see the instructor and each other if at all possible.
▶ An appropriate starting position should be selected for each exercise.
▶ Each exercise should be demonstrated or described clearly.
▶ The benefit of each exercise should be stated.
▶ The optimum number of repetitions for each exercise should be included.
▶ The practice of physical skills at home should be encouraged.

Many midwives will find themselves battling for floor space in crowded community clinics and may have to adapt some of the above criteria. Thought should be given to exercises which could be taught in other positions even though these might not be the first choice, e.g. pelvic tilting can be taught in sitting even though it is easier to learn in the lying position. Sometimes it may only be possible to demonstrate a position or to use visual aids to show it, if space is limited.

CLASSES

When should women begin physical preparation? The answer must be as early as possible as long as there is no risk of miscarriage. It is much easier to teach good posture and back care in early pregnancy rather than trying to relieve back problems in later pregnancy.

Two or three *early pregnancy classes* for couples at 3–4 months of pregnancy are extremely useful, though many hospitals/clinics have only the resources to provide one evening session at this time. In this case, the physical skills priorities would be posture, working positions and lifting techniques, pelvic tilting, pelvic floor and circulatory exercises.

Partners enjoy participating in the exercises and relaxation techniques at *couples classes*. They can be very supportive in helping with coping strategies and checking their partner's relaxation. It may be more appropriate on occasions to divide the couples so the women could cover such topics as pelvic floor problems whilst the men discussed their worries with another member of the antenatal team. Even if women have been attending daytime classes on their own, at least one evening session to practise coping strategies for labour should be provided for their partners.

Some women will prefer their antenatal preparation on a *one-to-one* basis because the group situation is not convenient or they have individual problems. In these cases the community midwife might provide the preparation in the woman's own home.

Any woman with *specific needs* for a physical disability should be referred to an obstetric physiotherapist if at all possible.

AQUANATAL SESSIONS

Aquanatal exercise is great fun both during pregnancy and afterwards. Many swimming pools offer special times for ante- and postnatal groups as well as sessions for baby too! The water temperature should be at least 30°C as cooler than this does not allow for relaxation to be included. However a hospital hydrotherapy pool at 37°C would be too warm.

The buoyancy of water supports the body weight, making it much easier to move and exercise without putting any additional strain on joints. It increases general muscle tone, improves venous return and respiratory co-ordination as well as giving the women a sense of well-being (McMurray *et al.*, 1990), freedom and weightlessness whilst in the water.

Women who swim may safely continue as long as they warm up gently beforehand and cool down afterwards. Some may find that breaststroke aggravates backache in pregnancy if they are in the habit of keeping their face out of the water, thus increasing the lumbar lordosis. These women may be happier on their backs.

There are certain safety recommendations and contraindications to aquanatal therapy in pregnancy which must be observed by any professional wishing to set up aquanatal classes.

Safety precautions

Adequate staffing levels are essential. At least two professional staff and one lifeguard are needed at every session unless one professional has life-saving qualifications. The professionals may be an obstetric physiotherapist and a midwife, or, if this is not possible, two midwives may run the sessions provided one has aquanatal qualifications. In the latter case, the exercise content should be discussed with an obstetric phsyiotherapist beforehand. The assistant midwife will be in the water with the women to facilitate and correct the exercises.

All women should be of at least 16 weeks gestation, have written permission from their obstetrician and have none of the contraindications listed below. Comprehensive records of appropriate personal and obstetric details of each participant should be kept available.

Strict observation of the group is necessary at all times so numbers should not exceed 10–12. To avoid fatigue and overheating, no more than 40 minutes of exercise should be performed which can be followed by relaxation if the temperature of the water is sufficient.

Exercises should avoid producing increased lumbar lordosis and should never cause pain. The pool surrounds must be safe and there must be access to an emergency telephone. Warm drinks after the session will prevent chilling.

Contraindications

Women participating in aquanatal classes, either ante- or postnatal, should be carefully checked for any of the following contraindications to group therapy in water: heart or lung disease, infections, diabetes mellitus or epilepsy.

Specific *pregnancy-related* conditions which would preclude women from antenatal classes in water include: history of spontaneous abortion, cervical cerclage, pregnancy-induced hypertension, antepartum haemorrhage, intrauterine growth retardation, ruptured membranes and history of preterm labour. However, if an earlier problem has settled and the obstetrician agrees in writing, then that woman may be included, but is carefully observed.

Postnatal contraindications would be an unhealed perineum, vaginal discharge or any infective condition.

If musculoskeletal problems present either ante- or postnatally the woman should be assessed by an obstetric physiotherapist before being accepted into the class.

EXERCISE-TO-MUSIC

There is a growing demand for exercise-to-music classes from women who are not usually 'exercisers', as well as from those who are health conscious and want to keep fit with specific safe and effective exercises designed for pregnancy. There are both physical and psychological gains from these group sessions which can be specially tailored for different stages of the childbearing year. During pregnancy the exercises can be gradually decreased in intensity then built up again in the postnatal weeks.

Special exercises for pregnancy, e.g. pelvic tilting and pelvic floor exercises, as described earlier in this chapter, can be incorporated into the classes. Circulation will be improved and a greater awareness of good posture and body image will be promoted. General exercises improve mobility and help to maintain a feeling of well-being.

Research is very limited in this area, but there is a growing acceptance of the gains from exercising to music and certainly women who are fit during pregnancy recover more quickly after the birth. Music can help motivation and increase the value of the exercise routine but needs to be a slower tempo than that used for normal movement to music classes for the non-pregnant population.

Classes should not be attended instead of preparation for parenthood classes but as well as them. They should be led by teachers who are qualified to teach the specific exercises which are safe and appropriate for each stage of the childbearing year. Recognized courses are run by the YMCA and Royal Society of Arts (RSA) to train teachers to lead such exercise-to-music sessions.

Conclusion

By teaching physical skills in the antenatal period, we can promote good health and a sense of well-being during pregnancy, increase the mother's confidence to cope in labour and facilitate a speedier return to normal after delivery. However, we should also encourage the mother to continue such skills as relaxation, back care and pelvic floor exercises for the rest of her life and to extend the message of good health to her family and friends.

References

Bush, A. (1992) Cardiopulmonary effects of pregnancy and labour. *J. Assoc. Chartered Physiother. Obstet. Gynaecol.* 71: 3.

Caldeyro-Barcia, R. (1978) The influence of maternal position on labour and the influence of maternal bearing-down efforts in the second stage of labour on fetal well-being. In Simpkin, P. & Reinke, C. (eds) *Kaleidoscope of Childbearing Preparation, Birth and Nurturing.* Seattle: Pennypress.

Calguneri, M., Bird, H.A. & Wright, V. (1982) Changes in joint laxity during pregnancy. *Ann. Rheum. Dis.* 41: 126.

Francis, W. (1960) The onset of stress incontinence. *J. Obstet. Gynaecol. Br. Empire* 67: 899.

Fry, D. (1992) Diastasis symphysis pubis. *J. Assoc. Chartered Physiother. Obstet. Gynaecol.* 71: 10.

Knight, K.L. (1989) Cryotherapy in sports injury management. In Grisogono, V. (ed.) *Sports Injuries.* Edinburgh: Churchill Livingstone.

McIntosh, J. (1988) Research in Reading into treatment of perineal trauma and late dyspareunia. *J. Assoc. Chartered Physiother. Obstet. Gynaecol.* 62: 17.

McMurray, R.G., Berry, M.J. & Katz, V. (1990) The beta endorphin response of pregnant women during aerobic exercise in water. *Med. Sci. Sports Exercise* 22(3): 298.

Noble, E. (1988) *Essential Exercises for the Childbearing Year,* 3rd edn. Boston: Houghton Mifflin.

Roberts, J.E., Mendez-Bauer, C. & Wodell, D.A. (1983) The effects of maternal position on uterine contractility and efficiency. *Birth* 10: 243.

Russell, J.G.B. (1982) The rationale of primitive delivery positions. *J. Obstet. Gynaecol.* 89: 712.

Sady, S.P. & Carpenter, M.W. (1989) Aerobic exercise during pregnancy. Special considerations. *Sports Med.* 7(6): 357.

Shepherd, A. (1980) Re-education of the muscles of the pelvic floor. In Mandelstam, D. (ed.) *Incontinence and its Management,* London: Croom Helm.

Weiss, G. (1984) Relaxin. *Ann. Rev. Physiol.* 46: 42.

Further Reading

Baum, G. (1987) *Aquarobics.* London: Faber.

Brayshaw, E. & Wright, P. (1994) *Teaching Physical Skills for the Childbearing Year.* Hale: Books for Midwives Press.

Brayshaw, E. & Wright, P. (1996) *Relaxation and Exercise for the Childbearing Year.* Hale: Books for Midwives Press.

Cullum, R. & Mowbray, L. (1986) *The English YMCA Guide to Exercise to Music.* London: Pelham Books.

Mitchell, L. (1988) *Simple Relaxation,* 2nd edn. London: John Murray.

Polden, M. & Whiteford, B. (1992) *The Postnatal Exercise Book.* London: Frances Lincoln.

Useful Addresses

Association of Chartered Physiotherapists in Women's Health (formerly Obstetrics and Gynaecology)
c/o The Chartered Society of Physiotherapy, 14 Bedford Row, London WC1R 4ED
Tel. 0171 242 1941

Royal Society of Arts (RSA)
Progress House, Westwood Way, Coventry CV4 8HS
Tel. 01203 470033

YMCA – London Central
112 Great Russell Street, London WC1B 3NQ
Tel. 0171 580 2989

Part Eight

From Pregnancy to Labour

26

The Biological Adaptations of the Fetus to Labour

The Adrenal Gland

Until about 35 weeks' gestation, the fetal adrenal gland is predominantly involved in the synthesis of dehydro-epiandrosterone sulphate (DHEAS). While *in vitro* studies have found a limited capacity for cortisol synthesis, measurements in the fetal circulation during the first half of pregnancy suggest that less than 5% of cortisol is of fetal origin. Since oestrogen stimulates most fetal tissues to convert cortisol to cortisone, maternal cortisol in the fetal circulation is thought to act within the hypothalamus to inhibit corticotrophin-releasing hormone (CRH), thereby delaying maturation of the fetal stress axis. Under these conditions, pituitary adrenocorticotrophic hormone (ACTH) remains low and does not activate the definitive, cortisol-producing zone of the adrenal gland (Pearson Murphy, 1979; Pepe and Albrecht, 1990; Pearson Murphy and Branchard, 1994; Pepe and Albrecht, 1995).

From the second half of pregnancy, levels of maternal cortisol decline in the fetal circulation due to the oestrogen-stimulated increase in placental conversion of cortisol to cortisone. Freed from the inhibitory effects of circulating cortisol, fetal synthesis of CRH begins to rise. The resulting increase in pituitary ACTH activates the definitive zone of the adrenal gland which enlarges and develops the capacity to synthesize the enzymes needed to convert pregnenolone to cortisol. At the same time oestrogen acts within most fetal tissues to convert cortisol to cortisone. Since cortisone is biologically inactive, it has no inhibitory effect on ACTH release from the anterior lobe of the pituitary gland. These findings suggest that oestrogen regulation of glucocorticoid metabolism within the placenta during the second half of pregnancy allows the structural development of the fetal stress axis in preparation for birth. Identical oestrogen regulation of glucocorticoid metabolism within the fetal compartment simultaneously mitigates the growth-retarding effects of cortisol on developing fetal tissues (Pearson Murphy, 1979; Pearson Murphy and Branchard, 1994; Pepe and Albrecht, 1995).

Cortisol and Fetal Maturation

The increased fetal adrenal capacity for cortisol synthesis during the latter part of pregnancy is accompanied by a rise in the capacity of selected fetal organs, particularly the liver, lungs and adrenal medulla, to convert cortisone to cortisol. In these tissues, cortisol acts with other hormones to induce a number of maturational adaptations that are important for the transition to extrauterine life. In the liver, cortisol increases glycogen synthesis and induces numerous hepatic enzymes required for the metabolism of carbohydrates, proteins and lipids. Hepatic glycogen increases rapidly from approximately 36 weeks' gestation to reach 50 mg/g at 40 weeks' gestation. In the first 12–24 hours following birth, maintenance of adequate blood glucose is largely dependent on the prior accumulation of hepatic stores of glycogen (Shelley *et al.*, 1975; Jones, 1989; Hawdon *et al.*, 1992; Kalhan, 1992).

Within the adrenal medulla, cortisol induces the synthesis of an enzyme complex that stimulates the conversion of noradrenaline to adrenaline. By this action, cortisol increases the ratio of adrenaline to noradrenaline as pregnancy advances. During the course of labour, the fetus releases a large surge of adrenaline that directly stimulates the absorption of lung liquid. This removal of lung liquid represents the culmination of a complex process of maturational changes in the lungs that are stimulated by a number of hormones including cortisol (Artal, 1980; Oliver, 1981; Jones, 1989).

Fetal Lung Maturation

Different cellular changes occur in pulmonary tissues during successive phases of lung development. Until approximately 17 weeks, terminal and respiratory bronchioles are lined with cuboidal epithelial cells that contain abundant amounts of glycogen. These stores are thought to provide energy and precursors for the subsequent synthesis of surfactant. By 24 weeks, some cuboidal epithelial cells differentiate into thin flat cells, called *type I pneumocytes*, that become more closely associated with expanding networks of surrounding capillaries. At the same time, a second type of cuboidal epithelial cell begins to differentiate within the emerging alveoli. These *type II pneumocytes* synthesize, store and secrete a complex substance called *surfactant* that is composed of a number of distinct glycerophospholipid and specialized protein molecules. As the secretion of surfactant increases,

cells lining the terminal sacs also become thinner, particularly during the last eight weeks of pregnancy. This allows the capillaries to intimately surround the entire alveoli, increasing the surface area potentially available for gas exchange, in preparation for the onset of respiration (Jobe, 1984; Snyder *et al.*, 1985; Pepe and Albrecht, 1995) (Figure 1).

When type II pneumocytes first appear they contain numerous glycogen granules. From approximately 18 weeks onwards, these stores begin to decrease through a process of glycogenolysis that seems to be stimulated by increasing concentrations of a lipid molecule called *platelet-activating factor* (PAF). PAF is thought to trigger the enzymatic reactions involved in the synthesis of surfactant-associated phospholipids within the endoplasmic reticulum. From approximately 24 weeks onwards, increasing quantities of PAF are stored in lamellar bodies in the cytoplasm. Secretion is evident from approximately 32 weeks, and levels progressively increase with advancing gestation. Relative concentrations of the principal phospholipids also change with advancing gestation. For example, surfactant that is initially secreted contains high levels of phosphatidylinositol (PI) and very low levels of phosphatidyglycerol (PG). This ratio is gradually reversed until term when very little PI is present. As secretion rates and maturation increases, surfactant forms a lipid monolayer lining around the lumen of the alveoli. This reduces surface tension of the terminal sacs and stabilizes the membrane which prevents them from collapsing following the onset of respiration (Jobe, 1984; Snyder *et al.*, 1985; Hoffman *et al.*, 1986; Pepe and Albrecht, 1995).

Hormonal Regulation

The differentiation of type II pneumocytes and the production of surfactant is closely associated with increasing levels of a number of different hormones, particularly cortisol, oestrogen, adrenaline, prolactin and thyroid hormone. In experimental studies, cortisol has been found to be involved in several aspects of lung maturation. These include growth of the alveolar diameter, regulation of glycogen metabolism, enhanced synthesis and activity of enzymes involved in lipid production and stimulation of beta-adrenergic receptors. As well as increasing secretion of an important phospholipid, these receptors stimulate the reabsorp-

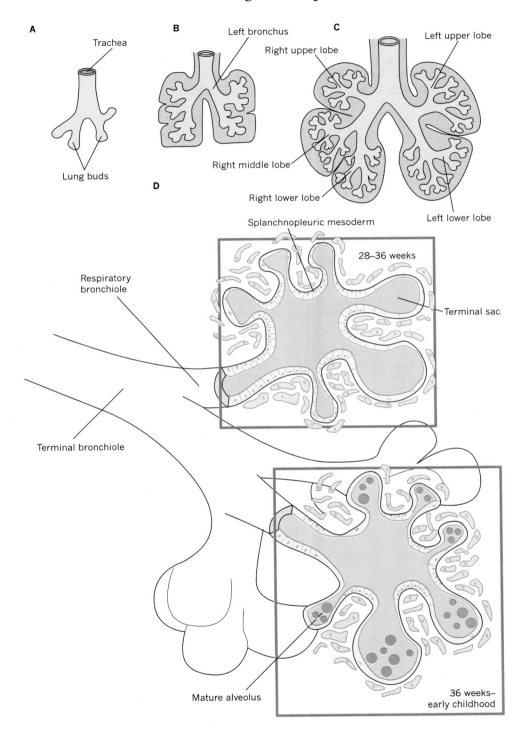

Figure 1   Successive stages in the development of the trachea and lungs. A, at 5 weeks; B, at 6 weeks; C, at 8 weeks; D, lung-tissue maturation. Terminal sacs (primitive alveoli) begin to form between weeks 28 and 36 and begin to mature between 36 weeks and birth. However, only 5–20% of all terminal sacs are formed prior to birth.

tion of lung fluid, particularly during labour. At present, prolactin and thyroid hormone are thought to act mainly by enhancing the stimulatory influences of cortisol. In recent experiments, the combined infusion of these three hormones has been found to have a greater effect on structural and secretory aspects of lung maturation compared to that produced by each hormone alone (Ballard, 1989; Rooney, 1992; Snyder and Dekowski, 1992; Smith and Post, 1994; Pepe and Albrecht, 1995).

References

Artal, R. (1980) Fetal adrenal medulla. *Clin. Obstet. Gynaecol.* **23**(3): 825–836.

Ballard, P.L. (1989) Hormonal regulation of pulmonary surfactant. *Endocrine Rev.* **10**(2): 165–181.

Hawdon, J.M., Ward Platt, M.P. & Aynsley-Green, A. (1992) Patterns of metabolic adaptation for preterm and term infants in the first neonatal week. *Arch. Dis. Childh.* **67**: 357–365.

Hoffman, D.R., Truong, C.T. & Johnston, J.M. (1986) The role of platelet-activating factor in human fetal lung maturation. *Am. J. Obstet. Gynecol.* **155**(1): 70–75.

Jobe, A. (1984) Fetal lung maturation and respiratory distress syndrome. In Beard, R.W. & Nathaniel, S.Z. (eds) *Fetal Physiology and Medicine*, pp. 317–351. New York: Marcel Dekker.

Jones, S.A. (1989) Fetal maturation in late pregnancy. In Turnbull, A. & Chamberlain, G. (eds) *Obstetrics*, pp. 119–127. Edinburgh: Churchill Livingstone.

Kalhan, S.C. (1992) Metabolism of glucose and methods of investigation in the fetus and newborn. In Polin, R.A. & Fox, W.W. (eds) *Fetal and Neonatal Physiology*, pp. 357–372. Philadelphia, W.B. Saunders.

Oliver R.E. (1981) Of labour and the lungs. *Arch. Dis. Childh.* **56**: 659–662.

Pearson Murphy, B.E. (1979) Cortisol and cortisone in human fetal development. *J. Steroid Biochem.* **11**: 509–513.

Pearson Murphy, B.E. & Branchard, C.L. (1994) The fetal adrenal. In Tulchinsky, D. & Little, A.B. (eds) *Maternal–Fetal Endocrinology*, pp. 275–296. Philadelphia: W.B. Saunders.

Pepe, G.J. & Albrecht, E.D. (1990) Regulation of the primate fetal adrenal cortex. *Endocrine Rev.* **11**(1): 151–176.

Pepe, G.J. & Albrecht, E.D. (1995) Actions of placental and fetal adrenal steroid hormones in primate pregnancy. *Endocrine Rev.* **16**(5): 608–648.

Rooney, S.A. (1992) Regulation of surfactant-associated phospholipid synthesis and secretion. In Polin, R.A. *et al.* (eds) *Neonatal and Fetal Medicine*, pp. 971–985. Philadelphia: W.B. Saunders.

Shelley, H.J., Basset, J.M. & Milner, R.D.G. (1975) Control of carbohydrate metabolism in the fetus and newborn. *Br. Med. Bull.* **31**(1): 37–43.

Smith, B.T. & Post, M. (1994) The influence of hormones on fetal lung development. In Tulchinsky, D. & Little, A.B. (eds) *Maternal–Fetal Endocrinology*, pp. 366–377. Philadelphia: W.B. Saunders

Snyder, J.M. & Dekowski, S.A. (1992) The role of prolactin in fetal lung maturation. *Seminars Reprod. Endocrinol.* **10**(3): 287–293.

Snyder, J.M., Mendelson, C.R. & Johnston, J.M. (1985) The morphology of lung development in the human fetus. In Nelson, G.H. (ed.) *Pulmonary Development Transition from Intrauterine to Extrauterine Life*, pp. 19–46. New York: Marcel Dekker.

27

Uterine Changes in Preparation for Labour

Uterine Activity

Current research findings point to the emergence of a nocturnal surge in uterine activity as an early indication of maternal changes that prepare for the onset of labour. Detailed studies on monkeys have demonstrated a circadian rhythm in uterine activity during the last trimester. This pattern of increased uterine contractility is accompanied by a nocturnal rise in plasma concentrations of oxytocin and an enhanced sensitivity of the myometrium to oxytocin. From 24 weeks' gestation, progressive nocturnal increases in myometrial activity have also been demonstrated in women and nocturnal peaks in plasma concentrations of oxytocin have been found in a study conducted between 37 and 39 weeks' gestation (Figueroa *et al.*, 1990; Fuchs *et al.*, 1992; Ducsay *et al.*, 1993; Germain *et al.*, 1993; Hirst *et al.*, 1993; Moore *et al.*, 1994).

Cervical and Myometrial Changes

From approximately 36 weeks onwards, structural alterations become apparent in cervical and myometrial tissues. Within the cervix, the composition and concentration of ground substance alters and this seems to

be accompanied by an increase in enzymes that degrade collagen. (Ground substance is the gel-like material in which connective tissue cells and fibres are embedded.) The concentration of ground substance relative to that of collagen is thought to reach maximum concentrations during the process of cervical softening prior to the onset of labour. This overall increase is characterized by the emergence of a higher proportion of molecules that have a weaker affinity for collagen fibrils. Towards the end of pregnancy, peak values have been reported in the concentration of specific molecules that demonstrate these features. A subsequent decline has also been found in molecules with a stronger binding capacity for collagen, that predominate during pregnancy (Uldbjerg, 1983; Granstrom *et al.*, 1989; Hillier, 1990; Jeffrey, 1991; Dessel, 1993).

These preparatory changes in cervical tissue in late pregnancy are followed by progressive dilatation of the external os during labour. This movement tends to occur slowly until approximately 4 cm and then more rapidly, until the cervix has passed over the presenting part of the descending fetus. Changes in cervical tissue during this period seem to be an acceleration of events in late pregnancy. During the latent phase of labour, a significant increase has been found in the concentration of a specific molecule called *hyaluronic acid*. In addition to its weak affinity for collagen, this molecule has a high water-binding capacity, which is thought to explain the swollen and fragile consistency of the cervix in labour. In addition, most studies report significant decreases in collagen content following labour and the duration of cervical dilatation is significantly correlated with cervical collagen content prior to the onset of labour (Jeffrey, 1991; Dessel, 1993).

In primiparous women, softening of cervical tissue proceeds alongside effacement. These events are thought to occur in response to an increase in the formation of *gap junctions* between adjacent cells in the myometrium. Gap junctions are composed of symmetrical portions of plasma membrane from adjacent cells. These form intercellular channels for the passage of ions and small molecules that facilitate rapid transmission of electrical impulses and chemical signals between cells. Gap junctions emerge in late pregnancy and undergo further increases in size and number during early labour. In animal studies the formation and permeability of gap junctions are stimulated by oestrogen and prostaglandins and inhibited by progesterone and relaxin (Tabb *et al.* 1991; Burghardt *et al.*, 1993; Lye *et al.* 1993; Chow and Lye, 1994).

By facilitating the propagation of action potentials from cell to cell, gap junctions synchronize myometrial activity. Tension is transmitted from the myometrium by the outer layer of muscle in the cervix and by localized pressure on the lower uterine segment, which is exerted by the fetus as the presenting part descends in the pelvis. These combined pressures produce a differential rate of tissue uptake in the cervix and the adjacent part of the uterus. Maximum uptake occurs at the lower peripheral end of the cervix, producing a gradual upward movement of soft cervical tissue that eventually merges with the lower uterine segment (Gee and Olah, 1993) (Figure 1).

In a recent study on women following induction and augmentation of labour, a number of significant features were associated with the presence or absence of cervical contractions in response to myometrial activity. Cervical contractions predominantly occurred in women with lower measures of cervical effacement and dilatation and a longer latent phase, compared to those in whom cervical contractions were absent. While these findings do not reflect the sequence of events during spontaneous labour, they highlight the importance of effacement and suggest that cervical muscle is actively involved in bringing it about (Olah *et al.*, 1993).

Current knowledge of biochemical changes in the

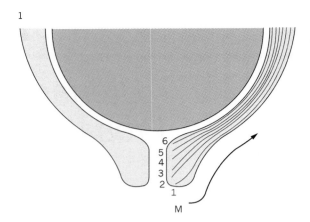

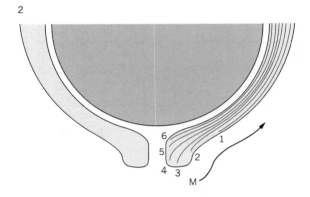

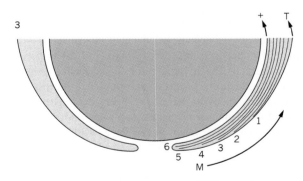

Figure 1　Diagram representing the differential movement of tissue planes at the time of cervical effacement and early dilatation. M, Direction of movement of collagen bundles; T, +, differential tension across the myometrium.

cervix have largely been put together from *in vitro* experiments on animals. While detailed knowledge exists of molecular changes in the different components of the cervix, the possible hormones involved in these events have not been clearly identified. Much of the work in this area suggests that while cervical changes may be stimulated under *in vitro* conditions by a variety of different hormones, these do not necessarily reflect the processes that occur *in vivo*.

For example, in *in vitro* experiments on rabbits, dehydroepiandrosterone sulphate (DHEAS) produces a moderate increase in the enzyme known to degrade collagen. But in this species, no change has been observed in collagen content between late pregnancy and postpartum. In women, use of prostaglandin E_2 (PGE_2) is associated with cervical maturation. Yet in recent *in vivo* experiments to induce cervical maturation, no increase in collagen breakdown occurred in response to PGE_2 treatment compared to cervices treated with a placebo. As recent *in vitro* experiments on women have found that PGE_2 treatment increases the turnover of specific polysaccharide chains, it is currently suggested that prostaglandins may regulate maturational changes in the ground substance and in this way indirectly influence the mechanical strength of collagen fibrils (Jeffrey, 1991).

However, changes in ground substance occur as part of an integrated process of tissue maturation that extends over late pregnancy and labour. In studies on women, a variety of hormone treatments seem to be involved in stimulating these events. These include oestrogen, relaxin, oxytocin, DHEAS, PGE_2 and $PGF_{2\alpha}$. At present, conflicting evidence exists with regard to progesterone. Studies in a variety of species have reported collagen breakdown and other maturational changes in response to antiprogestin treatments. However, studies using RU486 to induce labour at term in monkeys have found that progesterone withdrawal is associated with the absence of cervical dilatation and the orderly sequence of cervical and myometrial changes that occur with the spontaneous onset of labour (Evans *et al.*, 1983; Zuidema *et al.*, 1986; Haluska *et al.*, 1987; Hillier, 1990; Khalifa *et al.*, 1992; Dessel, 1993).

References

Burghardt, R.C., Barhoumi, R. & Dookwah, H. (1993) Endocrine regulation of myometrial gap junctions and their role in parturition. *Seminars Reprod. Endocrinol.* 11(3): 250–260.

Chow, L. & Lye, S.J. (1994) Expression of the gap junction protein connexin-43 is increased in the human mymometrium toward term and with the onset of labour. *Am. J. Obstet. Gynecol.* 170(3): 788–795.

Chwalisz K. (1994) The use of progesterone antagonists for cervical ripening and as an adjunct to labour and delivery, *Human Reprod.* 9, (Suppl. 1) 131–61

Dessel, T. van., Frijns, J.H. & Wallenburg, H.C. (1993) Prostaglandins and cervical dilatation. *Fetal Maternal Med. Rev.* 5: 79–88.

Duscay, C.A., Seron-Ferre, M., Germain, A.M. *et al.* (1993) Endocrine and uterine activity rhythms in the perinatal period. *Seminars Reprod. Endocrinol.* 11(3): 285–294.

Evans, M.J., Dougan, M.-B., Moawad, A.H. *et al.* (1983) Ripening of the human cervix with porcine ovarian relaxin. *Am. J. Obstet. Gynecol.* 147(4): 410–414.

Figueroa, J.P., Honnebier, B.O.M., Kenkins, S. *et al.* (1990) Alteration of 24-hour rhythms in myometrial activity in the chronically catheterized pregnant rhesus monkey after a 6-hour shift in the light-dark cycle. *Am. J. Obstet. Gynecol.* 163(2): 648–654.

Fuchs, A.-R., Behrens, O. & Liu, H.-C. (1992) Correlation of nocturnal increase in plasma oxytocin with a decrease in plasma estradiol/progesterone ratio in late pregnancy. *Am. J. Obstet. Gynecol.* 167(6): 1559–1563.

Gee, H. & Olah, K.S. (1993) Failure to progress in labour. *Progress in Obstetrics and Gynaecology*, 10: pp. 159–181. Edinburgh: Churchill Livingstone.

Germain, A.M., Valenzuela, G.J., Ivankovic, M. *et al.* (1993) Relationship of circadian rhythms of uterine activity with term and preterm delivery. *Am. J. Obstet. Gynecol.* 168(4): 1271–1277.

Granstrom, L., Ekman, G., Ulmsten, U. *et al.* (1989) Changes in connective tissue of corpus and cervix uteri during ripening and labour in term pregnancy. *Br. J. Obstet. Gynaecol.* 96: 1198–1202.

Haluska, G.J., Stanczyk, F.Z., Cook, M.J. *et al.* (1987) Temporal changes in uterine activity and prostaglandin response to RU486 in rhesus macaques in late gestation. *Am. J. Obstet. Gynecol.* 157(6): 1487–1495.

Hillier, K. (1990) Eicosanoids and the uterine cervix. In Mitchell, M.D. (ed.) *Eicosanoids in Reproduction*, pp 103–122. Boston: CRC Press.

Hirst, J.J., Haluska, G.J., Cook, M.J. *et al.* (1993) Plasma oxytocin and nocturnal uterine activity: maternal but not fetal concentrations increase progressively during late pregnancy and delivery in rhesus monkeys. *Am. J. Obstet. Gynecol.* 169(2): 415–422.

Jeffrey, J.J. (1991) Collagen and collagenase: pregnancy and parturition. *Sem. Perinatol.* 15(2): 118–126.

Khalifa R.M. Sayre B.L. Lewis B. (1992) Exogenous oxytocin dilates the cervix in ewes. *J. Anim. Sci.* 70: 38–42

Lye, S.J., Nicholson, B.J. & Mascarenhas, M. (1993) Increased expression of connexin-43 in the rat myometrium during labour is associated with an increase in the plasma estrogen : progesterone ratio. *J. Clin. Endocrinol. Metab.* 132(6): 2380–2386.

Moore, T.R., Iams, J.D., Creasy, R.K. *et al.* (1994) Diurnal and gestational patterns of uterine activity in normal human pregnancy. *Obstet. Gynecol.* **83**(4): 517–523.

Olah, K.S., Gee, H. & Brown, J.S. (1993) Cervical contractions: the response of the cervix to oxytocic stimulation in the latent phase of labour. *Br. J. Obstet. Gynaecol.* **100**: 635–640.

Osmers R. Werner R., Pflanz A *et al.* (1993) Glycosaminoglycans in cervical connective tissue during pregnancy and parturition. *Obstet. Gynecol.* **81**: 88–92.

Tabb, T.N., Garfield, R.E. & Thilander, G. (1991) Physiology of myometrial function: intercellular coupling and its role in uterine contractility. *Fetal Med. Rev.* **3**: 169–183.

Uldbjerg, N., Ulmsten, U. & Ekman, G. (1983) The ripening of the human uterine cervix in terms of connective tissue biochemistry. *Clin. Obstet. Gynecol.* **26**(1): 14–26.

Zuidema, L.J., Khan-Dawood, F. & Dawood, M.Y. (1986) Hormones and cervical ripening: Dehydroepiandrosterone sulphate, estradiol, estriol, and progesterone. *Am. J. Obstet. Gynecol.* **155**(6): 1252–1254.

28

Hormonal Interactions in Labour

Experimental findings on a variety of species suggest that maternal–placental–fetal interactions that actively support the fetus within the uterine cavity create gradual transformational changes that modify the accommodation of the fetus as pregnancy advances. While particular modifying changes have been identified in rats, sheep and other mammals, extensive research has failed to produce similar findings in humans and other primates. In these groups, preparatory transformational changes occur over a long time period and display a circadian rhythm that progressively evolves into labour and birth. A number of studies on women have reported that the onset of labour is most likely to occur from 21.00 to 03.00 and least likely from 13.00 to 14.00. A disproportionate number of births take place between 01.00 and 05.00 and lowest numbers between 14.00 and 18.00. As well as an increased frequency in the onset of labour during the hours of darkness, a shorter duration has also been reported in women that labour between 00.00 and 06.00 compared to those at other times of the day (Charles, 1953; Cooperstock *et al.*, 1987; Longo and Yellon, 1988; Figueroa *et al.*, 1990; Honnebier *et al.*, 1992; Germain *et al.*, 1993; Moore *et al.*, 1994).

Hormonal Regulation of Nocturnal Myometrial Activity

Experiments on rats and sheep have shown that the expression and storage of oxytocin in the hypothalamus and posterior pituitary increases during pregnancy under the stimulatory influences of oestrogen and progesterone. The pattern of increase found in these studies strongly indicates that central stores of oxytocin are augmented in preparation for labour and lactation. Other studies on monkeys have demonstrated that two distinct peaks occur ever 24 hours in circulating levels of oestrogen, during the latter half of pregnancy: a morning peak derived from maternal androgen secretion and a nocturnal peak derived from fetal secretion of dehydroepiandrosterone (DHEAS) (Caldwell *et al.*, 1989; Honnebier *et al.*, 1992; Broad *et al.*, 1993; Umezaki *et al.*, 1993).

From these findings, it has been suggested that the morning peak may stimulate the synthesis of gap junctions and oxytocin receptors in the myometrium, with a lag time of approximately 8–12 hours. Consequently, by the nocturnal peak in oestrogen secretion, the myometrium has become more sensitive to its direct stimulatory actions on the molecules that regulate contractions. Other studies on monkeys and humans have found a nocturnal peak in plasma concentrations of oxytocin and an enhanced sensitivity of the myometrium to oxytocin during the hours of darkness. Taken together, these experiments suggest that as central stores of oxytocin increase during the latter half of pregnancy, nocturnal relaxation releases the inhibitory influences on oxytocin which then acts in conjunction with oestrogen to stimulate episodes of increased myometrial activity (Honnebier *et al.*, 1992, 1993; Fuchs *et al.*, 1992; Hirst *et al.*, 1993a,b; Germain *et al.*, 1993; Umezaki *et al.*, 1993).

Tissue Changes and Inflammation

Local pro-inflammatory changes are thought to accompany the reorganization and stretching of cervical tissue that occurs in the latter part of pregnancy. The progressive release of a number of inflammatory mediators like prostaglandins and interleukin-1 may gradually overwhelm the selective suppression of inflammatory and immune responses that is established from the beginning of pregnancy. Current evidence suggests that the reorganization and stretching of the cervix and lower segment and the consequent disruption of fetal membranes is accompanied by local alterations in the relative activity of a number of mediators of inflammatory and anti-inflammatory reactions. These include a possible reduction in progesterone receptors and increased synthesis of inflammatory mediators including prostaglandins, without any change in prostaglandin dehydrogenase (PGDH), the enzyme stimulated by progesterone that inactivates prostaglandins throughout pregnancy (Siteri and Stites, 1982; Bennett *et al.*, 1992; Kelly 1994; How 1995; Schrey *et al.*, 1995).

Progesterone

In addition to its well-known inhibitory effects on the contractile responses of smooth muscle cells in the myometrium and vasculature, progesterone has a range of inhibitory effects on mediators of the immune/inflammatory response. A number of experiments have demonstrated that progesterone plays a critical role in preventing immune rejection of the feto-placental unit throughout pregnancy. While no reduction in plasma concentrations of progesterone has been demonstrated consistently in humans, recent findings indicate that uterine receptors for progesterone may decline towards term. This suggests that a local reduction in progesterone activity may occur at a time when tissue changes are stimulating a progressive rise in the synthesis of a large number of inflammatory mediators. Most research in this area has been focused on prostaglandins (Siteri and Stites, 1982; Cox *et al.*, 1993; Chwalisz, 1991; Kelly 1994; How 1995).

Prostaglandins

The placenta, decidua, myometrium and fetal membranes have varying capacities to synthesize prostaglandins, including $PGF_{2\alpha}$, PGE_2 and PGI_2. Both $PGF_{2\alpha}$ and PGE_2 stimulate myometrial contractions. Of the two, PGE_2 is 10 times more potent but unlike $PGF_{2\alpha}$ it has a dual action that simultaneously desensitizes the myometrium to its stimulatory effects. In contrast to these, PGI_2 is a potent vasodilator that relaxes smooth muscle. $PGF_{2\alpha}$ and PGE_2 are produced in varying amounts in the placenta, decidua and fetal membranes, while PGI_2 is predominantly produced by the myometrium and to a much lesser extent in the amnion (Fuchs and Fuchs, 1991).

Decidual prostaglandins

Current evidence suggests that the decidua is a major source of uterine prostaglandins during and after labour. In decidual cells obtained following spontaneous delivery, production rates of $PGF_{2\alpha}$ and PGE_2 are reported to be approximately 30 times greater than those obtained following elective Caesarean section, and this is accompanied by significantly greater concentrations of enzymes required for their production. Of the two groups, concentrations of $PGF_{2\alpha}$ are higher. This largely results from direct production of

PGF$_{2\alpha}$ with low conversion of PGE$_2$ to PGF$_{2\alpha}$ (Skinner and Challis, 1985; Cheung and Challis, 1989; Khan *et al.*, 1992).

The significance of decidual PGF$_{2\alpha}$ has also been confirmed by recent findings on the pattern of increase in its stable metabolite within the maternal circulation, during and after labour. Levels of 6-keto-PGF$_{1\alpha}$ and 13,14-dihydro-15-keto-PGF$_{2\alpha}$ (PGFM) progressively increase up to full dilatation and further increase at delivery of the fetal head. Between birth and placental separation, additional increases occur, producing values that are double those at full dilatation. Further increases occur after delivery, to reach highest levels at five minutes following placental separation (Fuchs *et al.*, 1982, 1983; Noort *et al.*, 1989) (Figure 1).

Amniotic prostaglandins

The amnion is composed of an epithelial layer, supported by a thick basement membrane composed of collagen and fibroblasts. This membrane produces mainly PGE$_2$, with much smaller amounts of PGF$_{2\alpha}$ and PGI$_2$. Reported increases of PGE$_2$ in association with labour are much lower than those of PGF$_{2\alpha}$ in the decidua. Basal output of PGE$_2$ in amniotic cells has been found to increase 3–4-fold between samples taken following elective Caesarean section and spontaneous

delivery (Skinner and Challis, 1985; Fuchs and Fuchs, 1991).

Unlike decidual prostaglandins, those from the amnion do not have direct access to the myometrium. Once produced, they are subject to distinct paracrine influences as they move across the chorion and the decidua. To gain an understanding of possible interactions during labour, a number of studies have attempted to examine these tissues in a way that reflects their interactions *in vivo* (McCoshen *et al.*, 1987, 1990; Collins *et al.*, 1992; Mitchell *et al.*, 1993; Germain *et al.*, 1994).

Amnion obtained following spontaneous labour at term has been found to produce higher levels of PGE$_2$, but no change in PGF$_{2\alpha}$ following exposure to term amniotic fluid, compared to membrane obtained following elective Caesarean section at term. However, these changes only appear on the fetal amniotic side of the membrane. Isolated chorion/decidual membranes obtained after labour produce significantly higher levels of PGE$_2$ and PGF$_{2\alpha}$, compared to membranes obtained at term. But this does not occur when these are studied as intact membranes, intimately associated with the amnion, as they exist *in vivo*. Exposure of laboured amnion to amniotic fluid *decreases* chorion/

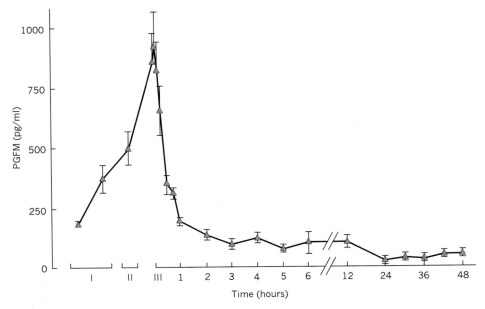

Figure 1   Plasma PGFM levels (pg/ml; mean ± SEM) I: in early labour and at full dilatation; II: at delivery of the fetal head; III: at placental separation; and up to 48 hours after placental separation. (Reproduced with permission from Noort *et al.*, 1989, p. 6.)

decidual release of PGE_2 and $PGF_{2\alpha}$ (McCoshen et al., 1987, 1990; Collins et al., 1992).

Action of the chorion

This difference seems to be due to varying levels of enzyme activity that metabolizes prostaglandins to their inactive metabolites. Amnion is characterized by a high capacity to synthesize and a low capacity to inactivate PGE_2. Chorion has a very low capacity to synthesize both PGE_2 and $PGF_{2\alpha}$ but, like the decidua, it contains high concentrations of PGDH that converts both groups of prostaglandins to inactive metabolites. The activity of this enzyme impedes the transfer of prostaglandins across intact amnio–chorio–decidua before and after the onset of labour (Germain et al., 1994).

The capacity of chorion to degrade prostaglandins is thought to be comparable to or greater than lung tissue which is known to be a rich source of PGDH. Research findings suggest that this membrane contains enzymes that degrade prostaglandins and other molecules that stimulate myometrial contractions. Experiments on dispersed chorion before and after spontaneous labour at term show a high level of $PGF_{2\alpha}$ metabolism but no net production of either PGE_2 or $PGF_{2\alpha}$. In a recent in vitro experiment, the specific activities of PGDH were not found to be significantly different in samples taken before and after the onset of labour. Similar findings have been reported in the decidua (Skinner and Challis, 1985; Casey et al., 1989; Germain et al., 1994).

In addition to PGDH and other similar enzymes, the chorion contains high concentrations of a protein called *gravidin* that has been found to inhibit the release of arachidonic acid from decidual cells. Recent experiments have found that the activity of this protein is significantly greater in chorion obtained following elective Caesarean section, compared to that following spontaneous delivery at term. *Phospholipase A_2* is an enzyme that directly releases arachidonic acid from plasma membranes. Within the decidua, concentrations of this enzyme have been found to increase three-fold during pregnancy. At the same time high concentrations of gravidin in the chorion may inhibit the activity of phospholipase A_2 in the adjoining decidua. Recent findings on gravidin suggest that with the onset of labour, this inhibitory regulation of decidual prostaglandins declines (Wilson et al., 1989).

Intact membranes

Experimental findings on the combined effects of intact membranes strongly indicate that they are ideally positioned to protect the fetus from locally produced prostaglandins and other inflammatory mediators that also have the capacity to stimulate the myometrium to contract. In a recent in vitro experiment, the presence of fetal membranes and decidua from term pregnancies following Caesarean section or vaginal delivery produced a 40% decrease in spontaneous contractions of adjacent muscle fibres. Studies on the accumulation of prostaglandins in different compartments of amniotic fluid before, during and after labour suggest that it occurs as a constituent part of local tissue changes that are an integral part of labour (Collins et al., 1993; MacDonald and Casey, 1993).

Rupture of the membranes

Findings on PGDH in decidua and chorion have led to suggestions that the increased production of PGE_2 in the amnion during labour may be involved in stimulating local changes that prepare the membranes for rupture and subsequent separation from the decidua following delivery. Recent experiments have found that amnion obtained from spontaneous deliveries is 42% heavier than that obtained following elective Caesarian sections. This is thought to result from PGE_2-stimulated increase in hydrolysis of collagen that results in increased uptake of water in the collagen matrix. This change is thought to facilitate the spontaneous rupture of membranes during labour (McCoshen et al., 1990).

Oxytocin

Receptors for oxytocin have been identified in the myometrium, decidua, placenta and fetal membranes. Those in the myometrium and decidua increase progressively from late pregnancy to labour, while increased binding to oxytocin has been demonstrated by those in the fetal membranes. Highest numbers have been found in early labour, when they reach two to three times above those at term. Within this overall increase, receptors are unevenly distributed in different parts of the uterus. During early labour, myometrial receptor concentrations are uniformly high in the upper segment and progressively lower in the isthmus and cervix. Those in the decidua are highest in the corpus, followed by the fundus and the isthmus (Fuchs *et al.*, 1984; Fuchs and Fuchs, 1991; Hirst *et al.*, 1993b).

Oxytocin receptors in the myometrium directly stimulate muscle contractions, while those in the remaining tissues may initiate synthesis of prostaglandins. The progressive formation of gap junctions in late pregnancy and early labour allows the activation of oxytocin receptors in the myometrium to stimulate synchronized contractions throughout the uterus. Experiments on the action of decidual receptors have found that the addition of oxytocin stimulates synthesis of PGE_2, and $PGF_{2\alpha}$ in decidual but not in myometrial tissue. Significantly higher basal and oxytocin-stimulated prostaglandin concentrations have been found in decidual samples obtained in early labour, compared to those at term. In contrast, no significant change occurs in myometrial concentrations over the same period (Fuchs *et al.*, 1982; Fuchs and Fuchs, 1991).

FETAL

Within the fetal membranes, increased oxytocin-receptor binding has been found between late pregnancy and labour, with highest increases detected in the amnion. This change appears to be a direct response to the increased release of fetal oxytocin during labour. Oxytocin in amniotic fluid is thought to directly flow from the umbilical circulation and from fetal urine. Concentrations of oxytocin in amniotic fluid are higher in samples taken at delivery than during late pregnancy. Following spontaneous labour and delivery, significantly higher levels of oxytocin have also been found in the umbilical artery than in the umbilical vein. In contrast, no significant differences have been found following elective Caesarean section (Dawood *et al.*, 1978a,b, Benedetto *et al.*, 1990).

During labour, increased amniotic fluid concentrations of oxytocin may stimulate production of PGE_2 within the amnion, while that in the umbilical circulation may stimulate prostaglandin synthesis within the placenta. However, the biological activity of fetal oxytocin remains to be defined. In rhesus monkeys, infusion of oxytocin into the fetal circulation results in a 60-fold rise in plasma concentrations, without affecting myometrial contractions or maternal plasma concentration of oxytocin. This implies that oxytocin from the fetal circulation may be degraded in the chorion and placenta, as both tissues contain high concentrations of oxytocinase which rapidly degrades oxytocin. In amniotic fluid samples obtained from women during

pregnancy, only 10% of oxytocin has been found to be biologically active (Roy *et al.*, 1986; Hirst *et al.*, 1993b; Germain *et al.*, 1994).

MATERNAL

Following its synthesis in hypothalamic nuclei, oxytocin is transported along axons that mainly terminate in the posterior lobe of the pituitary gland. From here it is released into a capillary network and carried by the systemic circulation to the uterus. During labour oxytocin is released in a pulsatile manner that continues during lactation. This discontinuous pattern of release has produced wide fluctuations and variations in serial samples obtained at different frequencies during labour (Leake *et al.*, 1981; Thornton *et al.*, 1992).

A more accurate picture has recently emerged from samples taken at one-minute intervals over 30 minutes during late pregnancy, labour and birth of the infant and placenta. *Group one* were at term but not in labour; *group two* were in spontaneous labour with cervical dilatation of 2–5 cm; and *group three* were at various points in the second and third stages of labour (Fuchs *et al.*, 1991) (Figures 2–4).

A highly individual pulsatile pattern is evident in all groups. Pulses are evident at irregular intervals with variable peak levels or amplitudes lasting 1–3 minutes. Mean pulse frequency and duration of pulses are lowest in group one and progressively increase as labour advances. No significant increase is evident in mean peak levels between labour and non-labour groups. Although highest peaks occur in the second and third stage of labour, these are highly variable and not uniformly associated with contractions, birth or delivery of

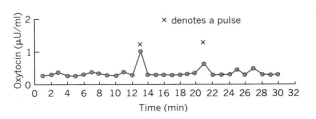

Figure 2 Plasma oxytocin level in a woman in late pregnancy not in labour. Samples were collected at one-minute intervals from indwelling catheter in right arm. (Reproduced with permission from Fuchs *et al.*, 1991, p. 1517.)

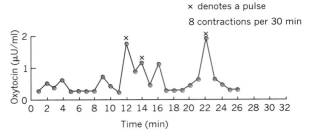

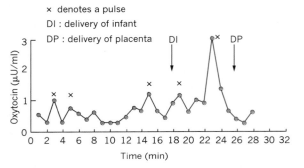

Figure 3 Plasma oxytocin level in a pregnant woman in the first stage of labour (cervix 2–5 cm dilated). (Reproduced with permission from Fuchs *et al.*, 1991, p. 1518.)

Figure 4 Plasma oxytocin level in a pregnant woman during the second and third stages of labour. DI, delivery of infant; DP, delivery of placenta. (Reproduced with permission from Fuchs *et al.*, 1991, p. 1519.)

the placenta. Similar findings at birth have also been reported in pigs (Fuchs *et al.*, 1991; Gilbert *et al.*, 1994) (Figure 5).

The release of oxytocin during labour is thought to occur in response to neuronal stimuli from the uterus, cervix and vagina. During pregnancy and labour, innervation is low in the body of the uterus and significantly higher in the cervix, vagina and adjacent parts of the pelvic cavity. Stretching and distension of these areas has been found to activate sensory afferent nerve pathways that transmit signals via the spinal cord and brainstem to oxytocin neurones in the hypothalamus. These respond with discrete bursts of accelerated discharge that transports the stored hormone along axons of hypothalamic neurones that mainly terminate in the posterior pituitary gland. From here oxytocin is released in a pulsatile manner into the general circulation (Luckman *et al.*, 1993; Antonijevic *et al.*, 1995; Johnson and Everitt, 1995) (Figure 6).

Recent findings on the lack of consistent association

between oxytocin pulses and uterine contractions at different phases of labour and birth has led to experiments on afferent pathways between the uterus and the hypothalamus and on other neuronal pathways that influence oxytocin in the hypothalamus and posterior lobe of the pituitary gland. At present, most detailed studies have been conducted in rats on the modulating influence of opioid neurones in the posterior pituitary gland (Leng *et al.*, 1988; Douglas *et al.*, 1993; Way *et al.*, 1993; Antonijevic *et al.*, 1995).

Endogenous Opioid Peptides

Plasma concentrations of β-endorphin rise significantly from 38 weeks to reach peak values during labour. This increased synthesis and release of β-endorphin occurs alongside that of ACTH and other related peptides from the anterior pituitary. In animal experiments, opioid-containing neurones and opioid receptors have also been identified in the posterior lobe of the gland (Chan *et al.* 1993; Douglas *et al.*, 1993; Leng *et al.*, 1994).

Opioids and the release of oxytocin

At present, direct evidence on the influence of opioid peptides during pregnancy and labour has been obtained in rats. In *in vitro* experiments, opioids have been found to inhibit the release of oxytocin by suppressing the electrical activity of hypothalamic neurones and by inhibiting electrically stimulated release from nerve terminals in the posterior pituitary. Studies on live animals have found that this inhibitory effect only operates during periods when oxytocin secretion is being stimulated (Dyer, 1988; Douglas *et al.*, 1993).

Recent studies on rats have identified the dynamic interactions that emerge between oxytocin and opioids during late pregnancy and labour. In this species, plasma concentrations of relaxin progressively increase from mid-pregnancy and undergo a further surge prior to the onset of labour. Relaxin has been found to increase plasma concentrations of oxytocin just prior to the onset of labour by directly stimulating oxytocin neurones in the hypothalamus. During late pregnancy and labour, this action of relaxin has been shown to *enhance* opioid modulation of oxytocin. In both periods, the naloxone-stimulated increase in oxytocin is significantly greater in animals that have not been deprived of ovarian release of relaxin. This implies that

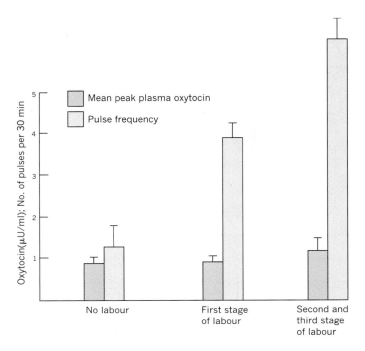

Figure 5   Mean oxytocin pulse frequency and amplitude determined in women at term, not in labour (*n* = 11), during first stage of labour (*n* = 13), and combined second and third stages of labour (*n* = 8). Oxytocin concentrations were measured by radioimmunoassay in samples collected at one-minute intervals for 30 minutes in each group; values greater than baseline ± 3 SD were considered a pulse. Means of all pulses in individual patients were calculated. Values given represent mean of these means ± SE; *n* = number of patients in each group. (Reproduced with permission from Fuchs *et al.*, 1991, p. 1520.)

the relaxin-induced release of oxytocin simultaneously enhances its opioid modulation (Way and Leng, 1992; Way *et al.*, 1993).

The stimulatory effects of relaxin on the release of both oxytocin and opioids are thought to be exerted via an afferent pathway to the hypothalamus, rather than at the level of nerve terminals in the posterior pituitary. This seems likely since the release of oxytocin during pregnancy and labour is known to be activated by sensory afferent nerve pathways that transmit signals via the spinal cord and brainstem to the hypothalamus. Supporting evidence for this thinking has emerged from the relaxin studies on rats and from similar studies that have identified the emergence, during late pregnancy, of a distinct pattern of opioid regulation in the posterior pituitary (Way and Leng, 1992; Douglas *et al.*, 1993; Way *et al.*, 1993).

During labour, rats have been found to release similar levels of oxytocin prior to naloxone stimulation, both in the presence and absence of relaxin. Despite this similarity, a smaller increase in oxytocin

concentration results from naloxone stimulation, only in animals that have been deprived of relaxin. This finding suggests that in these circumstances, opioids are specifically modulating the relaxin-induced increase in oxytocin neurones in the hypothalamus. Further studies have indicated that this enhanced opioid modulation of relaxin-stimulated increase in oxytocin is preceded in late pregnancy by a desensitization in opioid regulation of oxytocin from the pituitary. During this period, naloxone has been shown to have a diminished inhibitory effect on the release of oxytocin from nerve terminals in the posterior pituitary gland. From these combined results, it has been suggested that activation of oxytocin neurones in pregnancy induces an opioid inhibition that largely operates to limit its secretion and stores to accumulate prior to the onset of labour. In late pregnancy, the enhanced activation of oxytocin and opioid neurones in response to relaxin may lead to a gradual down-regulation of opioid receptors in the pituitary (Douglas *et al.*, 1993; Way *et al.*, 1993).

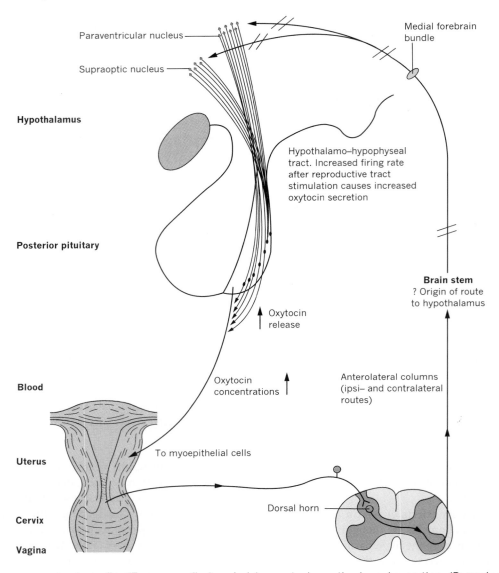

Paraventricular nucleus

Supraoptic nucleus

Hypothalamus

Posterior pituitary

Medial forebrain bundle

Hypothalamo–hypophyseal tract. Increased firing rate after reproductive tract stimulation causes increased oxytocin secretion

Brain stem
? Origin of route to hypothalamus

Oxytocin release

Blood

Oxytocin concentrations ↑

Anterolateral columns (ipsi– and contralateral routes)

Uterus

To myoepithelial cells

Cervix

Dorsal horn

Vagina

Figure 6   The neuroendocrine reflex (Ferguson reflex) underlying oxytocin synthesis and secretion. (Reproduced with permission from Johnson and Everitt, 1995, p. 299.)

This pattern of opioid regulation may play a part in initiating the storage of oxytocin during pregnancy and modulating its subsequent release in response to stimulatory and inhibitory influences in labour. During this process, oxytocin release is stimulated by the activation of sensory afferent nerve pathways and may also be inhibited by different forms of stress. Studies undertaken on rats have found that the rate of progress in labour is reduced in animals who are subjected to disturbance, compared to those left undisturbed. The opioid-induced nature of this effect is

indicated by the finding that progress returns to non-disturbed values following the injection of naloxone to the disturbed group (Newton *et al.*, 1968; Leng *et al.*, 1988).

These experimental findings on rats provide only general ideas about possible interactions in women. On present evidence, no comparable increases occur in plasma concentrations of relaxin during pregnancy and no direct information is possible on opioid regulation of oxytocin, either in the hypothalamus or the posterior pituitary gland. However, anecdotal evidence suggests that various forms of stress during labour tend to disrupt uterine activity and prolong the duration of labour (Peled, 1993).

Fetal Responses to Spontaneous Labour

The progressive nocturnal surge in uterine activity during the last trimester may gradually shift the fetus towards the lower pole of the uterus and allow the presenting part to descend into the pelvis. With successive contractions during labour, the fetus adopts a more flexed position and the presenting part descends further into the pelvis. As the presenting part meets the gutter-shaped angle of pelvic floor muscles with each contraction, it is gradually nudged in a more anterior direction, and when the vertex is presenting it becomes increasingly more flexed due to downward pressure of contractions and the simultaneous upward pull of the dilating cervix.

The fetus responds to these stimulatory influences with a significant rise in catecholamine output from the adrenal medulla and from extramedullary cells. Plasma levels have been found to rise from early labour and undergo a dramatic surge around the time of birth. Studies on the influence of labour on catecholamine production at term have found that umbilical arterial concentrations are four times higher in babies delivered vaginally, compared to those delivered by elective Caesarean section. Experimental findings in humans and other animals indicate that this large increase in catecholamine output produces a variety of cardiorespiratory and metabolic adaptations that occur during and after labour (Artal, 1980; Vyas et al., 1983; Faxelius et al., 1983; Lagercrantz and Slotkin, 1986; Lagercrantz and Marcus, 1991).

PULMONARY

The fetus is subject to many different forms of stimulation from hormonal and mechanical changes that facilitate the onset and progress of labour. During the last couple of days before labour begins, breathing activity is reduced and lung liquid is produced at a gradually decreasing rate. Experimental findings suggest that fetal breathing may be depressed by rising concentrations of PGE_2 while a decline in the volume of lung liquid is associated with increased production of catecholamines. In human studies, concentrations of catecholamines in amniotic fluid have been shown to rise from the second to the third trimester (Divers et al., 1981; Adamson, 1991; Bland, 1992).

In studies on lambs, rising concentrations of adrenaline during labour positively correlate with the progressive reabsorption of lung liquid. During labour, the composition of surfactant also matures and production levels increase following the administration of synthetic catecholamine preparations. The presence of similar changes in humans are evident from studies comparing lung function in infants born vaginally, to those delivered by elective Caesarean section. From measures taken at 30 and 120 minutes after birth, tidal volume, minute ventilation and dynamic lung compliance were found to be significantly lower in the Caesarean section group. Taken together these results indicate that higher levels of surfactant are produced and a more rapid elimination of lung liquid occurs in response to the stimulatory influences of labour (Oliver, 1981; Irestedt et al., 1982; Mortola et al., 1982).

CARDIOVASCULAR

Contractions induce transient reductions in uteroplacental perfusion that alter the pattern of feto-placental circulation. Ultrasonic studies on humans and monkeys suggest that at the beginning of a uterine contraction, maternal venous outflow is halted and the content of the uterine veins is expressed into the maternal circulation. At the same time arterial inflow that coincides with the onset of contractions is retained within the intervillous space. During contractions, this blood forms an increased pool that creates marked distension and vascular engorgement in the intervillous space. In this way, the transient reduction in uteroplacental perfusion during contractions may be partly compensated by the increased volume of maternal blood that is made available for gaseous exchange. To ensure the perfusion of the placenta, maternal blood pressure and cardiac output also rise in response to contractions. During the phase of uterine relaxation following each contraction an increased blood flow has been observed which may also compensate for decreased oxygen delivery during the preceding contraction (Ramsey et al., 1963; Smyth, 1973; Bleker et al., 1975; Robson et al., 1987).

Existing evidence suggests that the circulation of a healthy fetus in spontaneous labour is not compromised by contractions. The umbilical circulation does not appear to be altered by changes in intrauterine pressure or by short-term changes in fetal or maternal–placental blood flow that accompanies contractions. Fetal cardiac output rises in response to increased intrauterine pressure during contractions. This allows fetal blood pressure to maintain a relatively constant pressure difference between the inside and outside of its vascular system. At the same time, raised levels of fetal adrenaline specifically act to facilitate increases in heart rate and blood pressure, both of which serve to increase the rate of feto-placental blood flow between contractions. During the latter part of labour, selective pressure on the soft-walled umbilical vein has been reported to produce a net transfer of approximately 66 ml from fetus to placenta. While the fetal circulation remains attached to the high-capacity reservoir provided by the umbilical–placental unit, this redistribution of blood has no impact on the fetal circulation and only becomes relevant if the cord is clamped immediately after birth (Reynolds, 1955; Dunn, 1985).

The high fetal catecholamine levels that accompany spontaneous labour and normal pH values at birth are thought to be largely stimulated by pressure on the fetal head during contractions. Increased cranial pressure, particularly during the latter part of labour, is thought to be responsible for the late surge in catecholamines. This pressure may also produce central stimulation of parasympathetic fibres, particularly during active pushing following full dilatation of the cervix. Activation of the parasympathetic system inhibits cardiac pacemakers, resulting in decreased cardiac output, a slowing of the heart rate and reduced blood pressure. Slowing of the heart rate during contractions reduces the oxygen requirements of cardiac muscle. Parasympathetic influences on heart rate can be counteracted by adrenaline but not by noradrenaline. In the fetus at term, sufficient levels of adrenaline may be released to produce variable increases or decreases in heart rate, in response to uterine contractions (Reynolds, 1955; Lagercrantz and Slotkin, 1986).

References

Adamson S.L. (1991) Initiation of lung ventilation at birth. *Fetal Med. Rev.* **3**: 133–5.

Antonijevic, I.A., Leng, G., Luckman, S.M. *et al.* (1995) Induction of uterine activity with oxytocin in late pregnant rats replicates the expression of c-*fos* in neuroendocrine and brain stem neurons as seen during parturition. *Endocrinology* **136**(1): 154–163.

Artal, R. (1980) Fetal adrenal medulla. *Clin. Obstet. Gynecol.* **23**(3): 825–836.

Benedetto, M.T., Die Cicco, F., Rossiello, F. *et al.* (1990) Oxytocin receptor in human fetal membranes and term and during labour. *J. Steroid Biochem.* **35**(2): 205–208.

Bennett, P.R., Henderson, D.J. & Moore, G.E. (1992) Changes in expression of the cyclooxygenase gene in human fetal membranes and placenta with labour. *Am. J. Obstet. Gynecol.* **167**(1): 212–216.

Bland, R.D. (1992) Formation of fetal lung liquid and its removal near birth. In Polin, R.A. & Fox, W.W. (eds) *Fetal and Neonatal Physiology*, pp. 782–789. Philadelphia: W.B. Saunders Co.

Bleker, O.P., Kloosterman, G.J., Mieras, D.J. *et al.* (1975) Intervillous space during uterine contractions in human subjects: An ultrasonic study. *Am. J. Obstet. Gynecol.* **123**(7): 697–699.

Broad K.D., Kendrick K.M, Sitinathsinghji et al (1993) Changes in oxytocin immunoreactivity and mRNA expression in the sheep brain during pregnancy, parturition and lactation and in response to oestrogen and progesterone. *J. Neuroendocrinol.* **5**: 435–444.

Caldwell, J.D., Brooks, P.J., Jirikowski, G.F. *et al.* (1989)

Estrogen alters oxytocin mRNA levels in the preoptic area. *J. Neuroendocrinol.* **1**(4): 273–278.

Casey, M.L., Delgadillo, M., Cox, K.A. *et al.* (1989) Inactivation of prostaglandins in human decidua vera (parietalis) tissue: Substrate specificity of prostaglandin dehydrogenase. *Am. J. Obstet. Gynecol.* **160**(1): 3–7.

Chan, E.-C., Smith, R., Lewin, T. *et al.* (1993) Plasma corticotrophin-releasing hormone, b-endorphin and cortisol inter-relationships during human pregnancy. *Acta Endocrinol.* **128**: 339–344.

Charles, E. (1953) The hour of birth, a study of the distribution of times of onset of labour and of delivery throughout the 24 hour period. *Br. J. Preventative Social Med.* **7**: 43–59.

Cheung, P.Y.C. & Challis, J.R.G. (1989) Prostaglandin E₂ metabolism in the human fetal membrane. *Am. J. Obstet. Gynecol.* **161**(6): 1580–1585.

Collins, P.L., Goldfien, A. & Roberts, J.M. (1992) Exposure of human amnion to amniotic fluid obtained before labour causes a decrease in chorion/decidual prostaglandin release. *J. Clin. Endocrinol. Metab.* **74**(5): 1198–1205.

Collins, P.L., Idriss, E. & Moore, J.J. (1993) Human fetal membranes inhibit spontaneous uterine contractions. *J. Clin. Endocrinol. Metab.* **77**(6): 1479–1484.

Cooperstock, M., England, J.E. & Wolfe, R.A. (1987) Circadian incidence of labour onset hour in preterm birth and chorioamnionitis. *Am. J. Obstet. Gynecol.* **70**(6): 852–855.

Cox, S.M., King, M.R. & Casey, M.L. (1993) Interleukin-1β, -1α and -6 and prostaglandins in vaginal/cervical fluids of pregnant women before and during labour. *J. Clin. Endocrinol. Metab.* **77**(3): 805–815.

Dawood, M.Y., Raghavan, K.S., Pociask *et al.* (1978a) Oxytocin in human pregnancy and parturition. *Obstet. Gynecol.* **51**(2): 138–143.

Dawood, M.Y., Wang, C.F., Gupta, R. *et al.* (1978b) Fetal contribution to oxytocin in human labour. *Obstet. Gynecol.* **52**(2): 205–209.

Divers, W.A. *et al.* (1981) An increase in catecholamines and metabolites in the amniotic fluid compartment from middle to late gestation. *Am. J. Obstet. Gynecol.* **139**: 438–486.

Douglas, A.J., Dye, S., Leng, G. *et al.* (1993) Endogenous opioid regulation of oxytocin secretion through pregnancy in the rat. *J. Neuroendocrinol.* **5**: 307–314.

Dunn P.M. (1985) The third stage and fetal adaptation. In Clinch, J. & Matthews, T. (eds) *Perinatal Medicine: IX European Congress of Perinatal Medicine*, Dublin 1984, pp. 47–54. Lancaster: MTP Press.

Dyer, R.G. (1988) Oxytocin and parturition – new complications. *J. Endocrinol.* **116**: 167–168.

Faxelius, G., Hagnevik, K., Lagercrantz, H. *et al.* (1983) Catecholamine surge and lung function at delivery. *Arch. Dis. Childh.* **58**: 262–266.

Figueroa, J.P., Honnebier, B.O.M., Kenkins, S. *et al.* (1990) Alteration of 24-hour rhythms in myometrial activity in the chronically catheterized pregnant rhesus monkey after a 6-hour shift in the light–dark cycle. *Am. J. Obstet. Gynecol.* **163**(2): 648–654.

Fuchs, A.-F. & Fuchs, F. (1991) Physiology of parturition. In Gabbe, S.G. (ed.) *Obstetrics, Normal and Problem Pregnancies*, pp. 147–174. New York: Churchill Livingstone.

Fuchs, A.-F., Fuchs, F., Husselein, P. *et al.* (1982) Oxytocin receptors and human parturition: a dual role for oxytocin in the initiation of labour. *Science.* **215**: 1396–1398.

Fuchs, A.-F., Goeschen, K., Husslein, P. *et al.* (1983) Oxytocin and the initiation of human parturition. III Plasma concentrations of oxytocin and 13,14–dihydro–15–keto–prostaglandin $PGF_{2\alpha}$ in spontaneous and oxytocin–induced labour at term. *Am. J. Obstet. Gynecol.* **147**(5): 497–502.

Fuchs, A.-R., Fuchs, F., Husselein, P. *et al.* (1984) Oxytocin receptors in the human uterus during pregnancy and parturition. *Am. J. Obstet. Gynecol.* **150**(6): 734–741.

Fuchs, A.-R., Romero, R., Keefe, D. *et al.* (1991) Oxytocin secretion and human parturition: Pulse frequency and duration increase during spontaneous labour. *Am. J. Obstet. Gynecol.* **165**: 1515–1523.

Fuchs, A.-R., Behrens, O. & Liu, H.-C. (1992) Correlation of nocturnal increase in plasma oxytocin with a decrease in plasma estradiol/progesterone ratio in late pregnancy. *Am. J. Obstet. Gynecol.* **167**(6): 1559–1563.

Germain, A.M., Valenzuela, G.J., Ivankovic, M. *et al.* (1993) Relationship of circadian rhythms of uterine activity with term and preterm delivery. *Am. J. Obstet. Gynecol.* **168**(4): 1271–1277.

Germain, A.M., Smith, J., Casey, M.L. *et al.* (1994) Human fetal membrane contribution to the prevention of parturition: uterotonin degradation. *J. Clin. Endocrinol. Metab.* **78**(2): 463–470.

Gilbert, C.L., Goode, J.A. & McGrath, T.J. (1994) Pulsatile secretion of oxytocin during parturition in the pig: temporal relationship with fetal expulsion. *J. Physiol.* **475**(1): 129–137.

Hirst, J.J., Haluska, G.J., Cook, M.J. *et al.* (1993a) Plasma oxytocin and nocturnal uterine activity: maternal but not fetal concentrations increase progressively during late pregnancy and delivery in rhesus monkeys. *Am. J. Obstet. Gynecol.* **169**(2): 415–422.

Hirst, J.J., Chibbar, R. & Mitchell, B.F. (1993b) Role of oxytocin in the regulation of uterine activity during pregnancy and in the initiation of labour. *Seminars Reprod. Endocrinol.* **11**(3): 219–233.

Honnebier, M.B., Jenkins, S.I. & Nathanielsz, P.W. (1992) Circadian timekeeping during pregnancy: endogenous phase relationships between maternal plasma hormones and the maternal body temperature rhythm in pregnant rhesus monkeys. *Endocrinology* **131**(5): 2051–2058.

Honnebier, M.B., Mecnas, C.A., Jenkins, S.I. *et al.* (1993) Comparison of myometrial response to oxytocin during daylight with the response obtained during the early hours of darkness in the fetectomized rhesus monkey at 160–172 days gestational age. *Biol. Reprod.* **48**: 779–785.

How, H., Huang, Z.-H., Zuo, J. *et al.* (1995) Myometrial estradiol and progesterone receptor changes in preterm and term pregnancies. *Obstet. Gynecol.* **86**(6): 936–940.

Irestedt, L., Lagercrantz, H., Hjemdahl, P. *et al.* (1982) Fetal and maternal plasma catecholamine levels at elective caesarean section under general or epidural anaesthesia versus vaginal delivery. *Am. J. Obstet. Gynecol.* **142**(8): 1004–1010.

Johnson, M.H. & Everitt, B.J. (1995) *Essential Reproduction*, pp. 33–36. Oxford: Blackwell Science.

Khan, H., Ishihara, O., Sullivan, M.H. *et al.* (1992) Changes in decidual stromal cell function associated with labour. *Br. J. Obstet. Gynaecol.* **99**: 10–12.

Kelly, R.W. (1994) Pregnancy maintenance and parturition: the role of prostaglandin in manipulating the immune and inflammatory response. *Endo. Rev.* **15**(5): 684–706.

Lagercrantz H. & Marcus C. (1991) Sympathoadrenal mechanisms during development. In Polin R.A. *et al.* (eds) *Neonatal and Fetal Medicine*, pp. 160–169. Philadelphia: W.B. Saunders Company.

Lagercrantz, H. & Slotkin, T.A. (1986) The "stress" of being born. *Sci. Am.* **254**: 92–102.

Leake, R.D., Weitzman, R.E., Glatz, T.H. *et al.* (1981) Plasma oxytocin concentrations in men, nonpregnant women and pregnant women before and during spontaneous labour. *J. Clin. Endocrinol. Metab.* **53**(4): 730–733.

Leng, G., Mansfield, S., Bicknell, R.J. *et al.* (1988) Endogenous opioid actions and effects of environmental disturbance on parturition and oxytocin secretion in rats. *J. Reprod. Fertil.* **84**: 345–356.

Leng, G., Bicknell, R.J., Brown, D. *et al.* (1994) Stimulus-induced depletion of pro-enkephalins, oxytocin and vasopressin and pro-enkephalin interaction with posterior pituitary hormone release in vitro. *Neuroendocrinology.* **60**: 559–566.

Longo, L.F. & Yellon, S.M. (1988) Biological timekeeping during pregnancy and the role of circadian rhythms in parturition. In Kunzel, W. & Jensen, A. (eds) *The Endocrine Control of the Fetus*, pp. 173–192. Berlin: Springer-Verlag.

Luckman, S.M., Antonijevict, I., Leng, G., Dyer, S. *et al.* (1993) The maintenance of normal parturition in the rat requires neurohypophysial oxytocin. *J. Neuroendocrinol.* **5**: 7–12.

MacDonald, P.C. & Casey, M.L. (1993) The accumulation of prostaglandins (PG) in amniotic fluid is an after effect of labour and not indicative of a role for PGE_2 or $PGF_{2\alpha}$ in the initiation of human parturition. *J. Clin. Endocrinol. Metab.* **76**(5): 1332–1339.

McCoshen, J.A., Johnson, K.A., Dubin, N.H. *et al.* (1987) Prostaglandin E_2 release on the fetal and maternal sides of the amnion and chorion-decidua before and after term labour. *Am. J. Obstet. Gynecol.* **156**(1): 173–178.

McCoshen, J.A., Hoffman, D.R. & Kredenstser, J.V. (1990) The role of fetal membranes in regulating production, transport, and metabolism of prostaglandin E_2 during labour. *Am. J. Obstet. Gynecol.* **163**(5): 1632–1640.

Mitchell, B.F., Rogers, K. & Wong, S. (1993) The dynamics of prostaglandin metabolism in human fetal membranes and decidua around the time of parturition. *J. Clin. Endocrinol. Metab.* **77**(3): 759–764.

Moore, T.R., Iams, J.D., Creasy, R.K. *et al.* (1994) Diurnal and gestational patterns of uterine activity in normal human pregnancy. *Obstet. Gynecol.* **83**(4): 517–523.

Mortola, J.P., Fisher, J.T., Smith, J.B. *et al.* (1982) Onset of respiration in infants delivered by cesarean section. *J. Appl. Physiol.* **52**(3): 716–724.

Newton, N., Peeler, D. & Newton, M. (1968) Effect of disturbance on labour. *Am. J. Obstet. Gynecol.* **101**(8): 1096–1102.

Noort, W.A., van Bulck, B., Vereecken, A. *et al.* (1989) Changes in plasma levels of $PGF_{2\alpha}$ and PGI_2 metabolites at and after delivery at term. *Prostaglandins.* **37**(1): 3–12.

Oliver, R.E. (1981) Of labour and the lungs. *Arch. Dis. Childh.* **56**: 659–662.

Peled, G. (1993) Birth and the Gulf War. *MIDIRS Midwif. Dig.* **3**(1): 54.

Ramsey, E.M., Corner, G.W. & Donner, M.W. (1963) Serial and cincradioangiographic visualisation of maternal circulation in the primate (hemochorial) placenta. *Am. J. Obstet. Gynecol.* **86**(2): 213–225.

Reynolds, S.R.M. (1955) Circulatory adaptations to birth and their clinical implications. *Am. J. Obstet. Gynecol.* **70**(1): 148–161.

Robson S.C., Dunlop W., Boys R.J., et al (1987) Cardiac output during labour, *Br. Med. J.* **295** 1169–1172

Roy, A.C., Kottegoda, S.R., Viegas, O.A.C. *et al.* (1986) Oxytocinase activity in human amniotic fluid and its relationship to gestational age. *Obstet. Gynecol.* **68**(5): 614–617.

Schrey, M.P., Hare, A.L. & Ilson, S.L. (1995) Decidual histamine release and amplification of prostaglandin $F_{2\alpha}$ production by histamine in interleukin-1-β-primed decidual cells: potential interactive role for inflammatory mediators in uterine function at term. *J. Clin. Endocrinol. Metab.* **80**(2): 648–653.

Siteri, P.K. & Stites, D.P. (1982) Immunologic and endocrine interrelationships in pregnancy. *Biol. Reprod.* **26**: 1–14.

Skinner, K.A. & Challis, J.R.G. (1985) Changes in the synthesis and metabolism of prostaglandins by human fetal membranes and decidua at labour. *Am. J. Obstet. Gynecol.* **151**(4): 519–523.

Thornton, S., Davison, J.M. & Baylis, P.H. (1992) Plasma oxytocin during the first and second stages of spontaneous human labour. *Acta Endocrinol.* **126**: 425–429.

Umezaki, H., Valenzuela, G.J. & Hess, D.L. (1993) Fetectomy alters maternal endocrine and uterine activity rhythms in rhesus macaques during late gestation. *Am. J. Obstet. Gynecol.* **169**(6): 1435–1441.

Vyas, H., Milner, A.D. & Hopkin, I.E. (1983) Role of labour in the establishment of functional residual capacity at birth. *Arch. Dis. Childh.* **58**: 512–517.

Way, S.A. & Leng, G. (1992) Relaxin increases the firing rate of supraoptic neurones and increases oxytocin secretion in the rat. *J. Endocrinol.* **132**: 149–158.

Way, S.A., Douglas, A.J., Dye, S. *et al.* (1993) Endogenous opioid regulation of oxytocin release during parturition is reduced in ovariectomized rats. *J. Endocrinol.* **138**: 13–22.

Wilson, T., Liggins, G.C. & Joe, L. (1989) Purification and characterization of a uterine phospholipase inhibitor that loses activity after labour onset in women. *Am. J. Obstet. Gynecol.* **160**(3): 602–606.

29

Midwifery Care in the First Stage of Labour

Labour is the process by which the woman gives birth. It begins with the onset of regular uterine contractions and culminates in the delivery of the baby and the expulsion of the placenta and membranes. In normal labour the whole process is usually completed spontaneously within 18–24 hours and there are no complications. Nowadays, with modern management of labour, few women are in labour longer than 12–14 hours.

Stages of Labour

Labour is divided into three stages:

1 *First stage of labour*: From the onset of regular uterine contractions, accompanied by effacement of the cervix and dilatation of the os, to full dilatation of the os uteri.
2 *Second stage of labour*: From full dilatation of the os uteri to the birth of the baby.
3 *Third stage of labour*: From the birth of the baby to the expulsion of the placenta and membranes. This stage of labour also includes the control of haemorrhage.

The approximate time taken for each stage is shown in Table 1.

Such demarcations of the stages of labour are intended to aid clarity in understanding physiology and care for the professional care-giver. However, for the woman, labour is seen as a continuing physiological, psychological and emotional experience, the culmination and main focal point of the reproductive

Table 1   Approximate time taken for each stage of labour

	Primigravidae	Multigravidae
First stage	12–14 hours	6–10 hours
Second stage	60 minutes	Up to 30 minutes
Third stage	20–30 minutes or	20–30 minutes or
	5–15 minutes with active management	5–15 minutes with active management

process, where the above delineations acquire a different relevance and importance. The significance of labour, a biologically and socially creative life event, is reflected in the minutiae of detail women can recall about their particular labour(s). Such a picture may be readily recognized by midwives attempting to establish a woman's past maternity history, when events, relatively simple and usual from a midwife's perspective, acquire much meaning and importance in the eyes of the woman and her family. To maximize the potential for a satisfactory outcome of labour it is therefore essential that the care offered by the midwife during labour is sensitive to the needs of the woman and her family and underpinned by a sound knowledge base firmly rooted in research.

Factors Concerned with Labour

Causes of the onset of labour are discussed in Chapters 27 and 28.

The various factors concerned in labour are summarized in Table 2. A defect or delay at any stage or in any factor may result in complications.

Outline of the Physiology of the First Stage of Labour (Table 3)

There are two main physiological processes which take place in the first stage of labour:

▶ Effacement of the cervix.
▶ Dilatation of the os uteri.

These occur as a result of contraction and retraction of the uterine muscle.

Table 2   Factors concerned in labour

Muscular activity or powers	Involuntary: uterine muscle Voluntary: diaphragm thoracic muscles abdominal muscles
Birth canal or passages	Hard parts: bony pelvis Soft parts: lower uterine segment cervix uteri vagina pelvic floor
Uterine contents or passengers	Fetus Placenta, cord and membranes Liquor amnii
Hormones, e.g.	Prostaglandins Oxytocin Corticotrophin-releasing hormone Adrenocorticotrophic hormone Endogenous opioid peptides

(See Chapters 27 and 28)

Table 3   Summary of the physiological changes in the first stage of labour

Completion of effacement of the cervix and *dilatation of the os uteri* caused by *uterine activity*:

   Contraction and retraction of uterine muscle
   Fundal dominance
   Active upper uterine segment, passive lower segment
   Formation of the retraction ring
   Polarity of the uterus
   Intensity or amplitude of contractions
   Resting tone
Formation of the bag of *forewaters* and the *hindwaters*
Rupture of the membranes
Show

Effacement of the cervix

Effacement, or taking up, of the cervix may start in the latter two or three weeks of pregnancy. This occurs as a result of changes in the solubility of collagen present in cervical tissue. These changes are influenced by alterations in hormone activity, particularly oestradiol, progesterone, relaxin, prostacyclin and prostaglandins (Tucker-Blackburn and Loper, 1992). Braxton Hicks

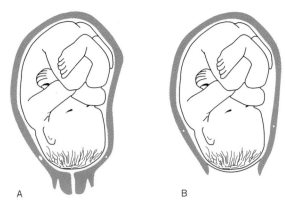

Figure 1 The uterus, showing **A**: cervix before effacement and **B**: effacement and dilatation of the cervix and the stretched lower uterine segment.

contractions, which become stronger in the final weeks of pregnancy, may also enhance the process. Cervical effacement is completed in labour. The cervix becomes shorter, dilates slightly and then becomes funnel-shaped as the internal os opens to form part of the lower uterine segment (Figure 1) (see Chapter 27).

Dilatation of the os uteri

Progressive dilatation of the os uteri (Figure 2) is a sign of true labour. It is assessed in centimetres by the midwife or doctor on examination per vaginam. When the os uteri is dilated sufficiently to allow the fetal head to pass through, full dilatation has been achieved. Although this is usually 10 cm, it may be more or less depending on the size of the fetal head.

In primigravidae, effacement of the cervix usually precedes dilatation of the os uteri, but in multigravidae effacement of the cervix and dilatation of the os uteri normally occur simultaneously.

Uterine contractions

Uterine contractions are responsible for achieving effacement and dilatation of the cervix and os uteri, and for the descent and expulsion of the fetus in labour. Contractions of the uterus in labour are:

▶ involuntary;
▶ intermittent and regular; and
▶ in most labours, painful.

The cause of the pain may be due, in part, to ischaemia developing in the muscle fibres during contractions. The backache which may accompany cervical dilatation is caused by stimulation of sensory fibres which pass via the sympathetic nerves to the sacral plexus.

Co-ordination of contractions

Contractions start from the cornua of the uterus and pass in waves, inwards and downwards. In normal uterine action the intensity is greatest in the upper uterine segment and lessens as the contraction passes down the uterus. This is called *fundal dominance*. The upper segment of the uterus contracts and retracts powerfully, whereas the lower segment contracts only slightly and dilates. Between contractions the uterus relaxes. Specific uterine pacemaker cells have not been identified. The co-ordinated uterine activity characteristic of normal labour occurs as a result of near-simultaneous contraction of all myometrial cells. During pregnancy increasing numbers of gap junctions form between the cells of the myometrium. These low-resistance communication channels enhance electrical conduction velocity and facilitate the co-ordination of myometrical contraction (Tucker-Blackburn and Loper, 1992) (see Chapter 27).

Retraction Retraction is a state of permanent shortening of the muscle fibres and occurs with each contraction (Figure 3). The muscle fibres therefore gradually become shorter and thicker, especially in the upper uterine segment. This exerts a pull on the less active lower uterine segment, the maximum pull being directed towards the weakest point, the cervix, and the os uteri. Hence the cervix is gradually taken up, or effaced, and the upward pull then dilates the os uteri, that is enlarges the opening. As the space within the upper uterine segment diminishes due to the contractions and retraction of the muscle fibres, the fetus is forced down into the lower segment and the presenting part exerts pressure on the os uteri. This not only aids dilatation, but also causes a reflex release of oxytocin from the posterior pituitary gland and thus promotes further uterine action.

Retraction ring A ridge gradually forms between the thick, retracted muscle fibres of the upper uterine segment and the thin, distended lower segment. This is called a retraction ring and is a normal physiological occurrence in every labour. Only in cases of obstructed labour when there is excessive contraction and retraction of uterine muscle is the retraction ring visible as a

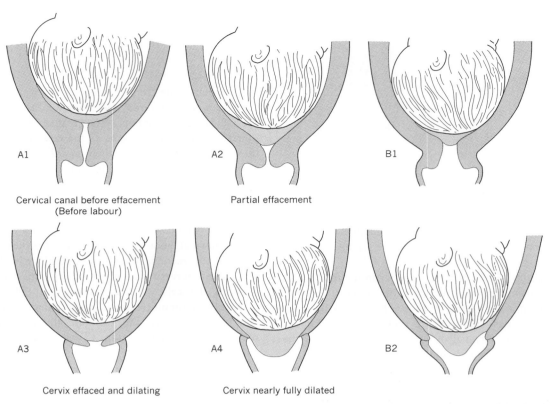

A1

Cervical canal before effacement
(Before labour)

A2

Partial effacement

B1

A3

Cervix effaced and dilating

A4

Cervix nearly fully dilated

B2

Figure 2 Effacement and dilatation of the cervix: **A**: in a primigravida; **B**: occurring simultaneously in a multigravida.

transverse ridge abdominally. It is then called a *Bandl's ring* and heralds imminent rupture of the uterus.

Polarity The co-ordination between the upper and lower segments is balanced and harmonious in normal labour. While the upper segment contracts powerfully and retracts, the lower segment contracts only slightly and dilates. This rhythmical co-ordination between the upper and lower uterine segments is called polarity.

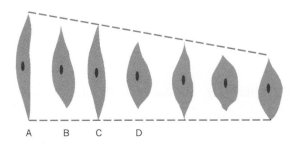

A   B   C   D

Figure 3 Retraction of the uterine muscle fibres.
A: Relaxed; **B**: contracted; **C**: relaxed but retracted;
D: contracted but shorter and thicker than those in B.

Intensity or amplitude Contractions cause a rise in intrauterine pressure. This is called the intensity or amplitude of contractions and can be measured by placing a fine catheter into the uterus and attaching it to an apparatus which records the pressure. Each contraction rises rapidly to a peak and then slowly declines to the *resting tone*. In early labour the contractions are weak, with an amplitude of about 20 mmHg. They last 20–30 seconds and occur infrequently, about every 20 minutes. As labour progresses the contractions become stronger, longer and more frequent. At the end of the first stage they are strong, with an amplitude of 60 mmHg, last 45–60 seconds and occur every 2–3 minutes.

Resting tone The uterus is never completely relaxed and in between contractions a resting tone can be measured. This is usually between 4 and 10 mmHg. During contractions the blood flow to the placenta is curtailed, thus oxygen and carbon dioxide exchange in the intervillous spaces is impeded. The period of relaxation between contractions when the uterus has a low resting tone is therefore vital for adequate fetal oxygenation (see cardiovascular section of Chapter 28).

Formation of the forewaters and hindwaters

As the lower uterine segment stretches and the cervix starts to efface, some chorion becomes detached from the decidua and both membranes form a small bag containing amniotic fluid; this protrudes into the cervix. When the fetal head descends on to the cervix, it separates the small bag of amniotic fluid in front, the *forewaters*, from the remainder, the *hindwaters*. The forewaters aid effacement of the cervix and early dilatation of the os uteri. The hindwaters help to equalize the pressure in the uterus during uterine contractions and thereby provide some protection to the fetus and placenta.

Rupture of the membranes

The membranes are thought to rupture as a result of increased production of PGE_2 in amnion in labour (McCoshen *et al.*, 1990) and the force of the uterine contractions, causing an increase in the fluid pressure inside the forewaters and a lessening of the support, as the os uteri dilates. In normal labour the membranes usually rupture towards the end of the first stage (see Chapter 28).

Show

The show is the operculum from the cervical canal which is shed per vaginam in labour. It is displaced when effacement of the cervix and dilatation of the os uteri occur. The show is recognized as a mucoid loss, slightly streaked with blood due to some separation of the chorion from the decidua around the cervix.

The reader is recommended to read Chapter 28 which explains the essential role of hormonal interactions in the process of labour.

Care in the First Stage of Labour

The first stage of labour is concerned with dilatation of the os uteri. It commences with the onset of regular uterine contractions and continues until full cervical dilatation is reached. For the woman it is the culmination of a long period of waiting accompanied by a variety of often conflicting emotions.

Aims of midwifery care in labour

The aims of midwifery care in labour are to achieve:

▶ the safe delivery of the mother;
▶ a live healthy baby; and
▶ a pleasurable, fulfilling experience of childbirth for both the mother and her partner.

To achieve these aims the midwife requires not only a knowledge of the anatomy of the reproductive tract and the physiology and management of labour, but also an understanding of human relations and skill in the art of communication. She must be competent to give good clinical care and skilled in procedures related to midwifery practice. The practice of midwifery should be based on valid research, where available, rather than on tradition.

The midwife also requires an understanding of the social and political context within which maternity care is planned and implemented. It is important that she has an appreciation of ethical issues surrounding childbirth and the confidence and ability to practise as an autonomous professional within a multidisciplinary team.

INDIVIDUALIZED CARE

Childbirth is an event of enormous biological and social significance to all women. Many now have high expectations and demand more autonomy in labour and greater emotional fulfilment. In order to give sensitive, individual care of a high standard, the midwife should:

1 assess the needs and expectations of each individual woman in labour;
2 plan care with each woman in labour tailored to meet her specific needs and expectations;
3 put the care plan into practice; and
4 evaluate the care given to measure its effectiveness.

The evaluation will provide information which can be of considerable value in improving quality of care. Evaluation of the care given takes place throughout labour and any necessary modifications are then made. It can also be helpful to visit the mother a day or two after delivery to discuss her labour. This not only gives the mother the opportunity to clear up any areas of confusion or concern, but also gives further feedback to the midwife which may be of value in her future practice. Such feedback is enhanced where continuity of midwifery care is offered. The Department of Health recommends in the report *Changing*

Childbirth (DOH, 1993) that at least 75% of women should know the professional(s) who will be assisting them in labour and at delivery.

If the midwife caring for the woman in labour has also been involved in her prenatal care she will be aware of the woman's wishes. Where this has not been possible, the midwife needs good communication skills in order to establish a rapport with the woman and her partner, gain their confidence and devise an appropriate plan of care.

Partnership in care

The relationship between the woman and her midwife is sometimes described as a partnership. Such a relationship, which (ideally) should begin in pregnancy, requires both members to have common aims and to seek ways of working together to achieve them.

The ultimate aims of both the woman and her midwife are likely to be the same, that is the safe delivery of a healthy baby. Evidence collected by a House of Commons Health Committee on the Maternity Services indicates that women attach great importance to continuity of care, choice of care and place of delivery and the right of control over their own bodies at all stages of pregnancy and birth (DOH, 1992).

These expectations require a social rather than a medical model of maternity care and include involvement of the woman and her partner in decision-making. Such involvement, implicit in a partnership approach to care, requires the woman to be able to voice her needs and wishes freely. The midwife should, therefore, strive to build a relationship of mutual trust and create an environment in which expectations, wishes, fears and anxieties can be readily discussed. This requires good communication, which results from a two-way interaction between equals. However, this may not be easy to achieve, as it has been suggested that women in labour do not always feel equal (Kirke, 1980). The woman may be reluctant to approach a midwife who appears to be very busy. In this situation she may seek information from others, who may be less well-informed (Kirkham, 1993).

Continuity of care(r) within a partnership approach to care facilitates the social support element of the midwife's role. The benefits of continuity and support appear to include both physical and emotional aspects such as a reduced requirement for analgesia, a lower episiotomy rate, less intervention and smoother adapta-

tion to motherhood (Flint *et al.*, 1987; Oakley *et al.*, 1990; Grant, 1992; Neilson, 1993).

Emotional and psychological care

It is important for the midwife to have a good understanding of a woman's feelings in labour. Attitudes and reactions to childbirth vary considerably and are influenced by differing social, cultural and religious factors. For a multigravida, the previous experience of birth will also be important. Many women anticipate labour with mixed feelings of fear and excitement. Some may eagerly anticipate the birth, confident in their ability to cope. They see birth as an emotionally fulfilling and enriching experience which possibly involves all immediate family members. They may have attended teaching sessions for natural or active childbirth and have a particular plan of action for their labour. Others may be excited at the prospect of actually seeing their baby, yet are fearful of labour and anxious about their ability to cope with pain and perform well. Some may consider labour to be a painful, unpleasant experience, controlled by obstetricians and midwives, and to be achieved with as little pain and active participation as possible.

The woman may be apprehensive about coming into an unknown, and often threatening, hospital environment. She may be concerned about relinquishing her personal autonomy and identity. In some instances expectations of labour may be unrealistic, and therefore be unfulfilled, and this may lead to disappointment and a sense of failure or loss. Multigravidae are often anxious about children they have left at home. The midwife can do much to alleviate these worries.

Husbands or partners, too, may have particular concerns which they feel unable to share. Such reservations may be influenced by the role society attributes to the male gender, that is, being strong and able to cope. However, on a more fundamental level, it may be simply fear of the unknown and concern for the person one loves. With a partnership and individual approach to care, particularly if established in the antenatal period, the midwife has a valuable opportunity to encourage the couple to voice their particular needs and anxieties, and explore and agree ways of dealing with them. Whatever the particular needs of the individual couple, they are usually influenced by the desire to do what is best for their baby and, if they have the confidence that the midwife will respect and comply with their wishes in normal circumstances, they will usually readily agree to modify expectations should problems arise.

Throughout labour there should be a free flow of information between the woman and her partner and the midwife, particularly in relation to examinations and their findings. Being fully informed and involved in decision-making helps the woman to retain a sense of autonomy and control (Flint et al., 1987). A survey conducted by Fleissig (1993) found that professionals have difficulty in communicating with single women and those belonging to minority ethnic groups. The midwife should be aware that not all individuals may feel sufficiently secure or able to freely express fears or anxieties during labour. Individual circumstances such as an unwanted pregnancy, fear or previously poor relationships with professional care-givers may engender feelings of unhappiness, hostility and resentment. The midwife needs to be particularly sensitive to non-verbal indicators of such feelings and give the necessary help and support so sorely needed by the woman (see Chapter 13).

The role of the birth supporter

Evidence from a number of studies indicates the positive effect of continuous support in labour (Holmeyr et al., 1991; Kennell et al., 1991). These studies indicated that women who had female support had shorter labours and less need for intervention. Although it is usual in the UK for a couple to support each other in labour, in some instances the woman may choose to have a relative, friend or labour supporter from a voluntary organization such as the National Childbirth Trust (NCT) as a labour companion. Whoever the chosen supporter is, the midwife should explore with them their experiences of childbirth, their role expectations during labour and their ability to undertake the agreed supporter role. It has been suggested that if chosen supporters have had negative childbirth experiences, these need to be addressed by the midwife if they are not to hinder the supporting relationship with the woman (Hayles, 1991).

The midwife should consider the birth supporter as part of the team, with a defined role. This may include sponging the woman's face, massaging her back, abdomen or legs, helping her with breathing awareness and relaxation and offering drinks and other means of sustenance. Such activities, during a highly anxious time, can be very valuable in helping the partner to feel usefully occupied and involved in the birthing

event. The presence of a birth supporter does not absolve the midwife from remaining with the woman. However, the midwife should also be sensitive to the possible need for personal space and privacy and will judge when, and if, it is appropriate to leave them alone. This is usually more acceptable in early labour but less so when labour is strong and well advanced, when to be left alone might be frightening. If the midwife must leave for a short period then she must ensure that the couple can summon help if necessary. The midwife must also be sensitive to the emotional needs of the partner and other members of staff and recognize that, particularly during a long labour, a short role break may be beneficial in helping to replenish energy levels.

The need for advocacy

For some women fear of the unknown, being cared for in hospital by unfamiliar people, greater pain than expected or the effect of analgesic drugs can give rise to feelings of vulnerability, loss of personal identity and powerlessness. Vulnerable individuals lose the ability to adequately express their needs, wishes, values and choices (Morrison, 1991) and therefore adopt a passive recipient role. In such circumstances, and as part of the supportive role, the midwife may need to adopt the role of advocate, in an attempt to ensure that personal needs are met (Keirse et al., 1989a). Such a role includes informing, supporting and protecting women, acting as intermediary between them and obstetric and other professional colleagues, and facilitating informed choice. It could be argued that a professional involved in the delivery of care cannot be sufficiently objective to fulfil the advocacy role. In order to act effectively as an advocate, the midwife must be professionally confident, have a clear awareness of the woman's needs, if possible determined prior to the stress of labour, and be able to communicate these to other colleagues to ensure effective collaboration. In addition, the midwife should empower the woman and her partner so that they feel sufficiently informed and confident to participate in decision-making during this important life experience.

RECOGNIZING THE ONSET OF LABOUR

Physiological changes that occur in late pregnancy have been described in Chapter 27. Such changes give rise to signs that herald the onset of labour. While recognizing that some women will follow a particular physiological pattern, allowance should be made for individual variations which may, for example, be associated with difference in pain perception and response, parity, and expectations of labour. These factors should be considered by the midwife in assisting the woman to recognize when she is in labour.

Show

This is a mucoid, often blood-stained, discharge which is passed per vaginam. It represents the passage of the mucoid operculum which previously occupied the cervical canal and is indicative of a degree of cervical activity, i.e. softening and stretching of tissues which causes separation of the membranes from the decidua around the opening of the internal os. The show is often the first sign that labour is imminent or has started.

Uterine contractions

Generally women will be aware of the painless, irregular, Braxton Hicks contractions of pregnancy which increase as pregnancy advances. In labour these will become regular and painful. Initially the woman may experience minimal discomfort and complain of sacral and/or lower abdominal pain, which she may not immediately associate with labour. Such discomfort may later be noted to coincide with tightening or tension of the abdomen, which occurs at regular 20–30 minute intervals and lasts for 20–30 seconds. These are uterine contractions and may be readily felt by the midwife on abdominal palpation. As labour progresses the contractions become longer, stronger and more frequent. This results in progressive effacement of the cervix and dilatation of the os uteri.

False labour

This occurrence, more common in multigravidae, is sometimes also described as spurious labour. It is recognized by failure of the os uteri to efface and dilate in the presence of regular painful uterine contractions. Appropriate care depends upon differentiation of false or spurious labour from a prolonged latent first phase. Unfortunately such a diagnosis can only be made in retrospect when contractions cease (Crowther et al., 1989). Little research has been done on this topic and subsequently there is no common approach to care. It is a distressing situation for the woman who feels she is in labour and the midwife will need to provide moral support, explanation and some means of pain relief.

Rupture of the membranes

Rupture of the membranes can occur before labour or at any time during labour (see Chapter 28). Although it is a significant occurrence it is not a true sign of labour unless accompanied by dilatation of the os uteri. It is estimated that 6–19% of women at term will experience spontaneous rupture of membranes before labour starts (Grant and Keirse, 1989). In 85% of women the membranes rupture spontaneously at a cervical dilatation of 9 cm or more (Schwarcz et al., 1977). The amount of amniotic fluid lost when the membranes rupture depends to a great extent on how effectively the fetal presentation assists in the formation of the forewaters. In the presence of a normal amount of amniotic fluid, if the head is not engaged in the pelvis and the presenting part is not well applied to the os uteri, rupture of the membranes is easily recognized by a significant loss of fluid. However, in the presence of an engaged head and well applied presenting part rupture of the forewaters may give rise to minimal fluid loss. This is usually followed by further seepage of amniotic fluid and may be mistaken for urinary incontinence which is not uncommon in late pregnancy.

Usually the woman's history, together with evidence of amniotic fluid, or the presence of vernix particles or discoloration from meconium confirms the rupture of the membranes. If in doubt, the fluid can be tested for protein and reaction. Protein is a normal constituent of amniotic fluid but not of urine. Urine *usually* gives an acid reaction but an alkaline reaction is inconclusive. The pH of the upper vagina increases from 4.5–6 to 7–7.5 in the presence of amniotic fluid. If a yellow nitrazine swab (sodium dinitrophenylazonaphthol disulphate) is placed in the upper vagina for 15 seconds, it will change to a blue/black colour, indicating an increase in vaginal pH and suggesting the presence of amniotic fluid. However, it has a false positive result of 15% which can result from exposure to tap water, antiseptic solutions, semen, cervical mucus, blood, and indeed alkaline urine (Friedman and McElwin, 1969). A negative result indicates the absence of amniotic fluid.

The hindwaters   If the forewaters are intact and there is minimal leaking of amniotic fluid, rupture of the hindwaters or a high water rupture may have occurred. Evidence is unclear as to whether or not hindwater rupture should be considered clinically different from forewater rupture. In the absence of such information, the only practical approach is to treat them in the same way.

Advice regarding rupture of membranes The woman should be advised to contact the midwife if she is in doubt as to whether or not the membranes have ruptured. Should rupture of the membranes precede uterine contractions, in the presence of a normal pregnancy and engagement of the fetal head, the woman may be advised to await the onset of uterine activity. Hospitalization is necessary if contractions do not commence within a few hours. If labour is not established within 12–24 hours the midwife will need to notify the obstetrician who will undertake a further assessment because of the increased likelihood of uterine infection. If the head is not engaged when the membranes rupture the midwife should also be aware of the risk of prolapse of the umbilical cord and assess the maternal and fetal condition.

CONTACT WITH THE MIDWIFE

Today, changing patterns of care enable more midwives to provide women with continuity of care. Consequently, there is an increased possibility that the woman will be cared for in labour, whether at home or in hospital, by a midwife known to her from the antenatal period. Indeed, in keeping with the suggested action points proposed by the Department of Health in the *Changing Childbirth* report (DOH, 1993), every women should have the name of the midwife who works locally and is known to her. She should, therefore, be advised to contact the midwife when regular contractions are recognized, when the membranes rupture, or should she be concerned for any reason. Clear and written instructions regarding relevant telephone numbers of the community or team midwives and where to locate them are necessary and useful for anxious partners and birth supporters. Such information should be given well in advance of the expected date of birth. Any particular information which relates to home birth and/or care should be clarified.

If the woman does not know the midwife, the midwife must be aware of the sensitivity of the first meeting and the importance of the initial interaction with the woman, which will form the basis for their future relationship. It is likely that the woman will be experiencing a variety of conflicting emotions such as excitement, anxiety or even fear for her own and the baby's safety. It may be her first time in hospital and this may be unsettling at best, and frightening at worst. Previous experiences may also influence the woman's feelings.

At this initial meeting the midwife must make a rapid assessment of the situation in order to prioritize her care. This will include taking a detailed history as discussed below. Information should be calmly and sensitively sought allowing sufficient time for the woman to express her feelings and identify needs.

Kirkham (1989) found that women gave lengthy replies to questions asked, but that proforma used by midwives required only short answers. It was noted that when the midwife filled in the form using brevity to reiterate the reply to the question, the woman's responses eventually become shorter. If the midwife can achieve a relaxed, confident and reassuring approach, while trying to acquire the necessary information and enable the woman to feel valued in her verbal contribution, it will do much to foster the desired supportive partnership in care. The presence and support of the woman's partner or birth supporter should be encouraged from the onset.

ASSESSMENT AT THE ONSET OF LABOUR

History

The midwife must read the woman's antenatal and other relevant records carefully. The records may show particular midwifery or obstetric risk factors, for example, a rhesus negative status which will influence the mode of care. It should include a *birth plan*, as advocated by the Department of Health in the report *Changing Childbirth* (DOH, 1993), which the woman has formulated with the midwife during the antenatal period. The birth plan should indicate the special needs and wishes of the woman and her partner and can assist in providing continuity of care. The woman has the reassurance of knowing that her particular needs and wishes are recorded for staff caring for her to see. Such plans may also be instrumental in enabling the woman to retain control of labour events and can provide the midwife with a valuable opportunity for health education in relation to birth.

If no birth plan has been prepared, the midwife should ascertain the woman's particular needs and wishes and attempt to incorporate these into safe and appropriate midwifery care. It must be acknowledged, however, that pregnancy and labour are dynamic processes and occasionally difficulties can arise which may require a departure from or modification of predetermined plans. If the relationship between the woman and midwife is one of confidence and trust and the woman feels she is included in the decision-making processes, such changes are more likely to be acceptable to her.

It is essential, therefore, that the midwife builds a relationship with the woman and her partner to encourage confidence in the care-givers. Then, should any problems arise in labour, they can be discussed openly and changes mutually agreed. An unhurried manner and good communication skills are essential.

The midwife should be aware that during admission the priority needs of the woman may differ from those of the midwife depending on whether problems are present. Whatever the situation, the woman needs to feel valued as a partner in care (Alexander *et al.*, 1990). The midwife should take every opportunity to inform and involve the couple in all procedures and examinations carried out. This helps to balance professional priorities with those of the woman and assists in the reduction of anxiety by promoting a sense of 'client' control.

Immediate assessment of labour

The midwife will need to make a speedy initial assessment of the stage of labour in order to determine the most appropriate action. This, and additional examinations outlined below, will provide a baseline against which further assessments can be measured. Unhurried discussion of the history of labour events should include the presence of a show, the state of the membranes and/or the time of rupture, the time contractions commenced, their length and frequency and the woman's perception of pain and her ability to cope.

While taking the history the midwife will be able to assess the pattern of uterine activity and also the woman's general demeanour, her ability to relax and cope with contractions, or any evidence of anxiety. Conversation will determine if the woman has been taught 'breathing awareness' and if this is proving helpful. The partner can be encouraged to assist and support the woman in her chosen method of relaxation. While helping the woman to undress, observations can be made of any vaginal discharge present on clothing and, if the membranes have ruptured, the colour and odour of the amniotic fluid.

Abdominal examination

A detailed abdominal examination is carried out, between contractions, to determine the lie, presentation, engagement and position of the fetus. It should be

a gentle process avoiding pain or discomfort and involving the couple as much as possible.

The *lie* should be longitudinal. An oblique or transverse lie will lead to obstructed labour and therefore requires prompt recognition. Unless corrected by the obstetrician an immediate Caesarean section will be necessary. It is also important to determine the *presentation* and whether or not it is, or will, *engage* in the pelvis. If the presentation is cephalic and not engaged, a head-fitting test as described in Chapter 19 can be undertaken.

Auscultation of the fetal heart completes the abdominal examination. It should be strong and regular with a rate of between 110 and 150 beats per minute.

Vaginal examination

This aseptic procedure may be gently carried out to confirm the onset of labour, the stage of cervical dilatation, and the station and position of the presenting part, if labour is sufficiently advanced.

Any evidence of amniotic fluid draining or abnormalities as previously described should be noted. Findings are plotted on a *partogram* (Figure 4) and these form a baseline against which progress in labour can be assessed when further examinations per vaginam are made, often at approximately 3–5 hourly intervals. Vaginal examination in labour is uncomfortable for the woman and also poses a potential risk of infection. Frequent examination should therefore be avoided.

General examination

The following general observations are made and recorded:

▶ *Temperature*: This is usually normal but a rise in temperature may indicate infection and further clinical assessment and investigations will be necessary.

▶ *Pulse*: Anxiety may initially cause a raised pulse rate. A continued rise of over 100 may indicate infection and will be associated with pyrexia. Tachycardia may also occur with ketonuria or haemorrhage.

▶ *Blood pressure*: A slight systolic rise may be associated with anxiety which usually decreases as apprehension lessens.

▶ *Urinalysis*: A midstream specimen is tested for protein, glucose and ketone bodies.

▶ *Protein*: A trace of protein may follow rupture of membranes or contamination from other vaginal discharges. A show may also contaminate the urine

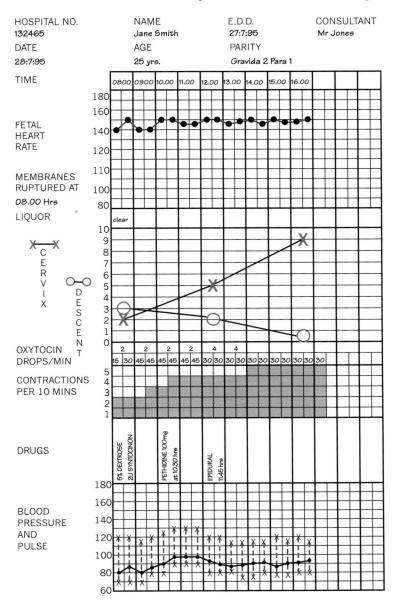

Figure 4 A partogram.

and cause a positive reaction to protein. Significant proteinuria may also be associated with a urinary tract infection or hypertensive disease of pregnancy, when it is usually associated with other clinical signs and symptoms. Both abnormalities require prompt attention and referral to the obstetrician.

▶ *Ketonuria*: A mild degree of ketonuria is considered common in labour and is due to the altered glycogenesis and ketogenesis of pregnancy (Grant, 1990).

▶ *Oedema*: A degree of ankle oedema is a normal physiological occurrence, particularly in late pregnancy. Pretibial, finger and facial oedema may be associated with hypertensive disease of pregnancy and must be recorded and reported to the doctor.

It is usual to ask if the woman has recently had, or been in contact with, any infection. Infectious conditions such as diarrhoea or chickenpox can be very harmful to newborn babies and isolation would be necessary to prevent cross-infection.

Preparation for labour

Unless contraindicated, the woman may appreciate a warm bath or shower. Ease of movement and comfort may be achieved by wearing a loose, comfortable cotton nightdress which should be changed as often as necessary to maintain cleanliness and comfort. The practice of routine shaving of the pubic, vulval and perineal areas and the giving of an enema has no value in contributing to a safe labour outcome (Romney and Gordon, 1981; Drayton and Rees, 1989). The discomfort caused by shaving is disliked by women and the procedure is likely to cause abrasions and discomfort (Oakley, 1979; Romney, 1980).

Records

All records must be fully completed following the admission procedure. The partogram (see Figure 4) is started and a care plan is prepared following discussion with the woman and her partner.

General Midwifery Care in Labour

Bladder care in labour

The woman is encouraged to empty her bladder every two hours. A full bladder is uncomfortable and may delay the progress of labour by inhibiting descent of the fetal head if it is above the ischial spines. This will reflexly inhibit efficient uterine contractions and cervical dilatation. Pressure on the distended bladder by the fetal head may give rise to oedema and bruising, leading to possible difficulties in micturition in the early days of the puerperium. Prolonged pressure can traumatize the bladder to such a degree that the resultant ischaemia may cause a vesico-vaginal fistula.

Retention of urine can occur in normal labour for reasons such as poor posture and lack of privacy. Simple measures such as privacy, use of the toilet rather than a bedpan and a warm bidet may induce emptying of the bladder. In late labour, when the advancing fetal head has displaced the bladder and is pressing against the urethra, the woman may be unable to pass urine spontaneously. In this event, using an aseptic technique, the midwife will need to catheterize the bladder to prevent trauma to the bladder as described above. All urine specimens obtained are tested for glucose, protein and ketone bodies and the urinary output is measured and recorded on the partogram or other record proforma.

Hygiene in labour

During labour a warm bath or shower may be much appreciated. Many women find a bath comforting and relaxing (Cammu et al., 1994) and the midwife may find this a useful opportunity to talk with the woman and establish rapport. If the membranes are ruptured and the presentation is not engaged and high, the potential risk of cord prolapse when ambulant must be considered. It is therefore considered safer for the woman to wash in bed or in the chair, until the presenting part is engaged.

During labour the woman will become hot and is likely to perspire. Hygiene measures in the form of a refreshing wash, sponge bath or shower may be repeated as often as necessary. Hair and mouth care may also be appreciated. If unable to bathe or shower a vulval wash will be required four hourly or at vaginal examination, and vulval pads and bed linen is changed when wet or soiled. As well as helping to keep the mother comfortable these simple hygiene measures may also serve to reduce the incidence of infection.

Activity in labour

The majority of women are more comfortable when encouraged to move freely in early labour and find the most comfortable position. Upright positions have proven physiological advantages in enhancing uterine activity and increasing cervical dilatation (Roberts et al., 1983, 1984). In addition, Abitol (1985) found that the supine position resulted in vena caval compression which affected maternal haemodynamics and caused a statistically significant increase in late decelerations of the fetal heart. In a review of the various trials it was noted that women who adopted an upright position had, on average, shorter labours, less need of narcotic analgesia and epidural anaesthesia, and required less oxytocic augmentation of labour. Apgar scores at one and five minutes were higher (Roberts, 1989).

Unless there is an obstetric reason which makes it inadvisable, the midwife should encourage women to be ambulant and to adopt a position or posture which assists comfort. Suggested positions for comfort are shown in Figure 5, or some women may find comfort in relaxing in a warm bath. As labour advances the woman may wish to recline in bed when contractions occur. This usually coincides with the increasing intensity of contractions and a cervical dilatation of 5–6 cm (Roberts, 1989). Others prefer to remain mobile and adopt alternative positions.

If in bed, the women should be assisted to lie on her side and maintain a semi-recumbent position, well-supported with pillows. This position will reduce the possibility of vena caval compression and supine hypotensive syndrome and will assist placental perfusion.

Many women find that having their back massaged over the sacral area during contractions reduces backache and aids relaxation. The use of touch can also be a means of communicating caring and the desire to help (Simkin, 1986). The partner, if present, can be encouraged to help with back rubbing and such activity may add to his feelings of involvement. A quiet, comfortable environment, dim lighting and implementing relaxation techniques may facilitate rest and enable the woman to sleep between contractions. This may be particularly welcome if labour has occurred at night and the woman is tired.

Prevention of infection

In labour both mother and fetus are vulnerable to infection, particularly when the membranes rupture. The possibility is increased when the immune response is undermined by suboptimal health, for example anaemia, malnourishment, chronic illness or when the women is exhausted by a long and arduous labour. The risk of infection is also increased when women are cared for in hospital and are thus exposed to a variety of unfamiliar organisms and possible sources of infection.

It is the professional responsibility of the midwife to ensure, as far as possible, a safe environment for the women and to prevent infection and cross-infection. Such measures include good standards of hygiene and care, correct handwashing on the part of the carers before and after attending the woman, frequent changing of vulval pads, and meticulous aseptic techniques when undertaking vaginal examination and other invasive procedures such as catheterization.

General measures such as limiting the flow of traffic within the delivery area, meticulous cleansing of communal equipment such as beds, baths, toilets and trolleys, and increasing staff awareness of the potential for, and prevention of, infection should all be observed. A formal mechanism for infection control within hospitals should also include maternity departments. In a survey published in 1992 (Evaldon *et al.*, 1992), surveillance of hospital-based obstetric and gynaecological infection showed a significant reduction in the incidence of infection when regular feedback to staff was implemented.

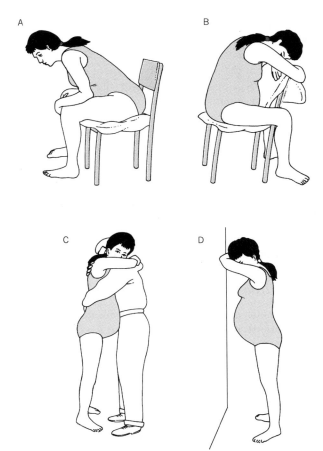

Figure 5 Resting positions in labour. **A**: In chair; **B**: astride chair; **C**: supported by partner; **D**: leaning. (Illustrations courtesy of Jim Morrin, 1993.)

Nutrition in labour

Labour is an energy-intensive activity which is estimated to require a similar calorific intake to that of an individual engaged in strenuous athletic activity (Hazle, 1986). If a suitable carbohydrate source is not available for conversion to glycogen, body fat will be utilized. As fatty acids are oxidized, the quantity of ketones in the tissue and blood increases, giving rise to ketoacidosis. In general, the women may wish to eat and/or drink in early labour but are less likely to want to eat in late labour, or when they have received narcotic analgesia.

Considerable differences of opinion exist in relation to whether or not oral fluid and food in labour should be given or withheld. A survey conducted on the policies of various maternity units in England and Wales (Michael *et al.*, 1991) indicated that 79.5% of units had a policy for oral intake in labour and that 96.4% of units allowed women some form of oral intake. However, only 38.8% allowed food and drink and, of these, 13.6% had a selection policy. Johnson and colleagues (1989) concluded that the risk of regurgitation and aspiration of gastric contents in labour is real and serious, and indeed this is a recognized cause of maternal mortality (DOH 1994). Such aspirations may include either food particles, which can obstruct the air passage and may result in atelectasis distal to the obstruction, with subsequent hypoxaemia, or aspiration of acidic stomach secretions and chemical burns of the airways (Mendelson's syndrome).

Whilst recognizing this risk it was also noted that incidences were almost entirely associated with the use of general anaesthetics and thus directly related to the frequency of general anaesthesia and the skill with which it is administered. Between 1991 and 1993 there were 8 maternal deaths which were directly attributable to anaesthesia (DOH, 1996).

The practice of imposed fasting in labour for all women is, however, questionable, particularly in the light of evidence which indicates that fasting in labour does not ensure an empty stomach or lower the acidity of stomach contents (Johnson *et al.*, 1989). It is also likely that such restrictions may lead to dehydration and ketosis with a resultant need for intervention. This should be weighed against the alternative course of allowing women to eat and drink as desired (Johnson *et al.*, 1989).

Advocates for providing oral nutrition in *normal* labour encourage frequent light meals, low in fat and roughage, which are easily absorbed (Grant, 1990, Johnson *et al.*, 1989). Such foods could include clear soup, jelly, ice cream, tea, toast and marmalade or jam, boiled egg, fruit juices or cooked fruit, or light cereals. These will provide the woman with a carbohydrate source which can be readily converted to glycogen and used as energy for the muscular activity of the uterus during labour, and for general levels of stamina. Fluids as desired should be given to replace fluid lost through perspiration and other biological functions and to prevent dehydration.

Grant (1990) suggests that a rational plan for nutrition in labour, in the light of current evidence, should include the following:

▶ Where no risk of general anaesthesia or instrumental delivery exists, the woman should be allowed to eat a light diet and drink as required.

▶ When narcotic analgesia has been given, oral food should be withheld, and only sips of water given.

In further attempting to reduce the very real risk of regurgitation and inhalation it is also common practice in some maternity units and by some obstetricians and anaesthetists to deploy pharmacological agents such as magnesium trisilicate, cimetidine or ranitidine to increase the pH of the stomach contents and drugs such as metachlorpropramide to alter the rate of gastric emptying. Johnson and colleagues (1989), however, state that utilizing such agents will not necessarily mean that the incidence and severity of Mendelson's syndrome will be reduced.

Intravenous carbohydrate-containing solutions have been used in the prevention or treatment of ketoacidosis. The effect of such intravenous therapy has been evaluated in a number of controlled trials. There may be undesirable effects such as fetal and early neonatal hyperinsulinaemia leading to a subsequent neonatal hypoglycaemia (Rutter *et al.*, 1980; Aynsley-Green and Soltesz, 1986; Johnson *et al.*, 1989).

Whether any degree of ketoacidosis in labour is physiological, or has pathiligical effects on uterine activity, is unclear (Dumoulin and Foulkes, 1984). Intravenous glucose solutions should be used with care in labour in order to avoid deleterious effects on the infant.

ONGOING ASSESSMENT OF LABOUR

Throughout labour the midwife will make regular observations of the maternal and fetal condition in order to determine that normal progress is being maintained. Observations are usually recorded on the partogram (Figure 4). The use of a partogram allows a structured graphical representation of labour events to be made. It is interesting to note that this widely used tool does not allow for psychological and emotional observations to be recorded. In order to provide a composite picture of the labour events, and the effect this has on the woman and her partner, the midwife should make additional notations as to the care provided and the woman's response to labour.

The woman's health – general observations

The temperature is recorded four hourly and the pulse hourly. In the active phase of the first stage the pulse is recorded every 30 minutes. Blood pressure is initially measured every 2–4 hours, then hourly as labour advances. Any changes arising, such as the onset of hypertension or the use of epidural anaesthesia, will need additional consideration and specific observations, which are addressed in the appropriate chapters.

All fluid intake and output is recorded and the midwife should be aware of the need to maintain the fluid balance.

The woman should be encouraged to empty her bladder two hourly. Each specimen of urine obtained is tested for protein, glucose and ketone bodies. It should be remembered that more than a trace of protein, particularly if accompanied by hypertension and generalized oedema, may be indicative of hypertensive disease of pregnancy and obstetric consultation will be necessary. A mild degree of ketonuria is considered common in labour, and is due to the altered glycogenesis and ketogenesis of pregnancy (Grant, 1990). Large amounts of ketone bodies in the urine indicate carbohydrate deficiency, depletion of glycogen stores and the utilization of fats in the absence of other energy sources.

Psychological assessment

As each person is different and unique, so also is each labour. Many factors influence the manner in which the woman and her birth supporter respond to and deal with the pain and process of labour. Such factors include cultural and social differences, physiological factors which may influence the length of labour, the woman's reaction to pain, the woman's confidence in her own ability to cope with labour, her trust in her carers, how welcome the pregnancy is or how much the labour process is feared or welcomed. The midwife should note how the woman copes with each contraction and how well she relaxes between contractions.

Additional relaxation techniques may be employed if relaxation during and between contractions is poor. The midwife should also be aware of the strain which may be experienced by the woman's partner or birth supporter and should determine ways by which the birth supporter may be included in the care of the woman without exacerbating stress. Occasional breaks for tea or a meal may be welcomed by the birth supporter.

Uterine activity

The patterns of uterine contractions provide valuable information on which to determine the progress of labour. The frequency, strength and duration of the contractions are assessed at increasingly frequent intervals until in the late first stage they are assessed every 15 minutes. As the initiation point for contractions is in the uterine fundus, contractions are assessed by placing the hand lightly on the fundus of the uterus which becomes increasingly firm as the contraction commences and reaches a peak, then diminishes. As the normal resting tone of the uterus is between 4 and 10 mmHg and pain is not felt until the contraction reaches 20 mmHg, the first and last few seconds of the contraction are pain free. Thus, the midwife will be able to feel the contraction for a few seconds before and after the woman feels pain. The total duration of the contraction can be timed.

In between contractions the fundus will be soft and relaxed. This is called the *resting tone* and enables placental perfusion to resume, thus facilitating fetal oxygenation. The resting tone of the uterus should be assessed at intervals throughout labour. There should be no significant increase. An abnormally high resting tone may precipitate fetal distress by reducing placental perfusion. The midwife can teach the woman and her birth supporter the characteristics of uterine contractions. This facilitates their participation in the labour process and enables them to incorporate the information into relaxation exercises or their use of self-administered methods of pain relief.

Frequency of the contractions is assessed by counting the interval from the onset of one contraction to the onset of the next. The strength of the contraction reflects the intrauterine pressure occurring at the time of contraction. Unless uterine activity is monitored mechanically, accurate measurement of intrauterine pressure, expressed in millimetres of mercury, will not be possible. However, the midwife can clinically assess strength by determining the degree of hardness exhibited by the uterus. This, coupled with the length of the contraction can provide the required information.

Loss per vaginam and rupture of the membranes

The time at which the membranes rupture should be recorded, together with the appearance of the liquor amnii. A greenish colour is indicative of meconium staining sometimes associated with fetal distress. A minor amount of blood-stained loss is consistent with a show or detachment of the membranes which occurs with increasing cervical dilatation. A copious mucoid blood-stained loss may herald full cervical dilatation, as can spontaneous rupture of the membranes in late labour. Frank bleeding per vaginam is abnormal, and if it occurs the midwife should consult with the obstetrician, who will ascertain the source, i.e. whether maternal or fetal, and determine the appropriate action.

Midwifery records

It is usual practice when labour is established to record all observations, examinations and any drug treatment on the partogram. The use of the World Health Organization partogram, which has been widely tested, clearly differentiates normal from abnormal progress in labour and identifies those women likely to require intervention (Kwast, 1994). The midwife's record of care constitutes a legal document and throughout labour accurate, concise and comprehensive records in accordance with the *Midwives' Rules* (UKCC, 1993a) and *Standards For Record Keeping* (UKCC, 1993b) must be maintained. Such notations should be made at, or as near the event as possible, and authenticated with the midwife's full and legible signature.

In addition to fulfilling the legal requirements, contemporaneous records are necessary to facilitate intelligent continuity of care in the event that care has to be transferred to another member of the team.

Assessing the Fetal Condition

The fetal response to the stress of labour may be assessed by clinical means and with the aid of ultrasound or electronic monitoring of the fetal heart. Tests used in labour to detect fetal compromise are only a tool to assist the practitioner in making a judgement about fetal well-being. The attendance of the same midwife during labour whenever possible is thought to be one of the most important aspects of monitoring fetal and maternal health.

The condition of the amniotic fluid

Observing the amniotic fluid for the presence of meconium can provide limited information regarding the condition of the fetus which *may* be suggestive of fetal compromise. Meconium is not usual prior to 35 weeks but is seen in 15% of pregnancies of 42 weeks duration (Gibb, 1988). The amount of meconium passed and the timing of the passage is directly associated with poor fetal outcome. Thick meconium at the onset of labour is associated with a five- to sevenfold risk of perinatal death (MacDonald *et al.*, 1985), as well as morbidity resulting from risk of meconium aspiration (McNiven *et al.*, 1994). Recent passage of meconium will give rise to dark greenish-black-coloured amniotic fluid, indicative of recent fetal compromise. In contrast, old or stale meconium gives rise to a paler green-brown discoloration.

The presence of fresh meconium requires reassessment of the fetal heart for any abnormalities indicative of distress. For surveillance purposes some authorities recommend routine assessment of the amniotic fluid by *amniotomy* or visualization with an *amnioscope* (O'Driscol and Meager, 1980). However, the presence of meconium alone is equivocal (Grant and Keirse, 1989). In the absence of other indicators of fetal compromise, such as cardiotocographic abnormalities, the advantages of amniotomy or amnioscopy should be weighed against the possible disadvantages of deliberate early rupture of membranes and the discomfort these procedures would cause to the woman. A randomized controlled trial of routine amniotomy on nulliparous women in spontaneous labour concluded that a policy of routine amniotomy had little effect on the important outcomes of labour and should not be recommended (UK Amniotomy Group 1994). In cases where amniotomy is performed the amnicot, a finger stall with a plastic hook on the end, has been found to cause less trauma to the fetal scalp than the amnihook, which is a long, rigid instrument (Harris and Cooper, 1993).

THE FETAL HEART AND MONITORING

In order to interpret the fetal response to labour it is essential that the midwife understands the mechanisms which control fetal heart response. The *cardioregulatory centre* of the brain, situated in the medulla oblongata, is influenced by many factors. Baroreceptors situated in the arch of the aorta and carotid sinus sense alterations in blood pressure and transmit information to the cardioregulatory centre. Similarly, chemo-receptors likewise situated in the carotid sinus and arch of the aorta will respond to changes in oxygen and carbon dioxide tensions.

The cardioregulatory centre is controlled by the autonomic nervous system and, in response to varying physiological factors, either the sympathetic or para-sympathetic nervous system will be stimulated. The sympathetic nervous system, via the sinoatrial node, causes an increase in heart rate while the parasympa-thetic nervous system causes a rate reduction. The continuous interaction of these two systems results in minor fluctuations in the heart rate which is recognized as variability.

Development of the sympathetic nervous system occurs early in fetal life, while the parasympathetic nervous response does not become pronounced until later in pregnancy. This accounts for the higher base-line rate of the fetal heart during early pregnancy and the lower rate at term.

Monitoring the fetal heart

The activity of the fetal heart may be assessed inter-mittently using the *Pinard fetal stethoscope*. This will provide the midwife with sample information relative to the rate and rhythm of the fetal heart. Using the Pinard stethoscope for one minute every 15 minutes during labour will, on average, sample the fetal heart activity for only 7% of the labour (Grant, 1989). Such intermittent auscultation is accessible only during a resting phase of the uterus, as it is difficult to hear the heart during a contraction and to persist would be uncomfortable for the woman.

Use of an *ultrasonic heart rate detector* provides additional information, in that the midwife can moni-tor the heart rate throughout the contraction phase and thus assess the fetal response to the reduced placental perfusion which accompanies the contraction. How-ever, as before, intermittent use will only sample the activity of the fetal heart at intervals.

Equipment is also available which enables the mid-wife to use *Doppler ultrasound* for intermittent moni-toring which will also produce an instant display of fetal heart activity. This equipment has the added advantage of being portable, easy to use, does not interfere with the woman's mobility and provides a ready picture of fetal heart activity and an accurate variability reading of the fetal heart.

Continuous fetal heart monitoring may be per-formed. However, when attempting to determine the value of continuous electronic fetal heart monitoring, Spencer (1994) states that results of randomized con-trolled trials show no significant perinatal advantage of electronic monitoring over intermittent ausculation. Grant (1989) questions the value of using continuous electronic fetal monitoring for all women in labour. Grant suggests that for the majority of labours where no contraindications exist, current evidence indicates that more intensive monitoring increases obstetric intervention and has no clear benefit to the fetus. Grant further suggests that the choice of technique for fetal heart monitoring has much wider ramifica-tions, which can interfere with the woman/midwife relationship, bringing an intensive care atmosphere to the delivery room, and affect the professional auton-omy of the midwife.

However, it is also acknowledged that departure from the accepted practice of universal monitoring which exists in some units may be difficult to imple-ment. The frequency with which the midwife decides to monitor the fetal heart will depend on the frequency and strength of the contractions and the effects on the fetus, and also any risk factors which are likely to affect fetal oxygenation (Dover and Gauge, 1995).

Intermittent auscultation of the fetal heart is usually undertaken hourly in early labour, every 15 minutes as contractions increase and after each contractions in the late first and second stages of labour (Gibb, 1988). The fetal heart should be auscultated for a full minute and, if using the Pinard stethoscope, immediately following the contraction. The rate normally ranges between 110 and 150 beats per minute, being lower in the term or post-term fetus, and higher in the preterm. The rhythm is normally regular with a typical coupled beat.

It is important to recognize that a marked change to an individual fetal heart pattern (i.e. of 20 beats or more, or irregularities of rhythm) are particularly sig-nificant and may indicate fetal compromise and require closer observation. Likewise any maternal changes, i.e. intrapartum bleeding, will require the midwife to monitor the fetal condition more closely. *Acute fetal hypoxia* (fetal distress) may manifest initially as a fetal tachycardia. Prolonged hypoxia will eventually mani-fest as fetal bradycardia. Slowing of the fetal heart rate with contractions may be significant.

Electronic monitoring

With present technology, uterine activity and fetal response can be electronically monitored either continuously or on an intermittent basis, i.e. for 15–30-minute periods over a given time (see Figure 6). The cardiotocograph simultaneously measures and records uterine and fetal heart activity and displays the findings in graphic form. Electronic monitoring enables the midwife to see how the fetal heart responds during the actual contraction, and throughout the labour.

There is considerable debate about the use of electronic fetal heart monitoring in labour because there is no clear evidence that it improves the outcome. It is also associated with a higher rate of medical intervention, including Caesarean section during the first stage of labour and instrumental delivery during the second (Neilson, 1993). To women the method of fetal heart monitoring has been found to be less important than the support they receive from staff and companions (Grant, 1992; Garcia *et al.*, 1985; Thornton and Lilford, 1994).

External electronic fetal heart monitoring using Doppler ultrasound is a less invasive method and relies on *transducers* placed firmly in contact with the abdomen (over the area where the fetal heart is most audible) to detect and record the rate and pattern of the fetal heart (Figure 7). The frequency and strength of contractions, and the resting phase and tone of the uterus is simultaneously assessed using a *tocodynamometer*. This is placed securely on the abdomen on the fundus of the uterus where it will respond to the increase and decrease in uterine pressure. Unfortunately, this method of monitoring can be disadvantaged by interference from fetal movements which may obscure the trace, giving a false picture of variability.

Monitoring by internal or direct means may also be carried out. This is an invasive procedure which requires the cervix to be 2–3 cm dilated and membranes ruptured prior to transcervical application of the fetal scalp electrode. To avoid fetal damage the electrode should be applied to the bony part of the fetal skull and not over the sutures or fontanelles. It is not suitable for use if there is a face presentation. The electrode is attached to the electronic monitoring appa-

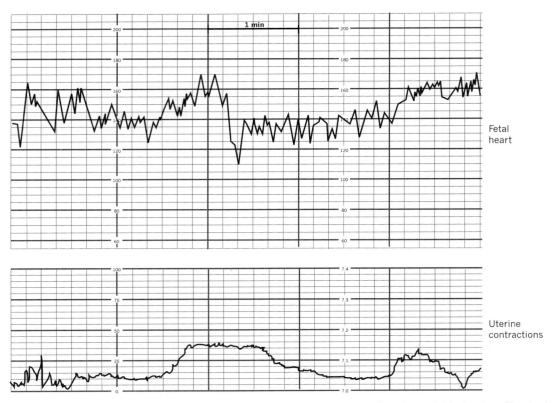

Figure 6   Normal cardiotocograph: the fetal heart rate is normal and reactive. (Courtesy of J.A. Jordan, Birmingham Maternity Hospital.)

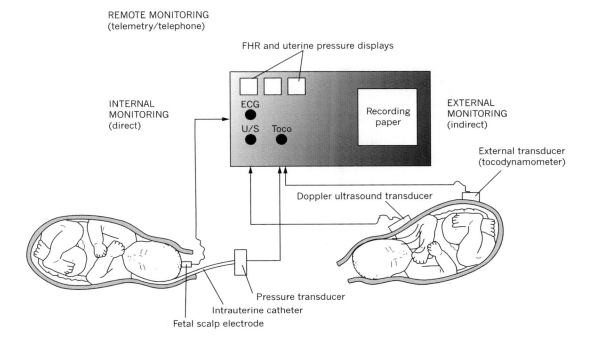

REMOTE MONITORING
(telemetry/telephone)

FHR and uterine pressure displays

INTERNAL
MONITORING
(direct)

ECG

U/S   Toco

Recording
paper

EXTERNAL
MONITORING
(indirect)

External transducer
(tocodynamometer)

Doppler ultrasound transducer

Pressure transducer
Intrauterine catheter
Fetal scalp electrode

Figure 7   Methods of monitoring fetal heart rate.

ratus and will produce a direct fetal electrocardiogram (Figure 7).

New techniques of assessing the fetal condition during labour are being developed, including *waveform analysis* of the electrocardiogram and *near-infrared spectroscopy* (Neilson, 1993). The latter directly measures fetal cerebral oxygenation and cerebral blood flow and would therefore improve the detection of fetal asphyxia in labour (O'Brien *et al.*, 1993).

Contractions may also be monitored by means of an *intrauterine catheter pressure device* which measures directly the pressure within the uterus during contractions, or alternatively, by the use of an external transducer described above. Some women find the apparatus uncomfortable and restrictive. It can interfere with their ability to move freely and adopt positions conducive to comfort. Where appropriate, the midwife may advise intermittent monitoring.

Common fetal heart patterns

The normal fetal heart   This has a *baseline rate* of between 100 and 150 beats per minute (bpm). The baseline rate refers to the heart rate present between periods of acceleration and deceleration (Sonicaid, 1987).

Baseline variability   This is the variation in heart rate of 5–15 bpm, which occurs over a time base of 10–20 seconds. Figure 8 demonstrates normal baseline variability. The presence of good variability is an important sign of fetal well-being (Sonicaid, 1987).

Variation in baseline variability   Prior to 34 weeks' gestation variability is less pronounced, the parasympathetic nervous system being less well-developed (Gibb, 1988). Reduced variability as in Figure 9 may occur when the fetus is in a 'sleep' state. This, however, is usually seen as recurrent 10–30-minute periods of reduced variability (Sonicaid, 1987). It may also be associated with the use of maternal narcotic analgesia, sedatives or antihypertensive agents (Gibb, 1988). Reduced baseline variability can also be a feature of fetal hypoxia and fetal viral infection. If present it requires further detailed analysis.

Acceleration pattern   Accelerations of the fetal heart of 15 bpm from the baseline as shown in Figure 10 are often associated with fetal activity and stimulation (Spencer, 1993) and are thought to be useful indicators of absence of fetal acidaemia in labour (Spencer, 1993). They are not considered to be clinically signifi-

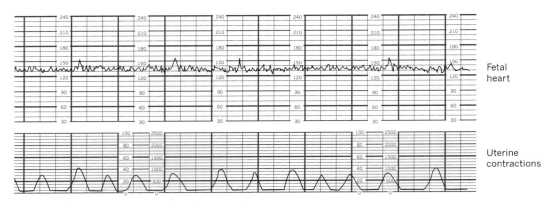

Figure 8 ECG trace showing baseline variability in fetal heart rate. (Courtesy of Sonicaid, Abingdon, Oxon.)

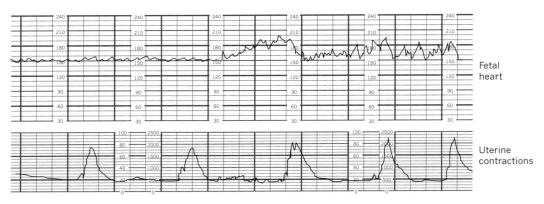

(Figure 9 Physiological reduction of baseline variability in fetal heart rate (left). Normal baseline variability (right). (Courtesy of Sonicaid, Abingdon, Oxon.)

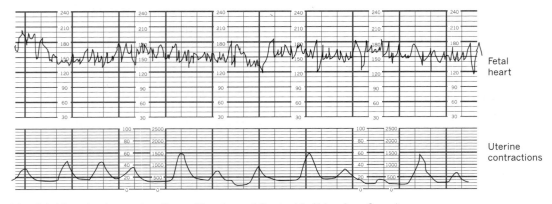

Figure 10 Fetal heart rate accelerations. (Courtesy of Sonicaid, Abingdon, Oxon.)

cant if they are of short duration, that is 15 seconds. When two are present within a 20-minute period the trace is described as 'reactive' (Gibb, 1988). This is considered to be a positive sign of fetal health indicating good reflex responsiveness of the fetal circulation.

Baseline bradycardia This refers to a consistent baseline rate of below 110 bpm as indicated in Figure 11. It is not considered abnormal if there is good baseline variability and reactivity, is not severe, that is below 100, and is not accompanied by deceleration or other abnormalities. The midwife should take care to ensure that the trace is truly of fetal origin as sometimes an incorrectly placed electrode or transducer can result in the maternal heart rate being recorded inadvertently.

Severe bradycardia is a more serious prognostic sign and indicates failure of the fetal compensatory mechanisms. It is thought that a bradycardia below 80 bpm will almost certainly result in fetal asphyxia.

Baseline tachycardia This refers to an increase in the baseline fetal heart rate of above 150 bpm (Figure 12). It is a feature of premature (less than 34 weeks' gestation) fetal heart activity which alters as the cardioregulatory centre of the brain matures. It is considered uncomplicated if it displays good baseline variability, reactivity and no decelerations. It may be associated with maternal pyrexia or early fetal hypoxia

(Sonicaid, 1987). Complicated tachycardia indicates fetal compromise and must be further assessed.

Early deceleration This is a decrease in the fetal heart rate of more than 15 bpm which is synchronous with the contraction. There is a return to a normal baseline when the contraction ends (Figure 13; Sonicaid, 1987). This reflexive response to the contraction is caused by head compression (Gibb, 1988) which induces a vagus nerve response.

Late decelerations The fetal heart slows after onset of the contraction (Figure 14). The lowest point of the deceleration is past the peak of the contraction. The longer the time lag (i.e. the time from the peak of the contraction to the lowest point of the deceleration) the more serious the concern. Initially, the deceleration may be quite shallow and not easy to recognize. This pattern is associated with uteroplacental insufficiency and a significant decrease in fetal cerebral oxygenation

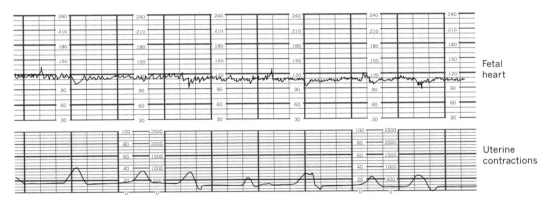

Figure 11 Normal baseline bradycardia. (Courtesy of Sonicaid, Abingdon, Oxon.)

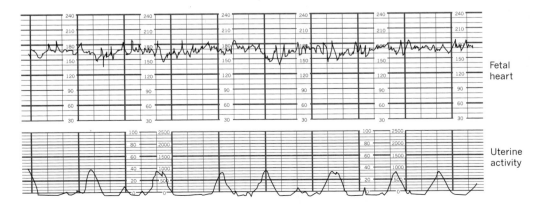

Figure 12 Uncomplicated baseline tachycardia. (Courtesy of Sonicaid, Abingdon, Oxon.)

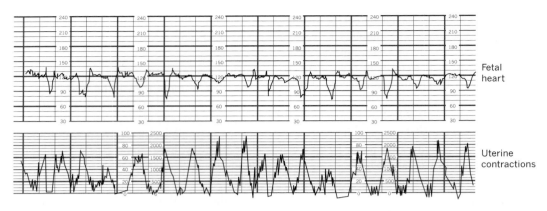

Figure 13   Early fetal heart rate decelerations. (Courtesy of Sonicaid, Abingdon, Oxon.)

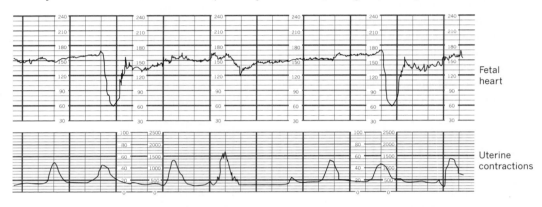

Figure 14   Late fetal heart rate decelerations. (Courtesy of Sonicaid, Abingdon, Oxon.)

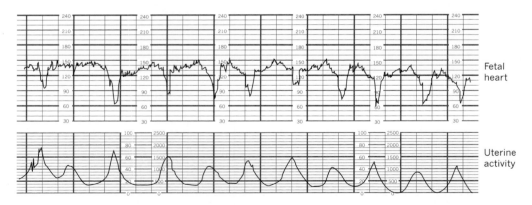

Figure 15   Variable fetal heart rate decelerations. (Courtesy of Sonicaid, Abingdon, Oxon.)

(Aldrich *et al.*, 1995), particularly when associated with reduced or abnormal variability, abnormal rate and with meconium-stained liquor (Gibb, 1988).

Variable decelerations   Fetal heart decelerations are variable in timing and frequency amplitude or shape

(Figure 15) hence the descriptive term of 'variable'. It is associated with cord compression in which venous flow is obstructed, resulting in a corresponding rise in fetal blood pressure. This pattern is not uncommon and the decelerations are usually of short duration. This pattern is usually benign but if the decelerations are below 60 bpm, or 60 bpm below the baseline fetal heart rate, or longer than 60 seconds, they can indicate fetal compromise and should be assessed further.

Unusual patterns

Sinusoidal pattern This is a rare pattern and manifests as a regular smooth trace with a frequency of 3–6 per minute and an amplitude range of 5–30 bpm. The cause is unknown but it has associations with rhesus iso-immunization, fetal anaemia and asphyxia (Figure 16).

Saltatory pattern This is characterized by the appearance of what appears to be excessive variability with an amplitude greater than 25 bpm. The cause and significance of this pattern is unclear, but it is thought to have some association with fetal acidosis.

FETAL BLOOD SAMPLING

Measurement of acid/base (pH) of the fetal blood is sometimes undertaken as an adjunct to electronic fetal monitoring, particularly when there is doubt as to the oxygenation status of the fetus. This usually follows the presence of an abnormal or suspicious fetal heart pattern and provides *current* evidence of fetal well-being. Grant (1989) postulates that evidence suggests that fetal blood sampling reduces the false positive and negative responses to abnormal fetal heart patterns, and is an essential adjunct to continuous electronic fetal heart monitoring and should be more widely used.

The procedure requires the informed consent of the woman, the membranes to be ruptured and cervical dilatation of at least 3 cm. An amnioscope of suitable size is passed transcervically and placed in contact with

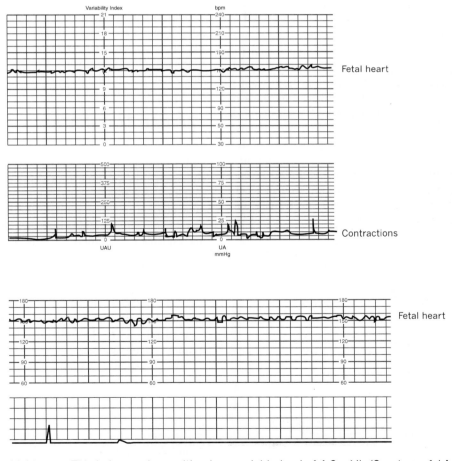

Figure 16 Sinusoidal traces. This baby was born with a haemoglobin level of 4.3 g/dl. (Courtesy of J.A. Jordan, Birmingham Maternity Hospital.)

the fetal scalp (Figure 17). The fetal scalp is sprayed with ethyl chloride to produce a reactive hyperaemia and a thin layer of silicone gel is applied which will allow the blood to form a droplet when a small scalp incision is made. Blood, free of air bubbles, is drawn into a heparinized capillary tube and an immediate estimation is made of blood gas tension, bicarbonate content and acidity. On completion of the procedure, pressure is applied to the fetal scalp wound to assist haemostasis.

A scalp pH of 7.25 and above is considered satisfactory. The fetal heart tracing should be observed and a further sample of fetal scalp blood analysed if deterioration occurs. A pH of 7.20–7.25 is borderline and the test should be repeated within 30 minutes. A pH of 7.20 or less indicates fetal acidosis and requires immediate delivery of the baby.

Assessment of Progress in Labour

The midwife will need to reassure herself – and the woman – that labour is progressing normally. Implicit in normal progress will be the ability of both woman and fetus to respond to the physiological demands of labour without abnormalities arising. Assessment of progress can be considered in the light of effective uterine action, facilitating continuing descent of the fetus and progressive cervical dilatation. The midwife acquires the necessary information by clinical assessment which includes incorporating the woman's perception of bodily sensations, e.g. uterine activity and perineal pressure.

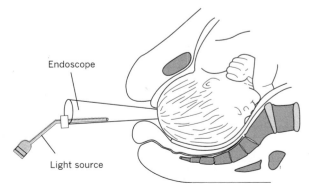

Endoscope

Light source

Figure 17   Fetal blood sampling.

UTERINE ACTIVITY AND THE DESCENT OF THE FETUS

Thus the character of the uterine contractions can give an indication of progress. When labour is established they become progressively longer, stronger, and more frequent until they occur every 2–3 minutes and last 50–60 seconds. On palpation the uterus will feel very hard, indicating the strength of the contraction. Such assessment of strength is not an accurate measure of changes in uterine pressure, but should an intrauterine pressure gauge be used it would show an amplitude of 60–80 mmHg. This is the most objective way of measuring uterine activity in labour, but does not appear to be associated with an improvement of outcome for mother or fetus (Gibb, 1993). The presence of pain-free periods at the onset and finish of the contraction together with good relaxation of the uterus between contractions indicate normalcy of action.

Descent of the fetus should take place throughout labour and is assessed by making regular examinations per abdomen and per vaginam. This is a particularly important observation when the head is not engaged at the beginning of labour and when normal progress in labour is not achieved.

VAGINAL EXAMINATION

This may be undertaken to determine the dilatation and condition of the cervix. It is preceded by an abdominal examination to determine the fetal lie, presentation, position, the engagement or otherwise of the presentation and to auscultate the fetal heart. In this way, the midwife can maximize the potential for acquiring valuable information.

Traditional practice observes a frequency of approximately 4–5 hours for vaginal examination. However, as there appears to be no firm basis for a hard and fast rule, the midwife should use her discretion to determine the frequency of vaginal examinations in relation to the individual labour, avoiding too frequent examinations.

Specific indications for vaginal examination in labour include:

▶ To confirm the onset of labour and to establish a baseline for further progress.
▶ To permit adequate assessment of labour progress and detect problems promptly.
▶ To exclude or diagnose cord prolapse when the membranes rupture in the presence of a non-

engaged or poorly fitting presenting part, or in the case of polyhydramnios.

▶ To confirm the onset of the second stage of labour.

▶ To diagnose the presentation, when this is in doubt.

▶ To determine the cause of undue delay in the second stage of labour.

▶ To apply a fetal scalp electrode.

▶ To rupture the membranes when necessary.

The midwife should be aware that this intimate and personal procedure can be a cause of embarrassment and discomfort to the woman, who, if in hospital, should be reassured as to the privacy of the examination. The midwife should prevent unnecessary interruption from other staff. A full explanation of the reason for and method of examination should be given, thus facilitating informed consent (Clement, 1994). To avoid undue discomfort the woman's bladder should be empty. The midwife must take precautions to prevent infection and cross-infection and use sterile/clean equipment and protective gloves.

Method The woman is made comfortable in a semi-recumbent or lateral position with her legs separated and as relaxed as possible. She can be encouraged to practice relaxation exercises. The vulval area is washed with an appropriate antiseptic lotion. To minimize the risk of ascending infection the midwife uses the hand which she will *not* use to insert into the vagina to cleanse the vulval and perineal area, swabbing forward from the labia and down and behind to the perineum. One swab is used once only and discarded. The examining fingers (index and forefinger) are generously lubricated with an appropriate antiseptic obstetric cream and gently inserted into the vagina.

Findings While gently separating the labia the midwife notes any abnormalities such as infective lesions, varicose veins, abnormal discharges, oedema or the presence of perineal scars indicative of past perineal trauma and repair. The tone of the pelvic floor muscles is noted as the examining fingers are inserted into the vagina. In multiparous women a *cystocele* (a prolapse of the bladder into the vaginal wall) or less commonly, a *rectocele* (a prolapse of the rectum into the vaginal wall) may be present.

The cervix is assessed for consistency, effacement and dilatation.

Consistency Prior to the onset of labour, under hormonal influences described in Chapter 27, the cervix is usually soft and pliable to the examining fingers. It may feel thick and is often described as having a consistency comparable to the lips.

Effacement Changes which bring about effacement have been detailed in Chapter 27. The cervical canal, which usually projects into the vagina, has become shorter, until no protrusion can be felt. This shortening is often referred to as the 'taking up' of the cervix which results from the dilatation of the internal cervical os, and the gradual opening out of the cervical canal. During and following effacement the consistency of the cervix alters and it becomes progressively thinner. Complete effacement may be present in primigravidae prior to the onset of labour and before the cervix begins to dilate. In the multiparous woman, although a degree of effacement may be present prior to labour, completion of the process occurs simultaneously with cervical dilatation as labour advances.

Cervical dilatation The rate of cervical dilatation is the most exact measurement of progress of labour. It is assessed and expressed in centimetres (cm). Prior to labour, particularly in multiparous women, the os uteri may admit one or two fingers. When labour is established there is progressive dilatation of the os uteri but the speed varies according to the period of the first stage.

The *latent phase* is the early part of the first stage. It is a concept poorly understood and which has given rise to much debate. Hendricks and colleagues (1970) consider it to be at the end of the prelabour period, while Koontz and Bishop (1982) argue that it is a definite part of the first stage of labour. Generally, however, the latent phase is recognized as being the period of time taken for the cervix to reach approximately 3–4 cm dilatation. In primigravidae this may last for 6–8 hours, while in a multigravida it may be less.

The latent phase is followed by the *active phase*, characterized by acceleration in the rate of cervical dilatation. The accepted dilatation rate of approximately 1 cm per hour in primigravidae and 1.5 cm in multigravidae is now being questioned, as many women who show slower rates of cervical dilatation proceed to normal uneventful delivery. It is suggested that a rate of 0.5 cm per hour might well be an acceptable lower limit for defining normal progress but that this too must be viewed in an individual context (Crowther *et al.*, 1989). Full dilatation is achieved when the fetal head can pass through the os uteri, usually at about 10 cm dilatation.

The rate of cervical dilatation may be charted using a cervicograph (Figure 18) and this assists the midwife to determine if the rate is within normal parameters. A shift to the right in the dilatation curve of about two hours indicates delayed cervical dilatation which requires further assessment prior to an action plan. As the finger is moved inside the rim of the cervix the consistency, thickness and application to the pre-senting part is noted. A soft, stretchy cervix, closely in contact with the presenting part, indicates potential for normal cervical dilatation. A tight, unyielding cervix or one loosely in contact with the presenting part is less favourable and may be associated with long labour.

The membranes   In early labour the membranes can be difficult to feel as they are usually closely applied to the head. During a contraction the increase in pressure may cause the bag of forewaters to become tense and bulge through the os uteri. The membranes may be

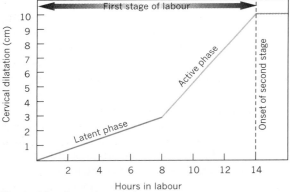

Figure 18   A cervicograph.

inadvertently ruptured if pressure is applied at this time. If the head is poorly applied to the cervix the bag of forewaters may bulge unduly early in the first stage and early rupture of membranes is likely to occur. This tends to occur with an occipitoposterior position. Spontaneous or deliberate rupture of the membranes can sometimes improve the fit between the presenting part and the cervix, thus assisting cervical dilatation, although whether the procedure confers more benefit than harm is debatable (Keirse *et al.*, 1989b). Thornton and Lilford (1994) found that routine amniotomy in labour has not been shown to have any important beneficial or adverse effects apart from shortening the duration of labour.

The presentation is normally the smooth round, hard vault of the head. Sutures and fontanelles can be felt with increasing ease as the os uteri dilates, thereby enabling confirmation of the presentation and determination of the position and attitude of the head. The degree of moulding of the fetal head can also be assessed. As labour continues, particularly if the mem-branes are ruptured, subsequent formation of a caput succedaneum may make recognition of sutures and fontanelles difficult and sometimes impossible. Rarely, a prolapsed cord may be felt as a soft loop lying in front of or alongside the fetal head. If the fetus is still alive the cord will be felt to pulsate.

The position   The position can be determined by identification of the fontanelles and the sutures (Fig-ures 19 and 20). An occipito-anterior position is iden-tified by feeling the posterior fontanelle towards the anterior part of the pelvis. In an occipitoposterior position the anterior fontanelle will be felt anteriorly.

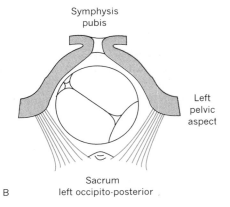

Figure 19   Identifying the position of the fetus. **A**: Left occipito-anterior: the sagittal suture is in the right oblique diameter of the pelvis. **B**: Left occipitoposterior: the sagittal suture is in the left oblique diameter of the pelvis.

The fontanelles are identified by the number of sutures which meet. The anterior fontanelle is the junction of four sutures, whereas the posterior fontanelle is the junction of three. The sagittal suture is one of the sutures identified. This is a long suture forming part of and linking both anterior and posterior fontanelle.

When the sagittal suture lies in the right oblique diameter of the pelvis (i.e. from the right posterior quadrant of the woman's pelvis to the left anterior quadrant) and the posterior fontanelle is felt anteriorly to the left, the position is the left occipito-anterior.

When the sagittal suture is felt in the left oblique diameter of the pelvis (i.e. from the left posterior quadrant of the woman's pelvis) and the posterior fontanelle anteriorly to the right, the position is the right occipito-anterior.

When the occiput is posterior the anterior fontanelle will be felt anteriorly. If the sagittal suture is in the right oblique with the anterior fontanelle lying anteriorly to the left, the position is a right occipitoposterior, whereas when the sagittal suture is in the left

oblique and the anterior fontanelle anteriorly to the right, the position is left occipitoposterior.

Occasionally the sagittal suture is found in the transverse diameter of the pelvis between the ischial tuberosities. It will be necessary to identify one or both fontanelles to determine the position. It may also be possible to feel an ear under the symphysis pubis and this may give an indication as to the position of the fetus. Prior to delivery, when the fetal head has rotated on the pelvic floor, the sagittal suture should be in the anteroposterior diameter of the pelvis. Again, the position of the fetus is determined by the position of the fontanelles.

Occasionally the posterior fontanelle is felt directly behind the symphysis pubis but more often it is felt towards either the right or left of the symphysis pubis denoting a left/right occipito-anterior position respectively. A summary of how to assess the position of the fetus is given in Table 4.

Flexion and station of the head   The fetal head may or may not be flexed at the onset of labour. However, in the presence of efficient uterine action and as a result of fetal axis pressure (Chapters 2 and 30) the fetal head usually flexes, further facilitating a well–fitting presenting part. Unless the pelvis is particularly roomy or the fetal head small, deflexion of the head is indicated if the posterior and anterior fontanelles can be felt. This may be associated with malposition of the fetal head, poor cervical stimulation and prolongation of labour.

The *station* or level of the presenting part refers to the relationship of the presenting part to the ischial spines. The maternal ischial spines are palpable as slight protuberances covered by tissue on either side of the bony pelvis (Figure 21). Descent in relation to

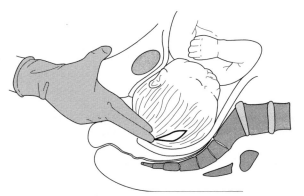

Figure 20   Identifying the sagittal suture and fontanelles during examination per vaginam.

Table 4   Assessing the position of the fetus

Position of sagittal suture	Position of fontanelle	Position of fetus
Right oblique	Posterior fontanelle anteriorly to the left	LOA
	Anterior fontanelle anteriorly to the left	ROP
Left oblique	Posterior fontanelle anteriorly to the right	ROA
	Anterior fontanelle anteriorly to the right	LOP
Transverse diameter of the pelvis	Posterior fontanelle to the left	LOL
	Posterior fontanelle to the right	ROL
Anteroposterior diameter of the pelvis	Posterior fontanelle felt anteriorly	OA
	Anterior fontanelle felt anteriorly	OP

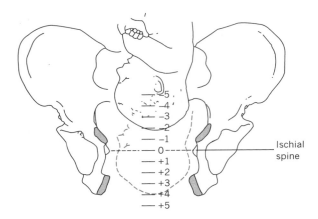

Ischial spine

Figure 21   The stations of the head. Descent in relation to the maternal ischial spines is expressed in centimetres.

the maternal ischial spines should be progressive and is expressed in centimetres as indicated in Figure 21.

The general shape of the pelvis   Before withdrawing her fingers the midwife should try to find out certain details of the bony pelvis. It may be obviously roomy or the fetal head may feel a tight fit. If the head is not engaged the curve of the sacrum should be

assessed. A well-curved sacrum is conducive to descent and rotation of the fetal head. The ischial spines are palpated for any undue prominence which could reduce the transverse diameter of the pelvic outlet and affect descent and rotation of the fetal head. The angle of the pubic arch is estimated, and a generous angle is indicated by the ability of the lower border of the symphysis pubis to accommodate the examining fingers easily. On withdrawal of the examining fingers, the intertuberous diameter is assessed by placing the knuckles on the perineum between the ischial tuberosities.

The examination is completed by cleansing and drying the vulva, applying a vulval pad, changing any soiled linen and making the woman comfortable. The fetal heart is auscultated. All findings are recorded and the midwife must now analyse these findings to establish a total picture on which to make an accurate assessment of the progress of labour and to forecast how the labour is likely to advance. Having done so, the midwife is then in a position to encouragingly relate to the woman and her partner the progress to date, and together review the original birth plan for any adjustments which the woman and the midwife feel are necesssary.

References

Abitol, M.M. (1985) Supine position in labor and associated fetal heart changes. *Obstet. Gynecol.* **65**: 481–486.

Aldrich, C.J., D'Antona, D. & Spencer, J.A. (1995) Late fetal heart decelerations and changes in cerebral oxygenation during the first stage of labour. *Br. J. Obstet. Gynaecol.* **102**(1): 9–13.

Alexander, J., Levy, V. & Roch, S. (eds) (1990) *Intrapartum Care – A Research-Based Approach.* London: Macmillan.

Aynsley-Green, A. & Soltesz, G. (1986) Metabolic and endocrine disorder, Part 1, Disorders of blood glucose homeostasis in the neonate. In *Textbook of Neonatology.* Edinburgh: Churchill Livingstone.

Cammu, H., Clasen, K. & Van Wettere, L. (1994) 'To bathe or not to bathe' during the first stage of labour. *Act Obstet. Gynecol. Scand.* **73**(6): 468–472.

Clement, S. (1994) Unwanted vaginal examinations. *Br. J. Midwifery* **2**(8): 368–370.

Crowther, C., Enkin, M., Keirse, M.J.N.C. & Brown, I. (1989) Monitoring the progress of labour. In Chalmers, I., Enkin, M. & Keirse, M.J.N.C. (eds) *Effective Care in Pregnancy and Childbirth*, Vol. 2, p. 841. Oxford: Oxford University Press.

DOH (Department of Health) (1992) *Health Committee, Second Report, Sessions 1991–1992, Maternity Services.* London: HMSO.

DOH (1993) *Changing Childbirth.* Report of the Expert Maternity Group, Part 1. London: HMSO.

DOH (1994) *Report on Confidential Enquiries into Maternal Deaths in the United Kingdom 1988–1990.* London: HMSO.

DOH (Department of Health) (1996) *Report on the Confidential Enquiries into Maternal Deaths in the United Kingdom 1991–1993.* London: HMSO.

Dover, S.L. & Gauge, S.M. (1995) Fetal monitoring – midwifery attitudes. *Midwifery* **11**(1): 18–27.

Drayton, S.M. & Rees, C. (1989) Is anyone out there giving enemas? In Alexander, J., Levy, V. & Roch, S. (eds) *Intrapartum Care – A Research-Based Approach.* London: Macmillan.

Dumoulin, J.G. & Foulkes, J.E.B. (1984) Ketonuria in labour. *Br. J. Obstet. Gynaecol.* **91**: 97–98.

Evaldon, G.R., Frederici, H., Jullig, C. *et al.* (1992) Hospital-associated infections in obstetrics and gynaecology. Effects of surveillance. *Acta Obstet. Gynaecol. Scand.* **71**(1): 54–58.

Fleissig, A. (1993) Are women given enough information by staff during labour and delivery? *Midwifery* **9**(2): 70–75.

Flint, C., Poulengeris, P. & Grant, A.M. (1987) The 'Know Your Midwife' scheme: a randomised trial of continuity of care by a team of midwives. *Midwifery* **5**: 11–16.

Friedman, M.L. & McElwin, T.W. (1969) Diagnosis of ruptured membranes: Clinical study and review of literature. *Am. J. Obstet. Gynecol.* **104**: 544–550.

Garcia, J., Corry, M., MacDonald, D., Elbourne, D. & Grant, A. (1985) Mothers' views of continuous electronic fetal heart monitoring and intermittent auscultation in a randomised controlled trial. *Birth* **12**: 79–85.

Gibb, D.M.E. (1988) *A Practical Guide to Labour Management.* London: Blackwell Scientific.

Gibb, D.M. (1993) Measurement of uterine activity in labour – clinical aspects. *Br. J. Obstet. Gynaecol.* **100**(Suppl. 9): 28–31.

Grant, A. (1989) Monitoring the fetus during labour. In Chalmers, I., Enkin, M. & Keirse, M.J.N.C. (eds) *Effective Care in Pregnancy and Childbirth*, Vol. 2. Oxford: Oxford University Press.

Grant, A.M. (1992) Electronic fetal heart monitoring (EFM) vs intermittent auscultation in labour. In Chalmers, I. (ed.) *Oxford Database of Perinatal Trials*, Version 1.3, disk issue 8, record 3884. Oxford: Oxford University Press.

Grant, J. (1990) Nutrition and hydration in labour. In Alexander, J., Levy, V. & Roch, S. (eds) *Intrapartum Care – A Research-Based Approach.* London: Macmillan.

Grant, J. & Keirse, M.J.N.C. (1989) Prelabour rupture of the membranes at term. In Chalmers, I., Enkin, M. & Keirse, M.J.N.C. (eds) *Effective Care in Pregnancy and Childbirth*, Vol. 2. Oxford: Oxford University Press.

Green, J.M., Coupland, V.A. & Kitzinger, J.V. (1990) Expectations, experiences and psychological outcome of childbirth: a prospective study. *Birth* **17**(1): 15–24.

Harris, M. & Cooper, E.V. (1993) Amnihook versus amnicot for amniotomy in labour. *Midwifery* **9**: 220–224.

Hayles, B. (1991) Supporting the supporter. *New Zealand Coll. Midwives J.* **5**: 15–16.

Hazle, N.R. (1986) Hydration in labor: is routine intravenous hydration necessary? *J. Nurse Midwifery* **31**: 171.

Hendricks, C.H., Brenner, W.E. & Kraus, G. (1970) Normal cervical dilatation pattern in late pregnancy and labour. *Am. J. Obstet. Gynecol.* **106**: 1065–1082.

Holmeyr, G.J., Nikodem, V.C. & Wolman, W.L. (1991) Companionship to modify the clinical birth environment: Effects on progress and perceptions of labour and breastfeeding. *Br. J. Obstet. Gynaecol.* **198**(8): 756–764.

Johnson, C., Keirse, M.J.N.C., Enkin, M. & Chalmers, I. (1989) Nutrition and hydration in labour. In Chalmers, I., Enkin, M. & Keirse, M.J.N.C. (eds) *Effective Care in Pregnancy and Childbirth*, Vol. 2. Oxford: Oxford University Press.

Keirse, M.J.N.C., Enkin, M. & Lumley, J. (1989a) Social and professional support in childbirth. In Chalmers, I., Enkin, M. & Keirse, M.J.N.C. (eds) *Effective Care in Pregnancy and Childbirth*, Vol. 2, pp. 805–814. Oxford: Oxford University Press.

Keirse, M.J.N.C., Enkin, M. & Lumley, J. (1989b) Augmentation of labour. In Chalmers, I., Enkin, M. & Keirse, M.J.N.C. (eds) *Effective Care in Pregnancy and Childbirth*, Vol. 2, pp. 952–956. Oxford: Oxford University Press.

Kennell, J., Klaus, M. & McGrath, S. (1991) Continuous emotional support during labour in a U.S. hospital: a randomized controlled trial. *J. Am. Med. Assoc.* **165**(17): 2197–2201.

Kirke, P.N. (1980) Mothers' view of obstetric care. *Br. J. Obstet. Gynaecol.* **87**: 1029–1033.

Kirkham, M.J. (1989) Midwives and information-giving during labour. In Robinson, S. & Thompson, A.M. (eds) *Midwifes, Research and Childbirth*, Vol. 1. London: Chapman & Hall.

Kirkham, M.J. (1993) Communications in midwifery. In Alexander, J., Levy, V. & Roch, S. (eds) *Midwifery Practice. A Research-Based Approach.* London: Macmillan.

Koontz, W.L. & Bishop, E.H. (1982) Management of the latent phase of labour. *Clin. Obstet. Gynecol.* **25**: 111–114.

Kwast, B. (1994) World Health Organisation partograph in management of labour. *Lancet* **343**: 1399–1404.

McCoshen, J.A., Hoffman, D.R. & Kredenster, J.V. (1990) The role of fetal membranes in regulating production, transport and metabolism of prostaglandin E_2 during labour. *Am. J. Obstet, Gynecol.* **163**(5): 1632–1640.

MacDonald, D., Grant, A., Sheridan-Perara, M. *et al.* (1985) The Dublin randomised trial of intrapartum fetal heart monitoring. *Am. J. Obstet. Gynecol.* **152**: 524–539.

McNiven, P., Roch, B. & Wall, J. (1994) Meconium-stained amniotic fluid. *Modern Midwife* **4**(7): 17–20.

Michael, S., Reilly, C.S. & Caunt, J.A. (1991) Policies for oral intake during labour. A survey of maternity units in England and Wales. *Anaesthesia* **46**(12): 1071–1073.

Morrison, A. (1991) The nurse's role in relation to advocacy. *Nursing Standard* **5**(41): 37–41.

Neilson, J.P. (1993) Cardiotocography during labour. *Br. Med. J.* **306**: 347–348.

Oakley, A. (1979) *Becoming a Mother.* Oxford: M. Robertson.

Oakley, A., Rajan, L. & Grant, A. (1990) Social support and pregnancy outcome. *Br. J. Obstet. Gynaecol.* **97**(2): 152–162.

O'Brien, P.M.S., Doyle, P.M. & Rolfe, P. (1993) Near infrared spectroscopy in fetal monitoring. *Br. J. Hosp. Med.* **49**(7): 483–487.

O'Driscoll, K., Meager, D. (1980) *Active Management of Labour.* London: W.B. Saunders.

Roberts, J. (1989) Maternal position during the first stage of labour. In Chalmers, I., Enkin, M. & Keirse, M.J.N.C. (eds) *Effective Care in Pregnancy and Childbirth*, p. 890. Oxford: Oxford University Press.

Roberts, J., Mendez-Bauer, C. & Wodell, D.A. (1983) The effects of maternal position on uterine contractility and efficiency. *Birth* **10**: 243–249.

Roberts, J., Mendez-Bauer, C., Blackwell, J., Carpenter, M.E. & Marchese, T. (1984) Effects of lateral recumbency and sitting on the first stage of labour. *J. Reprod. Med.* **29**: 477–482.

Romney, M.L. (1980) Pre-delivery shaving: an unjustified assault? *J. Obstet. Gynaecol.* **1**: 33–35.

Romney, M.L. & Gordon, H. (1981) Is your enema really necessary? *Br. Med. J.* **282**: 1269–1271.

Rutter, N., Spencer, A., Mann, N. & Smith, M. (1980) Glucose during labour. *Lancet* **2**: 115.

Schwarcz, R., Diaz, A.G., Fescina, R. & Caldeyro-Barcia, R. (1977) Latin American collaborative study on maternal posture in labour. *Birth Family J.* **6**(1): 1979.

Simkin, P. (1986) Stress, pain and catecholamines in labour. Part 2. Stress associated with childbirth events: a pilot survey of new mothers. *Birth* **13**: 234–240.

Sonicaid (1987) Fetal heart patterns and their clinical inter-pretation. Oxford: Sonicaid Ltd.

Spencer, J.A. (1993) Clinical overview of cardiotocography (Review)). *Br. J. Obstet. Gynaecol.* **100**(Suppl. 9): 4–7.

Spencer, J.A.D. (1994) Electronic fetal monitoring in the United Kingdom. *Birth: Issues in Perinatal Care and Education* **21**(2): 106–108.

Thornton, J.G. & Lilford, R.J. (1994) Active management of labour: current knowledge and research issues. *Br. Med. J.* **309**(6951): 366–369.

Tucker-Blackburn, S. & Loper, D.L. (1992) *Maternal, Fetal and Neonatal Physiology.* Philadelphia: W.B. Saunders.

UK Amniotomy Group (1994) Comparing routine versus delayed amniotomy in spontaneous first labour at term. A multicentre randomized trial. *Online J. Current Clin. Trials,* Doc. no. 122, April 1.

UKCC (1993a) *Midwives' Rules.* London: UKCC.

UKCC (1993b) *Standards for Records and Record Keeping.* London: UKCC.

UKCC (1994) *The Midwife's Code of Practice.* London: UKCC.

Further Reading

Axten, S. (1995) Is active management always necessary? *Modern Midwife* **5**(5): 18–20.

Hobbs, P. (1993) Infection control in the delivery suite and the role of protective clothing. *Br. J. Midwifery* **1**(4): 169–173.

Scullion, P. & McCalmont, C. (1995) Siblings in the delivery room. *Br. J. Midwifery* **3**(1): 39–42.

Stewart, P. & Spiby, H. (1989) Posture in labour. *Br. J. Obstet. Gynaecol.* **96**(11): 1258–1260.

Walsh, D. (1994) Management of progress in the first stage of labour. *Midwives Chronicle* **107**(1274): 84–88.

Midwifery Care in the Second Stage of Labour

The second stage of labour is the period from full dilatation of the os uteri to the birth of the baby. The physiological changes which take place are now concerned with the descent of the fetus through the birth canal and its expulsion.

Outline of Physiological Changes

Contractions

The character of the contractions in the second stage of labour is different from those in the first stage, since there is, in addition to the uterine contractions, a bearing down force on the part of the mother to overcome the resistance of the soft parts, vagina, pelvic floor and external parts. These expulsive contractions are strong, with an amplitude of 60–80 mmHg, occur every 2–3 minutes and last for 60–70 seconds. Marked retraction of the uterus further aids the descent of the fetus through the birth canal. There is no appreciable fall in the height of the fundus, however, because the fetal back tends to uncurl from its flexed attitude and the lower uterine segment stretches. The force of the uterine contractions and secondary powers is transmitted down the fetal spine to its head. This is called *fetal axis pressure* and helps the descent of the fetus through the birth canal.

Secondary powers

The expulsion of the fetus is further aided by the voluntary muscles of the diaphragm and abdominal wall. When the second stage is reached, the woman is compelled to bear down or push. As she holds her breath to push, the diaphragm is lowered and the abdominal muscles contract. These secondary powers increase the expulsive force of the uterine contractions.

Table 1   Summary of the physiological changes in the second stage of labour

1	The *contractions* are strong and expulsive in nature
2	The *secondary powers*, i.e. diaphragm and abdominal muscles, aid the expulsive effort
3	The *pelvic floor* is displaced by the advancing fetus
4	The *fetus* is expelled, making a series of passive movements before and during delivery called the *mechanism of labour*

Displacement of the pelvic floor

The advancing fetus greatly distends the vagina and displaces the pelvic floor. Anteriorly the pelvic floor is pushed up and the bladder is drawn up into the abdomen where it is less likely to be damaged. Posteriorly the pelvic floor is pushed down in front of the presenting part. The rectum is compressed thus any faecal contents will be expelled. The perineal body becomes elongated and paper-thin as it is flattened by the advancing fetus.

Expulsion of the fetus

This is the culmination of the second stage of labour. It is accompanied by marked retraction of the uterus which starts the process of placental separation. This is completed in the third stage of labour.

Mechanism of Labour

As labour progresses the fetus is moved through the birth canal and induced to make various twists and turns because of the forces acting upon him. These passive movements are called, collectively, the *mechanism of labour*. They are necessary because the fetus has to adapt to the changing shape of the mother's pelvis during his passage through the birth canal. The widest diameter of the brim of the pelvis is the transverse, whereas the widest diameter of the outlet is the anteroposterior. To make the best use of available space, therefore, the widest presenting diameter of the fetal head enters the pelvis in the transverse diameter. During its passage through the pelvis, first the fetal head and then the shoulders rotate to emerge in the anteroposterior diameter because that is the largest diameter of the pelvic outlet.

There is a mechanism for every presentation and position which can be delivered vaginally. The commonest presentation is the vertex and the commonest position either left or right occipito-anterior, thus this mechanism will be described.

The lie is longitudinal and the presentation is vertex. The attitude is one of flexion and therefore the denominator is the occiput. The engaging diameter is the suboccipitobregmatic which measures 9.5 cm. The position may be either right or left occipito-anterior.

Descent

Descent usually starts before the onset of labour when the fetal head becomes engaged in the pelvis (Figure 1). This is more likely in primigravidae. In multigravidae with lax uterine and abdominal muscles, engagement may not occur until labour is established. Further descent takes place throughout labour. The pressure of the uterine contractions on the fetus force him down the birth canal. When the membranes have ruptured, this pressure is directly on to the breech and the fetal axis pressure is transmitted down the spine to the occiput which must advance. Descent is especially marked in the second stage when the secondary powers, the diaphragm and the abdominal muscles, aid the expulsive effort.

Flexion

At the beginning of labour the head is in an attitude of natural flexion. Flexion is further increased as labour progresses when the head meets the resistance of the birth canal. Because the spine is joined to the head nearer to the back than to the front, fetal axis pressure is transmitted through the occiput rather than the forehead. As a result, the occiput is pushed down

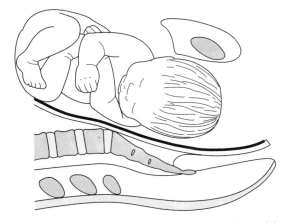

Figure 1   Descent of a well-flexed head into the pelvis. The sagittal suture is in the transverse diameter of the pelvis.

lower and the forehead is pushed upwards by the resistance of the soft parts, and so complete flexion is obtained.

Internal rotation

When the occiput meets the resistance of the pelvic floor it rotates forward 45°; that is, one-eighth of a circle (Figure 2). The slope of the pelvic floor aids this rotation forwards. Internal rotation allows the head to emerge in the longest diameter of the pelvic outlet; that is, the anteroposterior diameter (Figures 3 and 4). The occiput then escapes under the pubic arch and the head is crowned.

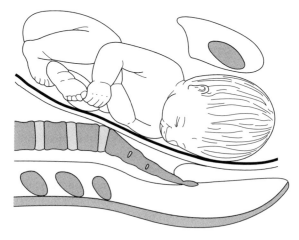

Figure 2   Internal rotation occurs. The sagittal suture is in the oblique diameter of the pelvis.

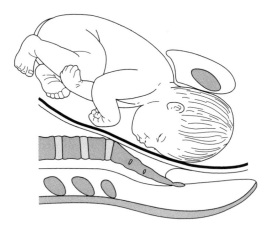

Figure 3   Internal rotation complete – further descent occurs. The sagittal suture is now in the anteroposterior diameter of the pelvis.

Crowning of the head

The head is crowned when it has emerged under the pubic arch and no longer recedes between contractions because the widest transverse diameter of the head (the biparietal diameter) is born (Figure 5).

Extension

Once the head is crowned, extension takes place to allow the bregma, forehead, face and chin to pass over the perineum (Figure 6).

Restitution

When the head is born it rights itself with the shoulders (Figure 7). During the movement of internal rotation the head is slightly twisted because the shoulders do not rotate at that time. The baby untwists his neck by restitution.

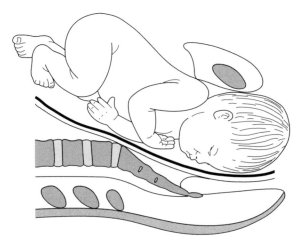

Figure 4   The head descended to the vulval outlet.

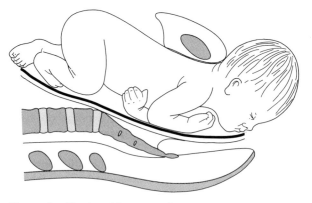

Figure 5   The head is crowned.

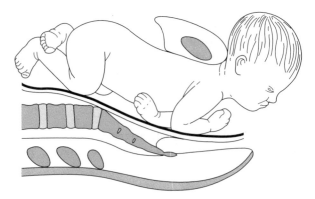

Figure 6   The face is delivered.

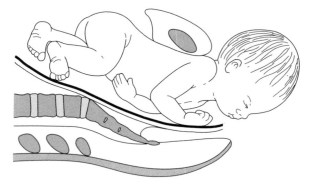

Figure 7   Restitution has taken place and internal rotation of the shoulders occurs

Internal rotation of the shoulders

The shoulders undergo an internal rotation similar to that of the head and then lie in the anteroposterior diameter of the outlet. The head, being free outside the birth canal, moves 45° at the same time, so internal rotation of the shoulders is accompanied by external rotation of the head. Rotation follows the direction of restitution; thus the occiput turns to the same side of the maternal pelvis as it was at the beginning of labour.

Lateral flexion

First the anterior shoulder is born under the pubic arch (Figure 8) then the posterior shoulder passes over the perineum (Figure 9). The trunk of the baby is born by bending sideways in order to pass through the curve of the birth canal.

An understanding of these movements is important to the midwife so that she can assess progress in labour, anticipate the movements of the fetus at delivery and recognize when assistance is required.

Care in the Second Stage of Labour

Throughout the first stage of labour the midwife has established a good, supportive relationship of partnership with the woman which engenders confidence and trust. This will enable them to work together in the second stage for the safe delivery of the baby. The woman's behaviour changes in the second stage of labour when the contractions become expulsive. She may acquire renewed energy and both she and her partner are totally focused on the birth of their baby. Constant observation and care is now necessary and the woman will need the emotional support and skilled care which the midwife is educated to give.

RECOGNIZING THE ONSET OF THE SECOND STAGE OF LABOUR

During the period of transition from first to second stage, some women may rest and doze for periods and appear to be in a trance-like state, while others appear to 'lose control' and become disorientated and nauseous (Inch, 1985). The woman may shake uncontrollably. If she has previously been coping quite well she may find this alteration disturbing. The midwife may need to employ supportive reasoning and reassuring measures to enable the woman to appreciate the meaning of this altered physiology and regain her equilibrium. At this stage, inhalational analgesia in the form of Entonox can be a useful short-term measure.

By definition, the second stage of labour begins with full dilatation of the cervix and culminates in the birth of the baby. Full dilatation of the cervix is described by Sleep *et al.* (1989) as the anatomical onset of the second stage, which may or may not coincide with the expulsive phase, when the woman desires to bear down. Roberts *et al.* (1987), in a descriptive study, found that up to two thirds of women experienced the desire to bear down prior to full dilatation of the cervix. However, some women may feel little or no desire to bear down when the cervix is fully dilated and this sensation does not develop until the fetal presentation descends to compress the tissues of the pelvic floor. This has led to a recognition of the need to distinguish between the early or passive phase of the second stage of labour, and the later active or perineal phase, when the woman experiences the irresistible urge to bear down (Morrin, 1985; Gibb, 1988).

During the second stage of labour the character of

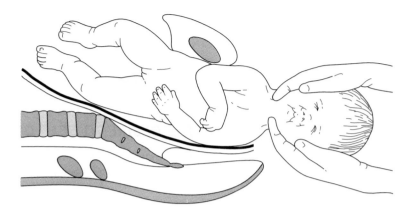

Figure 8   Gentle downward traction is applied to deliver the anterior shoulder.

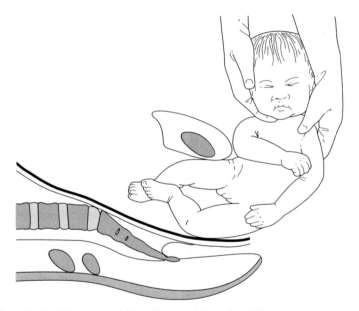

Figure 9   The posterior shoulder is delivered and then the trunk by lateral flexion.

uterine activity alters. Contractions become longer, stronger, more frequent and, in time, expulsive, although in some women there is a short period of reduced uterine activity initially. As the presenting part descends into the vagina at approximately 1 cm above the level of the ischial spines, pressure from the fetal presentation stimulates nerve receptors in the pelvic floor (*Ferguson's reflex*), and the woman experiences the desire to bear down (Figure 10). In addition to the uterine contractions, the bearing-down force on the part of the mother overcomes the resistance of the soft parts, the vagina and the pelvic floor. The voluntary muscles of the chest and abdominal wall act reflexly in concert with the uterine contractions. When the woman bears down her face becomes congested and she makes a characteristic grunting noise at the height of the contraction. These signs often precede the woman's conscious expulsive efforts and she may feel an urge to empty her bowels.

The midwife observes the vulval and perineal areas during contractions to note the *external signs of full dilatation*. The *perineum bulges* and is stretched thin as it is distended by the descending fetus. The *anus initially pouts* and then *dilates* with contractions. The

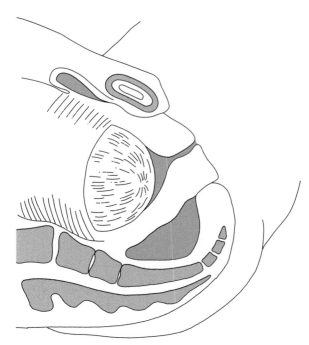

Figure 10   The os uteri is fully dilated and the head enters the vagina.

vagina begins to gape and finally the *presenting part is visible*. If in doubt about the onset of the second stage, the midwife can make an examination per vaginam to confirm full dilatation of the os uteri. No cervix will be felt. This is positive confirmation of the onset of the second stage of labour and the time is recorded.

The midwife should be aware of the rapidity with which the second stage can progress particularly in multiparous women, since sometimes it lasts only a few minutes. The woman should not be left alone in the late first or during the second stage of labour.

DURATION OF THE SECOND STAGE OF LABOUR

Evidence from research findings indicates that the traditional rigid time limitations set for the second stage are invalid and do not provide a sound guide for practice. It is now generally accepted that in the presence of effective uterine activity, where there is progressive descent of the presenting part and the condition of the mother and fetus does not give rise to concern, time alone does not provide sufficient grounds for curtailment of the second stage (Sleep *et al.*, 1989).

According to Watson (1994a) intervention should be based on the rate of progress rather than on the time which has elapsed since full dilatation of the cervix. Progress may be slower than expected in women who have had pethidine during the first stage of labour (Thomson and Hillier, 1994). Continuous observation is necessary in the second stage of labour to detect any alteration in the condition of the mother and fetus.

THE DESIRE TO BEAR DOWN

The woman will feel the urge to bear down when pressure from the presenting part activates Ferguson's reflex (McKay and Roberts, 1985). Organized sustained 'pushing' with contractions, which involves breath-holding (*closed glottis pushing*, known as the *Valsalva manoeuvre*) is still widely practised in the belief that it reduces the duration of the second stage of labour and therefore the period of highest risk to the fetus. This practice has been challenged intermittently since the late 1950s (Beynon, 1957). More recent research evidence indicates that sustained breath-holding during bearing down efforts predisposes to abnormalities of fetal heart activity and a depressed Apgar score (Martinez-Lopez *et al.*, 1984; Knauth and Haloburdo, 1986). Aldrich *et al.* (1995) found that maternal pushing leads to a significant decrease in fetal cerebral oxygenation, together with an increase in cerebral blood volume. *Open glottis pushing*, that is bearing down following exhalation, is advocated by Roberts *et al.* (1987), who suggest that if women are allowed to bear down spontaneously they will do so three to five times during a contraction, following exhalation, and for 4–6 seconds per bearing down effort. Roberts *et al.* (1987) suggest that this practice does not adversely influence the length of the second stage or have an adverse effect on mother or fetus (Paine and Tinker, 1992). This is further supported by Sleep *et al.* (1989) who advise that the modest decrease in the length of the second stage of labour obtained through 'closed glottis pushing' does not appear to confer any benefits but seems to compromise maternal–fetal gas exchange.

It is now considered appropriate to desist from this type of organized bearing down and to allow the woman to 'push' spontaneously when she feels the irresistible urge to do so and to a self-determined pattern. This has the additional advantages of ensuring that the woman does not waste valuable energy in bearing down before the active or perineal phase of the second stage of labour has begun and is less likely to contribute to fetal compromise.

General Midwifery Care

Care of the bladder

At the onset of the second stage the woman should be encouraged to pass urine unless she has recently done so. A full bladder will delay progressive descent of the presentation and the bladder may also be damaged by pressure from the advancing fetus. Occasionally, if the fetal head has descended deeply into the pelvis and has caused upward displacement of the urinary bladder, the woman may be unable to pass urine and the midwife may also find the passage of a catheter difficult. For this reason it is advisable to encourage micturition through-out labour and just prior to full cervical dilatation, before rapid descent of the presentation occurs.

Hygiene and comfort measures

The extreme exertion of the woman during the second stage of labour is likely to make her feel hot and sticky. She may appreciate having her face and hands sponged frequently to remove perspiration. However, some women find this distracting as it breaks their concentration: it is very much a matter of personal choice. If desired, the partner or birth supporter may wish to undertake this task and encouragement to do so is a practical means of encouraging involvement and promoting a sense of usefulness. The vulva is washed whenever necessary and is covered by a sterile pad between contractions. The woman may find sips of iced water welcome and refreshing, as bearing down can make her thirsty and her mouth dry. If oral fluids are contraindicated mouthwashes should be offered.

It is not uncommon for the woman to complain of leg cramps, particularly if she is tensing her muscles during bearing down efforts. This may be relieved by massage and by extending the leg and dorsiflexing the foot, that is, bending it upwards. During this highly charged period of maximum exertion, particularly for primigravidae, the woman should be praised for her efforts and both she and her partner kept fully informed of progress made. Information should be given between contractions, when the woman can relax and attend to what is being said. The midwife can help to promote confidence and allay anxiety by adopting a quiet, calm manner. This is further expressed in the midwife's tone of voice, tactile gestures and other non-verbal means of communication. Privacy is essential and unnecessary intrusion by other care-givers, which may interrupt the woman's concen-tration, should be avoided. It may help to have a 'do not disturb' sign on the door.

Observations

The second stage of labour is a very demanding time for both the woman and the fetus. It is a time when the possibility of fetal hypoxia increases as the alteration in uterine activity further reduces placental–fetal oxygenation (Katz et al., 1987). It is therefore important to assess the effect of contractions on both mother and fetus.

The woman's general condition is noted and her pulse taken at 15-minute intervals. An increase in pulse rate is likely to be due to the effects of bearing down and the excitement, anxiety or fear linked to the prospect of giving birth, but the pulse should remain regular and strong. Provided the blood pressure has been within normal limits it may be recorded every 15 minutes, between contractions. During contractions a rise in blood pressure of 30/25 mmHg can occur, followed by a compensatory fall at the end of the contraction. The frequency, strength and duration of uterine contractions are observed, as well as the relaxation of the uterus between contractions. At this stage the contractions are very strong, occurring every 2–3 minutes and lasting about 60 seconds. Any sustained loss of uterine activity will result in delayed progress and the midwife will need to reassess the situation to establish the likely cause and summon obstetric assistance.

The fetal heart is auscultated towards the end of each contraction. The use of a portable ultrasound monitor may make auscultation easier and is less disturbing to the woman than using the traditional Pinard's stethoscope. If continuous electronic fetal heart monitoring is in progress the cardiotocograph trace should be analysed and the midwife should assess its normality. The amniotic fluid is observed for meconium staining which is a sign of fetal hypoxia, except in a breech presentation when meconium is commonly passed at this stage due to the immense pressure exerted on the breech.

POSITIONS IN THE SECOND STAGE OF LABOUR

The woman is encouraged to adopt a position which is most comfortable and effective for her at this time. It is still common practice in the UK for women to deliver in bed, in a semi-recumbent position well-supported by pillows and perhaps a wedge. It is essential that if the woman chooses to adopt this position she should be well-supported to prevent her from sliding down and eventually adopting the dorsal position. Should this happen, the heavy gravid uterus is likely to compress the vena cava causing subsequent hypotension, reduced placental perfusion and fetal hypoxia (Humphrey et al., 1974; Johnstone et al., 1987).

Midwives and women are increasingly recognizing the value of alternative positions for delivery which promote comfort and pain relief. Many women are now requesting alternatives to the traditional delivery position and increasingly midwives are encouraging women to try alternative positions. A woman's choice of delivery position may vary from the left lateral in bed, to kneeling or squatting on the bed or on the floor, or supporting herself on her hands and knees. Others may elect to use a birthing chair, stool or bed and most maternity units have equipment which will meet some or all of these needs.

The effect of different positions on the length and outcome of labour has been the subject of much interest and investigation in recent years. In their exploration of the relevant research Enkin et al. (1989) have compared the upright posture – which may have been assisted by the use of specially designed wedges or chairs – with the recumbent position. They noted that in most instances the mean duration of labour was shorter with the upright position. It was also observed that, without exception, where maternal preference was elicited, the most frequent positive responses were from those women who had used an upright position (Sleep et al., 1989). They conclude that constraining women to adopt positions which they find awkward or uncomfortable can only be justified if there is good evidence to suggest that the policy has important health advantages for mother or baby. These findings are supported by other studies (Stewart, 1991; Watson, 1994b). Gardosi et al. (1989) found that kneeling was the most popular upright position as squatting is difficult to maintain.

Squatting

This is still the most common position for childbirth throughout the developing world. In Europe squatting and the use of a birth stool was widespread until the eighteenth century when medicalization of childbirth became acceptable. The recumbent position in bed was adopted as a more convenient position for the medical practitioners who were becoming increasingly involved

in attending women in childbirth and this gradually became accepted as the norm. In recent years the squatting position has started to regain favour in Europe and other Western countries, largely due to the work of Dr Michel Odent in France, who is a strong advocate of alternative positions for labour and delivery.

When squatting, the mother needs support with each contraction, usually from another person, or from some other form of stable, firm support. If this is unavailable she may support herself on her hands and knees. In a squatting position the woman flexes and abducts her thighs. This has a number of advantages. The thighs provide a measure of support for the abdominal muscles and the heavy gravid uterus. In an upright position gravitational force tilts the uterus forwards, thereby straightening the longitudinal axis of the birth canal. Fetal axis pressure is directed on to the presenting part, encouraging the maintenance of flexion and an anterior position (McKay, 1984). This, together with an increase in intra-abdominal pressure, results in increased expulsive efforts. The squatting position also leads to an increase in pelvic diameters (Golay et al., 1993; Maresh, 1987; Nelki and Bond, 1995).

Russell (1982) has shown that if the thighs are flexed and abducted, the weight of the body causes some separation of the lower end of the symphysis pubis with an outward movement of the innominate bones and a backward rotation of the sacrum. These changes have been observed radiologically and result in a 28% increase in the area of the pelvic outlet compared to the supine position. This can be a particularly valuable advantage if the pelvis is on the narrow side and the presentation a 'snug' fit. These changes would explain the association of the squatting position with a shorter duration for the second stage of labour and a reduction in the use of forceps to aid delivery. A further advantage is that, in the squatting position, vena caval compression and the resultant fetal compromise is less likely. Without antenatal preparation to strengthen the calf and thigh muscles the woman may find the position demanding (McKay, 1984).

To assist the woman who is delivering in the upright squatting position the midwife should place herself in front of the woman. Vision of the fetus and the perineum is sometimes difficult for the midwife with the woman in this position, but, if the woman has been well prepared for labour in the antenatal period and is in control of her delivery, then little assistance will be required from the midwife. The midwife should be aware of the need to guide the fetal head and shoulders in line with the pelvic curve in order to reduce the risk of perineal trauma. As vaginal and perineal pressure is evenly distributed in the squatting position, perineal stretching is maximized and the need for episiotomy is reduced (McKay, 1984).

Birthing chair

The electronically controlled birthing chair was introduced into the UK in 1981 and is now available in a number of maternity hospitals. Its introduction followed the increasing demand by women for greater mobility in labour and recognition of the disadvantages of being confined to bed. Although squatting is a most effective position for bearing down in labour, supporting a mother in a squatting position can be a problem and good vision and access to the fetus and perineum is not always easy. The birthing chair overcomes these problems, yet the mother still has the advantage of being in an upright position. The chair is electronically controlled and can be tilted back quickly and easily should the need arise. Procedures such as artificial rupture of the membranes, forceps and ventouse deliveries and perineal suturing can all be carried out with the mother in the chair. Should a general anaesthetic become necessary, however, the mother must be transferred to bed because in the chair she cannot be turned onto her side easily or placed in the Trendelenberg position.

An early study indicated that the use of a birthing chair reduced the incidence of instrumental delivery (Romney, 1983). However, the results of a large randomized controlled trial in nulliparous women indicate that there is no apparent reduction in operative delivery for fetal heart abnormalities and no beneficial effects on perineal trauma or post-delivery perineal pain (Crowley et al., 1991). Disadvantages of birthing chairs include an apparently higher mean blood loss and an increased incidence of postpartum haemorrhage in multigravidae (Waldenstrom and Gottvall, 1991; Stewart and Spiby, 1989). This may be a result of increased accuracy in collecting and measuring blood lost when delivery occurs in a birthing chair (Levy and Moore, 1985). However, blood loss from perineal trauma (as opposed to placental site bleeding) may be exacerbated by obstructed venous return resulting from pressure on the buttocks and perineum from the chair. Such pressure may be reflected in the obser-

vation of increased perineal oedema and a higher incidence of haemorrhoids in women who are upright in birthing chairs (Cottral and Shannahan, 1986). Sleep et al. (1989) note a higher incidence of low haemoglobin and an increased need for blood transfusion following this mode of delivery.

Delivery beds which can be converted into a chair position offer an alternative to the birthing chair.

Hands and knees or all-fours position

Some women like to be on their hands and knees during contractions and perhaps also for their delivery. It is a good position for bearing down and seems to give relief of pain to those suffering from backache. In between contractions the woman may wish to sit or lie down. Other advantages of this position are that it aids rotation and descent and causes less perineal trauma, although there is a possibility that it increases vulval trauma (Biancuzzo, 1991). In emergency situations such as prolapsed cord it relieves pressure on the cord and it may aid delivery of the shoulders in cases of shoulder dystocia (Glynn and Olah, 1994).

The all-fours position allows excellent vision of the fetus and perineum. Once the head and shoulders are delivered the trunk is delivered by lateral flexion between the mother's legs towards her abdomen. At this time the mother usually rises on to her knees and can receive the baby into her arms if she wishes. During the third stage the mother lies on her back in a semi-recumbent position, or she may prefer to squat.

The midwife should be able to adapt the principles of care in labour and management of delivery to whatever position the woman wishes to adopt. A summary of the positions which a woman may adopt for labour and delivery is shown in Table 2.

Preparation for the Birth

If the woman is a multigravida, the midwife should prepare for delivery as soon as she suspects that the second stage is imminent. The primigravida usually progresses more slowly and final preparations can therefore be made during the second stage.

The delivery room should be clean and warm for the birth of the baby. Privacy for the mother must be ensured because it is embarrassing and stressful for her to have people repeatedly entering her room. It has been suggested that stress during labour adversely

Table 2   Summary of alternative positions for labour/delivery

Position	Advantages	Disadvantages	Comments	References
Standing – includes supported and unsupported positions of an upright forward nature	Increased efficiency in expulsion of the fetus, especially where the fetus presents in a posterior position	Tiredness	Comfort of the mother, use of a thinner mattress on the floor	Sutton & Scott (1994)
	Less perineal trauma			Golay *et al.* (1993); Gardosi *et al.* (1989)
	Increased maternal involvement and pleasure			Golay *et al.* (1993); Waldenstrom & Gottvall (1991)
Squatting – includes supported squatting	Increased pelvic diameters	Tiredness, needs antenatal preparation	Need to discuss in antenatal period	Golay *et al.* (1993); Maresh (1987); Nelki & Bond (1995)
	Aids force of gravity	Requires support to maintain position for prolonged periods of time	Adaptation of equipment in a labour ward	
	Fewer assisted deliveries	Transient vulval oedema		
	Less perineal trauma			
All fours – includes kneeling	Aids rotation and descent	?Increased vulval trauma	Aids required for support and comfort of the woman	Biancuzzo (1991); Gardosi *et al.* (1989)
	Relieves backache			
	Relief of pressure on prolapsed cord			
	Aids delivery of shoulders in cases of shoulder dystocia			Glynn & Olah (1994)
	Less perineal trauma			
Birthing chairs	Facilitates upright maternal position without other aids or people giving support	Increased risk of post-partum haemorrhage		Waldenstrom & Gottvall (1991); Stewart & Spiby (1989)

Note: Adapted from table supplied by Patricia Simcock, PGCEA Student, University of Surrey, 1995.

affects uterine activity. However, not all authorities are in agreement on this (Odent, 1987; Newton, 1987). A sterile delivery trolley is prepared, including a sterile gown and gloves for the midwife who is to deliver the baby. To prevent contamination from blood or liquor splashes, and the risk of diseases contracted from body fluids, e.g. HIV, the midwife should also wear unobtrusive eye protection such as plain spectacles. Any other person likely to come into contact with blood or other body fluids should be similarly protected. Local anaesthetic and syringe are prepared in readiness for infiltration of the perineum prior to an episiotomy, should it be necessary. If active management of the third stage of labour is planned, a suitable oxytocic drug such as Syntometrine 1 ml or Syntocinon 5–10 units is checked and drawn up in readiness for use. A warm cot is prepared for the baby and resuscitation equipment is checked.

Conduct of Delivery

This is a time of great anticipation and it is now that the true value of the midwife–woman relationship and the skills of the midwife are demonstrated. If the midwife has established a good relationship with the woman and her partner, has enabled them to have trust and confidence in themselves and their carers, has taken care to help the woman to achieve satisfactory pain relief, and kept them informed of progress and what to expect in the second stage, then the woman and her supporter can approach the actual delivery with confidence. The atmosphere in the delivery room should be calm and unhurried, so that the woman and her supporter can reflect this calmness in their behaviour and the woman can emerge from the experience with positive memories and her self-respect intact. Some women may feel the desire to shout or scream with contractions. This may be contrary to the cultural expectations of the woman and her partner and both will need to be reassured that this does not mitigate against calmness but may serve as a positive action in the reduction of tension and breath-holding.

The midwife prepares to assist the delivery by putting on protective spectacles and thoroughly washing her hands. She puts on a sterile gown and gloves and organizes the equipment on the trolley for ease of use. Before the birth takes place the midwife washes the vulva with warm antiseptic lotion and covers the delivery area with sterile towels. A sterile pad is used to cover the anus to reduce the risk of infection from faecal contamination. The actual method of delivery can be learned only by experience. While methods may vary, the principles remain the same and can be applied to whatever position the woman adopts for delivery.

Good control of the head is essential to prevent sudden birth which might cause severe laceration of the perineum or intracranial injury to the baby. The delivery should be allowed to proceed slowly and steadily but the head should not be held back so long that, although obvious perineal lacerations are avoided, the deeper structures of the pelvic floor are over-stretched and torn. The midwife should be aware that pelvic floor and perineal trauma may have long-term implications for the woman and her partner (Sleep and Grant, 1987; Kitzinger, 1981). This includes the unnecessary use of episiotomy as well as prevention of lacerations. Many factors influence the maintenance of perineal integrity, including the condition of both mother and baby and the length of labour. Sleep *et al.* (1984) maintain that 69% of women will need some form of perineal repair.

Delivery should be encouraged to proceed slowly so that the fetal head can gradually distend and stretch the perineum. Perineal massage, the use of hot perineal compresses in labour and 'guarding' the perineum at delivery have all been used in the second stage of labour and may help to maintain the integrity of the pelvic floor (Floud, 1994a). However, there is currently no sound research evidence for their effectiveness. It has been suggested that some such techniques may cause damage to the vaginal and perineal tissues (Floud, 1994b).

As the head distends the perineum the midwife may decide that an episiotomy is necessary to prevent a severe perineal laceration. This intervention should only be performed if a third-degree laceration is likely. Second-degree lacerations heal as well as episiotomies, and cause less pain (Sleep *et al.*, 1984, 1986). An episiotomy is a surgical incision of the perineum to enlarge the vulval orifice. If an episiotomy is considered essential the perineum should be infiltrated with a local anaesthetic such as 10 ml of lignocaine 0.5% (i.e. 50 mg) before the episiotomy is performed (see Chapter 34).

The midwife controls the advance of the head, if necessary, and maintains flexion by placing the palm of her hand on the head with fingers pointing to the sinciput. Until the head crowns it will recede between contractions. It crowns when the widest transverse diameter, the biparietal diameter, distends the vulva and then it no longer recedes. During the delivery of the head the mother is asked to breathe steadily in and out to prevent the delivery taking place too quickly. She may use inhalational analgesia if required. Once crowned, the remainder of the head is born by extension. The midwife may change the position of her hand to grasp the parietal eminences to assist in extending the head, if necessary.

When the child's head is born the midwife slips her fingers over to the occiput to see if the cord is round the baby's neck. If so, it must be freed, or a loop made large enough for the shoulders to pass through. Failing this, two pairs of artery forceps must be applied 2–5 cm apart, and the cord cut between them and unwound. Mucus is then gently removed from the baby's nose and mouth and the eyes are swabbed, from within out, using one swab for each eye. At this stage some mothers like to be propped up to see their baby's head and watch, or perhaps assist with, the delivery of the trunk.

The birth of the trunk should not be hurried unless there is some special reason for doing so. The next contraction usually expels it. Following restitution and external rotation of the head, the shoulders should be in the anteroposterior diameter of the pelvis. Only then can they be delivered safely and without the risk of perineal trauma. To deliver the shoulders the midwife places her hands one each side of the baby's head. With the next contraction gentle downward traction is applied to the baby's head. The anterior shoulder then comes down below the symphysis pubis. As the anterior shoulder is delivered the mother may be given an intramuscular injection of Syntometrine 1 ml if active management of the third stage of labour is planned. The posterior shoulder is then delivered by guiding the head in an upward direction and the baby's trunk is carried towards the mother's abdomen, being born by lateral flexion. The baby can then be placed on the mother's abdomen, or in her arms, where she can immediately see and touch her baby. The time of delivery is noted.

If necessary an assistant will very gently clear the baby's pharynx and nostrils of any mucus and liquor, using swabs or a mucus extractor or electrical suction. For most babies naso-pharyngeal suctioning is unnecessary. Meanwhile the cord is clamped with artery forceps, approximately 7–12 cm from the umbilicus. It is cut between the clamps with blunt-ended scissors. The mother can then hold her baby more comfortably in her arms. It is important to ensure that he is gently dried and covered warmly to prevent excessive heat loss. This is a very thrilling moment for the parents and the midwife is privileged to share their joy in the birth of their baby.

Waterbirth

The therapeutic use of water in childbirth is a relatively new concept which has grown in popularity as some women seek alternative methods of relieving the pain and discomfort of labour. In response to women's requests for this way of labouring and giving birth, many maternity units have installed a purpose-built bath or pool in the labour area. If a home birth is planned, equipment can be hired, structure of the building permitting. Alternatively, use can be made of the domestic bath, although this may not allow maximum freedom of movement for the woman and may also restrict the midwife's activity because of its relatively small size. Many midwives have chosen to learn the particular skills necessary to assist the woman to deliver her baby with the help of water. However, there is little research into the practice of waterbirth and opinions differ as to the safety and efficacy of water as a method of pain relief and a medium for delivery. This lack of research was identified in the Report of the Expert Maternity Group (DOH, 1993), who noted the introduction of well-intentioned changes – not based on research findings – into maternity care. Where such practices are introduced into a maternity service or requested by women and their partners, the midwife must indicate what supporting evidence (or lack of) is available and discuss the implications with them. This will empower the couple to make an appropriately informed choice.

The amount of time a woman wishes to spend in the water varies and is governed by how comfortable she feels and the degree of pain relief she experiences. Some women may wish to spend most of their labour and delivery in the water pool, others choose to spend short periods and some women may wish to leave the water for the actual birth of the baby and delivery of the placenta. In 1991 waterbirths accounted for approximately 5% of all births (Burns and Greenish, 1993).

Background to waterbirth

Some early work was undertaken in the 1960s by Russian researcher Igor Tjarkovsky, whose work with animals led to further work with women (Lines, 1992). In the 1970s Michel Odent installed a water pool in the maternity unit in Pithivier, France, with the aims of helping women to cope in labour, reducing obstetric intervention and promoting the concept of 'gentle' birth.

The evidence in support of the benefits of waterbirth is mainly descriptive. McCraw (1989) suggests that the long-term benefits to the baby of such 'gentle birth' methods remain unproven by sound scientific research. Nevertheless, the increasing incidence of waterbirth is reflective of the desire to enable women to actively participate in labour and indicates a responsiveness to individual needs. In spite of the increasing practice of immersion in water during labour and/or birth there is no reliable information about its advantages, hazards or disadvantages. A recent survey concludes that there is no evidence that labour and delivery in water should not continue to be offered, but a randomized, controlled trial is required to address issues of concern (Alderdice *et al.*, 1995a,b).

Possible benefits of water immersion

Relaxation   It is suggested that the buoyancy and feeling of relative weightlessness produced by total or partial water immersion allows for ease of movement during the first stage of labour. This enables the woman to adopt a position most suited to comfort and facilitates the use of upright and kneeling positions (Balaskas and Gordon, 1992). Such relaxation, it is suggested, also reduces mental tension and this assists physical relaxation. It is also likely that the increased ability to relax may lower the woman's blood pressure (Church, 1989). Such relaxation may also contribute to increased emotional satisfaction with the labour and delivery experience.

Pain relief   This is thought to be achieved by several mechanisms. These include:

▶ a reduction in the intensity of uterine, abdominal and back muscle tone, thus aiding the ability to relax;
▶ decreased production of noradrenaline and other catecholamines, thus aiding the production of naturally occurring endorphins; and
▶ reduction of sensory stimuli and altered pain perception (Balaskas and Gordon, 1992).

Burns and Greenish (1993) suggest that their observations indicate a possible reduction in the need for pharmacological analgesia other than Entonox, implying possible benefits to both mother and fetus. However, in a previous study no noticeable reduction in labour pain was identified although it was thought that the first stage of labour may have been accelerated (Cammu *et al.*, 1992).

Enhanced cervical dilatation   This is thought to be assisted by the altered state of consciousness which reduces anxiety and assists the ability to relax and conserve energy, thereby facilitating normal uterine activity. Paradoxically, Balaskas and Gordon (1992) also suggest that because relaxation is maximized, too-early immersion in water may inhibit uterine activity. Therefore, unless the contractions are particularly strong or painful, the woman should refrain from entering the water before the os uteri is 4–5 cm dilated (Nightingale, 1994).

Perineal integrity

There is conflicting evidence on this issue. Church (1989) and Garland and Jones (1994) indicated that there was no difference in the incidence of perineal trauma, or it is possibly reduced, a finding not supported by the work of Burns and Greenish (1993) which indicated an increase in second-degree tears.

Effects on the fetus

No adverse fetal effects have been studied. In Odent's experience (1983) the majority of women leave the water to actually give birth, although some women, through choice or chance, deliver the baby underwater. Although midwives may feel more confident to assist the woman to deliver out of the water, underwater delivery is not known to have any detrimental effect on the fetus. Further research is required and the British Paediatric Surveillance Unit is conducting a survey on all babies who develop problems following labour and/or birth in water (Alderdice *et al.*, 1995b). Respiratory efforts are not initiated until the baby emerges from the water and experiences external stimuli (Jackson *et al.*, 1989). If the water is kept at a constant temperature of 36.5–37.5° C the baby will not lose body heat. Deans and Steer (1995) stress the importance of maintaining the correct temperature of the water in the pool.

Possible disadvantages or hazards of waterbirth

Because of the lack of research into the field of waterbirth, the midwife should be aware of the possible problems which may give rise to concern or pose a theoretical risk. Such risks include the following.

Infection of mother or baby   (George, 1990; Loomes and Finch, 1990; Rawal *et al.*, 1994.) It is possible that such risks may be reduced by using disposable tub linings where possible and by cleaning of the bath after use, in accordance with current methods of prevention of cross-infection, such as washing with a sanitizing agent and drying after use. Monitoring of cross-infection would also include regular swabbing of equipment and pipes etc. for bacteriological examination. Neither Odent nor Tjarkovsky, the pioneers of waterbirth, found infection to be a particular problem. It was not an issue when Burns and Greenish (1993) outlined their findings on the use of water. Gordon (1991) found no evidence of increased infection rates in the woman or baby.

Loomes and Finch (1990) and George (1990) discuss the possibility of infection when unacceptably high levels of bacteria have been isolated in water/pump heating equipment. However, this can be addressed by using normally heated tap water for filling the pool or bath, not allowing water to enter and exit from the same aperture, undertaking normal hygiene measures when cleaning the pool and by using disposable pool linings (Newton, 1992).

Rupture of the membranes   Once the membranes have ruptured the protection afforded by the intact amniotic sac is missed. Such a situation questions the safety of water immersion. A study undertaken by Waldenstrom and Nilsson (1992), using retrospective data, found that, although there was no statistical difference with respect to infection, respiratory difficulties and signs of maternal amnionitis, babies born more than 24 hours after rupture of the membranes had significantly lower Apgar scores than those born to women who had not had a waterbirth. Such findings, together with a lack of additional detail was influential in moderating the author's policy for criteria for water immersion in labour.

The question of HIV transmission has been raised by Gordon (1991), who suggests that, although there is a theoretical risk of HIV transmission to medical attendants, the water dilutes the infected liquor or blood and thus viral infectivity is diminished. He does propose that it may become necessary to screen all women for HIV status. However this would raise ethical concerns and is a debatable issue.

Water embolism   Although there is no evidence confirming the risk of water embolism (Jepson, 1989), in theory it may occur when maternal placental bed sinuses are torn in the third stage of labour. Water may then enter the circulation. For this reason it is deemed advisable for the third stage of labour to be conducted out of the water.

Perineal trauma   The possibility of perineal trauma should be borne in mind. The midwife should ensure that she is able to provide sufficient assistance within the pool to enable the woman to control her delivery, allowing the head and shoulders to emerge slowly during the perineal phase of the second stage of labour.

Additional disadvantages include a reduced choice of analgesia and the possibility of disappointment and unfulfilled birth expectations should labour not progress as anticipated.

Selection for waterbirth

The safety of the woman and her baby are of paramount importance. The midwife must also remember her professional responsibilities and accountability, as well as acknowledging potential medico–legal implications of new and unresearched birth techniques. The following selection criteria for waterbirth should be considered (Blair-Myers, 1989; Nightingale, 1994).

▶ The use of water must be at the woman's request.
▶ There should be no known or envisaged obstetric problems.
▶ Labour must not be pre- or post-term, that is, labour should have commenced between 37 and 40 weeks' gestation.
▶ The fetal heart trace, if recorded, must be normal.
▶ Labour should be established before the woman enters the water.
▶ The presentation must be cephalic.
▶ The maternal observations must be normal. If there are any abnormalities such as raised blood pressure, the midwife must seek the advice of an obstetrician.
▶ The woman and her partner must agree to leave the pool if requested to by the midwife.
▶ The midwife should be willing to undertake this type of care.

As there is as yet no firm research evidence to guide the midwife it will be necessary to determine the benefits and risks of waterbirth by a careful individual assessment of each woman. The midwife should also ascertain that there are no medical problems which might seriously affect the labour. In effect, the pregnancy should have been normal in all respects.

In accordance with the midwives' *Code of Practice* (UKCC, 1994a), the midwife must ensure that she is adequately prepared and competent to undertake this type of labour care. The midwife should also be familiar with the UKCC's *Position Statement on Waterbirths* (UKCC, 1994b).

Preparation for waterbirth

It is advisable to undertake a waterbirth in a tub or pool especially constructed for the purpose. These are usually larger than a domestic bath in order to allow freedom of movement for the woman and sufficient space for the midwife to undertake care adequately and comfortably. As one litre of water weighs a kilogram the midwife should ensure that the structure of the floor is able to support the considerable weight. If the birth is planned to take place at home this is the woman's responsibility. However, the midwife should ensure that the woman has given the matter consideration. The tub or pool should be equipped with a means of monitoring the water temperature. An adequate water supply should be available to allow easy removal and addition of water in order to maintain the desired temperature. Some purpose-built pools have a circulating pump which is able to maintain a regular temperature. Floor and bath surfaces should be non-slip to avoid accidents and the room should be warm and well-ventilated. A supply of dry, warm towels should be available. Soft lighting and soothing music may add to the atmosphere of relaxation. Privacy is essential. Toilet facilities should, ideally, be close by.

The tub should be filled sufficiently to allow the woman to immerse her body comfortably, as one would normally do when taking a bath. The amount of water will vary according to the size of the tub or pool, but the aims are to achieve buoyancy which will aid freedom of movement in adopting different positions and to utilize hydrostatic pressure, which is thought to reduce pain (Church, 1989). It may take 30 minutes to 1 hour to fill the pool, depending on its size and the water pressure. For this reason portable domestic pools take longer to fill than those in hospital. The water temperature must be carefully monitored to achieve adequate comfort and should be maintained at 36.5–37.5° C. This provides a neutral thermal environment and prevents wrinkling of the skin. A high water temperature is uncomfortable for the woman and may cause a fetal tachycardia (Nightingale, 1994). It must be checked and adjusted for the second stage of labour in order to provide the correct environment for the baby, as water which is too cool may induce respiration before the baby has been brought to the surface. Any faeces which contaminate the water should be removed using a simple plastic strainer. This should be disinfected after use. Fluids may be given freely as the woman requires, as she may perspire more in the warm water.

Monitoring maternal and fetal health

Observations of maternal and fetal well-being are made as for any labour. The fetal heart can be auscultated using an underwater ultrasonic monitor, or a Pinard's stethoscope. The woman should be asked to raise her abdomen clear of the water to aid auscultation. This may feel awkward and uncomfortable but close monitoring of the fetal heart is essential. Occasionally the midwife may advise the woman to leave the pool for intermittent electronic fetal heart monitoring which cannot be undertaken within water. When the membranes rupture the midwife should observe the liquor for the presence of meconium or any unusual blood loss. If these are noted then the midwife must make a careful assessment of the fetal and maternal condition and should summon medical assistance if necessary. The woman will need to leave the pool if continuous electronic fetal heart monitoring is thought necessary. Monitoring of the maternal pulse can be unobtrusive and the blood pressure can be taken without undue disturbance to the woman. Vaginal examination may be safely undertaken underwater.

Analgesia

Inhalational analgesia (Entonox) is a suitable means of providing additional pain relief during a waterbirth. The equipment should be placed close to the pool so that it is easily available to the woman. The woman should not be left unattended while using inhalational analgesia during a waterbirth. If narcotic analgesia is required the woman should leave the water as the drowsiness induced by the drugs compromises safety.

The second stage of labour

Two midwives should be present for the birth. This is a precautionary measure, should extra help be required or an emergency arise. Delivery is assisted in whichever position the woman finds the most comfortable. As with any birth, the midwife should ensure that the woman empties her bladder prior to the onset of the second stage of labour. If an episiotomy is necessary it may be performed underwater; although it can be awkward, visibility should be sufficiently favourable (Newton, 1992). The midwife and/or the woman control the fetal head to prevent sudden expulsion and risk of perineal tearing. Variations in position and difficulty in facilitating a slow, controlled delivery of the head may be factors influencing the differences in the incidence of perineal trauma discussed earlier. As with any birth directive bearing down efforts are best avoided.

The baby should be brought to the surface immediately after birth.

The umbilical cord should not be clamped and cut while the baby is still under water because the sudden reduction in placental–fetal blood flow may initiate respiration (Balaskas and Gordon, 1992). When the baby's head is above the surface of the water the cord may be divided. If the umbilical cord is found to be around the baby's neck during delivery it may be unwound if it is sufficiently loose. If this is not possible the woman should be asked to stand with the baby's head clear of the water so that the cord may be clamped and cut before delivery of the shoulders. A tight nuchal cord should not be divided underwater because of the risk of early inspiration and possible water inhalation by the baby. Similarly, should there be an emergency such as shoulder dystocia or haemorrhage the woman will need to leave the pool.

Delivery of the placenta

The third stage of labour should be conducted out of the water because of the theoretical risk of water embolus (Odent, 1983). Any oxytocic preparation, if used, should be given when the woman has left the water. The cord is then clamped and cut and delivery of the placenta and membranes achieved by controlled cord traction. If a physiological third stage is desired and is appropriate then the cord is not clamped and cut. If the woman stands in the pool to deliver the placenta the midwife should retrieve any blood clots which fall into the water and include these in the estimated blood loss. It may be difficult to make an accurate estimate of blood loss at a waterbirth and loss may be heavier than with a dry land delivery (Nightingale, 1994). The midwife should carefully monitor the woman's condition in the postnatal period and be alert for any signs of anaemia.

References

Alderdice, F., Renfrew, M., Garcia, J. & Marchant, S. (1995a) A national study of labour and birth in water. *Midwives* **108**(1284): 8.

Alderdice, F., Renfrew, M., Marchant, S. *et al.* (1995b) Labour and birth in water in England and Wales. *Br. Med. J.* **310**: 837.

Aldrich, C.J., D'Antona, D., Spencer, J.A. *et al.* (1995) The effect of maternal pushing of fetal cerebral oxygenation and blood volume during the second stage of labour. *Br. J. Obstet. Gynaecol.* **102**(6): 448–453.

Balaskas, J. & Gordon, Y. (1992) *Waterbirth.* London: Thornson Publishers.

Biancuzzo, M. (1991) The patient observer: does the hands and knees posture during labour help to rotate the occipitoposterior fetus? *Birth* **18**(1): 40–47.

Beynon, C.L. (1957) The normal second stage of labour: a plea for reform of its conduct. *J. Obstet. Gynaecol. Br. Empire* **64**: 815–820.

Blair-Myers, M. (1989) The lagoon room experience. *Nursing Times* **85** (November): 72–73.

Burns, E. & Greenish, K. (1993) Pooling information. *Nursing Times* **89**(8): 47–49.

Cammu, H., Clasen, K. & Van Wetteren, L. (1992) Is having a warm bath during labour useful? *J. Perinatal Med.* **20** (Suppl. 1): 104.

Church, L. (1989) Waterbirth: one centre's observation. *J. Nurse Midwifery* **34**(4): 165–170.

Cottral, B.H. & Shannahan, M.D. (1986) The effect of the birth chair on the duration of labour and maternal outcome. *Nursing Res.* **35**: 364–367.

Crowley, P., Elbourne, D., Ashurst, H. *et al.* (1991) Delivery in an obstetric chair: a randomised controlled trial. *Br. J. Obstet. Gynaecol.* **98**(7): 667–674.

Deans, A.C. & Steer, P.J. (1995) Labour and birth in water. Temperature of pool is important (letter). *Br. Med. J.* **311**(7001): 390–391.

DOH (Department of Health) (1993) *Changing Childbirth.* Report of the Expert Maternity Group. London: HMSO.

Enkin, M., Keirse, M. & Chalmers, I. (1989) *A Guide to Effective Care in Pregnancy and Childbirth.* Oxford: Oxford University Press.

Floud, E. (1994a) Protecting the perineum in childbirth 1: a retrospective view. *Br. J. Midwifery* **2**(6): 258–263.

Floud, E. (1994b) Protecting the perineum in childbirth 3: perineal care today. *Br. J. Midwifery* **2**(8): 356–361.

Garland, D. & Jones, K. (1994) Waterbirth: first stage immersion or non-immersion? Some outcomes of women's choice of birthing modality. *Br. J. Midwifery* **2**(3): 113–120.

George, R. (1990) Bacteria in birthing tubs. *Nursing Times* **86**(14): 14.

Gardosi, J., Sylvester, S. & B-Lynch, C. (1989) Alternative positions in the second stage: a randomised controlled trial. *Br. J. Obstet. Gynaecol.* **96**(11): 1290–1296.

Gibb, D.M.E. (1988) *A Practical Guide to Labour Management.* London: Blackwell.

Glynn, M. & Olah, K.S. (1994) The management of shoulder dystocia. *Br. J. Midwifery* **2**(3): 108–112.

Golay, J., Vedam, S. & Sorger, L. (1993) The squatting position for second stage of labour: effects on labour and on maternal and fetal well-being. *Birth* 20(2): 73–78.

Gordon, Y. (1991) Waterbirth – a personal view. *Maternal and Child Health* August: 245–250.

Humphrey, M.D., Chang, A., Wood, E.C. *et al.* (1974) A decrease in fetal pH during the second stage of labour when conducted in the dorsal position. *Br. J. Obstet. Gynaecol. British Commonwealth* 81: 600–602.

Inch, S. (1985) *Birthrights*. London: Hutchinson.

Jackson, V., Corsaro, M., Niles, C. *et al.* (1989) Incorporating waterbirths into nurse-midwifery. *J. Nurse Midwifery* 34 (4): 193–197.

Jepson, C. (1989) Water: can it help birth? *Nursing Times* 85(47): 74–75.

Johnstone, F.D., Aboelmagd, M.S. & Harouny, A.K. (1987) Maternal posture in second stage and fetal acid–base status. *Br. J. Obstet. Gynaecol.* 94: 753–757.

Katz, M., Lunenfeld, E., Meizner, I., Bashan, N. & Gross, J. (1987) The effect of the duration of the second stage on the acid–base of the fetus. *Br. J. Obstet. Gynaecol.* 94: 425–430.

Kitzinger, S. (1981) *Some Women's Experience of Episiotomy*. London: National Childbirth Trust.

Knauth, D.G. & Haloburdo, E.P. (1986) Effects of pushing techniques in a birthing chair on the length of the second stage of labour. *Nursing Res.* 35: 49–51.

Levy, V. & Moore, J. (1985) The midwife's management of the third stage of labour. *Nursing Times* 1(5): 47–50.

Lines, M. (1992) *Waterbirth: What I Need to Know*. M. Lines, 1 Mallard Close, Hordle, Lymington, Hampshire SO41 0FH.

Loomes, S. & Finch, R. (1990) Breeding ground for bacteria. *Nursing Times* 86(6): 14–15.

Maresh, M. (1987) Management of the second stage of labour. *Midwife, Health Visitor & Community Nurse* 23(11): 498–506.

Martinez-Lopez, V., de la Fanta, P., Iniguez, A. *et al.* (1984) Comparisons of two methods of bearing down during the second stage. Paper presented at the Society for Gynecologic Investigation, March, pp. 21–24.

McCraw, R. (1989) Recent innovations in childbirth. *J. Nurse Midwifery* 34(4): 206–210.

McKay, S. (1984) Squatting: an alternative position for the second stage of labor. *Am. J. Maternal-Child Nursing* 9 (May/June): 181–183.

McKay, S. & Roberts, J. (1985) Second stage of labour: what is normal? *J. Obstet. Gynecol. Neonatal Nursing* 14: 101–106.

Morrin, N. (1985) The second stage. *Nursing Mirror* 161(3): S7–S11.

Nelki, J. & Bond, L. (1995) Positions in labour: a plea for flexibility. *Modern Midwife* 5(2): 19–24.

Newton, C. (1992) Bath rights. *Nursing Times* 88(24): 34–35.

Newton, N. (1987) The fetal ejection reflex revisited. *Birth* 14(2): 106–108.

Nightingale, C. (1994) Waterbirth in practice. *Modern Midwife* January: 15–19.

Odent, M. (1983) Birth under water. *Lancet* December: 24/31.

Odent, M. (1987) The fetus ejection reflex. *Birth* 14(2): 104–105.

Paine, L.L. & Tinker, D.D. (1992) The effect of maternal bearing-down efforts on arterial cord pH and length of the second stage of labor. *J. Nurse Midwifery* 37(1): 61–63.

Rawal, J., Shah, A., Stirk, F. & Mehtar, S. (1994) Waterbirth and infection in babies. *Br. Med. J.* 309: 511.

Roberts, J.E., Goldstein, S.A., Gruener, J.S. *et al.* (1987) A descriptive analysis of involuntary bearing down efforts during the expulsive phase of labour. *J. Obstet. Gynecol. Neonatal Nursing* 16: 48–55.

Romney, M. (1983) Chair project. *Research and the Midwife, Conference Proceedings*, University of Manchester, pp. 69–80.

Russell, J.G.B. (1982) The rationale of primitive delivery positions. *Br. J. Obstet. Gynaecol.* 89: 712–715.

Sleep, J. & Grant, A. (1987) West Berkshire Perineal Management Trial: a three year follow-up. *Br. Med. J.* 295: 749–751.

Sleep, J., Grant, A., Garcia, J. *et al.* (1984) West Berkshire Perineal Management Trial. *Br. J. Med.* 289: 587–590.

Sleep, J., Grant, A., Garcia, J. *et al.* (1986) West Berkshire Perineal Management Study. *Br. Med. J.* 289: 587–590.

Sleep, J., Roberts, J. & Chalmers, I. (1989) Care during the second stage of labour. In Chalmers, I., Enkin, M. & Keirse, M. (eds) *Effective Care in Pregnancy and Childbirth*, Vol 2. Oxford: Oxford University Press.

Stewart, P. (1991) Influence of posture in labour. *Contemp. Rev. Obstet. Gynaecol.* 3: 152–157.

Stewart, P. & Spiby, H. (1989) A randomised study of the sitting position for delivery using a newly designed obstetric chair. *Br. J. Obstet. Gynaecol.* 96: 327–333.

Sutton, J. & Scott, P. (1994) Optimal fetal positioning. *MIDIRS Midwifery Digest* 4(3): 283–286.

Thomson, A.M. & Hillier, V.F. (1994) A re-evaluation of the effect of pethidine on the length of labour. *J. Adv. Nursing* 19(3): 448–456.

UKCC (United Kingdom Central Council for Nursing, Midwifery and Health Visiting) (1994a) *The Midwife's Code of Practice*. London: UKCC.

UKCC (1994b) *Position Statement on Waterbirths*. Annexe 1 to Registrar's Letter 16/1994, pp. 1–4. London: UKCC.

Waldenstrom, U. & Gottvall, K. (1991) A randomised trial of birthing stools or conventional semi-recumbent positions for second stage labour. *Birth* 18(1): 5–10.

Waldenstrom, U. & Nilsson, C.A. (1992) Warm tub bath after spontaneous rupture of membranes. *Birth* 19(2): 57–63.

Watson, V. (1994a) The duration of the second stage of labour. *Modern Midwife* 4(6): 21–22.

Watson, V. (1994b) Maternal position in the second stage of labour. *Modern Midwife* 4(7): 21–24.

Further Reading

Chapman, V. (1994) Waterbirths: breakthrough or burden. *Br. J. Midwifery* **2**(1): 17–19.

Cosner, K.R. & de Jong, E. (1993) Physiologic second stage labor. *MCN – Am. J. Maternal/Child Nursing* **18**(1): 38–43.

Floud, E. (1994) Protecting the perineum in childbirth 2: risk of laceration. *Br. J. Midwifery* **2**(7): 306–310.

Howard, S., McKell, D., Mugford, M. & Grant, A. (1995) Cost-effectiveness of different approaches to perineal suturing. *Br. J. Midwifery* **3**(11): 587–590.

McKay, S. & Barrows, T. (1991) Holding back – Maternal readiness to give birth. *MCN – Am. J. Maternal/Child Nursing* **16**(5): 251–254.

Parnell, C., Langhoff-Roos, J., Iversen, R. *et al.* (1993) Pushing method in the expulsive phase of labor: a randomised trial. *Acta Obstet. Gynecol. Scand.* **72**(1): 31–35.

Sagady, M. (1995) Renewing our faith in second stage. *Midwifery Today* **33** (March): 29–31, 41–43.

Wagner, V. (1995) Question of the quarter (circumstances when a midwife should intervene and tell a woman not to push). *Midwifery Today* **33** (March): 26.

31

Midwifery Care in the Third Stage of Labour

The third stage of labour is the period following delivery of the baby until expulsion of the placenta and membranes. The process is concerned with separation and delivery of the placenta and membranes and the control of bleeding from the placental site. The third stage of labour is the most hazardous for the woman because of the possibility of complications such as haemorrhage occurring. It is the time when the midwife's knowledge and skill can assist the physiological processes that occur and this is crucial in reducing complications and the resultant maternal mortality and/or morbidity.

The risk of complications may be minimized by helping the woman to achieve maximum health in pregnancy, so that when she goes into labour she is not anaemic and will not be debilitated by blood lost during the third stage. Good midwifery care in labour should aim to avoid a prolonged first or second stage, both of which can lead to maternal exhaustion and dehydration and resultant poor uterine action. The woman should not enter the third stage of labour with a full bladder as this may impede the normal processes of separation, descent and control of bleeding.

The method of conducting the third stage of labour (that is, active or expectant/physiological management) will be influenced by many factors, including the woman's informed preference, the midwife's skill and confidence in the selected method, the absence of a previous history of third-stage complications and the normality of the present pregnancy and labour. Complications during labour have been significantly associated with an increased incidence of postpartum haemorrhage (Gilbert *et al.*, 1987). Haemorrhage is the commonest cause of maternal death in the world and good antenatal, intranatal and postnatal care are required to decrease this serious complication (WHO, 1994).

Outline of the Physiology of the Third Stage of Labour

MECHANISM OF PLACENTAL SEPARATION

Separation of the placenta usually begins with the contraction which delivers the baby's trunk and is completed with the next one or two contractions. As the baby is delivered there is a marked reduction in the size of the uterus due to the powerful contraction and retraction which takes place. The placental site therefore greatly diminishes in size. When the placental site is diminished by half, the placenta, being inelastic, becomes wrinkled and is shorn off the uterine wall. This happens because it is tightly compressed by the contracted uterus; some fetal blood is pumped back into the baby's circulation, and maternal blood in the intervillous spaces is forced back into the veins in the deep spongy layer of the decidua basalis. The blood in these veins cannot return to the maternal circulation because of the contracted and retracted state of the myometrium. The result is that the congested veins rupture and this small amount of extravasated blood shears off the villi from the spongy layer of the decidua basalis, thereby separating the placenta (Inch, 1985). Bleeding is controlled by the action of the interlacing spiral fibres, the so-called 'living ligatures', which contract around the torn maternal vessels to prevent further blood loss. This process causing separation of the placenta occurs very rapidly after the birth of the baby. Brandt (1933) studied 30 women during the third stage with the aid of radiology and found that in all cases the placenta had completely separated from the uterine wall within three minutes of the baby's birth and was lying in the lower uterine segment.

With modern management of the third stage of labour the cord is usually clamped immediately after the birth of the baby. Fetal blood is therefore retained in the placenta rather than returning to the fetal circulation and this extra volume prevents the placenta being so tightly compressed by the uterus. As a result

contraction and retraction of the uterus may be less effective, thereby resulting in more oozing from the torn maternal vessels and the formation of a large retroplacental clot (Inch, 1985). Under these circumstances the retroplacental clot aids placental separation. Botha (1968) does not consider the formation of a large retroplacental clot a physiological process. Rather it occurs as a result of intervention, in this case the clamping of the cord.

When separation is complete, the upper uterine segment contracts strongly, forcing the placenta into the lower segment and then into the vagina. Detachment of the membranes begins in the first stage of labour, when separation occurs around the internal os. In the third stage of labour complete separation of the membranes takes place assisted by the weight of the descending placenta, which peels them from the uterine wall (Figure 1).

There are two methods by which the placenta separates from the uterine wall:

1 *Schultze method*: In the majority of cases separation starts in the centre of the placenta and this part descends first. The fetal surface therefore appears at the vulva with the membranes trailing behind. The retroplacental clot is contained within the inverted sac; thus there is minimal visible blood loss. Akiyama *et al.* (1981), using ultrasound, found that over 80% of placentae separate by the Schultze method (Figure 1).
2 *Matthew Duncan method*: Less commonly separation starts at the lower edge of the placenta. The placenta therefore slips down sideways and the maternal surface appears first at the vulva. This method of separation is usually accompanied by some bleeding per vaginam, since blood from the placental site escapes immediately; thus a retroplacental clot does not form. As this method results in slower separation of the placenta (no retroplacental clot to aid separation) bleeding is also likely to be more profuse.

CONTROL OF BLEEDING

Following separation of the placenta, bleeding from the large, torn maternal sinuses in the placental site is controlled by:

1 the powerful contraction and retraction of the uterus, especially the action of the interlacing

muscle fibres, sometimes known as 'living ligatures', which constrict the blood vessels running through the myometrium (Figures 2 and 3);

2   pressure exerted on the placental site by the walls of the uterus, which becomes firmly contracted, with the walls in apposition, once the placenta and membranes have been delivered;

3   the blood clots at the placental site, in the sinuses and torn blood vessels.

Management of the Third Stage of Labour

EXPECTANT OR PHYSIOLOGICAL MANAGEMENT

This method of delivering the placenta and membranes is sometimes chosen by women and midwives who

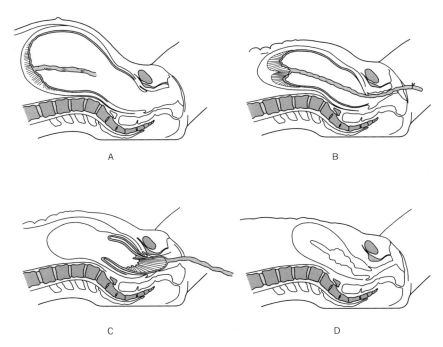

A

B

C

D

Figure 1   The mechanism of placental separation. **A**: The placenta before the child is born. **B**: The placenta partially separated immediately after the birth of the child. **C**: The placenta completely separated. **D**: The placenta expelled and the uterus strongly contracted and retracted.

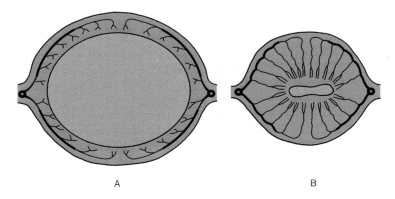

A

B

Figure 2   Transverse sections of the uterus. **A**: Relaxed before the third stage. **B**: Contracted and retracted after the third stage – blood vessels are compressed and bleeding arrested.

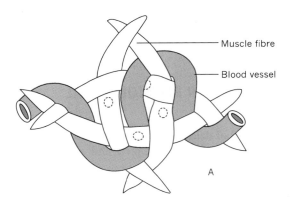

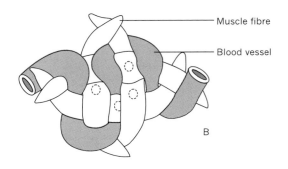

Figure 3   How the blood vessels run between the interlacing muscle fibres of the uterus. **A**: Muscle fibres relaxed and blood vessels not compressed. **B**: Muscle fibres contracted, blood vessels compressed and bleeding arrested.

support a non-interventionist approach to childbirth. It allows placental separation to occur physiologically, without the use of oxytocic drugs, after which expulsion is achieved by maternal effort. Using expectant management, the average length of the third stage is 15 minutes (Prendiville *et al.*, 1988) but it may take up to 30 minutes. A controlled trial comparing outcomes of active and physiological management indicated that the length of the third stage was shorter, averaging five minutes in the actively managed group (Prendiville *et al.*, 1988). The results also indicated that the postpartum haemorrhage rate was reduced with active management, being 5.9%, compared with 17.9% in those women who had expectant or physiological management.

This difference in the postpartum haemorrhage rate is a cause of concern; however, the authors acknowledge that not all midwives involved in the trial were experienced in physiological management of the third stage of labour, and this may have had a significant influence on the findings. The authors further state that the trial should be replicated in units where expectant management is the norm. In 1986–1988 at Hinchingbrooke Hospital, Huntingdon, where physiological management is commonly practised, the postpartum haemorrhage rate was 7% in those women who had a physiological management of the third stage as opposed to the overall rate of 7.6% (Levy, 1990). A more recent prospective randomized controlled trial, studying the amount of blood lost in the third stage of labour, found no difference in blood loss between those women who had active management of the third stage of labour and those where the third stage was managed by expectant means (Thilaganathan *et al.*, 1993).

Division of the umbilical cord

In accordance with the principle of non-intervention in physiological management, Inch (1985) maintains that the cord should be left unclamped. This enables compaction and compression of the placenta and retraction of muscle fibres to occur unhindered. Clamping of the cord causes fetal blood to be trapped within the placenta and this produces a counterpressure which impedes the physiological process. If the cord is left undivided until after the placenta has been expelled, delay in placental separation and excessive blood loss will be avoided. This view is not fully supported by Prendiville and Elbourne (1989) who, from their review of the literature, state that early clamping of the cord reduces the length of this part of labour. The practice of delayed clamping of the cord should be avoided in rhesus negative women because it increases the risk of feto-maternal transfusion. The midwife should also be aware that delayed cord clamping will cause placental–fetal transfusion of between 20 and 50%, depending on when the cord is clamped and whether the baby is positioned at a level higher or lower than the placenta in the uterus (Enkin *et al.*, 1989).

Delay in cord clamping may be beneficial to the preterm baby. In a study conducted by Kinmond *et al.* (1993), a 30 second delay in cord clamping with the infant held 20 cm below the introitus is associated with an improved outcome for the baby. It results in a higher initial packed cell volume and therefore a reduced need for red cell transfusions. Higher arterial–alveolar oxygen tensions were also noted in the first 24 hours which indicates less right-to-left shunting of deoxygenated blood.

Maternal posture

While the woman may adopt whatever position she finds the most comfortable, the dorsal position is best avoided as it may prove difficult for the woman to expel the placenta against the force of gravity. If the woman has delivered in the supported semi-recumbent position she may wish to remain undisturbed. The woman may adopt a squatting position (or a variation of the squatting position) and, to be comfortable, she will need some form of support such as those described for delivery. Squatting is thought to be particularly effective for placental delivery as descent and expulsion are aided by gravity and increased intra-abdominal pressure (Botha, 1968). If the woman wishes, she may put the baby to the breast. The release of oxytocin which follows suckling will assist the physiological process of placental separation and expulsion.

Placental separation

With expectant management of the third stage of labour the midwife must wait and observe for signs of placental separation and descent. She must also watch carefully for any signs of relaxation of the uterus and excessive blood loss. The longer the placenta remains within the uterine cavity, the greater the possibility of bleeding. The midwife should place her hand gently on the fundus to note the contraction and position of the uterus and ensure it is not relaxing and filling with blood. Any manipulation of the uterus must be avoided, as this interrupts the regular, rhythmic contractions which occur in a physiological third stage and predisposes to delayed separation and bleeding. The midwife observes the woman's general condition and notes any blood loss per vaginam. The following signs indicate separation and descent of the placenta:

▶ *Signs of separation*: A trickle of blood: as the uterus continues to contract and retract and placental separation begins a small amount of fresh blood loss occurs.
▶ *Signs of descent*: The uterus becomes smaller, narrower and rounder. The fundus rises in the abdomen, is harder and more freely mobile. This indicates that the placenta has separated and occupies the lower uterine segment. The cord lengthens. Once separation and descent of the placenta have occurred the placenta can be expelled.

Expulsion of the placenta

At this point, as the weight of the placenta causes a sensation of pressure in the vagina, the woman may feel a desire to bear down. This is more likely to happen if she is in a squatting position. In response to this sensation, the woman may push the placenta out without prompting. If this does not occur, the midwife, having *ascertained separation and descent* of the placenta and that the *uterus is well contracted*, may encourage the woman to bear down as she did for the birth of the baby. If the woman needs assistance to expel the placenta, as may happen if she is lying in the dorsal position, the midwife may assist her by placing her hand flat on the woman's abdomen while the woman bears down. This provides counterpressure to compensate for poor abdominal muscle tone. The midwife may need to ease the trailing membranes out of the vagina by grasping them with a pair of artery forceps, or by holding the placenta in cupped hands and rotating it so that the membranes are twisted into a 'rope' and therefore strengthened. Gentle traction may then be applied to tease the membranes through the os uteri and vagina, to prevent tearing and subsequent retention of pieces of membrane.

Fundal pressure

If the woman cannot expel the separated placenta by maternal effort, fundal pressure may be used (Figure 4). It is important to ensure that the placenta is separated if the procedure is to be successful. To facilitate correct direction of fundal pressure the woman should lie in the supported semi-recumbent position. The woman relaxes; the midwife puts her left hand on the fundus of the well-contracted uterus and pushes downwards and backwards. The uterus is pushed against the placenta and the placenta emerges from the vagina. This action is similar to pushing the piston of a syringe against the fluid in the barrel, which in turn is forced out of the syringe. This method of placental expulsion is not without problems. In unskilled hands it can cause considerable pain to the woman, and bruising of the tissues of the uterus. This bruising may interfere with uterine contractions and thus predispose to postpartum haemorrhage. Fundal pressure also places strain on the supporting ligaments of the uterus. If used vigorously and if the uterus is not well-contracted, it may cause acute inversion of the uterus, a serious obstetric emergency.

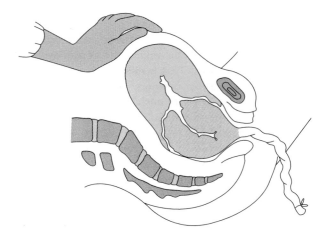

Figure 4   Expulsion of the placenta by fundal pressure.

ACTIVE MANAGEMENT

This method of management involves the administration of an oxytocic drug at the end of the second stage of labour to enhance uterine contraction and retraction and thereby placental separation. This is combined with controlled traction on the umbilical cord which hastens the process of separation and delivery of the placenta and reduces blood loss. Until recent years this was the most common method of third stage management in the UK (Turnbull, 1976; Garcia *et al.*, 1987). However, physiological management of the third stage appears to be increasingly practised in some units (Levy, 1990).

Active management of the third stage of labour is recommended by the WHO (1994) to reduce the incidence of postpartum haemorrhage, especially in the developing world where it is the commonest cause of maternal death. In the UK postpartum haemorrhage is less of a problem because most women are healthy and medical facilities are easily available. Therefore women who make an informed choice for a physiological third stage normally have their wish, provided there are no complications and the midwife or doctor is competent to conduct the third stage in this way.

Oxytocic drugs

Oxytocic drugs stimulate the uterus to contract. Used before, during or after the third stage of labour, they hasten placental separation and reduce blood loss. It has become common practice in the UK to manage the third stage of labour by giving the woman an oxytocic preparation during the birth of the baby and, when the uterus responds by contracting, to deliver the placenta by controlled cord traction. The general acceptance of active management as a means of accelerating the third stage of labour and preventing postpartum haemorrhage is reflected in a survey which showed that maternity units in England that had a policy for management of the third stage practised active management (Garcia *et al.*, 1987).

While recognizing the benefits of oxytocic drugs in *controlling* atonic postpartum haemorrhage, their routine use in *preventing* the problem has been the subject of much debate and various clinical trials. In their study of several controlled trials Enkin *et al.* (1989) conclude that there is evidence to support the routine use of oxytocic drugs in the third stage of labour because of a likely reduction in the risk of postpartum haemorrhage in the order of 30–40%. Prendiville and Elbourne (1989), in considering the benefits of different oxytocic preparations, state that there is little justification for the sole use of ergot preparations (such as ergometrine) in the third stage of labour. They support the use of Syntometrine, as opposed to oxytocin alone, as being most effective in reducing the rate of postpartum haemorrhage.

A recent randomized double-blind comparison of Syntometrine and Syntocinon in the management of the third stage of labour was conducted on a sample of 1000 women. The authors concluded that Syntometrine is a better choice than Syntocinon. The use of Syntometrine resulted in a reduced blood loss, a lower risk of postpartum haemorrhage and minimal maternal side-effects. It is reported that hypertension did not appear to be a significant problem in this study (Yuen *et al.*, 1995).

However, in a large randomized controlled trial conducted by McDonald *et al.* (1993) to compare the use of intramuscular oxytocin (10 IU) alone and intramuscular oxytocin with ergometrine (Syntometrine 1 ml) for the active management of the third stage of labour, there was no significant difference in the rate of postpartum haemorrhage between the two groups, but the use of Syntometrine was associated with nausea, vomiting and increased blood pressure. These findings were confirmed by a later study conducted in the United Arab Emirates by Khan *et al.* (1995).

Ergometrine is known to cause nausea and vomiting which can be distressing for the woman and may detract from the pleasure of the birth. It also has a vasopressor action which may result in hypertension. Occasionally this effect may be very pronounced and so it should not be given to any woman with pre-existing hypertension (DOH, 1994). Other reported complications include cardiac arrest, pulmonary oedema and cerebral haemorrhage. It has also been associated with reduced serum prolactin levels (Prendiville and Elbourne, 1989) which may interefere with breast milk production and successful breastfeeding. Begley's study (1990) did not confirm this effect upon prolactin levels, although she noted that women who had not received ergometrine were likely to breastfeed for longer.

Intravenous oxytocin may cause a transient but marked *fall in blood pressure* (Hendricks and Brenner, 1970), with tachycardia and an increased stoke volume, which increases cardiac output. It also has an anti-diuretic action and when given in large doses (over 100 units) over a few hours it can cause serious water intoxication. The chances of this occurring are diminished if the woman is given a crystalloid as opposed to dextrose in water infusion (Baskett, 1991).

Midwives may use the following oxytocic drugs:

Intramuscular Syntometrine 1 ml   This preparation is usually given with the birth of the anterior shoulder. Syntometrine contains ergometrine 500 μg and oxytocin 5 units in 1 ml. The oxytocin fraction will induce strong, rhythmic contraction of the muscle fibres of the upper segment of the uterus within 2–3 minutes of administration. Its effect lasts for approximately 5–15 minutes (Baskett, 1991). This rapid-acting, short-duration component is designed to initiate strong uterine action, which is sustained by the action of the ergometrine fraction, which will induce a strong, non-physiologic spasm of uterine muscle within 6–8 minutes (Sorbe, 1978). The effect of ergometrine is maintained for approximately 60–90 minutes (Baskett, 1991). Because of the spasm-inducing properties of ergometrine there is a theoretical risk of retained placenta and therefore the midwife should aim to deliver the placenta before the ergometrine takes effect.

Oxytocin (Syntocinon)   This may be given in doses of 5 units intravenously or 5–10 units intramuscularly. It may be given after the birth of the head or with the delivery of the anterior shoulder. Intramuscular oxytocin acts within 2–3 minutes of administration. It is considered the oxytocic drug of choice if there is a pre-existing hypertension (DOH, 1994). It was thought to be less effective in preventing blood loss and postpartum haemorrhage than intramuscular Syntometrine 1

ml (Dumoulin, 1981), but recent studies refute this (McDonald *et al.*, 1993; Khan *et al.*, 1995).

Intramuscular ergometrine 500 μg   This will cause a strong, sustained uterine contraction, as described above. If intramuscular ergometrine is administered instead of Syntometrine it is given a little earlier, at the crowning of the head, as it takes longer to act, 6–8 minutes.

Intravenous ergometrine 250–500 μg   This takes effect approximately 45 seconds after administration. It is usually given by a doctor but may be given by the midwife in an emergency situation, usually to control postpartum bleeding.

A simple alternative to parenteral oxytocics for the third stage of labour is *nipple stimulation* which, according to Irons *et al.* (1994), tended to reduce the length of the third stage and the amount of blood loss. This was a small study, however, and larger trials are required.

Maternal posture

The mother may be semi-recumbent in the dorsal position in bed, or sitting on a birthing chair or stool or in a squatting position for the delivery of the placenta and membranes. The mother usually has the baby in her arms and warmth will be provided by a light covering or an overhead heater.

Controlled cord traction

After rinsing her hands in an antiseptic lotion, the midwife places a receiver close to the vulva to catch any blood and liquor that may escape from the vagina. The end of the cord is placed in the receiver. A sterile towel is draped over the abdomen and the midwife places her left hand on the fundus of the uterus to await a contraction. The oxytocic drug, usually Syntometrine 1 ml, will have been given with the birth of the anterior shoulder or the crowning of the head. As soon as the *uterus contracts* the midwife prepares to undertake *controlled cord traction* (Figure 5). The left hand is moved from the fundus and placed just above the symphysis pubis, with palm facing towards the umbilicus, and thumb on one side of the midline and fingers on the other. This hand is at the level of the junction of the upper and lower uterine segments and is used to push the uterus upwards, towards the umbilicus. At the same time the midwife grasps the umbilical cord with the right hand and applies steady, sustained traction on the cord in a downward direction. If this attempt to deliver the placenta fails, controlled cord traction is repeated in 2–3 minutes with a contraction (Spencer, 1962). When the placenta becomes visible, traction is exerted in an upward direction, thereby following the curve of the birth canal. As the placenta emerges from the vagina it is delivered into a receiver. Sometimes the membranes are not completely separated and have to be eased out gently to prevent tearing. Twisting the placenta to form the membranes into a rope or grasping the membranes with artery forceps and moving them gently up and down may help to separate them. Great care must be taken to avoid tearing the membranes.

Although controlled cord traction, as described by Spencer (1962), should be commenced as soon as the uterus contracts in order to reduce the mean blood loss, Levy (1990) suggests waiting until signs of separation are present before applying traction to the cord. This recommendation is based on the fact that the study undertaken by Spencer, in which signs of separation were not awaited, was not a controlled trial, thus making comparisons impossible. Levy's recommendation is supported by the results of a study of management of the third stage of labour conducted by Levy and Moore (1985). This showed that more than half the midwives involved in the study waited for signs of placental separation before starting controlled cord traction. Despite this, there was no significant difference in the incidence of postpartum haemorrhage, or the length of the third stage, between those who started controlled cord traction as soon as the uterus contracted and those who waited for signs of separation. However, the rate of postpartum haemorrhage

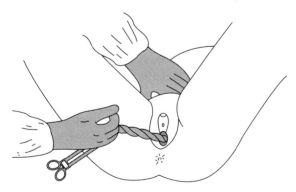

Figure 5 Controlled cord traction.

appeared to be significantly higher when the midwife *unsuccessfully* used controlled cord traction without awaiting signs of separation.

After the Third Stage of Labour

The midwife must make sure that the uterus is well-contracted and that blood loss per vaginam is not excessive. The perineum and vulva must be inspected in a good light to identify the presence of any lacerations. These should be repaired as soon as possible. Many midwives in the UK are now skilled in perineal repair, but if the laceration is extensive and the midwife anticipates difficulty in repairing it, then the help of an experienced doctor should be sought. The vulva and perineum are gently cleaned with an antiseptic solution and a sterile vulval pad is applied. Soiled linen is removed, the woman is covered warmly and made comfortable. She is again given her baby to cuddle while the midwife makes a careful examination of the placenta and membranes.

EXAMINATION OF THE PLACENTA AND MEMBRANES

The placenta and membranes are carefully examined as soon after delivery as possible. If the couple wish, and are interested, they may like to observe the midwife's examination of the placenta. The midwife should wear gloves and other protective clothing, as she did for the delivery. The main purposes of this examination are:

▶ to determine whether or not the placenta and membranes are complete; and
▶ to detect other abnormalities which might provide retrospective information about an intrauterine problem. This may be helpful in planning care for the neonate.

First wash the placenta in running water, remove the clots and then hold it up firmly by the cord to see if the membranes are complete. If they are, there will be one hole through which the fetus has passed. Then strip the amnion from the chorion and see if both membranes are present. Next, turn the placenta over, with the fetal surface resting upon the hand, and let the membranes hang over the forearm, so that the position that the placenta occupied in the uterus may be seen. Examine the maternal surface and see if all the lobes are complete. Notice if the maternal surface seems ragged. If all the lobes are present there will be no spaces whatever. Note also any areas of infarction which are recognized as rather firm whitish patches. Then examine the edge of the placenta to see if the blood vessels run into the membranes; if so, they lead to a *placenta succenturiata*, or accessory placenta (Figure 6), which has developed away from the main placenta. Occasionally one vessel only is seen, which comes back into the placenta; this is called an *erratic vessel*.

Next, examine the umbilical cord, noting the insertion of the cord, its length and the number of umbilical vessels. Usually the cord insertion is central and the length is approximately 50 cm. Occasionally only one umbilical artery is present and this may be associated with congenital anomalies, especially renal agenesis. The paediatrician should be informed and a detailed examination of the newborn requested. The placenta is usually weighed and the weight at term should be approximately one-sixth of the weight of the baby. If clamping of the umbilical cord was not delayed the placenta will contain a greater residual blood volume and will therefore weigh slightly more (Prendiville and Elbourne, 1989).

Finally, measure all blood loss which has been collected and add this amount to the *estimated* amount of unmeasurable loss which has soaked into linen and pads. A realistic assessment of the blood loss is essential in order to determine whether the loss was excessive and is likely to have a detrimental effect on maternal well-being. However, accurate measurement of blood loss is hindered by the fact that blood soakage and spillage is difficult to estimate. Blood loss up to 300 ml is usually fairly accurately assessed, but the greater the loss, the greater the error in estimation (Levy and Moore, 1985). These findings support previous work by Brant (1967) and Haswell (1981) and this has led to the practice recommendation that blood loss of 500 ml and above should be doubled in order to make a more accurate assessment (Levy, 1990).

The findings of the examination of the placenta and membranes and an estimate of the blood loss are recorded in the mother's notes. It is important to report to the doctor immediately if it is thought that a piece of placental tissue has been retained, since postpartum haemorrhage is likely at any time while it remains in the uterus. It also predisposes to puerperal sepsis. If some membrane is retained, it is usually passed spontaneously within a few days, but again may predispose to puerperal sepsis.

IMMEDIATE CARE OF THE WOMAN AND BABY

The midwife now attends to the woman and her baby. The midwife should gently palpate the uterus to reas-

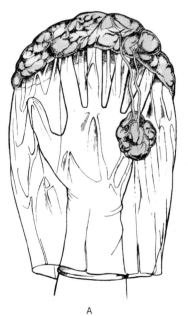 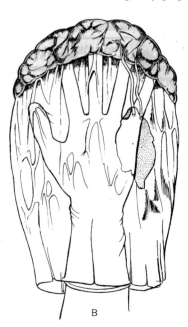

A   B

Figure 6   **A**: Succenturiate placenta. **B**: The torn membrane – the missing lobe is in the uterus.

sure herself and the woman that the uterus is still well-contracted and blood loss per vaginam is normal. The woman's temperature, pulse and blood pressure are taken and recorded. These should all be within the normal range. The woman and her birth supporter may welcome a warm drink at this point and it is an ideal time for the midwife to share the couple's delight with their baby and to encourage any questions regarding the labour or about the baby. This can be a good opportunity for health education and may also facilitate the development of parent/baby attachment. The couple should be encouraged to cuddle and explore their baby. Most women will welcome this early contact with their baby and there is evidence that early and unhurried contact between mother and baby during the first hour after birth significantly affects maternal emotional well-being when measured at six weeks after delivery (Ball, 1994).

The father too usually wishes to share this time with his partner and new baby and should be encouraged to do so. It is the responsibility of the midwife to ensure that the parents' emotional needs as well as their physical needs are taken care of. She should also realize that the unfamiliar institutional environment may inhibit the parents' response to their baby and therefore needs to try and create a calm, unhurried atmosphere where they can relax and enjoy this time together with their baby. Restricted time and interaction between mother and baby may result in less affectionate maternal behaviour (Anisfeld and Lipper, 1983; Gomes-Pedro et al., 1984). The midwife should therefore facilitate this early period of contact between mother, father and their baby, giving it priority over the many routine procedures which can safely be carried out later.

Sensitivity is required in caring for women who appear to show little interest in their baby at birth, sometimes because they are in pain or under the influence of drugs administered in labour, or because their social or cultural patterns dictate particular birth customs or rituals. A good relationship and communications between the mother and midwife will help the midwife to understand the mother's reaction to her baby and enable her to facilitate timely maternal–infant attachment in the appropriate way.

Mothers who plan to breastfeed should be encouraged to give the baby a feed soon after birth, usually within the first hour or so. At this time the baby usually displays a strong urge to suck and a successful feed benefits both mother and baby. The mother is encouraged in her ability to breastfeed and the baby receives a feed of colostrum which has a high protein content, including anti-infective agents, and is easily digested. There is also evidence to suggest that women who breastfeed their baby soon after birth continue to breastfeed for a longer period of time (Salariya, 1978). An additional benefit of this early feed is that oxytocin is released from the posterior pituitary gland during suckling which stimulates uterine contractions and therefore helps to maintain haemostasis.

It cannot be emphasized too strongly that, during the hour after delivery, the midwife should frequently feel the uterus to determine that it is well-contracted, and check the lochia. The woman is encouraged to pass urine as a full bladder predisposes to a relaxed uterus and heavy blood loss. If the uterus does relax, the midwife must massage the fundus with her fingers to stimulate it to contract, and, when contracted, apply fundal pressure to expel blood clots. A warm vulval wash is given and the vulva is covered with a sterile pad. The woman will usually appreciate a shower or a blanket bath, and the opportunity to clean her teeth, comb her hair and change into clean nightwear.

During this period the midwife must closely observe the baby, noting colour, respiration, and general activity. The umbilical cord must be observed at frequent intervals to ascertain that the cord clamp is firmly in place and that there is no bleeding.

Care should be taken to ensure that the baby does not become chilled and body temperature can be maintained if the baby is warmly wrapped and cuddled by the parents. It has been demonstrated that the postnatal fall in body temperature of the neonate can be effectively reduced by skin-to-skin contact (Gardiner, 1987). If necessary, an overhead heater may be used. The woman and her baby should remain in the birthing room for at least one hour after delivery. In the community the midwife must not leave until at least one hour after delivery. In practice she is unlikely to do so, as cleaning up and attending to the woman and baby will take longer than this.

RECORDS

A complete and accurate account of labour must be recorded. Such notations must be sufficiently comprehensive to enable other carers to have a clear picture of events, thus facilitating communication and avoiding discontinuity of care (UKCC, 1993).

Statute requires that a birth notification form be

completed. This is normally undertaken by the midwife and sent, within 36 hours of the birth, to the medical officer of the district in which the birth took place (UKCC, 1994).

The Placenta at Term

At term the placenta is flat and round or oval in shape. It is 18–20 cm in diameter and about 2.5 cm thick in the centre, becoming thinner towards the edges. Its weight is about 600 g, or one-sixth of the weight of the fetus. The placenta is usually situated on the anterior or posterior wall of the uterine cavity, near the fundus. The placenta has two surfaces, *maternal* and *fetal*.

Maternal surface

This surface is attached to the uterine decidua, is deep red in colour and divided by deep grooves or sulci into about 15–20 irregular lobes. These lobes are cotyledons and they contain masses of chorionic villi. On examination after birth a thin greyish layer, part of the basal decidua, can be seen (Figure 7).

Fetal surface

This surface lies adjacent to the fetus. From the insertion of the cord, which is usually situated centrally, blood vessels can be seen radiating to the periphery, like the roots of a tree, where they disappear from sight. These vessels give off branches which penetrate into the substance of the placenta, each cotyledon having its own supply of fetal blood. In the centre of each cotyledon there is a main branch of the umbilical artery and vein.

The fetal surface of the placenta is covered with amnion.

ABNORMALITIES OF THE PLACENTA

Succenturiate lobe

A succenturiate lobe (Figure 8) is a small portion or lobe of placenta separated from the main body, which is formed from some of the villi of the chorionic membrane which have continued to develop instead of becoming atrophied. It is attached to the main placenta by blood vessels which cross the intervening membrane, these vessels running from the edge of the placenta. There is a possibility of this cotyledon's being retained in the uterus after the main placenta has been expelled. A retained cotyledon is a very serious matter and gives rise to postpartum haemorrhage and sepsis. When there is a small hole in the fetal membranes, with placental vessels running towards it, it indicates the retention of a placental lobe corresponding in size to the hole in the membrane.

Circumvallate placenta

In this type of placenta the chorion is attached not to the edge of the placenta, but to the fetal surface at some distance from the edge (Figure 9).

Bipartite placenta

This is a placenta divided into two main lobes.

Placenta accreta

This is a placenta which becomes abnormally adherent to the uterine muscle over the whole or part of its surface. It is very rare.

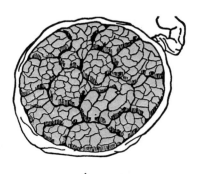
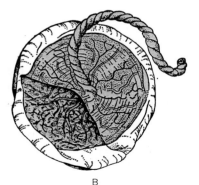

A   B

Figure 7   The placenta. **A**: The maternal surface, showing the cotyledons. **B**: The fetal surface.

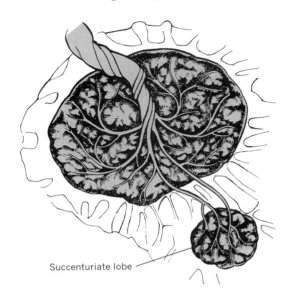

Succenturiate lobe

Figure 8   Succenturiate placenta.

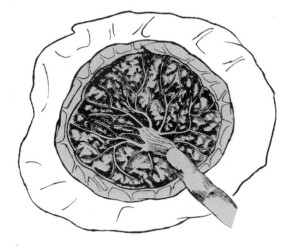

Figure 9   Circumvallate placenta.

Infarcts

These are red or white patches sometimes seen on the maternal surface of the placenta. They are caused by localized death of placental tissue due to interference with the blood supply.

Infarcts are red at an early stage of their development; later they become white and appear as patches of white fibrous tissue. They may be seen occasionally in any placenta, but they are often associated with pre-eclampsia.

Calcification

On the maternal surface of the placenta small greyish-white patches are often to be seen, particularly on the post-mature placenta. These are deposits of lime salts. They convey a gritty sensation to the fingers and are not of any significance.

Fetal Membranes

There are two fetal membranes: the *chorion* and the *amnion*.

Chorion

The chorion is the outer membrane, continuous with the edge of the placenta and derived from the tropho-blast. It is opaque, thick but friable and roughened by tiny pieces of decidua adherent to it. It lines the uterine cavity.

Amnion

The amnion is the inner membrane, derived from the inner cell mass. It is smooth, transparent and the stronger membrane of the two. The two membranes lie over each other, but can be separated from each other; the amnion may be stripped back to the insertion of the cord, where it continues as the covering of the cord. The amnion secretes the amniotic fluid or liquor amnii which at term measures 1000–1500 ml.

Umbilical Cord

The umbilical cord (Figure 10) or funis connects the placenta to the fetus. The cord is about 50 cm in length and 2 cm in thickness. It is composed of a jelly-like substance known as *Wharton's jelly*; this is a primitive connective tissue, primary mesenchyme. The cord is covered externally by amnion. It supports and protects three blood vessels: one large *umbilical vein* carrying oxygenated blood to the fetus, and two *umbilical arteries* winding around the vein carrying deoxygenated blood from the fetus to the placenta. The absence of a vessel may be associated with fetal abnormalities such as renal agenesis (absence of kidneys). The cord has a spiral twist; this torsion gives a certain amount of protection from pressure.

The function of the cord ceases as the lungs start to function immediately after birth and pulmonary

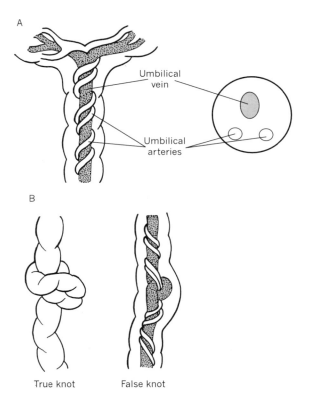

Figure 10   **A**: The umbilical cord in side view and cross-section, showing the one umbilical vein with the two umbilical arteries twisting spirally around it. The vein and arteries lie in Wharton's jelly; the cord is enclosed within the amnion. **B**: True and false knots.

respiration is established. The cord is clamped and cut; the circulation in the cord ceases and, as the small portion attached to the baby's umbilicus receives no further blood supply, it becomes dead tissue and immediately begins to atrophy. Great care is required to prevent bacteria gaining access to it. About the fifth day after birth it should separate, leaving a dry and healthy surface.

ABNORMALITIES OF THE UMBILICAL CORD

The cord may be too short, causing, occasionally, delay in descent of the head and difficulty at delivery, or too long, when prolapse of the cord is more liable to occur. Occasionally it is very thick or very thin; in either case great care is required in tying the cord and subsequently watching for haemorrhage. Rarely a piece of fetal intestine may protrude into the cord, but the possibility of this abnormality will be suspected if the cord is swollen close to the umbilicus, the size of the swelling depending on the amount of intestine which has protruded. Knots are caused by movements of the fetus before birth, the baby slipping through a loop of the cord. False knots may be due to the blood vessels being longer than the actual cord, and so doubling back upon themselves in the Wharton's jelly, or to irregularities and the formation of nodes.

Abnormalities of insertion

The cord may be attached to one side of the placenta (an *eccentric insertion*) or to the margin of the placenta

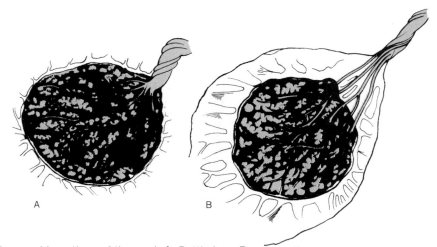

Figure 11   Abnormal insertions of the cord. **A**: Battledore; **B**: velamentous.

(a *battledore insertion*), or the vessels of the cord may break up and run into the membrane before reaching the placenta (a *velamentous insertion*) (Figure 11). This is particularly dangerous if the unprotected blood vessels should lie near the internal os. This very rare condition is called *vasa praevia* (vessels in advance of the fetus). Should a blood vessel so situated be compressed when the membranes rupture, the fetus will suffer hypoxia. If such a vessel should actually rupture, the fetus will lose blood from his own vessels in the membrane. Such fetal haemorrhage is dangerous and could lead to stillbirth.

References

Akiyama, H., Kohzu, H. & Matsuoka, M. (1981) An approach to detection of placental separation and expulsion with new clinical signs: a study based on haemodynamic method and ultrasonography. *Am. J. Obstet. Gynecol.* 5: 505–511.

Anisfeld, E. & Lipper, E. (1983) Early contact, social support and mother–infant bonding. *Pediatrics* 72(1): 79–83.

Ball, J.A. (1994) *Reactions to Motherhood*. Hale: Books for Midwives Press, 113–115.

Baskett, T. (1991) *Essential Management of Obstetric Emergencies*. Bristol: Clinical Press.

Begley, C.M. (1990) The effect of ergometrine on breastfeeding. *Midwifery* 6(2): 60–72.

Botha, M.A. (1968) The management of the umbilical cord in labour. *S. African J. Obstet. Gynaecol.* 25: 662–667.

Brandt, M.L. (1933) The mechanism and management of the third stage of labour. *Am. J. Obstet. Gynecol.* 25: 662–667.

Brant, H.A. (1967) Precise estimation of postpartum haemorrhage: difficulties and importance. *Br. Med. J.* 1: 398–400.

DOH (Department of Health) (1994) *Confidential Enquiries into Maternal Deaths in the UK 1988–90*. London: HMSO, p. 32.

Dumoulin, J.G. (1981) A reappraisal of the use of ergometrine. *J. Obstet. Gynaecol.* 1: 178–181.

Enkin, M., Keirse, J.N.C. & Chalmers, I. (1989) *A Guide to Effective Care in Pregnancy and Childbirth*. Oxford: Oxford University Press.

Garcia, J., Garforth, A. & Ayers, S. (1987) The policy and practice of midwifery study: introduction and methods. *Midwifery* 3: 2–9.

Gardiner, S. (1987) The mother as an incubator – after delivery. *J. Obstet. Gynaecol. Neonatal Nursing* May/June: 174–176.

Gilbert, L., Porter, W. & Brown, V.A. (1987) Postpartum haemorrhage – a continuing problem. *Br. J. Obstet. Gynaecol.* 94(1): 67–71.

Gomes-Pedro, J., Bento de Almeida, J., Silveria da Costa, C. & Barbarosa, A. (1984) Influence of early mother and baby contact on dyatic behaviour during the first month of life. *Devel. Med. Child Neurol.* 26: 657–664.

Haswell, J.N. (1981) Measured blood loss at delivery. *J. Indiana State Med. Assoc.* 74(1): 34–36.

Hendricks, C.H. & Brenner, W.E. (1970) Cardiovascular effects of oxytocic drugs used postpartum. *Am. J. Obstet. Gynecol.* 108: 751–760.

Inch, S. (1985) *Birthrights*. London: Hutchinson.

Irons, D.W., Sriskandabalan, P. & Bullough, C.H. (1994) A simple alternative to parenteral oxytocics for the third stage of labour. *Int. J. Gynaecol. Obstet.* 46(1): 15–18.

Khan, G.Q., John, I.S., Chan, T. *et al.* (1995) Abu Dhabi third stage trial: oxytocin versus Syntometrine in the active management of the third stage of labour. *Eur. J. Obstet. Gynecol. Reprod. Biol.* 58(2): 147–151.

Kinmond, S., Aitchison, T.C., Holland, B.M. *et al.* (1993) Umbilical cord clamping and preterm infants: a randomised trial. *Br. Med. J.* 306: 172–175.

Levy, V. (1990) The midwife's management of the third stage of labour. In Alexander, J., Levy, V. & Roch, S. (eds) *Midwifery Practice – Intrapartum Care – A Research Based Approach*. Basingstoke: Macmillan.

Levy, V. & Moore, J. (1985) The midwife's management of the third stage of labour. *Nursing Times* 81(39): 47–50.

McDonald, S.J., Prendiville, W.J. & Blair, E. (1993) Randomised controlled trial of oxytocin alone versus oxytocin and ergometrine in active management of labour. *Br. J. Med.* 307(6913): 1167–1171.

Prendiville, W.J. & Elbourne, D. (1989) Care during the third stage of labour. In Chalmers, I., Enkin, M. & Keirse, M. (eds) *Effective Care in Pregnancy and Childbirth*, Vol. 2. Oxford: Oxford University Press.

Prendiville, W.J., Harding, J.E., Elbourne, D.R. & Stirrat, G.M. (1988) The Bristol Third Stage Trial: Active versus physiological management of the third stage of labour. *Br. Med. J.* 297(6659): 1295–1300.

Salariya, E.M., Easton, P.M. & Cater, J.I. (1978) Duration of breast feeding after early initiation and frequent feeding. *Lancet* ii: 1141–1143.

Sorbe, B. (1978) Active pharmacologic management of the third stage of labor. *Obstet. Gynecol.* 52: 694–697.

Spencer, P.M. (1962) Controlled cord traction in the management of the third stage of labour. *Br. Med. J.* 1: 1728–1732.

Turnbull A.C. (1976) Obstetrics: traditional use of ergot compounds. *Postgrad. Med. J.* 52 (Suppl. 1): 15–16.

Thilaganathan, B., Cutner, A. & Latimar, J. *et al.* (1993) Management of the third stage of labour in women at low risk of postpartum haemorrhage. *Eur. J. Obstet. Gynaecol. Reprod. Biol.* 48(1): 19–22.

UKCC (UK Central Council for Nursing, Midwifery and Health Visiting) (1993) *Standards for Records and Record Keeping*. London: UKCC.

UKCC (1994) *The Midwife's Code of Practice*. London: UKCC.

WHO (World Health Organization) (1994) *Mother–Baby Package. Implementing Safe Motherhood in Developing Countries.* Maternal Health and Safe Motherhood Programme, Division of Family Health, WHO, Geneva, WHO/FHE/MSM/94:11.

Yuen, P.M., Chan, N.S.T., Yim, S.F. & Chang, A.M.Z. (1995) A randomised double blind comparison of Syntometrine and Syntocinon in the management of the third stage of labour. *Br. J. Obstet. Gynaecol.* **102**: 377–380.

Further Reading

Begley, C.M. (1990) A comparison of 'active' and 'physiological' management of the third stage of labour. *Midwifery* **6**(1): 3–17.

Dombrowski, M.P., Bottoms, S.F., Saleh, A. *et al.* (1995) Third stage of labor: analysis of duration and clinical practice. *Am. J. Obstet. Gynecol.* **172**(4): 1279–1284.

Enkin, M., Keirse, M., Renfrew, M. & Neilson, J. (1995) *A Guide to Effective Care in Pregnancy and Childbirth*, 2nd edn. Oxford: Oxford University Press.

Herman, A., Weintraub, Z., Bukovsky, I. *et al.* (1993) Dynamic ultrasonographic imaging of the third stage of labor: new perspectives into third stage mechanisms. *Am. J. Obstet. Gynecol.* **168**(5): 1496–1499.

Inch, S. (1989/90) Bristol third stage trial: commentary. *AIMS Q. J.* **1**(4): 8–10.

Logue, M. (1990) Management of the third stage of labour: a midwife's view. *J. Obstet. Gynaecol.* **10** (Suppl. 2): S10–S12.

Lamont, R.F. (1990) Management of the third stage of labour: is prophylaxis still necessary and what would be the best agent? *J. Obstet. Gynaecol.* **10** (Suppl. 2): S7–S9.

Prichard, K., O'Boyle, A. & Hodgen, J. (1991) Third stage of labour. Outcomes of physiological third stage of labour care in the homebirth setting. *New Zealand Coll. Midwives J.* **12** (April): 8–10.

Relief of Pain in Labour

Pain is a complex, personal, subjective, multifactorial phenomena which is influenced by psychological, biological, sociocultural and economic factors and, although pain is universally experienced and acknowledged, it is not completely understood (Walding, 1991). It has three components: *sensodiscriminatory* (perception), *affective-motivational* (emotional and behavioural) and *cognitive* (past experiences, learned behaviour, conditioned responses and individual situational analysis and interpretation) (Boss and Goloskov, 1983). It may be described by location, intensity, temporal aspects, quality, impact and meaning for the person involved (Royal Colleges of Surgeons, and Anaesthetists, 1990). This is very evident when caring for women in labour whose perception and reaction to pain is diverse, and may be influenced by some or all of these factors.

In the late 1960s Grantly Dick Read (1969) studied the subject of pain in childbirth and concluded that fear increases the amount of pain experienced. He advocated antenatal education and preparation for childbirth to reduce the cycle of fear, tension and pain associated with childbirth in Western culture. In a recent paper, Walding (1991) tends to confirm a relationship between pain, anxiety and powerlessness and agrees that active participation by the woman may reduce the perception of pain. It has been shown in carefully controlled laboratory conditions that instead of differing pain thresholds, there is, in fact, a uniform sensation threshold (Sternbach and Tursky, 1965). It is other factors such as cultural values, anxiety, attention and suggestion which can cause this sensation threshold to be interpreted as differing pain thresholds.

In particular, the anticipation of pain increases anxiety levels and hence the pain experienced. Where pain is caused by sudden severe injury it may not be felt at the time. This is referred to as *episodic analgesia* (Melzack and Wall, 1988).

Pain may cause an increase in both adrenaline secretion and catecholamine levels, which affect the cardiac, respiratory, genitourinary, gastrointestinal and skeletal systems (Read *et al.*, 1983). The result is an increase in cardiac output, heart rate and rhythm, and blood pressure, and this gives rise to hyperventilation which decreases cerebral and uterine blood flow by vasoconstriction. Acid–base balance may also be altered, giving rise to maternal alkalosis (which may cause fetal hypoxia), nausea and vomiting, interfere with uterine action by decreasing contractions (catecholamines) and interfere with bladder function (Heywood and Ho, 1990). Hayward (1975) shows that giving information reduces anxiety and pain significantly and antenatal education for childbirth helps to reduce anxiety and hence the pain experienced in labour. This may be linked with the 'locus of control' theory, which states that women having an internal locus of control (where events are influenced by actions taken by the individual) are more likely to cope effectively with their anxiety (Walding, 1991). Attention to pain is also likely to increase its intensity: hence the value of distractive techniques for women in labour.

Individual perceptions of pain, particularly pain tolerance levels, meaning, expression of pain, coping mechanisms and communication about pain, vary markedly in different cultural groups and these affect the degree and quality of pain experienced. These factors are important to the midwife who should be aware of sociocultural diversity and examine personal beliefs about pain in order to avoid misconceptions and misunderstandings and to give sensitive and effective care to women in labour. Health care professionals have an important role in influencing the experience and expression of pain (Davitz and Davitz, 1980).

The Physiology of Pain

The sense organs for pain are receptors (*nociceptors*) which are free nerve endings. These receptors are branching, bushy networks which overlap each other and are found in almost every tissue of the body, many in the skin. Following stimulation, which may be mechanical, electrical, thermal or chemical, the receptors transmit nerve impulses along sensory nerve fibres. These include large, myelinated A beta and small, myelinated A delta fibres which conduct sharp, well-defined localized pain at a fast rate, or unmyelinated C fibres which conduct diffuse, intense pain at a slow rate to the dorsal root of the spinal nerve (first neurone fibre). There the sensory nerve patterns (or pain) synapse in the marginal zone of the dorsal horn (the substantia gelatinosa, laminae 2 and 3) with a second neurone which arises in the posterior horn, crosses over within the spinal cord and ascends through the medulla to the third neurone in the thala-

mus. This transmits the sensory impulse to the sensory cortex, where it is translated and passed to a deeper portion of the brain. This is the *dorsal column* or *lemniscal direct pathway*. Pain is also conveyed by two spinal cord brainstem pathways, the *direct* (lateral) *spinothalamic* and the *indirect* (ventral) *spinothalamic* (Ganong, 1985).

Damage to tissue results in the release of a coded pattern of nerve impulses from many fibres entering the spinal cord. The sensory patterns may be modified before they pass from the spinal cord neurons along nerve fibres to the brain. Stimulation of the receptors does not mark the beginning of the pain process. There is a pre-existent context and stimulation produces nerve impulses which enter an active nervous system which, in the adult, is already affected by past experience, culture, anxiety, anticipation and other such influences (Melzack and Wall, 1988). Conditioning affects the perception of pain and the individual's response to it. As early as 1927 and 1928 Pavlov showed that stimulation of the receptors is localized, identified and evaluated before there is any response to it.

Theories of Pain

A number of theories have been described, including specificity, two pathway, pattern and central summation, gate control theory, endogenous opiate, sensory interaction and behaviourist theory (Melzack and Wall, 1988). Of these the one most quoted is the *gate theory* by Melzack (1973) and Melzack and Wall (1988). It is proposed that a neural mechanism in the dorsal horns of the spinal cord acts like a gate which can increase or decrease the flow of nerve impulses from peripheral fibres to the central nervous system. The gating mechanism is thought to be in the substantia gelatinosa (laminae 2 and 3) which extend for the length of the spinal cord on each side. It is the position of the gate which determines how much information is freely transmitted to the brain and therefore the amount of pain generated. If it is partly open or closed, some or no information passes through, whereas if wide open, information is freely transmitted to the brain. The position of the gate depends on the activity of the large and small afferent fibres and on the nerve impulses which come from the brain. Activity in the large fibres tends to inhibit the transmission of information (i.e. closes the gate), hence the generation of pain is lessened, whereas activity in the small fibres facilitates transmission (i.e. opens the gate) and the generation of pain is increased. In normal circumstances the activity of the large fibres predominates, hence transmission is inhibited.

Activity in the central nervous system may also facilitate or inhibit the passage of information. Influences such as anxiety, anticipation, suggestion and attention exert a powerful influence on the pain process. For instance, heightened anxiety in labour causes the gate to open and increases the level of pain experienced by the mother. The skilled midwife will try to reduce the mother's anxiety and in so doing lessen the pain experienced by her. Conversely the higher centres may have an inhibitory effect which closes the gate. Psychological processes arising from past experience and emotion may also influence the perception of pain and the individual's response to it by acting on the gating mechanism. Some psychological factors open the gate whilst others close it. The main advantage of the gate control theory of pain, which is complex and continually being developed, is that, unlike some of the earlier theories, it acknowledges that pain perception is influenced by the psychological state of the individual (Walding, 1991). According to Green (1993), anxiety about pain of labour is a strong predictor of negative experiences during labour, lack of satisfaction with the birth and poor emotional well-being in the postnatal period.

In recent years studies have also revealed the presence of endogenous pain-relieving substances which are produced by the brain. They are peptides known as *encephalins* and *endorphins*, which appear to produce analgesia by acting on morphine-binding sites in the brain and spinal cord. This principle is the basis of the use of *transcutaneous electrical nerve stimulation (TENS)*.

An adequate understanding of pain and of the factors which affect it should enable the midwife to provide more effective antenatal preparation for childbirth and promote greater pain relief in labour. The process of labour and the various methods of pain relief available should be discussed with parents during the antenatal period so that they can make an informed choice. Anxiety levels may then be reduced and the woman can look forward to labour with confidence. Recent evidence suggests that the perception of midwives and of women as to the effectiveness of pain relief methods in labour are not in accord. Lack of

communication and understanding by the midwife of the woman's need for choice and involvement in decision-making is implicated (Rajan, 1993).

Pharmacological Methods of Pain Relief

Much of the satisfaction or otherwise with childbirth as an experience for women is focused around their perception of having some control over the process, including relief of pain in labour (Green *et al.* 1989). It is recommended that more encouragement and support for the woman's own choice of pain relief should be given. The value to women of methods over which they have some control should be recognized, together with consideration of cultural and individual differences and preferences. Inhalational analgesia (Entonox), narcotics (pethidine) and regional blocks (epidural analgesia) remain the commonest pharmacological methods of pain relief in the UK. Decisions made by the professionals caring for women in labour and constraints such as availability of an epidural service within the system tend to dominate the choice of pain relief open to women (Rajan, 1993).

Pharmacological pain relief is made more effective by good midwifery care. Imparting accurate, research-based information, giving support and opportunity for self-control by the mother, attention to individual pain relief needs, and non-stereotyping can do much to relieve pain in labour (Mander, 1992; Rajan, 1993). This facilitates a relationship of trust and confidence which is considered essential to care given during labour. In addition to hygiene and physical needs, e.g. bladder care, women need constant support to help overcome fear and tension, reassurance and help with relaxation, breathing awareness and position changes. Non-pharmacological methods of pain control such as massage, counterpressure, touch, effleurage, application of heat and cold may be effective and between contractions women should be encouraged to relax and rest.

SYSTEMIC ANALGESIA

Analgesia is defined as reduced sensibility of pain, without loss of consciousness and sense of touch being necessarily affected (Dickersin, 1989). The objective of using analgesic drugs in labour is to achieve an acceptable level of pain relief whilst not compromising the health of mother or fetus. There should be minimal effect on physiological processes, such as uterine activity, and minimal side-effects. Availability of a specific antagonist may be important. A number of systemic narcotic analgesics have been used, the opioids being the commonest, usually given in the first stage of labour. Of these, *pethidine* is the most commonly administered. This is a synthetic controlled drug, introduced in 1939, which is a powerful analgesic, sedative and antispasmodic drug. It has been shown to be effective in labour and is relatively safe. Its effect is rapid, and lasts for approximately 3–4 hours. It may be given intramuscularly or as an intravenous injection or in an infusion which may be self-administered. The dose ranges from 50 to 200 mg and is dependent on the route of administration, the mother's weight, the degree of pain, the stage of labour and the rate of progress. The side-effects may be nausea, loss of self-control, reduction in blood pressure and sweating. It may not be effective with some women. It crosses the placenta and depresses the fetal respiratory centre. Changes in fetal heart rate pattern and a loss of base-line variability may be noted within 40 minutes of maternal administration. To avoid the greatest depressant effect on the fetus it should not be given to the mother within 2–3 hours of delivery. Least effect on the fetus is when delivery is within one hour or there has been more than six hours since maternal administration (Clyburn and Rosen, 1993).

Pethidine tends to result in respiratory depression in the baby at birth but the peak effects of the drug on the baby were observed on and after the 7th day of age (Redshaw and Rosenblatt, 1982). The babies were found to be less alert, quicker to cry when disturbed, more difficult to quieten and less able to settle themselves. There is a specific antagonist, *naloxone hydrochloride* (Narcan), which may be administered either to the mother prior to delivery or to the baby at birth. The neonatal dose is 0.01 mg/kg, which may be given intramuscularly or into the umbilical vein.

Meptazinol is an analgesic drug which has partial opiate antagonistic properties. It has little effect on cardiovascular and respiratory function. The usual dose is 100–150 mg and it is administered intramuscularly (Heywood and Ho, 1990). Some preliminary trials have shown that meptazinol gives better analgesia than pethidine and causes no known adverse effects on the fetus (Jackson and Robson, 1980, 1983). However, a comparative study by Sheikh and Tunstall (1986) showed no significant differences in the analgesic effects and side-effects of the two drugs, although meptazinol is more likely to cause vomiting in the mother.

TRANQUILLIZERS

This group of drugs are very occasionally given in conjunction with pethidine in labour. Tranquillizers are anti-emetic, potentiate the analgesic and relieve anxiety and apprehension. Those used most commonly are promazine 25–50 mg (Sparine), promethazine 25–50 mg (Phenergan) and diazepam. Diazepam may cause an increase in fetal heart rate and loss of beat-to-beat variation.

INHALATIONAL ANALGESIA

Inhalation of a low concentration of an anaesthetic agent, usually nitrous oxide, gives analgesia but not anaesthesia with partial relief of pain. The use of inhalation analgesia for pain relief in childbirth originated from the work of James Young Simpson of Edinburgh in 1847 who introduced chloroform for anaesthetic purposes (Ostheimer, 1992). In 1853 Queen Victoria availed herself of chloroform during the birth of her seventh child, Prince Leopold, and was greatly pleased with the relief it gave. The anaesthetic thus became known as '*chloroform à la reine*' and was much in demand. However, anaesthesia not only relieves pain but also produces loss of consciousness with its associated risks (Ostheimer, 1992). Midwives are not permitted to administer anaesthetics but may administer inhalational analgesics, subject to guidelines issued by the UKCC (1990).

A midwife is required to have special instruction in the essentials of obstetric analgesia and to be proficient in the use of the apparatus approved by the UKCC (1990). There are now four apparatus for the administration of Entonox gas approved by the UKCC for use by midwives on their own responsibility. These are (UKCC, 1995):

1   the original BOC Entonox apparatus;
2   the PneuPac apparatus;
3   SOS Nitronox – the midwifery model;
4   the Peacemaker apparatus.

UKCC (1995) draws attention to European Community requirements for checking apparatus, taking effect 13 June 1998, but this will not affect existing approvals.

The midwife is also responsible for ensuring that the apparatus has been properly maintained (UKCC, 1993). Maintenance is carried out at prescribed intervals and documentation should be issued which provides evidence of such maintenance. In the NHS a midwifery manager or an administrator may be responsible for sending the equipment away for maintenance at the prescribed times, but this does not absolve the midwife who is using the apparatus from ensuring that proper maintenance has been carried out. The independent midwife is responsible for ensuring that her apparatus is maintained regularly.

Most women are medically fit to receive inhalational analgesia in labour. In cases of doubt, usually due to the presence of a relevant medical condition, the midwife should seek a medical opinion.

Nitrous oxide and oxygen (Entonox)

Entonox is a mixture of equal parts of nitrous oxide and oxygen (pre-mixed) which may be available by cylinder or as a piped supply from a central cylinder store. Nitrous oxide has low lipid solubility, provides rapid onset of analgesia, is inexpensive and has no specific odour. Where it is provided in a portable cylinder the nitrous oxide and oxygen are pre-mixed and delivery is made by means of a reducing and a demand flow valve connected by corrugated tubing to a face mask or disposable mouthpiece (Figure 1). This mixture has the advantage of combining 50% nitrous oxide, which gives relatively effective pain relief, with 50% oxygen, which is beneficial to fetal oxygenation (Dickersin, 1989).

The apparatus is quite easily portable and the mix-

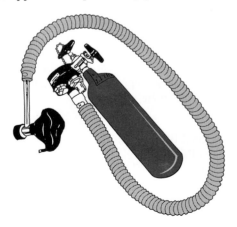

Figure 1   The Entonox inhaler.

ture is stable at normal temperatures. If the cylinders are stored at temparatures of $-8°C$ or less, however, the two gases may separate, the heavier nitrous oxide sinking to the lower part of the cylinder and the oxygen rising to the top. The emergent gas in these circumstances would be oxygen initially and when this is exhausted almost pure nitrous oxide, with danger to the mother and fetus. The gases remix when the cylinder is warmed and then inverted three or four times and this is a necessary precaution when cylinders are cold. Stringent precautions are laid down for the handling and storage of pre-mixed gas cylinders (Moir and Thorburn, 1986).

Although Entonox is considered to be safe, recent evidence suggests that it may result in post-childbirth fatigue in women over 30 years of age. This may be due to metabolism of vitamin B_{12}, although this is not yet established (MacArthur *et al.* 1991).

Technique of administration   The woman should be instructed in the use of the apparatus in the antenatal period. She should be assured that she will not lose consciousness at any time and will be fully aware of the birth of her baby, but that the pain and discomfort will be considerably lessened. It is important to explain to women the limitations of Entonox as an analgesic to avoid disappointment if it is ineffective (Moir and Thorburn, 1986). Entonox is best commenced in labour according to individual needs, not too early but neither should it be withheld if the mother is distressed. Many women require it towards the end of the first stage of labour, when it is too late to give systemic analgesia. Earlier in the first stage it may be used as an interim expedient, until systemic or regional analgesia takes effect, or during a vaginal examination prior to giving systemic analgesia.

The midwife should show the mother how to place the mask over her face so that it fits closely which is essential for effective analgesia. Many women prefer to use a mouthpiece rather than a mask. Nitrous oxide takes about 40 seconds to achieve full analgesic effect and for effective pain relief the mother should breathe into the mask as soon as she suspects that a contraction is about to begin. It is important to start inhaling the gas early so that analgesia is greatest when the contraction is at its height. It may be administered during the second stage of labour and used as an aid to suturing the perineum in conjunction with local anaesthetic.

After use, the mask, if used, should be washed well and dried; the mouthpiece should be discarded. The

Entonox machine should be tested, cylinders changed if appropriate and the apparatus then turned off. Women who use Entonox only in labour are generally more satisfied than those who used other methods of pain relief (Green, 1993).

REGIONAL AND LOCAL ANALGESIA

Increasing use is being made of regional analgesia for relief of pain in labour. This includes epidural, spinal, pudendal, very occasionally caudal or paracervical block and local infiltration.

Epidural analgesia

Epidural analgesia is an invasive procedure performed by an experienced anaesthetist whereby a local anaesthetic is introduced into the epidural space. It is regarded by some as the 'gold standard' of pain relief in labour (Dickersin, 1989). Women should be informed and given accurate information during the antenatal period on the methods of pain relief available, including epidural analgesia, so that they are able to make decisions based on choice (Crawford, 1985). Further information may be required in labour, however.

For an epidural a single dose of local anaesthetic may be given or, more commonly, a continuous technique is used in which a catheter is inserted into the epidural space so that further doses of local anaesthetic may be given as required (Carrie, 1989). Continuous epidural analgesia gives effective pain relief to 80% of women in labour who use this method. Approximately 8% of women experience only partial relief of pain due to unblocked segments giving pain between contractions, usually in the right groin. In most cases this pain is relieved by the injection of 3–4 ml of local anaesthetic with the woman lying on the affected side. Approximately 21% of women may have unilateral analgesia, and in about 5% of cases the epidural will be ineffective. Such difficulties are usually due to simple technical reasons such as an inadequate amount of local anaesthetic or insertion of an excessive length or catheter into the epidural space. These may be overcome by injecting more local anaesthetic or partial withdrawal of the epidural catheter with the woman lying on the affected side, as appropriate (Moir and Thorburn, 1986).

To give a full and safe epidural service, 24-hour cover by experienced anaesthetists is required, in addition to skilled and adequately trained midwives for the

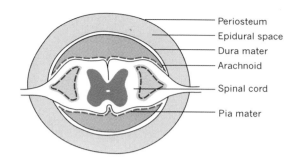

Periosteum
Epidural space
Dura mater
Arachnoid
Spinal cord
Pia mater

Figure 2   The epidural space.

constant supervision of women undergoing epidural (Moir and Thorburn, 1986). In a study Frank *et al.* (1988) reported that many of these requirements are not being met in the UK and they suggest the setting of standards for accepted practices.

The choice of epidural analgesia as a method of pain relief in labour by women may be on the decline since, in a recent study, Green (1993) reported that 79% of the women asked did not want epidural analgesia. However, it is the preferred choice for Caesarean section by 42% of women (Green *et al.* 1989).

Routes for epidural analgesia   The epidural space is a small space 4 mm wide surrounding the dura mater which is the outermost layer of the meninges (Figure 2). It contains blood vessels, fatty tissue and nerves which enter and arise from the spinal cord. The local anaesthetic may be introduced into the epidural space either by the lumbar or by the caudal route.

Lumbar epidural analgesia   In this procedure the needle may be inserted between L1 and L2, L2 and L3, or L3 and L4 (Figure 3). Rarely, the L4 and L5 interspace is used (Bevis, 1984). The procedure is similar to a lumbar puncture, except that the meninges must not be punctured. This is the route most commonly used for epidural analgesia in labour.

Caudal epidural analgesia   This is a technique whereby local anaesthetic is injected via the sacral hiatus into the caudal canal. It has largely been replaced by lumbar epidural analgesia. The needle is inserted through the sacral hiatus (the opening at the lower end of the sacrum (Figure 4)). This is a quicker but more painful approach, requires a higher dose of anaesthetic, and thus the risk of toxicity and placental transfer of the local anaesthetic is increased. It also has a higher failure rate, between 10 and 20%. Since the

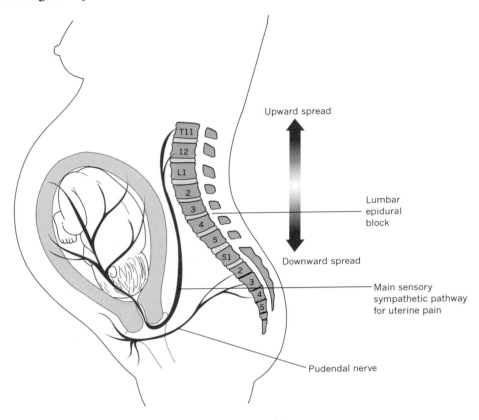

Figure 3   Nerve supply in relation to epidural anaesthesia during labour.

sacral nerves are blocked, perineal sensation is lost and the mother loses the reflex urge to bear down in the second stage of labour. The need for forceps delivery is therefore more likely. Accidental injection of the local anaesthetic into the presenting part of the fetus may occur with fatal results (Moir and Thorburn, 1986).

Sensory fibres from the uterus and the upper third of the vagina enter the spinal cord at the level of the 10th, 11th and 12th thoracic segments. Lumbar epidural block usually anaesthetizes T10–T12 and is thus most effective for the pain of the first stage of labour. Pain sensations from the lower two thirds of the vagina and perineum are transmitted to S2, S3 and S4 nerve roots, so the caudal route is most suitable for perineal pain in the second stage of labour. Complete relief of pain from the birth canal can be achieved, however, by using either the lumbar or the caudal route.

Preparation for epidural analgesia   The procedure, including the risks, are fully explained to the mother by the anaesthetist before obtaining her

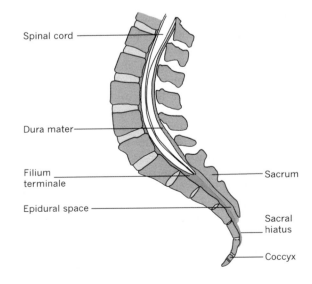

Figure 4   The epidural space and sacral hiatus.

informed consent. Temperature, pulse, blood pressure and fetal heart rate are taken and recorded and the mother is encouraged to empty her bladder. An intravenous infusion is commenced using 500–1000 ml of a crystalloid solution such as Hartmann's before the epidural is established. This pre-load is to reduce the risk of hypotension due to the vasodilation which occurs in the lower part of the body with an epidural block. Moir and Thorburn (1986) state that a fall in systolic blood pressure to 90 mmHg or lower is likely in 4–5% of mothers having epidural analgesia. It is caused by loss of peripheral vascular resistance due to the sympathetic block which occurs together with the sensory and motor block when local anaesthetic is injected into the epidural space. The situation may be exacerbated by hypovolaemia (a low circulating blood volume) due to pooling in the peripheral vessels and aortocaval occlusion which may occur when the mother is in the dorsal position and the weight of the gravid uterus compresses these vessels. The intravenous therapy will be continued throughout the period of the epidural analgesia to maintain an adequate circulating volume of fluid. It will be prescribed by the anaesthetist and may include Hartmann's solution and dextrose solutions (Moir and Thorburn, 1986).

Resuscitation equipment and drugs should be readily available and will include vasopressor drugs such as ephedrine to treat hypotension. Ephedrine is given in cases of severe hypotension as it increases maternal blood pressure, heart rate and cardiac output and, in spite of being associated with transient fetal tachycardia and increased beat-to-beat variation, it is still the drug of choice (Armand *et al.*, 1993). Recent evidence suggests that to avoid vasoconstriction, which may affect uterine vessels, the blood level of ephedrine should be maintained at low levels, especially in cases of pregnancy-induced hypertension (Hollmen, 1993).

The procedure is carried out with the mother positioned on her side, usually the left, or sitting up. Whichever position is adopted the mother is asked to flex her back as much as possible by placing her chin on her chest and by flexing her thighs and knees and drawing them up to her abdomen. This helps to separate the vertebrae. The mother's flexed back should be near the edge of the bed if she is in the lateral position.

Procedure   The procedure is carried out using a strict aseptic technique. The skin is cleaned and the area draped with sterile towels. A small amount of local anaesthetic is usually injected into the skin before inserting a 16G Tuohy needle. This needle is specially designed for epidural use and consists of a blunt needle and a stilette. It is gradually advanced until it reaches the resistance of the ligamentum flavum just before entering the epidural space. The stilette is usually removed at this stage and a syringe containing air or normal saline is attached to the needle. Further slight advance of the needle brings it into the epidural space which is recognized by a loss of resistance when the plunger of the syringe is depressed. Occasionally the needle is advanced too far and enters the subarachnoid space. Leakage of cerebrospinal fluid would indicate that a dural tap has occurred with its associated problems (Stride and Cooper, 1993)

If no cerebrospinal fluid or blood is seen, the epidural catheter is gently threaded through the Tuohy needle until the tip is in the epidural space. A test dose of 3–4 ml of local anaesthetic is then injected slowly. Rapid onset of paraesthesia (a feeling of pins and needles) or anaesthesia of the legs and hypotension would indicate that the catheter is probably in the subarachnoid space. If there are no adverse signs and symptoms after five minutes the catheter is securely strapped in place. A filter designed to prevent bacterial contamination entering the epidural space is attached to the end of the catheter. The remainder of the initial dose of local anaesthetic and all subsequent injections are then given via the bacterial filter.

Positioning of the mother during and after the procedure will be determined by the mother and the preference of the anaesthetist. Some doctors like to give the injection with the mother lying on her back to promote equal distribution of the local anaesthetic, whilst others prefer to give half the dose with the mother lying on one side and, after about five minutes, the remainder of the dose with her on the other side. The latter regimen not only reduces the risk of the uterus compressing the inferior vena cava which causes a reduction in cardiac output and thereby a fall in blood pressure, but also enables the doctor to assess the effect of the dose of local anaesthetic proposed. For pain relief at the end of the first stage and in the second stage of labour, the mother may sit up during and after injection of local anaesthetic.

Drugs   Bupivacaine (Marcain 0.25% or 0.5% solution) is commonly used as it is longer acting than lignocaine 1–2%, even when adrenaline 1 in 200 000 is added to lignocaine. The dose varies but is usually between 8 and 16 ml of bupivacaine 0.25% or 4–8 ml of bupivacaine 0.5% The effect usually lasts 2–3 hours. Top-up doses of local anaesthetic may then be given, if required.

Observations and midwifery care

After the administration of the first dose and of any subsequent top-up doses of local anaesthetic, the blood pressure and pulse should be measured and recorded every five minutes for 20–30 minutes and then every 30 minutes. The mother may sit up in bed once it is established that the blood pressure is stable, but should be tilted to one side to prevent caval occlusion. Her position should then be changed from side to side throughout labour to avoid pressure. The fetal heart is usually monitored electronically using a scalp electrode. Lindblad *et al.* (1984) measured fetal blood flow by ultrasound before and after maternal epidural analgesia and found that there was no appreciable change.

The mother will be unaware of a full bladder, so the midwife must ensure that the woman is encouraged to empty her bladder regularly. Similarly she will not feel uterine contractions, nor a desire to bear down in the second stage of labour, so close observation of progress in labour is necessary. Uterine activity may be electronically monitored.

There has been considerable debate about whether epidural analgesia adversely affects uterine activity, thereby increasing the duration of the first stage of labour. Crawford (1982) suggests that, provided there is no hypertension or hypovolaemia, uterine contractions are unaffected and therefore the duration of labour is not increased. However, Read and Hunt (1983) found that epidural analgesia delays progress in labour, especially if given early, in the latent phase.

Examinations per vaginam are made regularly to assess progress, especially before top-up injections are administered.

It is generally accepted that the duration of the second stage is increased in women who have epidural analgesia because of the absence of *Ferguson's reflex* (i.e. urge to bear down with contractions), with resultant effect on uterine action in the second stage (Carrie, 1989). This is associated with an increase in instrumental deliveries. Dickersin (1989) suggests the use of a more liberal approach to the length of the second stage, provided that the fetal condition is not compromised and is carefully monitored, and advises careful timing of top-ups to mitigate this situation. However, the issue is a controversial one.

A study by Darman and Wright (1983) concludes that unless the head is descended to within 3 cm of the introitus and sensation is returning before active pushing starts, spontaneous delivery is unlikely in primigravidae. Maresh *et al.* (1983) also studied the effect of delayed pushing in the second stage and found that there was no adverse effect on the fetus and more likelihood of a spontaneous delivery. There is thus considerable evidence to support the practice of allowing the fetal head to descend and some maternal sensation to return before encouraging active pushing in the second stage of labour (Reynolds, 1991). Careful monitoring of the fetal heart, electronically if possible, is essential to detect any signs of fetal hypoxia.

Indications for epidural analgesia

Pain relief   Hospitals with a 24-hour epidural service usually offer epidural analgesia to women in labour on request. However, this form of pain relief is not readily available to all women (Hibberd and Scott, 1990) and a number of constraints, including availability of an anaesthetist, physical condition of the mother and staff shortages may affect the provision of epidural analgesia (Rajan, 1993).

Hypertensive conditions   Although epidural analgesia is not considered to be a means of lowering the blood pressure, blood pressure is less likely to rise and, indeed, a slight fall may occur (Moir and Thorburn, 1986). Also, effective analgesia prevents distress which could result in a rise in blood pressure. Another advantage of lumbar epidural block for women with severe pre-eclampsia is that the intervillous blood flow is significantly improved, thus reducing the risk of fetal hypoxia in labour (Jouppila *et al.*, 1982). However, it may be contraindicated in severe pregnancy-induced hypertension complicated by coagulopathy.

Preterm labour   Narcotic drugs which depress the fetal respiratory centre can be avoided when the mother has an epidural block. It offers good analgesia for an elective instrumental delivery which may be performed to reduce the risk of intracranial injury due to poor ossification of the fetal skull. The relaxed pelvic floor is also thought to reduce the risk of intracranial injury. In spite of these benefits, recent evidence suggests that the use of epidural for preterm labour is disappointingly low (Chamberlain *et al.*, 1993).

Prolonged labour   An oxytocic infusion is usually prescribed to accelerate labour when it is prolonged and an epidural block gives relief from the painful contractions which ensue. The freedom from pain also allows the mother to rest and sleep, thereby avoiding exhaustion.

Hypertonic uterine action The severe pain associated with these contractions is relieved and uterine activity tends to revert to normal following an epidural block.

Malpresentation An epidural block is usually considered the analgesia of choice for a breech presentation as it prevents premature pushing and provides good analgesia for any necessary manoeuvres and the application of forceps to the aftercoming head. Chadha *et al.* (1992), however, found that the significant decrease in uterine contractions associated with epidural anaesthesia results in an increased incidence of breech extraction or Caesarean section.

Malposition An occipitoposterior position is associated with a prolonged and painful labour. Epidural block gives good relief from pain and allows the mother to rest. The reduction in tone of the pelvic floor may delay the rotation of the head, however, and a manual or instrumental rotation and delivery may be necessary.

Multiple pregnancy Epidural analgesia allows any necessary manipulations and instrumental deliveries to be carried out without delay. The second and subsequent babies can therefore be delivered more promptly and this reduces morbidity and perinatal mortality.

Cardiac and respiratory disease Epidural analgesia is preferable to narcotic drugs which depress the respiratory centre. It also provides good analgesia in the second stage when an elective instrumental delivery may be performed to minimize maternal stress. Epidural analgesia is likely to prevent hyperventilation which may precipitate wheezing in the asthmatic and it is noted that in any neurological condition, where a rise in intracranial pressure may be dangerous, it is recommended (Macdonald, 1990).

Operative deliveries Epidural analgesia is suitable for all types of operative delivery, including Caesarean section in most cases. An increasing number of Caesarean sections are now carried out under epidural block due to awareness of the risks of general anaesthesia. This requires meticulous attention to technique to prevent and manage hypotension and give adequate block for pelvic surgery. It has many benefits, including significant reduction in blood loss with reduced maternal morbidity, improved condition of the infant at birth and a satisfying experience for staff and parents (Moir and Thorburn, 1986). In many hospitals the partner is allowed to be with the mother during the operation to share the experience with her and give support. Together they can see, hear and usually hold their baby at birth and this gives most couples great emotional satisfaction.

Expected difficulties with intubation The HMSO (1991) report on maternal deaths in the United Kingdom suggests that this is an important indication for epidural analgesia. Intubation may be difficult in the presence of laryngeal oedema which may occur in hypertensive disorders in pregnancy, or in other cases, e.g. achondroplasia where it may be impossible (Macdonald, 1990).

Contraindications

Maternal reluctance If the mother does not wish to have an epidural block and withholds her consent, her wishes must be respected (Carrie, 1989). Other methods of pain relief will be offered instead.

Sepsis at the site of injection This is a contraindication because of the risk of transmitting infection directly into the central nervous system.

Systemic sepsis Epidural analgesia is not recommended in cases of herpes simplex virus (HSV) type 2 primary genital herpes, due to risks of viraemia. Secondary infection is not a problem unless the lesions are in the lumbar area. It is recommended that women who are HIV positive are carefully assessed and, if systemic manifestations of AIDS are present, epidural should not be used. Caution is required in the use of epidural morphia which may reactivate HSV-1 virus (Macdonald, 1990).

Haemorrhagic disease/clotting disorder In these cases there is a risk of a haematoma developing which could cause cord compression and paraplegia. Epidural analgesia is contraindicated in women with severe pregnancy-induced hypertension when the platelet level is less than 100 000, and in women taking aspirin if the bleeding time is above 10 minutes. Macdonald (1990) recommends that the potential risk of low-dose aspirin administration should not be ignored.

Spinal deformity The anaesthetist may wish to examine the mother before making a decision. Difficulties in achieving an epidural block often arise when there is a spinal deformity.

Neurological disease   Conditions such as disseminated sclerosis are usually considered contraindications for epidural analgesia. They tend to become worse after pregnancy and labour and the mother may attribute the deterioration to the epidural analgesia.

Hypovolaemia/hypotension   This is a contraindication because the ability of blood vessels to vasoconstrict in response to a fall in blood pressure may be impaired.

Chronic back trouble   Women with back problems may not be suitable for epidural analgesia. Research has shown a connection between epidurals and long-term backache (MacArthur *et al.*, 1991).

Presence of a uterine scar   This is not an absolute contraindication to epidural as pain associated with impending uterine rupture usually 'breaks through' the epidural block; the so called 'epidural sieve' effect (Carrie, 1989). However, meticulous monitoring of the maternal and fetal condition is essential to recognize any early signs of impending uterine rupture.

Complications

Hypotension   This is the commonest complication and occurs in more than 5% of women (Moir and Thorburn, 1986). Prevention is aided by maintenance of an adequate volume of circulating fluid and by placing the mother in a lateral position to prevent aortocaval compression. A foam rubber wedge may be used to help maintain a lateral tilt of 15–30 degrees. If hypotension occurs, the mother is turned on to her left side immediately to avoid aortocaval compression, given oxygen by face mask and her legs are raised on pillows. The foot of the bed may be raised and the infusion rate increased. Recordings of blood pressure, pulse and fetal heart sounds are made and the anaesthetist is informed. In severe cases intravenous ephedrine, a synthetic predominant beta-adrenergic agent and vasopressor, may be given by the anaesthetist to increase maternal blood pressure, heart rate and cardiac output (Armand *et al.*, 1993).

Dural tap   This occurs when the Tuohy needle or possibly the catheter accidentally punctures the dura and causes a leakage of cerebrospinal fluid, thereby reducing the intracranial pressure. This occurs in 1% of cases. The mother is likely to develop a *postdural puncture headache* (PDPH) occurring within 1–3 days,

but this may be delayed, and persisting for about a week. The headache is related to position, the upright position exacerbates it whilst recumbency alleviates it. The woman is therefore nursed lying flat during labour and often also during the first 24–48 hours of the postnatal period. The diagnosis may be confirmed by applying abdominal compression which relieves the headache immediately by compressing the vena cava, causing engorgement of the epidural veins which displaces cerebrospinal fluid into the cranium (Reynolds, 1993a) An elective forceps delivery may be indicated to prevent straining and further loss of cerebrospinal fluid.

After delivery the anaesthetist may decide to infuse normal saline into the epidural space with the aid of an infusion pump over a period of 24 hours. This helps to maintain pressure in the epidural space and thereby reduces the loss of cerebrospinal fluid. Mild laxatives are given to prevent constipation and straining which could result in an increased loss of cerebrospinal fluid. Gradually the punctured dura will heal and the volume of cerebrospinal fluid will be restored.

If the headache persists the anaesthetist may offer the mother an *epidural blood patch* (Stride and Cooper, 1993). This procedure is carried out by a skilled anaesthetist and an assistant, both practising full aseptic technique. The anaesthetist passes the Tuohy needle into the epidural space whilst the assistant withdraws a venous blood sample of 10–20 ml from the mother. This blood is injected slowly into the epidural space via the Tuohy needle. The needle is withdrawn and a dressing applied to the injection site. It is thought that when the blood clots it seals the puncture site in the dura mater. This treatment often gives the mother instant relief from her headache. She can gradually sit up after about half an hour and can then be mobilized. Undue exertion and straining must be avoided, however, because of the risk of dislodging the blood clot. It is important to observe the woman closely for any sign of infection following this treatment. It is recommended that autologous blood patch be avoided in the presence of maternal fever or septicaemia (Gutsche, 1990).

There is evidence to suggest that the use of epidural opioids and the direction of the needle bevel (facing laterally to create a smaller hole in the dura by splitting the fibres) may reduce the incidence of post-dural puncture headache (Stride and Cooper, 1993). Gutche (1990) recommends three aspects to management: prevention, accurate diagnosis and prompt effective treatment. Other methods of treatment which may be used are abdominal binder, fluids, oral and intravenous, intravenous caffeine and sodium benzoate, dextran 40 and analgesics (Gutsche, 1990; Stride and Cooper, 1993).

Toxic reaction to local anaesthetic This may be caused by a high dose of local anaesthetic or following an intravascular injection. A mild toxic reaction may cause restlessness, dizziness, tinnitus and drowsiness. A serious toxic reaction which causes convulsions may be preceded by premonitory twitchings and may lead to coma and respiratory arrest.

Retention of urine This is caused by the lack of sensation which is the result of an epidural block. The mother should be encouraged to pass urine before each 'top-up' or two hourly in labour. After delivery care must be taken to ensure that the mother continues to empty her bladder regularly. If she is unable to do so and her bladder is unduly distended it will be necessary to pass a urinary catheter.

Horner's syndrome This is a temporary, harmless complication following epidural which gives rise to miotic pupils and ptosis. The explanation is unclear (Moir and Thorburn, 1986).

Inadequate epidural block This is a situation which is distressing for the woman and is probably due to unblocked segments giving rise to pain between contractions, often in the right groin. Unilateral analgesia may occur and is due to the insertion of excessive length of catheter into the epidural space, or the presence of an anterior septum. Both situations may be remedied by a further injection of 3–4 ml of local anaesthetic, with the woman lying on the affected side, and by partial withdrawal of the catheter to ensure 1–2 cm only in the epidural space in cases of unilateral block (Moir and Thorburn, 1986).

Infection This is a rare complication since a strict aseptic technique is used for epidural analgesia.

Fetal bradycardia This may occur as a result of uncorrected maternal hypotension, supine hypotensive syndrome or the use of high dosages of local anaesthetic.

Total spinal anaesthetic This is a rare but serious complication which occurs if a full dose of local anaesthetic is accidentally injected into the subarachnoid space. It will lead to marked hypotension and respiratory arrest. Artificial ventilation and vasopressor drugs must be administered urgently or death may ensue. It may follow the initial or a top-up injection and early recognition is mandatory. Midwives need to be vigilant in recognizing the signs of a fall in maternal arterial pressure and ascending muscle weakness and notify the anaesthetist immediately (Moir and Thorburn, 1986).

Bloody tap This results from the puncture of a blood vessel in the epidural space, usually by the catheter. It may be necessary to resite the epidural (Moir and Thorburn, 1986).

Sense of deprivation Although this is perhaps not a complication, it is a feeling experienced by many mothers who have pain-free labours with epidural analgesia. In 1976 Billewicz-Driemel and Milne studied the sense of deprivation experienced by mothers following epidural analgesia. They suggest that some mothers are emotionally prepared for pain in labour and feel deprived if it is obviated. Morgan *et al.* (1982) consider that epidural analgesia did not give as much satisfaction with childbirth as less effective forms of pain relief. Haddad *et al.* (1985) report that women with a high tendency to anxiety are more likely to require oxytocin to augment uterine contractions in labour. As a consequence they often require epidural analgesia because the augmented contractions tend to be more painful.

In a study of a consumer view of epidural analgesia, Williams *et al.* (1985) found that although it is a much more effective form of pain relief, there is a greater incidence of intervention in labour and of minor problems during the early postnatal period. These problems include dizziness, backache, painful perineum and difficulty in passing urine and occur at an important time for the development of maternal–infant bonding.

Oakley (1980) suggests that there is a link between epidural analgesia and postnatal blues. It has been suggested that this could be linked to the effect of bupivacaine on the neonate, causing unresponsiveness to the mother during the critical bonding period after birth (Klaus and Kennel, 1976; Murray *et al.*, 1982; Rosenblatt *et al.*, 1981). Women whose choice of analgesia was epidural and who did not have complete pain relief as expected were both disappointed and angry (Green, 1993).

Topping-up of epidural blocks

Topping-up of epidural blocks refers to the administration of subsequent doses of local anaesthetic to achieve continuous relief of pain. The doctor gives the test dose and first injection but a midwife may give the following top-up injections if certain criteria are met. The UKCC (1971) specifies that the following safeguards must be observed:

1   that the ultimate responsibility for such a technique should be clearly stated to rest with the doctor;
2   that written instructions as to the dose should be given by the doctor concerned;
3   that in all cases the dose given by the midwife should be checked by one other person;
4   that instructions should be given by the doctor concerning details such as the posture of the patient at the time of injection, observation of blood pressure and measures to be taken in the event of any side-effects;
5   that the midwife be thoroughly instructed in the technique so that the doctor is satisfied as to her ability.

Procedure   The woman is encouraged to empty her bladder and an examination per vaginam may then be made to assess the progress of labour. The blood pressure, pulse and fetal heart are measured and recorded. The prescribed dose of local anaesthetic is ascertained from the records, checked by a second person and, under strict aseptic conditions, the dosage is injected slowly through the bacterial filter attached to the catheter between uterine contractions (during a contraction the epidural space is reduced). The top-up dose may be ordered and given in divided doses to allow for assessment of the effects of the initial dosage before proceeding, for increased safety in administration. Following the injection the blood pressure is measured and recorded every five minutes for 20–30 minutes and then every 30 minutes, as indicated earlier. Midwives need to be aware of the complications which may arise and be skilled in their management of these complications. Earlier evidence suggested that this may not be the case in all midwifery units (Frank *et al*, 1988).

Removal of the epidural catheter   If removed by the midwife on completion of the analgesia, the catheter must be carefully examined and checked by a second person to ensure that the tip is complete. This fact is recorded in the mother's notes.

Epidural opiates   Epidural opiates used alone have not been found to be an effective form of analgesia in labour, except to give incomplete but adequate analgesia in cases where local anaesthetics are contraindicated, e.g. cystic fibrosis. The use of dilute combinations of local anaesthetic with the opiate is reported to be effective. It gives a rapid-onset, more profound analgesia and has a longer lasting effect, with less motor blockade, because the local anaesthetic blocks the A delta fibres whilst the opiates work on the impulses generated by the C fibre stimulation. The drugs most commonly used are fentanyl with bupivacaine. Epidural opioids have a number of side-effects such as pruritis, urinary retention, postural hypotension, nausea, vomiting and respiratory depression (Wild and Coyne, 1992).

The mixture of bupivacaine with fentanyl may be administered by epidural infusion rather than by bolus. It reduces the motor block, allows careful mobilization of the woman into a chair, reduces blood pressure swings and allows active participation by the mother in the second stage of labour. It is contraindicated in women who have had an opiate administered within two hours of the epidural, those in whom delivery is anticipated within one hour of the epidural and in women who want total numbness. Monitoring of fetal and maternal condition is similiar to the standard epidural but, in addition, maternal respiratory rates are checked hourly. If less than 12 respirations per minute are recorded the anaesthetist is informed. Hourly assessment of the height of the block with ethyl chloride spray is required to ascertain the level of the block in relation to the umbilicus. The rate of the infusion can then be adjusted to avoid the block spreading too high, and to give adequate pain relief. In the event of respiratory depression naloxone may be used. This has also been found to reduce the incidence of pruritis.

Paracervical nerve block

This is a simple and effective procedure which is performed in established labour whereby local anaesthetic is injected into the Lee–Frankenhauser's plexus through the lateral vaginal fornices (Figure 5). It is a method of pain relief which may be used in the first stage of labour.

Paracervical nerve block is unpopular in the UK due to the high and very variable reported incidence (2–70%) of fetal bradycardia, which may be severe, occurring within minutes of the block, taking up to 30 minutes to resolve, and associated with fetal acido-

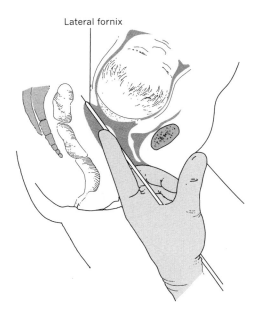

Figure 5   Paracervical nerve block.

sis and occasionally fetal death (Dickersin, 1989). Bupivacaine is the local anaesthetic agent of choice, in spite of reducing uteroplacental blood flow, because it is longer acting than lignocaine and reduces the need to repeat the block frequently. A dose of 5–10 ml of 0.25% solution is injected at 3 and 9 o'clock in relation to the cervical os. The needle is introduced through a special guard which is pressed into the lateral fornix of the vagina, the needle is then advanced 0.5–1 cm. To reduce the adverse fetal effects, possibly caused by inadvertent intravascular injection of local anaesthetic into the uterine artery which lies in close proximity to Lee–Frankenhauser's plexus, it is recommended that the needle is inserted 3 mm only and a maximum of 10 ml of local anaesthetic be given using two injection sites in each fornix (Moir and Thorburn, 1986).

Bilateral paracervical block is effective in eliminating the pain of cervical dilatation, but the uterine contractions and perineal stretching can still be felt. Another disadvantage of this method is the limited area affected and the short period of pain relief. It may be employed if other methods of pain relief are not available but requires continuous monitoring of fetal heart rate and uterine contractions and facilities for fetal blood sampling to measure the pH. It is recommended that this procedure is not employed in the case of placental insufficiency or pre-term labour (Moir and Thorburn, 1986).

Recent evidence suggests this method may be having a resurge of popularity due to the use of chlor-procaine, a rapidly hydrolysed anaesthetic agent which is less toxic than amide-linked agents such as bupiva-caine, but has a short duration of action (Dickersin, 1989).

Pudendal nerve block

A local anaesthetic agent is used to infiltrate an area around the pudendal nerve, which is derived from the anterior roots of the S2–S4 nerves, and is a mixture of motor and sensory nerves, usually by a transvaginal route as it passes across the ischial spine (Figure 6). This provides analgesia of the lower vagina and perineum and is suitable for forceps delivery, breech delivery and repair of episiotomies. The woman is placed in the lithotomy position and two fingers are introduced into the vagina to locate the ischial spine. A pudendal block needle with guide is then introduced, guided by the two fingers, and advanced until it penetrates the vaginal wall at the level of and behind the ischial spines to a depth of 1.25 cm. The needle should be felt to have entered the tough sacro-spinous ligament. It is recommended that aspiration for blood be performed as puncture of the adjacent pudendal vessels may occur with a serious toxic reaction. Just below each ischial spine, 10 ml of 1% lignocaine is injected. To avoid toxicity the dosage is usually limited to 20 ml of the 1% solution of lignocaine.

Pudendal block does not relieve pain of uterine origin, nor does it adversely affect the neonate pro-

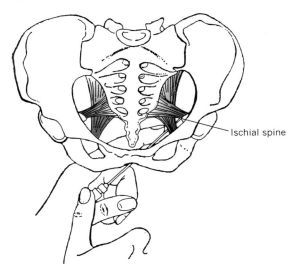

Figure 6   Pudendal nerve block.

vided dosages are adhered to and intravascular injection is avoided.

Perineal infiltration

A local anaesthetic is used to infiltrate the perineal region prior to the performance and repair of episiotomies and repair of perineal lacerations. A fan-like distribution of injections is made from the centre point of the fourchette using a total of 10 ml of plain lignocaine 0.5% solution. Precautions are taken to avoid intravascular injection of the local anaesthetic. The midwife is permitted by the UKCC to infiltrate the perineum before making an episiotomy and prior to suturing.

Transcutaneous Electric Nerve Stimulation (TENS)

Massage has psychological, mechanical and physiological effects and may be used to reduce pain in labour. Similarly transcutaneous electrical nerve stimulation (TENS) may be used for pain relief (Wall, 1985). TENS is the application of pulsed electrical current through surface electrodes placed on the skin. The electrodes are usually placed parallel to and on each side of the spine. The first pair reaches from the 10th thoracic to the 1st lumbar vertebra and treats the pain associated with the first stage of labour, and the second pair extends from the 2nd to the 4th sacral vertebra and treats the pain of the second stage (Figure 7).

TENS works through the gate control theory. Stimulation of the large peripheral nerve fibres closes the gate to pain. It is said to stimulate release of cerebrospinal endorphins (Simkin, 1989).

The advantages of TENS are that it is a non-invasive form of pain management and can be used effectively whether the mother is in bed or mobile. There is no depression of respiration or sedation and the pain relief is continuous. Special obstetric apparatuses are now produced with a demand switch which is operated by the mother herself. She can therefore boost the current by bringing the high-frequency current into play as well as the low-frequency one during contractions, thus obtaining maximum pain relief. There is no depression of the fetus due to drugs and Apgar scores have proved to be satisfactory. Finally the apparatus is relatively inexpensive and easy to use.

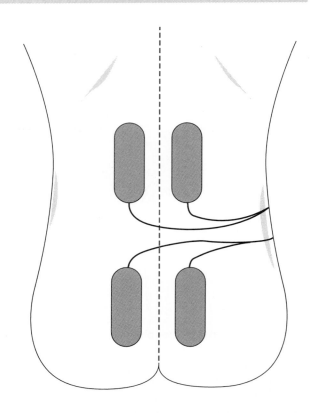

Figure 7   Positions of TENS electrodes for pain relief in labour.

In 1991 the UKCC approved that midwives may, on their own responsibility, manage pain relief in labour by the use of TENS provided that:

▶ they have received adequate and appropiate instruction, which is a matter to be determined by agreed local policy; and
▶ safety standards conform to those laid down by the Department of Health Medical Devices Directorate in England, or equivalent body in Scotland, Wales or Northern Ireland.

For best results TENS should be introduced to the mother in late pregnancy so that she is familiar with the apparatus and understands how to use it. The time to begin using TENS in labour is early on in the first stage to encourage the release of endorphins and raise the mother's pain threshold. It takes about 40 minutes for the maximum endorphin level to be reached (Salar *et al.*, 1981). When the mother feels she needs extra pain relief she can then depress the booster button which will bring the high-frequency current into play during the contraction. At the end of the contraction, she depresses the booster button once more, to return to the low-frequency current. Once the electrodes have been placed in position the mother controls the use of the apparatus herself. This gives her autonomy and helps her achieve greater emotional fulfilment from the experience of childbirth (Cluett, 1994).

TENS is reported to be reasonably effective in early labour but limited trials do not suggest significant benefit in advanced labour (Harrison *et al.*, 1986). Many women using TENS have to resort to other methods such as epidural analgesia and Entonox (Reynolds, 1993b). In the National Survey conducted by the National Birthday Trust only 5.5% of women reported using TENS (Chamberlain *et al.*, 1993).

Concern has been expressed that the fetal heart rate and fetal monitoring might be affected, but it is reported that, provided the electrodes are positioned in the lumbar region, no adverse effects were proven.

TENS has also been used post-operatively following Caesarean section. The electrodes can be placed above the incision or on the back over the nerve roots supplying the dermatomes of the affected area. A constant low-frequency current seems to give effective pain relief.

Refer to Chapter 22 for the use of complementary therapies for the relief of pain in labour and Chapter 25 for physical preparation for labour.

References

Armand, S., Jasson, J., Talafre, M.L. & Ameil-Tison, C. (1993) The effects of regional analgesia on the newborn. In Reynolds, F. (ed.) *Effects on the Baby of Maternal Analgesia and Anaesthesia.* London: W.B. Saunders.

Bevis, R. (1984) *Anaesthesia in Midwifery.* London: Baillière Tindall.

Billewicz-Driemel, M. & Milne, M.D. (1976) Long term assessment of extradural analgesia for relief of pain in labour: sense of 'deprivation' after extradural analgesia in labour: relevant or not? *Br. J. Anaesth.* 48: 139.

Boss, B.J. & Goloskov, J.W. (1983) Pain. In Lewis, S.M. & Collier, I.C. (eds) *Medical and Surgical Nursing: Assessment and Management of Clinical Problems.* New York: McGraw-Hill.

Carrie, L.E.S. (1989) Epidural analgesia in obstetrics. *J. Continuing Education for GPs* June, 38 (11): 1257–1263.

Chadha, Y.C., Mahmood, T.A., Dick, M.J. *et al.* (1992) Breech delivery and epidural analgesia. *Br. J. Obstet. Gynaecol.* 99: 96–100.

Chamberlain, G., Steer, P. & Wraight, A. (1993) *The 1990 Pain Relief in Labour Survey.* London: National Birthday Trust Fund.

Cluett, E. (1994) Analgesia in labour: A review of the TENS method. *Prof. Care Mother Child* 4(2): 50–52.

Clyburn, P.A. & Rosen, M. (1993) The effects of opioid and inhalation analgesia on the newborn. In Reynolds, F. (ed.). *Effects on the Baby of Maternal Analgesia and Anaesthesia.* London: W.B. Saunders.

Crawford, J.S. (1982) The effect of epidural block on the progress of labour. In Studd, J. (ed.) *Progress in Obstetrics and Gynaecology*, Vol. 2. Edinburgh: Churchill Livingstone.

Crawford, J.S (1985) The midwife's contribution to epidural analgesia for labour and delivery. *Midwifery* 1: 24–31

Darman, F.M. & Wright, J.T. (1983) A prospective study on the second stage of labour following epidural analgesia in labour. *J. Obstet. Gynaecol.* 4: 40–41.

Davitz, L.L. & Davitz, J.R. (1980) *Nurses Response to Patient's Suffering.* New York: Springer-Verlag.

Dickersin, K. (1989) Pharmacological control of pain during labour. In Chalmers, I., Enkin, M. & Keirse, M.J.N. (eds) *Effective Care in Pregnancy and Childbirth*, Vol. 2. Oxford: Oxford University Press.

Frank, M., Heywood, A. & Macleod, D.M. (1988) Survey of the practice of epidural analgesia in a regional sample of obstetric units. *Anaesthesia* 43: 54–58.

Ganong, W.F. (1985) *Review of Medical Physiology.* Los Altos: Lange Medical.

Green, J.M. (1993) Expectations and experiences of pain in labour: Findings from a large prospective study. *Birth* 20 (2): 65–72.

Green, J.M., Coupland, V.A. & Kitzinger, J.V. (1989) *Great Expectations.* Cambridge: Child Care and Development Group, University of Cambridge.

Gutsche, B. (1990) Lumbar epidural analgesia in obstetrics: taps and patches. In Reynolds, F. (ed.) *Epidural and Spinal Blockade in Obstetrics.* London: Baillière Tindall.

Haddad, P.F., Morris, N.F. & Spielberger, C.D. (1985) Anxiety in pregnancy and its relation to use of oxytocin and analgesia in labour. *J. Obstet. Gynaecol.* 6: 77–81.

Harrison, R.F., Woods, T., Shore, M., Matthews, G. & Unwin, A. (1986) Pain relief in labour using transcutaneous electrical nerve stimulation (TENS). A TENS/TENS placebo controlled study in two parity groups, *Br. J. Obstet. Gynaecol.* 93: 739–746.

Hayward, J. (1975) *Information – A Prescription Against Pain.* London: Royal College of Nursing.

Heywood, A.M. & Ho, E. (1990) Pain relief in labour. In Alexander, J., Levy, V. & Roch, S. (eds) *Intrapartum Care: A Research Based Approach.* London: Macmillan.

Hibberd, B.M. & Scott, D.B. (1990) The availability of epidural anaesthesia and analgesia in obstetrics. *Br. J. Obstet. Gynaecol.* 97: 402–405.

HMSO (1991) *Report on Confidential Enquiries into Maternal Deaths in the United Kingdom 1985–87.* London: HMSO.

Hollmen, A.I. (1993) The effects of regional and anaesthesia on utero- and fetoplacental blood flow. In Reynolds, F. (ed.) *Effects on the Baby of Maternal Analgesia and Anaesthesia.* London: W.B. Saunders.

Jackson, M.B.A. & Robson, P.J. (1980) Preliminary experience of the use of meptazinol as an obstetric analgesia. *Br. J. Obstet. Gynaecol.* **87**: 296–301.

Jackson, M.B.A. & Robson, P.J. (1983) Preliminary clinical and pharmacokinetic experience in the newborn when meptazinol is compared with pethidine as an obstetric analgesic. *Postgrad. Med. J.* **59** (Suppl. 1): 47–51.

Jouppila, P., Joupilla, R., Hollmen, A. & Koivula, A. (1982) Lumbar epidural analgesia to improve intervillous blood flow during labour in severe pre-eclampsia. *Obstet. Gynecol.* **59**(2): 158–161.

Klaus, M.H. & Kennel, J.H. (1976) *Maternal–Infant Bonding: Impact of Early Separation and Loss on Family Development.* St Louis: Mosby.

Lindblad, A., Marsal, K., Vernersson, E. & Renck, H. (1984) Fetal circulation during epidural analgesia for caesarean section. *Br. Med. J.* **228**: 1329–1330.

MacArthur, C., Lewis, M. & Knox, E.G. (1991) *Health After Childbirth.* University of Birmingham, London: HMSO.

MacDonald, R. (1990) Indications and contraindications for epidural blockade in obstetrics. In Reynolds, F. (ed.) *Epidural and Spinal Blockade in Obstetrics.* London: Baillière Tindall.

Mander, R. (1992) The control of pain in labour. *J. Clin. Nursing* 1: 219–223.

Maresh, M., Choong, K.H. & Beard, R.W. (1983) Delayed pushing with lumbar epidural analgesia in labour. *Br. J. Obstet. Gynaecol.* **90**: 623–627.

Melzack, R. (1973) The puzzle of pain mechanisms: a new theory. *Science* **150**: 971.

Melzack, R. & Wall, P. (1988) *The Challenge of Pain.* London: Pelican.

Moir, D. & Thorburn, J. (1986) *Obstetric Anaesthesia and Analgesia.* London: Baillière Tindall.

Morgan, B.M., Bulpitt, J., Clifton, P. & Lewis, P.J. (1982) Analgesia and satisfaction in childbirth. (The Queen Charlotte's 100 Mother Survey). *Lancet* **11** (8302) 9 October: 808–810

Murray, A.D., Dolby, R.M., Nation, R.L., Thomas, D.B. & Read, M.D. (1982) Effects of epidural anaesthesia on newborns and their mothers. *Child Devel.* **52**: 803–810.

Oakley, A. (1980) *Women Confined.* Oxford: Martin Robinson.

Ostheimer, G.W. (1992) *Manual of Obstetric Anaesthesia.* New York: Churchill Livingstone.

Pavlov, I.V. (1928) *Conditioned Reflexes.* Oxford: Oxford University Press.

Rajan, L. (1993) Perceptions of pain and pain relief in labour: the gulf between experience and observation. *Midwifery* **9**: 136–145.

Read, G.D. (1969) *Childbirth Without Fear.* London: Pan.

Read, M.D., Hunt, L.P. & Lieberman, B.A. (1983) *Psychological Aspects of Pregnancy.* London: Longman.

Read, M.D. & Hunt, L.P. (1983) Epidural block and the progress and outcome on labour. *J. Obstet. Gynaecol.* **4**: 35–39.

Redshaw, M. & Rosenblatt, D.B. (1982) The influence of analgesia in labour on the baby. *Midwife, Health Visitor and Community Nurse* **18**: (4): 126–132.

Reynolds, F. (1991) Pain relief in labour. In Studd, J. (ed.) *Progress in Obstetrics and Gynaecology*, Vol. 9. Edinburgh: Churchill Livingstone.

Reynolds, F. (1993a) Dural puncture and headache. *Br. Med. J.* **306**: 874–875.

Reynolds, F. (1993b) Pain relief in labour. *Br. J. Obstet Gynaecol.* **100**: 979–983.

Rosenblatt, D., Belsey, E.M., Lieberman, L., Smith, R.L. & Beard, R.W. (1981) The influence of maternal analgesia on neonatal behaviour: II Epidural bupivacaine. *Br. J. Obstet. Gynaecol.* **88**: 407–413.

Royal College of Surgeons of England & The College of Anaesthetists (1990) *Report on the Working Party on Pain after Surgery.* London: RCOS.

Salar, G., Job, I., Mingrino, S., Bosio, A. & Trabucchi, M. (1981) Effect of transcutaneous electrical nerve stimulation. A prospective matched study. *Acta Obstet. Gynecol. Scand.* **60**: 459–468.

Sheikh, A. & Tunstall, M.E. (1986) Comparative study of meptazinol and pethidine for the relief of pain in labour. *Br. J. Obstet. Gynaecol.* **93**: 264–269.

Simkin, P. (1989) Non-pharmacological methods of pain relief during labour. In Chalmers, I., Enkin, M. & Kierse, M.J.N.C. (eds) *Effective Care in Pregnancy and Childbirth*, vol. 2, pp. 893–912. Oxford: Oxford University Press.

Sternbach, R.A. & Tursky, B. (1965) Ethnic differences among housewives in psychophysical and skin potential responses to electric shock. *Psychophysiology* **1**: 241.

Stride, P.C. & Cooper, G.M. (1993) Dural taps revisited. A 20 year survey from Birmingham Maternity Hospital. *Anaesthesia* **48**: 247–255.

UKCC (1971) *Statement of Policy. The Maintenance of Epidural Block by Midwives.* London: UKCC.

UKCC (1990) Registrar's letter 14/1990, *Approval of Apparatus for the Administration of Inhalational Analgesia by Midwives.* London: UKCC.

UKCC (1991) Registrar's Letter 8/91, *Transcutaneous Nerve Stimulation for the Relief of Pain in Labour.* London: UKCC.

UKCC (1993) *Midwives' Rules.* London: UKCC.

UKCC (1995) Registrar's letter 31/1995, *Approval of Apparatus for the Administration of Inhalational Analgesia by Midwives.* London: UKCC.

Walding, M.F. (1991) Pain, anxiety and powerlessness. *J. Adv. Nursing* **16**: 338–397.

Wall, P.D. (1985) The discovery of transcutaneous nerve stimulation. *Physiotherapy* **71**(8): 348–350.

Wild, L. & Coyne, C. (1992) The basics and beyond, epidural analgesia. *Am. J. Nursing* April: 26–30

Williams, S., Hepburn, M. & McIlwaine, G. (1985) Consumer view of epidural anaesthesia. *Midwifery* **1**: 32–36.

33

Community Midwifery and Home Birth

Community Midwifery: A Historical Perspective

The role of the midwife working in the community in Britain has been constantly changing since the first Midwives Act was passed in 1902. At this time, the majority of midwives were working as independent practitioners in the community, taking responsibility for the total care of women who hired their services. Most babies were born at home and, on the whole, general practitioners were only called by midwives when problems occurred. Whilst antenatal care was virtually non-existent, the new professional midwives placed emphasis on the postnatal care of mothers and babies. Women were strictly 'confined to bed' for at least ten days and postnatal care was characterized by elaborate, time-consuming rituals such as routine bed bathing (Leap and Hunter, 1993).

By 1937, the numbers of births at home had decreased as the percentage of births in institutions rose. Campbell and Macfarlane (1994: 13) cite government records: in 1927, 15% of births took place in institutions. This rose to 24% in 1932 and to almost 35% by 1937. At this time an Act had been passed which would radically change the working lives of most midwives working in the community. The Midwives Act of 1936 charged local authorities in England and Wales with providing an adequate salaried midwifery service. Most midwives became employees of local authorities and no longer had to purchase their own uniforms and equipment. For the first time they had 'off-duty', annual leave, pensions and financial security (Towler and Bramall, 1986: 226). However, until the establishment of the National Health Service in 1948, midwives still had to collect fees for their services from their clients, albeit on behalf of the local authorities.

After the Health Service Reorganisation Act of 1973 (implemented in 1974), community midwives were no longer employed by local authorities. Together with hospital midwives, they became employees of health authorities. The concept of the midwife being part of a team was developed and many community midwives became 'general practitioner (GP) attached' (Towler and Bramall, 1986: 271). This reorganization resulted in a loss of autonomy for many community midwives.

Throughout the 1970s and 1980s the home birth rate continued to decline until by the late 1980s, only 1% of births occurred at home. This meant that the focus of the community midwife's work centred on statutory postnatal visits. Some were able to develop their own antenatal clinics and in many areas the 'Domino' ('Domiciliary Midwife In and Out') scheme enabled community midwives to provide intrapartum care in hospital with an early transfer home.

In the 1990s, the role of the community midwife continues to change. Early transfer home from hospital has become normal practice for the majority of women and thus the number of postnatal visits for each community midwife has increased. The burden of the increased workload has to some extent been ameliorated in the last decade by changes in the *Midwives' Rules* (UKCC, 1993). Midwives no longer have to follow prescriptive rules about statutory visits and there is scope for flexible decision-making based on the needs of individual mothers and babies.

The concept of midwifery practices based in the community with midwives providing continuity of care for women, regardless of place of birth, was first suggested in *The Vision*, a document published by the Association of Radical Midwives (ARM, 1986). These themes were reiterated in *Towards a Healthy Nation*, published by the Royal College of Midwives (RCM, 1987, 1991).

In their book *Who's Left Holding the Baby?*, Ball *et al.* (1992) proposed a framework for change that would maximize midwifery skills. The establishment of midwifery group practices where midwives have caseloads would be a key feature in the framework for change. Already, there is evidence of the benefits of such practice. For example, an audit of over 1000 births attended by independent midwives between 1980 and 1991 described beneficial outcomes for the women involved (RCM, 1993). Almost 90% of the women had a spontaneous vaginal birth, 95% of the women

breastfed, 75% of the women gave birth at home and all the women received continuity of care, including those transferred to hospital. The perinatal mortality rate was 7.7 per 1000 for the whole audit population. Although this study has some shortcomings, such as incomplete data from the midwives' birth registers and arguably an unrepresentative sample of the general population, it is an example of the benefits of one pattern of midwifery care.

There is a move towards a more integrated role, with midwives moving between hospital and community providing a service which enables women to have more choice, control and continuity of care in childbirth. Such themes were first proposed by the Welsh Planning Forum (1991) and were further developed by the Winterton Report (House of Commons, 1992).

The government responded to the Winterton Report by asking Lady Cumberlege, Parliamentary Under Secretary of State for Health, to set up a committee 'to review policy on NHS maternity care, particularly during childbirth, and to make recommendations' (DOH, 1993a). The report of this Expert Maternity Group, *Changing Childbirth* (DOH, 1993a), sets objectives and action points for both purchasers and providers of maternity care. Community-based care and active user involvement in planning and reviewing services are central themes of this report: 'services should be based on an understanding of local health, social and cultural needs' (DOH, 1993a: 83).

Initiatives in the Community

Examples of some early community-based schemes include the Sighthill Scheme in Edinburgh (McKee, 1984). Initiated in 1975, this scheme was primarily concerned with addressing the poor uptake of antenatal services and the high perinatal mortality rate. Subsequent changes in the organization of care brought about a more community-based service that met the needs of local women as well as providing more satisfaction for the midwives, general practitioners and obstetricians involved. The proportion of women that 'booked' early in pregnancy was increased and appointments were better attended. Moreover, there were improved outcomes of labour and a significant fall in the perinatal mortality rate over the next five years.

In a similarly socially deprived area in Newcastle-upon-Tyne, a Community Midwifery Care project was set up in 1983 to assess the impact of midwives providing additional care to women in their own homes. The evaluation of the project revealed an improvement in client satisfaction coupled with a greater partnership in care by the women. Furthermore, a survey of case notes revealed a reduction in the incidence of preterm labour and a reduction in the births of low birthweight babies (Davies, 1992).

The 'Know Your Midwife' ('KYM') scheme (Flint et al., 1989) marked a significant shift in emphasis in antenatal care, from a service characterized by clinical interventions to one that stressed the importance of social care (Oakley, 1992: 62). Flint et al. (1989) demonstrated that the provision of continuity of care by midwives based in the community resulted in greater satisfaction, control and information compared to a control group. Also, quantitative data revealed that the women in the 'KYM' group had fewer antenatal admissions, more spontaneous labours and less analgesia in labour than those in the control group.

Some of the more recent community-based schemes have included those in the Rhondda, Wales (Keats, 1993), in West London (Stone, 1990), in Leicester (O'Brien, 1993; MacVicar et al., 1993) and in Oxford (Watson, 1990; Williams, 1991). In Midwifery Teams and Caseloads, Caroline Flint (1993) has outlined some of the research findings related to these and other initiatives offering continuity of carer.

The Department of Health commissioned a survey of team midwifery that was carried out in England and Wales during the spring of 1992 (Wraight et al., 1993). This survey, Mapping Team Midwifery, identified that, 'the concept of team midwifery encompasses a very broad range of definitions and a wide variety of working practices'. The report highlighted the need for careful, ongoing evaluation of new schemes particularly in light of the fact that over 25% had been discontinued within their first year. This was due to problems such as rushed implementation and insufficient collaboration with clinical midwives at the planning stage. Moreover, only a third of the schemes reviewed sought to include women's views of their care in the evaluation process.

It has been suggested by some midwives that caseload practice is an ideal way to provide woman-centred continuity of midwifery care (Leap, 1994). In 1994 the South East London Midwifery Group Practice became the first group of self-employed midwives to be contracted into the NHS. This group is one of three pilot schemes aimed at providing examples of how caseload practice can be implemented within a community setting (Reid, 1994).

Schemes such as those described above have demonstrated that midwifery practices based in the community provide an arena in which the midwife is able to use and develop all her skills. Each of these schemes have developed a particular idea of how to practice but there is no organizational blueprint. In setting up practices, midwives need to take into consideration the needs of their local community, both socially and culturally. Undoubtedly, the community provides an ideal environment in which to develop new ways of working and the chance for midwives to develop more flexible and satisfying working patterns.

Working in the Community

NETWORKING

There is a well-recognized need for midwives working in the community to liaise with other health workers and social workers. They are also well-placed to forge links with community workers, youth workers and voluntary organizations. For example, this may mean that midwives become involved with the work of local organizations such as women's groups and welfare rights projects. In Britain, it could mean getting involved in the work of a Community Health Council (CHC), a Maternity Services Liaison Committee (MSLC), a local branch of the National Childbirth Trust (NCT) or the Stillbirth and Neonatal Death Society (SANDS).

Midwives also have a responsibility to encourage women to get involved with such organizations, enabling them to make their voices heard in places where change can be effected. This may mean pursuing funding for expenses and crêche facilities so that user attendance at meetings can be representative of the local community.

For midwives, networking is not only about building up their own relationships in the community or about using agencies; it is also about putting people in touch with each other. It is about linking people, particularly new mothers, in similar circumstances. Antenatal and postnatal groups provide an ideal forum for networking between women.

Questions you might like to ask could include:

▶ Is there a local directory of voluntary/statutory organizations? If not, does the MIDIRS *Directory of Maternity Organisations* (MIDIRS, 1991) provide me with national contacts from whom I may be able to find local contacts?

▶ Are there any community centres or youth clubs or young mothers' groups/hostels in this area?

ANTENATAL AND POSTNATAL EDUCATION/SUPPORT GROUPS

In recent years the conventional model of 'parentcraft' has been challenged and there is a move away from formal antenatal 'classes' towards a more facilitative style within groups (Murphy-Black and Faulkner, 1988; Priest and Schott, 1991; Leap, 1991; MacKeith *et al.*, 1991). Hospitals are no longer the primary setting for such groups and they may be successfully run in youth and community centres, health centres, leisure centres or in the midwife's home.

Women who have made friendships within an antenatal group are well-motivated to continue to meet where provision exists in the postnatal period (Leap, 1991). Alternatively, midwives can support the establishment and continuation of postnatal groups run by voluntary organizations or by women themselves. This may reduce the isolation, loneliness and depression that many new mothers experience (Protrykus, 1990; Grevatt, 1992).

Antenatal and postnatal groups provide an opportunity for women to share their experiences and to learn from each other. Women set the agenda and they are encouraged to see themselves as 'the experts'. The midwife's skill in facilitating the group lies in listening and in ensuring that everyone is introduced and included. She needs to know when to provide guidance and information and when it is more appropriate to enable group members to respond to each other (Kindred, 1985; Leap, 1991; Priest and Schott, 1991).

In responding to local need, midwives may need to consider establishing women-only groups, evening groups that partners or friends can attend, or other groups such as those for young women (MacKeith *et al.*, 1991) or for women who need interpreters.

In her work, the midwife needs to have an awareness of the social and cultural stereotyping of women (Green *et al.*, 1990; Bowler, 1993). Consideration needs to be given to using images and audiovisual aids that are racially and culturally appropriate. There is also a need to resist using words and phrases that can trivialize or disempower women such as 'old wives' tales' and 'confinement'; and referring to women as 'girls' or 'ladies' (Leap, 1992b).

POSTNATAL CARE

In Britain midwives attend women and their babies in the postnatal period for 'a period of not less than ten and not more than twenty-eight days' (UKCC, 1993). Such a relatively short time with a woman and her family needs to be used effectively.

The key to postnatal care lies in providing support and encouragement to new parents, thus building self-confidence and minimizing dependency on professionals. The midwife can encourage parents to rely on their own commonsense and intuition. She can enable them to believe in their own ability to care for their child and to make decisions around parenting.

Where the midwife sees the mother as her baby's expert, she will avoid gratuitous advice and instructions. A directive approach may be appropriate in certain situations, such as when the mother asks for information or where there is a safety issue. For example, midwives need to inform mothers about the link between babies' sleeping positions, overheating and sudden infant death syndrome (SIDS) (DOH, 1993b). In many instances there are no definite answers and midwives will encourage women to explore a wide range of possibilities in most situations.

Some questions you may like to ask yourself could include:

▶ What are the appropriate ways to phrase questions to a woman and what do I want to find out?

▶ How am I going to find out about support without making assumptions about a woman's lifestyle?

▶ What are the ways in which I can find out how well a woman, her baby and her partner are, both physically and emotionally?

▶ How well do I use open-ended questions in conversation with new parents and how sensitive am I to their cues?

▶ Do I always need to do a daily physical examination of a woman and her baby? Do I need to wake a sleeping baby?

Home Birth

ISSUES OF SAFETY

> There is no convincing and compelling evidence that hospitals give a better guarantee of the safety of the majority of mothers and babies. It is possible, but not proven, that the contrary may be the case.
>
> (House of Commons Health Committee, 1992: xii)

In the 1920s, 15% of women in England and Wales gave birth in institutions. By the 1950s the percentage of births in hospital had increased to 65% and the rate rose steadily over the following three decades. In 1992 96.5% of women gave birth in hospital (Campbell and Macfarlane, 1994).

This decline in the home birth rate was advocated by successive government reports such as the Cranbrook Report (Ministry of Health, 1959), the Peel Report (Standing Maternity and Midwifery Advisory Committee, 1970) and the Short Report (Social Services Committee, 1980). The overall message of such reports was that birth in hospital is safer than birth at home and that the reduction in stillbirths and neonatal deaths could be attributed to the increase in hospitalization for childbirth.

In a study of the personal registers of 300 midwives working during the years 1948–1972, Julia Allison analysed data on 35 000 home births (Allison, 1992). She identified that the rate of stillbirth and neonatal death were consistently less at home than in hospital despite the fact that 50% of women who gave birth at home would be considered 'unsuitable' for home birth by current criteria. Also, as the percentage of these deaths fell at a similar rate for both home and hospital, she suggests that socio-economic factors played a more important role than place of birth.

The statistics about the safety of home birth were first challenged in the late 1970s, particularly by statistician Marjorie Tew (1978). A comprehensive summary of her analysis of the data is presented in *Safer Childbirth* (Tew, 1990). Although Tew's methodology has been challenged by Campbell and Macfarlane (1994), they also questioned the prevailing assumptions that had underpinned government policy since the 1960s. Their conclusions included the following statements:

> There is no evidence to support the claim that the safest policy is for all women to give birth in hospital (p. 119).

> The statistical association between the increase in the proportion of hospital deliveries and the fall in the crude perinatal mortality rate seems unlikely to be explained either wholly or in part by a cause and effect relationship (p. 119).

> There is some evidence, although not conclusive, that morbidity is higher among mothers and babies cared for in an institutional setting. For some women, it is possible but not proven, that the iatrogenic risk associated with institutional delivery may be greater than any benefit conferred (p. 120).

Campbell *et al.* (1984) addressed the importance of distinguishing between planned and unplanned home births when interpreting data. They noted a difference in perinatal mortality according to the intended place of birth, ranging from 4.1/1000 in those booked for birth at home compared with 196.6/1000 unbooked home birth. They recognized that women booking a home birth are a selected group and that those transferred to hospital during labour would not have been included in the survey. Nevertheless, they concluded that perinatal mortality among births booked to occur at home was low, particularly for parous women.

When supporting women in making choices about the place of birth, midwives may like to consider the words of Nancy Stewart of the Association for Improvements in Maternity Services (AIMS):

> All of living involves some risk, and this applies to giving birth and being born, wherever the birth takes place. . . . It is important to go beyond the statistics, to consider the real influences on safety for you and your baby. . . . Where to give birth is not a matter of physical safety versus feelings. They are inextricably wrapped up together and you can trust the wisdom of your feelings in choosing where your baby is to be born.
>
> (AIMS Information Booklet,
> *Choosing a Home Birth*)

FACILITATING HOME BIRTH

The Winterton Report (House of Commons, 1992) recognized that many women would like to give birth at home but reported that:

> We have had considerable evidence that women who wish to have a home birth not infrequently find themselves in a confrontational situation with the

team of professionals who are available to give them care.

(House of Commons Health Committee, 1992: para. 76)

In the section on home birth in *The Midwife's Code of Practice* (UKCC, 1994: 20), it is made clear that midwives have a statutory duty to liaise with the supervisor of midwives in any situation where 'risk factors have been identified' and medical assistance is not available or is refused by the woman or her partner. In such situations midwives are advised to 'agree and record appropriate arrangements to provide advice and support as necessary'.

Questions you might like to ask yourself could include:

▶ Are strict criteria for those considered suitable for home birth appropriate in a situation where women can make informed choices about the place of birth?
▶ As midwives, which situations would we want to avoid at home and how would we cope if they arose?
▶ How will I update my skills in coping with emergencies, such as neonatal resuscitation?

Why home birth?

Reasons given by women for choosing to give birth at home have included (Wesson, 1990; Kitzinger, 1991; Leap, 1992a):

▶ Family tradition.
▶ Personal control and privacy.
▶ Comfortable surroundings and an unhurried, relaxed environment.
▶ Safety and security.
▶ Fear of hospitals, especially when unable to understand English, and fear of unnecessary, routine intervention.
▶ Knowing the midwives/continuity of carer.
▶ Intimacy with children and partners.
▶ Emotional and physical spontaneity.

Midwives who regularly attend home births have noted that women are less likely to require pharmacological analgesia when they labour and give birth in their own homes (Cronk and Flint, 1989: 61; RCM, 1993). Various authors have described the significance of the social environment of birth and its impact on labour (Odent, 1984; Simkin, 1986; Gaskin, 1990). Arguably home birth provides the optimum chance for physiological processes to take place without disturbance. These may be among the reasons for the reported favourable outcomes for planned home births in the Western world (Ford *et al.*, 1991; Tew and Damstra-Wijmenga, 1991; Durand, 1992).

PREPARATION FOR BIRTH AT HOME

When planning to attend a woman who has chosen to give birth at home, the midwife needs to notify her intention to practise to the supervisor of midwives for the area in which the woman lives if she has not already done so (UKCC, 1993). It is courteous anyway to inform the supervisor of midwives of any bookings that you make for home birth and you may need her support at any stage. The supervisor of midwives may wish to inspect the midwife's methods of practice, records, equipment and premises as part of her statutory duty. She will ensure that the midwife has access to referral for any screening tests that are necessary and will provide forms such as the birth notification. She may also facilitate referral to an obstetrician or paediatrician when problems arise where the midwife does not have arrangements for direct referral. If the midwife is not an employee of the hospital she may ask the supervisor to organize a contract to enable her to continue to provide midwifery care to the woman should transfer become necessary.

Midwives attending home births may find the following checklist useful when discussing preparations for birth at home with a woman and her supporters in the antenatal period:

▶ An immediate source of heating, light, running water, an extension lead and access to phone.
▶ Sanitary towels, plastic sheets, bin liners and clean sheets for the bed.
▶ Towels, blankets and clothing for the baby.
▶ Arrangements for other children.
▶ Preparation of a bag in case transfer to hospital is necessary, or a list of items to pack in a hurry.
▶ Other midwives who might attend the birth and whether the woman has had a chance to meet them.
▶ Other items for additional comfort, e.g. hot water bottle, fruit juices, ice cubes, food for labour and for afterwards.

A more detailed list may be drawn up which can then become the focus of discussion for exploring the possibilities around labour and birth. The midwife also needs to clarify that she will bring all the equipment in order to cope with emergencies. This would include equipment for neonatal resuscitation, drugs to control haemorrhage and equipment for administering intravenous fluids. She also needs to be clear about the procedures and arrangements for transfer to hospital should this be necessary.

Equipment

A midwife needs to consider what equipment she considers to be necessary to take to a home birth. An example of some of the equipment that will be needed for attending home births is set out below:

Instruments: cord scissors, two artery forceps, episiotomy scissors

Stethoscope	Sphygmomanometer
Pinard's stethoscope	Doppler/'Sonicaid'
Sterile gloves	Oxytocic drugs
Mucus extractor	Urinary catheter
Amnihook	Urine testing equipment
'KY' jelly	Torch
Needles and syringes	Tourniquet
Equipment for suturing	Blood and urine bottles
Bendy straws	Spare pens
'Incopads'	Paracetemol
IV equipment and IV fluids	Cord clamp/dental floss
Tape measure	Scales
Thermometers	Bedpan
Entonox	Mirror
Measuring jug	Birth notification forms
Sterile gauze	

Since preventing heat loss in newborn babies is very important, midwives may like to consider carrying a small electric heating pad, which is easily obtainable from large chemist shops. The use of such a heating pad also means that there is no rush to wrap the baby to keep it warm. Skin-to-skin contact can therefore be prolonged with full access to the baby's body for the mother.

Midwives attending home births will have considered where they will get support from during the labour, particularly if events do not progress in a straightforward fashion. She needs to remember Rule 40 in the *Midwives' Rules* (UKCC, 1993) which states that:

> In any case where there is an emergency or where she detects in the health of a mother and baby a deviation from the norm, a practising midwife shall call to her assistance a registered medical practitioner and shall forthwith report the matter to the local supervising authority.
>
> (UKCC, 1993)

DURING THE BIRTH

The midwife's primary responsibility during the labour lies in ensuring that the woman can labour in a safe environment that encourages the normal physiological processes to work without disturbance. It is not about 'managing' the labour. It is about listening, watching, thinking, picking up cues and responding. At home women are often less inhibited about moving around, making noise and behaving instinctively. This enables midwives to develop their skills in assessing the progress of labour without resorting to routine vaginal examinations.

The midwife can minimize disruption at a home birth by not turning the woman's home into a 'mini labour ward'. Non-essential equipment can often be left out of the immediate vicinity chosen by the woman for labour and birth. Since women often decide at the last minute where they will give birth, it can be practical to place all the essential equipment on a tray so that the midwife can follow the woman to the place of her choice. As part of the midwife's role is to ensure safety, she may need to improvise at a home birth, particularly where heating is concerned. For example, towels may be warmed on a hot water bottle, a radiator or a heating pad.

Points that you may need to consider include:

▶ How might I know that labour is progressing well and what do I do in this situation?
▶ How might I know that labour is not progressing well and what might I do about it?

THE EXPERIENCE OF HOME BIRTH

Women describe feeling empowered by giving birth at home. They also speak of a shift in the balance of power where the midwife is an invited guest in their homes:

> When you go into hospital it's their place, they know where the loo is and all that and you're standing around waiting for them to tell you what to do. Whereas at home, it's your place, you know where everything is and they have to ask you where things are.
>
> (Leap, 1992a)

The midwife can facilitate a safe and satisfying experience for women who choose to give birth at home. This is also the experience for many women when transfer to hospital has been necessary:

> The hospital were absolutely brilliant. We were seen to really well. . . . I think people who choose a home birth have to deal with how you would go to hospital. . . . I was a bit sacred . . . but they were wonderful, they welcomed us with open arms. . . . so I had to go to hospital and I didn't have my home birth, but I'd go so far as to say that it was really quite wonderful, the whole experience.
>
> (Leap, 1992a)

As the proposals outlined in *Changing Childbirth* (DOH, 1993) are implemented, more midwives will be providing care for women whom they know in the community. Midwifery care will follow the woman regardless of whether she needs or wants to give birth in hospital. Increasingly, midwives will encourage women to see home birth as a safe choice for uncomplicated childbirth. Final decisions about the place of birth can be left for the woman to make during labour, thereby ensuring that she keeps all her options open. Inevitably this will mean an increase in the rate of home birth. It will also mean that midwives move more freely between hospitals and the community. Thus the conventional 'community midwife', as discreetly different from her hospital counterpart, may disappear.

References

AIMS (Association for Improvements in Maternity Services) (undated) *Choosing a Home Birth*. London: AIMS.

Allison, J. (1992) Midwives step out of the shadows. *Midwives Chronicle* 105(1254): 167–174.

ARM (Association of Radical Midwives) (1986) *The Vision: Proposals for the Future of the Maternity Services*. ARM, 62 Greetby Hill, Ormskirk, Lancashire, L39 2DT.

Ball, J., Flint, C., Garvey, M., Jackson-Baker, A. & Page, L.A. (1992) *Whose Left Holding the Baby? An Organisational Framework for Making the Most of Midwifery Services*. University of Leeds: The Nuffield Institute for Health Services Studies.

Bowler, I.M.W. (1993) Stereotypes of women of Asian descent in midwifery: some evidence. *Midwifery* 9(1): 7–16.

Campbell, R. & Macfarlane, A. (1994) *Where to be Born?: The Debate and the Evidence*, 2nd edn. Oxford: National Perinatal Epidemiology Unit.

Campbell, R., MacDonald Davies, I., Macfarlane, A. & Beral, V. (1984) Home Births in England and Wales, 1979: perinatal mortality according to intended place of delivery. *Br. Med. J.* 289: 721–724.

Cronk, M. & Flint, C. (1989) *Community Midwifery: A Practical Guide*. London: Heinemann Medical Books.

Davies, J. (1992) The role of the midwife in the 1990s. In Chard, T. & Richards, M.P.M. (eds) *Obstetrics in the 1990s*. London: MacKeith Press.

DOH (Department of Health) (1993a) *Changing Childbirth*. Report of the Expert Maternity Group. London: HMSO.

DOH (1993b) *Report of the Chief Medical Officer's Expert Group on Sleeping Position of Infants and Cot Death*. London: HMSO.

Durand, A.M. (1992) The safety of home birth: the Farm study. *Am. J. Public Health* 82(3): 450–453.

Flint, C. (1993) *Midwifery Teams and Caseloads*. Oxford: Butterworth Heinemann.

Flint, C., Poulengeris, P. & Grant, A. (1989) The 'Know your Midwife' Scheme – a randomised control trial of continuity of care by a team of midwives. *Midwifery* 5: 11–16.

Ford, C., Iliffe, S. & Franklin, O. (1991) Outcome of planned home births in an inner city practice. *Br. Med. J.* 303: 1517–1519.

Gaskin, I.M. (1990) *Spiritual Midwifery*, 3rd edn. Summertown, TN: The Book Publishing Company.

Green, J.M., Kitzinger, J.V. & Coupland, V.A. (1990) Stereotypes of childbearing women: a look at some evidence. *Midwifery* 6(3): 125–132.

Grevatt, H. (1992) The baby blues club. *Nursing Times* 88(39): 46–47.

House of Commons Health Committee (1992) *Maternity Services Second Report* (Winterton Report) (Chairman, Sir Nicholas Winterton). London: HMSO.

Keats, J. (1993) The team approach to giving midwifery care for the 1990s. *Midwives Chronicle* 106(1261): 46–48.

Kindred, M. (1985) *Once upon a Group*. Available from the author at 20 Dover Street, Southwell, Notts NG25 0EZ (£4.50 & 50p p&p).

Kitzinger, S. (1991) *Homebirth and Other Alternatives to Hospital*. London: Dorling Kindersley.

Leap, N. (1991) *Helping You to Make Your Own Decisions – Antenatal and Postnatal Groups in South East London*. VHS Video and Video Notes. Available from SELMGP, The Albany, Douglas Way, Deptford, London SE5 4AG.

Leap, N. (1992a) *Home Birth Your Choice*. VHS Video and Video Notes. Available from SELMGP, The Albany, Douglas Way, Deptford, London SE5 4AG.

Leap, N. (1992b) The power of words. *Nursing Times* 88(21): 60–61.

Leap, N. (1994) Caseload practice within the NHS: are midwives ready and interested? *Midwives Chronicle* 107 (1275): 130–135.

Leap, N. & Hunter, B. (1993) *The Midwife's Tale: An Oral History From Handywoman to Professional Midwife*. London: Scarlet Press.

MacKeith, P., Phillipson, R. & Rowe, A. (1991) *45, Cope Street: Young mothers learning through group work An evaluation report*. Nottingham Community Health, Memorial House, Standard Hill, Nottingham, NG1 6FX (£5 & £1 p&p).

MacVicar, J., Dobbie, G., Owen-Johnstone, L., Jagger, C., Hopkins, M. & Kennedy, J. (1993) Simulated home delivery in hospital: a randomised controlled trial. *Br. J. Obstet. Gynaecol.* **100**: 316–323.

McKee, I.H. (1984) Community antenatal care: the Sighthill Community Antenatal Scheme. In Zander, L. & Chamberlain, G. (eds) *Pregnancy Care for the 1980s*. London: Royal Society of Medicine, Macmillan Press.

MIDIRS (Midwives Information and Resource Service) (1991) *Directory of Maternity Organisations*, 4th edn. MIDIRS, 9 Elmdale Road, Clifton, Bristol, BS8 1SL.

Ministry of Health (1959) *Report of the Maternity Services Committee* (Cranbrook Report) (Chairman, Lord Cranbrook). London: HMSO.

Murphy-Black, T. & Faulkner, A. (1988) *Antenatal Group Skills Training: A Manual of Guidelines*. Chichester: John Wiley & Sons.

Oakley, A. (1992) *Social Support and Motherhood*. Oxford: Blackwell.

O'Brien, C. (1993) Division of labour. *Nursing Times* **89**(14): 48–50.

Odent, M. (1984) *Birth Reborn: What Birth Can and Should Be*. London: Souvenir Press.

Priest, J. & Schott, J. (1991) *Leading Antenatal Classes*. Oxford: Butterworth Heinemann.

Protrykus, C. (1990) Post natal depression: does it exist? *Health Visitor* **63**(5): 154–155.

RCM (Royal College of Midwives) (1987) *Towards a Healthy Nation*. RCM, 15 Mansfield Street, London W1M 0BE.

RCM (1991) *Towards a Healthy Nation*, 2nd edn. RCM, 15 Mansfield Street, London W1M 0BE.

RCM (1993) *Audit of Independent Midwifery 1989–1991*. RCM, 15 Mansfield Street, London W1M 0BE.

Reid, T. (1994) A bid for independence. *Nursing Times* **90**(30): 18.

Social Services Committee (1980) *Perinatal and Neonatal Mortality. Second Report from the Social Services Committee* Session 1979–80, vol. 1 Cmmd 663–I (Short Report) (Chairman, Renee Short). London: HMSO.

Simkin, P. (1986) Stress, pain and catecholamines. *Birth* **13**(4): 227–240.

Stone, Y. (1990) Riverside midwifery team approach. *Maternity Action* **44**: 6–7.

Standing Maternity and Midwifery Advisory Committee (1970) *Domiciliary Midwifery and Maternity Bed Needs* (Peel Report) (Chairman, Sir John Peel). London: HMSO.

Tew, M. (1978) The case against hospital deliveries: the new statistical evidence. In Kitzinger, S. & Davis, J.A. (eds) *The Place of Birth*. Oxford: Oxford University Press.

Tew, M. (1990) *Safer Childbirth? A Critical History of Maternity Care*. London: Chapman & Hall.

Tew, M. & Damstra-Wijmenga, S.M.I. (1991) Safest birth attendants: recent Dutch evidence. *Midwifery* **7**(2): 55–63.

Towler, J. & Bramall, J. (1986) *The Midwife in History and Society*. London, Croom Helm.

UKCC (United Kingdom Central Council for Nursing Midwifery and Health Visiting) (1993) *Midwives' Rules*. London: UKCC.

UKCC (1994) *A Midwife's Code of Practice*. London: UKCC.

Watson, P. (1990) *Report of the Kidlington Midwifery Scheme*. Institute of Nursing, Radcliffe Infirmary, Woodstock Road, Oxford OX2 6HE.

Welsh Planning Forum (1991) *Protocol for Investment in Health Gain – Maternal and Child Health*. Welsh Office.

Wesson, N. (1990) *Home Birth: A Practical Guide*. London: Optima.

Williams, J. (1991) Day by day. *Professional Care of Mother and Child* **1**(3): 124.

Wraight, A., Ball, J., Seccombe, I. & Stock, J. (1993) *Mapping Team Midwifery*. Brighton: Institute of Management Studies.

34

The Pelvic Floor and its Injuries

The Pelvic Floor

The structures filling in the bony outlet of the pelvis and extending from the peritoneum above to the skin below are known collectively as the pelvic floor. In midwifery practice the most important of these structures are those which support the pelvic organs and prevent them from prolapsing. These are sheets of overlapping muscle fibres which line the walls and floors of the pelvic cavity. The pelvic floor muscles support the pelvic organs and are critical for the long-term health and functional capacity of the uterus, vagina, bladder and rectum. During labour, spontaneous pushing, without any additional downward pressure from conscious forced contractions of abdominal muscles, has been shown to increase the incidence of spontaneous delivery and to minimize damage to the pelvic floor and its attached organs following childbirth.

The bony pelvis is lined by muscles. The posterior wall of the pelvis is lined by the pyriformis and ischio-coccygeus muscles. The larger, superior section of the lateral walls are lined by the obturator internus and the pyriformis muscles, while the inferior sections are lined by the levator ani. The obturator internus muscle is covered by heavy fascia that gives rise to the levator ani. Most of the pelvic floor is formed by the levator ani.

STRUCTURE

From above, downwards, the pelvic floor consists of the following layers.

Pelvic peritoneum

This is described as hanging over the uterus and uterine tubes, like a sheet over a clothes line. In front, it forms the *uterovesical pouch* and covers the upper surface of the bladder; at the back, it dips down behind the posterior vaginal fornix, forming the *pouch of Douglas* and then passes over the rectum. The peritoneal coverings of the uterine tubes are called the *broad ligaments*, but in spite of their name they do not act as supports.

Pelvic fascia

The connective tissue which fills in the space between the pelvic organs condenses to form strong ligaments which support the uterus.

Transverse cervical ligaments These ligaments are also known as the *cardinal* and *Mackenrodt's ligaments*. They extend fan-wise from the cervix and vagina to the side walls of the pelvis. These are the principal direct supports of the uterus.

Uterosacral ligaments These run backwards and upwards from the cervix, encircling the rectum to attach to the anterior part of the sacrum.

Pubocervical ligaments These run from the cervix passing beneath the bladder to attach to the pubic bones.

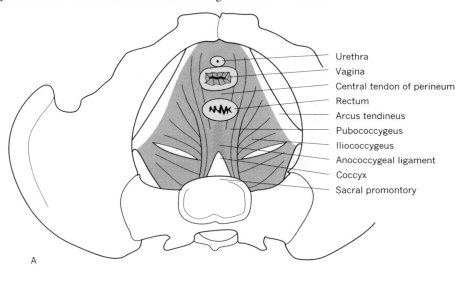

Urethra
Vagina
Central tendon of perineum
Rectum
Arcus tendineus
Pubococcygeus
Iliococcygeus
Anococcygeal ligament
Coccyx
Sacral promontory

A

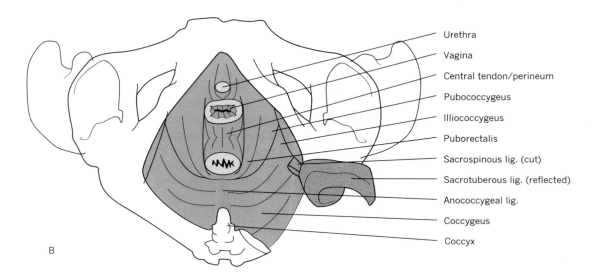

Urethra
Vagina
Central tendon/perineum
Pubococcygeus
Illiococcygeus
Puborectalis
Sacrospinous lig. (cut)
Sacrotuberous lig. (reflected)
Anococcygeal lig.
Coccygeus
Coccyx

B

Figure 1 Muscles of the pelvic diaphragm. **A**: Superior view; **B**: inferior view. (Reproduced with permission from Gabbe, S.G., Niebyl, J.R. & Simpson, J.L. (eds) (1991) *Obstetrics: Normal and Problem Pregnancies*, pp. 6–7. New York: Churchill Livingstone.)

These three pairs of ligaments act as a kind of hammock, holding the uterus at the level of the supra-vaginal cervix, so that while it is quite mobile, it cannot prolapse.

Round ligaments   These originate near the fundus of the uterus, passing through the inguinal canal and anterior abdominal wall to end in the labia majora. They assist in keeping the uterus in its normal ante-verted (forward tilted) anteflexed (bent on itself) position.

Deep muscle layer

The deep muscle layer consists of two *levator ani* muscles (Figure 1). Each arises from the back of the pubic bone, along the 'white line' of the obturator fascia, and from the ischial spine. They pass down-wards and backwards around the vagina to meet in the perineal body, then around the anal canal, finally being inserted in the coccyx and lower sacrum. The two muscles thus form a strong muscular sling which effectively supports the vaginal walls, and, indirectly, the uterus. The anal canal is also strongly supported, and the bladder receives some support. In these two levator ani muscles, then, lies the main strength of the pelvic floor.

They are divided into three individual muscles: the pubococcygeus, iliococcygeus and ischiococcygeus:

► Each *pubococcygeus* muscle forms the more anterior section of the levator ani. They arise from the posterior surface of the pubic bone and pass back-wards on either side of the urethra, the lowest third of the vagina and the anal canal before the longest fibres are inserted into the anococcygeal body and the coccyx.

► Each *iliococcygeus* muscle forms a broad posterior section of the levator ani. They arise from the white line of pelvic fascia and pass downwards and inwards to be inserted into the anococcygeal body and the coccyx.

► Each *ischiococcygeus* muscle arises from the ischial spines and passes downwards and inwards to be inserted into the coccyx and lower part of the sacrum.

Superficial perineal muscles

These muscles, though small, contribute appreciably to the total strength of the pelvic floor (Figure 2).

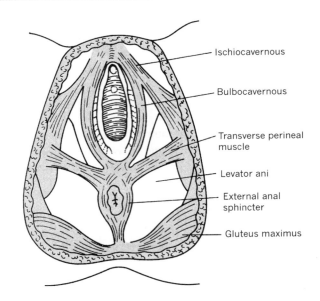

Figure 2   The perineal muscles.

► The two *bulbocavernosus muscles* extend from the perineal body around the vagina to the clitoris. They act like a sphincter around the vagina and urethra.

► The two *ischiocavernosus muscles* pass from the ischial tuberosities to the clitoris. Their fascia extends across the pubic arch to form the *triangular ligament*, which supports the neck of the bladder and assists in the control of micturition.

► The *transverse perineal muscles* pass from the ischial tuberosities to the perineal body. They provide additional support transversely across the perineal region.

► The *external anal sphincter* surrounds the anal orifice, being embedded in front in the perineal body and attached behind to the coccyx. It controls the passage of faeces and flatus.

► The *membranous sphincter of the urethra* is formed by two bands of muscle which arise from one pubic bone and pass above and below the urethra and are inserted into the other pubic bone.

Superficial fascia and fat and skin

Neither of these has any supporting function.

BLOOD, LYMPH AND NERVE SUPPLY

Blood is supplied from branches of the internal iliac arteries and venous drainage is into corresponding veins. Lymph drains into the internal iliac glands.

Fibres from the third and fourth sacral nerves and the pudendal nerve supply the pelvic floor.

FUNCTIONS

The pelvic floor (Figure 3) forms a diaphragm which closes the outlet of the bony pelvis, and its primary function is to act as a support for the pelvic organs, namely the vagina, the uterus, the bladder and the rectum.

The pelvic floor counteracts changes of intra-abdominal pressure which occur when the abdominal muscles contract, as they do in coughing, laughing or lifting heavy objects. If, through childbearing, the bladder and urethral supports are weakened, coughing and sneezing will cause urine to dribble involuntarily from the bladder (*stress incontinence*). This is a common complication following childbirth (MacArthur *et al.*, 1993). In a large study of 1278 respondents to a questionnaire survey conducted 6–7 months after delivery, one in five women reported that they had experienced stress incontinence, and three quarters of these women were still symptomatic (MacArthur *et al.*, 1993).

During the course of pregnancy the pelvic floor becomes softened and relaxed. This, incidentally, makes pelvic examinations, if required, easier for the midwife or doctor and less uncomfortable for the woman when made in late pregnancy rather than in the early stages; however, the purpose of this relaxation is to permit the tremendous amount of stretching which must occur in labour to allow the fetus to be born. Because of its remarkable elasticity, the pelvic floor is able, after labour, to resume its original sup-porting function in a surprisingly short time. Postnatal exercises promote the return to effective function and help to prevent any long-term urinary problems and prolapse (Brayshaw and Wright, 1994).

PERINEAL BODY

The perineal body is a wedge-shaped mass of muscular and fibrous tissue lying between the lowest part of the vagina and the anal canal. It is an integral part of the pelvic floor, since it is the central point where both the levator ani and most of the superficial muscles unite. Injury to the perineal body thus weakens the pelvic floor as a whole, and even apparently trivial injuries should be regarded seriously.

The perineal body is triangular in shape, the base being the skin and the apex pointing upwards. Each side of the triangle measures approximately 3.8 cm in length. It consists of an outer layer of skin and the following superficial and deep muscles of the pelvic floor:

Bulbocavernosus	
Transverse perinei }	Superficial muscles
Pubococcygeus	Deep muscle

The perineal body assists in defecation and in childbirth. Blood is supplied by the pudendal arteries and venous drainage is into the corresponding veins. Lymph drains into the inguinal and external iliac glands. The nerve supply is derived from the perineal branch of the pudendal nerve.

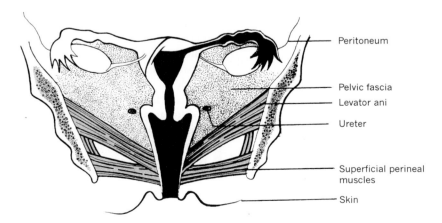

Peritoneum
Pelvic fascia
Levator ani
Ureter
Superficial perineal muscles
Skin

Figure 3   The layers of the pelvic floor.

Perineal Trauma

Perineal trauma may be caused by:

► Perineal laceration.
► Episiotomy.

LACERATIONS OF THE GENITAL TRACT

Perineal lacerations

Lacerations of the perineum may be classified as follows:

► *First-degree laceration* involves the skin of the fourchette only.
► *Second-degree laceration* (and episiotomy) involves the skin of the fourchette, the perineum and perineal body. The superficial muscles involved are the bulbocavernosus and the transverse perinei and the deep muscle, the pubococcygeus.
► *Third-degree laceration* involves the skin of the fourchette, the perineum, the perineal body and the anal sphincter.
► *Fourth-degree laceration* includes all the above structures and extends into the rectal mucosa.

Some classify perineal lacerations into three categories only, the third including both the anal sphincter and any involvement of the rectal mucosa.

Labial lacerations

Lacerations of the labia are very superficial, but, like skin grazes, rather painful. They are not sutured but kept clean and dry, and analgesics are given for the discomfort, if required.

Vaginal and cervical lacerations

If these occur they are sutured immediately as they can cause serious bleeding. There is no further treatment other than good vulval hygiene to reduce the risk of infection.

EPISIOTOMY

An episiotomy is an incision through the perineum and perineal body, equivalent to a second-degree laceration. It is performed immediately prior to delivery, where indicated, to enlarge the vulval outlet for the birth. The UKCC permits the midwife to perform an episiotomy, following the infiltration of the perineum if time permits. The rate of episiotomy rose considerably in the 1970s and 1980s and reached a level of approximately 50% of all deliveries (Sleep, 1984a,b). In some maternity hospitals in the UK a rate as high as 90% was suggested (Reading *et al.*, 1982; Buchan and Nicholls, 1980). The West Berkshire Perineal Management Trial (Sleep *et al.*, 1984) compared the liberal and restrictive use of episiotomy for maternal indications in otherwise normal deliveries. The findings provide little support for the liberal use of episiotomy in otherwise normal deliveries and it is therefore recommended that its use should be restricted to fetal indications only. These findings are supported by the study conducted by Harrison *et al.* (1984). In the Sleep study (Sleep *et al.*, 1984) women were followed up after delivery and it was found that both the liberal and restricted groups experienced a comparable amount of pain assessed at 10 days and three months postpartum, and there were no differences in the reported incidence of dyspareunia or of urinary symptoms three months after delivery. Since the publication of these and other reports (Begley, 1986), and the widespread publicity, there has been a marked reduction in the episiotomy rate in the UK.

Begley (1987) conducted a further study six months after her first to ascertain whether any change had taken place in episiotomy, laceration and intact perineum rates following the dissemination of the findings of her previous study. There had been a significant reduction in episiotomy rate from 54% to 34% for primigravidae, from 25% to 7% for those in the para 1 group, and from 5% to 2% for those of greater parity. No increase in lacerations requiring sutures was found.

A more recent study in Denmark also found that a reduction in the episiotomy rate increased the incidence of women with an intact perineum, without a concomitant rise in tears of the anal sphincter (Henriksen *et al.*, 1994). An episiotomy rate of no lower than 20–30% is recommended in this study to avoid an increase in tears of the anal sphincter.

Nowadays women should be well-informed about episiotomy at delivery and many will make an informed choice about this intervention which is recorded on their birth plan. The midwife should support the woman in her choice and have established a good relationship of mutual trust and co-operation with her so that, if unexpected events occur in labour, they are fully explained and any necessary changes in the plan are agreed.

Indications

The indications for episiotomy should be mainly for fetal complications, which include the following:

▶ To speed delivery when the fetal head is on the perineum and there is evidence of fetal distress.
▶ To reduce the risk of intracranial damage to the fetus in preterm labour and breech delivery.

Other possible indications (but each should be assessed individually):

▶ To reduce the effort involved in bearing down in cases of hypertensive or cardiac disease.
▶ To expedite delivery in cases of maternal distress.
▶ To aid delivery if there is *serious* delay in the second stage of labour. Occasionally this is due to a rigid perineum.
▶ To prevent perineal trauma following previous major surgical repair of the pelvic floor, e.g. third or fourth degree tear, fistula or bladder repair. An elective Caesarean section may be preferable in these cases.

Discussion

One of the commonest reasons given for performing an episiotomy is to prevent a perineal laceration, the rationale behind this being that a clean cut heals better than an uncontrolled tear. However, research carried out by Sleep (1984a,b) and Harrison *et al.* (1984) disproves this reason for making an episiotomy. The findings in Sleep's study show that the policy of using episiotomy to prevent tears does not result in less trauma, improved healing and fewer maternal problems such as urinary incontinence and dyspareunia. Nor do spontaneous tears cause less discomfort than an episiotomy. Harrison *et al.* (1984) also found that the degrees of pain, bruising and swelling, and the administration of analgesics were no greater in mothers who had sustained a second-degree tear than in those who had had an episiotomy. Healing of the perineal wound was similar in the two groups. Other studies question the benefits of episiotomy (Gass *et al.*, 1986; Thorp and Bowes, 1989; Larsson *et al.*, 1991; Henriksen *et al.*, 1992). The high level of pain experienced by women after episiotomy (Reading *et al.*, 1982) has led others to express the need for firm evidence that this procedure is of benefit to women.

Wilkerson (1984) suggests that the practice of setting a time limit on the second stage is a common reason for midwives performing an episiotomy. Her study indicates that there are wide variations in practice amongst midwives, some performing episiotomy more frequently than others, regardless of the condition of mother and baby. Many midwives now are being encouraged to audit their practice and justify the decisions and actions they take.

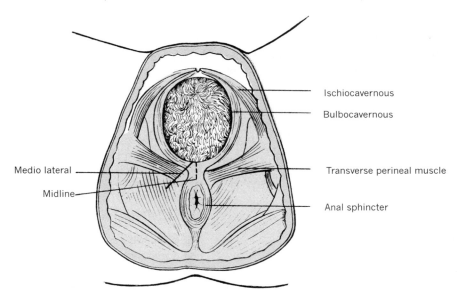

Figure 4   Episiotomy.

Anatomical structures

When an episiotomy is made the scissors cut through the fourchette, posterior vaginal wall, perineal muscles and skin. The midwife must be able to locate the position of the muscles in this area when the perineum is distended and to know with certainty where the external anal sphincter muscle, which extends for 2.5 cm around the anus, and the Bartholin's glands lie (Figure 4).

Types of incision

There are two main types of incision:

1 *Mediolateral episiotomy* (sometimes called postero-lateral): This incision starts at the midline and runs backwards to a point midway between the ischial tuberosity and anus. This is the method most commonly used in the UK because it avoids damage to Bartholin's gland and is thought to be more unlikely to extend and involve the anal sphincter, although this is questionable. In a study conducted by Sultan *et al.* (1994) on women who had sustained a third-degree tear, 42% of the women had had a posterolateral episiotomy.

2 *Midline episiotomy*: This is a midline incision, easy to do, but considered more likely to lead to a third-degree tear if it extends during delivery. A study in the USA found that more third-degree tears occurred in women who had a midline episiotomy than in those who had a mediolateral episiotomy (Coats *et al.*, 1980). An advantage of the midline episiotomy is that it bleeds very little; it is also easy to repair and women seem to experience less discomfort in the puerperium from this type of episiotomy.

Further research is required to establish the advantages and disadvantages of these two methods of episiotomy.

Infiltration of the perineum

This should be carried out before an episiotomy is made. The requirements are:

Lignocaine solution 0.5% or 1%;
10 ml syringe;
Gauge 21 needle 4 cm in length.

After cleansing the skin with an antiseptic solution, the gloved first and second fingers of the left hand are inserted into the vagina to protect the fetal head from the local anaesthetic. Lignocaine 10 ml of 0.5% or 5 ml

of 1%, is usually used for the local anaesthetic. The needle is inserted at the fourchette and, for a medio-lateral episiotomy, is directed at an angle of about 45° from the midline for 4–5 cm, usually on the mother's right side, at the same depth below the skin (Figure 5). The piston is withdrawn before injection of the local anaesthetic to check whether the needle is in a blood vessel. If blood is withdrawn the needle must be repositioned and further checks made until no blood is withdrawn. Then the lignocaine can be injected as the needle is slowly withdrawn. Some practitioners inject all the local anaesthetic along the line for the proposed incision in this way. It is thought to be more effective, however, if only 3–4 ml of the local anaesthetic are injected initially and then, before the tip of the needle is fully withdrawn, it is redirected to first one side of the initial injection for more local anaesthetic to be given and then to the other, so that lignocaine is injected on each side of the first injection in a fan-shape. At least four minutes should elapse to give time for the analgesia to become effective before making the incision.

Incision

Straight, blunt-ended Mayo episiotomy scissors are usually used, or occasionally the doctor may prefer to use a scalpel. The two fingers are inserted as for infiltration to protect the fetal head. The blades are opened and one blade is passed flat along the fingers. They are then rotated so that a deliberate cut can be made 4 cm long through the infiltrated area (Figure 5). The cut should be bold and deliberate and is best made during a contraction when the perineum is well-stretched, bleeding is reduced and, if the local anaesthetic is not fully effective, pain is minimized. Delivery is likely to follow immediately and the midwife must be prepared to control the head to prevent sudden expulsion which may cause an extension of the episiotomy. If there is any delay in the delivery, pressure should be applied to the episiotomy between contractions to control bleeding, which may be considerable.

SUTURING THE PERINEUM

Midwives who have been taught to suture the perineum and pronounced proficient may carry out the procedure (Figure 6). However, they should be aware of any limitations imposed on their practice by their employing authority. Many midwives feel that whoever performs the delivery should carry out any perineal

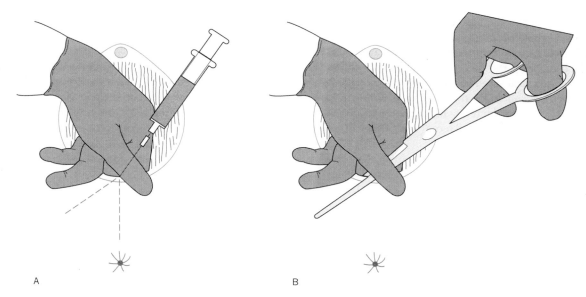

Figure 5   **A**: Infiltration of the perineum. **B**: Making a mediolateral incision.

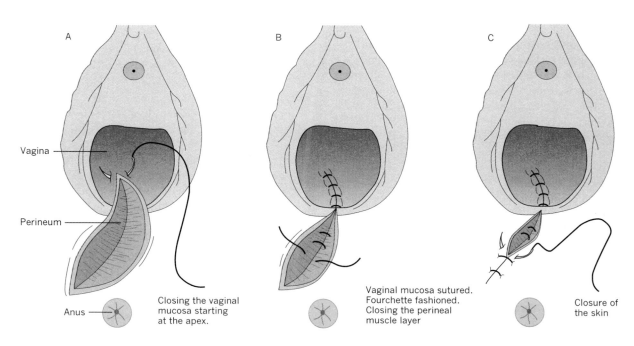

Vagina

Perineum

Anus

Closing the vaginal mucosa starting at the apex.

Vaginal mucosa sutured. Fourchette fashioned. Closing the perineal muscle layer

Closure of the skin

Figure 6   Suturing the perineum. **A**: Closing the vaginal mucosa, starting at the apex. **B**: Vaginal mucosa sutured, fourchette fashioned, closing the perineal muscle layer. **C**: Closure of the skin.

suturing that is required as this gives continuity of care (Cunningham, 1984). An advantage of the midwife suturing the perineum is that it is often carried out more promptly than when the doctor has to be summoned.

Technique

The repair is carried out under aseptic conditions with the mother in lithotomy position under a good light. In situations where lithotomy position is not possible, the woman can lie sideways across a bed with her buttocks at the edge of the bed and her legs wide apart with her feet on chairs. An antiseptic such as chlorhexidine is usually used to clean the perineal area, but a recent study comparing the use of tap water with chlorhexidine for perineal cleansing before delivery and perineal suturing concludes that tap water is as effective, and there was no increase in perineal infections or neonatal eye infections (Hervé and Parkin, 1994). Further studies are required.

After cleansing the perineal area and applying sterile drapes a local anaesthetic, usually 10–30 ml of lignocaine 0.5 or 1%, is injected into the perineal muscles and under the skin. Adequate time must be allowed for it to take effect fully, usually four minutes or so. If the mother has an epidural in progress local infiltration will not be necessary, but the epidural may need to be topped-up to give effective analgesia. A taped vaginal tampon is usually inserted into the vagina to prevent blood oozing down and obscuring the wound. The tape should be attached to the drapes with a pair of forceps to remind the midwife to remove the tampon on completion of the suturing. A record is made of the insertion of the tampon, and later of its removal.

The extent of the wound is explored by parting the tissues with the fingers, or with the aid of artery forceps, to expose the upper limit. If, on examination, the midwife finds extensive vaginal lacerations or a third-degree tear, she should call an experienced doctor who will be responsible for the repair.

Suture materials

The choice of suturing material should be based on current research. Chalmers *et al.* (1989) reviewed absorbable suture materials used for perineal suturing and concluded that polyglycolic acid sutures such as Dexon or Vicryl should be used for perineal repair of both the deep layers and the skin, rather than chromic or plain catgut. One of the main advantages of polyglycolic acid suturing materials is that women have less perineal pain in the early puerperium, but it is frequently necessary to remove the sutures within the first 10 days after delivery because of irritation and tightness (Mahomed *et al.*, 1989). Resuturing, however, was less common when polyglycolic acid suturing materials were used (Banninger *et al.*, 1978; Mahomed *et al.*, 1989). Another study compared the use of repairing all layers of the perineum with glycerol–impregnated catgut and chromic catgut (Grant *et al.*, 1989). The use of glycerol–impregnated catgut was found to be asso-

ciated with significantly more pain 10 days after delivery and a higher incidence of dyspareunia three months after delivery. Grant *et al.* (1989) found in a three-year follow-up study that dyspareunia persisted in women who had been sutured with glycerol-impregnated catgut. An overview of studies comparing the use of absorbable skin sutures with those which are non-absorbable found that polyglycolic acid sutures (absorbable) again are associated with less pain in the early puerperium than both silk and polyamide nylon (non-absorbable) sutures (Grant, 1989).

A further study comparing Vicryl (polyglycolic material) and the use of black silk for perineal skin suturing after delivery has been conducted by Roberts *et al.* (1993). In this study the mothers were followed up at five days and three months after delivery. The results concluded that perineal pain at five days was reduced with subcuticular polyglactin 910 (Vicryl). At three months sexual problems (persistent dyspareunia and non-resumption of sexual intercourse) were also reduced, although these findings were not statistically significant. These results support the use of subcuticular polyglactin 910 (Vicryl) for repair of the perineum. The strength of this study was the high rate of follow-up at three months (92%) by the three midwife researchers in the team.

The wound is repaired in three layers, taking care to ensure correct anatomical apposition (Figure 6).

1 Starting at the apex of the wound, the vaginal submucosa is sutured and continued down to the level of the fourchette. A review of studies on perineal suturing techniques (Chalmers *et al.*, 1989) concludes that continuous, subcuticular sutures are associated with less pain in the early postnatal period than interrupted transcutaneous sutures (Banninger *et al.*, 1978; Isager-Sally *et al.*, 1986; Mahomed *et al.*, 1989). There appears to be no significant differences between the two suturing techniques with regard to long-term pain and dyspareunia. Careful suturing is essential to avoid dead space where blood can collect.

2 Next the deeper perineal muscles are sutured, preferably using continuous, subcuticular sutures in the light of the above findings.

3 Finally the skin is sutured using a similar technique, using polyglycolic acid sutures such as Dexon or Vicryl which are absorbable, in preference to other suturing materials (see above).

It is important to ensure that the sutures are not too tight, otherwise they will be very painful.

On completion of the suturing the vaginal pack is removed and the vagina should easily admit two fingers. A gloved finger is also inserted into the rectum to detect any sutures which have inadvertently extended to involve the rectal tissues. If present they must be removed and the perineum resutured. On completion the suture line is cleaned and covered with a sterile pad.

The midwife records the procedure in the mother's notes, including the number of skin sutures inserted and the removal of the vaginal tampon.

THIRD- AND FOURTH-DEGREE TEARS

Third- or fourth-degree tears occur in about 0.6% of vaginal deliveries (Haadem *et al.*, 1991; Sultan *et al.*, 1994). They are severe perineal injuries which must be repaired by a senior obstetrician under an epidural or a general anaesthetic. Anal incontinence is a serious complication. Risk factors associated with third- or fourth-degree tears are:

▶ forceps delivery, which has a higher risk of resulting in severe perineal trauma than vacuum extraction (Johanson *et al.*, 1993; Sultan and Kamm, 1993; Sultan *et al.*, 1994);
▶ primiparous women;
▶ birthweight greater than 4 kg;
▶ occipitoposterior position at delivery (Sultan *et al.*, 1994).

A third- or fourth-degree tear may occur, however, without the presence of any of these risk factors.

Sultan *et al.* (1994) found in their study of 50 women who had sustained a third- or fourth-degree tear over a two and a half year period that a significant number had residual sphincter defects and about half were experiencing anal incontinence due to persistent anatomical sphincter disruption. In all cases the tears had been repaired by an obstetrician immediately after delivery. Nearly three quarters of the women (72%) in this study had had a posterolateral episiotomy. This study highlights the need to prevent severe perineal injury and review the methods employed for sphincter repair.

After care

A full explanation of the injury sustained must be given to the woman and she will require considerable support and understanding as she will no doubt be anxious and perhaps upset. A broad-spectrum antibiotic is usually prescribed for a week because the risk of infection is high. An aperient to soften the stools, such as lactulose, is also prescribed for 1–2 weeks.

Complications include infection, the development of a fistula and defecatory problems which may be long-term. Psychological problems may also occur. Follow-up is essential to detect any long-term sequelae. Many women are embarrassed to say that they have faecal incontinence and so should be asked directly about this symptom at their postnatal examination.

Careful assessment of the integrity of the anal sphincter by physiological tests and ultrasound should be made in a subsequent pregnancy on women with long-term defecation problems and the mode of delivery decided on the findings of this examination, as well as on other factors.

PROLAPSE

Prolonged, repeated or extreme stretching of the pelvic floor muscles causes permanent damage in that they never regain their former tone and elasticity. If these muscles fail to support the pelvic organs, prolapse results. This may occur in the course of a prolonged or difficult labour, especially if the baby is very large. More commonly it occurs in women who have had many deliveries (*grande multiparae*).

In *uterovaginal prolapse*, the vaginal walls are weakened and the uterus lies lower than normal. In *cystocele* the upper anterior vaginal wall is lax and allows the bladder to bulge into the vagina. In *urethrocele* the urethra bulges into the lower anterior vaginal wall. In *rectocele*, the posterior vaginal wall is damaged and the rectum bulges into the vagina. Surgical repair is usually required.

The mode of delivery in a subsequent pregnancy will be carefully considered to try to minimize further damage.

References

Banninger, V., Buhrig, H. & Schreiner, W.E. (1978) A comparison between catgut and polyglycolic acid sutures in episiotomy repair. *Geburtshilfe Frauenheilkd* **30**: 30–33.

Begley, C.M. (1986) Episiotomy – use or abuse? *Nursing Rev.* **4**: 4–7.

Begley, C.M. (1987) Episiotomy – A change in midwives' practice. *Irish Nursing Forum and Health Services* **5**(6): 12–14.

Brayshaw, E. & Wright, P. (1994) *Teaching Physical Skills for the Childbearing Year*, pp. 82–83. Hale: Books for Midwives Press.

Buchan, P.C. & Nicholls, J.A.J. (1980) Pain after episiotomy – a comparison of two methods of repair. *Gen. Pract.* **30**: 297–300.

Chalmers, I., Enkin, M. & Keirse, M.J.N.C. (1989) *Effective Care in Pregnancy and Childbirth*, Vol. 2, pp. 1136–1137 & pp. 1173–1179. Oxford: Oxford University Press.

Coats, P.M., Chan, K.K., Wilkins, M. & Beard, R.J. (1980) A comparison between midline and mediolateral episiotomy. *Br. J. Obstet. Gynaecol.* **87**: 408–412.

Cunningham, A. (1984) Perineal damage in childbirth. *Nursing Mirror* **158**(11): Suppl. i–ix.

Gass, M.S., Dunn, C. & Stys, S.J. (1986) Effect of episiotomy on the frequency of vaginal outlet lacerations. *J. Reprod. Med.* **31**: 240–244.

Grant, A. (1986) Repair of episiotomy and perineal tears. *Br. J. Obstet. Gynaecol.* **93**: 417–419.

Grant, A. (1989) The choice of suture materials and techniques for repair of perineal trauma: an overview of the evidence from controlled trials. *Br. J. Obstet. Gynaecol.* **96**: 1281–1289.

Grant, A., Sleep, J., Ashurst, H. & Spencer, J.A.D. (1989) Dyspareunia associated with the use of glycerol-impregnated catgut to repair perineal trauma – report of three-year follow-up study. *Br. J. Obstet. Gynaecol* **96**: 741–743.

Haadem, K., Dahlstrom, J.A. & Lennart, A. (1991) Anal sphincter competence in healthy women: clinical implications of age and other factors. *Obstet. Gynecol.* **78**: 823–827.

Harrison, R.F., Brennan, M., North, P.M., Reed, J.V. & Wickham, E.A. (1984) Is routine episiotomy necessary? *Br. Med. J.* **288**: 1971–1975.

Henriksen, T.B., Bek, K.M., Hedegaard, M. & Secher, N.J. (1992) Episiotomy and perineal lesions in spontaneous vaginal deliveries. *Br. J. Obstet. Gynaecol.* **99**: 950–954.

Henriksen, T.B., Bek, K.M., Hedegaard, M. & Secher, N.J. (1994) Methods and consequences of changes in use of episiotomy. *Br. Med. J.* **309**: 1255–1258.

Hervé, J. & Parkin, J. (1994) Perineal cleansing with tap water prior to normal and forceps delivery and perineal suturing.

In *MIRIAD, 1994*, pp. 247–249. Hale: Books for Midwives Press.

Isagar-Sally, L., Legarth, J., Jacobson, B. & Bustofte, E. (1986) Episiotomy repair – immediate and longterm sequelae. A prospective randomized study of three different methods of repair. *Br. J. Obstet. Gynaecol.* **93**: 420–425.

Johanson, R.B., Rice, C., Doyle, M. *et al.* (1993) A randomised prospective study comparing the new vacuum extractor policy with forceps delivery. *Br. J. Obstet. Gynaecol.* **100**: 524–530.

Larsson, P.G., Platz-Christensen, J.J., Bergman, B. & Walstersson, G. (1991) Advantage or disadvantage of episiotomy compared with spontaneous perineal laceration. *Gynecol. Obstet. Invest.* **31**: 213–216.

MacArthur, C., Bick, D. & Lewis, M. (1993) Persistent health problems after childbirth and their effect on women's quality of life. *Research and the Midwife*, Conference Proceedings, Manchester, pp. 18–21.

Mahomed, K., Grant, A., Ashurst, H. & James, D. (1989) Southmead perineal suture trial. *Br. J. Obstet. Gynaecol.* **96**: 1272–1280.

Reading, A.E., Sledmore, C.M., Cox, D.N. & Campbell, S. (1982) How women view post-episiotomy pain. *Br. Med. J.*, **284**: 243–246.

Roberts, M., Richardson, L., Johnson, D., Coleman, S. & Michael, E.M. (1993) A comparison of subcuticular polyglactin 910 (Vicryl) and interrupted black silk for perineal skin closure. *Online J. Curr. Clin. Trials* (serial outline) 1993 September (Doc. No. 90).

Sleep, J. (1984a) Episiotomy in normal delivery, 1. *Nursing Times* **80**(47): 29–30.

Sleep, J. (1984b) Episiotomy in normal delivery, 2. Management of the perineum. *Nursing Times* **80**(48): 51–54.

Sleep, J.M., Grant, A., Garcia, J. *et al.* (1984) West Berkshire perineal management trial. *Br. Med. J.* **289**: 587–590.

Sultan, A.H., Kamm, M.A., Hudson, C.N. & Bartram, C.I. (1994) Third degree obstetric and sphincter tears: risk factors and outcome of primary repair. *Br. Med. J.* **308**: 887–891.

Sultan, A.H. & Kamm, M.A. (1993) Ultrasound of the anal sphincter. In Schuster, M.M. (ed.) *Atlas of Gastrointestinal Motility in Health and Disease*, pp. 115–121. Baltimore: Williams & Wilkins.

Thorp, J.N. Jr. & Bowes, W.A. Jr. (1989) Episiotomy: can its routine use be defended? *Am. J. Obstet. Gynecol.* **160**: 1027–1030.

Wilkerson, V.A. (1984) The use of episiotomy in normal delivery. *Midwives Chronicle* and *Nursing Notes*, April: 1984: 106–110.

The Puerperium and Midwifery Practice

35

The Anatomy of the Breast

The breasts are situated on the anterior chest wall on either side of the midline. They lie above the pectoralis muscle. At birth they consist of a nipple and a few rudimentary ducts. No further development occurs until puberty, when under the influence of the ovarian hormones the breasts enlarge and take on the characteristic rounded contour. Full maturity is reached only during pregnancy and lactation. After the menopause the breasts tend to atrophy and much of their adipose tissue is lost.

The mature breast extends from the second to the sixth rib and from the sternum to the axilla (Figure 1). It is hemispherical in shape, radiating upwards and outwards in a tail-like structure called the *axillary tail*. It is this tail that often becomes swollen during the early puerperium causing discomfort. It is also this tail that necessitates the extensive area removed in a radical mastectomy. About the centre of each breast is an area of sensitive erectile tissue, the *nipple*, which is pink in colour but darkens in pregnancy. The nipple is surrounded by a pinkish area known as the *areola*.

Structure

In adult life, the mammary gland is composed of *glandular* and *contractile* cells lying within a supportive framework of *connective* and *adipose* tissue that carries the vascular supply, nerve cells and lymphatic vessels. *Glandular tissue* is organized into numerous ducts that drain clusters of 10–100 alveoli that are formed into lobules. *Contractile tissue* is made up of myoepithelial cells covering the alveoli and small ducts, together with smooth muscle that surrounds the large ducts and blood vessels. The small ducts are lined by secretory cells, whereas larger ducts and sinuses are lined by non-secretory cuboidal epithelium. Each *alveolus* consists of a hollow ball of secretory cells surrounded by a network of contractile myoepithelium and capillaries (Figure 2A). Between 20 and 40 *lobules* – collections of alveoli (Figure 2B) – are grouped into *lobes* and drain into a single *lactiferous duct*. Adjacent lobes are separated by layers of connective and adipose tissue. In the non-pregnant state, this component makes up the largest part of the gland (Figure 3).

The nipple contains openings for approximately 15–20 lactiferous ducts that form into lactiferous sinuses and act as small reservoirs of milk during lactation. This area is covered by stratified squamous epithelium, with numerous papillae or elevations that allow the rich supply of nerve endings to lie close to the skin surface. The surrounding area of pigmented aerola that accommodates sweat and sebaceous glands becomes darker and more pronounced during pregnancy. Beneath the skin, the nipple is composed of connective tissue, smooth muscle fibres and, on the surface, the small

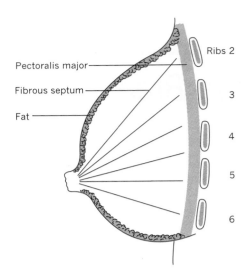

Pectoralis major ——

Fibrous septum ——

Fat ——

Ribs 2

3

4

5

6

Figure 1   The supporting structures of the breast.

openings of sebaceous glands. The latter are known as *Montgomery's glands*. These become enlarged during pregnancy and lubricate the nipple during lactation (Lawrence, 1989; Fuchs, 1991).

The glandular tissue is the functioning part of the breast. It is capable of selecting from the blood in the breast the necessary constituents for preparing milk. The structure of the breast is sometimes referred to as resembling a bunch of grapes closely packed together, the grapes and the stalks corresponding to the groups of secreting glands and the ducts.

There is a rich blood supply from the internal and external mammary and upper intercostal arteries. Blood drains from the breast into a circular vein behind the nipple and thence into the internal mammary and axillary veins. The lymphatic drainage is extensive and the lymphatic drainage systems of the two breasts communicate freely; this accounts for the rapid spread of malignant growth from one breast to another. The breast has a poor nerve supply and its function is controlled by hormones (see Chapter 36).

Changes During Pregnancy

At about the sixth week of pregnancy the breasts become nodular and lumpy due to the growth and enlargement of the ducts and alveoli. Oestrogens are responsible for the growth of the duct system and progesterone for the increase of alveoli. The mother often complains of tenderness and tingling similar to that experienced before a menstrual period. Vascularity increases and the veins are more apparent.

By the 12th week the nipples have become more prominent and the primary areola has become pigmented. Approximately 18 small swellings appear in the areola; these are *Montgomery's tubercles*, enlarged sebaceous glands which lubricate and protect the nipple during suckling. Colostrum is present at 16 weeks and in a primigravida this is diagnostic of pregnancy. By the 24th week there is further pigmentation

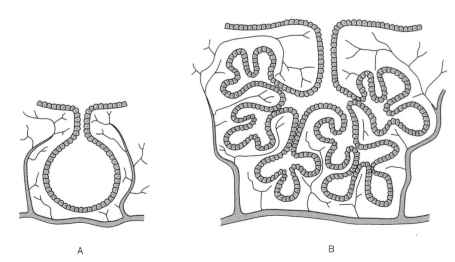

A

B

Figure 2   The structure of the breast. **A**: Single alveolus; **B**: one lobule.

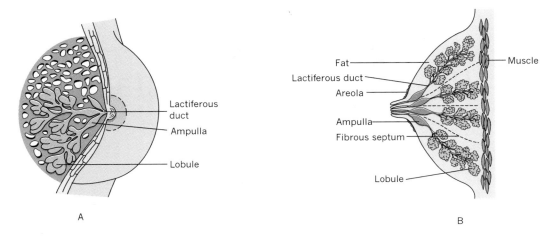

Figure 3   The breast. **A**: The lobes seen from the front; **B**: sagittal section.

around the primary areola known as the secondary areola. The breasts usually enlarge about 5 cm overall and increase by 1400 g in weight; these two factors must be taken into account when buying a brassière.

The brassière needs to be 10 cm larger than usual and the straps at least 2 cm wide to support the weight without cutting the shoulders.

References

Fuchs, A.F. (1991) Physiology and endocrinology of lactation. In Gabbe, S.G., Niebyl, J.R., Simpson, J.L. (eds) *Obstetrics, Normal and Problem Pregnancies*, pp. 175–205. New York: Churchill Livingstone.

Lawrence, R.A. (1989) *Breastfeeding*. St Louis: C.V. Mosby Co.

Further Reading

Carola, R., Harley, J.P. and Noback, C.R. (1992) *Human Anatomy and Physiology*. New York: McGraw-Hill.
Green, J.H. (1981) *Introduction to Human Anatomy*. Oxford: Oxford University Press.
Thirobeau, G.A. and Patton, K.T. (1993) *Anatomy and Physiology*, 2nd edn. St Louis: Mosby.

Verrall, S. (1993) *Anatomy and Physiology Applied to Obstetrics*, 3rd edn. Edinburgh: Churchill Livingstone.
Wilson, K.J.W. (ed.) (1990) *Ross and Wilson's Anatomy and Physiology in Health and Illness*, 7th edn. Edinburgh: Churchill Livingstone.

36

The Physiology of Lactation

The contact established between mother and infant during lactation simultaneously provides for their distinct emotional, sensory and physical needs. For the mother, infant suckling lowers responses to stress; induces feelings of well-being and contentment; enhances the use of energy stores built up in pregnancy; and improves the quality of sleep. For the infant, skin contact provides sensory stimuli that enhances growth and other measures of well-being, while the array of nutritive and non-nutritive substances in milk make up for his or her own immaturities and supply ongoing developmental requirements (Darmady and Postle, 1982; Lebenthal, 1989; Patton *et al.*, 1990; Chiodera *et al.*, 1991; Altemus *et al.*, 1995; Farquharson *et al.*, 1995).

The Initiation of Lactation

Developments in pregnancy and labour set up the conditions needed for lactation. Maternal hormonal and metabolic changes stimulate growth of the mammary gland and the uptake and storage of lipids and other components of milk, particularly in the third trimester. During the latter part of labour, the amplitude of oxytocin pulses increase and both maternal and fetal catecholamine levels are elevated. Over the same period, the stimulatory influence of placental oestrogen on prolactin seems to be overridden by an independent mechanism that is thought to involve a stress-induced rise in dopamine. Circulating levels of prolactin fall sharply and reach lowest levels approximately two hours prior to birth. This pattern is followed by a dramatic rebound that lasts for approximately 2–3 hours after birth. In the absence of any further stimulation by placental oestrogen, prolactin levels subsequently decline. This proceeds rapidly and then more slowly, over a period of 14–26 days, unless secretion is stimulated by infant suckling (Rigg and Yen, 1977).

These hormonal changes indicate that labour and birth stimulate a hormonal profile that enhances the capacity of mother and infant to communicate with each other, particularly in the period immediately following birth. During this time, high levels of catecholamines induce a state of mutual alertness, while oxytocin enhances maternal behaviour. Over the same period, prolactin levels remain elevated and are easily stimulated by short periods of suckling (Figure 1).

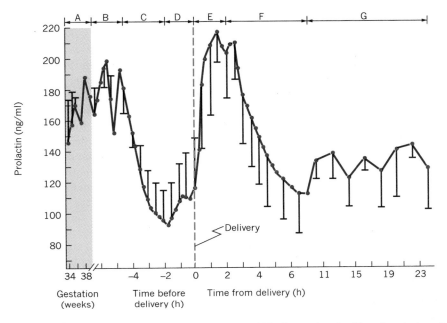

Figure 1   Prolactin levels in maternal blood (mean ± SEM; *n* = 4) in the periparturitional period centred around the time of vaginal delivery (*t* = 0) and divided into time phases(A–G). (Reproduced with permission from Rigg and Yen, 1977, p. 216.)

Somatosensory Pathways

Infant suckling triggers neuronal impulses from a high density of sensory nerve endings that lie beneath the areola and the nipple. These ascend in the spinal cord and are transmitted via a series of interconnected neurones. Although the exact route has not been fully identified in any species, existing evidence suggests that they follow the spinocervical tract through diffuse pathways in the brainstem that converge in the midbrain region. From here, impulses reach the hypothalamus by two distinct routes that independently regulate the release of prolactin and oxytocin. Current experimental evidence on cows suggests that the suckling-induced release of prolactin is completely dependent on the somatosensory route, while oxytocin release is not diminished by complete disconnection of the sensory nerve pathways (Barofsky *et al.*, 1983; Friedman *et al.*, 1983; Ben-Jonathan *et al.*, 1989; Laudon *et al.*, 1990; Fuchs, 1991; Hill *et al.*, 1993; Williams *et al.*, 1993; Wakerley *et al.*, 1994).

Neurohormonal Regulation

PROLACTIN

Unlike most other hormones from the anterior pituitary, prolactin does not have a specific target organ and is not therefore subject to feedback regulation from the periphery. Under general physiological conditions, the release of prolactin is predominantly regulated from the hypothalamus by tonic inhibition that is modified by the selective action of less potent stimulatory factors. These hypothalamic influences are coupled with additional stimulation from ovarian oestrogen, which is evident during the late follicular and luteal phases of the cycle. In the hypothalamus, dopamine has been identified as the primary inhibitor of prolactin release. Under a variety of physiological conditions, it is thought to operate in conjunction with other less potent inhibitors and stimulators that act within the hypothalamus and at the level of the pituitary gland (Friedman *et al.*, 1983; Abe *et al.*, 1985; Malarkey *et al.*, 1987; Ben-Jonathan *et al.*, 1989; Chiocchio *et al.*, 1991).

Immediately after childbirth, the anterior pituitary retains the pregnancy-induced changes in the relative size and secretory capacity of lactotrophs and gonadotrophs. The resulting increase in the capacity for prolactin secretion is accompanied by low basal levels of luteinizing hormone (LH) and follicle-stimulating hormone (FSH) and by an absent or limited pituitary responsiveness to exogenous gonadotrophin-releasing hormone (GnRH) stimulation. During this period, the ovaries are also characterized by low basal secretion of oestrogen and progesterone and most studies also report a refractory ovarian response to exogenous FSH and LH stimulation (Andreassen and Tyson, 1975; Keye and Jaffe, 1976; De La Lastra and Llados, 1977; Miyake et al., 1978; Sheehan and Yen, 1979; Marrs et al., 1981; Jacobs, 1991).

Patterns of prolactin release

Under general physiological conditions, prolactin is released from the anterior pituitary gland in pulses of varying amplitude, superimposed on a pattern of basal secretion that displays marked variability during the 24-hour clock. Plasma concentrations are minimal during morning and noon hours. A rise occurs during late afternoon and a major nocturnal increase begins after the onset of sleep and culminates around midsleep. Studies on prolactin concentrations during daytime sleep and following shifts of the sleep–wake cycle suggest that secretion is regulated by sleep and by an intrinsic circadian rhythm. Studies during daytime sleep have not demonstrated a consistent relationship between prolactin increases and short periods of sleep. In studies that have imposed a seven-hour advance on the sleep–wake cycle, only modest elevations occurred after sleep onset in the new time zone, and maximum levels were reached only after wakening, at a time which coincided with anticipated sleep onset, before the imposed time shift (Desir et al., 1982; Rossmanith et al., 1993).

Suckling and prolactin

Suckling is the most potent natural stimulus for prolactin release. Prolactin concentrations rise significantly within 10 minutes of the onset of suckling and further rises positively correlate with the duration of each suckling episode. Prolactin concentrations peak at 30 minutes following each feed and return to baseline levels within 3–4 hours. In keeping with the circadian rhythm of prolactin release, the suckling-induced increment is minimal in the morning and greatest at night (McNeilly et al., 1983; Glasier et al., 1984a; Glasier, 1990; Fuchs, 1991).

Longitudinal studies on breastfeeding women have found a significant decline in basal and suckling-induced prolactin concentrations over the first postpartum year. Both measures of prolactin release are negatively influenced by the elapse of time following birth and by the gradual decline in the frequency and duration of suckling. Time duration and suckling frequency appear to contribute in different degrees to basal and stimulated components of prolactin release. All studies have found that the degree of prolactin increase in response to similar periods of suckling progressively diminishes with the elapse of time following birth. But studies on basal prolactin have found that its gradual decline is negatively correlated with suckling frequency, during the first postpartum year (Figures 2 and 3) (Johnston and Amico, 1986; Diaz et al., 1989; Glasier, 1990; Uvnas-Moberg et al., 1990).

No relationship has been found between milk yield and prolactin concentrations. In longitudinal studies, the progressive decline in basal and suckling-induced prolactin is not accompanied by any diminution in milk yield. In cross-sectional studies, large individual variations in prolactin responses to suckling have been found in women demonstrating a similar objective capacity to breastfeed. Varying sensitivity of the mammary gland may account for differences observed between individuals, while the fall in individual concentrations over time suggests increases in prolactin receptors in the mammary gland, or the involvement of other hormones in milk production during established lactation (Howie et al., 1980; Diaz et al., 1989).

Suckling-induced regulation of prolactin

The neuroendocrine mechanisms that mediate the suckling-induced increase in prolactin have largely been studied in rats. Until the 1980s, most of this work focused on identifying various modulating factors in the hypothalamus that were thought to have direct and indirect influences on prolactin-releasing cells in the anterior pituitary. More recent evidence suggests that suckling may predominantly activate neuronal links between the hypothalamus and the posterior lobe of the pituitary. Within the intermediate and neural components of the posterior pituitary, a series of neurohormonal interactions have been identified that enhance the secretory capacity of prolactin-

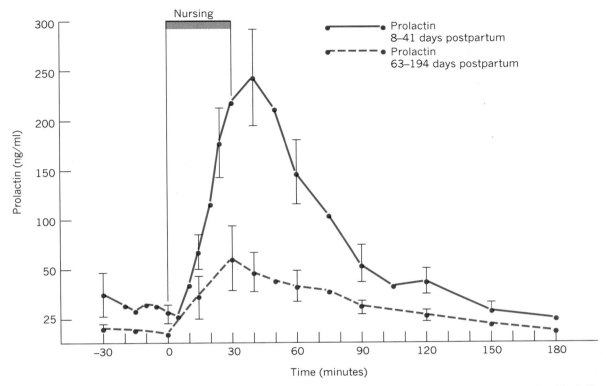

Figure 2   Plasma prolactin concentrations during feeding in postpartum women at two different periods of lactation. (Adapted from Noel *et al.* (1974), p. 415.)

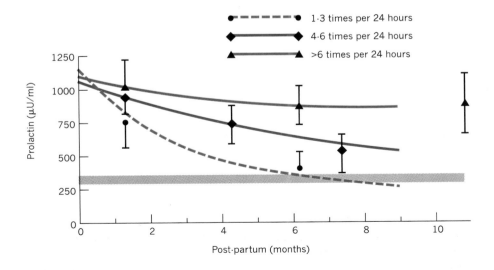

Figure 3   Relationship of mean serum prolactin levels to the duration of lactation and frequency of suckling in groups of African women. Shaded area represents the mean prolactin levels for a group of 25 non-lactating women. (Adapted with permission from Delvoye *et al.* (1977) p. 449.)

releasing cells in the anterior lobe of the gland. Although some of these findings have been confirmed in women, current evidence from rats can only be used as a general indication of what may happen in women (Bower *et al.*, 1974; Leong *et al.*, 1983; Laudon *et al.*, 1990; Mori *et al.*, 1990; Hill *et al.*, 1991, 1993; Murburg *et al.*, 1993).

The hypothalamus contains two major dopamine pathways that project from cell bodies in the arcuate nucleus. The *tuberoinfundibular* (TIDA) pathway sends short projections to the external layer of the median eminence, where dopamine is released into the long portal vessels that supply the anteror lobe of the pituitary. In contrast to this vascular route, the *tubero-hypophyseal* (THDA) pathway sends long projections that directly innervate the neural and intermediate lobes of the gland (Figure 4) (Ben-Jonathan *et al.*, 1989).

Experiments have explored the possibility that suckling stimulates a prolactin-releasing factor, either in the hypothalamus or in the anterior pituitary. In this area of investigation, a large number of substances have been found to stimulate prolactin release, but only a few have been clearly shown to operate as a physiological prolactin-releasing factor during lactation. This cate-

gory includes vasoactive intestinal peptide (VIP), thyrotrophin-releasing hormone (TRH) and oxytocin. All have been found to stimulate prolactin release. However, TRH does not increase during suckling, nor does it demonstrate any significant capacity to improve lactation, and passive immunization against VIP and oxytocin only delays or reduces prolactin release (Yli-korkala *et al.*, 1980; Plotsky and Neill, 1982; Riskind *et al.*, 1984; Abe *et al.*, 1985; Sampson *et al.*, 1986; Israel *et al.*, 1990; Chiocchio *et al.*, 1991; Parker *et al.*, 1991).

More recent evidence suggests that the suckling-induced rise in prolactin is mediated by a complex neuroendocrine axis involving midbrain and hypothalamic neurones that innervate the neural and intermediate lobe of the pituitary. Afferent pathways from the spinal cord carrying sensory inputs from the areola and the nipple synapse on serotonin neurones in the midbrain that send projections to the hypothalamus. Neurotoxin lesions placed on specific serotonin neurones in the midbrain have been shown to significantly deplete both hypothalamic concentrations of serotonin and the suckling-induced release of prolactin (Barofsky *et al.*, 1983; Lindley *et al.*, 1988; Laudon *et al.*, 1990; Hill *et al.*, 1993).

Within the hypothalamus, the suckling-induced activation of serotonin seems to stimulate selective interactions involving serotonin, β-endorphin and dopamine neurones. While hypothalamic β-endorphin appears to decrease the turnover and release of TIDA neurones, the predominant effect seems to be on the synthesis and release of dopamine from THDA neurones that innervate the intermediate and neural lobe of the pituitary gland. Surgical removal of the posterior lobe of the pituitary has been shown to produce a 3–4-fold increase in basal plasma prolactin but to completely abolish the suckling-induced rise in prolactin. This finding confirms the predominance of the hypothalamic–posterior-pituitary axis in regulating release of prolactin during suckling but it does not identify the neourohormonal interactions involved (Ben-Jonathan *et al.*, 1991; Laudon *et al.*, 1990).

The stimulatory influence of β-endorphin on suckling-induced prolactin has traditionally been thought to occur in the hypothalamus or in the anterior lobe of the pituitary. However, more recent evidence indicates that melanocyte-stimulating hormone (MSH) and β-endorphin are co-released from the intermediate lobe in response to suckling. In experiments on lactating rats, secretory activity in the intermediate lobe has been found to increase significantly following only

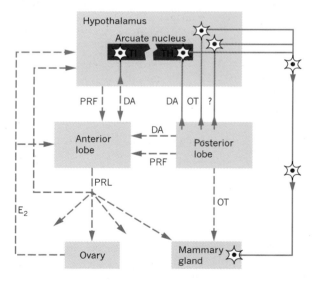

Figure 4 A model depicting the neuroendocrine regulation of prolactin secretion. TH, Tuberohypophysial; TI, tuberoinfundibular; OT, oxytocin; E_2, oestradiol; PRF, prolactin-releasing factor; PRL, prolactin; DA, dopamine. (Reproduced with permission from Ben-Jonathan *et al.*, 1991, p. 28.)

one minute of suckling. The timing of this response differed markedly from that of prolactin which did not rise significantly until 10 minutes after the onset of suckling. The rate of prolactin increase in this study is in agreement with other findings in a variety of species, including humans. In a recent study on women, plasma concentrations of β-endorphin have been shown to rise significantly in response to suckling in the absence of any change in cortisol. This indicates that suckling stimulates peripheral increases in a form of β-endorphin that is not derived from the anterior lobe of the pituitary (Franceschini *et al.*, 1989; Hill *et al.*, 1993; Murburg *et al.*, 1993).

Incomplete evidence exists on the ways in which MSH and β-endorphin may influence the release of prolactin. *In vitro* experiments have shown that β-endorphin blocks the dopamine inhibition of prolactin release, while MSH has been found to stimulate the release of prolactin in the presence of *very low* concentrations of dopamine and other known prolactin-stimulating factors, including angiotensin II and TRH. Taken together, this evidence suggests that following the initial inhibitory actions of serotonin and β-endorphin on both TIDA and THDA neurones in the hypothalamus, the tonic inhibitory control of MSH is removed. This frees the intermediate lobe to release MSH and β-endorphin which are transported to the anterior lobe via the short portal vessels. Prolactin release is enhanced by the dopamine-blocking action of β-endorphin, while MSH operates in conjunction with the new *reduced levels* of dopamine, to alter the capacity of lactotrophes to respond to a variety of stimulatory influences (Nagy and Frawley, 1990; Porter *et al.*, 1994).

OXYTOCIN

Suckling and oxytocin

The active expulsion of milk is regulated by a receptor-mediated action of oxytocin on contractile tissues within the mammary gland. Myoepithelial cells surrounding the alveoli contract in response to the pulsatile release of oxytocin. This action compresses the sacs, raising intra-alveolar pressure that propels milk along the ducts. The subsequent contraction of smooth muscle fibres in the ducts shortens and widens the ductal system, making it easier for milk to flow into the lactiferous sinuses (Fuchs, 1991).

Studies taking frequent blood samples have found that the pattern of oxytocin release varies considerably from that of prolactin. Oxytocin concentrations are invariably increased immediately prior to suckling and in some women, maximum concentrations have been found during this period. When feeding commences, the pattern of release is characterized by variable pulsatile increases that coincide with the duration of suckling. Longitudinal studies suggest that the pulsatile release of oxytocin is enhanced and more defined as lactation continues. In exclusively breast-feeding women, more consistent increases in oxytocin have been found at 4 and 11 weeks, compared to the first week postpartum and significantly higher peak levels have been found at 15–24 weeks compared to those at 2–4 and 5–14 weeks postpartum (McNeilly *et al.*, 1983; Johnston and Amico, 1986; Uvnas-Moberg *et al.*, 1990).

Regulation of oxytocin release

During lactation, oxytocin neurones are subject to a variety of stimulatory and inhibitory influences. In a number of studies, pulsatile release of oxytocin occurs in association with the sight and sound of the infant immediately prior to suckling and to a lesser extent during feeding. Episodic pulses of oxytocin also occur between periods of suckling, which are thought to be triggered by fleeting images of suckling or from sounds of other crying babies (McNeilly *et al.*, 1983; Wakerley *et al.*, 1994).

Experimental evidence suggests that oxytocin is sensitive to a variety of inhibitory and stimulatory influences from large areas of the brain that respond to stressful and emotional states. In rats, direct findings indicate that inhibitory and stimulatory pathways exist between oxytocin neurones in the hypothalamus and a variety of interconnected neurones within the fore-brain. In women, observational studies have consistently reported that milk-ejection is readily disrupted by anxiety, stress or embarrassment, particularly during early lactation (Wakerley *et al.*, 1994).

The neuroendocrine mechanisms that facilitate these interactions have largely been studied in rats. Densely packed clusters of oxytocin neurones have been identified in the supraoptic, paraventricular and in smaller accessory nuclei within the hypothalamus. Most axons project to the posterior pituitary and smaller numbers innervate the median eminence and the brainstem.

During lactation, oxytocin cells become larger and demonstrate significant increases in membrane oppositions between adjacent cell bodies and dendrites, both within and between the two major nuclei. Increases have also been found in the number of nerve terminals that make contact with two or more postsynaptic elements. Recordings of oxytocin cells during suckling suggest that these connections produce a progressive activation of cells within each nuclei and simultaneous firing of paired cells in the supraoptic and paraventricular nuclei (Wakerley et al., 1994).

As milk-ejection is subject to a range of stimulatory and inhibitory influences, anatomical studies have predictably revealed that complex neural pathways and chemical transmitters regulate the release of oxytocin. Sensory connections from the mammary gland are relayed to the hypothalamus by a series of multisynaptic pathways. Neurotransmitters including noradrenaline, β-endorphin, serotonin and dopamine impinge at different points along the route, from ascending transmission in the spinal cord, to the point of oxytocin release in the posterior pituitary (Wakerley et al., 1994).

Most afferents from the nipple terminate in the dorsal horn of the spinal cord. Observational studies of the effects of spinal lesions on milk-ejection suggest that from the dorsal horn the stimulus ascends via the spinocervical tract, which relays within the lateral cervical nucleus, in the cervical segment of the spinal cord. From this point, ascending fibres cross into the brainstem, where the suckling stimulus is thought to be relayed by diffuse pathways that converge in different regions of the midbrain. Final links connecting sensory input to the midbrain and the hypothalamus are thought to follow subthalamic pathways that enter the posterior hypothalamus near the third ventrical (Wakerley et al., 1994).

Neural pathways that mediate conditioning and inhibition of milk-ejection are thought to project to the hypothalamus from different regions of the forebrain. Excitatory and inhibitory effects on oxytocin cells have been observed following electrical stimulation of cells in the amygdala, hippocampus and septum. Collectively known as the *limbic system*, this region has widespread reciprocal connections between its different components and is known to co-ordinate emotional responses to a variety of environmental cues (Wakerley et al., 1994).

These complex controls over oxytocin release from higher brain centres may be more influential than the somatosensory pathway from the mammary gland. Current evidence on the pattern of oxytocin release

in relation to suckling coupled with the lack of influence of denervation strongly indicates the importance of understanding the emotional states that are conducive to its enhanced release as lactation continues (Newton and Newton, 1967; McNeilly et al., 1983; Chiodera et al., 1991; Williams et al., 1993).

Recovery of Reproductive Capacity

After birth a major shift occurs in the concentrations of placental hormones in the maternal circulation. Following delivery of the placenta, human placental lactogen (hPL) disappears within hours. Progesterone and oestrogen decline over several days and reach early follicular phase concentrations by day 5 and 7 respectively (Martin et al., 1980). Combined measurements of human chorionic gonadotrophin (hCG)/LH suggest that hCG disappears from the circulation by approximately 18 days postpartum (Liu et al., 1983).

In non-lactating women, the duration of time that elapses before the resumption of regular ovulatory cycles is determined by the recovery times required by different components of the hypothalamic–pituitary–ovarian axis. Two main approaches have been used to identify the changing activity levels and degrees of interaction between the hormones, neurotransmitters and endocrine organs involved. Some studies have attempted to understand the pace and variation of overall functional recovery by longitudinal measures of pituitary–ovarian hormones. Various methods have been used, including direct measurement of pituitary LH content, plasma values of gonadotrophins and urinary assays of oestrogen and progesterone. Other studies have attempted to identify distinct patterns of hypothalamic, pituitary and ovarian recovery by measuring hormonal responses to synthetic GnRH at various intervals. In general, results have been limited by small sample sizes, different methods of pituitary–ovarian stimulation, infrequent and imprecise measurements of pituitary–ovarian function and lack of data on pituitary and ovarian hormone levels over the same time period (Marrs et al., 1981; Liu et al., 1983; Glasier et al., 1986).

Direct findings from post-mortem studies suggest that by the end of pregnancy, the pituitary content of LH is dramatically low compared to that found in women during the menstrual cycle. This evidence of reduced capacity for gonadotrophin secretion is gen-

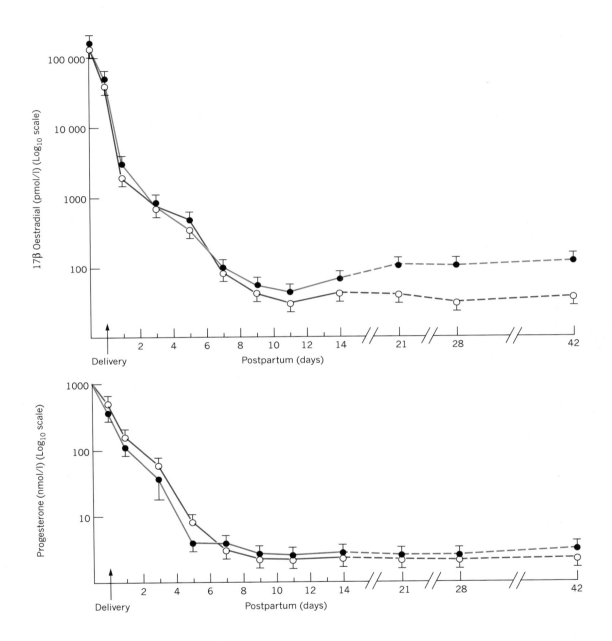

Figure 5   Mean (± SEM) serum concentrations of 17β-oestradiol and progesterone in lactating and nonlactating subjects. Lactating subjects (*n* = 10) o–o; nonlactating subjects (*n* = 9) •–•.

erally confirmed by serial sampling of LH and FHS in the peripheral circulation. Studies using weekly daytime sampling suggest that baseline concentrations of LH remain at follicular phase levels until approximately seven weeks postpartum. More recently, weekly sampling of LH has been undertaken at 20-minute intervals over periods of 12–24 hours. These more detailed findings suggest that unchanging mean values of LH are accompanied by significant sleep-related nocturnal increases in pulse amplitude in some women, from approximately three weeks postpartum. In contrast, most studies on FSH have found that basal concentration rise significantly by approximately three weeks postpartum and no change has been observed in pulse amplitude during nocturnal sleep. At present, the functional significance of nocturnal changes in LH have not been identified. Evidence from small samples suggests that it is not consistently associated with a corresponding rise in plasma oestrogen or with lower nocturnal levels of prolactin, up to three weeks postpartum (Liu *et al.*, 1983; Glasier *et al.*, 1984b; Liu and Park, 1988).

Recovery of pituitary–ovarian activity has also been studied using steroid and LH measurements on daily morning urine samples over the first three menstrual episodes. In a sample of 22 women, the first day of menstrual bleeding ranged from 30 to 53 days postpartum and the first inferred ovulation from 25 to 49 days postpartum. These large individual variations in the timing of recovery were accompanied by greater consistency in the level of recovery with each successive cycle. Strong evidence of disturbances in ovulation and the luteal phase occurred in 82% of all first postpartum cycles, compared to 37% in second and third cycles (Gray *et al.*, 1987).

Other measures of pituitary–ovarian recovery have been obtained by injecting women with varying doses of synthetic GnRH, over different time periods. In these studies, functional capacities have been assessed by measuring the degree of pituitary–ovarian hormonal responses over time and by comparing response levels to those obtained from women during different phases of the cycle.

Data obtained from studies points to a gradual process of pituitary–ovarian recovery over the first 12 weeks postpartum. Results on individual profiles suggest that while the timing of recovery is highly variable, the levels of recovery show a fairly consistent pattern between first and subsequent cycles (LeMarie *et al.*,

1974; Keye and Jaffe, 1976; Miyake *et al.*, 1978; Sheehan and Yen, 1979).

SUCKLING AND REPRODUCTION

In a number of different species, lactation is associated with considerable delay in the resumption of reproductive cycles. In women, regular suckling prolongs pituitary–ovarian recovery but the period of delay is extremely variable, both between and within different populations. Over a wide range of studies, lactational amenorrhoea has been reported to last from two months to four years. While a number of epidemiological studies have found a strong statistical association between the frequency of suckling and the duration of amenorrhoea, recent hormonal profiles on fully breastfeeding women suggest that similar feeding patterns are maintained by varying responses of the neuro-hormonal reflex to suckling (Campbell and Gray, 1993; Diaz *et al.*, 1989; Gray *et al.*, 1990; Smith *et al.*, 1989; Smith *et al.*, 1990; Short *et al.*, 1991).

A clear understanding remains to be gained of the mediating links between suckling-induced hormonal changes and hypothalamic–pituitary–ovarian inhibition. Extensive research has revealed that both systems are regulated by complex neuroendocrine pathways that vary considerably between species. While high levels of prolactin are generally thought to be involved, its possible sites and modes of action on the reproductive axis have not been identified (Garcia *et al.*, 1985; McNeilly *et al.*, 1994; McNeilly, 1994).

Studies on the influence of lactation on pituitary–ovarian recovery suggest that basal LH levels gradually increase to the lower limits of normal by three weeks postpartum. Throughout the remaining period of lactational amenorrhoea, women are reported to have LH patterns that are lower or similar to those in the follicular phase of the cycle. Most studies report that basal FSH increases to follicular phase levels by three weeks postpartum. Serial measurements of ovarian hormones generally suggest that levels of oestrogen and progesterone remain low throughout the period of lactational amenorrhoea (Figure 5). Although brief elevations in oestrogens have been reported in association with increased pulsatile secretion of LH, gonadotrophs are thought to be more sensitive to the negative feedback mechanism from the ovary. In this way, so long as LH levels remain inhibited by the hormonal effects of suckling, any small increases in oestrogen will inhibit further LH secretion and prevent normal follicular development (McNeilly *et al.*, 1994; McNeilly, 1994).

In women, suckling is associated with the inhibition of gonadotrophin secretion, particularly the pulsatile release of LH. A variety of studies have found that prolonged amenorrhoea is positively associated with suckling frequency in fully breastfeeding women. More recently, this finding has been qualified by results showing that women who produce higher basal and suckling-induced levels of prolactin are more likely

to remain amenorrhoeic than women from the same cohort who maintain similar nursing patterns with lower levels of prolactin. Although both of these findings imply that suckling-induced prolactinaemia mediates the suppression of LH, the latter study suggests that individual variations exist in the sensitivity of the breast–hypothalamic–pituitary axis in response to similar patterns of suckling. Further work is obviously needed before women can use lactation as a reliable means of contraception (Diaz *et al.*, 1989).

References

Abe, H., Engler, D., Molitch, M.E. *et al.* (1985) Vasoactive intestinal peptide is a physiological mediator of prolactin release in the rat. *Endocrinology* 116(4): 1383–1390.

Altemus, M., Deuster, A., Galliven, E. *et al.* (1995) Suppression of hypothalamic-pituitary-adrenal axis responses to stress in lactating women. *J. Clin. Endocrinol. Metab.* 80(10): 2954–2959.

Andreassen, B. & Tyson, J.E. (1975) Role of the hypothalamic-pituitary-ovarian axis in puerperial infertility. *J. Clin. Endocrinol. Metab.* 42(6): 114–122.

Barofsky, A-I., Taylor, J. & Massari, J. (1983) Dorsal raphe-hypothalamic projections provide the stimulatory serotonergic input to suckling-induced prolactin release. *Endocrinology* 113(5): 1894–1983.

Ben-Jonathan, N. Arbogast, L.A. & Hyde, J.F. (1989) Neuroendocrine regulation of prolactin release. *Prog. Neurobiol.* 33: 399–477.

Ben-Jonathan, N., Laudon, M. & Garris, P.A. (1991) Novel aspects of posterior pituitary function: regulation of prolactin secretion. *Frontiers Neuroendocrinol.* 12(3): 231–277.

Bower, A., Hadley, M.C. & Hruby, V.J. (1974) Biogenic amines and control of melanocyte stimulating hormone release. *Science* 184: 70–72.

Campbell, O.M.R. & Gray, R.H. (1993) Characteristics and determinants of postpartum ovarian function in women in the United States. *Am. J. Obstet. Gynecol.* 169: 55–60.

Chiocchio, S.R., de las Nieves Parisi, M. & Leiza Vitale, M. (1991) Suckling-induced changes of vasoactive intestinal peptide concentrations in hypothalamic areas implicated in the control of prolactin release. *Neuroendocrinol.* 54: 77–82.

Chiodera, P., Salvarani, C. & Bacchi-Modena, A. (1991) Relationship between plasma profiles of oxytocin and adrenocorticotrophic hormone during suckling or breast stimulation in women. *Hormone Res.* 35: 119–123.

Darmady, J.M. & Postle, A.D. (1982) Lipid metabolism in pregnancy. *Br. J. Obstet. Gynaecol.* 89: 211–215.

De La Lastra, M. & Llados, C. (1977) Luteinizing hormone content of the pituitary gland in pregnant and non-pregnant women. *J. Clin. Endocrinol. Metab.* 44(5): 921–923.

Delvoye, P., Demaegd, M. & Delogne-Desnoek, J. (1977) The influence of the frequency of nursing and of previous lactation experience on serum prolactin in lactating mothers. *J. Biosocial Sci.* 9: 447–451.

Desir, D., Van Cauter E., L'hermite M. *et al.* (1982) Effects of 'jet lag' on hormonal patterns. III. Demonstration of an intrinsic circadian rhythmicity in plasma prolactin. *J. Clin. Endocrinol. Metab.* 55(5): 849–857.

Diaz, S., Seron-Ferre, M., Cardenas, H. *et al.* (1989) Circadian variation of basal plasma prolactin, prolactin response to suckling, and length of amenorrhea in nursing women. *J. Clin. Endocrinol. Metab.* 68(5): 946–955.

Farquharson, J., Jamieson, E.C., Abbasi, K.A. *et al.* (1995) Effect of diet on the fatty acid composition of the major phospholipids of infant cerebral cortex. *Arch. Dis. Childh.* 72: 198–203.

Franceschini, R., Venturini, P., Cataldi, A. *et al.* (1989) Plasma beta-endorphin concentration during suckling in lactating women. *Br. J. Obstet. Gynaecol.* 96: 711–713.

Friedman, E., Krieger, D.T., Mezey, E. *et al.* (1983) Serotonergic innervation of the rat pituitary intermediate lobe: decrease after stalk section. *Endocrinology* 112(6): 1943–1947.

Fuchs, A.-R. (1991) The physiology of lactation. In Gabbe, S.G., Niebyl, J.R. & Simpson, J.L. (eds) *Obstetrics, Normal and Problem Pregnancies*, pp. 75–205. New York: Churchill Livingstone.

Garcia, A., Herbon, L., Barkan, A. *et al.* (1985) Hyperprolactinemia inhibits gonadotrophin-releasing hormone (GnRH) stimulation of the number of pituitary GnRH receptors. *Endocrinology* 117(3): 954–959.

Glasier, A. (1990) Physiology of lactation. *Baillière's Clin. Endocrinol. Metab.* 4(2): 379–395.

Glasier, A., McNeilly, A.S. & Howie, P.W. (1984a) The prolactin response to suckling. *Clin. Endocrinol.* 21: 109–116.

Glasier, A., McNeilly, A.S. & Howie, P.W. (1984b) Pulsatile secretion of LH in relation to the resumption of ovarian activity post partum. *Clin. Endocrinol.* 20: 415–426.

Glasier, A., McNeilly, A.S. & Baird, D.T. (1986) Induction of ovarian activity by pulsatile infusion of LHRH in women with lactational amenorrhoea. *Clin. Endocrinol.* 22: 243–252.

Gray, R.H., Campbell, O.M. & Zacur, H.A. *et al.* (1987) Postpartum return of ovarian activity in nonbreastfeeding women monitored by urinary assays. *J. Clin. Endocrinol. Metab.* 64(4): 645–650.

Gray, R.H., Campbell, O.M. & Apelo, R. (1990) Risk of ovulation during lactation. *Lancet* 335: 25–29.

Hill, J.B., Nagy, G.M. & Frawley, L.S. (1991) Suckling unmasks the stimulatory effect of dopamine on prolactin release: possible role for α-melanocyte-stimulating hormone as a mamotrope responsiveness factor. *Endocrinology* 129(2): 843–847.

Hill, J.B., Lacy, E.R., Nagy G.M. *et al.* (1993) Does α-melanocyte-stimulating hormone from the pars intermedia regulate suckling-induced prolactin release? Supportive evidence from morphological and functional studies. *J. Clin. Endocrinol. Metab.* 133(6): 2991–2997.

Howie, P.W., McNeilly, A.S., McArdle, T. *et al.* (1980) The relationship between suckling-induced prolactin response and lactogenesis. *J. Clin. Endocrinol. Metab.* 50(4): 670–673.

Israel, M.J., Kukstas, L.A. & Vincent, J.-D. (1990) Plateau potentials recorded from lactating rat enriched lactotroph cells are triggered by thyrotrophin releasing hormone and shortened by dopamine, *Neuroendocrinology* 51: 113–122.

Jacobs, H.S. (1991) The hypothalamus and pituitary gland. In Hytten, F. & Chamberlain, G. (eds) *Clinical Physiology in Obstetrics*, pp. 345–356. Oxford: Blackwell Scientific.

Johnston, J.M. & Amico, J.A. (1986) A prospective longitudinal study of the release of oxytocin and prolactin in response to infant suckling in long term lactation. *J. Clin. Endocrinol. Metab.* 62(4): 653–657.

Keye, W.R. & Jaffe, R.B. (1976) Changing patterns of FSH and LH response to gonadotrophin releasing hormone in the puerperium. *J. Clin. Endocrinol. Metab.* 42(6): 1133–1138.

Laudon, M., Grossman, D.A. & Ben-Jonathan, N. (1990) Prolactin-releasing factor: cellular origin in the intermediate lobe of the pituitary. *Endocrinology* 126(6): 3185–3192.

Lebenthal, E. (ed.) (1989) *Textbook of Gastroenterology and Nutrition in Infancy.* New York, Raven Press.

LeMarie, W.J., Shapiro, A.G., Riggall, F. *et al.* (1974) Temporary pituitary insensitivity to stimulation by synthetic LRF during the postpartum period. *J. Clin. Endocrinol. Metab.* 38(5): 916–918.

Leong, D.A., Frawley, L.S. & Neill, J.D. (1983) Neuroendocrine control of prolactin secretion. *Ann. Rev. Physiol.* 45: 109–127.

Lindley, S.E., Gunnet, J.W., Lookingland, K.J. *et al.* (1988) Effects of alterations on the activity of tuberohypophysial dopaminergic neurons on the secretion of α-melanocyte stimulating hormone. *Proc. Soc. Exp. Biol. Med.* 188: 282–286.

Liu, J.H. & Park, K.H. (1988) Gonadotrophin and prolactin secretion increases during sleep during the puerperium and nonlactating women. *J. Clin. Endocrinol. Metab.* 66(4): 839–845.

Liu, J.H., Rebar, R.W. & Yen, S. (1983) Neuroendocrine control of the postpartum period. *Clin. Perinatol.* 10(3): 723–736.

Malarkey, W.B., Zvara, B.J. & DeGroff, V.L. (1987) Angiotensin II promotes prolactin release from normal human anterior pituitary cell cultures in a calcium dependent manner. *J. Clin. Endocrinol. Metab.* 64(4): 713–717.

Marrs, R.P., Kletzky, O.A. & Mishell, D.R. (1981) Functional capacity of the gonadotrophs during pregnancy and the puerperium. *Am. J. Obstet. Gynecol.* 141(6): 658–661.

Martin, R.H., Glass, M.R., Chapman, C. *et al.* (1980) Human α-lactalbumen and hormonal factors in pregnancy and lactation. *Clin. Endocrinol.* 13: 223–230.

McNeilly, A.S. (1994) Suckling and the control of gonadotrophin secretion. In Knobil, E., Neill, J.D., Greenwald, G.S. *et al.* (eds). *The Physiology of Reproduction*, New York, Raven Press Ltd, 1179–1212.

McNeilly, A.S., Robinson, I.C.A.F., Houston, M.J. *et al.* (1983) Release of oxytocin and prolactin in response to suckling. *Br. Med. J.* 286: 257–259.

McNeilly, A.S., Tay, C.C.K. & Glasier, A. (1994) Physiological mechanisms underlying lactational amenorrhea. *Ann. NY Acad. Sci.* 709: 145–155.

Mori, M., Vigh, S., Miyata, A. *et al.* (1990) Oxytocin is the major prolactin releasing factor in the posterior pituitary. *Endocrinology* 126(2): 1009–1013.

Miyake, A., Tanizawa, O., Aono, T. *et al.* (1978) Pituitary LH response to LHRH during puerperium. *Obstet. Gynaecol.* 51(1): 37–40.

Murburg, M.M., Wilkinson, W., Raskind, M.A. *et al.* (1993) Evidence for two differentially regulated populations of peripheral β-endorphin-releasing cells in humans. *J. Clin. Endocrinol. Metab.* 77(4): 1033–1044.

Nagy, G. & Frawley, L.S. (1990) Suckling increases the proportions of mammotropes responsive to various prolactin-releasing stimuli. *Endocrinol.* 127(5): 2079–2084.

Newton, N. & Newton, M. (1967) Psychological aspects of lactation. *N. Eng. J. Med.* 277(22): 1179–1188.

Noel, G.H., Suh, H.K. & Frantz, A.G. (1974) Prolactin release during nursing and breast stimulation in postpartum and nonpostpartum subjects. *J. Clin. Endocrinol. Metab.* 38(3): 413–423.

Parker, S.L., Armstrong, W.E., Sladek, C.D. *et al.* (1991) Prolactin stimulates the release of oxytocin in lactating rats: evidence for a physiological role via an action at the neural lobe. *Neuroendocrinology* 53: 503–510.

Patton, S., Canfield, L.M. & Huston, G.E. *et al.* (1990) Carotenoids of human colostrum. *Lipids* 25(3): 159–165.

Plotsky, P.M. & Neill, J.D. (1982) Interactions of dopamine and thyrotrophin-releasing hormone in the regulation of prolactin release in lactating rats. *Endocrinology* 111(1): 168–173.

Porter, T.E., Grandy, D. & Bunzow, J. *et al.* (1994) Evidence that stimulatory dopamine receptors may be involved in the regulation of prolactin secretion. *Endocrinology* 134(3): 1263–1268.

Rigg, L.A. & Yen, S.S.C. (1977) Multiphasic prolactin secretion during parturition in human subjects. *Am. J. Obstet. Gynecol.* 128(2): 215–218.

Riskind, P.N., Millard, W.J. & Martin, J.B. (1984) Opiate modulation of the anterior pituitary response during suckling in the rat. *Endocrinology* 114(1): 589–593.

Rossmanith, W.G., Boscher, S. & Ulrich, U. *et al.* (1993) Chronobiology of prolactin secretion in women: diurnal and sleep-related variations in the pituitary lactotroph sensitivity. *Neuroendocrinology* 58: 263–271.

Sampson, W.K., Lumkin, M.D. & McCann, S.M. (1986)

Evidence for a physiological role for oxytocin in the control of prolactin secretion. *Endocrinology* **119**(2): 554–560.

Sheehan, K.L. & Yen, S.S.C. (1979) Activation of pituitary gonadotrophic function by an agonist of luteinizing hormone-releasing factor in the puerperium. *Am. J. Obstet. Gynecol.* **135**(6): 755–758.

Short, R.V., Lewis, P.R. & Renfree, M.B. *et al.* (1991) Contraceptive effects of extended lactational amenorrhoea: beyond the Bellagio Consensus. *Lancet* **337**: 715–717.

Smith, M.S., Lee, L.R. & Pohl, C.R. (1989) Neuroendocrine basis of lactational acyclicity. In Delemarre-van de Waal, H.A., Plant, T.M., van Rees G.P. *et al.* (eds) *Control of the Onset of Puberty III*, pp. 285–293. Oxford: Elsevier Science.

Smith, M.S., Lee, L-R. & Pohl, C.R. (1990) Inhibitory effects of the suckling stimulus on hypothalamic GnRH release and pulsatile LH secretion, in Yen S.S.C., Vale, W.W. (eds). *Neuroendocrine Regulation of Reproduction*, Seronon Symposia, Massachusetts, 39–46.

Uvnas-Moberg, K., Widstrom, A-M. & Werner, S. *et al.* (1990) Oxytocin and prolactin levels in breast-feeding women. *Acta Obstet. Gynaecol. Scand.* **69**: 301–306.

Wakerley, J.B., Clarke, G. & Summerlee, A.J.S. (1994) Milk ejection and its control. In Knobil, E., Neill, J.D., Greenwald, G.S. *et al.* (eds). *The Physiology of Reproduction*, New York, Raven Press, 1131–1377.

Williams, G.L., Mcvey, W.R. & Hunter, J.F. (1993) Mammary somatosensory pathways are not required for suckling-mediated inhibition of luteinizing hormone secretion and delay of ovulation in cows. *Biol. Reprod.* **49**: 1328–1337.

Ylikorkala, O., Kivinen, S. & Kauppila, A. (1980) Oral administration of TRH in puerperial women: effect on insufficient lactation, thyroid hormones and on the responses of TSH and prolactin to intravenous TRH. *Acta Endocrinol.* **93**: 413–418.

37

Postnatal Care

After childbirth, the processes of recovery and adjustment to the reality of motherhood begin during the puerperium. The word 'puerperium' means the period belonging to the child, and it is defined as the time from immediately after the end of labour until the reproductive organs have returned as near as possible to their pre-gravid condition, a period of 6–8 weeks. For some women adaptation to motherhood and sometimes full physical recovery take much longer and they may need support and care beyond the puerperium (MacArthur *et al.*, 1993a; Ball, 1994) (see Chapter 38).

In the *Midwives' Rules* (UKCC, 1993) the *postnatal period* 'means a period of not less than ten and not more than 28 days after the end of labour, during which time

the continued attendance of a midwife on the mother and baby is requisite'. These definitions only focus on periods of time and, in the case of the puerperium, physiological changes. Yet one of the main aims of postnatal care is to help the mother adapt and successfully fulfil the role and responsibilities of motherhood. A major part of the midwife's role in postnatal care is therefore concerned with the provision of appropriate emotional, psychological and educational support which should be tailored to meet the particular needs of each mother. Such support and a facilitative style of parent education helps to build up the woman's confidence in her mothering ability, especially in the key areas of developing a relationship with her baby and establishing successful feeding.

Physiological Changes
(see Chapter 36)

During the puerperium certain physiological changes take place:

► Involution of the uterus and other soft parts of the genital tract.
► Secretion of milk in the breasts (Chapter 36).
► Physiological changes in other systems of the body.

Involution

The term 'involution' means the return of the uterus to its normal size, tone and position (Figure 1). The vagina, the ligaments of the uterus and the muscles of the pelvic floor also return to their pre-pregnant state during the process of involution. If the ligaments of the uterus and the muscles of the pelvic floor do not return to normal and are permanently weakened, a prolapse may occur later. During the process of involution the lining of the uterus is cast off in the *lochia* and is later replaced by new endometrium. After the birth of the baby and the expulsion of the placenta, the muscles of the uterus constrict the blood vessels, so that the blood circulating in the uterus is considerably reduced. This is known as *ischaemia*.

Redundant muscle, fibrous and elastic tissue has to be disposed of. The phagocytes of the bloodstream deal with the last two by phagocytosis, but the process is

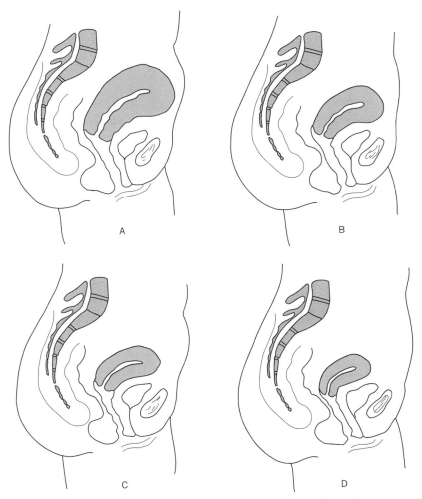

Figure 1   Involution of the uterus. **A**: At the end of labour; **B**: one week after delivery; **C**: two weeks after delivery; **D**: six weeks after delivery.

usually incomplete and some elastic tissue remains, so that a uterus which has once been pregnant never returns to its nulliparous state. Muscle fibres are digested by proteolytic enzymes, a process known as *autolysis*. The lysosomes of the cells are responsible for this process. The waste products then pass into the bloodstream to be eliminated by the kidneys.

The decidual lining of the uterus is shed in the lochia. The new endometrium grows from the basal layer, beginning to be formed from about the 10th postnatal day and is completed in about six weeks.

The process of involution takes at least six weeks to complete; during this time the weight of the uterus decreases from 1000 to 60 g and its size decreases from $15 \times 11 \times 7.5$ cm to $7.5 \times 5 \times 2.5$ cm. At the end of a week the uterus weighs about 500 g and the cervix is reforming and closing and will admit one finger.

The rate of involution can be assessed by the rate of descent of the uterine fundus. On the first day the height above the symphysis pubis is just over 12 cm. There is a steady decrease in the height of the fundus of about 1 cm a day so that by the seventh day the fundal height is about 5 cm; by the 10th day the fundus is barely palpable at the level of the symphysis pubis.

The rate of involution varies from one mother to another and is thought to be slower in a woman of high parity. Ultrasonic studies on primiparous and multiparous women found some correlation between the birthweight of the baby and uterine size postnatally (Lavery and Shaw, 1989) but did not demonstrate that parity affected the rate of uterine involution, nor did they state that grande multiparous women were included in the study (Rodeck and Newton, 1976; Lavery and Shaw, 1989). Further research is therefore needed to substantiate or refute the widely accepted theory that there is a slower rate of involution in women of high parity. Involution may be unduly slow if there is retention of placental tissue or blood clot, particularly if it is associated with infection.

By feeling the uterus each day, the midwife may note the steady decrease in its size. The practice of daily measuring and charting the fundal height, once popular, is declining. Careful palpation of the uterus and observation of the lochia, preferably by the same midwife each time, should reveal whether or not involution is progressing normally.

Lochia

The lochia are discharges from the uterus occurring after childbirth and persisting for the first 3 or 4 weeks of the puerperium. The changes in the lochia have been described in three stages: *lochia rubra*, *lochia serosa* and *lochia alba*; names which describe the changes in colour of the lochia. The lochia consist at first of blood, coming chiefly from the placental site, mixed with shreds of decidua (lochia rubra). After a few days the lochia become brownish in colour, consisting of altered blood and serum and containing leucocytes and organisms (lochia serosa). Towards the end of the second week the discharge is yellowish-white in colour consisting of cervical mucus, leucocytes and organisms (lochia alba).

Occasionally, however, the lochia remain slightly blood-stained for over three weeks before finally ceasing. There may be some slight increase of blood during the second week, but no special treatment is required for this unless it is excessive or associated with abnormal signs and symptoms. The most important point to note is whether there is persistent excessive loss or sudden profuse loss. This is almost always due to retained placental tissue and must be reported to the doctor. Normal lochia are not offensive. Offensive lochia and pyrexia may indicate uterine infection and will require investigation by the doctor.

Ovaries and uterine tubes

The ovaries and uterine tubes become pelvic organs again. Following the delivery of the placenta, the levels of oestrogens and progesterone fall. Eventually a negative feedback mechanisms triggers off the ovarian-menstrual cycle. Ovulation takes place before menstruation, so that a woman may become pregnant again before she has a period.

Breasts

Lactation is initiated by the secretion of prolactin by the anterior pituitary gland. There is a steady rise of serum prolactin levels throughout pregnancy. The milk comes into the breasts about the third day after delivery. Once lactation starts it is maintained by the baby suckling, since prolactin is produced at this time (see Chapters 36 and 64).

Changes in other systems

Urinary tract   There is a marked diuresis after delivery which lasts for 2–3 days. This is due to the reduction in blood volume which occurs at this time. The dilatation of the urinary tract which occurs in pregnancy due to increased vascular volume resolves and the renal organs gradually return to their pre-gravid state.

Alimentary tract Following the expulsion of the placenta the level of progesterone falls, hence smooth muscle tone gradually improves throughout the body. Heartburn therefore improves but constipation may continue to be troublesome during the first few days of the puerperium. It is probably due to inactivity and perhaps reflex inhibition of defecation by a painful perineum.

Circulatory system The blood volume decreases to pre-gravid levels and the blood regains its former viscosity. Smooth muscle tone in the vessel walls improves, cardiac output returns to normal and the blood pressure returns to its usual level.

Respiratory system Full ventilation of the basal lobes of the lungs is again possible since they are no longer compressed by the enlarged uterus.

Endocrine system After the expulsion of the placenta the circulating levels of oestrogens and progesterone fall. Hence the negative feedback mechanism comes into action and promotes the release of follicle-stimulating hormone and luteinizing hormone which are responsible for the resumption of the ovarian–menstrual cycle (see Chapter 36).

The enlarged thyroid gland regresses to its former size and the basal metabolic rate returns to normal.

Musculoskeletal system (see Chapter 12) The softened pelvic joints and ligaments of pregnancy gradually return to normal over a period of about three months.

The abdominal and pelvic floor muscles gradually regain their tone with the assistance of postnatal exercises. Occasionally, however, the rectus abdominal muscles remain separated in the midline. This is called *diastasis recti* and is most likely to occur in grande multiparous women or in those who have had a multiple pregnancy or polyhydramnios.

Psychological state

Emotional lability (swing of mood) is very common during the early days of the puerperium. After delivery most women experience a feeling of elation, but a few days later they may be depressed and tearful. This

is a transient phase and is probably a reaction to the physical and mental stress of childbirth, coupled with the marked physiological changes which are taking place at that time. Anxiety about the baby and perhaps a feeling of inadequacy as a mother may also be responsible for this period of depression (see Chapter 58).

The Psychology of the Puerperium and Psychosocial Support

Major emotional changes take place in the majority of women during the puerperium but there is wide variation in the amount of distress caused by these changes. It takes between 6 and 12 weeks for most women to return to their normal emotional state.

0–3 days after delivery

This is known as the latent period because functional mental illness is very unlikely to occur at this time. The woman is normally in a state of euphoria, excitement and restlessness. She may not take enough rest during the day and tends to have difficulty with sleeping at night. Because she feels so well there is a tendency to minimize the physical effects of childbirth. Consequently she may do too much, especially when she is transferred home early from hospital. Midwives should be alert to this problem and strongly advise the mother to rest for periods during the day, and to avoid taking over household duties too soon. Help should be available to take over the domestic duties for at least the first week of the puerperium. This enables the mother to rest and concentrate on her baby at this time.

3–10 days

The 'blues' may occur at any time between the third and tenth postnatal day (Swyer, 1985). Although sometimes called the 'third day blues', the commonest day for this condition to occur is on the fifth postnatal day. It is considered a normal reaction to childbirth and affects about 70–80% of all postnatal mothers (Ball, 1994). Paykel *et al.* (1980) describe the blues as a transient, self-limiting condition with no known serious after-effects. Although most women recover from the blues within a day or two, Cox *et al.* (1982) consider that a serious episode may be an important predictor of the onset of postnatal depression. This is a serious condition which may last for months or even years.

The timing of the blues (3–10 days) coincides with the timing of the onset of most puerperal psychoses. This according to Kendell (1985), suggests that whatever trigger mechanism is responsible for the blues may also precipitate psychoses in susceptible women (see Chapter 58). According to Levy (1984) the blues is also experienced by women following gynaecological and other surgery.

Despite the fact that this condition will have been discussed with most women during the antenatal period, the majority are totally unprepared for it. They are overwhelmed by feelings of tearfulness, inadequacy and perhaps a feeling of panic. Often they fear that there is something dreadfully wrong with them or their baby and tend to lose all sense of proportion. Problems with establishing breastfeeding and/or the onset of neonatal jaundice often occur at this time and add to the emotional turbulence of the blues. Feelings of embarrassment about their behaviour only serve to increase their distress.

It is at this distressing time that a caring, competent and understanding midwife, especially one well-known to her, can be of invaluable help to the mother. The blues responds to physical comfort and emotional support and reassurance. The mother may be tired and upset by the discomforts of the early postnatal period, worried about her baby, miss her husband and other children if she is in hospital, and, in many cases, it is a trivial factor that triggers off her distress. The midwife offers patient and expert help and tries to elicit from the woman the cause of her distress. She listens carefully to the mother's fears and problems, gives reassurance where possible and helps her to work out her own solutions. If the problem is related to the baby it is fully discussed and the midwife tries to build up the mother's confidence in her ability to care for her baby, and reassure her about minor problems such as physiological jaundice which may occur at this time. A good sleep often helps the mother recover more quickly from an episode of the blues and so help with breastfeeding to ensure that the baby has a good feed before settling mother and baby down to sleep is often very helpful. With support and skilled help most mothers recover from the blues within 24 hours or so.

1–12 weeks

During this period of time the mother's emotional state gradually returns to normal. Primiparous women take time to adjust to the experience of caring for a young baby, especially as in most cases this is their first real contact with a newborn infant. To most mothers the baby seems fragile, vulnerable and totally dependent and at times they find the responsibilities of motherhood overwhelming. The often unpredictable and, indeed, confusing behaviour of the newborn only adds to their anxiety and even leads to feelings of panic. Mothers worry and feel guilty that they are not caring for their baby correctly, or doing all they should. These worries are often paradoxical in that one minute they are anxious about overfeeding and the next about starving their child. Similarly they worry about the baby crying and not sleeping and then, when the baby is asleep, wake it up to make sure that it is still alive.

These problems of coping with motherhood in the early weeks are often exacerbated by lack of sleep. Rarely will the breastfeeding mother sleep for more than 3–4 hours at a stretch for the first 6–8 weeks after the birth of her baby. Constantly feeling tired and, at times, absolutely exhausted diminishes her normal coping resources. Most new mothers remain easily upset and vulnerable at this time. They are oversensitive to criticism and easily lose their sense of proportion. Feelings of inadequacy persist and they tend to burst into tears for no apparent reason, especially when particularly tired.

Amongst all these problems of early motherhood there are times of great joy and happiness, sometimes almost frightening in intensity. But there are also times when the mother experiences feelings of anger, frustration and even resentment towards her child. She may feel that no matter how hard she tries her baby does not appreciate it, or show any sign of love, but just cries and demands more and more attention. These transient feelings of antagonism towards her child can be very frightening and make her feel that she is deviant or might even harm her own baby.

Some mothers vividly imagine harm coming to their baby and naturally find these thoughts very distressing. Such thoughts are obsessional (that is, unwanted and recognized as being silly), yet they are difficult to overcome and cause considerable distress. Other forms of obsessional behaviour may also occur in the mother during the puerperium. It may be revealed in various ways such as the mother's need to check her baby repeatedly, or wash her hands. Some mothers set themselves routines and standards which are well nigh impossible to achieve. Failure only accentuates their feelings of inadequacy, anxiety and guilt. Feelings of doubt, uncertainty and indecisiveness are also common in such mothers.

Initially most new mothers feel extremely possessive about their babies and do not like to be separated from them. They often dislike other people handling the baby, even members of their own family. If the father or grandmother of the infant appear to the mother to be more competent in handling the baby than she is, then the mother may experience intense feelings of jealousy. The emotionally fraught mother may also feel jealous if her partner appears to pay more attention to the baby than to her. Her fear is that the infant has usurped her position in his affections. Fathers, too, experience these feelings of jealousy when they feel left out of the close relationship developing between mother and child.

It is usual for women to be preoccupied with thoughts about their labour and delivery for some weeks after the event. They relive the experience in their mind and like to talk about it in detail repeatedly. A pleasurable, fulfilling confinement can be emotionally helpful to the mother at this time whereas a disappointing, traumatic experience can make the mother feel angry and upset and she may find these emotions difficult to cope with. The midwife can therefore see how important it is to do everything possible to help mothers have a pleasurable, fulfilling experience of childbirth. Also, every woman should be given the opportunity to discuss her labour within a day or two of the event with the midwife who attended her, so that explanations can be given, if required, and the mother can be reassured if she has any feelings of failure, or of not coping as well as she hoped.

Many women are surprised to find how lonely and socially isolated they are when caring for a young baby alone at home all day. They miss the companionship of friends and colleagues and, no matter how much they love their baby, find it difficult to adjust to such loneliness. They may also miss the intellectual stimulation of a busy career and to some women this is a great problem. Nowadays there are postnatal support groups in some areas where mothers can meet, share experiences and make new friends. If the midwife knows of such groups she should inform mothers about them so that they can contact the appropriate person if they wish to join. Some midwives have actually started such groups.

Difficulty with concentration often continues for 4–6 weeks after delivery, thus the mother may experience difficulty with intellectual tasks at this time. To some extent this is caused by lack of sleep and may result in poor memory and difficulty in making decisions.

Resolution

It takes 6–12 weeks for the mother to recuperate from childbirth. By this time she knows her baby and he is usually more settled. Her sleep pattern is less disturbed, although she may continue to feel tired for some considerable time, especially if she is breastfeeding. Loneliness may still be a problem, however, and even though her baby is more responsive this does not make up for the loss of adult companionship. The mother may still feel a sense of loss for her lifestyle before the birth of her baby.

Libido often takes some time to return. Sexual activity may be resumed as early as 2–3 weeks after delivery, although for many couples it is later, up to 6–12 weeks. Dyspareunia is a problem for a significant number of women after childbirth (Sleep *et al.*, 1984; MacArthur *et al.*, 1993a) and professional help may be required in some cases. For some women it takes a year or more before a real interest in sexual activity returns (see Chapter 59).

PSYCHOSOCIAL SUPPORT

Raphel-Leff (1992) describes the period following birth as 'a state of inner disequilibrium and external upheaval quite unlike any other encountered in adult life'. Most mothers are totally unprepared for the depth and extent of this change in their feelings and their lives and react in a number of different ways. Some try and take positive action in an attempt to cope with the stress of the situation, but this is not always easy when they are in a tired and vulnerable state and the behaviour of their baby is unpredictable. Others do their best to avoid the situation, or sink into apathy which, according to Lazarus (1966), can be seen as a symptom of depression. This may occur more commonly in women who lack control over their lives, perhaps due to social problems, and inadequate family support (Brown and Harris, 1978). Lazarus (1966) describes coping as coming to terms with a situation, whereas adjustment is exerting mastery over it. Those who come to terms with their situation eventually become adjusted to it.

The support given to mothers in the postnatal period may help them to cope with their feelings and have a significant contribution to their emotional well-being and adaptation to motherhood. The midwife therefore has a vital role in giving support to the postnatal mother, and in helping the woman's partner understand how important his support is to her. Oakley (1994) describes social support as listening, responding, informing when asked, and helping whenever and however appropriate. To achieve this the midwife must make time to talk to the mother and listen, actively listen, to her concerns, and respond appropriately. This aspect of postnatal care is equally important to the well-being of the mother and her family as the routine observations which are carried out on well women, many of which have never been evaluated. Weiss (1976) defines effective support as that given by a person, either professional or lay, who is accepted as an ally by the distressed person. The midwife needs to build up a good relationship with the mother, prove to be her advocate and show her care and concern if she is to be considered an ally by her. Support from the midwife in the postnatal period helps the mother to move from the stage of physical, emotional and parenting dependence to the independence of a woman who has fully recovered from the physical and emotional effects of childbirth and is a confident and happy mother (Rickitt, 1987).

Some women who lack social support at home may need extra care and support from both the midwife and social worker during the postnatal period, especially if there are social problems such as poor housing and financial difficulties. These problems should be identified in the antenatal period, whenever possible, so that there is time to explore ways of best helping the woman and start making any necessary arrangements before she has her baby. Those with disabilities also have additional problems to overcome and may require special help and arrangements to enable them to care for their baby at home.

Mothers from different cultural backgrounds and ethnic groups have different attitudes, beliefs and customs about childbirth which need to be understood and respected by all those involved in their care. Knowledge and understanding of these beliefs and customs, good communications and individualized care should enable any special needs to be met. In many cases, however, communication is a problem if the woman does not speak English. Interpreters need to be available in these situations and, where possible, a carer who can communicate with the mother should be involved in her care.

Care During the Puerperium

THE ROLE OF THE MIDWIFE

The role of the midwife in caring for the mother and baby during the postnatal period demands great skill because, unlike caring for the woman in labour, her feelings and needs may not be immediately obvious. Most women have little or no difficulty in explaining how they are feeling physically, but may be more reticent about revealing their feelings of inadequacy as a mother, inability to cope or, for some, their perceived lack of maternal instinct, all of which can be very distressing for the woman. The midwife needs the sensitivity and insight to understand how the woman is feeling about herself and her ability to cope with the demands of motherhood, and the skill and wisdom to help the woman adapt to her new role and develop confidence in her mothering ability.

Nowadays, with the increasing number of schemes designed to give the woman continuity of care and carer, the mother may be cared for in hospital and at home by the same midwife, or one of a small team, whom she has known since booking in the antenatal period. Over this length of time the midwife often becomes a trusted friend, as well as a professional carer, and this facilitates a good supportive relationship which helps the woman to adjust to her changed role and lifestyle and cope with the stress which often accompanies such changes. It is at times of change and stress that people are more susceptible to the influence of others and the quality of support offered by midwives as well as family and friends can affect the outcome (Ball, 1994).

The midwife also promotes and monitors the health of the mother and baby during the postnatal period, giving health education as appropriate and building up the woman's confidence in her mothering abilities. Any deviations from the normal will be detected and medical advice sought.

The aims of postnatal care can therefore be summarized as follows:

1   To promote and monitor the mother and baby's physical well-being.
2   To promote and monitor the mother's psychological, emotional and social well-being and provide appropriate support.
3   To help the mother establish a successful infant feeding regime.

4   To foster the development of good maternal–infant relationships and the acceptance of the new baby within the family.
5   To enhance the mother's confidence in her ability to fulfil her mothering role.
6   To promote health education, including education for planned parenthood.

Patterns and Delivery of Postnatal Care

In recent years there has been increasing concern about the patterns and delivery of postnatal care which have been based on a medical model with fixed routines and resulted in a fragmented and task-orientated approach to care. Postnatal care has often been described as the Cinderella of the maternity services because most emphasis and resources have been placed on ante- and intranatal care, perhaps because most mothers appear to make a good physical recovery after delivery and few serious complications arise. An increasing number of studies carried out in the last decade, however, have revealed that there are significant levels of both physical and psychological morbidity associated with childbirth, and that the patterns of postnatal care have a considerable impact on postnatal recovery and the adaptation process which the new mother has to make (Garcia and Marchant, 1993; MacArthur et al., 1993a; Ball, 1994; Garcia et al., 1994; Murphy-Black, 1994).

Most women start their postnatal recovery in hospital and, for mothers who have had an uncomplicated birth, their length of stay ranges from about six hours to 2 or 3 days. According to Rush et al. (1989), the promotion of very early postnatal transfer home is sometimes for the needs of the institution rather than to meet the wishes of the mother. The report Changing Childbirth (DOH, 1993) recommends that, as far as is practicable, the length of time spent in a postnatal ward should be discussed and agreed between the woman, the midwife and other professionals as necessary. Firm decisions should not be made until after delivery and even then there needs to be flexibility to meet the changing needs of mother and baby. Some women are anxious to return home as soon as possible, whereas others prefer to spend a few days in hospital to start their recovery from pregnancy and childbirth, and learn to care for their new baby with the guidance of

the midwife readily available both day and night. A review of trials on early versus standard postnatal discharge from hospital concluded that early discharge from hospital is feasible and apparently safe, but it is neither clearly beneficial nor wanted by the majority of women (Hay-Smith, 1994a).

The environment of the postnatal ward can influence the mother's satisfaction with her postnatal experience. Field (1985) found that poor physical surroundings were the most important issue that adversely affected the mother's degree of satisfaction with her postnatal stay in hospital. Hospital routines and many procedures which may be necessary for those who are ill are inappropriate for postnatal mothers. Freedom to use flexible patterns of care and approaches which are tailored to meet the needs of individuals, rather than fit into hospital routines and practices, is essential if midwives are to be empowered to give woman-centred care to new mothers and their babies. All the staff on postnatal wards need to help create a friendly, relaxed and caring atmosphere in which the new mothers can recuperate happily and learn to care for themselves and their babies.

After transfer home from hospital the mother will be visited by a midwife, preferably by her named midwife who has been responsible for her ante-, intra- and early postnatal care in hospital. The midwife visits the mother for a minimum of 10 days and for a maximum of 28 days (UKCC, 1994), after which she discharges the mother to the care of the health visitor. Midwives used to visit daily for 10 days, but now there is more flexibility in visiting which is adjusted to try and meet the particular needs of each mother. In a recent study conducted by Garcia et al. (1994) it was found that policies on postnatal home visiting by midwives had changed to be selective, rather than routine, up to the 10th postnatal day in all but 20% of English NHS districts. Mothers who have a home delivery continue to receive care from their midwife during the postnatal period. Again postnatal visiting may be selective rather than daily, depending on the needs of the mother and her baby.

Admission to the postnatal ward
The mother and baby in hospital are usually transferred to the postnatal ward within an hour or two of delivery. At home the midwife remains with the mother for the same length of time and when she leaves gives the mother a telephone number where she can contact

her, if required. On admission to the postnatal ward the mother is welcomed and introduced to her named midwife who will be responsible for her care, if she is not already known to her. She is also introduced to other staff and the mothers in the vicinity of her bed. The layout of the ward is explained and information is given about meals and other services, thereby helping the mother to orientate herself to her new surroundings and feel more at ease. The midwife will observe the mother's general physical and mental condition, palpate the uterus to note whether it is contracted or not and observe the lochia. If the mother has not passed urine since delivery she may be helped to the lavatory or, if she has had a complicated labour, may be offered a commode by the bed or a bedpan. The baby is also checked by the midwife, noting in particular colour, respiration, temperature, condition of the cord and name labels. Many women are hungry after delivery and, unless a meal is imminent, should be offered a snack before having a time of undisturbed rest. Some women are too excited to sleep at this time but appreciate a period of rest and quiet with their baby in its cot beside them.

Sleep and rest

For many mothers insufficient sleep is the most common and distressing problem in the postpartum period and, indeed, during the first few months of motherhood (Turton, 1980). A study by Salzarulo and Rigoard (1987) found that sleep problems associated with childbirth may be the starting point of long-lasting sleep disturbances in women. During the early weeks of motherhood therefore rest and sleep should be considered a priority and practical steps need to be taken by staff of postnatal wards and later by relatives and the midwife visiting at home to enable mothers to have undisturbed sleep. These steps include providing a quiet, comfortable environment, appropriate remedies, including analgesics if required, for a painful perineum and other discomforts, and ensuring that the mother is not disturbed unnecessarily. Sleeping mothers should only be disturbed for breastfeeding. Routine procedures and meals can wait until the mother awakes. Adequate help should be given to mothers in postnatal wards who are breastfeeding at night (as well as during the day) so that they remain calm and relaxed and the baby feeds well, and then both mother and baby are more likely to go back to sleep.

Inability to sleep for no obvious reason should be investigated. It may be caused by anxiety, often about the baby, and the midwife should encourage the mother to talk through her problems and give appropriate support, as required. Only rarely are mild hypnotics such as temazepam 10–20 mg, a short-acting benzodiazepine, required. Unexplained sleeplessness can be associated with puerperal psychosis, thus careful observation of the mother's behaviour is necessary and hypnotics may be prescribed.

Ambulation

Mothers who have had an uncomplicated delivery usually get up almost immediately to use the toilet and have a shower or a bath. They may need assistance at this early stage as some women feel dizzy or faint when they first get up after delivery. Early ambulation reduces the incidence of thromboembolic disorders and most mothers derive a feeling of well-being from this early activity. For some Asian women, however, the need to stay in bed with their baby for rest and recuperation after childbirth is central to their concept of postnatal care and they may find it unacceptable to be expected to be ambulant at this early stage. Ethnicity and cultural attitudes towards the postnatal care of the mother and her baby need to be considered (Woollett and Dosanjh-Matwala, 1990).

Ambulation will be delayed in women who have had an epidural until full sensation returns and then they will require more help initially.

Diet and fluids

The mother should continue having a good, mixed diet, as advised in pregnancy. The woman's appetite usually returns very quickly after labour is ended and she has had some sleep. Foods rich in iron and vitamin C will help improve the haemoglobin level in women who are found to have iron-deficiency anaemia (see Chapter 42).

The only special advice which may be required by breastfeeding mothers is to avoid foods which may upset the baby via her breast milk, such as highly spiced dishes or excess fruit which may cause diarrhoea.

The daily fluid intake should be about 2.5 litres in breastfeeding mothers or sufficient to quench their thirst. Many mothers like to have a drink within reach whilst they are breastfeeding.

Hygiene and perineal care

The first bath or shower after delivery should be supervised as the mother is often a little unsteady at this time. Thereafter she takes a bath or shower once or twice daily and uses the bidet when she has used the lavatory. The vulval and perineal area is then dried with soft toilet paper and a clean pad is applied. A large study conducted by Sleep and Grant (1988) on a sample of postnatal mothers 10 days after delivery concludes that the practice of adding salt or Savlon bath concentrate to baths for postnatal mothers is ineffective in terms of reducing perineal discomfort and improving healing. However, 93% of the mothers in the trial reported that bathing in the first 10 days after delivery had eased perineal discomfort, the results being similar whether or not an additive was added to the bath.

The large placental site is a potential site for infection and because of this the cleanliness of baths, showers, lavatories and bidets is of the utmost importance. These facilities should be cleaned by domestic staff at intervals throughout the day and, in addition, by the mothers before and after use on each occasion. Reports published in the last decade have highlighted several outbreaks of puerperal sepsis in modern maternity units in the UK and Sweden caused by Lancefield groups A, C and G haemolytic streptococci (Claesson and Claesson, 1985; Haynes *et al.*, 1987; Teare *et al.*, 1989; Gordon and Lochhead, 1994). Toilet facilities, including automated douche, toilet and shower heads, were implicated in the spread of infection in all these reports (Gordon and Lochhead, 1994). Maternal deaths occurred following infection in some cases (Acharya *et al.*, 1988; Kavi and Wise, 1988).

If for any reason the mother is confined to bed, she may need help with washing, including her vulval and perineal toilet, until she is well enough to get up and use the facilities.

The perineum must be inspected daily if there are sutures to see that healing is taking place and to detect any signs of infection. Non-absorbable sutures are removed on the fifth or sixth day.

Many women suffer high levels of pain following perineal trauma and suturing and effective methods of pain relief are required. Intensive pelvic floor exercises have been found to significantly reduce perineal pain. A survey of midwives' management of postpartum perineal pain revealed that the first line of management in most cases was oral analgesia, most commonly paracetamol. Ice was the most popular form of local treatment, but gives short-term pain relief only. Other local applications to the perineum for the relief of pain include witch hazel, which again only gives short-term pain relief, and pramoxine and hydrocortisone spray (Epifoam), which one study indicates is associated with more cases of wound breakdown (Greer and Cameron, 1984), probably due to the inclusion of steroids in the spray. Its effectiveness as an analgesic is inconclusive because the studies reviewed by Grant and Sleep (1989) and Harris (1992) give conflicting results. Local anaesthetics may be applied to the perineum for pain relief and a review of the literature concludes that local anaesthetics alone (without the addition of steroids) are useful for the relief of perineal pain in the immediate postpartum period. Aqueous 5% lignocaine spray or lignocaine gel are recommended (Grant and Sleep, 1989).

Electrical therapies such as ultrasound and pulsed electromagnetic energy may also be used to relieve perineal pain, but their effectiveness is not yet proven. If paracetamol fails to give adequate pain relief, a non-steroidal, anti-inflammatory agent such as ibuprofen may be given as an alternative. Drugs containing codeine are avoided during the postnatal period because of their constipating effect. In some cases, when measures to relieve severe perineal pain are not effective, oral opioids may be required.

Long-term problems such as dyspareunia may follow perineal trauma and should be diagnosed at the postnatal examination. Referral for expert help can then be offered (see Chapter 38).

Micturition and bowels

Most women pass urine without difficulty after delivery, especially when they can get up and use the toilet. Early and regular emptying of the bladder encourages the uterus to remain well-contracted which helps to control uterine bleeding. A diuresis occurs during the first few days after delivery and the mother will pass urine more frequently. Occasionally, however, the bladder is numbed by injury or pressure during labour, and the woman is unaware that it needs emptying. The bladder can contain only a certain amount of urine even when distended; when that capacity has been reached the sphincter of the bladder relaxes and urine escapes. This condition is known as *retention with overflow*. However, retention should never be allowed to progress to this state. The midwife should suspect that retention is present by the woman's complaint of difficulty or inability to pass urine. Examination of the abdomen may show the presence of a soft rounded suprapubic swelling which often displaces the uterus upwards and to the right side. Catheterization may be necessary, but it should be avoided if possible; however excellent the technique, there is a risk that infection may be introduced.

It is usually 2 or 3 days after delivery before the woman has a bowel movement, epecially if she has painful perineal sutures or has had an operative delivery. It is common practice to offer the mother a mild aperient a day or two after delivery if she has not had a bowel movement, but a review of trials to assess the effect of postpartum laxatives on maternal and infant morbidity concludes that laxatives are not necessary in most cases (Hay-Smith, 1994b). Senokot was found to be associated with an unacceptably high level of maternal discomfort and also diarrhoea in breastfed babies. In the few cases when laxatives are required therefore, bulk-forming rather than irritant laxatives are recommended.

The presence of haemorrhoids is not uncommon and the pain they cause may be eased by an anaesthetic cream such as Anacal (Hay-Smith, 1994c) or a suppository. If they have prolapsed an ice-pack may help to reduce their size.

MANAGEMENT OF BREASTFEEDING

Breastfeeding should be a happy, satisfying experience for both the mother and her baby. The mother who is keen to breastfeed and has the support of her partner is most likely to succeed, especially if she has the skilled help and support of her midwife. Some mothers are uncertain whether to breastfeed or not, but decide to give it a try. In these cases the midwife's attitude, help and support have a most important influence on whether breastfeeding is successful. Other factors which promote success are a healthy baby who fixes well at the breast and feeds on demand. This means that the frequency and duration of feeds is determined by the baby both day and night. No complementary feeds (that is artificial feeds in addition to breastfeeding) or supplementary feeds (feeds instead of breast milk) should be given. Finally the mother needs sufficient rest, a good diet to promote her own health and feeling of well-being, and the assurance that help and support are available from the midwife when she needs it.

The first feed

This should be given soon after birth, within the first hour preferably, and should always be supervised by a midwife, usually the midwife who was present at the birth and knows the mother. Most babies show signs of being ready to feed within an hour of birth (Widstrom et al., 1987) and a successful first feed is most encouraging for the mother and appears to have a positive effect on breastfeeding (Salariya et al., 1978; Chateau, 1980). Salariya's study indicated that babies who breastfed early were likely to remain breastfed for longer, an important consideration when 65% of women start breastfeeding, but only 26% are still feeding at four months (Martin and White, 1988).

Breastfeeding technique

After the first feed the baby should be fed on demand and there should be no limit to the frequency and duration of feeds. Initially the mother will require help and supervision from the midwife to position her baby correctly at the breast. The baby should be held close to the mother with his head and shoulders facing her breast, head slightly extended and nose at the level of her nipple. As he opens his mouth and begins to root he is moved on to the breast with his mouth wide open and lower lip well below the nipple so that he grasps as much of the breast tissue as possible. The nipple and as much of the areola as possible should be in the baby's mouth. This is because the ampullae, where the milk is stored, lie within the areola and it is the rhythmical, rolling action of the baby's tongue on the ampullae that expresses the milk into the baby's mouth. The nipple lies passively well back in the baby's mouth at the junction of the hard and soft palate and, when correctly positioned there, is not damaged by any friction from the gums (Inch, 1990). Nipple damage is unlikely to occur if the baby is attached correctly, as described above, and there should be no pain during feeding. If pain is experienced it is essential to remove the baby from the breast and check that both the position of the baby and attachment to the breast are correct, otherwise nipple damage will ensue. Also, the baby will obtain insufficient milk and this will not only result in a hungry, unsettled baby but, if allowed to continue, also leads to a reduction in the production of milk.

Feeding should start on alternate breasts at each feed and continue on the first breast until the baby comes off spontaneously. The fat content of the hindmilk is higher than that of the foremilk and therefore the baby obtains a higher calorific intake when the breast is emptied (Lucas *et al.*, 1979), and also more fat-soluble vitamins such as vitamin K (Kries *et al.*, 1987). The second breast is offered but very often the baby is satisfied with only one side.

After feeds breast pads may be applied to absorb any leakage of milk and most women appreciate the comfort of a well-fitting bra. It is not considered necessary to wash the breasts before and after feeds because too much washing removes natural skin oils and soreness is then more likely (Newton, 1952). The application of creams or sprays to the nipples has been shown to be ineffective in the prevention of soreness (Herd and Feeney, 1986; Inch and Fisher, 1987). The midwife should examine the nipples and areola if the woman complains of pain or soreness and also observe the baby feeding to ensure that positioning and attachment are correct, because it is incorrect positioning and attachment which are the causes of nipple damage.

The early days of breastfeeding are often very tiring for the mother because, after the first day or two of birth, the baby usually feeds very frequently for the next few days, sometimes as often as every hour or two (Saint *et al.*, 1984; Carvahlo *et al.*, 1984). Unless the midwife explains to the mother that this is normal behaviour at this time, she may think that her milk is insufficient, or of inferior quality, and be tempted to give up breastfeeding. After a few days the frequency of feeds gradually decreases but may still be very irregular for the next few weeks. Studies have demonstrated that babies who are completely demand-fed with no restrictions imposed on them gain weight more quickly (Carvahlo *et al.*, 1983) and breastfeed for longer (Martin and Monk, 1982) than those who are restricted. The fact that the baby gains weight well is very reassuring and encouraging for the mother, but her tiredness may be a source of great stress and she should be encouraged to try and have some sleep during the day when the baby is asleep.

Conflicting advice about feeding is another major source of stress for breastfeeding mothers and efforts must be made by all professionals involved in their care to prevent this occurring. With a named midwife and continuity of carer this problem should be lessened. Ball (1989) noted that conflicting advice had an adverse effect on the woman's self-image in relation to feeding her baby and that the mother needs encouragement and praise to build up her confidence, rather than a confusing array of advice which leaves her anxious and

further lacking in confidence (Murphy-Black, 1994). Inch (1982) considers that more women give up breastfeeding as a result of destroyed confidence and sore nipples than insufficient milk. It is always wise to check what advice the mother has had from others and ensure that any further advice is not in conflict with what she has already received. Discussing problems and possible options with the mother, and then helping her to make her own decisions, and supporting her in those decisions, will help to build up her confidence.

Most women are transferred home early in the postnatal period now and, in a review of two trials which compared the effect of early versus late discharge from hospital on breastfeeding success, it was found that women who were discharged early (i.e. within 48 hours) were more likely to be breastfeeding at six months postpartum, especially multiparae, than those who remained in hospital for four days or longer. Also the babies of the early discharge group were less likely to have supplementary fluids in the first week of life (Renfrew and Lang, 1994).

Mothers may need to be reassured that the return of menstruation makes no difference to breastfeeding. The mother should be aware, however, that breastfeeding alone is not a safe method of contraception. The combined contraceptive pill which contains oestrogen as well as progesterone should be avoided because it inhibits lactation.

On discharge from the midwife between 10 and 28 days the mother can consult the health visitor or general practitioner with any problems. In many areas now there are breastfeeding support groups where mothers can help and support each other with breastfeeding.

SUPPRESSION OF LACTATION

Lactation is suppressed in women who do not want to breastfeed, or if breastfeeding is contraindicated in any way. It may be suppressed by natural methods or by the use of drugs.

Natural methods

Initially milk is produced, but because the baby is not put to the breast the release of prolactin gradually ceases and the breasts stop secreting milk. On the third or fourth day after delivery the breasts become engorged with blood and this causes pressure on the cells which produce milk, the acini cells. Milk engorgement may follow venous engorgement. If the woman is very uncomfortable a little milk may be expressed from her breasts to relieve the discomfort. This practice does not increase lactation because prolactin levels remain low. It reduces the incidence of mastitis and subsequent breast abscess.

Whilst lactation is being suppressed the breasts should be well supported with a well-fitting bra or, if this is not available, a firm binder, for comfort and to prevent stasis in the dependent areas of the breast. Mild analgesics may be required for a day or two.

Drugs

Bromocriptine This drug inhibits the release of prolactin by the pituitary gland. The dose is 2.5 mg on the first day and then 2.5 mg twice daily for 14 days. Mothers treated with bromocriptine are likely to start ovulating earlier than would otherwise be the case and so should be given appropriate family planning advice. Renfrew (1994a) reviewed eight trials to assess the effects of bromocriptine and found that it reduces lactation, breast pain and breast engorgement in the first week postpartum, but in some trials the mothers reported side-effects such as dizziness, and rebound lactation occurred in a number of women after the course of treatment had stopped.

Cabergoline This is another drug which may be prescribed for the suppression of lactation. In Renfrew's (1994b) review of cabergoline versus bromocriptine for the suppression of lactation, there were less side-effects and a lower incidence of rebound lactation with cabergoline and therefore it is recommended as the drug of choice.

Oestrogens These have now been superseded by bromocriptine and cabergoline. Although they inhibit lactation, they are associated with an increased risk of embolism and should therefore be avoided.

POSTNATAL PAIN

Many women experience significant pain and discomfort in the puerperium, even after an uncomplicated delivery (Dewan *et al.*, 1993; MacArthur *et al.*, 1993a). In the first 3 or 4 days after delivery the problems are mainly uterine cramps, perineal pain, dysuria and neck or shoulder muscle pain, the latter occurring mainly in women who have had a general anaesthetic. After three days or so breast and nipple pain may become more severe.

The main forms of pain relief for the conditions described above are paracetamol or mefenamic acid. In the study conducted by Dewan *et al.* (1993), mefenamic was rated a more effective analgesia than paracetamol, but still did not provide adequate pain relief for a significant number of women. Some women continue to have significant morbidity for some weeks or months after childbirth, and this is discussed in Chapter 38.

Another cause of postnatal pain is symphysis pubis pain which occurs 8–60 hours after delivery and may be serious enough to inhibit mobility (Driessen, 1987). Treatment includes bedrest with hips adducted and some relief of pain may be achieved by the application of a pelvic binder, an elasticated support bandage or trochanteric belt. A side-lying position in bed may help to reduce separation of the symphysis. Effective analgesics will be required. As the pain subsides, mobility is gradually resumed, often with the use of elbow crutches or a walking frame to minimize weight bearing. The woman will need help and support from her family and friends for some weeks until she is fit enough to resume all her normal activities, especially as she also has a young baby to care for (see Chapter 20).

OBSERVATIONS AND RECORDINGS

Many of the observations which are made routinely on the mother in the postnatal period are now under scrutiny because their value in preventing or predicting complications has never been evaluated (Rush *et al.*, 1989). Individualized care involves the midwife assessing each mother in her care and making professional judgements about the observations and examinations which are required. Until recently, postnatal care focused almost entirely on physical examinations and care, and on the establishment of a satisfactory pattern of infant feeding. Nowadays there is greater awareness of the need for psychological and emotional assessment and support, and of the long-term problems which can ensue if these aspects of care are neglected. Psychological disorders such as postnatal depression, inadequate maternal/infant attachment and puerperal psychosis cause considerable disruption to the woman and her family (Cogill *et al.*, 1986; Murray, 1988). It is therefore essential that the midwife's assessment of the postnatal mother focuses on her psychological and emotional condition as well as her physical progress and well-being.

Mental state

The mother's attitude to her baby and her perception of how her baby is behaving and feeding gives some insight into her mental and emotional state. It is very important that the midwife gives the mother quality time and encourages her to express any concerns she may have about herself or her baby. This is where the midwife's communication skills are of paramount importance, especially the ability to listen attentively, not only to what the mother is saying, but also to what she is evading or omitting (Laryea, 1984). Only then can the mother's emotional and psychological needs be identified and discussed in a supportive and empathic way. Care should be directed towards helping the mother develop a good relationship with her baby, and helping other members of the family accept the new baby and give the mother the help and support which she needs at this vulnerable time. Learning to care for a newborn baby is a daunting prospect for many mothers and an important aspect of the midwife's role is to educate the parents in such a way that they quickly develop confidence in their parenting abilities and enjoy their new role and responsibilities.

Discussing problems and the implications of different courses of action, and encouraging the mother to make her own decisions about the care of her baby and, indeed, her own care, helps to build up her confidence. The midwife supports the mother and gradually 'stands back' as she develops confidence and skill in her mothering role. Inevitably the mental and physical condition are closely intertwined and the first week of the puerperium is often a time of particular instability when the mother is recovering from the birth, has many physical discomforts and is also beginning to adjust to the demands of motherhood. After the first 2 or 3 days of euphoria, the most equable woman is readily depressed and dispirited over small matters and the more highly strung mother is in an agony of apprehension about her baby's most trivial setback. Periods of depression and tearfulness are common about 4–5 days after childbirth. A kindly, sensible midwife can do much to comfort and support the mother through this time. More serious forms of mental illness can occur and the midwife therefore observes the mother's general behaviour, her sleeping and eating habits, her attitude to her baby and any change in her relationships with family, staff and other mothers.

Physical examination

Temperature and pulse   The temperature and pulse rate are taken for the first few days, and thereafter only if the mother appears unwell, and/or there are signs of complications such as infection, haemorrhage or thromboembolic disorders. A significant rise in either would necessitate referral to the doctor.

Blood pressure   The blood pressure is recorded soon after delivery and then, if normal and there is no history of hypertension in pregnancy or other complications, it need not usually be taken again after the first 24 hours. Women who have a history of hypertension in pregnancy, or other obstetric complications, will have their blood pressure closely monitored postpartum for as long as it is considered necessary.

Urinary output and bowels   The midwife makes a point of asking the mother if she is passing urine normally and whether she has any discomfort or stress incontinence. The problem of stress incontinence after childbirth, if not detected and treated, usually by an intensive programme of pelvic floor exercises supervised by a physiotherapist, may be a long-term problem (MacArthur et al., 1993b). A marked diuresis is normal during the first 2 or 3 days after delivery but there should be no dysuria.

Regular bowel movements should be resumed within 2–3 days of delivery and routine aperients should not be required (Hay-Smith, 1994b). Women with perineal sutures are often fearful of rupturing their stitches during a bowel movement and may be more comfortable if they support the sutured perineum with a pad or wad of tissue paper during the first bowel action after delivery.

Breasts   The breasts are examined, usually at the time of a feed if the mother is breastfeeding, to note their tension and consistency, any signs of infection and, in breastfeeding mothers, the amount and flow of milk and the condition of the nipples and areola. During the examination the midwife discusses the progress of feeding with the mother, giving her time to express any anxieties, no matter how trivial, and helps her to decide the course of action she wishes to take from the various options available to her. Sometimes the mother only requires confirmation and reassurance that what she is doing is safe and appropriate.

Abdomen and involution of the uterus
With the woman lying flat on her back and having just passed urine, the midwife palpates the abdomen just above the symphysis pubis to note whether or not the bladder is palpable. A palpable bladder in a woman who has just passed urine would suggest retention of urine with overflow.

The midwife also notes the condition of the abdominal muscles and, on the first day or two after delivery, examines the abdomen for *diastasis recti*. This is a condition where a gap of 3 cm (two fingers) or more appears between the two rectus muscles (Brayshaw and Wright, 1994). It is diagnosed by pressing the fingers into the abdomen just above or below the umbilicus and asking the mother to raise her head and shoulders from the bed. Normally the taut rectus muscles can be felt on either side of the fingers, but if they cannot be felt until two or more fingers are inserted and 'peaking' of the recti is seen, this is diagnostic of diastasis recti (see later in this chapter and Chapter 25). If this condition is diagnosed or suspected the mother should be referred to a physiotherapist for appropriate exercises and treatment. It causes constant backache which can be very debilitating, but responds to support and special exercises.

The uterus is usually assessed daily to note the rate of involution, either by palpation or by using a tape measure to estimate the height of the uterine fundus above the upper border of the symphysis pubis. The accuracy of these methods is not known, especially when carried out by different practitioners (Montgomery and Alexander, 1994). There should be no uterine tenderness and it should be well-contracted, central and involute gradually at the rate of about 1 cm daily during the first 7–10 days of the puerperium. Thereafter involution occurs more slowly and is completed within 6–8 weeks of delivery.

Although this examination may be common practice during the postnatal period, a review of the literature conducted by Montgomery and Alexander (1994) indicated that there is no evidence that any form of external measurement of uterine involution in the early postnatal period has either preventive or predictive value. Research is therefore required to evaluate the practice of assessing uterine involution during the postnatal period (Rush *et al.*, 1989; Montgomery and Alexander, 1994).

Lochia
The lochia are inspected to note the colour, amount and consistency. If involution of the uterus is proceeding normally, the lochia are likely to be normal, whereas if involution is abnormal, this is likely to be reflected in the lochia.

Perineum
The perineum is inspected for any bruising or oedema and if the woman has sutures, the wound is observed for cleanliness and healing. Pain relief is assessed and alternative methods discussed and tried if relief is inadequate. During this part of the examination haemorrhoids may be noted and appropriate treatment advised.

Legs
Finally the midwife examines the mother's legs for oedema, inflammation and pain, especially after operative delivery or if for any reason the woman is confined to bed. Any abnormality may be caused by superficial or deep vein thrombosis and thus should be reported to the doctor immediately.

Postnatal exercises
These are taught, usually the day after an uncomplicated delivery, and the mother encouraged to perform them daily for a period of six weeks (see later in this chapter).

Haemoglobin estimation

Anaemia is common in the puerperium, especially in women who were anaemic before delivery or had more than an average blood loss at delivery. In a survey conducted by Campbell and Holbrook (1992) to assess the value of routine haemoglobin estimation during the postnatal period, it was found that anaemia was diagnosed in nearly 10% of those who had a normal predelivery haemoglobin and normal estimated blood loss at delivery. Many authorities therefore advocate routine haemoglobin estimations between 3 and 5 days after delivery to ensure that anaemia is diagnosed and treated. Earlier testing than this reduces the value because of the haemodilution of pregnancy. If anaemia is diagnosed iron tablets are prescribed. A study to assess the effects of a low haemoglobin on postnatal women found that at 10 days after delivery it was related to physical symptoms of low energy, breathlessness, faintness and dizziness, painful sutures and tingling in the fingers and toes. Tiredness was found to persist to six weeks after delivery (Paterson *et al.*, 1994). If the mother complains of these symptoms, especially in areas where routine haemoglobin estimates are no longer carried out, the midwife should suspect anaemia and arrange for her haemoglobin to be checked so that anaemia can be diagnosed and treated.

HEALTH EDUCATION AND MOTHERCRAFT TEACHING

A most important aspect of the midwife's role in the postnatal period is to promote health education and help the mother to learn and develop confidence in her mothering skills. She should listen patiently to the fears the mother expresses, answer her questions and, throughout, give her encouragement, reassurance and praise for her achievements.

Postnatal teaching should be a continuation of the mother's antenatal education. The importance of adequate rest and sleep is stressed and the mother should continue taking a good, well-balanced diet. If she is anaemic advice is given on foods which are rich in iron and also iron tablets will be prescribed. High standards of personal hygiene will be emphasized and the mother is taught how to care for herself and her baby. Postnatal exercises will be taught and the mother encouraged to continue practising them for at least 6 weeks.

Primiparae, in particular, may be anxious about the care of their baby. Nowadays mothers who have had an uncomplicated delivery start to care for their baby soon after delivery, with the help of their midwife, and this early contact helps them to develop confidence more quickly. Those who have had a complicated delivery will require more time to recuperate before they are ready to start caring for their baby and so the midwife will undertake this care, until she judges that the woman is well enough to start taking an active part in the care. The midwife teaches the mother all the basic principles of infant care. These include hygiene, prevention of infection, cord care, feeding, how to interpret and cope with crying, and the importance of getting to know her baby, of talking to him and giving him love and a sense of security. The mothers may express concerns about their baby, for instance, general behaviour, erratic sleep patterns or the unpredictability of the daily schedule. This gives the midwife an opportunity to examine the baby to ensure that all is well and educate the mother about the normal range of behaviour patterns, changing patterns of behaviour to be expected and abnormal behaviours which require medical advice. Sometimes the mother only requires reassurance that her baby's behaviour is normal, but if there is a problem the midwife may suggest various strategies which the mother could employ to try and resolve it. Very often the mother also has concerns about her own fatigue and physical problems and again the midwife can offer help and health education to try and alleviate her problems (Field, 1991). It is essential that the midwife gives mothers time and the opportunity to discuss these concerns, listens and answers their questions and supports their actions rather than taking over the care of their baby.

Health education also includes discussion of emotional problems which commonly arise during the puerperium and of relationships within the family. The arrival of a new baby has an effect on all members of the family, including other children, and the multiparous mother may be concerned about their reaction and how best to cope with sibling jealousy. Fathers also have important adjustments to make, especially after the birth of their first child, and may feel neglected and jealous on occasions if their partner appears to have little time for them. They have a vital role to play in supporting their partner and in sharing the care of their baby and perhaps other children, and so where possible should be included in health education and discussions about baby care.

Sexual problems may also be discussed, especially during the latter part of the postnatal period when the couple are usually resuming sexual relations. For some women dyspareunia after childbirth is a long-term problem (MacArthur et al., 1993a) and expert advice may be required.

Family planning is considered and the parents are given information on the methods available so that they can make an informed choice. The mother may be referred to her general practitioner or to a family planning clinic. In some cases this may be combined with the postnatal examination.

CARE AFTER CAESAREAN SECTION

Care after a Caesarean section is initially the same as for any woman after a major abdominal operation, but the postnatal mother also has her baby to consider, and may be very anxious if the infant is separated from her because it needs special or intensive care in a neonatal unit. Sometimes the Caesarean section follows a complicated labour and the woman has to recover from the physical and mental stress of this event as well as from a major abdominal operation.

During the first 24 hours frequent observations will be made on vital signs, including temperature, and the lochia and wound will be observed for bleeding. Other observations are as for women after an uncomplicated delivery. Antibiotics are often prescribed as a prophylactic measure to reduce the risk of infection. Initially good pain relief and an adequate fluid intake will be required. Pain relief may be achieved by intramuscular or intravenous opiates, the latter sometimes administered on a demand basis, or by regional analgesia in the form of an epidural. After 24 hours or so, oral analgesics are usually prescribed. An intravenous infusion will be maintained for the first 12–24 hours until the woman is taking sufficient oral fluids. A light diet may also be started, unless the surgeon prefers the woman to delay food intake until bowel sounds are heard because of the risk of paralytic ileus.

Soon after delivery the woman should see and, if possible, hold her baby. If she wishes to breastfeed this may be started, provided the baby is well, with the mother in a comfortable position, usually with the baby alongside her supported on a pillow so that his weight is not on her abdomen. The midwife's help will be required to help the mother breastfeed until she is more mobile and free from pain, and the mother and baby have learnt the art of correct attachment to the breast.

Deep breathing and leg exercises should be taught whilst the mother is in bed and she should be encouraged to do them frequently to reduce the risks of thromboembolic disorders, which are higher following an operative delivery. Within the first 24 hours of delivery the mother should be helped out of bed and into a chair and, if she is well enough, to the bathroom and lavatory. She will require help with her personal toilet for the first 2 or 3 days, or until she is well enough to manage alone.

Urinary output should be noted for the first 24 hours, or until the mother is passing urine normally. Abdominal pain due to gas or air in the intestinal tract may be a source of considerable pain during the first 48 hours or so and measures to try and relieve it include passing a flatus tube, giving suppositories and gentle exercises like bending forward from the waist several times. Postnatal exercises may also help, and should be gradually introduced after the first day or two.

During the first 48 hours or so after the Caesarean section the midwife will care for the baby, but when the mother is well enough she gradually becomes involved until she is fully caring for her infant with the support of the midwife, as necessary. Abdominal sutures are removed according to the surgeon's wishes, usually about the fifth day.

The mother will require considerable help and support after discharge from hospital, preferably for some weeks, as morbidity is higher after Caesarean section and adequate rest is difficult to achieve with the care of a young baby.

DISCHARGE FROM HOSPITAL

Before leaving the hospital the mother is usually examined by her midwife to make sure that she is fit for discharge and the baby may be examined by a paediatrician, although the report *Changing Childbirth* recommends that midwives should be taught how to examine the normal newborn (DOH, 1993). All records are completed and, if anaemic, the mother may be given iron tablets to take. The importance of the postnatal examination is explained and the mother is either given a hospital appointment or asked to make an appointment with her general practitioner for about six weeks after delivery. If she is menstruating at the time of the postnatal examination she should telephone and defer her appointment for a week or two.

The midwife explains that she, or another midwife, will visit the woman at home the next day and thereafter at intervals to be agreed for a minimum of 10 days, and the mother is given a telephone number where she can contact her midwife if problems arise in between her visits. The provision of a 24-hour telephone helpline to the maternity unit for parents of young babies is very reassuring (Hay-Smith, 1994d), especially when problems arise in the middle of the night and the parents are reluctant to disturb their midwife or general practitioner who have been working all day. Medical care after transfer home from hospital is provided by the mother's general practitioner.

The Postnatal Examination

The postnatal examination is carried out either by the general practitioner or, following a complicated delivery, usually by the obstetrician at about six weeks after delivery. By this time the reproductive organs should have returned to their pre-gravid state and the mother should have made a good recovery from childbirth. Many women, however, have long-term morbidity which should be detected at the postnatal examination and appropriate help can then be given.

The examination includes an assessment of the woman's general physical and mental health and a medical examination. The mother should be invited to bring the baby too and the doctor enquires about the progress of the baby, observes the maternal/infant relationship and gives the mother the opportunity to discuss any problems that may be concerning her (Metcalfe and Rathbone, 1988). Assessment of her mental state is very important, as a significant number of women are suffering from postnatal depression at this time.

The mother is weighed, her urine is tested and her blood pressure is recorded. An examination of breasts, abdomen, vulva, perineum and legs is then carried out by the doctor. This is followed by an examination per vaginam to note the condition of the cervix, the size and position of the uterus and the muscle tone of the genital tract, including the pelvic floor. A cervical smear may be taken.

The doctor should enquire about stress incontinence as many women are too embarrassed to discuss this problem (MacArthur et al., 1993b). Another issue which they may be reticent about broaching is the resumption of sexual intercourse, especially if they have problems, and so tactful enquiry should be made. Postnatal loss of libido is a very common condition which can threaten the stability of the marriage if it continues for too long (Tobert, 1990). Very often it is associated with childhood experiences as well as the overwhelming fatigue of the puerperium and, in many women, dyspareunia. If it is not resolved within a few weeks the mother can be offered specialist help.

A specimen of blood may be taken for haemoglobin estimation if the mother is thought to be anaemic, or was anaemic earlier in the puerperium.

Family planning is discussed and the mother is given information, as required. Menstruation recommences at the end of the puerperium or within the next month or two, but may be delayed when the woman is breast-feeding owing to high prolactin levels. Ovulation takes place before menstruation and therefore pregnancy could occur before the resumption of menstruation.

If the examination proves satisfactory the mother will be discharged. Otherwise she will be given a further appointment or be referred to an appropriate specialist.

Many women do not attend for a postnatal examination, especially those in socioeconomic groups III, IV and V and those who have experienced abnormal deliveries (Bowers, 1984).

According to Bowers' study, the problems most worrying to the mothers at this examination were haemorrhoids, backache, vaginal discharge and depression. Dyspareunia was not reported in this study, perhaps because only 53% of male general practitioners raised the issue of sexual relations with the mother. Coats et al. (1980) followed up women who had episiotomies at delivery and found that 45% complained of pain at intercourse more than four weeks after resuming sexual activity and 15% more than eight weeks. These findings have been substantiated by other studies (Kitzinger and Walters, 1981; Sleep et al., 1984; MacArthur et al., 1993a).

Bowers (1984) found in her study that women regarded the discussion as being the most important part of the postnatal examination, yet it was often unsatisfactory. It seems that again more emphasis on the social and psychological aspects of care is required, and time needs to be allowed for this.

Postnatal Support Groups

In some areas postnatal support groups have been formed where mothers can meet together for company and share their problems. Many mothers feel isolated and lonely at home caring for a young baby and find the companionship and support of such a group of great benefit. Some groups are established by midwives and health visitors while others are self-help groups arranged by the mothers themselves, often comprising the same group who met for antenatal education.

The National Childbirth Trust runs postnatal groups and also offers a personalized service in some areas, whereby a new mother is put in touch with a support person who has also recently become a mother. Other support groups such as the Meet-a-Mum Association (MAMA) developed following television personality Esther Rantzen's awareness of the problems of isolation and loneliness of new mothers (Smith, 1987).

Physical Rehabilitation

Many physical changes take place during pregnancy and it is important to ensure that the effects of these changes resolve gradually without causing any long-term problems. Exercises and advice will not only help to reduce physical problems but will give the woman an improved sense of well-being.

The main aims of physical rehabilitation in the postnatal period are to:

▶ improve circulation and ventilation
▶ restore the pelvic floor muscles to full function and to avoid urinary problems, for example, stress incontinence
▶ strengthen the abdominal muscles to restore their function as prime movers of the trunk, supporters of the spine and the abdominal contents and maintainers of intra-abdominal pressure
▶ ensure adequate care of the back
▶ speed up resolution of postnatal musculoskeletal problems, for example, diastasis recti, symphysis pubis dysfunction.

The benefits of each exercise should be explained to the mother as well as the long-term problems which may result if the pelvic floor and abdominal muscles do not fully recover.

The pelvic floor muscles play a part in the maintenance of continence (Nielsen et al., 1988). Wilson et al. (1996) claimed that as many as one in three women suffered from some degree of urinary incontinence three months postpartum. The pelvic floor muscles have two types of muscle fibres namely slow twitch and fast twitch (Gilpin et al., 1989). The slow twitch fibres are the postural fibres capable of sustaining action whilst the fast twitch fibres can be activated quickly to prevent an 'accident'. Both types of fibres need re-educating postnatally to restore full function.

The abdominal muscles play a significant role in supporting the spine and preventing backache. Back problems in women occurring even several years after childbirth have been identified as resulting from weak abdominal muscles (Nouwen et al., 1987; Panjabi et al., 1989). Like the pelvic floor muscles the abdominals have both slow and fast twitch fibres and it is the former which play the larger part in maintaining correct posture (Richardson, 1992). The deeper transversus abdominis and internal oblique muscles are seen as the most important stabilisers of the lumbar spine (Richardson et al., 1990) as they are closest to the spine and take attachment from the lumbar fascia thus forming a complete corset of support (Jull and Richardson, 1994). The transversus muscle is composed of nearly all slow twitch type fibres. Previously the longitudinal rectus muscles were considered the most important to exercise after childbirth as they

control the tilt of the pelvis and consequent alignment of the lumbar spine and these were the main abdominals to be rehabilitated postnatally often at the expense of the deeper transverse abdominals. However the recti have more fast twitch than slow twitch fibres and are not as concerned in preventing back problems. Both groups need rehabilitating to restore full function.

FOLLOWING NORMAL DELIVERY

Immediately postpartum, exercises to improve the circulation should be encouraged to lessen the risk of deep venous thrombosis and reduce any residual oedema.

Circulatory exercises

The mother should be encouraged to circle both ankles vigorously at least 15 times in each direction as often as possible during the first 48 hours postdelivery (or even longer if any oedema persists). This can be done under or on top of the bedclothes or sitting on a chair with feet and legs supported on a stool or similar. The ankle circling should be followed by at least 10 tightenings of the leg muscles by pulling up both feet at the ankles and pressing the back of both knees down onto the support and holding the legs taut for approximately 5 seconds. Breathing should be normal throughout the exercise.

If any swelling persists postdelivery the mother may lie with her feet elevated higher than her hips whilst sleeping, resting and performing her circulatory exercises. Even if there is no oedema she should be discouraged from sitting or lying with her legs crossed and from standing for long periods of time when this is unnecessary.

It must be remembered that deep breathing also improves the circulation, especially venous return, by the pumping action of the diaphragm on the inferior vena cava. Three or four deep breaths at a time are sufficient as more could induce hyperventilation. Deep breathing will also ensure full expansion of the lung bases following the upward pressure of the diaphragm during pregnancy.

Pelvic floor exercise

Because the pelvic floor muscles and nerves have been stretched during delivery and pain or numbness of the perineum may be present, pelvic floor exercises will be quite difficult to perform at first. It is important that they are encouraged as the exercise will become easier and repeated practice will help the healing process of the perineum post-episiotomy. The easiest position in which to do the exercise is sitting on the toilet or on a chair but it can be performed in any position and whilst feeding, nappy changing, bathing baby etc.

The mother is asked to close and squeeze the muscles round her back and front passages as though preventing the loss of wind and urine and then lift up all three passages inside. This 'squeeze and lift' should be held for as long as possible up to 10 seconds breathing normally throughout. The mother should aim to repeat the exercise up to 10 times altogether though this may take a few weeks to achieve. This strengthens the deep slow twitch fibres of the pelvic floor muscles. To retrain the fast twitch fibres of the pelvic floor the routine should be followed by up to 10 quick 'squeeze and lifts' without holding.

The mother should be advised to brace her pelvic floor when coughing, squatting or lifting as these activities all raise the intra-abdominal pressure and leaking of urine could result. She should test her pelvic floor muscles about 8–12 weeks postdelivery to ensure that her muscles have regained full function (see Chapter 25).

Abdominal exercises

Exercise for the transverse and rectus muscles can be commenced as soon as the woman feels up to it. The oblique muscles which insert into the linea alba (see Chapter 25) should not be exercised until a check to ensure there is no undue gap between the two rectus muscles has been carried out. This procedure is explained in Chapter 25. As this check is not accurate before the third day postdelivery (fifth day post LSCS) exercises for the oblique abdominal muscles should **not** be commenced before then because of the shearing effect they may have on the linea alba increasing the gap between the recti (Noble, 1988). If the linea alba separates, the muscles inserting into it and into the rectus sheath also separate and there is no protection anteriorly except for skin, subcutaneous fat and peritoneum (see Figure 7 in Chapter 25). A diastasis of 4+ fingers width will result in severe backache due to lack of anterior support for the lumbar spine and the woman will experience the sensation that her abdominal contents are going to fall out in front. This is most distressing and must be treated as a priority. Support for the whole length of the abdominals and lumbar spine can be provided in severe cases by two thicknesses of size 'J' or 'K' Tubigrip long enough to extend from under the bra to below the buttocks – approximately 22 inches in length.

Special exercises to close the diastasis must be started as soon as the diagnosis is made and continued as long as is necessary (see later in this section).

Abdominal retraction

This exercise to strengthen the deep transversus muscles can be done kneeling on all fours (not after LSCS), sitting, standing or side- back- or prone-lying. The mother should be asked to breathe in and whilst breathing out to draw the bottom part of her abdomen in towards her spine keeping her back flat. The contraction should be held for up to a count of 10 whilst breathing normally and repeated up to 10 times several times during the day. Like the pelvic floor contraction this exercise can be performed whilst doing activities with the baby.

Pelvic tilting

This can be practised in back-lying with knees bent up. The mother is asked to pull in her abdominal muscles, tighten her buttock muscles and press the small of her back downwards onto the bed. The contraction should be held for up to a count of 10 and repeated up to 10 times whilst breathing normally. Other positions in which to practice are sitting, kneeling, and standing.

Pelvic tilting should become a habit on assuming an upright posture after lying or sitting to ensure the correct pelvic tilt after pregnancy. If the anterior tilt is allowed to persist the muscles of the back may shorten giving disparity between the length of the spinal muscles and the length of the abdominal muscles. This is a major cause of backache and may lead to mechanical back problems (Panjabi *et al.*, 1989). The mother will feel much slimmer and flatter if she performs the pelvic tilting whenever she stands.

Oblique abdominal exercises

These will strengthen the internal and external oblique abdominal muscles and may only be progressed if there is no significant diastasis of the recti on testing (less than 2 fingers width) and no peaking or doming of the abdomen occurs on performance of the exercises. Straight curl-ups, knee rolling and hip updrawing are described and illustrated in Chapter 25 and may be commenced after the third day.

FOLLOWING CAESAREAN DELIVERY

Circulatory exercises are extremely important following Caesarean delivery as the pelvic circulation has been interrupted. Deep breathing will help the venous return as well as loosening chest secretions. If the mother needs to cough she will be most comfortable sitting over the edge of the bed with her knees bent and supporting her wound with her hands to reduce pain and tension.

Early ambulation is encouraged to improve both circulation and ventilation. The mother should be taught how to get out of bed correctly by bending her knees up, rolling over onto her side and pushing herself up into a sitting position using her underneath elbow and hands. When walking an upright posture must be adopted and pelvic tilting can be practised in this position.

Pelvic tilting and abdominal retraction in lying may ease the back discomfort that many post-Caesarean mothers experience especially after epidural anaesthesia and may be commenced when she feels comfortable.

Pelvic floor exercises are still important because of the hormonal effect on the pelvic floor during pregnancy, but may be left for a few days. Other abdominal exercise may be started after the diastasis check has been performed on the fifth day or later (see Chapter 25).

Because post-Caesarean mothers have experienced major surgery as well as childbirth they need a lot of practical help and support at home. The midwife is the ideal person to explain this to relatives and friends.

FOLLOWING ASSISTED DELIVERY

An assisted delivery often causes painful perineal bruising and oedema and these mothers will require adequate pain relief before mobilising. Circulatory and pelvic floor exercises are important as early as possible, but if the mother is in a lot of distress she may need local pain relief to the perineum before commencing pelvic floor exercises (see Chapter 25). Prone lying with pillows under the hips and the head is a comfortable resting position.

POSTNATAL BACK CARE

Immediately postpartum the mother's pelvic ligaments are still lax and her abdominal muscles stretched so her joints have little protection. She must be advised of this

situation and urged to avoid lifting if at all possible and to delegate strenuous housework such as vacuuming for several weeks. Optimum positions for feeding, bathing and nappy changing should all be discussed with the mother (see Figure 11 in Chapter 25).

FURTHER EXERCISE AND SPORT

Before rejoining keep fit or aerobic classes the mother should be encouraged to practise stronger exercises for the abdominal, back and hip muscles (Brayshaw and Wright, 1996). General exercise such as walking, swimming and cycling should be promoted but more strenuous activities and competitive sports should be left for up to 10-12 weeks or longer if any musculoskeletal or pelvic floor problems persist. **NB** Double leg lifts and sit-ups with straight legs should never be performed.

POSTNATAL MUSCULOSKELETAL PROBLEMS

Diastasis recti and symphysis pubis dysfunction are postnatal problems which require special attention postnatally to encourage early resolution.

Special exercises for diastasis recti

Specific exercises to reduce a diastasis are a priority if the gap between the rectus bellies is 3 fingers width or more. The woman should lie flat on her back with only one pillow, knees bent up, feet flat on the bed and hands crossed over her abdomen so the palm of her left hand is over the right rectus muscle belly and the palm of her right hand is over the left rectus muscle belly. She is asked to pelvic tilt and draw the two rectus muscle bellies towards midline by pulling both hands towards each other. She should hold this position for up to 10 seconds breathing normally throughout. This should be repeated at least 5 times followed by 6 repetitions of the same exercise together with lifting the head only (not shoulders) from the pillow whilst pelvic tilting. When able to perform the 6 repetitions of each exercise the number may be increased up to 10 repetitions. The head should never be lifted before tilting the pelvis as this could cause further diastasis as could lifting the shoulders. Doming or peaking of the muscles must not occur. Exercising the transverse abdominal muscles will help to stabilise the linea alba and protect the lumbar spine. Six to ten abdominal retractions may be performed in any position the mother finds comfortable. The routine of pelvic tilts, pelvic tilts with head lifts and abdominal retractions should be performed several times a day until the gap is less than 2 fingers width. The advice of an obstetric physiotherapist should be sought if a diastasis of 4 or more fingers width is found. She will review the diastasis at regular intervals for as long as necessary and ensure full rehabilitation of the abdominal muscles. The diastasis will recur in future pregnancies and the woman should be advised to wear some support during those pregnancies and to seek referral to the obstetric physiotherapist postdelivery.

Rehabilitation of symphysis pubis dysfunction (SPD)

Diastasis of the symphysis pubis, now known as symphysis pubis dysfunction, is a very distressing problem which appears to be more prevalent in recent years though no obvious cause has been found for this (Fry, 1992). During pregnancy the joint can increase in width from 4 to 9 mms but more than this causes a gliding action on weight-bearing which is extremely painful. Some mothers suffer from SPD during pregnancy which continues postdelivery, others may have become aware of pain and tenderness over the symphysis during labour or immediately postdelivery. On rare occasions pain does not become apparent for several hours

postdelivery (Dreissen, 1987) but this is caused by an inflammatory process which usually subsides fairly quickly.

In the case of a true diastasis bedrest postdelivery is essential until the acute pain subsides. Circulatory exercises must be encouraged to reduce the risk of DVT. Adequate pain relief is necessary and local pain relief may be administered by the physiotherapist in the form of therapeutic ultrasound, pulsed electromagnetic energy, TENS or ice. The mother must be told to press her knees firmly together before rolling over and to bend both her knees up together. She will need a lot of support and help especially with the baby but should be able to breast feed in side-lying. A trochanteric belt or binder (see Figures 1 and 2 in Chapter 20) may give the mother some support and pain relief. As well as circulatory exercises, pelvic tilting, pelvic floor and abdominal retractions can and should be performed in side- or back-lying with knees bent.

In severe cases an orthopaedic referral may be appropriate if the condition persists. The Association of Chartered Physiotherapists in Women's Health has produced a guideline for treatment of symphysis pubis dysfunction in pregnancy, labour and post-partum for medical, midwifery and therapy staff (ACPWH, 1996).

References

Acharya, U., Lamont, C.A. & Cooper, K. (1988) Group A beta-haemolytic streptococcus causing disseminated intravascular coagulation and maternal death. *Lancet* i: 595.

ACPWH (1996) *Symphysis Pubis Dysfunction Guideline*. London: Association of Chartered Physiotherapists in Women's Health.

Ball, J.A. (1989) Postnatal care and adjustment to motherhood. In Robinson, S. & Thomson, A. (eds) *Midwives, Research and Childbirth*, Vol. I, pp. 154–175. London: Chapman & Hall.

Ball, J.A. (1994) *Reactions to Motherhood. The Role of Postnatal Care*. Hale: Books for Midwives Press.

Bowers, J. (1984) The six week postnatal examination. Parts I and II. *Research and the Midwife*, Conference Proceedings, University of Manchester, pp. 28–30.

Brayshaw, E. & Wright, P. (1994) *Teaching Physical Skills for the Childbearing Year*. Hale: Books for Midwives Press.

Brayshaw, E. & Wright, P. (1996) *Relaxation and Exercise for the Childbearing Year*. Hale: Books for Midwives Press.

Brown, G. & Harris, T. (1978) Social origins of depression. In *Reactions to Motherhood. The Role of Postnatal Care*, p. 13. Hale: Books for Midwives Press.

Campbell, C. & Holbrook, A. (1992) Routine postnatal haemoglobin screening: a critical review. *Modern Midwife* May/June: 8–9.

Carvahlo, M., Robertson, S., Friedman, A. & Klaus, M. (1983) Effect of frequent breast feeding on early milk production and infant weight gain. *Pediatrics* 72: 307–311.

Carvahlo, M., Robertson, S. & Klaus, M. (1984) Does the duration and frequency of early breast feeding affect nipple pain? *Birth* 11(2): 81–84.

Chateau, P. de (1980) The first hour after delivery: its impact on synchrony of parent–infant relationship. *Paediatrics* 9: 151–168.

Claesson, B.E.B. & Claesson, U.L.E. (1985) An outbreak of endometritis in a maternity unit caused by spread of group A streptococci from a shower head. *J. Hosp. Infect.* 6: 304–311.

Coats, P.M., Chan, K.K., Wilkins, M. & Beard, R.J. (1980) A comparison between midline and mediolateral episiotomies. *Br. J. Obstet. Gynaecol.* 87: 408–412.

Cogill, S., Alexandra, H., Mordecai Robson, K. & Kumar, R. (1986) Impact of maternal postnatal depression on cognitive development of young children. *Br. Med. J.* 292: 1165–1167.

Cox, J.L., Connor, Y. & Kendell, R.E. (1982) Prospective study of the psychiatric disorders of childbirth. *Br. J. Psychiat.* 140: 111–117.

Dewan, G., Glazener, C. & Tunstall, M. (1993) Postnatal pain: a neglected area. *Br. J. Midwifery* 1(2): 63–66.

DOH (Department of Health) (1993) *Changing Childbirth*,

Report of the Expert Maternity Group, Part 1. London: HMSO.

Driessen, F. (1987) Postpartum arthropathy with unusual features. *Br. J. Obstet. Gynaecol.* **94**: 870–872.

Field, P. (1985) Parents reactions to maternity care. *Midwifery* **1**: 37–46.

Field, P.A. (1991) Teaching and support: nursing input in the postpartum period. *Int. J. Nursing Stud.* **28**(2): 131–144.

Fry, D. (1992) Diastasis Symphysis Pubis. *J. Assoc. Chartered Physiother. Obstet. Gynaecol.* **71**: 10–13.

Garcia, J. & Marchant, S. (1993) Back to normal? Postpartum health and illness. *Research and the Midwife*, Conference Proceedings, University of Manchester, pp. 2–9.

Garcia, J., Renfrew, M. & Marchant, S. (1994) Postnatal home visiting by midwives. *Midwifery* **10**: 40–43.

Gilpin, S.A., Gosling, J.A., Smith, A.R.B. & Warrell, D.W. (1989) The pathogenesis of genitourinary prolapse and stress incontinence of urine. A histological and histochemical study. *Br. J. Obstet. Gynaecol.* **96**: 15–23.

Gordon, G. & Lochhead, D. (1994) An outbreak of group A haemolytic streptococcal puerpural sepsis spread by communal use of bidets. *Br. J. Obstet. Gynaecol.* **101**: 447–448.

Grant, A. & Sleep, J. (1989) Relief of perineal pain and discomfort after childbirth. In Chalmers, I., Enkin, M. & Keirse, M.J.N.C. (eds) *Effective Care in Pregnancy and Childbirth*, Vol. 2, p. 1351. Oxford: Oxford University Press.

Greer, I.A. & Cameron, A.D. (1984) Topical pramoxine and hydrocortisone foam versus placebo in relief of postpartum episiotomy symptoms and wound healing. *Scot. Med. J.* **29**: 104–106.

Harris, M. (1992) The impact of research findings on current practice in relieving postpartum perineal pain in a large district general hospital. *Midwifery* **8**: 125–131.

Haynes, J., Anderson, A.W. & Spence, W.N. (1987) An outbreak of puerperal fever caused by group G streptococci. *J. Hosp. Infect.* **9**: 120–125.

Hay-Smith, J. (1994a) Early vs standard postnatal discharge from hospital. In Enkin, M.W., Keirse, M.J.N.C., Renfrew, M.J. & Neilson, J.P. (eds) *Pregnancy and Childbirth Module.* Cochrane Database of Systematic Reviews: Review no. 02735. Cochrane Updates on Disk, Disk Issue 1. Oxford: Update Software.

Hay-Smith, J. (1994b) Postpartum laxatives. In Enkin, M.W., Keirse, M.J.N.C., Renfrew, M.J. & Neilson, J.P. (eds) *Pregnancy and Childbirth Module.* Cochrane Database of Systematic Reviews: Review no. 03663. Cochrane Updates on Disk, Disk Issue 1. Oxford: Update Software.

Hay-Smith, J. (1994c) 'Anacal' ointment for puerperal haemorrhoid. In Enkin, M.W., Keirse, M.J.N.C., Renfrew, M.J. & Neilson, J.P. (eds) *Pregnancy and Childbirth Module.* Cochrane Database of Systematic Reviews: Review no. 07428. Cochrane Updates on Disk, Disk Issue 1. Oxford: Update Software.

Hay-Smith, J. (1994d) Provision of hospital telephone service for new parents. In Enkin, M.W., Keirse, M.J.N.C., Renfrew, M.J. & Neilson, J.P. (eds) *Pregnancy and Childbirth Module.* Cochrane Database of Systematic Reviews: Review no. 07321. Cochrane Updates on Disk, Disk Issue 1. Oxford: Update Software.

Herd, B. & Feeney, J.G. (1986) Two aerosol sprays in nipple trauma. *The Practitioner* **120**: 31–38.

Inch, S. (1982) *Birth Rights: A Parents' Guide to Modern Childbirth.* London: Hutchinson.

Inch, S. (1990) Postnatal care relating to breast feeding. In Alexander, J., Levy, V., Roch, S. (eds) *Postnatal Care*, p. 23. London: Macmillan.

Inch, S. & Fisher, C. (1987) Antiseptic sprays and nipple trauma. *The Practitioner* **230**: 1037–1038.

Jull, G.A. & Richardson, C.A. (1994) Rehabilitation of Active Stabilisation of the Lumbar Spine, in: Eds Twomey, L.T. & Taylor, R.J. *Physical Therapy of the Low Back.* New York; chap 9, 251–273.

Kavi, J. & Wise, R. (1988) Group A beta-haemolytic streptococcus causing disseminated intravascular coagulation and maternal death. *Lancet* **i**: 993–994.

Kendell, R.E. (1985) Emotional and physical factors in the genesis of mental disorders. *J. Psychosomat. Res.* **29**(1): 3–11.

Kitzinger, S. & Walters, R. (1981) *Some Women's Experience of Episiotomy.* London: National Childbirth Trust.

Kries, R. von, Shearer, M., McCarthy, P.T., Haug, M., Harzer, G. & Gobel, U. (1987) Vitamin K1 content of maternal milk: influence of the stage of lactation, lipid composition and vitamin K1 supplements given to the mother. *Paediat. Res.* **22**: 513–517.

Laryea, M.G.G. (1984) *Postnatal Care – The Midwife's Role.* Edinburgh: Churchill Livingstone.

Lavery, J.P. & Shaw, L.A. (1989) Sonography of the puerperal uterus. *J. Ultrasound Med.* **8**: 481–486.

Lazarus, R.S. (1966) Psychological stress and the coping process. In Ball, J. (1994) *Reactions to Motherhood*, pp. 11–14. Hale: Books for Midwives Press.

Levy, V. (1984) The third day 'blues'. *Midwives' Chronicle* November: xiv–xv.

Lucas, A., Lucas, P.J. & Baum, J.D. (1979) Patterns of milk flow in breastfed babies. *Lancet* **ii**: 57–59.

MacArthur, C., Bick, D. & Lewis, M. (1993a) Persistent health problems after childbirth and their effect on women's quality of life. *Research and the Midwife*, Conference Proceedings, University of Manchester: 18–21.

MacArthur, C., Lewis, M. & Bick, D. (1993b) Stress incontinence after childbirth. *Br. J. Midwifery* **1**(5): 207–215.

Martin, J. & Monk, J. (1982) *Infant Feeding 1980.* London: HMSO.

Martin, J. & White, A. (1988) *Infant Feeding.* London: HMSO.

Metcalfe, E.M. & Rathbone, A.R. (1988) The postnatal examination. *Update* 1 March: 1868–1875.

Montgomery, E. & Alexander, J. (1994) Assessing postnatal uterine involution: a review and a challenge. *Midwifery* **10**(2): 73–86.

Murphy-Black, T. (1994) Care in the community during the postnatal period. In Robinson, S. & Thomson, A.M. (eds) *Midwives, Research and Childbirth.* London: Chapman & Hall.

Murray, L. (1988) Effects of postnatal depression on infant development: direct studies of early mother–infant interactions. In Kumar, R. & Brockington, I.F. (eds) *Motherhood and Mental Illness.* London: Wright, Butterworth & Co.

Newton, M. (1952) Nipple pain and nipple damage. *J. Pediatr.* **41**: 411–423.

Nielsen, C.A., Sigsgaard, I., Olsen, M., Tolstrup, M., Danneskiold-Samsoee, B., & Bock, J.E. (1988) Trainability of the pelvic floor. *Acta Obstet. Gynecol. Scand.* **67**: 437–440.

Nouwen, A., Van Akkerveeken, P.F., & Versloot, J.M. (1987)

Patterns of muscular activity during movement in patients with chronic low back pain. *Spine.* **12**: 777–782.

Oakley, A. (1994) Giving support in pregnancy: the role of research midwives in a randomised controlled trial. In Robinson, S. & Thomson, A.M. (eds) *Midwives, Research and Childbirth.* Vol. 3. London: Chapman & Hall.

Panjabi, M., Abumi, K., Duranceau, J., & Oxland, T. (1989) Spinal stability and intersegmental muscle forces: A biomechanical model. *Spine.* **14**: 194–200.

Paterson, J.A., Davis, J., Gregory, M. *et al.* (1994) A study on the effects of low haemoglobin on postnatal women. *Midwifery* **10**(2): 77–86.

Paykel, E., Emms, E., Fletcher, J. & Rassaly, E. (1980) Life events and social support in puerperal depression. *Br. J. Psychiat.* **136**: 339–346.

Raphel-Leff, J. (1992) *Psychological Processes of Childbearing.* London: Chapman & Hall.

Renfrew, M.J. (1994a) Bromocriptine for lactation suppression. In Enkin, M.W., Keirse, M.J.N.C., Renfrew, M.J. & Neilson, J.P. (eds) *Pregnancy and Childbirth Module.* Cochrane Database of Systematic Reviews: Review no. 03384. Cochrane Updates on Disk, Disk Issue 1. Oxford: Update Software.

Renfrew, M.J. (1994b) Cabergoline versus bromocriptine for lactation suppression. In Enkin, M.W., Keirse, M.J.N.C., Renfrew, M.J. & Neilson, J.P. (eds) *Pregnancy and Childbirth Module.* Cochrane Database of Systematic Reviews: Review no. 06471. Cochrane Updates on Disk, Disk Issue 1. Oxford: Update Software.

Renfrew, M.J. & Lang, S. (1994) Early versus late discharge for breast feeding mothers. In Enkin, M.W., Keirse, M.J.N.C., Renfrew, M.J. & Neilson, J.P. (eds) *Pregnancy and Childbirth Module.* Cochrane Database of Systematic Reviews: Review no. 08283. Cochrane Updates on Disk, Disk Issue 1. Oxford: Update Software.

Richardson, C., Jull, G., Toppenberg, R., & Comerford, M. (1992) Techniques for active lumbar stabilisation for spinal protection: A pilot study. *Australian Journal of Physiotherapy.* **38**(2): 105–112.

Richardson, C., Toppenberg, R., & Jull, G. (1990) An initial evaluation of eight abdominal exercises for their ability to provide active lumbar stabilisation for the lumber spine. *Australian Journal of Physiotherapy.* **36**(1): 6–11.

Rickitt, C. (1987) Stress in the puerperium. *Midwives' Chronicle* November: 347–350.

Rodeck, C.H. & Newton, J.R. (1976) Study of the uterine cavity by ultrasound in the early puerperium. *Br. J. Obstet. Gynaecol.* **83**: 795–801.

Rush, J., Chalmers, I. & Enkin, M. (1989) Care of the new mother and baby. In Chalmers, I., Enkin, M. & Keirse, M.J.N.C. (eds) *Effective Care in Pregnancy and Childbirth,* pp. 1339–1349. Oxford: Oxford University Press.

Saint, L., Smith, M. & Hartmann, P.E. (1984) The yield and nutrient content of colostrum and milk of women giving birth to one month postpartum. *Br. J. Nutr.* **52**: 87–95.

Salariya, E.M., Easton, P.M. & Cater, J.I. (1978) Duration of breast feeding after early initiation and frequent feeding. *Lancet* ii: 1141–1143.

Salzarulo, M.D. & Rigoard, M.T. (1987) Long-lasting sleep disturbances in women after childbirth. *J. Reprod. Infant Psychol.* **5**: 245–246.

Sleep, J. & Grant, A. (1988) Relief of perineal pain following childbirth: A survey of midwifery practice. *Midwifery* **4**: 118–122.

Sleep, J., Grant, A., Garcia, J., Elbourne, D., Spencer, J.A.D. & Chalmers, I. (1984) West Berkshire perineal management trial. *Br. Med. J.* **289**: 587–590.

Smith, P. (1989) Postnatal concerns of mothers: an update. *Midwifery* **5**: 182–188.

Smith, S. (1987) Postnatal – who cares? *J. R. Coll. Gen. Pract.* January: 1–2.

Swyer, G.I.M. (1985) Postpartum mental disturbances and hormone changes. *Br. Med. J.* **20**: 1232–1233.

Teare, E.L., Smithson, R.D., Efstratiou, A., Devenish, W.R. & Noah, N.D. (1989) An outbreak of puerperal fever caused by group C streptococci. *J. Hosp. Infect.* **13**: 337–347.

Tobert, A. (1990) Sexual problems in pregnancy and the postnatal period. *Midwife, Health Visitor & Community Nurse* **26**(5): 177–179.

Turton, P. (1980) Sleep and comfort during pregnancy and after birth. *Nursing*: 863–865.

UKCC (United Kingdom Central Council for Nursing, Midwifery and Health Visiting) (1993) *Midwives' Rules.* London: UKCC.

UKCC (1994) *The Midwife's Code of Practice.* London: UKCC.

Weiss, R.S. (1976) Transition states and other stressful situations: their nature and programs for their management. In Caplan, G. & Killelia, M. (eds) *Support Systems and Mutual Help,* pp. 211–232. New York: Grune & Stratton.

Widstrom, A.M., Ransjo-Arvidson, A.B., Christensson, H.K., Mattiesen, A.S., Winberg, J. & Uvnas-Moberg, K. (1987) Gastric suction in healthy newborn infants: effects on circulation and developing feeding behaviour. *Acta Paediat. Scand.* **76**: 566–572.

Wilson, P.D., Herbison, R.M. & Herbison, G.P. (1996) Obstetric practice and the prevalence of urinary incontinence three months after delivery. *Br. J. Obstet. Gynaecol.* **103**: 154–161.

Woollett, A. & Dosanjh-Matwala, N. (1990) Postnatal care: the attitudes and experiences of Asian women in east London. *Midwifery* **6**: 178–184.

Morbidity Associated with Childbirth

Traditionally, the six-week examination marks the end of the puerperium and a woman's routine postnatal contact with the health services. After this the health visiting service is available but in practice this focuses much more on the welfare of the child than on the health of the mother. It is known that occasionally women suffer from childbirth-related problems after this time, some even requiring re-admission to hospital, and the persistence of postnatal depression is well documented, but until recently there have been few systematic investigations of longer term morbidity following childbirth.

Two large-scale studies, in Birmingham (MacArthur *et al.*, 1991) and in Aberdeen (Glazener *et al.*, 1993, 1995) have recently carried out a general investigation into health problems associated with childbirth. Both have identified enormous numbers of cases of postpartum ill-health, many of which go unreported to the health professionals. Some smaller studies have had similar findings (Johansen *et al.*, 1993; Garcia and Marchant, 1993). There have also been a few studies investigating individual symptoms or groups of symptoms, which will be referred to where relevant.

Extent of Longer Term Morbidity

The study in Birmingham obtained data from postal questionnaires completed by 11 701 women who had delivered their youngest child in a large maternity hospital between 1978 and 1985. Questionnaires were sent in 1987, deliveries having occurred 1–9 years earlier, thus allowing the reporting of problems with long durations. Questionnaires from the women were linked, using hospital registration number, to their computerized maternity case-notes so that associations could be made between the symptoms and various obstetric circumstances and procedures.

Almost half of the women in the sample (47%) reported at least one new symptom, starting for the first time within three months of the birth and lasting for more than six weeks. Including recurrent symptoms as well, this total rose to almost two-thirds of the sample (64%). Most symptoms lasted much longer than six weeks: 35% of the women reported new symptoms lasting over a year and 31.5% still had unresolved symptoms at the time of questioning, indicating the chronicity of much of this childbirth-related morbidity.

Examples of the reported problems were backache; headache and other musculoskeletal symptoms; bladder problems; haemorrhoids; depression and fatigue; paraesthesias and other sensory disturbances, all of which are discussed individually later in this chapter.

Another follow-up study is currently underway in Birmingham to find out more about the severity and impact of these long-term symptoms on the women's lives. The preliminary results of this have confirmed the extensiveness of morbidity after childbirth, and have shown that many of the symptoms present daily, that some can be severe and that many affect aspects of the women's lives (Bick and MacArthur, 1995a).

The study in Grampian, Scotland, recruited a 20% sample of all births between 1990 and 1991 in the region and surveyed women three times. First, they were asked to complete a questionnaire whilst in hospital, then at eight weeks post-delivery, thus obtaining data on shorter term problems. At 12–18 months post-delivery half the group ($n = 438$) completed a further postal questionnaire, providing information on longer lasting problems. This survey was more detailed than the Birmingham study, although of a smaller group, but again identified an enormous amount of childbirth-related morbidity. Seventy-six per cent of the women surveyed 12–18 months after the birth reported one or more problems that had persisted after the completion of their eight-week questionnaire.

Medical Consultation

Even though so many women reported health problems after childbirth, most did not consult a doctor. The exact proportions varied according to the particular symptoms, but on average only a third of the symptoms reported to the researchers in the Birmingham study had been reported to a doctor. There could be many reasons for this lack of consultation. The symptom might only be mild or occur infrequently; the problem might be considered by the woman as 'normal' after having children so must be endured; or she

may think that there is nothing that a doctor could do. Whatever the reason, the effect of this lack of consultation is that the full extent of the postpartum morbidity experienced by women has previously remained unrecognized by the medical profession.

Backache

It has long been known that backache during pregnancy is common, occurring in around half of women and resulting from the hormonal effects of relaxed ligaments, altered posture and extra weight (Mantle *et al.*, 1977; Ostgaard *et al.*, 1991). Short-term backache occurring after childbirth has also been reported (Grove, 1973; Berg *et al.*, 1988). Investigations showing the existence of persistent post-delivery backache are more recent.

In the Birmingham sample described above, 14% complained of backache starting after delivery and lasting over six weeks, rising to 23% when women who had also had backache previously were included. Two-thirds of these symptomatic women still had backache at the time of questioning, 1–9 years later. A similar proportion (20%) of women with backache lasting for more than eight weeks after childbirth was found in the sample from Grampian. Russell *et al.* (1993), specifically assessing postpartum backache, found that in a group of 1051 women delivering their first baby 29.5% had backache lasting for more than six months after delivery, and for 15.4% this was new backache starting after the birth.

Epidural anaesthesia during labour has been found to be closely associated with subsequent long-term backache (MacArthur *et al.*, 1990; Russell *et al.*, 1993; MacLeod *et al.*, 1995), except where the epidural was given for an elective section. Reports from women to the National Childbirth Trust (NCT) about problems following epidural also highlighted persistent backache (Kitzinger, 1987). The postulated mechanism to account for this association relates to stressed positions, which can occur anyway during labour, but are exacerbated by epidural anaesthesia due to muscular relaxation, the abolition of pain inhibiting the desire to move and inability to move unaided. A woman can remain without immediate discomfort for some time in a potentially damaging position. Randomized controlled trials are underway to determine whether this backache–epidural relationship is causal, or whether it is accounted for by some other factors, for example differences in the types of women who choose to have an epidural.

A recent study conducted in Boston, USA, found no excess backache after epidural analgesia in a group of women surveyed two months after delivery (Breen, 1994) and followed up at 12–18 months postpartum (Groves *et al.*, 1994). However, the epidurals differed from those in the UK. The epidural was administered by constant infusion and lower concentrations of anaesthetic agents used, which allowed the majority of women to remain mobile. Further research is urgently required to assess whether differences in mobility whilst under epidural are related to subsequent backache.

Russell *et al.* (1993) have suggested that women receiving epidural analgesia must be carefully positioned during labour and that advice on posture in the weeks afterwards should be given. It is likely that a position which gives support to the lumbar-sacral region of the back during labour would be advantageous but there have been no investigations of the longer term benefits of different positions.

Headache

Like backache, the occurrence of postpartum headaches of short duration, in at least a quarter of women, has been reported in the literature (Pitt, 1973; Grove, 1973; Stein *et al.*, 1984) but the existence of longer lasting headaches has only recently been examined.

MacArthur *et al.* (1991) asked about frequent headaches and migraine, allowing women to define these for themselves: 3.6% reported frequent headaches and 1.4% migraine as new postdelivery symptoms lasting over six weeks; and a further 4.7% and 5.7% respectively had also had the same symptoms before. Almost two-thirds of the symptomatic women still had their headache symptoms 1–9 years later.

Russell *et al.* (1993) found similar proportions with headache (not specifically frequent headaches) lasting more than six months after delivery: 3.7% reported new headaches, with a further 4.0% reporting recurrent headaches. Glazener *et al.* (1993) found that 15% of the sample had headaches (new plus recurrent) lasting over eight weeks.

Epidural anaesthesia was associated with frequent headaches in the Birmingham study (MacArthur *et al.*, 1991), but Russell *et al.* (1993) found no association. In the National Childbirth Trust study (Kitzinger, 1987) 3% of women felt that their persistent headaches represented long-term side-effects of their epidural. Dural puncture which occurs accidentally in about 1% of epidurals typically produces severe postural headaches and it is possible that these might also persist (Scott and Hibbard, 1990; MacArthur *et al.*, 1993a).

Headache is a common complaint which most people experience at times irrespective of having a baby and can be generally related to stress and fatigue. The additional responsibilities and activities associated with caring for babies and children are likely to be influential factors irrespective of the childbirth process. Social support in the postnatal period is important here.

Other Musculoskeletal Symptoms

New *neckache* and *shoulderache* were reported by around 2% of women after delivery, a further 2% reporting recurrent symptoms. MacArthur *et al.* (1992) found that persistent neckache was more common after epidural analgesia, but Russell *et al.* (1993) found no relationship.

Neckache and shoulder pain were also associated with having Caesarean section under general anaesthesia, although only small numbers of women were affected by this (MacArthur *et al.*, 1990). Dewan *et al.* (1993) have confirmed this association for short-term neck and shoulder pain. This could be due to the posture associated with section, where the neck is positioned to facilitate intubation and is unprotected by muscle tone.

Pains and weakness in the arms and legs starting after birth and persisting for weeks, months or years were each reported by between 1–2% of the women in the Birmingham sample, and this was much more common among the women of Asian origin. This could result from differences in cultural reporting but might be accounted for by vitamin D deficiency, commonly found among Asians resident in the UK (Brooke *et al.*, 1980), accentuated by the extra demands and postural stresses of pregnancy and delivery (MacArthur *et al.*, 1993b).

Overall, the skeletal system of the parturient woman seems to be extraordinarily sensitive to various forms of long-term injury, probably because of the laxity of ligaments resulting from the effects of relaxin. Great care should be taken over positioning during labour and delivery, although research is needed to assess the benefits of different positions.

Bladder Problems

Urinary *stress incontinence* is widely experienced among middle-aged women (Thomas *et al.*, 1980; Yarnell *et al.*, 1981), with childbirth generally considered the most common cause. The precise role of pregnancy and of different delivery factors remains unclear, but it is generally linked to pelvic floor innervation damage (Snooks *et al.*, 1984; Allen *et al.*, 1990). The predictors of this damage and the extent to which the symptom occurs and persists long after birth has only recently been examined.

Sleep and Grant (1987a), in a trial of perineal management, followed women up three years after the birth, at which time almost a third reported stress incontinence. This was not affected by whether or not the woman had had an episiotomy. Other studies have found that around 20% of women complained of stress incontinence 2–3 months postpartum (Sleep and Grant, 1987b; Garcia and Marchant, 1993). In the Birmingham study 21% of women reported stress incontinence lasting over six weeks, 15% having new stress incontinence first starting after the birth. As many as 70% of these symptomatic women still had the problem at questioning, 1–9 years later. It was clearly chronic, yet only 14% had consulted a doctor. An examination of predictive factors showed that long-term stress incontinence was more common in older mothers, after a long second stage of labour and in the vaginal delivery of a bigger baby. It was around half as likely after caesarean section. When delivery was by section, the size of the baby had no effect on symptoms, but the relationship with older age remained (MacArthur *et al.*, 1991, 1993c).

Chronic stress incontinence as a result of delivering a child is much more common than previously assumed, but there is almost no information on the severity of this problem. Among the symptomatic women in the study by Sleep and Grant (1987a) most (62%) said they had experienced stress incontinence less than once in the past week, although more than a quarter found the problem sufficiently severe to have to wear a pad at some time. An ongoing study in Birmingham is examining the severity of a number of postpartum symptoms and their effect on the women's lives 6–9 months after delivery. Preliminary results show that 22% of the women experienced stress incontinence (either new or recurrent) and of these more than a quarter had this at least every day; just under a third said it had an effect on their activities; and as many as 47% had needed to wear pads at some time (Bick and MacArthur, 1995a).

Pelvic floor exercises are often taught to women postnatally in order to strengthen the perineal muscles and minimize the likelihood of stress incontinence. A randomized controlled trial of additional education on pelvic floor exercises found no differences in subsequent incontinence between the groups at three months postpartum (Sleep and Grant, 1987b). Many women however practise pelvic floor exercises ineffectively, if at all, since they compete with all the other demands in the immediate postnatal period. Further research to measure the effectiveness of these physiotherapeutic techniques is underway.

Other postpartum bladder problems include *difficulties in voiding* and *urinary frequency*. Difficulty in passing urine is generally considered an immediate postdelivery complication but Glazener *et al.* (1993) found that in 2% of women it lasted between 1 and 8 weeks. In the same study, 5% of women complained of a urinary tract infection within the first postpartum year. MacArthur *et al.* (1991) found that new postpartum urinary frequency was experienced by 5% of the sample and 4% had similar recurrent symptoms. For three-quarters of the symptomatic women this remained unresolved.

The possibility of low-grade *urinary tract infections* needs to be considered. At present few women have a urine test at their postnatal examination. Only 37% of 1158 women who attended for their six-week postnatal check reported having received a urine test (Bick and MacArthur, 1995b).

Bowel Problems

Constipation is common during pregnancy due to the hormonal relaxation of the bowel, and this, together with pelvic pressure and straining during the second stage of labour, can result in *postpartum haemorrhoids*. These can be extremely painful but it has generally been considered that most cases will regress within a few days of the birth.

More recently, however, studies have shown that childbirth-associated haemorrhoids can be much longer lasting. Glazener *et al.* (1993) in the Grampian study and Garcia and Marchant (1993) in a London sample have found that two months after the birth between 15 and 20% of women still had haemorrhoids. In the Birmingham sample 18% reported haemorrhoids lasting longer than six weeks, half of which were new symptoms starting after the birth, and two-thirds of these women had unresolved haemorrhoids 1–9 years later. It is now clear that after only one baby a large proportion of women will develop haemorrhoids that become chronic.

A long second stage of labour, a forceps birth and the delivery of a bigger baby, were more likely to result in haemorrhoids (MacArthur *at al.*, 1991), showing a clear relationship with pelvic trauma. Glazener *et al.* (1995) found haemorrhoids were more than twice as common after instrumental delivery. Women delivered by Caesarean section were much less likely to experience haemorrhoids afterwards. With an abdominal delivery only 4% reported haemorrhoids starting for the first time afterwards. Others have also found low rates of haemorrhoids (3%) persisting after Caesarean section (Hillan, 1992). Some will eventually need surgical treatment. Dietary advice and the avoidance of constipation and straining are important.

The likely association between obstetric injury and *faecal incontinence* is increasingly being noted (Snooks *et al.*, 1984; Corman, 1985; Swash, 1993) and there have been incidental findings reported from studies of other problems. Sleep and Grant (1987b), in their study of urinary incontinence, did note that at one year after delivery 3% of the sample reported occasional faecal loss. In a German study (Rageth *et al.*, 1989) of long-term sequelae of different types of episiotomy compared with no episiotomy, there was an overall rate of 6.6% of women reporting the occasional involuntary passage of faeces, although only 1% had this lasting more than six months. Postpartum faecal continence has only recently, however, been the subject of specific investigation.

The results of recent studies using techniques developed to investigate physical and neurological damage to the anal sphincters (endosonography and manometry) now suggest that structural damage to the anal sphincters associated with childbirth has a more adverse effect than neurological factors affecting the pelvic floor (Kamm, 1994). Sultan and colleagues (1993) examined 202 women at 34 weeks gestation and 6–8 weeks postpartum to investigate associations between injury, physiological function and type of delivery. Anal endosonography showed no antenatal sphincter defects among the primiparous women who had a vaginal delivery, but 35% had defects at 6–8 weeks postpartum; 40% of multiparae had antenatal defects and 44% at postnatal follow-up. It seems, therefore, that most anal sphincter damage occurs following a first delivery. Anal sphincter damage was found to be more common after a forceps delivery.

An ongoing study in Birmingham examined the occurrence of faecal continence problems 6–9 months after delivery. Information was obtained through sensitive questioning by midwife-interviewers and showed that 36 (4%) of 906 women interviewed reported new faecal continence problems. Most had a feeling that they needed a bowel movement and had to rush to the toilet, others had soiling and staining of their underwear and a few had episodes of frank incontinence. Hardly any of the women had consulted their doctor or talked to their health visitor about these unpleasant symptoms. Instrumental delivery was again found to be a risk factor for these symptoms.

Perineal Problems

Perineal pain after trauma sustained during vaginal delivery is experienced by most women in the few days following the birth, and repair of the perineal floor is one of the most common surgical procedures carried out in the UK (Doyle *et al.*, 1993). Few studies have been conducted into ways of minimizing perineal pain felt by women and its extent as a persistent problem is less well documented. The study of postpartum health in the Grampian region found that as many as 10% of women had suffered perineal pain lasting for longer than eight weeks (Glazener *et al.*, 1993).

Episiotomy is common and is performed in a significant proportion of deliveries, although rates differ widely in different units (Logue, 1991). The rationale is to avoid severe lacerations thus protecting the perineal musculature. Descriptions from women have suggested that there is more discomfort following an episiotomy than a perineal tear (Kitzinger and Walters, 1981). However, the results from a randomized trial of 'liberal' compared with 'restrictive' episiotomy policy found no differences in pain experienced three months later, at which time 8% of the women still experienced perineal pain (Sleep *et al.*, 1984; Sleep, 1991). Similar results have been found in other randomized studies (Harrison *et al.*, 1984; Thranov *et al.* 1990) suggesting that there is little evidence to justify episiotomy as a means of limiting postpartum perineal pain. The findings of a recent study from North America has confirmed this conclusion (Klein *et al.*, 1994).

Different suture materials (glycerol-impregnated compared with chromic catgut) also had no effect on the incidence of perineal pain three months later (Grant *et al.* 1989a), nor did ultrasound treatment and pulsed electromagnetic energy therapy (Grant *et al.*, 1989b), nor did different bath additives, although women reported that bathing did ease their pain (Sleep and Grant, 1988).

A continuous subcuticular stitch to close the perineal skin was shown to reduce the incidence of perineal pain at three months postpartum (Isgar-Sally *et al.* 1986) provided that the person carrying out the repair was experienced in the technique (Grant, 1989).

Dyspareunia (pain on intercourse) can be embarassing to women, lower their feelings of well-being and affect their relationship with their partner. Long-term dyspareunia has been little researched and women are often reluctant to initiate medical consultation about it. By the time of the six-week postnatal check half will have attempted intercourse and potential long-term problems of dyspareunia will not be apparent (Buchan and Nicholls, 1980).

Like perineal pain, descriptive studies had suggested that women who have an episiotomy are more likely to suffer dyspareunia than those who had a perineal laceration (Kitzinger and Walters, 1981). The randomized trial of different perineal management regimes, however, found no difference in the reporting of dyspareunia three months or three years postpartum, although more women in the restrictive episiotomy group had resumed intercourse within a month of the birth (Sleep *at al.*, 1984; Sleep and Grant, 1987a; Sleep, 1991). Johansen *et al.* (1993) found a 21% prevalence of dyspareunia among women who had normal vaginal deliveries, followed up 15–24 months later. More problems (37%) were reported after instrumental vaginal deliveries.

The type of suture material used to close the perineum was associated with dyspareunia, women sutured with softgut being more likely to experience dyspareunia at both three months and three years postpartum (Grant *et al.*, 1989b).

There is some scope, therefore, for the midwife to select the way in which the perineum is closed in order to reduce long-term perineal pain and dyspareunia. Episiotomy does not reduce perineal problems and its use should be limited to essential indications only (Harrison *et al.*, 1984). Midwives should be encouraged to monitor and vary their practice in the light of research findings (Logue, 1991).

Fatigue

Tiredness after having a child is to be expected due to the strain of pregnancy, the delivery, the additional childcare load and the sleeplessness associated with night feeding. However many women report *exhaustion* as a persistent problem, which can have a significant effect on their relationships, their social and occupational activities and their psychological health.

Glazener *et al.* (1993) found that just over half of their sample reported tiredness lasting for more than eight weeks after the birth. MacArthur *et al.* (1991) asked about *extreme tiredness* and found that 17% reported this lasting more than six weeks, with 12% never having had such extreme fatigue before. Half of the women who complained of fatigue said it had lasted for longer than a year. Extreme tiredness within the year after childbirth has been noted in other smaller studies (Field *et al.*, 1983) and after Caesarean sections (Hillan, 1992).

The Birmingham study looked at predictors of fatigue and found that older women, those who were unmarried, those with twins and those who breastfed were more likely to report extreme tiredness. Different levels of practical and social support in the year after birth are relevant here. There was no relationship with the type of delivery the women had (section, forceps or spontaneous vaginal) but those who had a postpartum haemorrhage reported more tiredness (MacArthur *et al.*, 1991). This could be related to undiagnosed or inadequately treated *anaemia*. Haemoglobin testing is not a routine practice at the six-week postnatal examination and many women are discharged from hospital so early after the birth that it is not tested there either. In the Grampian study 7% of women had anaemia at some time between 2 and 18 months after the birth (Glazener *et al.*, 1993).

Women rarely consulted a doctor about postpartum fatigue (MacArthur *et al.*, 1991; Field *et al.*, 1983; Glazener *et al.*, 1993), perhaps because they see it as 'normal' or because they think the doctor would do nothing, the cause not being a 'medical' one. Without specific investigation, therefore, the presence of postpartum anaemia will remain unknown. Paterson and colleagues (1994) from Bedford studied the effects of low haemaglobin during the first six weeks. They showed a clear link between low haemoglobin and symptoms, including fatigue. These researchers suggested the need for a review of policies for postnatal haemoglobin testing.

Fatigue is commonly reported in association with *depression* (MacArthur *et al.*, 1991; Glazener *et al.*, 1993) although which problem came first is not known. It is likely that in some cases at least it is relentless physical exhaustion that affects a woman's psychological health. Psychiatric disorders *per se* are the subject of a separate chapter in this book.

Other Problems

Varicose veins are associated with childbirth, generally starting in pregnancy due to hormonal action, increased venous pressure and additional weight. They may regress afterwards but typically become worse with successive pregnancies and can become permanent. In the Birmingham sample, 7% had varicose veins still unresolved at the time of questioning, 1–9 years after the birth. In subsequent years some women will require surgical treatment.

Tingling in the hands or fingers, starting after the birth were experienced by 2.5% of the sample in the Birmingham study, and in two-thirds of cases these had never resolved. They were associated with epidural anaesthesia. These symptoms are not uncommon during pregnancy and can be due to carpel tunnel syndrome, but their onset afterwards has not previously been documented.

Paraesthesias in the legs, buttocks and lower back have been reported as side effects of epidural anaesthesia (Kitzinger, 1987). In the Birmingham study paraesthesias in the back and legs were not included as listed but 26 women mentioned this in the open-ended symptom category. All but three of these women had had an epidural (MacArthur *et al.*, 1991).

Dizziness/fainting and *visual disturbances* were reported as new long-term problems after the birth by 1.5% and 1.8% respectively of the women in the Birmingham sample. Both were more common after epidural. Both symptoms were also associated with spinal and with general anaesthesia and visual disturbances with pethidine as well. Except for a kind of sensory confusion reported by one or two women as long-term side-effects in a National Childbirth Trust study of problems after epidural (Kitzinger, 1987), this relationship has not been documented elsewhere and deserves further investigation.

Implications for Midwives

Health problems following childbirth continue far beyond the six-week postnatal check and this has implications for midwifery in developing strategies to identify and provide for the health needs of postpartum women.

Different methods of predicting and subsequently reducing the impact of postpartum morbidity must be researched and evaluated. Discharge criteria for example, based on a woman's duration of labour, mode of delivery, analgesia in labour and the weight of baby might be used to predict potential health problems. Discharge planning based on individual needs would result in a better provision of subsequent care.

Women should be provided with the contact numbers of the various voluntary organizations, such as the National Childbirth Trust, La Leche League, that are aimed at supporting postpartum women, making it clear that it is appropriate and acceptable to obtain further help and support. The establishment of local postnatal support groups, facilitated by midwives and health visitors could also have an important effect.

Community midwives presently have a statutory duty to attend a postpartum woman for a minimum of 10 days, up to a maximum of 28 days, the former being the norm. The role of the midwife might appropriately be extended beyond this period to make provision for the huge amount of longer term childbirth-related morbidity. Women are clearly reluctant to initiate consultations about their own health so that careful, sensitive questioning from suitable professionals is required, followed by referral and treatment where necessary. It seems important now that new recording schedules are devised, collecting systematic information on all of the health problems described in this chapter, with the same concern and uniformity traditionally undertaken for antenatal care, so that women do not feel abandoned by the maternity services at a stage at which we now know they are by no means ready.

References

Allen, R.E., Hosker, G.L., Smith, A.R.B. & Warrell, D.W. (1990) Pelvic floor damage and childbirth: a neurophysiological study. *Br. J. Obstet. Gynaecol.* **97**: 770–779.

Berg, G., Hammar, M., Moller-Neilsen, J., Linsden, U. & Thorbald, J. (1988) Low back pain during pregnancy. *Br. J. Obstet. Gynaecol.* **71**: 71–75.

Bick, D.E. & MacArthur, C. (1995b) Attendance, content and relevance of the six week postnatal examination. *Midwifery* **11**: 69–73.

Bick, D.E. & MacArthur, C. (1995a) The extent, severity and effect of health problems after childbirth. *Br. J. Midwifery* **3**(i): 27–31.

Breen, T.W., Ransil, J., Groves, P.A. *et al.* (1994) Factors associated with back pain after childbirth. *Anesthesiology* **81**: 29–34.

Brooke, O.G., Brown, I.R.F., Bond, C.D.M. *et al.* (1980) Vitamin D supplementation in pregnant Asian women: effects on calcium status and fetal growth. *Br. Med. J.*: 751–754.

Buchan, P.C. & Nicholls, J.A.J. (1980) Pain after episiotomy – a comparison of two methods of repair. *J. Coll. Gen. Pract.* **30**: 297–300.

Corman, M.L. (1985) Anal incontinence following obstetrical injury. *Dis. Colon Rectum* **28**: 86–89.

Dewan, G., Glazener, C. & Tunstall, M. (1993) Postnatal pain: a neglected area. *Br. J. Midwifery* **1**(2): 63–66.

Doyle, P.M., Geetha, T. & Wilkinson, P. (1993) A prospective randomised controlled trial of perineal repair after childbirth, comparing interrupted chromic catgut to subcuticular prolene for skin closure. *Br. J. Obstet. Gynaecol.* **100**: 93–94.

Field, S., Draper, J., Kerr, M. & Hare, M.J. (1983) Women's illness in the postnatal period. *Mat. Child Health* **8**(7): 302–304.

Garcia, J. & Marchant, S. (1993) Back to normal? Postpartum health and illness. In: Robinson, S. *et al.* (eds) *Research and the Midwife Conference Proceedings, 1992, University of Manchester.* pp. 2–9.

Glazener, C., Abdalla, M., Russell, I. & Templeton, A. (1993) Postnatal care: a survey of patient's experiences. *Br. J. Midwifery* **1**: 67–74.

Glazener, C.M.A., Abdalla, M., Shroud, P. *et al.* (1995) Postnatal maternal morbidity: extent, causes, prevention and treatment. *Br. J. Obstet. Gynaecol.* **102**(4): 282–287.

Grant, A. (1989) Repair of perineal trauma. In Chalmers, I. *et al.* (eds) *Effective Care in Pregnancy and Childbirth.* Oxford: Oxford University Press.

Grant, A., Sleep, J., Ashurst, H. & Spencer, J. (1989a) Dyspareunia associated with the use of glycerol-impregnated catgut to repair perineal trauma. Report of a 3 year follow-up study. *Br. J. Obstet. Gynaecol.* **96**: 741–743.

Grant, A., Sleep, J., McIntosh, J. & Ashurst, H. (1989b) Ultrasound and pulsed electromagnetic energy treatement for perineal trauma. A randomised placebo controlled trial. *Br. J. Obstet. Gynaecol.* **96**: 434–439.

Grove, L.H. (1973) Backache, headache and bladder dysfunction after delivery. *Br. J. Anaesth.* **45**: 1147–1149.

Groves, P.A., Breen, T.W., Ransil, J. *et al.* (1994) Natural history of postpartum backpain and its relationship with epidural anaesthesia. *Anesthesiology* **81A**: 1167.

Harrison, R.F., Brennen, M., North, P.M., Reed, J.V. & Wickham, E.A. (1984) Is routine episiotomy necessary? *Br. Med. J.* **288**(June): 1971–1975.

Hillan, E.M. (1992) Short term morbidity associated with Caesarean delivery. *Birth* **19**: 190–194.

Isgar-Sally, L., Legarth, J., Jacobson, B. & Bostofte, E. (1986) Episiotomy repair – immediate and long-term sequelae. A prospective randomised study of three different methods of repair. *Br. J. Obstet. Gynaecol.* **93**: 420–425.

Johansen, R., Wilkinson, P., Bastible, A. *et al.* (1993) Health after childbirth. *Midwifery* **9**(3): 161–168.

Kamm, M. (1994) Obstetric damage and faecal incontinence. *Lancet* **ii**(344): 730–733.

Kitzinger, S. (1987) *Some Women's Experiences of Epidurals. A Descriptive Study.* London: National Childbirth Trust.

Kitzinger, S. and Walters, R. (1981) *Some Women's Experiences of Episiotomy.* London: National Childbirth Trust.

Klein, M.C., Gauthier, M.D., Robbins, J.M. *et al.* (1994) Relationship of episiotomy to perineal trauma and morbidity, sexual dysfunction, and pelvic floor relaxation. *Am. J. Obstet. Gynecol.* **171**: 591–598.

Logue, M. (1991) Putting research into practice: perineal management during delivery. In Robinson, S. & Thomson, A.M. (eds) *Midwives, Research and Childbirth.* London: Chapman & Hall.

MacArthur, C., Lewis, M., Knox, E.G. & Crawford, J.S. (1990) Epidural anaesthesia and long-term backache following childbirth. *Br. Med. J.* **301**: 9–12.

MacArthur, C., Lewis, M. & Knox, E.G. (1991) *Health After Childbirth.* London: HMSO.

MacArthur, C., Lewis, M. & Knox, E.G. (1992) Investigation of long-term problems after obstetric epidural anaesthesia. *Br. Med. J.* **304**: 1279–1282.

MacArthur, C., Lewis, M. & Knox, E.G. (1993a) Accidental dural puncture in obstetric patients and long-term symptoms. *Br. Med. J.* **306**: 883–885.

MacArthur, C., Lewis, M. & Knox, E.G. (1993b) Comparison of long-term health problems following childbirth in Asian and Caucasian women. *Br. J. Gen. Pract.* **43**: 519–522.

MacArthur, C., Lewis, M. & Bick, D. (1993c) Stress incontinence after childbirth: predictors, persistence, impact and medical consultation. *Br. J. Midwifery* 1(5): 207–215.

MacLeod, J., MacIntyre, C., McClure, J.H. & Whitfield, A. (1995) Backache and epidural analgesia. *Int. J. Obstet. Anaesth.* 4(1): 21–25.

Mantle, M.J., Greenwood, R.M. & Currey, H.L.F. (1977) Backache in pregnancy. *Rheumatol. Rehabil.* 16: 95.

Ostgaard, H.C., Andersson, G.B.J. & Karlsson, K. (1991) Prevalence of back pain in pregnancy. *Spine* 16: 549–552.

Paterson, J., Davis, J., Gregory, M. *et al.* (1994) A study of the effects of low haemoglobin on postnatal women. *Midwifery* 10: 77–86.

Pitt, B. (1973) Maternity blues. *Br. J. Psych.* 122: 431–433.

Rageth, J.C., Buerklen, A. & Hirsch, H.A. (1989) Spatkomplikationen nach episiotomie. *Z. Geburtsh U. Perinat.* 193: 233–237.

Russell, R., Grove, P., Taub, N., O'Dowd, J. & Reynolds, F. (1993) Assessing long-term backache after childbirth. *Br. Med. J.* 306: 1299–1303.

Scott, D.B. & Hibbard, B.M. (1990) Serious non-fatal complications associated with extradural block in obstetric practice. *Br. J. Anaesth.* 64: 537–541.

Sleep, J. (1991) Perineal care: a series of five randomised controlled trials. In Robinson, S. & Thompson, A.M. (eds) *Midwives, Research and Childbirth*, Vol. 2. London: Chapman & Hall.

Sleep, J. & Grant, A. (1987a) West Berkshire perineal management trial: three year follow-up. *Br. Med. J.* 295: 749–751.

Sleep, J. & Grant, A. (1987b) Pelvic floor exercises in postnatal care. *Midwifery* 3: 158–164.

Sleep, J. & Grant, A. (1988) Effect of salt and Savlon bath concentrate postpartum. *Nursing Times Occasional Paper* 84: 55–57.

Sleep, J., Grant, A., Garcia, J. *et al.* (1984) West Berkshire perineal management trial. *Br. Med. J.* 298: 587–590.

Snooks, S.J., Swash, M., Setchell, M. & Henry, M.M. (1984) Injury to innervation of pelvic floor sphincter musculature in childbirth. *Lancet* 8 September: 546–550.

Stein, G.S., Morton, J., Marsh, A. *et al.* (1984) Headaches after childbirth. *Acta Neurol. Scand.* 69: 74–79.

Sultan, A.H., Kamm, M.A., Hudson, C.N. *et al.* (1993) Anal sphincter disruption during vaginal delivery. *New Eng. J. Med.* i(329): 1905–1911.

Swash, M. (1993) Faecal incontinence. Childbirth is responsible for most cases. *Br. Med. J.* 307: 636–637.

Thomas, T.M., Plymat, K.R., Blannin, J. & Meade, T. (1980) Prevalence of urinary incontinence. *Br. Med. J.* 281: 1243–1245.

Thranov, I., Kringelbach, A., Melchior, E., Olsen, O. & Darnsgaard, M. (1990) Episiotomy or tear at vaginal delivery. *Acta Obstet. Gynecol. Scand.* 69: 11–15.

Yarnell, J.W.G., Voyle, G.J., Richards, C.J. & Stephenson, T.P. (1981) The prevalence and severity of urinary incontinence in women. *J. Epidemiol. Community Health* 35: 71–75.

39

Vomiting

Nausea and vomiting is a common 'minor' disorder of pregnancy, affecting up to 70% of the pregnant population (Weigel and Weigel, 1989). Indeed it is often regarded as a normal occurrence and is taken to be a presumptive sign of pregnancy.

Vomiting occurs when one of the two centres in the brain is stimulated: the *emetic centre* in the medulla or the *chemoreceptor trigger zone*, situated on the lateral wall of the fourth ventricle (Billett, 1992). The cause of vomiting in pregnancy is unclear and several explanations have been proposed. The rising levels of pregnancy hormones are widely accepted as a causative factor, as both human chorionic gonadotrophin (hCG) and oestrogen stimulate the chemoreceptor trigger zone in the brain. Serum levels of hCG are higher in women who experience nausea and vomiting in pregnancy (Masson *et al.* 1985). Other explanations include the following (Thorp *et al.*, 1991; Boyce, 1992; Tucker-Blackburn and Loper, 1992):

▶ *Physiological changes* of pregnancy such as reduced gastric motility, reflux oesophagitis.
▶ *Metabolic changes* such as carbohydrate deficiency, vitamin B deficiency, alteration in serum lipids and lipoproteins.
▶ *Genetic incompatibility*
▶ *Position of the corpus luteum*: A corpus luteum situ-

ated in the right ovary may cause high concentrations of sex steroids in the hepatic portal system, leading to nausea and vomiting. Excision of a right-sided corpus luteum has been used for the treatment of hyperemesis gravidarum, but with variable results.
▶ *Psychological factors* such as rejection of, or ambivalence about the pregnancy, psychological conflict regarding gender role or maternal role.

The condition is commoner in young and primigravid women and is strongly associated with multiple pregnancy, hydatidiform mole and severe pre-eclampsia. The midwife should remember that vomiting may occur as a result of incidental conditions such as gastroenteritis, hiatus hernia, duodenal ulcer, appendicitis, pyelonephritis or cerebral lesions. Such conditions are more difficult to diagnose in pregnancy but other signs such as pain or pyrexia will be present. Psychological disturbance should not be assumed to be a cause of vomiting in pregnancy unless pathological causes have been excluded and there are frank signs of psychoneurosis. In these rare cases psychotherapy may be beneficial (Beischer and Mackay, 1986).

Vomiting in pregnancy is associated with a decreased risk of spontaneous abortion and seems to have no adverse effects on the length of gestation, birthweight, placental weight or head circumference (Weigel and Weigel, 1989).

Mild Vomiting in Pregnancy

This is a transient and self-limiting condition, although unpleasant for the woman. Classically, it appears in the fourth week of pregnancy although it may commence earlier. It resolves by the 14th week when hCG levels are falling and the body is becoming habituated to the rising levels of oestrogen. It may occasionally recur in the third trimester. The woman often feels nauseated on waking and vomiting occurs on rising from bed. The symptoms usually recede during the day although nausea may be persistent. The sense of smell is heightened and some women develop food aversions at this time, commonly to substances such as tea, coffee, alcohol, fatty foods and tobacco. This may be a physiological defence mechanism designed to reduce exposure of the embryo to potential teratogens. On examination the woman does not appear dehydrated and the urine does not contain ketones. The midwife can reassure her that the condition will improve in time.

Dietary modification may help to reduce the woman's discomfort. Meals should be taken more frequently and should be small and light. Fatty, spicy or strong-smelling food should be avoided. Fresh fruit and savoury foods are usually acceptable. A milky drink at bedtime and dry toast or a biscuit before rising often alleviates the early morning nausea; carbonated drinks such as soda water or non-alcoholic dry ginger are useful if nausea persists during the day. *Medication* is not usually required. The woman should be advised to *rest* as much as possible as tiredness and stress will exacerbate the vomiting.

Complementary remedies have become popular and some are used to treat morning sickness. Vitamin B_6 may be useful (Sahakian *et al.*, 1991) but vitamin supplements should be used with caution as over-dosage may cause fetal damage. The woman can be advised to eat foods which are rich in vitamin B_6, such as tuna, mackerel, banana, avocado, raisins, sunflower seeds and hazelnuts. Ginger has been used and has recognized anti-emetic properties (Fischer-Rasmussen *et al.*, 1990). It may be taken as powdered ginger root capsules, crystallized stem ginger or in biscuits or drinks.

Acupuncture and acupressure have been shown to relieve vomiting in pregnancy (Dundee *et al.*, 1988; Belluomini *et al.*, 1994) and acupressure wristbands designed to prevent motion sickness have been used by some women (Stannard, 1989). Success has also been claimed for aromatherapy and homoeopathic remedies. The midwife herself may not use any complementary therapy for her clients unless she is properly qualified in that field as some complementary medicines and techniques can be harmful in pregnancy (UKCC, 1992). The midwife also has a duty to advise the woman if she believes that any remedy or treatment the woman is using may be harmful to the pregnancy.

Empathic support is an important part of the care of the woman with mild vomiting in pregnancy. Although not clinically ill, the woman often feels miserable and her symptoms should not be regarded as trivial.

Moderate Vomiting in Pregnancy

This is more serious as the woman will be vomiting several times during the day, often after meals. The dietary advice described above may help but often the woman continues to vomit and will begin to show signs of dehydration. There may be some weight loss and ketones will appear in the urine. The woman will usually be feeling very anxious about her condition and that of the fetus. The midwife should contact the doctor and arrange for the woman to be admitted to hospital. Examinations to exclude any underlying pathology will be carried out and the doctor may prescribe a drug such as promethazine (Phenergan) to control the vomiting.

Medication should be used with caution, especially in the first trimester when organogenesis is taking place. Many drugs are teratogenic and the human embryo is particularly susceptible to damage during the early weeks of pregnancy. Intravenous fluids may be required to correct dehydration. The midwife should keep a careful record of fluid balance. She should give support and reassurance to the woman and her relatives. The vomiting usually ceases quickly and once the woman is tolerating a normal diet she may be discharged home.

Hyperemesis Gravidarum

This is the pathological form of vomiting in pregnancy. It is a serious disorder which may lead to maternal death. The vomiting usually begins in the first 10 weeks of pregnancy and is continuous and severe. Ptyalism may accompany the symptoms. The woman rapidly shows signs of dehydration such as sunken eyes, loss of skin elasticity, parched mouth and lips, fetor oris (offensive odour of the breath) and oliguria. Urinalysis reveals a marked ketosis. The woman loses weight and becomes hyponatraemic and hypochloraemic. Any woman with a history of hyperemesis gravidarum or who has a pre-existing liver disease is at increased risk.

The precise cause is unknown but may be related to thyroid function and hormonal activity during pregnancy, or psychosocial stress such as an unwanted pregnancy or short inter-pregnancy interval.

There is an association between *thyroid activity* in pregnancy and hyperemesis gravidarum: women who are hyperemetic·tend also to have significantly higher thyroxin concentrations (Lao *et al.*, 1988). The thyroid-stimulating hormone (TSH)–like activity of human chorionic gonadotrophin may cause a transient relative thyrotoxicosis. Thyroid function returns to normal during the puerperium.

The woman's condition will deteriorate rapidly unless the disease is treated swiftly. Liver and renal damage may occur and the woman may become jaundiced. Vitamin B_1 deficiency will cause neurological symptoms such as polyneuritis. *Wernicke's encephalopathy* is a rare but serious complication. In this condition small petechial haemorrhages occur in the hypothalamus and upper brainstem. Signs include disturbance of consciousness and memory, abnormalities of eye movements, ataxia and polyneuropathy. The hypothalamic lesions may cause temperature instability, particularly hypothermia. Wernicke's encephalopathy may lead to coma and death unless treated; the condition responds well to thiamine (Johnson, 1988).

Oesophageal tears (Mallory-Weiss syndrome) and *haematemesis* may occur in women with severe and persistent vomiting. If the maternal weight loss is greater than 5% of the pre-pregnancy weight there is an increased risk of *intrauterine growth retardation*, probably due to the disruption of the fetal growth pattern by the maternal metabolic disturbances (Gross *et al.*, 1989). There appear to be no other serious fetal effects.

CARE

The midwife should contact a doctor and the woman must be admitted to hospital at once. She should be nursed in a single room if possible to avoid undue disturbance. Nothing is given by mouth until the vomiting stops – ice may be given to suck.

A blood sample is taken to estimate urea and electrolyte levels and for liver function tests. The urine is tested for ketones, bile, protein and glucose. A midstream specimen of urine is sent for culture in order to exclude pyelonephritis. An intravenous infusion is commenced to correct the dehydration. Dextrose and Hartmann's solution, with added potassium, are used to restore the electrolyte balance.

Slow-drip enteral feeding and *total parenteral nutrition* (TPN) have been used in the management of hyperemesis gravidarum (Levine and Esser, 1988; Boyce, 1992). Both methods carry risks: persistent vomiting during enteral feeding may cause aspiration pneumonia if vomit is inhaled; TPN used for the management of hyperemesis gravidarum has been associated with cardiac tamponade and maternal and fetal death (Greenspoon *et al.*, 1989).

The doctor will prescribe an anti-emetic drug such as prochlorperazine (Stemetil) or metaclopramide (Maxolon). Vitamin B injections may also be prescribed. Hypnotherapy may occasionally be of use (Torem, 1994).

The midwife should make frequent records of the woman's temperature, pulse, blood pressure and urinalysis. An accurate record of fluid balance is essential. The woman's care will also include attention to personal and oral hygiene. The midwife should inform the doctor at once if the woman exhibits neurological symptoms such as disorientation, drowsiness, abnormal eye movements or ataxia.

Termination of the pregnancy is only considered if the vomiting is intractable and signs of major organ failure appear, such as persistent pyrexia or hypothermia, persistent tachycardia, jaundice, persistent proteinuria, polyneuritis or encephalopathy.

Once the vomiting ceases, oral fluids and food may be gradually reintroduced. The midwife should provide psychological support for the woman as this condition affects her self-image and also her confidence in her body's ability to bear a child. The partner also needs the midwife's communication and counselling skills as he will be very anxious. The woman may be discharged when she is taking a normal diet and gaining weight. The midwife should be aware that this condition may recur later in the pregnancy. In future pregnancies 25% of these women will suffer hyperemesis gravidarum again (Llewellyn-Jones, 1986).

The more serious consequences of hyperemesis gravidarum are fortunately rare and some cases may be avoidable if the vomiting is treated promptly and effectively. The midwife should inform the doctor of any woman found to have ketones in her urine.

References

Beischer, A. & Mackay, E. (1986) *Obstetrics and the Newborn*. London: Baillière Tindall.

Belluomini, J., Litt, R., Lee, K. & Katz, M. (1994) Acupressure for nausea and vomiting of pregnancy: a randomised, blinded study. *Obstet. Gynecol.* 84(2): 245–248.

Billett, J. (1992) A closer look at pregnancy sickness. *Professional Care of Mother and Child* November–December: 310–311.

Boyce, R. (1992) Enteral nutrition in hyperemesis gravidarum: a new development. *J. Am. Dietetic Assoc.* 92(6): 733–736.

Chalmers, L., Enkin, M. & Kierse, M. (1989) *Effective Care in Pregnancy and Childbirth*. Oxford: Oxford University Press.

Creasy, R. & Resnik, R. (1989) *Maternal–Fetal Medicine: Principles and Practice*, 2nd edn. London: W.B. Saunders.

Dundee, J., Sourial, F., Ghaly, R. & Bell, P. (1988) P6 Acupressure reduces morning sickness. *J. R. Soc. Med.* 81(8): 456–457.

Fischer-Rasmussen, W., Kjaer, S., Dahl, C. & Asping, U. (1990) Ginger treatment of hyperemesis gravidarum. *Eur. J. Obstet. Gynaecol. Reprod. Biol.* 38(1): 19–24.

Greenspoon, J., Masak, D. & Kurz, C. (1989) Cardiac tamponade in pregnancy during central hyperalimentation. *Obstet. Gynecol.* 73(March): 465–466.

Gross, S., Librach, C. & Cecutti, A. (1989) Maternal weight loss associated with hyperemesis gravidarum: a predictor of fetal outcome. *Am. J. Obstet. Gynecol.* 160(4): 906–909.

Johnson, R. (1988) Autonomic failure in alcoholics. In Bannister, R. (ed.) *Autonomic Failure*. Oxford: Oxford University Press.

Lao, T., Chin, R., Mak, Y. & Panesar, N. (1988) Plasma zinc concentration and thyroid function in hyperemetic pregnancies. *Acta Obstet. Gynecol. Scand.* 67(7): 599–604.

Levine, M. & Esser, D. (1988) Total parenteral nutrition for the treatment of severe hyperemesis gravidarum: maternal nutritional effects and fetal outcome. *Obstet. Gynaecol.* 72(1): 102–107.

Llewellyn-Jones, D. (1986) *Fundamentals of Obstetrics and Gynaecology*, Vol. 1: *Obstetrics*, 4th edn. London: Faber & Faber.

McGregor, A. (1991) The thyroid gland in pregnancy. In Phillip, E. & Setchell, M. (eds) *Scientific Foundations of Obstetrics and Gynaecology*. London: Butterworth-Heinemann.

Masson, G., Anthony, F. & Chau, E. (1985) Serum chorionic gonadotrophin (HCG), Schwangerschafts protein 1 (SP1), progesterone and oestradiol levels in patients with nausea and vomiting in early pregnancy. *Br. J. Obstet. Gynaecol.* 92(3): 211–215.

Sahakian, V., Rouse, D. & Sipes, S. (1991) Vitamin B6 is effective therapy for nausea and vomiting of pregnancy: a randomised, double-blind, placebo-controlled trial. *Obstet. Gynecol.* 78(1): 33–36.

Stannard, D. (1989) Pressure prevents nausea. *Nursing Times* 85(4): 25 January: 33–34.

Tisserand, M. (1990) *Aromatherapy for Women*. London: Thorsons.

Thorp, J., Watson, W. & Katz, V. (1991) Effect of corpus luteum positions on hyperemesis gravidarum, a case report. *J. Reprod. Med.* 36(10): 761–762.

Torem, S. (1994) Hypnotherapeutic techniques in the treatment of hyperemesis gravidarum. *Am. J. Clin. Hypnosis* 37(1): 1–11.

Tucker-Blackburn, S. & Loper, D.L. (1992) *Maternal, Fetal and Neonatal Physiology: a Clinical Perspective*. London: W.B. Saunders.

UKCC (1992) *Standards for the Administration of Medicines*. London: UKCC.

Weigel, M. & Weigel, R. (1989) Nausea and vomiting of early pregnancy and pregnancy outcome. An epidemiological study. *Br. J. Obstet. Gynaecol* 96: 1304–1311.

Further Reading

Iancu, I., Kotler, M., Spivak, B., Radwan, M. & Weizman, A. (1994) Psychiatric aspects of hyperemesis gravidarum. *Psychother. Psychosomatics* 61(3–4): 143–149.

Newman, V., Fullerton, J. & Anderson, P. (1993) Clinical advances in the management of severe nausea and vomiting during pregnancy. *J. Obstet. Gynecol. Neonatal Nursing* 22(6): 483–490.

Ohkoshi, N., Ishii, A. & Shoji, S. (1994) Wernicke's encephalopathy induced by hyperemesis gravidarum, associated with bilateral caudate lesions on computed tomography and magnetic resonance imaging. *Eur. Neurol.* 34(3): 177–180.

Wilson, R., McKillop, J., MacLean, M. *et al.* (1992) Thyroid function tests are rarely abnormal in patients with severe hyperemesis gravidarum. *Clin. Endocrinol.* 37(4): 331–334.

40

Bleeding in Pregnancy

Bleeding from the genital tract is usually considered in two groups, depending on whether it occurs before or after the 24th week of pregnancy (Barron, 1995).

Bleeding from the genital tract in early pregnancy, that is before the 24th week, may be caused by:

▶ Implantation bleeding.
▶ Abortion.
▶ Hydatidiform mole.
▶ Ectopic pregnancy.
▶ Cervical lesions.
▶ Vaginitis.

Any bleeding per vaginam is considered abnormal and should be reported to a doctor.

Implantation Bleeding

There may be a little bleeding when the trophoblast embeds into the endometrial lining of the uterus. The bleeding is usually bright red and of short duration. As implantation is taking place 8–12 days after fertilization the bleeding will occur just before the menstrual period is due and, if mistakenly thought to be a menstrual period, will confuse the expected date of delivery. A careful menstrual history is therefore essential to detect probable implantation bleeding, thereby avoiding miscalculation of dates.

Abortion

SPONTANEOUS ABORTION

At least 15% of confirmed pregnancies end in spontaneous abortion, most of these occurring before the 12th week of pregnancy. The true rate of pregnancy loss is much higher as it is not known how many unrecognized pregnancies are lost. Spontaneous abortion is commoner in women having their first pregnancy (Lewis and Chamberlain, 1990).

Causes of abortion

There are many causes of abortion, including the following.

Maldevelopment of the conceptus The most common cause of spontaneous abortion is a defective conceptus. Chromosomal abnormalities account for approximately 70% of defective conceptions, although spontaneous mutations may arise (Lewis and Chamberlain, 1990). Other causes are defective implantation and a hydatidiform mole.

General maternal disease Any acute illness, particularly with a high temperature, may cause abortion. This may be due to the general metabolic effect of a high fever or the result of transplacental passage of viruses. Conditions such as influenza, rubella, appendicitis, pyelonephritis, pneumonia, toxoplasmosis, cytomegalovirus, listeriosis, syphilis and brucellosis may all cause abortion. Other medical disorders which may cause abortion include diabetes, thyroid disease, renal disease and hypertensive disorders.

Endocrine abnormalities These include poor development of the corpus luteum, inadequate secretory endometrium and low serum progesterone levels. Endocrine deficiency may cause recurrent abortion.

Maternal immune response The feto-placental unit develops from both maternally and paternally derived origins. In order to avoid a host–graft rejection reaction the maternal immune system is relatively suppressed in pregnancy. It is possible that the stimulus to the change in maternal immune response is trophoblastic in origin. Defective adaptation of the maternal immune response will allow activation of host immune defences and the pregnancy will be rejected. This is thought to be a factor in some cases of recurrent abortion.

Uterine abnormalities The majority of the female genital tract arises from the two Müllerian ducts which form during embryonic life. Failure of development may cause structural abnormalities such as double uterus, unicornuate, bicornuate, septate or subseptate uterus. Such structural uterine abnormalities are implicated in approximately 15% of early pregnancy losses. Sometimes the uterus fails to develop to the full adult size, remaining infantile. Pregnancy in such a uterus may also end in abortion. A uterus containing fibroids

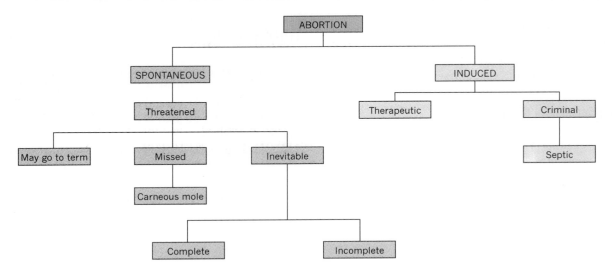

Figure 1 The classification of abortion.

may be the cause. Retroversion of the uterus does not itself cause abortion. As the uterus enlarges it will usually rise into the abdomen. If it fails to do so, vaginal and abdominal manipulation to correct the retroversion is much more likely to cause an abortion.

A deep laceration of the cervix or undue stretching of the internal cervical os, produced by a previous abortion or childbirth, may allow the membranes to bulge through the cervical canal and rupture to produce abortion. This condition, an *incompetent cervix*, may be the cause of repeated late abortions. A nylon tape inserted and tied around the cervix at about the 14th week may prevent this. This is called cervical cerclage. The tape must be removed before the onset of labour.

Environmental factors   Some external influences may cause abortion. These include environmental teratogens such as lead and radiation, and teratogenic substances such as drugs and alcohol. Smoking has been linked with spontaneous abortion but research findings are inconsistent. Maternal passive smoking may be at least as damaging as an established tobacco habit (Windham *et al.*, 1992). In recent years there has been concern about the safety of visual display units (VDUs) but these are not now thought to increase the likelihood of abortion.

Stress   A severe emotional upset may cause abortion by disrupting hypothalamic and pituitary functions (Llewellyn Jones, 1990).

Paternal causes   Environmental teratogens may affect the quality of male sperm. The father may be the cause of transmission of chromosomal abnormalities, particularly in cases of recurrent abortion.

In vitro fertilization (IVF) pregnancy   About 21% of IVF pregnancies abort spontaneously (Healy and Wood, 1989).

Despite detailed investigations no cause for abortion can be found in the majority of cases.

Threatened abortion

Slight bleeding may occur, usually during the first three months of pregnancy. It may be painless or associated with slight lower abdominal pain or backache, but there is no cervical dilatation.

No aperient or enema should be given and no vaginal examination should be made by the midwife, for a threatened abortion may easily become an actual abortion. The treatment is bedrest until the bleeding ceases. A mild sedative may be prescribed by the doctor. The woman may be admitted to hospital where ultrasound scans may be carried out to monitor the growth of the pregnancy. Heavy or increasing bleeding is an ominous sign and may precede inevitable abortion. Declining serum progesterone levels may indicate doubtful viability of the pregnancy (Lewis and Chamberlain, 1990).

Inevitable abortion

The key feature of inevitable abortion is cervical dilatation. As the name suggests, the outcome is unavoidable pregnancy loss. The bleeding is more severe than in a threatened abortion and the woman may collapse from blood loss. The gestation sac separates from the uterine wall and the uterus contracts to expel the conceptus. The uterine contractions cause discomfort similar to that of labour contractions. If a vaginal examination were made the doctor would find the cervix dilating, possibly with products of conception protruding through it. The gestation sac may be expelled complete (*complete abortion*) or part, usually placental tissue, may be retained (*incomplete abortion*).

Should the midwife be the first to arrive she should swab the vulva, using full aseptic precautions, and apply a sterile pad. This will enable the doctor to estimate the amount of blood lost in a given time. Whatever is passed must be saved for the doctor's inspection, so as to ascertain if any part of the conceptus has been expelled. The midwife should make the woman comfortable while awaiting the doctor.

If the abortion is complete and the condition of the woman is good, the doctor will probably give ergometrine maleate 500 μg or Syntometrine 1 ml and she can be cared for at home. If the abortion is incomplete or if there has been much blood loss the woman may be transferred to hospital after ergometrine has been given, provided her condition is good. If haemorrhage is severe, it is much wiser to call for emergency help. This is usually a paramedic team from the Ambulance Service. They will resuscitate the woman, if necessary giving a blood transfusion. When her condition has improved she may then be transferred to hospital. In hospital, evacuation of retained products of conception from the uterus may be carried out and a blood transfusion given if blood loss has been severe.

Medical management of inevitable or incomplete abortion is possible, using mifepristone and misoprostal (Macrow and Elstein, 1993; Henshaw *et al.*, 1993).

The midwife's responsibility will be to observe the pulse, blood pressure and vaginal loss, prepare the requirements for the doctor and give support and reassurance to the woman and her partner.

Once the uterus is empty, vulval hygiene is important to prevent infection and the woman should be advised to clean the vulval area twice daily, using a bidet or shower if possible.

If the breasts begin to secrete the woman should be advised to wear a well-fitting brassière in order to minimize discomfort. Bromocriptine may be given to suppress lactation.

If the woman is rhesus negative anti-D gammaglobulin 50–100 μg is given within 60 hours of abortion to prevent iso-immunization and potential rhesus problems in subsequent pregnancies. Women who are non-immune to rubella may be given rubella vaccination at this time and advised to avoid the risk of pregnancy for the next three months.

Missed abortion

This is also known as carneous mole, blood mole or fleshy mole. At an early stage in pregnancy a threatened abortion occurs, i.e. haemorrhage without expulsion of the uterine contents. Bleeding occurs between the gestation sac and the uterine wall and the embryo dies. Layers of blood clot are formed, later becoming organized. The uterus does not increase in size and as the presence of the mole appears to inhibit menstruation the woman is apt to think that her pregnancy is continuing, although other signs of pregnancy have disappeared. The bleeding from the vagina may only be a trickle or there may be none at all, but usually there is a brownish discharge.

Gradually the signs of pregnancy disappear and some women become aware that all is not well. The diagnosis is confirmed by ultrasound and the woman is admitted for evacuation of the uterus. The uterus would eventually expel the mole spontaneously, but this may not occur for many weeks. Many women find the idea of a dead fetus *in utero* very distressing and there is also the risk of disseminated intravascular coagulation. If the size of the uterus is less than 12–13 weeks the uterus may be evacuated per vaginam with a suction curette. Alternatively, medical abortion may be induced with oral mifepristone 600 mg followed 36–48

hours later with oral misoprostol 600 μg, in divided dose (el-Rafaey *et al.* 1992). If the uterus is larger than 13 weeks a combination of vaginal prostaglandins and intravenous Syntocinon may be used to empty the uterus (Lewis and Chamberlain, 1990). If a well-formed dead fetus is retained *in utero* it will become flattened and mummified (fetus papyraceous) rather than being reabsorbed.

Recurrent abortion

This is a term used when three or more consecutive abortions have occurred. The term 'habitual abortion' is no longer used. Careful investigation should be undertaken to find the cause. Occasionally the causative factors are different for each abortion, with no clear single factor associated. However some conditions may be implicated in recurrent abortion:

▶ *Structural abnormality* of the uterus.
▶ *Incompetent cervix.*
▶ *Maternal systemic disease.*
▶ *Genetic causes:* These account for up to 13% of cases of recurrent abortion. The majority of defects are translocation. In cases of consanguinous or cousin marriage a lethal recessive gene may cause recurrent abortion.
▶ *Uterine infection,* especially toxoplasmosis or *Ureaplasma urealyticum.*
▶ *Hormonal deficiency* (although not all authorities accept this as a cause of recurrent abortion).
▶ *Low maternal birthweight:* Women suffering recurrent abortion are significantly more likely to have been of low birthweight themselves. This may indicate a genetic tendency to pregnancy failure or poor fetal growth.
▶ *Maternal immune response:* The stimulus to suppression of the maternal immune response may come from the developing trophoblast. Specific blocking IgG antibodies are found in the maternal circulation in pregnancy and these are thought to be a factor in preventing rejection of the fetal allograft. Women with a history of recurrent abortion may lack these antibodies. This may be overcome in some cases by injecting the woman with paternal or donor lymphocytes before pregnancy (Mowbray, 1988; Lewis and Chamberlain, 1990; Llewellyn Jones, 1990; Stirrat, 1990; Christiansen *et al.*, 1992; Tucker *et al.*, 1992).

Treatment varies according to the cause. Infections are treated with the appropriate antibiotic. An incompetent cervix may be closed by insertion of a suture (cervical cerclage). The suture is removed just before term or earlier if labour commences. Fetal allograft rejection may be treated with lymphocyte injections as described above. Hormonal deficiency may be treated by the administration of 17-α-hydroxyprogesterone hexanoate (Proluton Depot) 250–500 mg weekly during the first 14–16 weeks of pregnancy. However, there is no real evidence that this treatment is effective. Intramuscular injections of human chorionic gonadotrophin (hCG) 10 000 IU twice weekly have been used with some success. The injections continue until the 16th week of pregnancy. hCG stimulates development of the corpus luteum and early feto-placental endocrine activity and thus supports the pregnancy (Harrison, 1988).

Psychological effects of abortion

Many women experience a marked grief reaction following abortion and may require much counselling and support. Psychological distress may be severe and some women become clinically depressed. Those most at risk are single women and those who have suffered repeated losses (Friedman and Gath, 1989). Staff should treat the parents with sensitivity and should avoid referring to the lost pregnancy as an abortion as some parents will find this distressing: the term 'miscarriage' is generally kinder and carries no overtones of a deliberate action. The couple may wish to see the fetus and staff should take account of their wishes. The guidelines written by the Stillbirth and Neonatal Death Society (Sands, 1991) and Kohner (1992) are useful.

The midwife should remember that the legal age of fetal viability is 24 weeks as defined by the Stillbirth (Definition) Act 1992. After the end of the 24th week of pregnancy the infant must be registered as a stillbirth. Many maternity hospitals offer a funeral or memorial service for pre-viable fetuses and will provide a decent burial. In this situation the hospital chaplain may be a valuable source of support and advice. The couple may wish to discuss future pregnancies with the doctor and in some cases may be referred for genetic counselling. The midwife may give the couple the address of the Miscarriage Association, whose members provide support for those who have undergone a spontaneous abortion.

INDUCED ABORTION

Induced abortions are divided into therapeutic and criminal.

Therapeutic abortion

Therapeutic abortion has been legal in the United Kingdom since 1967 when the Abortion Act became law. This Act allows termination of a pregnancy if two registered medical practitioners are of the opinion that continuance of the pregnancy:

1 involves risk to the life of the pregnant woman;
2 involves risk of injury to her physical or mental health;
3 involves risk to any existing children of her family, greater than if the pregnancy were terminated; or
4 carries a substantial risk that if the child were born it would suffer from such physical or mental abnormalities as to be seriously handicapped.

On 1 April 1991 the Abortion Law was changed as a result of the Human Fertilisation and Embryology Act 1991, and the upper gestation limit for legal termination was defined as the end of the 24th week. The only circumstances in which therapeutic abortion may be carried out after the 24th week are:

1 if there is a risk to the woman's life;
2 if there is a risk of grave permanent damage to the woman's physical or mental health; or
3 if there is a substantial risk that the child would be seriously handicapped.

The law also allows for selective fetal reduction in multifetal pregnancy, if continuance of the pregnancy with that number of fetuses would threaten the health or life of the woman, or if one or more of the fetuses were seriously abnormal (Paintin, 1991).

A termination of pregnancy must be carried out in an approved institution and all terminations are notified to the Chief Medical Officer of the Department of Health. Staff are allowed to refuse to advocate or take part in abortions on moral or conscientious grounds.

Abortions after 24 weeks may only be carried out in NHS hospitals.

Adequate counselling should be available before a woman undergoes termination of pregnancy so that she is able to make an informed decision, without undue influence of medical opinion or pressure from relatives.

Methods of therapeutic abortion during the first trimester

Mifepristone (RU 486, Mifegyne)   This drug blocks the action of progesterone. It is licensed for use in the termination of pregnancy up to nine weeks' gestation and effects a complete abortion in 96% of cases. The woman must be under 35 years old and no more than a light smoker. Oral mifepristone 600 mg is given and the woman may go home two hours later. She is readmitted 36–48 hours later and a gemeprost vaginal pessary (1 mg) is inserted. The majority of women (96%) will abort within eight hours (Heard and Guillebaud, 1992; Roussel Laboratories Ltd, 1992).

Suction evacuation   This is carried out under general anaesthesia. Although this is generally a safe method, complications such as haemorrhage, infection, cervical damage and perforated uterus may still occur. The cervix is dilated and the uterus emptied by suctioning and curettage (Figure 2).

Menstrual extraction   This may be used if the woman's period is late, whether or not pregnancy has been confirmed. A fine plastic cannula is passed through the cervix into the uterine cavity and suction is applied with a 50 ml syringe. This removes the endometrium. However, there is a risk that the conceptus will be missed and the pregnancy continue. This method is also open to potential criminal abuse (Tindall, 1987).

Methods of therapeutic abortion during the second trimester

Prostaglandin E_1, E_2 or F_2 alpha   These compounds may be administered as an intra-amniotic or extra-amniotic infusion (Figure 3), or as vaginal pessaries or gel. Intra-amniotic infusion is by a fine polythene catheter introduced into the amniotic sac through the abdominal wall. The uterus may take up to five days to expel its contents.

This method has been largely superseded by extra-amniotic prostaglandins (Tindall, 1987). Extra-amniotic infusion is achieved by passing a 14 French gauge Foley catheter through the cervix into the uterus and infusion of the drug into the extra-amniotic area. Intra-amniotic prostaglandins may be combined with urea and intravenous Syntocinon for greater effectiveness. A laminaria tent may be inserted into the cervix prior to administration of prostaglandins.

Suction evacuation   This method may be used in pregnancies of up to 18 weeks' gestation, if the operator is trained in the technique. The cervix is prepared with a prostin pessary prior to the operation. A Foley catheter or laminaria tent may be used to reduce the risk of cervical damage. The liquor amnii is aspirated with a suction curette and the fetus and placenta are removed with sponge forceps (Savage, 1989; el-Rafaey *et al.*, 1994).

Intra-amniotic saline   This method is rarely used now as there is a considerable risk of coagulopathy, major organ damage and death if the solution accidentally enters the circulation.

Hysterotomy   This operation is rarely performed as the scar which results is in the upper uterine segment and may rupture in a subsequent pregnancy.

Placental expulsion may be delayed when second trimester abortion is performed and the woman may require a manual removal of the placenta.

Contraceptive advice must be given before the woman is discharged as fertility returns very quickly following termination of pregnancy and an unplanned pregnancy may result if the woman is unaware of this.

Selective fetal reduction   This technique is sometimes employed in a higher order (four or more) multiple pregnancy. It may be performed if one of the fetuses is found to be abnormal. More usually it is carried out to reduce the number of fetuses and therefore decrease the risk to the woman's health.

A needle is inserted, under ultrasound guidance, through the abdominal wall and into the amniotic sac. The needle is then introduced into the fetal chest and a small dose of potassium chloride is injected. Cardiac

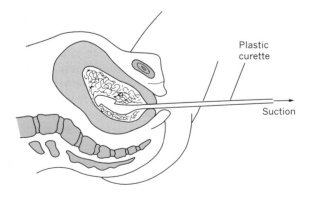

Plastic curette

Suction

Figure 2   Vacuum aspiration.

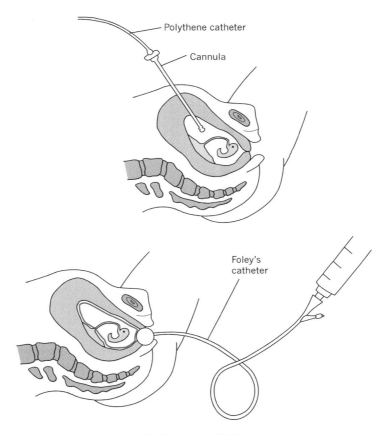

Figure 3 Intra-amniotic (above) and extra-amniotic (below) instillation.

activity usually ceases within 2 minutes (Evans and Fletcher, 1992). If the procedure is carried out in early pregnancy the tiny fetus will be reabsorbed; if later in pregnancy the fetus may become papyraceous and will be discovered among the membranes at delivery. Selective fetal reduction raises some difficult ethical issues.

The midwife should remember that termination of pregnancy may have profound psychological effects. Depression and feelings of guilt are not uncommon in the weeks that follow and may be re-awakened when the woman becomes pregnant again. The emotional pain may be particularly severe if the termination was for fetal abnormality. The midwife may be able to provide the woman and her partner with emotional support and counselling when pregnancy is terminated (Bewley, 1993). She can also provide parents with details of the charitable organization SATFA (Support Around Termination For Fetal Abnormal-

ity), which offers support for those undergoing this painful ordeal (see later).

Criminal abortion

This is the evacuation of the uterus by unauthorized persons and is an offence punishable by law. The abortion may have been induced either by the woman herself or by some other person. Drugs or instruments may have been used. Whether successful or not the action is illegal. The methods used may cause sudden death from haemorrhage, air embolus or vagal inhibition. Because of lack of asepsis infection readily occurs and may lead to chronic ill-health or salpingitis and sterility. Midwives should always remember that they are vulnerable members of society and may be asked for advice and help when bleeding occurs. The woman should be immediately referred to a doctor. Any involvement in a case of criminal abortion may render the midwife liable to prosecution.

SEPTIC ABORTION

Uterine infection may occur after any abortion and has been reported after invasive procedures such as chorionic villus sampling (Garden *et al.*, 1991). It more commonly follows criminal abortion or spontaneous abortion where there are retained products of conception. The incidence of septic abortion has declined in countries which allow legal termination of pregnancy. Causative organisms include *Staphylococcus aureus*, *Clostridium welchii*, *Escherichia coli*, *Klebsiella*, *Serratia* and occasionally group A haemolytic *Streptococcus* (Pearlman and Faro, 1990; Dotters and Katz, 1991).

The woman will feel acutely ill with fever, tachycardia, headache, nausea and general malaise. On examination signs of pregnancy such as breast changes may be evident. The uterus may be tender and the vaginal loss is offensive. The woman should be isolated. A high vaginal swab is sent for microscopy and blood cultures are taken. The obstetrician will prescribe antibiotics. These are usually commenced before any surgical intervention is undertaken and may be given intravenously if the woman is very ill.

When her condition allows, the woman is taken to theatre and the uterus is emptied. The midwife must be aware that severe infection may cause septicaemia and endotoxic shock. There is a risk of disseminated intravascular coagulation. Liver and renal damage may occur and the midwife must make careful observations in order to detect signs of organ damage such as oliguria and jaundice. The damage caused by pelvic infection may result in adhesion formation, salpingitis and infertility.

Hydatidiform Mole

This condition occurs as a result of degeneration of the chorionic villi at an early stage of pregnancy (Figure 4). Usually the embryo dies and is reabsorbed, but occasionally a hydatidiform mole may be found alongside a fetus. Triplet pregnancy has been reported, consisting of dizygotic female twins and a complete vesicular mole. The pregnancy aborted spontaneously at 19 weeks' gestation (Azuma *et al.*, 1992).

The incidence of hydatidiform mole in the UK is approximately one in 1000 pregnancies. It is more common in:

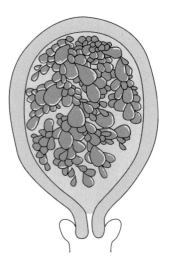

Figure 4 A hydatidiform mole.

▶ women under 20 or over 40 years old;
▶ multiparous women;
▶ smokers; and
▶ women with a previous history of hydatidiform mole (although not all authorities agree that this is a risk factor).

There are also geographical variations in that the condition is commoner in Asia, South-East Asia and Mexico (Beischer and Mackay, 1986; Lewis and Chamberlain, 1990; Parazzini *et al.*, 1991; Symonds, 1992).

The appearance of a hydatidiform mole has been likened to grapes or whitecurrants. The villi become distended with fluid and may measure 1 cm in diameter. The outer layer of the villi is trophoblastic tissue and this may later become malignant if it is not completely removed. A hydatidiform mole may be partial or complete. A *complete mole* shows degeneration of all villi. The karyotype is almost always 46XX but the chromosomes are of paternal origin. The ovum nucleus has been lost and the full complement (46XX) is achieved by duplication of the chromosomes of the X-bearing haploid sperm which penetrated the ovum. Occasionally an anucleate ovum is penetrated by two haploid sperm (X and Y) to give a chromosome complement of 46XY (Szulman, 1988). *Partial moles* occur when some vesicles develop within an otherwise normal placenta. The fetus is usually present. The chromosome complement of partial moles is usually triploid (69XXX, 69XXY or 69XYY). This occurs when a normal haploid ovum (23X) is fertilized by a two haploid sperm or one single diploid sperm (Lewis and Chamberlain, 1990; Tucker *et al.*, 1992).

Signs and symptoms

The woman may complain of intermittent bleeding per vaginam from around the 12th week of pregnancy. When the mole begins to abort there may be profuse haemorrhage. Pre-eclampsia may develop even in the early weeks of pregnancy and severe nausea and vomiting is common. On abdominal examination the uterus is usually large for the period of gestation and may feel soft and doughy to the fingers. No fetal parts are palpable and the fetal heart is absent. There may be signs of mild thyrotoxicosis due to the thyroid-stimulating hormone (TSH)-like activity of human chorionic gonadotrophin which is secreted in large amounts by the molar vesicles. The diagnosis is suggested by the clinical findings and is confirmed by an ultrasound scan which will reveal no fetal parts but only a diffuse vesicular effect (Llewellyn Jones, 1990). Urinary or serum hCG levels are higher than those of a multiple pregnancy. Occasionally molar pregnancies may be detected through maternal serum screening ('triple test') for Down's syndrome (Cuckle *et al.*, 1992).

Treatment

Once the diagnosis is confirmed, the uterus must be completely evacuated at once. If the mole has begun to abort the process may be encouraged by the use of a Syntocinon infusion or prostaglandins. Following expulsion of the molar mass a careful curettage is performed under general anaesthesia. If the mole is detected before it has begun to detach from the uterine wall the woman is taken to theatre and the uterus emptied by suction evacuation followed by curettage under general anaesthesia. Following evacuation of the uterus, a Syntocinon infusion is used to maintain uterine contraction and avoid haemorrhage. The woman is then registered at a specialist follow-up centre (Crawford and Pettit, 1986a).

After treatment for hydatidiform mole careful observation is required for at least one year as approximately 3% of these women will develop malignant trophoblastic disease (*choriocarcinoma*). Beta hCG levels are monitored fortnightly for two months then monthly for a year. Serum assays are more accurate but urine samples are commonly used as these are easier to collect. If any molar tissue remains in the uterus it will continue to grow and may invade the myometrium.

Perforation of the uterine wall is then likely and this will cause major internal haemorrhage. Signs that the mole is continuing to grow are indicated by the persistence of high hCG levels 24 hours after uterine evacuation and high levels one month after treatment. If the serum or urinary hCG fails to return to normal levels within six months or begins to rise again the woman is at risk of malignant trophoblastic disease (Crawford and Pettit, 1986a).

The woman must avoid another pregnancy until she has been discharged from the follow-up programme. The use of hormonal contraception before the disease is eliminated may increase her chance of developing malignant trophoblastic disease and thus requiring antineoplastic treatment. Therefore she must not use the contraceptive pill until the hCG levels have returned to normal (Crawford and Pettit, 1986a). The midwife may need to advise the couple on barrier methods of contraception.

Choriocarcinoma

Choriocarcinoma is a malignant disease of trophoblastic tissue. It follows approximately 3% of hydatidiform moles and may occasionally occur following a normal term pregnancy although this is rare, the incidence being between one in 50 000 and one in 100 000 (Crawford and Pettit, 1986b). The pregnancy test will become strongly positive again and bleeding occurs.

Estimation of serum concentrations of inhibin may be useful in detecting both hydatidiform mole and choriocarcinoma. Inhibin is a glycoprotein hormone secreted by the ovaries and testes. It is also produced by the placenta and levels begin to rise in early pregnancy. Concentrations of inhibin are significantly elevated in cases of hydatidiform mole. Once the uterus is completely emptied of the molar tissue the serum levels fall. Should they remain high it is strongly suggestive of incipient choriocarcinoma. Inhibin is thought to be a more accurate marker for these conditions than human chorionic gonadotrophin, the values of which tend to overlap those of normal pregnancy (Yohkaichiya *et al.*, 1989).

As the growth infiltrates the uterus and vagina pain increases. The condition will be rapidly fatal unless treated and the *Report on Confidential Enquiries into Maternal Deaths in the United Kingdom (1991–1993)* reported one death from choriocarcinoma (DOH,

1996). The disease spreads by local invasion and via the bloodstream; metastases may occur in the lungs, liver and brain. Fetal metastases may occur during pregnancy but this is very rare. The infant may be stillborn. If it is live born it will show signs of the disease within the first six months of life. No affected infant has survived beyond 8 months of age (Flam *et al.*, 1989; Chandra *et al.*, 1990; Chen *et al.*, 1994).

Choriocarcinoma responds extremely well to chemotherapy. Cytotoxic drugs such as methotrexate, etoposide and actinomycin-D are used and a cure is effected in almost every case. Follow-up surveillance of urinary hCG is required for life. The woman should avoid another pregnancy for at least one year after the completion of treatment and should not use the oral contraceptive pill as this may encourage the disease to persist (Crawford and Pettit, 1986b).

Ectopic or Extrauterine Gestation

Ectopic pregnancy was first clearly described by the Arabian writer Abulcasis (AD 936–1013) (Dimitry and Rizk, 1992). It occurs when the fertilized ovum implants outside the uterine cavity. In 95% of cases the site of implantation is the uterine tube and these are known as *tubal pregnancies*. Occasionally the site may be the ovary, the abdominal cavity or the cervical canal but these are rare. The incidence of tubal pregnancy is one in 150. There is a geographical effect in the distribution of ectopic gestation: in the West Indies one pregnancy in 28 is ectopic; abdominal pregnancy is much commoner in African countries than in the Western world and cervical pregnancy is commoner in Japan (Lewis and Chamberlain, 1990; Stabile and Grudzinskas, 1990). Ectopic pregnancy is the major cause of maternal death before 20 weeks' gestation in the industrialized world.

TUBAL PREGNANCY

This is the commonest type of ectopic pregnancy and the incidence is increasing: a two- to three-fold rise has been reported in the last 25 years (Kadar, 1992). This is thought to be largely due to the increasing incidence of sexually transmitted disease, widespread use of both the progestogen-only oral contraceptive pill and the intrauterine contraceptive device, and the current trend towards delaying the first pregnancy until comparatively late in reproductive life. Tubal pregnancy

occurs when there is a delay in the transport of the zygote along the fallopian tube. This may be due to a congenital malformation of the uterine tubes or more commonly to tubal scarring following pelvic infection. The ovum implants and begins to develop in the lining of the tube. The ampulla is the commonest site (Figure 5).

The conceptus is frequently abnormal and there is a higher incidence of blighted ovum. This may reflect poor conditions within the tube (Stabile and Grudzinskas, 1990).

Although tubal pregnancy may occur in the absence of any significant history there are certain risk factors (Stabile and Grudzinskas, 1990; Dimitry and Rizk, 1992; Kadar, 1992):

- ▶ Older mother.
- ▶ Women of low gravidity or parity.
- ▶ History of previous tubal pregnancy.
- ▶ Tubal surgery.
- ▶ Hormonal stimulation of ovulation.
- ▶ Salpingitis, especially chlamydial.
- ▶ Intrauterine contraceptive device.
- ▶ *In-vitro* fertilization.
- ▶ Tubal endometriosis.
- ▶ History of pelvic inflammatory disease.
- ▶ Appendicectomy.
- ▶ Pelvic or abdominal surgery.
- ▶ Progestogen-only pill (this appears to have a detrimental effect on tubal ciliation).

Diagnosis

Diagnosis may be difficult as the clinical picture may appear similar to pelvic inflammatory disease or threatened abortion. Delay in diagnosis and treatment may contribute to maternal mortality and morbidity. Hor-

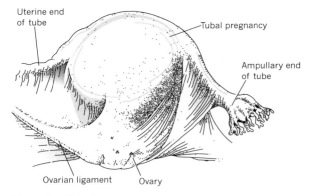

Figure 5   Tubal pregnancy.

monal assays may assist detection of ectopic pregnancy as serum progesterone levels tend to be low. Ultrasound scanning may reveal fluid in the pelvis, an adnexal mass and the absence of an intrauterine pregnancy. This, together with low or falling hCG levels, is strongly suggestive of ectopic gestation (Clancy and Illingworth, 1989; Nager and Murphy, 1991).

As the conceptus develops and grows the tube distends to accommodate it. Initially the woman will experience the usual signs of pregnancy such as nausea and breast changes, although amenorrhoea is not always present. The uterus will soften and enlarge under the influence of the pregnancy hormones. As the tube becomes further distended the woman will experience abdominal pain and some vaginal bleeding. The blood loss is uterine in origin and signifies endometrial degeneration. If the site of implantation is the narrower proximal end of the tube, tubal rupture is likely to occur between the 5th and 7th weeks of pregnancy (Figure 6).

If the pregnancy is located in the wider ampullary section the gestation may continue until the 10th week. Occasionally the gestation sac is expelled from the fimbriated end of the tube as a tubal abortion (Figure 7).

As the ovum separates from its attachment to the ampullary part of the tube, layers of blood clot may be deposited around the dead ovum to form a mass of blood clot similar to a uterine carneous mole; this is called a *tubal mole*. It may remain in the uterine tube or be expelled from the fimbriated end of the tube as a *tubal abortion*.

When the tube ruptures there will be severe intraperitoneal haemorrhage and the woman will experience intense abdominal pain. There may also be referred shoulder tip pain on lying down as blood tracks up towards the diaphragm (Lewis and Chamberlain, 1990). The woman will appear pale, shocked and nauseated and may collapse. The abdomen is tender and may be distended. Pelvic examination is usually exquisitely tender, especially on movement of the cervix. Ruptured ectopic pregnancy is an acute surgical emergency and requires immediate treatment.

Management

An intravenous infusion is inserted to correct hypovolaemia and blood is taken for cross-matching. The woman is taken to theatre as soon as possible where a salpingectomy will be performed. This may be achieved via a laparoscopic technique. If the condition

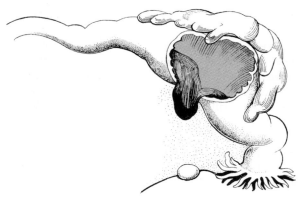

Figure 6   Rupture of the uterine tube.

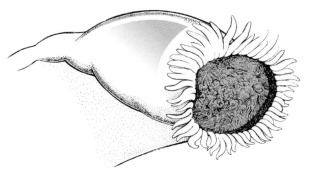

Figure 7   Tubal abortion.

is detected in the early stages and before tubal rupture supervenes, conservative management may be attempted with local injections of prostaglandin F_2-alpha or systemic prostaglandin E_2. Methotrexate may also be used but this may be of most value in cornual pregnancy (Stabile and Grudzinskas, 1990; Dimitry and Rizk, 1992; Lundorff, 1992).

Symptoms of tubal abortion

A woman who has a tubal abortion also suffers pain which may be colicky in nature at first (Beischer and Mackay, 1986). The condition is not so acute because the bleeding is less and although surgical treatment may be given the emergency is not so great.

SECONDARY ABDOMINAL PREGNANCY

Very rarely, when rupture of a tubal pregnancy occurs, there may be partial extrusion of the ovum into the peritoneal cavity, but with enough chorionic villi remaining attached to the tube to ensure that the embryo does not die. Chorionic villi on the surface of the ovum then become attached to the neighbouring abdominal organs and the pregnancy continues with the fetus developing free within the abdominal cavity. The fetus is at risk of severe growth retardation because of the relatively poor placentation and may also suffer pressure deformities as there is no protective uterine wall. This condition is usually detected on ultrasound scanning but may be suggested by a persistently abnormal fetal lie and the fact that fetal parts are unusually easy to palpate. Delivery is by laparatomy. The placenta is usually left *in situ* to be absorbed, as an attempt to detach it may cause uncontrollable haemorrhage.

Bleeding from Associated Conditions

The following conditions may cause bleeding although, strictly speaking, they are not early bleedings of pregnancy since the bleeding is not from the site of the pregnancy.

Cervical polyp

This is a small red gelatinous growth attached by a pedicle to the cervix, close to the external os. It may give rise to slight irregular bleeding.

Ectropion of the cervix

A cervical erosion is formed when the columnar epithelium lining the cervical canal proliferates due to the action of the pregnancy hormones. The ectropion forms a reddish area on the cervix, extending outwards from the external os. It may give rise to a blood-stained discharge from the vagina. No treatment is necessary and the ectropion will recede during the puerperium.

Carcinoma of the cervix

Invasive cervical carcinoma is rarely seen in pregnancy, although cervical intraepithelial neoplasia (CIN) may occasionally be discovered if a cervical smear is taken. If the cervical cytology report suggests precancerous changes, colposcopy is performed to identify the affected areas and a small cervical biopsy may be carried out. Treatment is deferred until after delivery if the condition is not invasive.

Invasive cervical cancer is very serious as the disease may progress quickly. On vaginal examination the cervix is hard and irregular and bleeds when touched. There may also be a purulent vaginal discharge. If the condition is discovered in the first trimester the pregnancy may be terminated and treatment initiated. In the third trimester the fetus is viable and will be delivered by Caesarean section. Once the infant is born the obstetrician may carry out a radical hysterectomy (*Wertheim's hysterectomy*). A dilemma arises if the condition is discovered in the second trimester as the fetus is unlikely to survive if delivered yet any significant delay will severely compromise the woman's chance of survival (Lewis and Chamberlain, 1990).

Any history of vaginal bleeding during pregnancy should be reported to the doctor.

Bleeding After the 24th Week – Antepartum Haemorrhage

Antepartum haemorrhage is defined as bleeding from the genital tract after the 24th week of pregnancy and before the birth of the baby. Bleeding which occurs during labour is sometimes referred to as intrapartum haemorrhage.

Antepartum haemorrhage is a serious complication which may result in the death of the mother or the baby.

There are two main varieties of haemorrhage:

1 *Placenta praevia* (unavoidable or inevitable haemorrhage) is bleeding from separation of an abnormally situated placenta. (The placenta lies partly or wholly in the lower uterine segment and bleeding is inevitable when labour begins.)
2 *Abruptio placentae* (placental abruption) is bleeding from separation of a normally situated placenta.

Extraplacental bleeding

Incidental or associated bleeding sometimes occurs. This is vaginal bleeding from some other part of the birth canal, e.g. a cervical polyp, as described above.

Placenta Praevia

The incidence of placenta praevia at term ranges from 0.5 to 1%. In grandmultiparity the incidence may be as high as 2% (Mabie, 1992). It is usually detected on ultrasound scanning in early pregnancy and may be seen in as many as one quarter of all pregnancies in the second trimester. As the lower segment grows and stretches the placental site appears to rise up the uterine wall, away from the internal os uteri, until at term in the majority of cases the placenta no longer occupies the lower segment. Those cases where the placenta overlies the internal os in early pregnancy are at highest risk of haemorrhage (Sanderson and Milton, 1991). The classification of placenta praevia is shown in Table 1. This is a standard classification and the distinction between types III and IV is purely academic. The types are illustrated in Figure 8.

Table 1 Classification of placenta praevia

Type I	Placenta mainly in the upper segment but encroaching on the lower segment
Type II	Placenta reaches to, but does not cover, the internal os
Type III	Placenta covers the internal os when it is closed but not completely when it is dilated
Type IV	Placenta completely covers the internal os

Causes

The cause of placenta praevia is unknown but the following factors are known to be associated (Cunningham *et al.*, 1989; Williams *et al.*, 1991a; Mabie, 1992; Nimrod, 1992; Williams and Mittendorf, 1993; Taylor *et al.*, 1994; Handler *et al.*, 1994):

► *Multiparity*: The increased size of the uterine cavity following repeated childbearing may predispose to placenta praevia.
► *Multiple pregnancy*: The larger placental site is more likely to encroach on the lower segment of the uterus.
► *Age*: Older mothers are more at risk than younger ones.
► *Scarred uterus*: One previous Caesarean section doubles the risk of placenta praevia.
► *A history of myomectomy.*
► *Smoking*: The exact mechanism is unclear but the relative hypoxia induced by smoking may cause enlargement of the placenta in order to compensate for the reduced oxygen supply. Pregnant women who smoke more than 20 cigarettes a day are twice as likely to develop placenta praevia.

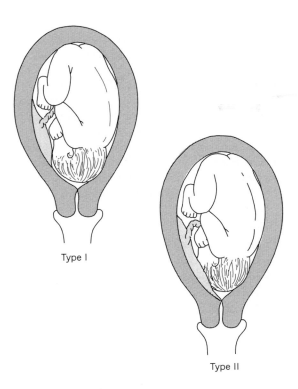

Type I

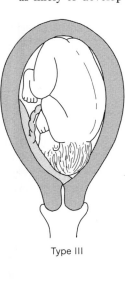

Type II

Type III

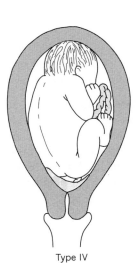

Type IV

Figure 8 Placenta praevia, types I to IV.

▶ *Placental abnormality*: Bipartite and succenturiate placentae may cause placenta praevia. Placenta membranacea (placenta diffusa) may also be a cause. This is a rare developmental abnormality of the placenta where all the chorion is covered with functioning villi. The placenta develops as a thin membraneous structure, covering an unusually large surface of the uterus. The condition may be diagnosed on ultrasound. In pregnancy it may cause severe haemorrhage possibly requiring hysterectomy. It may not separate readily in the third stage of labour. Fetal nutrition appears to be relatively undisturbed in cases of placenta membranacea.

There may be an association between male fetal sex and placenta praevia (Jakobovits and Zubek, 1989).

Associated conditions

A low-lying placenta puts the woman and her fetus at risk of other complications. The most serious of these is *placenta accreta*. This usually occurs where the previous delivery was Caesarean section. The combination of the relatively thin decidua in the lower segment and the presence of scar tissue increases the likelihood of trophoblastic invasion of the myometrium.

Intrauterine growth retardation may occur, possibly as a result of repeated small haemorrhages (Mabie, 1992).

Signs and symptoms

As placenta praevia is normally diagnosed on ultrasound scanning in early pregnancy the midwife will usually be aware of any woman in her care who has a low-lying placenta. However, not all women choose to have an ultrasound scan and the midwife must be aware of the signs which indicate a possible placenta praevia:

▶ *Malpresentation of the fetus*: Although the presentation may be cephalic often it is not. The placenta occupies space in the pelvis and the midwife may find that the breech presents, as there is more room for the head in the fundus, or that the lie is oblique and the fetal shoulder presents.

▶ *Non-engagement of the presenting part*: This is especially likely with a type III or IV placenta praevia.

▶ *Difficulty in identifying fetal parts on palpation*: An anterior placenta praevia (especially type I and II) lies between the fetus and the midwife's hand like a cushion. This makes the fetal parts relatively difficult to identify.

▶ *Loud maternal pulse below the umbilicus*: An anterior placenta praevia (especially type I and II) may often be detected by the presence of loud maternal arterial sounds from the placental bed. This is more easily heard with an electronic fetal heart monitor (Doppler). The fetal heart sounds may be difficult to detect as they are muffled by the placenta, especially in a cephalic presentation.

An anterior type I or II placenta praevia will cushion some of the fetal movements and the woman may mention that she only feels fetal movement above the umbilicus.

When bleeding occurs it usually begins after the 24th–28th week of pregnancy, although it may occur earlier. In the third trimester of pregnancy the lower segment is completing its development, Braxton–Hicks contractions are increasing and towards the end of pregnancy, the cervix is becoming effaced. Bleeding is caused by detachment of the placenta which cannot stretch to adapt to these changes in uterine structure. As the placenta is in the lower pole of the uterus the blood escapes easily, thus giving rise to the classical fresh, painless bleeding of placenta praevia. 'Warning haemorrhages' are associated with placenta praevia. These are small, recurrent, fresh and painless haemorrhages occurring during the third trimester. Each episode of bleeding indicates further placental detachment. If the placenta is torn, some fetal bleeding will occur and this will further compromise the condition of the fetus. Torrential maternal haemorrhage may occur at any time but is more likely once labour begins and the cervix dilates.

It is impossible to predict the course of events in a case of placenta praevia and even in the absence of bleeding the condition is regarded as a major and life-threatening complication of pregnancy.

Management

At home   A midwife who is called to a woman who is bleeding must visit at once. The woman should be helped to lie down, in bed if possible. If bleeding is profuse she should lie on her side or with a pillow or towel wedged under the right hip to achieve a slight pelvic tilt and avoid supine hypotensive syndrome. The doctor must be called and the midwife should indicate the severity of the bleeding and the woman's condition, which will be in direct proportion to the blood loss.

If, as is probable, the initial loss is small, her blood pressure and pulse rate will be normal and she will appear well, though probably a little anxious. Should the loss be severe she will present the typical picture of a woman who has had a haemorrhage: pale, sweating, restless, thirsty, with a rising pulse rate and falling blood pressure. In this event the midwife should herself call for emergency obstetric help since the woman is now in urgent need of resuscitative treatment before she is moved. A paramedic team from the Ambulance Service will transport the woman to hospital. The midwife should make quarter-hourly recordings of pulse and blood pressure until medical help arrives. The blood loss should be noted and a vulval pad applied. All soiled material should be saved so that the total loss may be estimated. In any case of this kind *no vaginal examination should be made in the woman's home.* If this is a case of placenta praevia, a vaginal examination could precipitate a disastrous haemorrhage. Rectal examinations are similarly dangerous: even examining the abdomen, which often provokes Braxton Hicks contractions, might cause further bleeding. In fact, whatever the degree of haemorrhage, the less the woman is disturbed the better. The midwife should tell the woman that she will need to be admitted to hospital.

In hospital   On admission to hospital the woman is made comfortable in bed. She will give a history of sudden, unexpected painless bleeding. Occasionally the bleeding occurs following coitus but usually there is no apparent cause. There may be a recent history of slight 'spotting'. Abdominal examination will reveal a soft, non-tender uterus which corresponds in size to the period of gestation. There is often a malpresentation or an unstable lie and the presenting part is high. The fetus is normally in good condition.

It may be difficult to differentiate placenta praevia from abruptio placentae. In abruptio placentae there is often associated pre-eclampsia, while the presentation and engagement of the fetal head are normal. Thus, an absence of pre-eclampsia and a high or abnormal presenting part would be evidence in favour of placenta praevia.

Observation   Temperature, pulse, blood pressure and fetal heart should be observed. The pulse and blood pressure are recorded as frequently as the woman's condition dictates: quarter-hourly if the bleeding is continuing. The fetal heart should be continuously monitored by external cardiotocography whilst bleeding persists. The urine is tested for protein and, if bleeding is severe, a catheter specimen may be required. Blood is taken for haemoglobin estimation and Kleihauer test if she is rhesus negative, and at least two units of donor blood are cross-matched for use in the event of a sudden severe haemorrhage. An intravenous infusion of Hartmann's solution will be commenced if bleeding is persistent. Intravenous access will be maintained until the bleeding ceases. The abdominal girth is sometimes measured and recorded. Finally the blood loss is estimated and recorded. The woman should remain in bed until the bleeding ceases.

Conservative management   When slight to moderate bleeding occurs before the 38th week of pregnancy and the maternal and fetal conditions are satisfactory, conservative treatment aims to maintain the pregnancy until as near the 38th week as possible to avoid prematurity. When the bleeding ceases the doctor may carry out a speculum examination to exclude incidental causes of bleeding. The placental site will be identified by ultrasound examination. If the placenta is found to be normally situated the woman may be allowed to go home when the bleeding has ceased, provided her condition, and that of the fetus, is good. If placenta praevia is diagnosed the implications of this condition should be discussed with her. The woman will usually be advised to remain in hospital for the rest of her pregnancy as the risk of further and severe haemorrhage is very real.

The midwife may need to involve the social worker if there are childcare arrangements to be made. In the absence of active bleeding the woman should not be confined to her bed and should be encouraged to wear her usual clothes during the day. Women who find themselves in this situation can very quickly become demoralized by the prospect of having to spend some weeks in hospital. The midwife should make every effort to maintain the woman's morale; the effects of separation from the family may be reduced by allowing unrestricted visiting.

Following antepartum haemorrhage, tests to assess fetal well-being will be carried out because premature separation of the placenta may result in impaired placental function. Fetal growth will be assessed by ultrasound and periods of continuous fetal heart monitoring will be performed. Women who are rhesus negative should be given Anti-D gammaglobulin after each episode of bleeding.

Delivery   If no serious haemorrhage has made it imperative to act before, the woman will be delivered at about 38 weeks' gestation. Delivery at this stage avoids the problems of prematurity for the infant.

If the placental location is unclear an examination under anaesthetic may be carried out in theatre, with the woman anaesthetized and the theatre set up in readiness for a Caesarean section. An intravenous infusion is commenced and cross-matched blood is at hand. With the woman in the lithotomy position the obstetrician makes a very gently and cautious vaginal examination, passing a finger through the cervix into the lower pole of the uterus. If the placenta is palpable the obstetrician will immediately perform a Caesarean section. If the placenta is not palpable in the lower segment the membranes may be ruptured and the woman allowed to labour. This procedure avoids unnecessary Caesarean section for women in whom placenta praevia is not confirmed. However, nearly all women have access to ultrasound scanning and the diagnosis is usually clear. Vaginal delivery is usually possible in cases of type I placenta praevia, although some authorities believe that Caesarean section should be the mode of delivery in any case of placenta praevia (Fraser and Watson, 1989).

Active management   In cases where bleeding first occurs at 38 weeks or later, conservative treatment is not appropriate as the fetus is mature. Active management is also necessary in cases where labour has started, if bleeding is severe or there are signs of fetal distress. An intravenous infusion is commenced and the woman's condition is stabilized if necessary. The obstetrician performs an emergency Caesarean section under general anaesthesia. A paediatrician should be present to attend to the baby which may be asphyxiated at birth.

Third stage   Postpartum haemorrhage may complicate the third stage of labour since there are few oblique muscle fibres to control bleeding from the placental site in the lower uterine segment.

Placenta accreta may occur in women who have had a previous Caesarean section and torrential haemorrhage may result from attempts to separate the placenta. Hysterectomy will be required and this may be preceded by ligation of the internal iliac arteries in order to control the haemorrhage.

It cannot be emphasized too strongly that vaginal examination in placenta praevia is an extremely danger-ous procedure and should not be attempted, except with the precautions described above.

Abruptio Placentae

Abruptio placentae is bleeding due to the separation of a normally situated placenta (Figure 9). It is sometimes referred to as placental abruption or accidental bleeding. Placental abruption may occur at any stage of pregnancy, or during labour.

Causes

The cause of the placental separation cannot always be satisfactorily explained. In the majority of abruptio placentae, particularly when the bleeding is slight, no cause can be found. However, the following risk factors have been associated with the condition (Fraser and Watson, 1989; Lowe and Cunningham, 1990; Voigt *et al.*, 1990; Hoskins *et al.*, 1991; Williams *et al.*, 1991b):

▶ Essential hypertension.
▶ Pre-eclampsia.
▶ Sudden decompression of the uterus such as may follow spontaneous rupture of the membranes in cases of polyhydramnios.
▶ Preterm prelabour rupture of the membranes.
▶ Previous history of placental abruption.
▶ Trauma, for example following external cephalic version, road traffic accident, a fall or a blow.
▶ Smoking.
▶ Illegal drug abuse, e.g. cocaine, crack, marijuana.
▶ Folic acid deficiency (although this has not been confirmed).

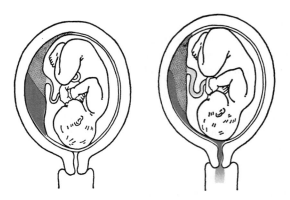

Figure 9   Abruptio placentae.

Maternal hypertension is the most consistent finding in cases of placental abruption.

The bleeding may be revealed, concealed or partially revealed (Figure 10):

▶ *Revealed bleeding*: This occurs when the site of detachment is at the placental margin. The blood thus dissects between the membranes and the decidua and escapes through the os uteri. With revealed placental abruption the degree of shock is in proportion to the visible vaginal blood loss.

▶ *Concealed bleeding*: This occurs when the site of detachment is close to the centre of the placenta. The blood cannot escape and a large retroplacental clot forms. The blood may infiltrate the myometrium, sometimes as far as the peritoneal covering. This is called a *Couvelaire uterus*. There is no visible blood loss but the pain and shock may be severe as the intrauterine tension rises.

▶ *Partially revealed bleeding*: This occurs when some of the blood trickles between the membranes and the decidua to become visible as vaginal bleeding. Not all the blood escapes and a variable amount remains concealed. In this situation the bleeding and thus the degree of shock will be much more severe than the visible loss suggests.

The severity of placental abruption may be classified as mild, moderate or severe:

▶ *Mild abruptio placentae*: The loss is usually slight and the bleeding may be entirely concealed,

although often there is a slight trickle per vaginam. The mother may experience no more than mild abdominal pain, the uterus is not tender and the fetus is alive. There is no sign of maternal shock.

▶ *Moderate abruptio placentae*: The blood loss is heavier, the abdominal pain more severe and, on palpation, the uterus may be tender and firm. The mother may be hypotensive and have a tachycardia and usually there are signs of fetal distress.

▶ *Severe abruptio placentae*: This is an obstetric emergency. More than half the placenta will have separated, the blood loss will exceed 1 litre and the mother will be very shocked. Abdominal pain will be severe. On palpation the uterus will be hard ('woody') and tender and on auscultation the fetal heart sounds will not be heard. A posteriorly sited placenta may cause backache when bleeding occurs and this may confuse the diagnosis (Fraser and Watson, 1989).

It is essential to rembember that the amount of bleeding per vaginam is no guide to the degree of placental separation.

Management of mild abruptio placentae

At home When the mother reports the bleeding the midwife will visit her and call a doctor, all in the manner described for placenta praevia above. No pelvic examination is carried out, no final diagnosis is made, although the differential diagnosis from placenta praevia may be suspected as described below. The mother is quickly transferred to hospital.

In hospital On admission to hospital the woman is made comfortable in bed. She must still be treated as having a placenta praevia although there may be some features which help in making a diagnosis. The woman may relate the bleeding to trauma or strenuous activity which may have caused a rise in her blood pressure. There may be pain, especially if blood is retained within the uterus, and there will be no history of 'warning' haemorrhages (see Table 2). Often the distinction is not clear; it is particularly difficult if the mother has had a small revealed haemorrhage but no pain, no apparent cause for the bleeding and no signs of pre-eclampsia. She is therefore treated exactly as described for placenta praevia: rest in bed, haemoglobin estimation and Kleihauer test if she is rhesus negative; cross-matching of blood; speculum examination to exclude cervical or vaginal lesions. The midwife

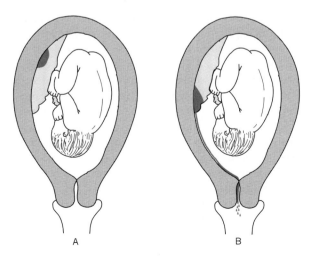

Figure 10   **A**: Concealed abruptio placentae.
B: Revealed abruptio placentae.

Table 2 Differential diagnosis with placenta praevia

Clinical sign	Placenta praevia	Abruptio placentae
Pain	No pain	Uterine pain, may be severe; backache if placenta is posterior
Colour of blood loss	Bright, fresh	May be darker
'Warning' haemorrhage	Yes	No
Onset of bleeding	Possibly following coitus, otherwise unexpected	May follow exertion, trauma
Degree of shock	In proportion to visible loss	May be more severe than visible loss suggests
Consistency of uterus	Soft, non-tender	Increased uterine tone, may be tense, rigid, 'woody'
Palpation	Fetus usually fairly easy to palpate	Tense uterus makes palpation difficult
Presentation	May be a malpresentation	Probably cephalic
Engagement	Not engaged	May be engaged
Fetal heart	Probably present	May be absent
Abdominal girth	Equivalent to gestation	May increase due to concealed haemorrhage

must remember that the discovery of a cervical lesion (e.g. an ectropion) does not eliminate the possibility of abruptio placentae as a diagnosis. The placental site will be confirmed by ultrasound scan. If the placenta is localized in the upper uterine segment and both maternal and fetal condition is satisfactory the woman may be discharged home once the bleeding ceases. The pregnancy will be closely monitored with ultrasound scans and regular cardiotocography to assess fetal growth and well-being. It would be unwise to allow the pregnancy to proceed beyond term.

Management of moderate or severe abruptio placentae

At home Emergency medical help is called. Pillows are removed and the woman should be on her side or with a small wedge under the right hip, which achieves a slight left tilt, and thus helps to avoid supine hypotensive syndrome. Pulse and blood pressure are recorded every 15 minutes. Any urine passed is carefully measured and saved. The obstetrician will order morphine 15–20 mg intramuscularly to relieve the pain. An intravenous infusion is commenced and group O rhesus negative blood is given. Plasma expanders such as Haemaccel, Gelofusine or Hetastarch preparations (Hespan) may be used. When the woman's condition has improved she is transferred to hospital by a paramedic team from the Ambulance Service.

In hospital The aim is to restore blood loss and thus improve the mother's general condition, to get her baby delivered as quickly as possible and to avoid the dangerous complications of renal failure and blood coagulation disorders. The woman is admitted to the Delivery Unit. Blood is taken for group and cross-matching. Other tests include haemoglobin estimation, platelet count, urea and electrolytes, clotting studies and fibrin degradation products. Central venous pressure is monitored to avoid the dangers of over- or under-transfusion. The mother's blood pressure, pulse and respiratory rate are recorded frequently and a Foley urinary catheter is inserted. The urinary output is closely monitored, a marked decrease being a grave sign. The blood transfusion is continued – several units of donor blood may be required as much has been lost.

The most important treatment is to empty the uterus. If fetal condition permits, labour is induced by rupturing the membranes and an oxytocic infusion is commenced. Vaginal delivery may be possible. If the fetus is in poor condition delivery will be by Caesarean section unless the woman is already in the second stage of labour, when a forceps delivery will be performed. Caesarean section is not carried out if there is evidence of fetal death. Ergometrine 500 µg is given intravenously at delivery to control haemorrhage in the third stage of labour. It is usual to continue the Syntocinon infusion for some hours after delivery in order to maintain uterine contraction.

The best treatment for severe haemorrhage and defective coagulation is the transfusion of fresh blood. If fresh blood is not available, fresh frozen plasma should be given as this contains fibrinogen, platelets and clotting factors III, V and VIII.

Fibrinogen concentrate used to be the treatment of

choice but nowadays it is resorted to only if neither fresh blood nor fresh frozen plasma is available as it could aggravate the clotting disorder.

Complications

Blood coagulation disorders When tissue damage occurs there is a release of thromboplastins from the local cells. Thromboplastins activate the clotting mechanism and this results in the conversion of fibrinogen into fibrin. The sticky web of fibrin traps the cellular components of the blood and a clot forms, sealing off the bleeding point. The clot is later dispersed by plasmin which is the active product of the fibrinolytic system. When a clot is broken down fibrin degradation products (FDPs) are formed. Clot dispersal is a protective mechanism to prevent capillary blockage.

The system of initial clot formation followed by fibrinolysis is normally delicately balanced. If the coagulation system fails bleeding will persist, while if the fibrinolytic system fails clotting will persist.

Occasionally tissue damage is so severe or widespread that there is a massive release of thromboplastins into the general circulation. Widespread clotting will then occur throughout the body. This condition is known as *disseminated intravascular coagulation* (DIC). It is extremely dangerous as the microthrombi generated by the thromboplastins will occlude small blood vessels. This results in ischaemic tissue damage within the body organs: the damaged tissue releases thromboplastins, which stimulates further clotting. Thus a vicious circle of tissue damage and uncontrolled clotting occurs. Any body organ may be affected: renal damage will result in oliguria or anuria; liver damage will lead to jaundice. If the lungs are affected dyspnoea and cyanosis will occur and convulsions or coma indicate cerebral involvement. Microthrombi in the retina may cause blindness; if the pituitary gland is affected Sheehan's syndrome may occur.

Eventually the available circulating platelets are depleted. Clotting factors such as prothrombin (Factor II), thromboplastin (Factor III), proaccelerin (Factor V), anti-haemophilic factor (Factor VIII) and fibrinogen (Factor I) are exhausted. No further coagulation can take place: bleeding becomes apparent. This may take the form of oozing from venepuncture sites, mucous membrane bleeding, petechiae and uncontrollable uterine haemorrhage.

DIC is always a secondary event, that is it occurs as a result of massive tissue damage and thromboplastin release. It may complicate conditions such as severe pre-eclampsia, septicaemia or amniotic fluid embolism. It may also occur following abruptio placentae when thromboplastins are released from the damaged placental, decidual and myometrial tissue. Unless DIC is recognized and treated promptly the condition may become uncontrollable and maternal death is almost inevitable. The midwife must be aware of any woman who is at risk of DIC and be alert for the signs of coagulation failure. All Maternity Units should have an emergency protocol for dealing with such cases. Any woman with an abruptio placentae should have screening tests for coagulation defects. These tests include (Brandjes *et al.*, 1991; Sipes and Weiner, 1992):

- ▶ Partial thromboplastin time (normally 35–45 seconds).
- ▶ Prothombin time (normally 10–14 seconds).
- ▶ Thrombin time (normally 10–15 seconds).
- ▶ Fibrinogen levels (2.5–4 g/l).
- ▶ Fibrin degradation products.
- ▶ Whole blood film and platelet count.

More sensitive tests such as antithrombin III and α_2-antiplasmin may be carried out to detect subclinical DIC.

Fresh frozen plasma, packed cells and platelets are used in the treatment of disseminated intravascular coagulation. Heparin is rarely used as it may exacerbate the haemorrhage, especially if the uterus is not empty.

Acute renal failure This may occur following severe shock in cases of abruptio placentae.

Sheehan's syndrome Sheehan's syndrome, or anterior pituitary necrosis, is a rare complication of severe and prolonged shock. The earliest sign is failure to lactate followed by amenorrhoea. The activity of the thyroid and adrenal glands is gradually diminished, hence the woman becomes lethargic and complains of feeling cold, coarsening of hair and skin and loss of libido. The secondary sexual characteristics are affected: the genitalia and the breasts will atrophy (Lewis and Chamberlain, 1990). Recognition of the condition and treatment is essential if serious ill-health or possible death is to be avoided.

Postpartum haemorrhage Following severe abruptio placentae postpartum haemorrhage is most likely to be caused by a blood coagulation disorder, whereas following placenta praevia it is due to the inability of the lower uterine segment to contract effectively. Aortic compression may be necessary to control cases of intractable haemorrhage.

Infection Sepsis is likely owing to the woman's lowered resistance following a state of severe shock, a large blood transfusion, more interference in labour and anaemia.

Anaemia The haemoglobin must be checked and anaemia corrected in the puerperium.

Psychological disturbances/psychoses Psychological disorders after childbirth are more likely following complications of pregnancy and labour.

Vasa Praevia

This unusual condition may result in vaginal bleeding. It is associated with velamentous insertion of the cord. One of the fetal vessels traverses the membranes in the region of the internal os, in front of the presenting part. When the membranes rupture the vessel is torn and severe fetal bleeding occurs. The perinatal mortality associated with this condition is high. Diagnosis is difficult but a pulsating vessel may be felt on vaginal examination. Vasa praevia has been diagnosed by transvaginal and colour flow Doppler ultrasound (Nelson *et al.*, 1990).

If the midwife suspects the presence of a vasa praevia she should leave the membranes intact and inform the doctor. Delivery will be by emergency Caesarean section if vasa praevia is diagnosed during the first stage of labour. In the second stage of labour delivery is expedited by an episiotomy and forceps. Vaginal bleeding with sudden severe fetal distress following rupture of the membranes should alert the midwife to the possibility of a ruptured vasa praevia. A sinusoidal fetal heart trace on cardiotocography is also suggestive of fetal bleeding. The blood loss may be tested for the presence of fetal cells using the alkalidenaturation test, which will determine whether the blood is fetal or maternal in origin. However, it is unlikely that there will be time for this as delivery must be immediate if there is to be any hope of saving the fetus. If born alive, the baby will require expert resuscitation and a paediatrician should be present at the delivery. A blood transfusion will be given to correct hypovolaemia and anaemia. The midwife should be aware that there is a much higher incidence of velamentous insertion of the cord in IVF pregnancies and therefore the risk of a vasa praevia is greater (Healy and Wood, 1989).

Conclusion

Bleeding in pregnancy remains a major cause of maternal mortality. The midwife must be familiar with local policy and should also read the guidelines for the management of massive obstetric haemorrhage recommended in the Report on Confidential Enquiries into Maternal Deaths in the United Kingdom 1985–1987 (DOH 1991), and the revised guidelines in the subsequent Report for 1988–1990 (DOH, 1994).

References

Azuma, C., Saji, F., Takemura, M. *et al.* (1992) Triplet pregnancy involving complete hydatidiform mole and two fetuses: genetic analysis by deoxyribonucleic acid finger print. *Am. J. Obstet. Gynecol.* **166**(2): 664–667.

Barron, S. (1995) Bleeding in pregnancy. In Chamberlain, G. (ed) *Turnbull's Obstetrics.* Edinburgh: Churchill Livingstone.

Beischer, N. & Mackay, E. (1986) *Obstetrics and the Newborn.* London: Baillière Tindall.

Bewley, C. (1993) The midwife's role in pregnancy termination. *Nursing Standard* 8(12): 25–28.

Brandjes, D., Schenk, B., Buller, H. & ten Cate, J. (1991) Management of disseminated intravascular coagulation in obstetrics. *Eur. J. Obstet. Gynecol. Reprod. Biol.* **42**: 587–589.

Chandra, S., Gilbert, E., Viseskul, C., Strother, C. & Hasing, R. (1990) Neonatal intracranial choriocarcinoma. *Arch. Pathol. Lab. Med.* **114**(10): 1079–1082.

Chen, R.J., Huang, S.C., Chow, S.N., Hsieh, C.Y. & Hsu, H.C. (1994) Persistent gestational trophoblastic tumour with partial hydatidiform mole as the antecedent pregnancy. *Br. J. Obstet. Gynaecol.* **101**: 330–334.

Christianson, O., Mathieson, O., Lauritsen, J. & Grunnet, N. (1992) Study of the birthweight of parents experiencing unexplained recurrent miscarriages. *Br. J. Obstet. Gynaecol.* **99**: 408–411.

Clancy, M. & Illingworth, R. (1989) The diagnosis of ectopic pregnancy in an Accident and Emergency Department. *Arch. Emergency Med.* **6**: 205–210.

Crawford, M. & Pettit, D. (1986a) Hydatidiform mole and choriocarcinoma. *Nursing Times* 3 December: 38–39.

Crawford, M. & Pettit, D. (1986b) Treatment schedules hydatidiform mole and choriocarcinoma. *Nursing Times* 10 December: 40–42.

Cuckle, H., Densem, J. & Wald, N. (1992) Detection of hydatidiform mole in maternal serum screening programmes for Down's syndrome. *Br. J. Obstet. Gynaecol.* **99**: 495–497.

Cunningham, F., MacDonald, P. & Gant, N. (1989) *Williams Obstetrics*. London: Prentice Hall.

Dimitry, E. & Rizk, B. (1992) Ectopic pregnancy: epidemiology, advances in diagnosis and management. *Br. J. Clin. Pract.* **46**(1): 52–54.

DOH (Department of Health) (1991) *Report on Confidential Enquiries into Maternal Deaths in the United Kingdom 1985–1987*. London: HMSO.

DOH (1994) *Report on Confidential Enquiries into Maternal Deaths in the United Kingdom 1988–1990*. London: HMSO.

DOH (1996) *Report on Confidential Enquiries into Maternal Deaths in the United Kingdom 1991–93*. London: HMSO.

Dotters, D. & Katz, V. (1991) Streptococcal toxic shock associated with septic abortion. *Obstet. Gynecol.* **78**(3)(2): 549–551.

el-Rafaey, H., Hinshaw, K., Henshaw, R., Smith, N. & Templeton, A. (1992) Medical management of missed abortion and anembryonic pregnancy. *Br. Med. J.* **305** (5 December): 1399.

el-Rafaey, H., Calder, C., Wheatley, D. & Templeton, A. (1994) Cervical priming with prostaglandin E1 analogues, misoprostol and gemeprost. *Lancet* **343**(8907): 1207–1209.

Evans, M. & Fletcher, J. (1992) Multifetal pregnancy reduction. In Reece, E., Hobbins, J., Mahoney, M. & Petrie, R. (eds) *Medicine of the Fetus and Mother*. Philadelphia: J.B. Lippincott.

Flam, F., Lundstrom, V. & Silfversward, C. (1989) Choriocarcinoma in mother and child. Case report. *Br. J. Obstet. Gynaecol.* **96**(2): 241–244.

Fraser, R. & Watson, R. (1989) Bleeding during the latter half of pregnancy. In Chalmers, R., Enkin, M. & Keirse, M. (eds) *Effective Care in Pregnancy and Childbirth*. Oxford: Oxford University Press.

Friedman, T. & Gath, D. (1989) The psychiatric consequences of spontaneous abortion. *Br. J. Psychiat.* **155**: 810–813.

Garden, A., Johnston, M. & Davis, N. (1991) Intra-uterine infection and miscarriage following transabdominal chorionic villus sampling. Case report. *Br. J. Obstet. Gynaecol.* **98**: 413.

Handler, A., Mason, E., Rosenberg, D. & Davis, F. (1994) The relationship between exposure during pregnancy to cigarette smoking and cocaine use and placenta praevia. *Am. J. Obstet. Gynecol.* **170**(3): 884–889.

Harrison, R. (1988) Early recurrent pregnancy failure: treatment with human chorionic gonadotrophins. In Beard, R. & Sharp, F. (eds) *Early Pregnancy Loss, Mechanisms and Treatment. Proceedings of the Eighteenth Study Group of the Royal College of Obstetricians and Gynaecologists*. London: RCOG.

Healy, D. & Wood, C. (1989) Extracorporeal fertilisation (IVF). In Turnbull, A. & Chamberlain, G. (eds) *Obstetrics*. Edinburgh: Churchill Livingstone.

Heard, M. & Guillebaud, J. (1992) Medical abortion. *Br. Med. J.* **304** (25 January): 195–196.

Henshaw, R., Cooper, K., El-Refaey, H., Smith, N. & Templeton, A. (1993) Medical management of miscarriage: Non-surgical uterine evacuation of incomplete and inevitable spontaneous abortion. *Br. Med. J.* **306** (3 April): 894–895.

Hoskins, I., Friedman, D., Frieden, F., Ordorica, S. & Young, B. (1991) Relationship between antepartum cocaine abuse, abnormal umbilical artery Doppler velocity and placental abruption. *Obstet. Gynecol.* **78**(2): 279–282.

Jakobovits, A. & Zubek, L. (1989) Sex ratio and placenta praevia. *Acta Obstet. Gynecol. Scand.* **68**: 503–505.

Kadar, N. (1992) Ectopic and heterotopic pregnancies. In Reece, E., Hobbins, J., Mahoney, M. & Petrie, R. *Medicine of the Fetus and Mother*. Philadelphia: J.B. Lippincott.

Kohner, N. (1992) *A Dignified Ending*. London: Stillbirth and Neonatal Death Society.

Lewis, T. & Chamberlain, G. (1990) *Obstetrics by Ten Teachers*. Sevenoaks: Hodder & Stoughton.

Llewellyn Jones, D. (1990) *Fundamentals of Obstetrics and Gynaecology*, Vol. I, *Obstetrics*, 5th edn. London: Faber & Faber.

Lowe, T. & Cunningham, F. (1990) Placental abruption. *Clin. Obstet. Gynecol.* **33**(3): 406–413.

Lundorff, P. (1992) Modern management of ectopic pregnancy. *Acta Obstet. Gynecol. Scand.* **71**: 158–159.

Mabie, W. (1992) Placenta praevia. *Clin. Perinatol.* **19**(2): 425–435.

Macrow, P. & Elstein, M. (1993) Managing miscarriage medically. *Br. Med. J.* **306** (3 April): 876.

Mowbray, J. (1988) Success and failures in immunisation for recurrent spontaneous abortion. In Beard, R. & Sharp, F. (eds) *Early Pregnancy Loss, Mechanism and Treatment. Proceedings of the Eighteenth Study Group of the Royal College of Obstetricians and Gynaecologists*. London: RCOG.

Nager, C. & Murphy, A. (1991) Ectopic pregnancy *Clin. Obstet. Gynecol.* **34**(2): 403–411.

Nelson, L., Melone, P. & King, M. (1990) Diagnosis of a vasa praevia with transvaginal and colour flow Doppler ultrasound. *Obstet. Gynecol.* **76**(3)(2): 506–509.

Nimrod, C. (1992) Third trimester bleeding. In Reece, E., Hobbins, J., Mahoney, M. & Petrie, R. (eds) *Medicine of the Fetus and Mother*. Philadelphia: J.B. Lippincott.

Paintin, D. (1991) The implications of the new legislations on abortion. *Maternal and Child Health*. July: 221–224.

Parazzini, F., Mangili, G., La Vecchia, C., Negri, E., Bocciolone, L. & Fasoli, M. (1991) Risk factors for gestational trophoblastic disease: A separate analysis of complete and partial hydatidiform mole. *Obstet. Gynecol.* **78**(6): 1039–1045.

Pearlman, M. & Faro, S. (1990) Obstetric septic shock: A pathophysiologic basis for management. *Clin. Obstet. Gynecol.* **33**(3): 482–491.

Roussel Laboratories Ltd (1992) *Medical Termination of Early Pregnancy with Mifegyne: Information for Health Care Professionals*. Uxbridge, Middlesex: Roussel Laboratories Ltd.

Sanderson, D. & Milton, P. (1991) The effectiveness of ultrasound screening at 18–20 weeks' gestational age for prediction of placenta praevia. *J. Obstet. Gynaecol.* **11**(5): 320–323.

SANDS (Stillbirth and Neonatal Death Society) (1991) *Guidelines for Professionals.* London: SANDS.

Savage, W. (1989) Therapeutic abortion. In Turnbull, A. & Chamberlain, G. (eds) *Obstetrics.* London: Churchill Livingstone.

Sipes, S. & Weiner, C. (1992) Coagulation disorders in pregnancy. In Reece, E., Hobbins, J., Mahoney, M. & Petrie, R. (eds) *Medicine of the Fetus and Mother.* Philadelphia: J.B. Lippincott.

Stabile, I. & Grudzinskas, J. (1990) Ectopic pregnancy: A review of incidence, etiology and diagnostic aspects. *Obstet. Gynaecol. Surv.* 45(6): 335–345.

Stirrat, G. (1990) Recurrent miscarriage II: clinical associations, causes and management. *Lancet* 336 (22 September): 728–733.

Symonds, E. (1992) *Essential Obstetrics and Gynaecology,* 2nd edn. Edinburgh: Churchill Livingstone.

Szulman, A. (1988) The biology of trophoblastic disease: complete and partial hydatidiform moles. In Beard, R. & Sharp, R. (eds) *Early Pregnancy Loss, Mechanism and Treatment. Proceedings of the Eighteenth Study Group of the Royal College of Obstetrics and Gynaecologists.* London: RCOG.

Taylor, V., Kramer, M., Vaughan, T. & Peacock, S. (1994) Placenta praevia and prior caesarean delivery: how strong is the association? *Obstet. Gynecol.* 84(1): 55–57.

Tindall, V.R. (1987) *Jeffcoate's Principles of Gynaecology.* London: Butterworths.

Tucker, Blackburn, S. & Loper, D.L. (1992) *Maternal Fetal and Neonatal Physiology.* London: W.B. Saunders Co.

Voigt, L., Hollenbach, K., Krohn, M., Daling, J. & Hickok, D. (1990) The relationship of abruptio placentae with maternal smoking and small for gestational age infants. *Obstet. Gynecol.* 75(5): 771–774.

Williams, M. & Mittendorf, R. (1993) Increasing maternal age as a determinant of placenta praevia. More important than increasing parity? *J. Reprod.* 38(6): 425–428.

Williams, M., Mittendorf, R., Lieberman, E., Monson, R., Schoenbaum, S. & Genest, D. (1991a) Cigarette smoking during pregnancy in relation to placenta praevia. *Am. J. Obstet. Gynecol.* 165(1): 28–32.

Williams, M., Leiberman, E., Mittendorf, R., Monson, R. & Schoenbaum, S. (1991b) Risk factors for abruptio placentae. *Am. J. Epidemiol.* 134(9): 965–972.

Windham, G., Swan, S. & Fenster, L. (1992) Parental cigarette smoking and risk of spontaneous abortion. *Am. J. Epidemiol.* 135(12): 1394–1403.

Yohkaichiya, T., Fukaya, T., Hoshiai, H., Yajima, A. & de Krester, D. (1989) Inhibin: a new circulating marker of hydatidiform mole. *Br. Med. J.* 298(6689): 1684–1686.

Further Reading

Biskup, I. & Malinowski, W. (1994) Ultrasound in abruptio placentae praecox of the second twin. 'Boomerang phenomenon'. *Acta Obstet. Gynecol. Scand.* 73(6): 515–516.

DiPierri, D. (1994) RU 486, Mifepristone: a review of a controversial drug. *Nurse Pract.* 19(6): 59–61.

Evans, M., Dommergues, M., Timor-Tritsch, I. *et al.* (1994) Transabdominal versus transcervical and transvaginal multifetal pregnancy reduction: international collaborative experience of more than one thousand cases. *Am. J. Obstet. Gynecol.* 170(3): 902–909.

Mouer, J. (1994) Placenta praevia: antepartum conservative management, inpatient versus outpatient. *Am. J. Obstet. Gynecol.* 170(6): 1683–1685.

Rashid, A., Moir, C. & Butt, J. (1994) Sudden death following caesarean section for placenta praevia and accreta. *Am. J. Forensic Med. Pathol.* 15(1): 32–35.

Regas, L. (1991) Recurrent miscarriage. *Br. Med. J.* 302 (9 March): 543–544.

Stirrat, G. (1990) Recurrent miscarriage I: definition and epidemiology. *Lancet* 336 (15 September): 673–675.

Tabsh, K. (1993) A report of 131 cases of multifetal pregnancy reductions. *Obstet. Gynecol.* 82(1): 57–60.

Thomas, A., Alvarez, M., Friedman, F. *et al.* (1994) The effect of placenta praevia on blood loss in second-trimester pregnancy termination. *Obstet. Gynecol.* 84(1): 58–60.

World Health Organization Task Force on Post-Ovulatory Methods of Fertility Regulation (1993) Termination of pregnancy with reduced dose of Mifepristone. *Br. Med. J.* 307 (28 August): 532–537.

Useful Addresses

The Miscarriage Association
c/o Clayton Hospital, Northgate, Wakefield, West Yorkshire WF1 3JS

Tel. 01924 200799
(24 hour service – out of hours answerphone)

Support Around Termination for Fetal Abnormality (SATFA)

73 Charlotte Street, London W1P 1LB

Tel: 0171 631 0280

0171 631 0285 (Helpline)

41

Hypertensive Disorders of Pregnancy

Hypertensive disorders in pregnancy accounted for 20 deaths in the United Kingdom between 1991 and 1993 (DOH, 1996) confirming them as a major cause of maternal death. Although referred to as hypertensive disorders, hypertension is but one major characteristic of these multisystem disorders. In this chapter, consideration is given to terminology, aetiology, predisposing factors, screening, identification, treatment and outcomes.

Terminology

Throughout the years various terms have been applied to a condition arising in pregnancy which is characterized by a rise in blood pressure, presence of proteinuria, possibly oedema, and convulsions. Gestosis, pre-eclampsia, toxaemia and toxicosis are names which have been applied to these conditions (Wallenburg, 1989) and this variety of names has led to difficulties in the epidemiology of the disease and the establishment of clinical trials. In this chapter, the term *hypertensive disorders of pregnancy* has been adopted, with the term *pregnancy-induced hypertension* used to indicate a hypertensive disorder in a woman who was previously normotensive and non-proteinuric. Bearing in mind that the convulsive state which may ensue is known as *eclampsia*, the term *pre-eclampsia* has been retained to denote a condition in which a pregnant woman exhibits hypertension in conjunction with proteinuria, with or without oedema.

On the subject of terminology, as Chamberlain (1991) observes, the semantics are of far less importance than the ability of health professionals to recognize the features of a life-threatening disorder of pregnancy.

CLASSIFICATION

A number of authorities have attempted to classify hypertensive disorders which occur in pregnancy (Wallenburg, 1989) but their validity is questionable since many conditions are only classified retrospectively, either from post-mortem following maternal death, or from follow-up investigations postnatally. Despite the dubious value of classification, greater understanding of the number and forms of hypertensive conditions occurring during pregnancy may be achieved by the use of some form of classification. In addition, a standard classification may provide a common foundation on which research can be based and results assessed.

The classification shown in Table 1 (Davey and MacGillivray, 1988) sparked off debate and discussion concerning its usefulness (Editorial, 1989a) when it first appeared; however, it provides a clear overview of the complex nature of hypertensive disorders occurring in pregnancy, and illustrates the combinations in which the four major features of the condition may appear.

Wallenburg (1989) suggests that there are at least two distinct aetiological types of pregnancy hypertension:

1   a hypertensive disorder induced by pregnancy but resolved within ten days following delivery; and
2   a pre-existing hypertensive disorder which may be diagnosed for the first time during pregnancy and upon which pre-eclampsia may be superimposed.

Pregnancy-induced Hypertension (Gestational Hypertension)

There are some differences in the definition of this condition. In this text gestational hypertension or pregnancy-induced hypertension without proteinuria is defined as follows:

> The occurrence of a blood pressure of 140/90 mmHg or more and/or an increase in diastolic pressure of 20 mmHg or more after the 20th week of pregnancy on at least two separate occasions more than 24 hours apart in a woman known to be previously normotensive.
>
> (Broughton Pipkin, 1981)

When hypertension is associated with significant *proteinuria* the disease is considered to be severe and a diagnosis of *pre-eclampsia* or gestational proteinuric hypertension is made. Oedema used to be included as one of the three cardinal signs of pre-eclampsia. Nowadays, however, it is considered a feature of normal pregnancy (Thomson *et al.*, 1967). Although oedema is usually present in cases of pre-eclampsia, it is difficult to quantify and is only considered of significance in the presence of proteinuria.

Aetiology of pre-eclampsia (gestational proteinuric hypertension)

Despite much research, the cause of pre-eclampsia remains uncertain. It has been called the 'disease of theories'. Widespread endothelial damage is known to occur and is associated with an ischaemic placenta, but the cause of this is unknown. Possible causes advanced include conditions associated with a large placenta, hormones, the renin–angiotensin system, and factors influencing the retention of salt and water such as the antidiuretic/vasopressin hormones from the pituitary gland and aldosterone from the adrenal gland. Immunological factors are being studied and there is increasing evidence that genetic dissimilarity of father and mother plays an important role (Symonds, 1980; Alderman *et al.*, 1986). MacGillivray (1981) reports a familial tendency to the condition and racial tendencies have also been observed (Davies, 1971). Geographical location has been considered and there is some evidence that eclampsia may be more common in humid rather than dry conditions (Neutra, 1974).

The latest aetiological theory which holds credence suggests that there is a basic maladaptation of the maternal circulatory system in response to the fetal trophoblast. This maladaptation arises when physiological dilatation of the spiral arterioles fails to occur; instead of maternal blood pooling in the placental bed creating a shunt which leads to a lowering of blood pressure, it is raised by being forced through the constricted arterioles. The muscle coating of the spiral arterioles is further damaged leading to arteriosclerosis and local platelet aggregation, causing a further rise in blood pressure (Chamberlain, 1991).

This failure in the reduction of peripheral resistance is further complicated by an increased sensitivity to angiotensin II, leading to vasospasm in the spiral arterioles. Normally, in pregnancy a delicate balance is maintained between prostacyclin and thromboxane which prevents this aggravated response to angiotensin II (Chamberlain, 1991). Recent studies on the use of low-dose aspirin in hypertensive disorders of pregnancy, discussed later in this chapter, are based on the theory that the antiplatelet properties of aspirin act to maintain the prostacyclin/thromboxane ratio.

Predisposing causes

Certain pregnant women have a predisposition to pre-eclampsia. It is sometimes called a disease of primigravidae because it is far more common in primigravidae

Table 1   Clinical classification of hypertensive disorders of pregnancy

A.	**Gestational hypertension and/or proteinuria**

Hypertension and/or proteinuria developing during pregnancy, labour, or the puerperium in a previously normotensive non-proteinuric woman subdivided into

1. *Gestational hypertension (without proteinuria)*
   a. Developing antenatally
   b. Developing for first time in labour
   c. Developing for first time in the puerperium
2. *Gestational proteinuria (without hypertension)*
   a. Developing antenatally
   b. Developing for the first time in labour
   c. Developing for first time in puerperium
3. *Gestational proteinuric hypertension (pre-eclampsia)*
   a. Developing antenatally
   b. Developing for first time in labour
   c. Developing for first time in puerperium

B. **Chronic hypertension and chronic renal disease**

Hypertension and/or proteinuria in pregnancy in a woman with chronic hypertension or chronic renal disease diagnosed before, during, or after pregnancy subdivided into

1. *Chronic hypertension (without proteinuria)*
2. *Chronic renal disease (proteinuria with or without hypertension)*
3. *Chronic hypertension with superimposed pre-eclampsia*
   Proteinuria developing for first time during pregnancy in a woman with known chronic hypertension

C. **Unclassified hypertension and/or proteinuria**

Hypertension and/or proteinuria found either

At first examination after 20th week of pregnancy (140 days) in a woman without known chronic hypertension or chronic renal disease

or

During pregnancy, labour, or the puerperium where information is insufficient to permit classification is regarded as unclassified during pregnancy and is subdivided into

1. Unclassified hypertension (without proteinuria)
2. Unclassified proteinuria (without hypertension)
3. Unclassified proteinuric hypertension

D. **Eclampsia**

The occurrence of generalized convulsions during pregnancy, during labour, or within 7 days of delivery and not caused by epilepsy or other convulsive disorders

Notes on classification:

A. Hypertension and/or proteinuria at the first visit before the 20th week of pregnancy (in the absence of trophoblastic disease) is presumed to be caused by either
   1. Chronic hypertension (hypertension only)

or

   2. Chronic renal disease (proteinuria with or without hypertension)
B. Unclassified hypertension and/or proteinuria may be reclassified after delivery
   1. If the hypertension and/or proteinuria disappears into
      a. Gestational hypertension (without proteinuria)

or

      b. Gestational proteinuria (without hypertension)

or

      c. Gestational proteinuric hypertension (pre-eclampsia)
   2. If the hypertension and/or proteinuria persists after delivery or other tests confirm the diagnosis into
      a. Chronic hypertension (without proteinuria)

or

      b. Chronic renal disease (proteinuria with or without hypertension)

or

   3. Chronic hypertension with superimposed pre-eclampsia
C. Gestational proteinuric hypertension may be regarded as synonymous with 'pre-eclampsia'. 'Gestational hypertension' is often regarded as synonymous with 'pregnancy-induced hypertension', but the term 'pregnancy-induced hypertension' is reserved in this classification for that form of hypertension that commonly but not exclusively occurs in primigravid women and is primarily caused by an abnormality of pregnancy, which if it is severe or progresses is associated with the development of proteinuria and other features of 'pre-eclampsia'.

Source: From Davey and MacGillivray, 1988.

than in multigravidae. Even if the first pregnancy results in abortion, especially induced abortion, there is a reduced incidence of pre-eclampsia in the second pregnancy. However, the degree of protection is not as great as that following a first, term pregnancy (Beck, 1985). A small study of 1011 consecutive pregnant women in the UK suggested that an extended period of cohabitation with a partner prior to conception may also protect against pre-eclampsia (Robillard *et al.*, 1994).

The condition is more likely to develop in young teenagers and in women over 35 years of age (Mac-Gillivray, 1983). Obesity seems to be a predisposing factor (Treharne *et al.*, 1979), and women with essential or renal hypertension may develop a superimposed pre-eclampsia. It occurs in polyhydramnios and in conditions where the placenta is enlarged, such as multiple pregnancy, diabetes, hydrops fetalis and hydatidiform mole. In hydatidiform mole it may develop early in pregnancy. More commonly it arises later, after 32 weeks, but it may occur as early as 20 to 24 weeks in rare instances.

Familial tendencies have been described (Kilpatrick *et al.*, 1989) showing a higher rate of pre-eclampsia amongst sisters suggesting a genetic susceptibility connected with *HLA-DR4*; however this single-gene hypothesis is disputed by Thornton and Onwude (1991), whose study of identical female parous twins failed to confirm a genetic link, at least on the maternal side.

Dietary aspects have also been considered, and some studies suggest that there is a link between low dietary calcium and pregnancy-induced hypertension (Belizan *et al.*, 1988; Lopez-Jaramillo *et al.*, 1989, 1990; Marcoux *et al.*, 1990). The role of calcium in the prediction of pregnancy-induced hypertension is considered an important area for investigation (Wallenburg, 1989) since hypocalciuria appeared more common in women with pregnancy-induced hypertension than in those who were normotensive. O'Dent (1994) reviews the role of calcium in prevention of pre-eclampsia, and offers a complex, but plausible connection between long-chain ϖ-3 fatty acids (present in oily fish), low-dietary calcium, and the development of pre-eclampsia.

Complications

The two common features in the pathology of pre-eclampsia are:

1 arteriolar vasoconstriction;
2 disseminated intravascular coagulation.

The effects of these two features are seen in the kidney, liver and the placental bed. Abruptio placentae may occur due to arteriolar vasoconstriction and spasm resulting in ischaemia and subsequent rupture of arterioles. Disseminated intravascular coagulation (see Chapter 40) is caused by the release of thromboplastic material into the circulation. In pre-eclampsia and eclampsia the source of thromboplastin is probably the damaged placental tissue, whether or not it is associated with abruptio placentae.

Severe pre-eclampsia may lead to eclampsia which is characterized by epileptiform convulsions. In severe pre-eclampsia and eclampsia the effects of arteriolar vasoconstriction and disseminated intravascular coagulation are widespread and include cerebral haemorrhage, cardiac failure with pulmonary oedema, acute renal failure from tubular or cortical necrosis and hepatic failure.

Pre-eclampsia also adversely affects the well-being of the fetus since it may cause placental dysfunction. Complications such as intrauterine growth retardation, intrauterine hypoxia and intrauterine fetal death may occur. The perinatal mortality is raised not only because of these conditions but also because of prematurity since early delivery is necessary for severe pre-eclampsia and eclampsia. In the *1988–90 Report on Confidential Enquiries into Maternal Deaths in the United Kingdom* the perinatal mortality was 13.1%, a marked fall from the previous report (DOH, 1994).

Diagnosis

Hypertension A reading of 140/90 mmHg is regarded as the upper limit of normal, but a rise in diastolic blood pressure of 15–20 mmHg or more above the level recorded in the early weeks of pregnancy is always regarded with suspicion. A woman whose blood pressure is normally 90/60 mmHg may have quite severe pregnancy-induced hypertension with a blood pressure of 120/80 mmHg, especially if accompanied by proteinuria. The diastolic pressure is of more significance than the systolic because it is not affected by posture and other factors such as stress and excitement. It should be measured at the 'muffling' stage and not at the disappearance of sounds.

Many women with a diastolic pressure of 90 mmHg or more, often with oedema, have perfectly normal pregnancies and deliver babies of a good birthweight, whereas others, albeit a minority, develop severe pre-eclampsia which may lead to convulsions (eclampsia).

Oedema Oedema is no longer considered one of the cardinal signs of pregnancy-induced hypertension because it is so often a feature of normotensive as well as hypertensive pregnancies (Thomson *et al.*, 1967). Indeed, it is associated with above average weight babies unless proteinuria develops (MacGillivray, 1985). Similarly a high weight gain in pregnancy is not always associated with pregnancy-induced hypertension, unless proteinuria develops. It is also associated with large babies. Despite this, both marked oedema and high weight gain may be premonitory signs of pre-eclampsia, and thus cannot be disregarded. Severe oedema affects the feet, legs, hands, face and abdominal wall. Excessive weight gain may be due to occult oedema. During the latter half of pregnancy normal weight gain is approximately 0.5 kg per week. Weight gain significantly in excess of this which is accompanied by hypertension and proteinuria is likely to be associated with pre-eclampsia.

Proteinuria Proteinuria is usually the last sign of pre-eclampsia to be manifested and it is *always* serious. When proteinuria is present together with hypertension both the perinatal mortality rate and the incidence of low birthweight babies are increased (MacGillivray and Campbell, 1980). The risk of the mother developing eclampsia is also increased.

Protein may be found in urine which is contaminated by vaginal discharge due to infection, amniotic fluid or blood and in urinary tract infection, since pus is present and pus contains protein. If, however, a midstream specimen which looks crystal-clear contains protein, this is almost certainly 'true' proteinuria, that is the kidneys are damaged and plasma proteins are leaking from the blood into the urine.

Diagnostic tests Hypertension and proteinuria are not the only signs of pre-eclampsia, or necessarily the most important. Diagnostic tests to assess *renal function*, *thrombocytopenia* and *liver enzymes* are necessary to diagnose the extent to which the maternal system is affected by the disease (Douglas and Redman, 1994; BEST Report, 1994).

The midwife's responsibility

The diagnosis of pregnancy-induced hypertension is usually made on physical signs and not on symptoms. This is important, since a woman may have severe pregnancy-induced hypertension and yet feel well. It is only when eclampsia is imminent that the woman develops symptoms and begins to feel ill. Thus, since early diagnosis is essential, all antenatal women need regular blood pressure estimations, examinations for signs of marked oedema and urine tests to detect proteinuria.

Although hypertension and proteinuria, with or without oedema occur in pre-eclampsia, the severity of these signs varies considerably and a small number of women present with symptoms such as *headache*, *visual disturbances* or *epigastric pain* which are all indicative of serious systemic complications, and may be soon followed by eclampsia (Barry *et al.*, 1994). It may be only after the woman complains of these symptoms that hypertension and proteinuria are diagnosed. If a woman complains of these symptoms, therefore, the midwife must take her blood pressure and test the urine for protein, and then refer her to an obstetrician immediately, even if her blood pressure is not significantly raised, because it is now known that convulsions may precede hypertension or proteinuria (Redman, 1994).

The midwife's work in the detection of pregnancy-induced hypertension must begin with an accurate recording of the woman's history to identify risk factors. Blood pressure screening must be carried out accurately, preferably using a standardized technique. Research indicates that widely differing methods of obtaining blood pressure readings are adopted, leading to gross variability of results (Brown and Simpson, 1992). It is recommended that the diastolic measurement is taken at the 'muffling' or IV stage of the Korotkov sounds since, during pregnancy, there may not be complete disappearance of sound. Maternal position should be such that the sphygmomanometer cuff is at the same level as the left atrium. Large size cuffs should be available for those women who need them; Mahomed and James (1988) suggest a larger cuff size for women weighing more than 85 kg.

Although automated blood pressure devices may be useful, a small study of 40 normotensive women and 17 with pre-eclampsia carried out in the USA suggested that automated blood pressure recording machines may underestimate blood pressure by as much as 30 mmHg (Quinn, 1994).

It is essential to assess the severity of pregnancy-induced hypertension since this, together with the period of gestation, will determine the management and the likely outcome.

Gestational hypertension without proteinuria (mild pregnancy-induced hypertension) The diastolic blood pressure is usually less than 100 mmHg and there is no proteinuria. Oedema is difficult to quantify and may not exceed that found in a normotensive woman. Close antenatal supervision will be required with the mother usually at home. The midwife is involved with women being treated at home, and, if at the next antenatal visit the blood pressure is raised again, further self-monitoring at home and community care by the midwife will be required, often with visits to the antenatal assessment unit for tests and monitoring (Haley, 1995; Morris de Lassalle, 1994). The condition often recurs and this shows clearly that pregnancy-induced hypertension is not cured before delivery.

In some cases the condition worsens, with the diastolic blood pressure rising to 100 mmHg or more and there may be slight proteinuria, up to about 0.5 g/litre. Once proteinuria develops admission to hospital is required. In some women the blood pressure remains elevated. In these women labour may be induced at 38 weeks or earlier if tests indicate intrauterine growth retardation or failing placental function, or if there is a significant deterioration in the mother's condition and persistent proteinuria supervenes.

Gestational proteinuric hypertension (pre-eclampsia) The diastolic blood pressure is usually over 100 mmHg (often over 110 mmHg) and there is generalized oedema and persistent proteinuria, usually over 1 g/litre. Pregnancy is normally terminated to avoid the risks to mother and fetus, especially if signs of imminent eclampsia develop. Only if severe pre-eclampsia occurred early in pregnancy, before about 28–30 weeks, would conservative management be considered for a week or two to allow the fetus to mature a little more before delivery. In this case close observation of mother and fetus is essential and if there are any signs of deterioration in their condition pregnancy is terminated, usually by Caesarean section. Delivery is the only known cure for pregnancy-induced hypertension. The disease usually resolves within 48–72 hours of delivery.

Dangers of pregnancy-induced hypertension

▶ *Maternal*: eclampsia, placental abruption, disseminated intravascular coagulation, maternal death.

▶ *Fetal*: intrauterine growth retardation, fetal hypoxia (especially in labour), intrauterine death.

Management

The aim of management is to deliver the baby before complications occur which threaten the life or health of mother or fetus. Difficulties arise when the disease occurs in the second or early third trimester of pregnancy and the problems of an immature baby have to be weighed against the risks of continuing the pregnancy. Nowadays, with skilled neonatal intensive care, it is often safer for both mother and baby to expedite the delivery, especially if diagnostic tests indicate that maternal systems are being adversely affected by the disease and/or there are fetal complications such as growth retardation.

Bedrest Bedrest has always been advised for the expectant mother with pre-eclampsia. It is thought to decrease the blood pressure and oedema and to increase urinary output and placental blood flow (Editorial, 1981). However, many studies have now been carried out which question the value of bedrest. Mathews *et al.* (1971) found ambulatory management and self-monitoring at home to be effective in those women with no proteinuria and no evidence of placental insufficiency. In this study there was a decrease in both the incidence of eclampsia and the number of perinatal deaths. Other studies, some with pregnant women in hospital, have shown bedrest to be of little or no benefit for the woman with pregnancy-induced hypertension or for her fetus (Beischer and O'Sullivan, 1972; Letchworth *et al.*, 1974; Hauth *et al.*, 1976; Chew et al., 1976; Mathews, 1977; Mathews *et al.*, 1980). Cartwright *et al.* (1992) suggest that when blood pressure is monitored serially, there is no difference in anxiety levels between women monitored at home or in hospital.

MacGillivray (1985) states that there is no good evidence to suggest that bedrest is of benefit but undue activity should obviously be avoided. Many centres now offer facilities for assessment on an outpatient basis (Mahomed and James, 1988), with mothers actively involved in their own screening programmes. It must be emphasized, however, that women who develop proteinuria in the absence of chronic renal disease require admission to hospital. In particular proteinuria in a woman with essential hypertension signifies a superimposed pre-eclampsia and not a worsening of essential hypertension. Therefore again admission to hospital is essential.

Drugs   If the blood pressure remains high in cases of severe pregnancy-induced hypertension and immediate delivery seems inadvisable, the doctor may prescribe *antihypertensive drugs* to control the blood pressure, although they do not improve the underlying effects of the disease. Control of the blood pressure reduces the risk of cerebral haemorrhage and eclampsia, however, and thereby the risk of maternal death.

Methyldopa given intravenously or orally is commonly used to treat hypertension in pregnancy; it acts centrally by inhibiting sympathetic outflow and the overview of clinical trials on its use suggests that it significantly reduces the risk of developing severe hypertension (Collins and Wallenburg, 1989).

Labetolol, a combined α- and β-antagonist acts to reduce peripheral resistance and cardiac output, thereby reducing blood pressure, but in common with β-adrenoceptor antagonists such as propanolol and atenolol, it may result in severe fetal and neonatal bradycardia (Collins and Wallenburg, 1989). Nevertheless, it is suggested that it is generally as safe and effective as methyldopa (Plouin *et al.*, 1988), and that its antihypertensive action may be more controlled than hydralazine (Collins and Wallenburg, 1989).

Hydralazine has long been the choice of drug in cases of severe hypertension; it is a vasodilator and may be given orally or intravenously. It is an effective antihypertensive drug, but when given intravenously may lead to sudden maternal hypotension. It should not be given intramuscularly due to its unpredictable rate of absorption.

Calcium antagonists such as nifedipine lower blood pressure by the inhibition of calcium ion activity in the smooth muscles of blood vessels, resulting in a decrease in peripheral vascular resistance.

Despite the implication of angiotensin II in hypertensive disorders of pregnancy, the use of agents to inhibit angiotensin-converting enzyme (*ACE inhibitors*) is associated with prematurity, low birthweight and sudden unexplained fetal death (Editorial, 1989b), and is therefore not recommended for use during pregnancy.

Aspirin has been the subject of clinical trials (CLASP – Collaborative Low-dose Aspirin Studies in Pregnancy) to assess its use in the prevention and treatment of pregnancy-induced hypertension. The results of earlier trials (deSwiet and Fryers, 1990)

suggest that aspirin is most effective when low doses (60 mg per day) are given to women considered at higher risk of developing pregnancy-induced hypertension, rather than for the treatment of those who actually develop these disorders. In addition, low-dose aspirin may be of value in the treatment of intrauterine growth retardation. However, despite hopes for a significant beneficial role, aspirin has not yielded the definite results which were indicated by the initial small trials (Bellin, 1994). In a large multicentre study of 9354 pregnant women, randomly allocated 60 mg aspirin daily or matching placebo, there was no significant reduction in pre-eclampsia, intrauterine growth retardation, stillbirth or neonatal death (CLASP, 1994). There was a slight, but significant reduction in preterm delivery, and an indication that low-dose aspirin may be beneficial before 20 weeks' gestation for women who have a previous history of early pre-eclampsia.

Diuretics are no longer prescribed for the treatment of pregnancy-induced hypertension. They are not effective in controlling the blood pressure and cause a reduction in circulating blood volume and increased blood viscosity (Lang *et al.*, 1984).

Sedatives are not normally prescribed. They would be indicated only if the woman seemed particularly anxious or was not sleeping well.

Diet   A normal, well-balanced diet is given, and there is no indication for restriction of salt intake.

Observations and investigations

Blood pressure   This is recorded twice daily or, if very high, four-hourly or more frequently.

Fluid balance   The fluid intake and urinary output are measured and recorded. Oliguria can then soon be detected. It is also important to avoid intravenous fluid overload since the volume of the vascular bed is markedly reduced in severe pre-eclampsia. The administration of intravenous fluids should be controlled by an expert, since pulmonary complications due to intravenous overload accounted directly for one maternal death in the 1988–90 triennium (DOH, 1994) and was evident in six cases in the 1991–93 triennium (DOH, 1996). Pulmonary oedema was also a factor in some of the nine deaths due to adult respiratory distress syndrome (DOH, 1991, 1994, 1996). Although as previously stated, diuretics are not used to control hypertension in pregnancy-induced hypertension (gestational hypertension), in severe cases where intensive therapy is given, and where a central venous pressure line is *in situ*, diuretics may be used where pulmonary overload is suspected.

Urine analysis   Urine is tested daily; the volume and concentration of urine affects random readings and protein excretion is variable according to time of day (Davey and MacGillivray, 1988). Twenty-four-hour urine collections may provide a more accurate measurement of proteinuria, although Wallenburg (1989) suggests that random dipstick sampling, together with estimation of specific gravity provide acceptable methods of screening.

Urine should also be tested to exclude infection.

Oedema   Although 85% of women with pregnancy-induced hypertension will develop oedema, it is not possible to differentiate between physiological and pathological oedema (Wallenburg, 1989). Nevertheless, it may be uncomfortable and distressing for women who develop it and for that reason it is important to observe its development and to discuss the significance with the woman.

Weight   The whole issue of whether weighing pregnant women is of any value is discussed in Chapter 19. Smooth weight gain associated with some degree of oedema bodes for a more favourable fetal outcome, whereas in pre-eclampsia there may be a rapid weight gain due to a sudden increase in oedema.

Assessment of renal function   In cases of moderate and severe hypertension in pregnancy renal function should be assessed. Investigations include estimations of:

▶ plasma electrolytes,
▶ blood urea, and
▶ creatinine and uric acid,

which will all be elevated if renal function is sufficiently impaired. Creatinine clearance to detect impaired renal function and serum proteins may be decreased. Serial tests are required to monitor renal function.

A specimen of urine is also sent to the laboratory for microscopy and culture.

Assessment of liver function   Serial measurements of *liver enzymes* and *liver function tests* should be carried

out in women with moderate or severe hypertensive disease in pregnancy. Hepatic complications can then be diagnosed at an early stage and appropriate management instituted.

Assessment of coagulation complications   Repeated investigations to detect the development of coagulation complications should also be performed. These investigations include:

▶ blood film,
▶ platelet count, and
▶ coagulation studies

to detect the development and/or degree of disseminated intravascular coagulation in cases of severe pre-eclampsia.

The multisystem nature of the condition is reflected in changes which take place in the blood and may give rise to the *HELLP* syndrome, characterized by Haemolysis, Elevated Liver proteins and Low Platelets.

Biochemical tests, described above, are essential to diagnose this serious condition.

Assessment of fetal well-being   (see Chapters 21 and 46) Pre-eclampsia is associated with a reduction in maternal placental blood flow which results in intrauterine growth retardation and hypoxia of the fetus. Careful monitoring of the fetus is therefore of paramount importance and any deterioration in the fetal condition will influence the management. Investigations to assess the fetal condition include:

1   abdominal examination to note fetal growth and the amount of amniotic fluid and to ausculate the fetal heart sounds;
2   cardiotocography;
3   a record of fetal movements (kick chart);
4   ultrasound scanning for:

▶ record of fetal breathing movements,
▶ cephalometry,
▶ measurement of abdominal girth,
▶ length of femur,
▶ Doppler studies;

Placental function tests are no longer carried out in the UK.

Delivery

Pregnancy-induced hypertension will resolve only when pregnancy is terminated. Many obstetricians therefore induce labour at term, that is at 38 weeks or more. Others induce labour only when there is evidence of deterioration in the maternal and/or fetal well-being. The disease usually resolves within 48–72 hours of delivery.

In cases where the disease develops before term, unless severe, the treatment is usually conservative, allowing the pregnancy to mature as near to 38 weeks as possible, thereby avoiding the risks associated with an immature baby. According to the *Report on Confidential Enquiries into Maternal Deaths in the UK, 1991–93* (DOH, 1996), however, attempts to secure a more mature fetus must not lead obstetricians to underestimate the dangers of the disease which may be progressive, despite apparent control of the blood pressure by antihypertensive drugs.

IMMINENT ECLAMPSIA

In a few patients the condition worsens. The *hypertension* and *proteinuria* may increase and the patient for the first time begins to feel ill as she experiences definite symptoms:

1   Severe frontal *headache*, probably associated with cerebral oedema.
2   *Visual disturbances*, resulting from oedema of the retina. The vision may be dim or blurred, the patient saying that she cannot read her newspaper; or she may see spots or flashes of light.
3   *Vomiting*, which may be related to cerebral oedema or associated with (4).
4   *Epigastric pain* caused by haemorrhages under the liver capsule; this can be a warning that eclampsia is imminent. Barry *et al.* (1994) studied cases where upper abdominal pain was the first indication of pre-eclampsia and this symptom had been variously misdiagnosed as dyspepsia and urinary tract infection.
5   *Oliguria*, a diminished output of urine, is a most important sign. It may herald the onset of eclampsia or renal failure.
6   *Hyperpyrexia* is another important sign which may signify impending eclampsia.

It must not be supposed that every patient with severe pre-eclampsia presents all these symptoms and signs. Indeed any one symptom, with or without hypertension and proteinuria, is sufficient to indicate that the condition is worsening and that eclampsia is imminent.

Pre-eclampsia is, at present, not preventable but its severity can be lessened. Eclampsia is nearly, but not quite, preventable. It is important, therefore, to detect pre-eclampsia as early as possible in order to take action and thus try to prevent the disease from progressing to a more serious form.

Management

Effective sedation and antihypertensive drugs are given immediately to try to avert eclampsia and to lower the blood pressure. Labour is then induced or the pregnancy terminated by Caesarean section. Only when this condition arises before about 30 weeks may the doctor try conservative treatment in an attempt to delay the need for delivery until the fetus is a little more mature. The risks of eclampsia, placental insufficiency and abruption and intrauterine fetal death must be considered against those of prematurity. The management of patients with imminent eclampsia is as for those with eclampsia.

Twelve deaths were attributed to pre-eclampsia in the 1991–93 *Report on Confidential Enquiries into Maternal Deaths in the UK* (DOH, 1996).

Eclampsia

Eclampsia is the onset of convulsions in a pregnancy usually, but not always, complicated by pre-eclampsia. In a national study conducted in the UK in 1992, 38% of cases of eclampsia were not heralded by hypertension and proteinuria (Douglas and Redman, 1994). It occurs in the UK once in about 2000 births and carries serious risks for both mother and fetus. Douglas and Redman (1994) found that nearly one in 50 women who developed eclampsia died and one in 14 of their babies also died. Worldwide, 50 000 women die after suffering an eclamptic convulsion (Duley, 1994) and a multicentre trial is currently underway to assess the most appropriate drug to prevent and treat convulsions.

The convulsions may occur before, during or after labour. If antenatal care and care in labour are of a high standard, postpartum convulsions are more commonly seen. These can occur up to 48–72 hours after delivery. Monitoring of blood pressure and urine for proteinuria should therefore continue during the postpartum period.

Aetiology

In severe pre-eclampsia there is likely to be cerebral hypoxia due to intense vasospasm and oedema. Cerebral hypoxia leads to increased cerebral dysrhythmia and this may be the cause of the convulsions. Some patients have an underlying cerebral dysrhythmia and therefore convulsions may occur following less severe forms of pre-eclampsia.

There is one sign of eclampsia, namely, the *eclamptic convulsion*, four phases of which are recognized.

1 *Premonitory stage*: This transient stage may be missed if the mother is not under constant observation. The woman rolls her eyes, while her facial and hand muscles twitch momentarily.
2 *Tonic stage*: Almost immediately her muscles go into violent spasm. Her fists are clenched and her arms and legs are rigid. She clenches her teeth and she may bite her tongue. Since her respiratory muscles are in spasm, she stops breathing and her colour becomes deeply cyanosed. This spasm continues for perhaps 30 seconds.
3 *Clonic stage*: As the spasm ceases, jerky muscular movements begin and become increasingly violent. Her whole body is thrown restlessly from side to side, while frothy, often blood-stained saliva appears on her lips. The breathing is stertorous and she may inhale mucus or blood from her mouth. The convulsive movements gradually subside. This restless phase lasts up to two minutes and is followed by a period of coma.
4 *Comatose stage*: The woman is deeply unconscious and perhaps breathing noisily. The cyanosis fades, but her face may remain swollen and congested. Sometimes she regains consciousness in a few minutes or the coma may persist for hours.

Table 2 Causes of death in cases of severe pre-eclampsia and eclampsia in the UK in 1991–93 (DOH, 1996)

Causes of death	No. of women who died
Cerebral	
Haemorrhage – intracerebral	5
Pulmonary	
Adult respiratory distress syndrome	8
Oedema	3
Other	4
Total	20

Dangers

Maternal The convulsions are extremely exhausting and, if they recur frequently, heart failure will develop. If hypertension is greatly increased, the woman may have a cerebral haemorrhage. Patients with massive oedema and oliguria can develop pulmonary oedema or renal failure. Inhalation of blood or mucus may lead to asphyxia or pneumonia. Hepatic failure may occur.

Any of these complications may be fatal. The number of maternal deaths from eclampsia in the UK in 1991–93 was 11. In over half these deaths women died after only one or two fits. The immediate cause of death was as shown in Table 2.

Fetal In antenatal eclampsia the fetus may be affected by placental insufficiency. This leads to intrauterine growth retardation and hypoxia. During the fit when the mother stops breathing the fetal oxygen supply, already impaired, is further reduced. The perinatal mortality rate is as high as 15%. Intrapartum convulsions are also very hazardous to the fetus because intrauterine hypoxia is already increased due to the uterine contractions.

Management

If pre-eclampsia is recognized early and treated promptly, eclampsia will hardly ever occur. Very rarely, a fulminating form of pre-eclampsia may begin and proceed rapidly to eclampsia between regular and frequent antenatal examinations. If the woman is outside hospital when a convulsion occurs, ambulance paramedics should be called immediately to give expert attention before transfer to hospital.

Management during a convulsion The essentials are to:

▶ Maintain a clear airway
▶ Protect the woman from injury.

The woman should be turned on to her side and her convulsive movements restrained, all this being done as gently as possible and not forcibly. The mouth is cleared of mucus and blood with suction apparatus. Oxygen is then given, as it will benefit both mother and fetus. At the earliest opportunity medical aid should be summoned.

Subsequent management The principles of management are:

▶ Control of convulsions.
▶ Control the blood pressure.
▶ Deliver the baby.

Control of convulsions It is vital to control the convulsions, as the more convulsions the woman has, the greater the risk to her life and that of her fetus. Sedation is given immediately to reduce the excitability of the nervous system. The drug of choice for the treatment of eclampsia is magnesium sulphate (Neilsen, 1995; Lucas, 1995).

1 *Magnesium sulphate* is an effective anticonvulsant and acts rapidly. The findings of the Collaborative Eclampsia trial, which were published in 1995, conclude that magnesium sulphate is more effective in reducing and preventing eclamptic convulsions than both diazepam and phenytoin (The Eclampsia Collaborative Trial Group, 1995). Women in the trial who received magnesium sulphate had a 52% lower risk of convulsions than those given diazepam, and a 67% lower risk than those given phenytoin. Magnesium sulphate is therefore recommended for the treatment of eclampsia. The World Health Organization is now recommending the use of magnesium sulphate for the treatment of eclampsia and advocating its inclusion in the Essential Drugs List (WHO, 1995). An initial intravenous injection of 4–5 g in a 20% solution may be given, followed by an infusion of 1–2 g/hour.

Magnesium sulphate has long been used to prevent and control convulsions in the USA; it is believed to inhibit presynaptic activity but does not have antihypertensive or sedative properties. It is administered intravenously and blood levels must be monitored regularly to ensure that they remain within the therapeutic range (2–4 mmol/l). Toxicity leads to loss of maternal reflexes and eventually muscle paralysis, respiratory arrest and cardiac arrest (Wallenburg, 1989).

2 An intravenous injection of *diazepam* 10–40 mg followed by an infusion of 20–80 mg in 500 ml of 5% dextrose at a rate of 30 drops a minute. The rate is adjusted according to the woman's response; thus it is increased if she is restless and decreased if she appears too drowsy. Diazepam exerts a direct depressant effect on the maternal thalamus and hypothalamus and is effective in controlling convulsions when given intravenously. However, it crosses the placenta readily and is slowly metabo-

lized by the fetus and the newborn. Its neonatal side-effects may include apnoea, delayed onset of respirations, hypotonia and poor sucking reflex (Wallenburg, 1989). Following the findings of the Eclampsia Collaborative Trial it should no longer be the drug of choice.

Other drugs such as morphine, tribromoethanal (Avertin), paraldehyde and lytic cocktail (a combination of pethidine, promethazine and chlorpromazine in an intravenous infusion of 5% dextrose solution) are not recommended nowadays. Phenytoin is widely used in the treatment of epilepsy and is currently enjoying renewed popularity in the management of pre-eclampsia. However, it is not effective in the control of eclamptic fits (The Eclampsia Collaborative Trial Group, 1995), and is considered as a prophylactic rather than a method of treatment (Howard, 1993).

Control of blood pressure Blood pressure is controlled by sedation and by the use of antihypertensive drugs such as hydralazine hydrochloride (Apresoline) 20 mg by intravenous injection initially, followed by 20–40 mg as an intravenous infusion, the rate being regulated according to the blood pressure.

Diuretic treatment is indicated when the urinary output is less than 20 ml/hour. Antibiotics may be prescribed to prevent pulmonary infection.

Biochemical tests to assess renal function, thrombocytopenia and liver enzymes are monitored to give information about the extent to which the maternal system is affected, and early warning of the HELLP syndrome.

Midwifery care Any stimulus may precipitate another fit, so external stimuli such as noise, bright lights and handling are reduced to a minimum. The woman is nursed in a quiet, single room and, until her convulsions are controlled, she must never be left alone. Anaesthetic instruments, suction apparatus and oxygen equipment must be beside the bed. Although bright sunshine should be excluded, the room should be light enough for the midwife to be able to assess the woman's condition without switching lights on and off. Only essential nursing procedures such as turning the patient two-hourly to avoid hypostatic pneumonia, mouth care and treatment of pressure areas are carried out initially, and then at a time when the patient is heavily sedated.

Observations   Vital observations include the following:

1 *Restlessness* or twitching may herald the onset of another convulsion.
2 *Colour* is observed and any cyanosis is an indication for the administration of oxygen. Because cyanosis is such an important sign of cardiorespiratory failure, patients must not be nursed in dark or semi-dark rooms.
3 The *temperature* is recorded four-hourly. Hyperpyrexia is a strain on the heart. This is especially important in hot climates. If there is no obvious sign of infection, the rise in temperature could be due to anoxic damage to the temperature-regulating centres in the midbrain.
4 *Pulse* and *respirations* may be recorded as often as every 15 minutes.
5 *Blood pressure* will be recorded frequently, probably half-hourly or hourly.
6 An accurate record of *fluid intake* and *output* is maintained. As oral fluids and nourishment cannot be given, intravenous fluids will be given and a second infusion may be required for the administration of drugs. The importance of avoiding intravenous overload cannot be overemphasized. A central venous pressure line should be established for an accurate measurement of fluid volume. A self-retaining catheter is inserted into the bladder and released hourly; thus urinary output can be measured accurately and the woman will not have to be disturbed to pass urine. A urinary output of less than 30 ml/hour suggests the onset of renal failure. Each specimen of urine is tested for the presence of proteins.
7 *Fetal heart* may be continuously monitored or auscultated at half-hourly or hourly intervals.
8 Signs of the *onset of labour* are observed, since labour may start spontaneously. Any loss per vaginam is noted and the fundus should be gently palpated if the woman appears to be restless at regular intervals because she could be disturbed by uterine contractions. A heavily sedated or comatose woman could progress to an advanced stage of labour unless the signs are recognized by an observant midwife.

Mode of delivery   As soon as the convulsions and blood pressure are under control, arrangements are made for delivery. If the fetus is alive an elective Caesarean section may be performed, or the doctor may prefer to induce labour by artificial rupture of the membranes followed by Syntocinon infusion.

Care in labour   In addition to the midwifery care already described, effective analgesia is essential and can best be achieved by epidural anaesthesia. It also has the advantage of lowering the blood pressure. Continuous monitoring of the fetal heart and uterine contractions should be carried out.

When the woman reaches the second stage of labour, pushing is inadvisable since it might cause a dangerous rise of blood pressure. For this reason elective episiotomy and forceps delivery are carried out when the os uteri is fully dilated. It is usual in such cases to prescribe Syntocinon only since ergometrine causes a rise in blood pressure and should therefore be withheld.

A paediatrician should be present to receive and resuscitate the baby at birth.

Management after delivery   Following delivery the woman is heavily sedated and sedation and antihypertensive drugs are continued for a further 48 hours, as postpartum fits may occur during this time. The special midwifery care and observations previously described are thus continued. After this time sedation is gradually withdrawn and the woman usually makes a rapid recovery. Within a few days, her blood pressure is normal, her output of urine, soon protein-free, is greatly increased and her oedema subsides.

It is essential to remember that convulsions may occur for the first time postpartum in women with pre-eclampsia, or may occur both ante- or intrapartum and postpartum. In any woman with a history of pre-eclampsia or eclampsia, close monitoring of blood pressure and urine for proteinuria must be continued after delivery. Symptoms such as headache, vomiting and epigastric pain should alert the midwife to seek help from a senior obstetrician. Unsatisfactory postpartum care accounts for a large part of the mortality from the hypertensive disorders of pregnancy. This was evident in 12 cases in the 1988–1990 *Report on Confidential Enquiries into Maternal Deaths in the United Kingdom* (DOH, 1994).

Eclampsia rarely occurs in a subsequent pregnancy, but pre-eclampsia may occasionally recur. It is not associated with a higher incidence of essential hypertension in later life.

Appropriate postpartum investigations should be

performed, for instance to assess renal function, in women who have suffered serious hypertensive disease in pregnancy. They may also be advised to obtain preconception advice and counselling before embarking on a future pregnancy.

It has been suggested that the subject of pre-eclampsia needs to be addressed nationally and its profile raised. The charity APEC (Action on Preeclampsia) seeks to inform all pregnant women of the risks of pregnancy-induced hypertension, emphasizing the fact that the disorder is largely asymptomatic and must be diagnosed by active screening. Whilst the charity welcomes the demedicalization of childbirth, it emphasizes the importance of informing women and securing their co-operation in all aspects of antenatal care (APEC, 1992). This informed and collaborative approach is also endorsed in the last two *Reports on Confidential Enquiries into Maternal Deaths* (DOH, 1991, 1994).

The *Report on Confidential Enquiries into Maternal Deaths* published in 1996 (DOH, 1996) notes that recent advances in detection and management of pregnancy-induced hypertension mean that few professionals will ever come across severe pre-eclampsia or eclampsia. In 16 of the 20 deaths (80%) from hypertensive disorders of pregnancy between 1991 and 1993, substandard care from health professionals was a factor. The Report reiterates the need for local specialized teams within Regions, who can act either in an advisory capacity, or within suitably equipped and staffed high-dependency units. It also stresses the need for a lead consultant and clear guidelines for the management of severe preeclampsia and eclampsia in each maternity unit.

Despite the strong recommendation in recent reports for a Regional Advisory Service, there is no record of help being sought from such a service in any of the deaths from hypertensive disorders in this report (DOH, 1996).

Essential Hypertension

Essential hypertension is a condition of permanently raised blood pressure in which no cause is usually apparent. Occasionally it is associated with renal disease, phaeochromocytoma or coarctation of the aorta. It tends to occur in families and, because it is fairly common in young people, it is seen quite frequently in pregnancy.

A woman attending the antenatal clinic is said to have essential hypertension if her blood pressure in early pregnancy is 140/90 mmHg or more. It is distinguished from pre-eclampsia by the fact that essential hypertension is present in the early weeks of pregnancy, long before pre-eclampsia normally arises, and there is no oedema or proteinuria.

During the middle weeks of pregnancy the blood pressure often falls to a normal level, rising again in the later weeks to its original point or even higher. If the woman books late, therefore, after the 18th week of pregnancy, it is more difficult to distinguish essential hypertension from pre-eclampsia.

Management

The woman will require very close antenatal supervision and is booked by a consultant obstetrician for hospital delivery. So long as the mother's blood pressure does not rise above 150/90 mmHg, the outlook is good. She is likely to have a normal pregnancy and labour but throughout pregnancy is advised to have extra rest and avoid putting on too much weight. Fetal well-being is monitored closely to detect growth retardation. The pregnancy is not allowed to go beyond term since postmaturity imposes an increased risk to the fetus of placental insufficiency. Earlier induction may be necessary if the blood pressure rises or there are signs of intrauterine growth retardation.

The outlook is less good if the blood pressure is very high. If it is 160/100 mmHg or more, she should rest in hospital under the care of both an obstetrician and a physician. Sedation and antihypertensive drugs may be prescribed to try and control the blood pressure. Investigations are carried out as described for pre-eclampsia. In addition urinary catecholamines or vanilmandelic acid (VMA) are usually measured because severe hypertension may be caused by phaeochromocytoma, a tumour of the adrenals.

The mother may develop a superimposed pre-eclampsia or have an abruptio placentae; renal failure is an occasional complication. If the blood pressure is exceptionally high, 200/120 mmHg or more, cerebral haemorrhage or heart failure may occur.

The fetus, too, is at risk, because the placental circulation is poor, hence intrauterine growth retardation and hypoxia may occur.

If the blood pressure cannot be controlled or there

are signs of fetal growth retardation or hypoxia, the obstetrician can avoid these serious risks only by hastening the delivery. Thus, labour is induced or, if the danger is more acute, or arises earlier, the obstetrician will deliver her by Caesarean section.

Renal Disease

Renal disease, usually chronic nephritis, is a rare but very serious problem when it occurs in pregnancy.

At the booking clinic a woman might give a typical history of a severe attack of scarlet fever and, subsequently, repeated bouts of 'kidney trouble', though sometimes there is no relevant medical history. She may or may not have hypertension and oedema. Nearly always the urine is of low specific gravity and contains protein. Laboratory tests will reveal that the blood urea is raised, the urine contains casts and the renal function tests (concentration and dilution test and urea clearance test) are deficient.

In severe nephritis, termination of pregnancy may be recommended. Nephritis is a cause of abortion, so the woman may miscarry spontaneously.

If renal function is not seriously impaired, pregnancy may proceed without complications. Throughout this time the mother is kept under close observation. She needs much extra rest and may have to spend long periods in hospital. The nephritis can become worse and renal failure may develop with the possibility of death from uraemia. A superimposed pre-eclampsia may develop, with the risk of placental abruption. Intrauterine death may occur as a result of placental insufficiency. Usually, therefore, labour is induced at about the 36th week, or in some cases a Caesarean section is carried out even earlier than this.

References

Alderman, B.W., Sperling, R.S. & Daling, J.R. (1986) An epidemiological study of the immunogenetic aetiology of pre-eclampsia. *Br. Med. J.* **292**: 372–374.

APEC (Action on Pre-eclampsia) (1992) APEC gets the official go-ahead. *APEC Newsletter* **2**: 1.

Barry, C., Fox, R. & Stirrat, G. (1994) Upper abdominal pain may indicate pre-eclampsia. *Br. Med. J.* **308**(6943): 1562–1563.

Beck, I. (1985) Incidence of pre-eclampsia in first full-term pregnancies preceded by abortion. *J. Obstet. Gynaecol.* **6**: 82–84.

Beischer, N.A. & O'Sullivan, E.F. (1972) The effect of rest and intravenous infusion of hypertonic dextrose on subnormal oestriol excretion in pregnancy. *Am. J. Obstet. Gynecol.* **113**: 771–777.

Belizan, J.M., Villar, J. & Pepke, J. (1988) The relationship between calcium intake and pregnancy induced hypertension: up-to-date evidence. *Am. J. Obstet. Gynecol.* **158**: 898.

Bellin, L. (1994) Aspirin and pre-eclampsia. *Br. Med. J.* **308** (6939): 1250–1251.

British Eclampsia Survey Team (BEST Report) (1994) Eclampsia in the United Kingdom *Br. Med. J.* **309**: 1395–1399.

Broughton Pipkin, F. (1981) Hypertensive disease in pregnancy. *Midwife, Health Visitor & Community Nurse* September: 365–368.

Brown, M.A. & Simpson, J.M. (1992) Diversity of blood pressure recording during pregnancy: implications for the hypertensive disorders. *Med. J. Austr.* **156**(5): 306–308.

Cartwright, W., Dalton, K.J., Swindells, H. *et al.* (1992) Objective measurement of anxiety in hypertensive pregnant women managed in hospital and in the community. *Br. J. Obstet. Gynaecol.* **99**(3): 182–185.

Chamberlain, G. (1991) Raised blood pressure in pregnancy. *Br. Med. J.* **302**: 1454–1458.

Chew, P.C.T., Mok, H. & Ratman, S.S. (1976) Plasma levels of oestradiol-17β, oestriol and human placental lactogen during bed rest. *Br. J. Obstet. Gynaecol.* **83**: 861–863.

CLASP (Collaborative Low-Dose Aspirin Study in Pregnancy) Collaborative Group (1994) *Lancet* **343**(8898): 619–629.

Collins, R. & Wallenburg, H.C.S. (1989) Pharmacological prevention and treatment of hypertensive disorders in pregnancy. In Chalmers, I., Enkin, M. & Keirse, M.J.N.C. (eds) *Effective Care in Pregnancy and Childbirth*. Oxford: Oxford University Press.

Davey, D.A. & MacGillivray, I. (1988) The classification and definition of the hypertensive disorders of pregnancy. *Am. J. Obstet. Gynecol.* **158**: 892–898.

Davies, A.M. (1971) *Geographical Epidemiology of the Toxemias of Pregnancy*. Springfield, IL: Thomas.

deSwiet, M. & Fryers, G. (1990) Review: the use of aspirin in pregnancy. *J. Obstet. Gynaecol.* **10**(6): 467–482.

DOH (Department of Health) (1991) *Report on Confidential Enquiries into Maternal Deaths in the United Kingdom 1985–87*. London: HMSO.

DOH (1994) *Report on Confidential Enquiries into Maternal Deaths in the United Kingdom 1988–90*. London: HMSO.

DOH (1996) *Report on Confidential Enquiries into Maternal Deaths in the United Kingdom 1991–93*. London: HMSO.

Douglas, K.A. & Redman, C.W.G. (1994) Eclampsia in the United Kingdom. *Br. Med. J.* **309**(6966): 1395–1400.

Duley, L. (1994) Maternal mortality and eclampsia: the eclampsia trial. *MIDIRS Midwifery Digest* **4**(2): 176–178.

Editorial (1981) Bed rest in obstetrics. *Lancet* i: 1137–1138.

Editorial (1989a) Classification of hypertensive disorders of pregnancy. *Lancet* **I**(8644): 935–936.

Editorial (1989b) Are ACE inhibitors safe during pregnancy? *Lancet* **II**(8661): 482–483.

Haley, J. (1995) Welcome to the antenatal day unit. *Modern Midwife* **5**(6): 27–30.

Hauth, J.C., Cunningham, F.G. & Whalley, P.J. (1976) Management of pregnancy-induced hypertension in nullipara. *Obstet. Gynecol.* **46**: 253–259.

Howard, R.J. (1993) The pharmacological treatment of hypertension in pregnancy. *Maternal & Child Health* January: 23–25.

Kilpatrick, D.C., Gibson, F. & Liston, W.A. (1989) Association between susceptibility to pre-eclampsia within families and HLA DR4. *Lancet* **II**(8671): 1063–1064.

Kwast, B.E. (1991) The hypertensive disorders of pregnancy: their contribution to maternal mortality. *Midwifery* **7**(4): 155–161.

Lang, G.D., Lowe, G.D.O., Walker, J.J., Forbes, C.D., Prentice, C.R.M. & Calder, A.A. (1984) Blood rheology in pre-eclampsia and intrauterine growth retardation: effects of blood pressure reduction with labetalol. *Br. J. Obstet. Gynaecol.* **91**: 438–443.

Letchworth, A.T., Howard, L. & Chard, T. (1974) Placental lactogen levels during bed rest. *Obstet. Gynecol.* **43**: 702–703.

Lopez-Jaramillo, P., Naravez, M. & Weigel, R.M. (1989) Calcium supplementation reduces the risk of pregnancy induced hypertension in an Andes population. *Br. J. Obstet. Gynecol.* **96**(6): 648–655.

Lopez-Jaramillo, P., Naravez, M., Felix, C. & Lopez, A. (1990) Dietary calcium supplementation and prevention of pregancy hypertension. *Lancet* **335**: 293.

Lucas, M.J., Leveno, K.J. & Cunningham, F.G.A. (1995) A comparison of magnesium sulphate with phenytoin for the prevention of eclampsia. *New Engl. J. Med.* **333**(4): 201–205.

MacGillivray, I. (1981) Raised blood pressure in pregnancy. Aetiology of pre-eclampsia. *Br. J. Hosp. Med.* **26**(2): 110–119.

MacGillivray, I. (1983) *Pre-eclampsia. The Hypertensive Disorders of Pregnancy*. Philadelphia: W. B. Saunders.

MacGillivray, I. (1985) Pre-eclampsia. *Midwifery* **1**: 12–18.

MacGillivray, I. & Campbell, D.M. (1980) In Bonnor, J., MacGillivray, I. & Symonds, E.M. (eds) *Pregnancy Hypertension*, p. 307. Baltimore, MD: University Park Press.

Mahomed, K. & James, D.K. (1988) Hypertension in pregnancy: Do we need to admit all mothers to hospital for assessment and management? *J. Obstet. Gynaecol.* **8**(4): 314–318.

Marcoux, S., Brisson, J. & Fabia, J. (1990) Calcium intake from dairy products and supplements and the risks of pre-eclampsia and gestational hypertension. *Am. J. Epidem.* **133**(12): 1266–1272.

Mathews, D.D. (1977) A randomised controlled trial of bed rest and sedation or normal activity and non-sedation in the management of non-albuminuric hypertension in late pregnancy. *Br. J. Obstet. Gynaecol.* **84**: 108–114.

Mathews, D.D., Patel, I.R. & Sengupta, S.M. (1971) Outpatient management of toxaemia. *J. Obstet. Gynaecol. Br. Commonwealth,* **78**: 610–19.

Mathews, D.D., Agarwal, V. & Shuttleworth, T.P. (1980) The effect of rest and ambulation on plasma urea and urate levels in pregnant woman with proteinuric hypertension. *Br. J. Obstet. Gynaecol.* **87**: 1095–1098.

Morris de Lassalle, S.H. (1994) The organisation and work of a fetal assessment day care unit. *Br. J. Midwifery* **2**(1): 20–25.

Neilsen, J.P. (1995) Magnesium sulphate: the drug of choice in eclampsia. *Br. Med. J.* **311**: 702–703.

Neutra, R. (1974) A case control study for estimating the risk of eclampsia in Cali Columbo. *Am. J. Obstet. Gynecol.* **117**: 894–903.

O'Dent, M. (1994) Effects of a combination of evening primrose oil (gamma linolenic acid) and fish oil (eicosapentaenoic + docahexaenoic acid) versus magnesium, and versus placebo in preventing pre-eclampsia. *MIDIRS Midwifery Digest* **4**(1): 44–45.

Plouin, P.F., Breart, G., Maillard, F. *et al.* (1988) Comparison of antihypertensive efficacy and perinatal safety of labetalol and methyldopa in the treatment of hypertension in pregnancy: a randomised controlled trial. *Br. J. Obstet. Gynaecol.* **95**(9): 868–876.

Quinn, M. (1994) Automated blood pressure measurement devices: a potential source of morbidity in pre-eclampsia. *Am. J. Obstet. Gynecol.* **170**(5:1): 1303–1307.

Redman, C. (1994) Pre-eclampsia: still a difficult disease. *Prof. Care of Mother and Child* **4**(1): 7–9.

Robillard, P.Y., Hulsey, T.C. & Perianin, J. (1994) Association of pregnancy induced hypertension with duration of sexual cohabitation before conception. *Lancet* **344**(8928): 973–975.

Symonds, E.M. (1980) Aetiology of pre-eclampsia: a review. *R. Soc. Med.* **73**: 871–875.

The Eclampsia Collaborative Trial Group (1995) Which anticonvulsant for women with eclampsia? Evidence from the Collaborative Eclampsia Trial. *Lancet* **345**: 1455–1463.

Thomson, A.M., Hytten, F.E. & Billewitz, Z. (1967) The epidemiology of oedema during pregnancy. *J. Obstet. Gynaecol. Br. Commonwealth* **74**: 1.

Thornton, J.G. & Onwude, J.L. (1991) Pre-eclampsia: discordance among identical twins. *Lancet* **303**(6812): 1241–1242.

Treharne, I.A.L., Sutherland, H.W., Stowers, J.M. & Sampher, M. (1979) In Sutherland, H.W. & Stowers, J.M. (eds) *Carbohydrate Metabolism in Pregnancy and the Newborn*, p. 479. Berlin: Springer-Verlag.

Wallenburg, H.C.S. (1989) Detecting hypertensive disorders of pregnancy. In Chalmers, I., Enkin, M. & Keirse, M.J.N.C. (eds) *Effective Care in Pregnancy and Childbirth*. Oxford: Oxford University Press.

Wallenburg, H.C.S., Dekker, G.A., Makovitz, J.W. & Rotman, P. (1986) Low-dose aspirin prevents pregnancy-induced hypertension and pre-eclampsia in angiotensin-sensitive primigravidae. *Lancet* i: 1–3.

World Health Organization (WHO) (1995) Magnesium sulphate is the drug of choice for eclampsia. *Safe Motherhood – A newsletter of worldwide activity.* Issue 18, 1995(2), pp. 3 & 13. Geneva: WHO.

42

Medical Conditions Complicating Pregnancy

Anaemia

Anaemia is a deficiency in the quality or quantity of red blood cells, with the result that the oxygen-carrying capacity of the blood is reduced. It is very commonly found to be present during pregnancy.

Physiology

During pregnancy the total blood volume increases and the increase is mainly in the plasma volume. While the red cell volume is increased this is proportionately lower than the increase in plasma volume. This results in a physiological haemodilution of the blood in preg-

nancy. Thus if a specimen of blood is tested the haemoglobin level is found to be lowered (see Chapter 21).

To prevent this fall in haemoglobin level iron was commonly given as a routine in pregnancy and some still continue to prescribe it. However, the benefit of iron supplementation is now questioned and some studies show that the routine administration of iron may be superfluous or even harmful (Hytten, 1976; Editorial, 1978; Hemminki and Starfield, 1978). Levels of haemoglobin traditionally regarded as pathological in the non-pregnant woman are, in fact, associated with good obstetric outcomes (Mahomed and Hytten, 1989; Steer *et al.*, 1995). The increase in plasma volume is essential to ensure perfusion of the vascular bed and maintenance of blood pressure and it is suggested that an increase in haemoglobin may result in a decrease of blood flow through tissues (Montgomery, 1990). There is a need to differentiate between physiological adaptation and a pathological condition. Routine supplementation in the absence of clinical indications is unnecessary, expensive and, especially when given in the first trimester, may exacerbate sickness and cause constipation or diarrhoea. Romslo *et al.* (1983) suggest that the aim of iron supplementation in normal pregnant women is not to elevate their haemoglobin but to refill their iron stores. A low serum ferritin value is indicative of depleted iron stores and the need for iron supplementation.

More iron is required for the extra haemoglobin in the increased blood volume and for uterine and fetal growth in pregnancy. During the last trimester of pregnancy the fetal demands for iron are particularly heavy.

The World Health Organization (WHO) (1979) considers anaemia to be present in the pregnant woman when haemoglobin is 11 g/dl or less. More arbitrary levels may be decided locally and usually range between 10 and 10.5 g/dl.

Types of anaemia

Anaemias can be classified according to their causes:

1 Iron-deficiency anaemia.
2 Folic acid deficiency anaemia.
3 Haemoglobinopathies, which include sickle cell disease and thalassaemia.
4 Anaemia as a result of blood loss or secondary to infection.
5 Aplastic varieties which are rare in pregnancy.

Effects on pregnancy

There are various effects associated with anaemia in pregnancy:

▶ It undermines the woman's general health.
▶ It lowers her ability to cope with infection.
▶ Minor disorders of pregnancy such as digestive problems may be exacerbated.
▶ In severe cases it may cause intrauterine hypoxia.
▶ The perinatal mortality is increased in severe anaemia.
▶ Antepartum and postpartum haemorrhage are rendered more serious.
▶ There is a higher risk of thromboembolic disorders.
▶ The maternal mortality is increased.

IRON-DEFICIENCY ANAEMIA

This is the commonest cause of anaemia in pregnancy in the UK. The anaemia may be present before pregnancy and is likely to occur in women who are poorly nourished or who lose excessive amounts of blood during menstruation. Repeated pregnancies, especially if close together, deplete the iron stores. The haemodilution of the blood and the increased demand for iron, as described above, predispose to anaemia in pregnancy. In a multiple pregnancy the demand for iron is further increased.

Malabsorption of iron may be associated with the intake of alkalis to relieve heartburn, or may be due to lack of vitamin C or to gastrointestinal disorders such as vomiting and diarrhoea. Iron is normally lost from the body in urine, sweat and bile. If there is further loss due to bleeding haemorrhoids or antepartum haemorrhage, anaemia is likely to develop. Chronic infections caused by conditions such as pyelonephritis may also lead to anaemia.

In developing countries, anaemia as defined by WHO is widespread. It may be associated with poor nutrition or may arise as a consequence of intestinal parasites or malaria.

Signs and symptoms

There is pallor of the mucous membranes and the woman generally complains of tiredness and perhaps dizziness and fainting. In more severe cases she may have dyspnoea on exertion, palpitations and oedema. Digestive upsets and loss of appetite commonly occur and tend to exacerbate the condition.

Investigations

After taking a detailed history about general health, diet, infection, blood loss and other relevant information the following investigations may be carried out.

▶ *Haemoglobin* is below 11 g/dl in anaemia. Investigations may also be carried out to detect abnormal haemoglobins such as sickle cell disease or thalassaemia.
▶ *Packed cell volume* (PCV) is the volume of red cells expressed as a fraction of the total volume of blood. It is normally 35–40% in pregnancy, but is reduced in anaemia.
▶ *Mean corpuscular volume* (MCV) is the average volume of a single red cell in cubic micrometres. It is normally about 90 μm^3 but is lower in anaemia.

▶ *Mean corpuscular haemoglobin* (MCH) is the average amount of haemoglobin in each red cell. It is normally about 30 pg and is reduced in anaemia.

▶ *Serum iron and total iron binding capacity*: In iron-deficiency anaemia the serum iron will be lower than 60 µg/100 ml (normal 60–120 µg/100 ml) and the total iron binding capacity over 400 µg/100 ml (normal 325–400 µg/100 ml). This indicates depleted iron stores. Iron is absorbed from the intestines and bound to a protein. Almost two-thirds of the protein is not combined with iron and this is the iron-binding-capacity of the blood. It rises in anaemia. NB. These tests as a reliable indicator of iron status in pregnancy have been called into question by Mahomed and Hytten (1989), who consider levels of ferritin a more reliable indicator.

▶ *Serum ferritin* below 10 µg/l indicates exhausted iron stores. The serum ferritin level falls up to the 28th–30th week of pregnancy. After that time it increases in women receiving iron supplementation but continues to fall in those not receiving iron therapy (Fenton *et al.*, 1977; Puolakka *et al.*, 1980a, b).

▶ *Serum B₁₂ and serum folate* may also be estimated.

▶ *Bone marrow puncture* may be carried out in cases of severe anaemia which do not respond to treatment.

▶ *A midstream specimen of urine* is sent to the laboratory to detect infection.

▶ *Faecal specimens* are obtained and examined in the laboratory for evidence of hookworm infestation in some immigrant patients.

Management

Where iron-deficiency anaemia has been diagnosed, oral iron 120–160 mg daily may be given as:

▶ *ferrous sulphate* – 200 mg tablet twice daily, giving 120 mg iron; or
▶ *ferrous gluconate* – 2 × 300 mg tablets twice daily, giving 140 mg iron.

The woman is given further advice about diet and the dose of oral iron and folic acid may be increased. In more severe cases of anaemia the woman may be given intramuscular injections of iron in the form of iron sorbital citrate complex known as Jectofer. The 2 ml ampoules contain 100 mg of iron and a dose of 1.5 mg per kilogram body weight is usually given daily for 10–20 days.

Iron may also be given in an intravenous infusion. An iron dextran complex (Imferon) is given in a total dose infusion over a few hours, the dose being calculated on body weight and the degree of anaemia. A test dose of 10 drops per minute is given for the first half hour and the woman is closely observed during this time as there is a risk of an anaphylactic reaction. If the woman tolerates the test dose, the infusion rate is then increased, but observations must continue every 15 or 30 minutes throughout the course of the infusion. It is two or three weeks after this treatment before the haemoglobin begins to rise.

Rarely is a blood transfusion necessary in pregnancy to treat anaemia, particularly given the current fears of HIV infection among the general population. A woman who is very anaemic in late pregnancy is more likely to be given a total dose infusion of iron. Blood should be cross-matched when the woman goes into labour and given if she has a postpartum haemorrhage. The woman will also need information about her condition and practical advice about diet appropriate to her social and cultural background, delivered in a way she can understand.

FOLIC ACID DEFICIENCY ANAEMIA

Folic acid is necessary for the formation of the nuclei in all the body cells. In pregnancy, when there is proliferation of cell formation, a deficiency is likely to occur unless the intake of folic acid is increased. In the bone marrow a deficiency of folic acid leads to the formation of *megaloblasts* (large red cells).

Megaloblastic anaemia is more common in women who are poorly nourished, in multiparous women and in those with a multiple pregnancy. It may also occur in women being treated with anticoagulant drugs, long-term sulphonamides or anticonvulsants, or in women drinking too much alcohol, as these substances interfere with folic acid metabolism. The anaemia is often fairly severe and fails to respond to iron therapy.

Diagnosis

The diagnosis of megaloblastic anaemia is usually made on examination of the peripheral blood. The red blood cells are large (*macrocytic*) and in severe cases there is *poikilocytosis* or irregularity in shape. The polymorphs are large and there may be a low platelet and white cell count. The serum folic acid is lower than 4 µg/ml.

Management

Dietary advice is important for those women considered to be at risk, for example, those with a multiple pregnancy. Dietary sources of folic acid are green leafy vegetables such as broccoli and spinach, which must not be overcooked (see Chapter 16). Following the demonstrated link between neural tube defects and intake of folic acid, all pregnant women, and those intending to become pregnant are advised to take 0.4–4 mg folic acid daily (DOH, 1992; Drugs and Therapeutics Bulletin, 1994).

Treatment of megaloblastic anaemia is by oral folic acid 5–10 mg daily. Occasionally, when the condition is very severe, folic acid may have to be given parenterally.

Megaloblastic anaemia may continue, or be diagnosed for the first time, during the puerperium. Treatment with iron and folic acid supplements should therefore continue until the haemoglobin has reached a satisfactory level.

Deficiency of vitamin B_{12} also produces a megaloblastic anaemia, but this is extremely rare in pregnancy. Since vitamin B_{12} is found exclusively in products of animal origin, including milk and cheese, women who are vegans are most likely to suffer from this deficiency.

HAEMOGLOBINOPATHIES

Haemoglobin is made up of two components:

▶ *Haem*: An iron-containing pigment of four pyrrole rings which are organic molecules joined by bridges. This structure then takes up an iron atom in the ferrous form, which it holds centrally.
▶ *Globin*: A protein consisting of a long chain of amino acids. In normal haemoglobin, four types of globin molecule exist, which are differentiated by slight changes in the amino acids. These four types are alpha (α), beta (β), delta (δ) and gamma (γ).

Each molecule of haemoglobin contains four globin chains; the globin chains occur in the following combinations which form the three major normally occurring haemoglobins:

Major adult haemoglobin	HbA	2 α plus 2 β
Minor adult haemoglobin	HbA	2 α plus 2 δ
Fetal haemoglobin	HbF	2 α plus 2 γ

Haemoglobinopathies are inherited conditions in which the normal adult haemoglobin, HbA, is wholly or partly replaced by one or more abnormal types. The main haemoglobinopathies which complicate pregnancy are *sickle cell disease* and *thalassaemia*. These conditions are complex in terms of genetics and inheritance and are presented here in a relatively simplified form. The section on Further Reading recommends sources of additional information.

Sickle cell trait and sickle cell disease

Abnormal haemoglobins (HbS) and/or HbC may be found in people who originate from Central and West Africa and parts of Asia. Their appearance is particularly associated with those whose ethnic origin lies in countries where malaria is endemic, since the sickle cell gene (in its trait form) is thought to provide some protection against malaria. More recently, however, population movement and the development of sexual relationships between members of different ethnic groups has resulted in a changed pattern of occurrence. In many areas, all women, regardless of ethnic origin are tested routinely, as are their babies. Both haemoglobins S and C are genetically inherited and thus there are heterozygous and homozygous forms of the disease. *Heterozygous* individuals inherit one normal and one abnormal haemoglobin, and thus have HbAS or HbAC, that is *sickle cell trait*. They are carriers of the disease but sickling does not usually occur. *Homozygous* individuals inherit abnormal HbS or HbC from both parents, and thus are HbSS or HbCC. Those with HbSS have *sickle cell anaemia* whereas those with HbCC have *homozygous CC disease*, where sickling does not occur because there is no S haemoglobin. In some cases an individual may inherit two different abnormal haemoglobins, HbS from one parent and HbC from the other, and thus be HbSC. In a non-pregnant patient this is a milder form of the disease than HbSS. However, in pregnancy,

Table 1 Haemoglobin combinations in sickle cell disorders

HbSS	Homozygous sickle cell disease (sickle cell anaemia)
HbSC	Heterozygous sickle cell disease (sickle cell C disease)
HbCC	Homozygous CC disease (*not* a sickling disorder)
HbS beta/thal	Sickle/beta thalassaemia
HbAS	Sickle cell trait

Table 2   Patterns of inheritance in sickle cell anaemia

	Mother			**Father**
	Sickle cell anaemia (HbSS)			Normal haemoglobin (HbAA)
Infants	HbAS	HbAS	HbAS	HbAS
		(All infants will have sickle cell trait)		
	Sickle cell anaemia (HbSS)			Sickle cell trait (HbAS)
Infants	HbAS	HbAS	HbSS	HbSS
	Sickle cell trait (HbAS)			Sickle cell trait (HbAS)
Infants	HbAA	HbAS	HbAS	HbSS

HbSC is the more hazardous to the mother (Tables 1 and 2).

In sickle cell disease the erythrocytes are sickle shaped and are easily haemolysed. This leads to chronic haemolytic anaemia because the lifespan of the abnormal red blood cells is shortened. In an effort to replace the short-lived red blood cells, the rate of haemoglobin synthesis in the bone marrow is increased and this may lead to folic acid deficiency. *Sickling* or alteration in shape of the abnormal red blood cells occurs when the oxygen tension is reduced. The high viscosity of the red blood cells which occurs with sickling slows the circulation and may lead to thrombosis and subsequent infarction. These acute episodes are known as crises and are precipitated by anaesthesia, infection, reduced oxygen tension as may occur in air travel and in pregnancy. Crises present with pain in bones, joints and abdomen, often accompanied by fever and vomiting.

Effect on pregnancy   The diagnosis is usually made in childhood and the patient has a history of haemolytic anaemia and chronic ill-health. Fertility is reduced but when pregnancy does occur it may be complicated by chronic ill-health, severe anaemia, crises, abortion and preterm labour. The perinatal and maternal mortality rates are increased.

Management

Pregnancy   All women at risk should be screened for haemoglobinopathies in early pregnancy by means of haemoglobin electrophoresis. Iron therapy should be avoided but folic acid is given routinely throughout pregnancy. Blood transfusions may be required to treat very severe anaemia and either direct or exchange transfusions may be carried out. The latter removes the abnormal HbS and replaces it with normal HbA. Heparin may also be given if a crisis develops to reduce the severity of bone pain and the incidence of thrombosis. Any infection should be treated with antibiotics.

Women with sickle cell disease may have poor appetites and should be encouraged to have regular small meals including meat, fish, eggs, cheese, fruit and wholemeal bread. Since dehydration may lead to crisis, plenty of fluids should be taken.

Labour   Dehydration, acidosis and infection all lead to sickling, so great care must be taken to avoid these complications in labour. Antiobiotics may be given prophylactically and blood is cross-matched in readiness for an emergency. The haemoglobin and packed cell volume are checked six-hourly and each specimen of urine is tested for proteinuria, since this may be a sign of an impending crisis.

Puerperium   Antibiotics are continued to avoid infection and the mother is closely observed for signs of a crisis. Anaemia is treated.

The midwife must be aware of sources of specialist help to which women and their partners may be directed, and of particular screening tests which may be offered during pregnancy and after delivery, to detect the presence of abnormal haemoglobins in the baby.

Thalassaemia

Thalassaemia is a condition in which there is an abnormal amount of HbA_2. It is most common in people of Mediterranean and Asian origin. The condition arises from defects in the alpha or beta globin chains and results in thin red cells, often misshapen and deficient in haemoglobin. They have a short lifespan and the patient suffers from profound anaemia. As with sickle cell trait, thalassaemia in its mild forms confers some protection against malaria.

The condition may be mild, moderate or severe, depending on the number of inherited defective genes; in *alpha thalassaemia major*, four defective alpha genes are inherited; this condition produces hydrops fetalis and is incompatible with extrauterine life.

In *beta thalassaemia major*, there are two defective beta genes; the condition usually presents between the ages of 3 and 18 months, when the child becomes pale and fails to thrive. Untreated, these children will die before the age of 8. Treatment is by regular blood transfusions, but excess iron builds up from red cell breakdown, causing damage to the heart and liver. Iron may be removed by Desferal, a chelating agent administered subcutaneously. With treatment, patients may survive into their childbearing years.

In *thalassaemia minor*, the alpha or beta chains may be affected, resulting in alpha thalassaemia minor (very rare in this country) or beta thalassaemia minor. These minor thalassaemias are often called traits and have significance for women who carry them in determining what screening tests should be carried out. Ideally, women and their partners should be screened before embarking on a pregnancy, since some thalassaemias are only detectable by blood testing and may coexist with iron deficiency, thereby confusing the diagnosis (Modell and Modell, 1990).

Management Since iron stores are likely to be overloaded, rather than depleted, iron supplements are not given unless iron deficiency is proved by measurement of iron stores. Folic acid is given throughout pregnancy, however, because the bone marrow is very active in replacing the short-lived red blood cells.

OTHER CAUSES

Glucose-6 phosphate dehydrogenase (G6PD) deficiency

This rare, X-linked inherited enzyme deficiency typically affects people of African, Asian and Mediterranean origin. Haemolytic crises occur if the affected person takes certain drugs, such as antimalarial preparations, sulphonamides, antibiotics (nitrofurantoin, nalidixic acid and possibly chloramphenicol) or if they eat broad beans. It may be implicated in cases of prolonged neonatal jaundice.

Secondary causes of anaemia include *blood loss* and *infection*, often a *urinary tract infection* which may be asymptomatic.

Some women may have a *hookworm infestation* which causes anaemia because blood is lost in the stools. When the ova of the hookworm are found in the stools bephenium hydroxynaphthoate (Alcopar) 5 mg is given on an empty stomach and may be repeated if required. Iron therapy will also be necessary.

Heart Disease

Heart disease is seriously complicated by pregnancy. The cause may be congenital heart disease such as atrial or ventricular septal defect or rheumatic heart disease such as mitral stenosis or incompetence. Rheumatic heart disease used to be the main problem but now more women with congenital heart disease are reaching childbearing age following the great advances which have been made in cardiac surgery.

Rheumatic heart disease Where there is mitral or aortic valve incompetence, arterial pressure is actually lowered in pregnancy, reducing strain on the heart. The major concern is prevention of endocarditis following infection.

Women who have had rheumatic fever in childhood may have been left with a permanently affected heart. The valves of the heart, particularly the mitral valve, may have been scarred following the infection. The scarred valve contracts, narrowing the opening. This is called *mitral stenosis*. While the heart is strong enough to drive the circulating blood through the narrowed opening no symptoms will occur and the condition is said to be compensated. When the heart muscle begins to fail, the woman will develop undue breathlessness and tachycardia on ordinary exertion. Finally even when resting in bed there is breathlessness, cyanosis and a rapid and perhaps irregular pulse. The heart is then said to be decompensated and heart failure is present. During pregnancy the extra weight, upward pressure of the uterus on the diaphragm, maintenance of the placental circulation and increased volume of circulating blood all throw additional strain on the heart muscle and may precipitate heart failure. The greatest strain on the heart occurs between the 28th and 36th week when the increased blood volume reaches its maximum.

Congenital heart disease   *Atrial septal defects, patent ductus arteriosus* and *ventricular septal defects* are the most commonly seen congenital lesions. Other more serious lesions include *Fallot's tetralogy* (ventricular septal defect, pulmonary stenosis, overriding aorta and right ventricular hypertrophy) and *Eisenmenger's syndrome* (ventricular septal defect, overriding aorta and right ventricular hypertrophy). Outcome of pregnancy is worst where pulmonary blood flow cannot be increased, and prognosis for the mother is especially poor in Eisenmenger's syndrome. Early termination of pregnancy may be advised for such women, since the maternal mortality rate is high.

Management of pregnancy

The aim of antenatal care is to detect heart failure and disturbances of cardiac rhythm. The woman is closely supervised during her pregnancy by an obstetrician and a cardiologist. Midwifery care is essential too as the woman and her partner need help and support during what may be a particularly anxious time.

Transport to the antenatal clinic will be arranged, if required, to reduce the fatigue of the more frequent visits which will be necessary. Extra rest is essential and the woman may require a home help to make this possible. Even if the pregnancy is uneventful all mothers are usually admitted to hospital for rest from one to four weeks before labour is anticipated.

Weight control is essential, so a high-protein, low-carbohydrate diet is recommended. Prevention of anaemia is important and the haemoglobin is estimated frequently.

Any *infection* must be treated vigorously with antibiotics to reduce the risk of the woman developing bacterial endocarditis. For this reason dental caries, which are a potential source of infection, should be treated early in pregnancy.

Cardiac failure   The major antenatal complications are *acute pulmonary oedema* and *congestive cardiac failure*. The woman who develops dyspnoea and a cough

must be admitted immediately for bedrest and sedation. She may require oxygen therapy, digitalization and a diuretic such as intravenous frusemide 20 mg. Digoxin in maternal therapeutic levels crosses the placenta but does not harm the fetus. Bronchial spasm may be relieved by intravenous aminophylline. If heart failure occurs in pregnancy the mother will remain in hospital under medical supervision until she is safely delivered.

Some more severely affected women may be found to be suitable for *mitral valvotomy*. This is an operation on the heart to increase the size of the narrowed mitral valve. Much improvement in the health of the mother may be produced by this operation. Women who have had valve replacements will be taking anticoagulants to reduce the risk of embolism. Oral anticoagulant therapy is continued throughout pregnancy until about two weeks before labour is anticipated. It is then replaced by subcutaneous or intravenous heparin which, unlike drugs such as warfarin, does not cross the placenta and therefore the risk of fetal haemorrhage during labour is reduced. Because the effects of heparin are easily reversed the possibility of postpartum haemorrhage is reduced should the patient go into labour.

Management of labour

Labour is conducted under medical supervision in hospital. Spontaneous onset of labour is desirable and cardiac patients are often noted to have a remarkably quick and easy labour. Induction of labour is carried out only when there is a good obstetric indication. To reduce the risk of infection and, in particular, bacterial endocarditis, antibiotics are usually given intramuscularly during labour.

Adequate sedation and analgesia are necessary to ensure that the woman obtains sufficient rest and is not distressed by pain. Epidural analgesia may be useful, but is contraindicated in women with Eisenmenger's syndrome, and women on anticoagulant therapy. Alternative, non-intervention methods of pain relief such as relaxation may be useful. The mother is usually most comfortable well propped up with pillows. The colour is observed and pulse and respiratory rates are recorded every 15 minutes. A pulse rate of over 110 per minute and a respiratory rate of over 24 per minute and any dyspnoea or cyanosis should be reported to the doctor immediately. Accurate fluid balance records must be maintained because of the risk of overload, which would cause cardiac embarrassment.

When cardiac failure occurs the outlook is serious. The patient should be digitalized, oxygen therapy is given and venesection may be required.

It is sensible to keep the strenuous second stage of labour as short as possible, but there is no reason for elective forceps or vacuum extraction if delivery is proceeding well. Excessive pushing should be avoided since it alters haemodynamics and may compromise cardiac activity. If the woman feels the urge to push, short pushes with the mouth open should be encouraged. Oxytocic drugs are given only with great caution. Sudden strong uterine contraction in the third stage may direct so much of the uterine circulation of blood to the systemic circulation that the impaired heart may become seriously embarrassed and congestive cardiac failure ensue. Intravenous ergometrine is therefore avoided, but there are conflicting opinions about the use of intramuscular Syntometrine; thus the doctor present should be consulted. Syntocinon may be used, unless the woman is in heart failure (deSwiet, 1989). Serious postpartum haemorrhage is treated in the usual way.

Management of the puerperium

As soon as labour is completed the mother should be well sedated and allowed to rest. Close observation will be necessary as heart failure may occur in the first few days of the puerperium. Mothers therefore require additional rest in bed for the first few days of the puerperium, but this should not mean complete immobilization. Physiotherapy will be necessary for those confined to bed to reduce the risk of thromboembolic disorders.

Any mother who has a cardiac lesion must be carefully protected from infection. Even a mild infection may be complicated by bacterial endocarditis, so prophylactic antibiotic therapy is continued.

There is usually no contraindication to breastfeeding.

The risk of congenital heart disease in the baby is increased and ranges from 1:4 in Fallot's tetralogy to 1:15 with atrial septal defects, therefore, careful examination of the neonate is essential.

The woman may need advice on family spacing methods; the intrauterine device with its associated risk of infection may not be appropriate; barrier methods may be used safely, as may the progesterone-only pill. Where the woman has completed her family, or where further pregnancy would severely compromise her health, she may wish to consider sterilization which is usually performed about 2–3 months after delivery.

The mother should be encouraged to stay in hospital until she is really rested and ready for discharge, since it is unlikely she will be able to get as much rest on returning to housework and the care of the baby. A home help may be arranged to enable the mother to have more rest at home. Follow-up care in the community is arranged, first with the community midwife and the general practitioner and then with the health visitor. The cardiologist will see the mother in hospital during the puerperium and arrange for her to attend clinic after her discharge.

Thyrotoxicosis

Severe thyrotoxicosis is associated with infertility but conception occurs quite commonly in less severe degrees of the disease which are treated. The condition does not appear to be made worse by pregnancy.

In mild cases thyrotoxicosis may be treated with rest and sedation only, but in moderate to severe degrees of the disease antithyroid drugs such as methyl thiouracil or carbimazole are the treatment of choice. These drugs cross the placenta and may affect the fetal thyroid, causing a goitre or even hypothyroidism in the fetus. Thyroid hormone supplements may be given to prevent fetal hypothyroidism. They do not cross the placenta. Ideally the woman will have had a thyroidectomy, so she can be given enough antithyroid drugs to control the fetal hyperthyroidism. If this renders her hypothyroid, she can take thyroxine which does not cross the placenta.

Inadequate treatment of the disease carries the risk of abortion, pre-eclampsia, prematurity and perinatal death.

Occasionally a subtotal thyroidectomy is considered necessary in pregnancy if the disease is difficult to control and in women with large goitres. The optimum time for such surgery in pregnancy is during the second trimester. These patients may be treated preoperatively with the β-adrenergic blocker propranolol which controls the peripheral effects of the disease.

Adequate rest and prevention of infection are

important for all women with thyrotoxicosis in pregnancy.

As a result of the transplacental transfer of long-acting thyroid stimulator from the mother to the fetus, the neonate will develop hyperthyroidism. It is therefore important to inform the paediatrician when a woman with hyperthyroidism is in labour. The baby's thyroid function will return to normal within three weeks.

Antithyroid drugs are excreted in the mother's breast milk and thus breastfeeding is contraindicated.

Hypothyroidism

Pregnancy will occur only if the condition is mild, as severe hypothyroidism causes infertility. If pregnancy does occur there is an increased risk of abortion. Patients who become pregnant while being treated for hypothyroidism require increased doses of thyroxine.

Renal Conditions in Pregnancy

PYELONEPHRITIS

This inflammatory state of the urinary tract is a bacterial infection generally involving the upper ureter, the renal pelvis and part of the kidney. It is particularly liable to arise in pregnancy because of the physiological changes which occur. The ureters and pelvis of the kidney become dilated in response to increased vascular volume and urinary stasis may occur. The dilatation of the ureters is further accentuated when the enlarging uterus presses on the ureters at the pelvic brim, particularly on the right side since the uterus inclines to the right. Other factors which predispose to infection are vesico-ureteric reflux of urine containing bacteria, urinary catheterization even with impeccable technique and abnormalities of the renal tract.

Pyelonephritis occurs in 1–2% of all pregnancies and is more common in women who exhibit bacteriuria (Dunlop and Davison, 1989).

Causative organisms

The organism usually responsible is *Escherichia coli*, which is a normal inhabitant of the intestines. The organisms may gain access to the urinary tract via lymphatics, from the colon or via the bladder. Occasionally other organisms such as *Proteus vulgaris*, *Streptococcus faecalis* or *Pseudomonas aeruginosa* are involved.

Signs and symptoms

The onset commonly occurs round about the 20th week of pregnancy and more frequently in primigravidae. The patient complains of pain from the loin to the groin, often on the right side, of headache, nausea and vomiting and, if there is an associated cystitis, as there often is, of pain and increased frequency of micturition. The temperature will be raised and the pulse rate increased. In severe infections the temperature may rise to 39° or 40°C, or more, and rigors may occur. The patient is often anaemic and urinary output may be diminished.

Diagnosis

The condition is diagnosed by the microscopical examination of a midstream specimen of urine. This will reveal the presence of pus cells and bacteriological examination will detect over 100 000 bacteria per millilitre. The urine is usually acid, has an offensive smell and contains some red blood cells and protein. Blood cultures may also be taken.

Management

The woman is admitted to hospital for bedrest, observation and treatment. After obtaining a midstream specimen of urine a broad-spectrum antibiotic such as ampicillin (500 mg every 6–8 hours) is usually prescribed, but when the bacteriological report is available the drug may have to be changed to one to which the organism is sensitive. Initially, intravenous administration will be more effective. At the same time the woman is encouraged to drink ample fluids and then urinary stasis will be avoided. An intake and output chart is maintained.

The woman is encouraged to lie on her unaffected side to relieve the pain and to assist drainage. Analgesics are prescribed as necessary. The temperature, pulse and respirations are recorded four-hourly and tepid sponging or an electric fan may be used if the temperature is very high. Further midstream specimens of urine are obtained at intervals for bacteriological examination until the urine is sterile and free of pus. The haemoglobin should be checked frequently because the risk of anaemia is increased.

A recurrence of the infection is likely in pregnancy or during the puerperium, so close follow-up is necessary. Antibiotic therapy is continued for a month, and in some cases is necessary throughout pregnancy. Three months or so after delivery when the renal tract has returned to normal, an intravenous pyelogram and other renal investigations may be carried out.

Effects on the fetus

The risk of abortion or preterm labour is increased and hyperpyrexia may result in intrauterine fetal death. The pain of uterine contractions associated with preterm labour may not be recognized if the mother is already in severe pain from the illness and labour may only be detected by cardiotocography. If the mother has a urinary tract infection at the time of delivery, the infant is at substantial risk of congenital infection.

CHRONIC RENAL DISEASE

Chronic renal disease may arise as a result of any of the following:

▶ Glomerulonephritis (acute or chronic).
▶ Polycystic renal disease.
▶ Chronic pyelonephritis.
▶ Diabetic nephropathy.
▶ Systemic lupus erythematosus.
▶ Scleroderma.
▶ Renal calculi.
▶ Congenital abnormality of the lower urinary tract.
▶ Solitary kidney.
▶ Nephrotic syndrome.

The outcome of pregnancy depends on the nature and severity of the disease, and the degree of loss of renal function. Outcome is best in women whose renal function is only moderately compromised, and where there is little or no hypertension. The outlook is worse where renal function is less than 50%.

In some cases of chronic renal disease, fertility may be impaired; women who are already being treated for a longstanding renal disease may have pre-pregnancy counselling in order to make a decision about conception, or the continuance of an unplanned pregnancy.

The aim of care during pregnancy is to avoid further deterioration in renal function. In addition to the normal care provided, more frequent antenatal visits are required for maternal and fetal surveillance. The woman may need extra rest and help with child-care and household work. She may need to be admitted to hospital for rest and observation of blood pressure, and assessment of renal function. Pre-eclampsia may be superimposed on the renal condition, and abortion or preterm labour may occur. Placental insufficiency may lead to intrauterine growth retardation, and in severe cases, fetal death. The course of the pregnancy will determine the mode and time of delivery; onset of labour and delivery may be spontaneous or labour may be induced. For some women, an elective Caesarean section may be performed, depending on maternal and fetal condition.

RENAL TRANSPLANT

Following a successful renal transplantation, pregnancy will occur in one in 50 women transplant patients of childbearing age (Dunlop and Davison, 1989). Pre-pregnancy counselling is essential for these women and, in general, the following advice is given (Dunlop and Davison, 1989):

▶ The woman must have been in good health for two years after transplantation.
▶ Her stature should not be one associated with adverse obstetric outcome.
▶ There should be no proteinuria and no significant hypertension.
▶ There should be no sign of rejection of the transplanted kidney.
▶ There should be no sign of distension of the renal pelvis or calyces.
▶ Plasma creatinine should be 200 μmol/l or less.
▶ Drug dosages should be at maintenance levels, e.g. prednisone, 15 mg/day or less and azathioprine 2 mg/kg body weight per day, or less.

The woman should be cared for by a nephrologist and an obstetrician; however, she still requires midwifery care and support.

The predisposition to urinary tract infection associated with pregnancy, coupled with immunosuppressive drugs taken by transplant patients renders the woman more likely to infection. She may also develop hypertension and she may become anaemic.

Labour may occur spontaneously unless there is an obstetric indication for intervention. Steroid therapy is increased and antibiotics must be given prophylactically for any surgical intervention, including episiotomy.

Neonatal problems include preterm delivery, intrauterine growth retardation, respiratory distress syndrome, adrenocortical insufficiency, thrombocytopenia, leucopenia, cytomegalovirus and other infections. Davison and Dunlop (1989) observe that where the mother has received multiple blood transfusions during haemodialysis, she may carry hepatitis B antigen, which may result in the neonate carrying the antigen.

Theoretically, breastfeeding is possible, but so many uncertainties surround the effects of some of the drugs used that it is not advised.

ACUTE RENAL FAILURE

A fall in urinary output is the first sign of acute renal failure. An output of less than 500 ml in 24 hours is considered a sign of renal failure.

Causes

Acute renal failure may occur in association with severe haemorrhage, eclampsia and septic abortion, particularly in a case of *Clostridium welchii* infection, and it may follow a mismatched blood transfusion or sulphonamide therapy. Though rare, it is extremely serious and, because the outcome is not predictable, it has been recommended that all women with renal failure should be transferred to a unit where renal dialysis is available in case of need.

It will be recalled that the kidneys have an abundant circulation of blood. As this large volume of blood flows through them the kidneys filter off water, containing waste materials such as urea and surplus amounts of materials such as potassium. Thus the blood is purified and its constituents are kept constant. If the renal blood vessels go into spasm, the blood flow through the kidneys is reduced almost to nothing. The kidneys can no longer excrete urea and potassium, so large amounts accumulate in the blood, making the woman dangerously ill. As she cannot excrete much water, she becomes oedematous. These results will also follow blockage of the renal tubules.

Management

It is important to be aware that acute renal failure can occur and to prevent its onset by adequate blood transfusion when conditions such as haemorrhage occur.

The aim of the treatment is to rest the kidneys since, given time, they may well recover. At the same time, the woman's blood urea must not rise too high or she will die of uraemia. Protein must be avoided as its end-product is urea. Thus she is given daily about 150 g of glucose and 500 ml water. This will just satisfy her need for food and fluid, without throwing unnecessary work on her kidneys. Vitamins are given intramuscularly.

The glucose solution can be given orally, when it may be more palatable in weak tea or coffee. It can be given as a continuous gastric infusion or, if vomiting is troublesome, as an intravenous infusion. This concentrated solution (30–40%) would cause clotting in small veins, so it is allowed to infuse into the inferior vena cava through a fine polythene tube introduced into the femoral vein.

The woman's fluid balance is carefully recorded, her blood urea and electrolytes are estimated daily and her physical and mental state observed carefully. At first only a few millilitres of urine are passed each day, sometimes none at all. Then, in favourable circumstances, the amounts increase to a large volume, while the blood urea and potassium level steadily decrease to normal. If this diuresis does not occur, the patient is in danger of death from uraemia, though with renal dialysis she may yet recover.

Diabetes Mellitus

Diabetes mellitus is a medical condition in which there is a total or relative lack of insulin produced by the pancreas for the requirements of the tissues. This means that glycolytic enzymes are inhibited and gluconeogenetic enzymes are activated, resulting in the liberation of additional glucose into the bloodstream. Without insulin, this additional glucose cannot be utilized for energy, since it is unable to cross the cell membrane into muscle and adipose tissue. The body therefore endeavours to utilize energy sources from fat and protein metabolism, breaking down amino acids for gluconeogenesis. Urea, a byproduct of amino acid metabolism, is excreted in large quantities in the urine.

Ketogenesis also takes place as fatty acids are liberated from adipose tissue in response to the body's requirements for energy. Ketones can be used by some body tissues as an energy source, but in uncontrolled diabetes, they may be produced in excess, resulting in their excretion in urine and through the lungs. Ketones are acidic substances and lower the body pH; in an effort to avoid acidosis, the body's buffer pool becomes exhausted, leading to possible shock (Crichton and Silverton, 1985).

Thus, blood glucose levels are high, and become increasingly higher as gluconeogenesis occurs; when insulin is absent or reduced, it is impossible for the body to utilize the high circulating levels of glucose for energy. This hyperglycaemia means that the transport maximum for reabsorption of glucose in the renal system is exceeded, and glycosuria results. Since glucose is osmotically active, it carries with it a corresponding amount of water as it is excreted in the urine, resulting in polyuria. As more and more water is excreted, so dehydration occurs, and the traditional picture is produced of the hyperglycaemic, dehydrated and ketotic patient with polyuria and polydipsia. Untreated, these symptoms will lead to acidosis, coma and death (Hinchliff and Montague, 1988).

Although the effects of diabetes mellitus are seen principally in relation to glucose metabolism, multiple metabolic pathways are disturbed and the disease exerts its effects on all systems of the body.

Diagnosis and classification

The diagnosis of diabetes is made by performing a glucose tolerance test which challenges the body's response to a glucose load. The fasting patient is given a drink containing 75 g glucose. Venous blood samples are obtained at regular intervals and compared with results within the normal range. The blood glucose levels rise initially, but should return to normal within two hours. Abnormal findings would be a fasting blood glucose of over 7 mmol/l, and a blood glucose level over 10 mmol/l after two hours. Where the two-hour figure is below 10 mmol/l, but greater than 7 mmol/l, glucose tolerance is said to be impaired (WHO, 1980).

The British Diabetic Association has adopted the World Health Organization (WHO) Classification of Diabetes Mellitus which is as follows:

Type I: insulin-dependent diabetes (formerly called clinical diabetes) The glucose tolerance test is abnormal and patients have signs and symptoms of the disease and require treatment. It is most common in juveniles, and is characterized by an almost complete lack of insulin, possibly due to a decrease in the number of beta cells in the islets of Langerhans. Hyperglycaemia, polyuria and ketosis are present, and this type of diabetes is insulin dependent.

Type II: non-insulin-dependent diabetes (formerly known as chemical diabetes) These women have

an abnormal glucose tolerance test but no symptoms. They are subject to the same complications as patients with overt clinical diabetes and the perinatal mortality is similarly increased. In this type of diabetes, there seems to be resistance in the tissues to the action of insulin; it is often diagnosed later in life, and frequently affects those who are obese. It is not dependent on insulin, and oral hypoglycaemic agents may be used to control it. It may also be controlled by diet alone.

Impaired glucose tolerance (IGT) (formerly latent diabetes) The glucose tolerance test is normal except in times of stress when the woman may develop diabetes. When this occurs in pregnancy it is known as gestational diabetes. Fifteen to twenty per cent of these women go on to develop insulin-dependent diabetes in later life, with the incidence rising to 70% if there is also obesity (Chamberlain, 1991).

Other This group would include potential diabetics who have a normal glucose tolerance test but because of certain risk factors have a higher incidence of diabetes than normal women. They may have:

▶ glycosuria on two occasions in the antenatal clinic;
▶ history of diabetes in first-degree relatives;
▶ previous baby weighing more than 4.5 kg;
▶ previous unexplained perinatal death;
▶ history of a baby with congenital malformations;
▶ polyhydramnios;
▶ obesity.

Gestational diabetes

This term has traditionally been applied to the condition in women who develop hyperglycaemia with an impaired glucose tolerance test during pregnancy. The association between gestational diabetes and adverse neonatal outcome led to active treatment by diet and insulin therapy for such women. Active screening, including random blood glucose estimation and glucose tolerance testing (in some centres for all pregnant women) aimed to detect and treat the condition in order to improve perinatal outcome.

A survey of perinatal complications in women with gestational diabetes suggests that even minute degrees of maternal hyperglycaemia may affect fetal outcome (Hod *et al.*, 1991).

Jarrett (1993) suggests that mass screening of pregnant women is unrealistic, as impaired glucose tolerance is simply a temporary condition associated with pregnancy; Hunter and Keirse (1989) also suggest that the glucose tolerance test itself is an unreliable screening tool, and that impaired glucose tolerance is a risk marker for adverse pregnancy outcome, rather than a cause in itself. They and others (Jacobson and Cousins, 1989; Green *et al.*, 1990) postulate that maternal age and weight influence glucose intolerance. However, Hunter and Keirse (1989) support the view that diet and insulin therapy can reduce the incidence of fetal macrosomia in pregnancies where glucose tolerance is impaired.

For midwives, the uncertainty surrounding diagnosis or even existence of gestational diabetes is confusing when it comes to providing care, since studies are inconclusive. Mass screening may result in unnecessary medicalization of otherwise uncomplicated pregnancies. In the absence of concrete evidence Hunter and Keirse (1989) recommend that all glucose tolerance testing be stopped, except for the purposes of further research and that women considered at risk should have repeated random blood glucose estimations throughout pregnancy.

As for the provision of midwifery care amidst this uncertainty, women with gestational diabetes and with pre-existing diabetes mellitus call for knowledgeable and skilled care, and a recognition of them as women in their own right rather than a reflection of a medical condition.

Pregnancy and diabetes

A number of hormonal and metabolic changes occur naturally as a result of pregnancy, and these changes, together with their accepted physiological norms have been well-documented (see Chapters 11 and 12).

Type I and Type II diabetes mellitus are complicated by the physiological changes which take place in glucose metabolism during pregnancy. In the first trimester of pregnancy, fasting blood glucose levels fall from 4 mmol/l until at term, the level may be as low as 3.6 mmol/l. However, the peak response to food is progressively higher and delayed as pregnancy progresses. In the non-diabetic, rises in insulin production maintain normoglycaemia (Jowett and Nichol, 1987) and there is considerable hypertrophy of the pancreatic islet cells in order to produce additional insulin in response to glucose stimulation. Maternal fat storage takes place in the first trimester, and is followed by fat mobilization in the later months as the fetus accelerates its use of glucose and amino acids. Thus, in non-

diabetic pregnancy, the metabolic state is altered to provide preferential perfusion of nutrients across the placenta to the fetus, to ensure embryogenesis, growth, maturation and survival (Hollingsworth, 1984).

Placental hormones exert an influence on the metabolic status both directly and indirectly; progesterones, oestrogens, human placental lactogen and increased free cortisol combine to produce a resistance to insulin (Jowett and Nichol, 1987). In this sense, pregnancy is said to be diabetogenic.

Glucose carried in plasma passes through the renal system, and is normally reabsorbed in the proximal convoluted tubule of the nephron. The transport system for glucose is linked to the active transfer of sodium ions, in a phenomenon known as co-transfer (Hinchliff and Montague, 1988).

There is a maximum amount of glucose which can be reabsorbed in this way (the *transport maximum*, or Tm), and in healthy persons, this means that when blood glucose levels are between 4.2 and 6.7 mmol/l, all glucose will be reabsorbed. However, the maximum rate for glucose reabsorption is 375 mg/min, and when plasma glucose levels exceed 10 mmol/l, the transport maximum is exceeded, therefore all the plasma glucose cannot be reabsorbed. Consequently, glucose is excreted in the urine, producing glycosuria. Normally, the action of insulin would prevent this.

In non-diabetic pregnancy, the glomerular filtration rate is increased, so that even when blood glucose levels are within normal limits, all glucose cannot be reabsorbed, and there may be glycosuria. In diabetic pregnancy, therefore, urinalysis is inadequate as a reflection of blood glucose.

In diabetes, episodes of hyperglycaemia cause haemoglobin to become irreversibly bound to glucose; this glycosylated haemoglobin (HbA1) normally constitutes 4–8% of the woman's total haemoglobin. This level may rise during hyperglycaemia, and a raised level is associated with fetal abnormalities in pregnancy (Hollingsworth, 1984; Drury, 1987; Reece and Coustan, 1988). Levels of HbA1 in the blood reflect blood glucose status up to three months previously, so that levels of HbA1 taken at ten weeks of pregnancy may reveal high blood glucose levels at the time of conception and embryogenesis.

Maternal complications

Although more complications occur in the pregnancies of diabetic mothers, the maternal mortality rate is no higher than 0.5%. In the pregnant diabetic woman, insulin requirements will obviously be greatly increased to cope with the relative fasting hypoglycaemia, and up to four times the usual dose of insulin will be required. Women with type II diabetes will also require insulin at this stage, although in both type I and type II diabetes, and in gestational diabetes, insulin requirements will return to normal immediately after delivery (Drury, 1987). Insulin-dependent diabetes becomes more unstable in pregnancy. The renal threshold for glucose is lowered in pregnancy and insulin requirements increase as pregnancy advances, so that diabetic control is more difficult.

Hyperglycaemia leads to glycosuria and ketoacidosis. Monilial vaginitis and urinary tract infections are commonly associated with hyperglycaemia whereas ketoacidosis may increase the severity of any nausea and vomiting in pregnancy. These metabolic changes can result in a period of instability in diabetic control for the pregnant woman, which may exacerbate existing complications of diabetes

There are conflicting views as to whether *diabetic retinopathy* worsens during pregnancy (Price *et al.*, 1984; Puklin, 1988). However, it is a progressive condition, and is the most frequent cause of blindness in type I diabetes (Puklin, 1988). It is advisable, therefore, that ophthalmic examinations of the fundi be carried out during each trimester (Drury, 1987). Women with retinopathy also experience a higher incidence of pre-eclampsia and perinatal complications, particularly preterm birth and low birthweight (Price *et al.*, 1984).

Likewise, *diabetic nephropathy* may be present, or may be detected during pregnancy (Kitzmiller, 1988), and may be complicated by a superimposed pre-eclampsia. Hollingsworth (1984) suggest that renal disease does not worsen during pregnancy, and this view is partially supported by Davison *et al.* (1985). However, Davison *et al.* (1985) observe that renal function will be severely impaired in a minority of women, with no improvement after delivery. Twenty-five per cent of pregnant women with diabetes will develop *polyhydramnios* (Brudenell, 1989); this may be associated with fetal abnormality, or may develop as a result of fetal polyuria in response to fetal hyperglycaemia.

There is an increased incidence of pre-eclampsia in diabetic women and it is made worse by poor diabetic control.

Diabetic mothers tend to have large babies (see Fetal complications), especially if the diabetic control is poor.

If there is any cephalopelvic disproportion a Caesarean section would be employed to avoid the risk of prolonged labour and a difficult vaginal delivery.

Fetal complications

Despite good diabetic control, Hunter (1989) observes that there is still a risk of fetal macrosomia (birthweight over 4000 g), with its attendant maternal and fetal risks. Macrosomia occurs for a number of reasons: maternal hyperglycaemia stimulates the fetus to produce insulin which results in deposition of fat and protein. Overproduction of the growth hormone from the anterior pituitary gland is also involved in the development of large babies. It is suggested that the fetus in diabetic pregnancy may have an increased potential for growth which is stimulated by relatively small increases in maternal blood glucose (Bradley, 1990). The major risk to the macrosomic fetus is birth trauma, principally brachial plexus injury, secondary to shoulder dystocia.

Intrauterine fetal death occurs frequently in the last 3–4 weeks of pregnancy but the cause is not really understood. It is particularly likely to occur when:

▶ the diabetes is not well controlled;
▶ there is marked polyhydramnios;
▶ the baby is very large; or
▶ the pregnancy is complicated by hypertension or impaired glucose tolerance.

The incidence of pre-eclampsia is increased in diabetic women and this may be partly responsible for the high perinatal mortality rate. Diabetic vascular disease, hyperglycaemia and ketoacidosis in the mother all increase the risk of fetal death. Studies suggest that chronic fetal hypoxia may be a cause of fetal death (Bradley, 1990); other causes may be related to fetal acidaemia and a compensatory fetal polycythaemia accompanied by thrombocytopenia (Salveson *et al.*, 1992). In the neonate, the higher haematocrit associated with polycythaemia predisposes the infant to jaundice.

The risks of birth trauma and fetal death resulted in a pattern of care which included elective Caesarean section at 36–37 weeks' gestation. This practice produced its own problems of prematurity and respiratory distress syndrome (related both to pulmonary immaturity and to the method of delivery). The trend now is to avoid intervention before term in an otherwise uncomplicated pregnancy and hope for spontaneous onset of labour (Hunter, 1989).

The incidence of malformations in diabetic pregnancy is four times higher than usual (Malins, 1978). Congenital abnormality is now the commonest cause of perinatal death in diabetic pregnancies (Brudenell, 1982). Cardiac anomalies occur four times as often in diabetic pregnancies; other congenital abnormalities include anencephaly and vertebral defects (Hunter, 1989). The perinatal mortality rate in diabetic pregnancy has greatly improved in recent years and is now below 5% (Essex and Pyke, 1979). This is largely due to the improved diabetic management of the pregnant diabetic mother. In cases where diabetic control is poor the perinatal mortality rate is likely to be higher (Hunter, 1989).

Prematurity is an important factor in perinatal mortality. Early delivery may be necessary because of the severity of the diabetes or the onset of complications. The newborn baby has a six-fold risk of developing respiratory distress syndrome.

Maternal and fetal complications affecting pregnant women with diabetes are summarized in Table 3.

Preconception care

Good diabetic control before and at the time of conception as well as throughout the antenatal period greatly improves the outcome of pregnancy. Women with diabetes mellitus should therefore discuss a proposed pregnancy with their doctor so that diabetic control can be improved, if necessary, before conception

Table 3 Maternal and fetal complications affecting pregnant diabetic women

Maternal complications

1   Unstable diabetic control
2   Ketoacidosis
3   Polyhydramnios
4   Pre-eclampsia
5   Preterm labour
6   Obstructed labour

Fetal complications

1   Congenital abnormalities
2   Macrosomia
3   Intrauterine death
4   Respiratory distress syndrome
5   Neonatal hypoglycaemia, hypocalcaemia, jaundice, polycythaemia

tion occurs, particularly given the association between fetal abnormality and hyperglycaemia during the period of fetal organogenesis. Women with diabetes may already be well-informed about their condition, and be aware of the importance of pre-pregnancy care. Associations such as the British Diabetic Association produce literature specifically related to pregnancy, and clinical nurse specialists in diabetic clinics should also be aware of the importance of periconception care.

Care during pregnancy

Collaborative care is essential for pregnant women who have diabetes; medical, obstetric and midwifery input, together with informed self-care by the woman can help to make the pregnancy as fulfilling for the expectant mother with diabetes as for her non-diabetic counterpart. Midwifery input must be knowledgeable and up to date, catering for all aspects of the woman's care during pregnancy, birth and the puerperium.

The woman is booked to have her baby in a consultant obstetric unit with a special care baby unit and is seen at least two-weekly, and more often if necessary.

Good diabetic control is essential if the fetal complications already described are to be minimized. Therefore it is important that the mother's diet and insulin requirements are adjusted and reviewed closely. The renal threshold for glucose falls in pregnancy, so assessment of diabetic control must be based on blood glucose levels rather than on urinary glucose.

Nowadays diabetic women with no obstetric complications are usually managed at home during the antenatal period rather than by repeated hospital admissions (Burke *et al.*, 1985). Regular monitoring of the blood glucose levels at home by the pregnant woman has proved successful in achieving good diabetic control and the safe delivery of normal babies (Stubbs *et al.*, 1980; Murphy *et al.*, 1984; Burke *et al.*, 1985).

Diet The carbohydrate energy content of the diet should be related to the energy requirements of the individual. In most cases it does not exceed 40%, but it can be higher without adverse effects (Metcalfe, 1984). Fat intake should be restricted because of the increased risk of arterial disease in diabetics. A high fibre intake is recommended because the slower gastric emptying delays the absorption of sugar into the bloodstream. Hypoglycaemia may exacerbate the effects of morning sickness; glucose and sugary foods should be avoided, and hypoglycaemia avoided by taking milk and a light snack. Glucagon should be available to women with diabetes, for use in emergencies.

Diabetes is particularly common in British women of Asian origin (British Diabetic Association, 1989). Dietary considerations for such women should avoid sweets such as gulab juman, halwa and jelabi and where the woman is also overweight, foods fried in ghee or oil should be reduced.

Insulin Insulin requirements usually increase in pregnancy due to the rise in energy requirements and the production of diabetogenic hormones from the placenta (Crichton and Silverton, 1985). The dose of insulin is carefully correlated to the glucose levels which are monitored daily. Better diabetic control is generally achieved if a combination of short and intermediate acting insulins are administered twice daily (Gillmer, 1983).

Continuous infusion of insulin may be maintained via a subcutaneous syringe pump, although this has not been shown to achieve better control than conventional multidose administration. Brudenell (1989) suggests the pump may be useful for women who, for whatever reason, find it difficult to cope with a multidose pattern; Hunter (1989) observes that the pump programme in itself may be difficult to master, but may be useful for women with very variable insulin requirements.

Three descriptions have been applied to control of blood glucose in pregnancy complicated by diabetes; very tight control, tight control and moderate control.

1 *Very tight control*: aims for blood glucose below 5.6 mmol/l.
2 *Tight control*: aims for blood glucose 5.6–6.7 mmol/l.
3 *Moderate control*: aims for blood glucose 6.7–8.9 mmol/l.

In normal pregnancy, blood glucose levels rarely exceed 6.6 mmol/l.

The effects of these degrees of control have not been thoroughly researched, but evidence suggests that tight control coupled with a holistic approach to the woman's care results in reduced incidence of macrosomia, urinary tract infection, respiratory distress syndrome, hypertension, preterm labour and perinatal mortality (Hunter, 1989).

The use of oral hypoglycaemic drugs is not recommended in pregnancy as they cross the placenta and may cause severe hypoglycaemia in the baby after birth

because of their slow metabolism in the infant's immature liver.

Assessment of blood glucose levels and glycosylated haemoglobin (HbA_1) Blood glucose levels are monitored four or six times on 2 or 3 days a week and the preprandial levels should be below 5.5 mmol/l. The woman has the use of a glucose monitor (reflectance meter) and is taught to monitor her own blood glucose levels and to change her treatment when necessary to remain normoglycaemic.

A reflectance meter is not essential, however, since the Dextrostix or BM (Böhringer Mannheim) stix can be used and read off against their respective standard charts. The mother also tests her first morning urine specimen for ketone bodies each day and charts this and her blood glucose levels. Ketoacidosis can be harmful to the fetus, resulting in an increased mortality rate (Brumfield and Huddleston, 1984).

Glycosylated haemoglobin (HbA_1) can also be measured and helps to assess diabetic control. It is a type of adult haemoglobin where one part of the beta chain has been combined with glucose. HbA_1 has been found to increase in diabetes, especially when the blood glucose control is poor (Crichton and Silverton, 1985). HbA_1 levels are not indicators of present diabetic status but of blood glucose levels during the preceding 1–3 months. Levels of 10% or lower are considered a sign of good control, while levels of more than 10% indicate poor control (Leslie *et al.*, 1978).

Fetal well-being In addition to careful supervision of the diabetes, fetal well-being is monitored closely throughout pregnancy. It may be assessed by kick counts and cardiotocography and growth is monitored by clinical examination and ultrasonography (see Chapter 21) (Gillmer, 1983). Biophysical profiles and Doppler blood flow studies may also be performed.

Obstetric care In addition to monitoring the diabetic condition the obstetric condition is carefully assessed. The frequency of attendance at the antenatal clinic varies but Gillmer (1983) suggests every two weeks until 32 weeks and then weekly. The incidence of pre-eclampsia is increased in women with diabetes, thus particular care is taken to record the blood pressure and examine the urine for protein. Hospitalization before 38 weeks is necessary only if complications such as pre-eclampsia, polyhydramnios, fetal growth retardation, infection or inadequate diabetic control occur.

At 37–38 weeks amniocentesis may be performed to estimate the lecithin–sphingomyelin ratio (see Chapter 21). This is because the incidence of respiratory distress syndrome is increased in babies of diabetic mothers. When the lecithin–sphingomyelin ratio is 2:1 respiratory distress syndrome in the newborn is unlikely to occur.

Pregnant women with well-controlled diabetes and no obstetric complications are usually delivered vaginally at 38 weeks. Those with poor diabetic control and/or obstetric complications will be delivered earlier to avoid the risk of intrauterine fetal death. They are usually delivered by Caesaeran section.

Care during labour

The midwife cares for the woman in labour in conjunction with medical and obstetric colleagues; labour onset may be spontaneous or induced, or delivery may be by elective Caesarean section.

Induction   Labour is usually induced by artificial rupture of the membranes and a scalp electrode is applied at that time. An oxytocin infusion is given using an infusion pump. One litre of 5% dextrose is infused every eight hours, and insulin is given on a sliding scale to maintain blood glucose levels at 4.5–5.5 mmol/l. Blood glucose levels are checked hourly.

During labour   Close fetal monitoring is essential, because of the increased risks of fetal distress and fetal hypoxia during labour. Satisfactory pain relief may be achieved by epidural anaesthesia. If progress is slow or fetal distress develops, a Caesarean section is carried out. Otherwise the mother proceeds to a vaginal delivery. After labour, insulin requirements usually revert to pre-pregnancy levels and women who began insulin therapy during pregnancy will not now require this.

Caesarean section   If an elective Caesarean section is to be performed the woman is starved on the day of operation and her usual morning dose of insulin is omitted. An intravenous infusion of dextrose 5% is started and soluble insulin is given subcutaneously, the dose being prescribed by the physician. The aim is to keep the blood glucose between 3.0 and 5.0 mmol/l and to avoid ketosis. After delivery, the insulin requirements fall steeply.

Care during the puerperium

The mother's insulin requirements fall sharply after delivery, so frequent blood glucose estimations are made to detect hypoglycaemia. The insulin dosage is reduced and the mother is gradually restabilized.

Breastfeeding is no longer contraindicated, although diabetic control is a little more difficult to achieve.

High standards of hygiene are necessary to combat the increased risk of infection in diabetic women.

Diabetic women require careful advice on family planning. If the mother wishes to have more children she is advised to do so quickly while she is relatively young.

The oral contraceptive pill may alter carbohydrate metabolism and a few mothers may need a higher dose of insulin. Younger mothers may take the oral contraceptive pill. However, they require careful review, and if they develop headaches or hypertension, may need alternative methods.

There is concern about the effectiveness of the intrauterine contraceptive device in diabetic women because of the risk of pelvic infection and also coating of the device with glucose deposits, so this method of contraception is less well-accepted. Barrier methods may be used by women for whom further pregnancy would not severely exacerbate diabetic complications. For some women with diabetes, sterilization may be a serious option which can be undertaken 3–6 months after delivery.

The baby of the diabetic mother

A paediatrician should be present at birth to receive the baby of the diabetic mother. In the past these babies were invariably large and plethoric but with better diabetic control the baby is more likely to be an appropriate weight for gestational age. Despite being large for gestational age the baby may be immature and require special care after birth, although routine separation of mother and baby for the simple purpose of observation is not required. These babies are particularly prone to respiratory distress syndrome and hypoglycaemia, so they require very close observation. In intrauterine life the hypertrophic islets of Langerhans produce more insulin in response to the high maternal blood sugar levels. After birth the pancreas continues to produce excess insulin initially, so the baby becomes hypoglycaemic. To prevent this, early feeding within two hours of birth is essential and the infant's blood glucose levels are measured with Destrostix two-hourly to detect hypoglycaemia.

Other complications to which this baby is particularly prone include skin infections, hyperbilirubin-aemia and bleeding from a very thick cord, and the incidence of congenital malformations is increased. Considerable weight loss occurs in the first week or so after birth and the baby tends to be lethargic, but then progress should be normal.

Respiratory Problems

TUBERCULOSIS

Pulmonary tuberculosis (TB) is responsible for 6% of all deaths worldwide, and available sources suggest that up to half the world's population is infected with the disease in either its latent or active form (Mays, 1993). Improvements in housing, nutrition and access to health care, coupled with a mass screening campaign in the 1950s, resulted in a significant decline in the disease in Great Britain. However, sources suggest that TB is becoming more prevalent, particularly among the homeless, in situations where there is overcrowding, and where there is exposure through contact with people from countries where the disease is widespread. Drug users and those infected with HIV are at increased risk of developing TB.

Classic symptoms are chronic cough and blood-streaked sputum, with fever, weight loss and night sweats occurring late in the disease. The onset is insidious and there is also a feeling of general malaise.

Diagnosis

Diagnosis is made by positive Mantoux test, presence of the causative organism (*Mycobacterium tuberculosis* or tubercle bacillus) in the sputum and by chest X-ray.

Women may become pregnant whilst being treated for TB, or may develop the disease during pregnancy.

Pregnancy care

Congenital TB is very rare, so the fetus is not at risk; if chest X-rays are needed, a lead apron is used to protect the mother's abdomen.

Care in pregnancy will be undertaken by an obstetrician and a physician specializing in respiratory disorders. Since social and economic factors feature in the care of women with TB, the midwife must liaise with a social worker where necessary so that any required improvements in social circumstances may be brought about. Help will be needed both during and after pregnancy with housework and childcare, since the woman will be fatigued. Liaison with other health care workers may be necessary since family members may need to be screened, and educated as to the nature of the disease and the steps needed to prevent its spread.

Drugs used to treat TB have side-effects for both mother and fetus (see Table 4); courses of treatment are long – 6–9 months or longer – but the symptoms of the disease resolve after only three weeks. Women must

Table 4   Drugs used for the treatment of active TB in pregnancy

Drug	Dose	Possible side-effects	
		Maternal	Fetal
Isoniazid	5 mg/kg/day Max. 300 mg	Hepatitis Peripheral neuropathy Agranulocytosis	None
Rifampicin	10 mg/kg/day Max. 600 mg	Hepatitis Decreased effectiveness of oral contraceptive	Increase in neural tube defects
Ethambutol	15–25 mg/kg/day Max. 2.5 g	Optic neuritis Visual problems	None
Pyrazinamide	15–30 mg/kg/day	Hepatitis Arthralgias	None

Note: Streptomycin is not given in pregnancy since it causes damage to fetal auditory and vestibular nerves be encouraged to continue treatment, otherwise there is the risk of drug-resistant strains developing.

Labour

Infection is spread by airborne transmission of droplet nuclei from a person with active TB. If the woman is infectious, she should be provided with a single room while she is in hospital. Crockery and cutlery are not involved in the transmission of infection and barrier nursing is not required.

In the absence of obstetric indications, labour onset is spontaneous and care during the first stage is as that of any normal labour. However, depending on the woman's respiratory function, nitrous oxide and oxygen (Entonox) may be contraindicated.

In order to avoid exhaustion of the mother, an elective forceps delivery or episiotomy may be performed. Blood loss may be minimized by active management of the third stage.

Postnatal period

This may be a very difficult time for the mother and her family; where the woman or any close family members have active pulmonary tuberculosis, particularly of a resistant strain, the baby is at risk of developing the disease and may need to be segregated from the family. The baby is vaccinated with the BCG (bacille Calmette–Guérin) vaccine and may be given syrup of isoniazid prophylactically, until a positive Mantoux reaction is obtained. If the disease is not active, the mother and baby are not separated, nor is breastfeeding contraindicated.

Additional help will be needed with housework and childcare, and this should be arranged in conjunction with the home help service.

Advice with family spacing methods will be needed, as the women with active TB should avoid pregnancy until there are no further signs of the disease, usually for a period of two years.

ASTHMA

The effect of pregnancy on asthma appears to be variable. Most mothers experience less asthmatic attacks, possibly due to the increased production of corticosteroids in pregnancy, but a few may have more. Schatz (1992) suggests that asthmatic women are more likely to develop hyperemesis gravidarum, chronic hypertension, pregnancy-induced hypertension and antepartum haemorrhage. The causes are

unknown but the conditions are less likely to arise where asthma is controlled well (Moore-Giloon, 1994). It is also suggested that maternal hypoxia during repeated asthmatic attacks results in intrauterine growth retardation. Treatment prescribed before pregnancy should be continued. This includes the use of steroids, though they would not normally be started for the first time during the first trimester of pregnancy.

If the woman is being treated with steroids, hydrocortisone should be given in labour. An elective forceps delivery is performed to shorten the second stage of labour. After delivery, the steroid requirements fall and thus the dosage of steroids is adjusted.

Epilepsy

Epilepsy is a condition of abnormal cerebral function in which characteristic, convulsive seizures occur. Seizures may be generalized (*petit mal* and *grand mal*), partial (*temporal lobe epilepsy*) or focal (*Jacksonian seizure*). Seizures frequently result in loss of consciousness, for periods of a matter of seconds, up to half an hour. In all cases abnormal, paroxysmal electrical discharges, recordable on EEG occur in the brain.

Status epilepticus is a serious condition in which seizures occur in rapid succession; it is most commonly associated with grand mal epilepsy in which the seizures follow a pattern of a warning aura, loss of consciousness, tonic spasm of the muscles followed by a clonic phase of jerking muscular contractions. In the pregnancy of a woman not known to have epilepsy, this could initially be mistaken for eclampsia.

Epilepsy may be controlled, but not cured, by the use of anticonvulsant drugs such as sodium valproate (Epilim) or phenytoin sodium (Epanutin). Phenobarbitone or benzodiazepines may also be given. Pregnancy has a variable effect on the pattern of seizures, but generally speaking, the more severe the disorder, the greater the effect on the pregnancy. Women who have epilepsy and who become pregnant, achieve successful pregnancy outcome in more than 90% of cases. Successful outcome relates to close monitoring of the epilepsy, co-operation of the woman in taking prescribed medication, and preferably preconception assessment and counselling (Brodie, 1990).

There is an increased incidence of congenital abnormalities in infants of women with epilepsy

(Drugs and Therapeutics Bulletin, 1990); some sources suggest that this is due to the teratogenic effects of anticonvulsant therapy and some that it is associated with the condition itself (Brodie, 1990; Chamberlain, 1991). Most common defects are cleft lip and cleft palate, spina bifida and heart disease. Abnormalities occur more often in women who receive combinations of anticonvulsants, so during pregnancy, treatment with one drug alone is recommended. Prophylactic folic acid for prevention of neural tube defects may reduce serum phenytoin levels thus affecting control of seizures in some women (Drugs and Therapeutics Bulletin, 1994). *Hydantoin syndrome* is a condition resembling fetal alcohol syndrome and may occur in infants of women taking hydantoin preparations.

This association between fetal abnormality and drug therapy highlights the importance of counselling for the woman. A balance needs to be maintained between preventing seizures, which in themselves may lead to intrauterine hypoxia and/or maternal injury, and maintenance of drug levels at the lowest maternal therapeutic doses possible. The physiological changes associated with pregnancy result in lower concentrations of anticonvulsant drugs (Brodie, 1990), which may need to be increased, subject to estimations of plasma levels. These drugs alter the absorption of folic acid and 5 mg/day should be given as a prophylactic precaution. For the same reason, vitamin K clotting factors may be inhibited in the neonate, who should receive vitamin K.

During pregnancy, the woman and her partner need full information about the incidence of congenital abnormalities and the screening tests available to them. They may also need individualized parenting programmes to help them devise strategies for coping safely with their baby. Midwives should be aware of the effects of phenytoin toxicity, which are nystagmus and ataxia in the woman.

In the absence of obstetric complications, labour and delivery will be spontaneous.

All anticonvulsants are secreted in breast milk, but as long as the maternal dosage is not excessively high, there is no contraindication to breastfeeding. If the mother has received high doses of phenobarbitone, primidone or benzodiazepines during pregnancy, the baby may be hyperactive, restless, reluctant to suckle and may have vomiting or diarrhoea for up to a month (Brodie, 1990).

Parents need extra support postnatally; the woman may be afraid that she will have a seizure while holding or bathing her baby and the strategies devised antenatally can be put into practice.

References

Bradley, R. (1990) Diabetic pregnancy. *Br. J. Hosp. Med.* **44**(6): 386–390.

British Diabetic Association (1989) *Pregnancy Pack*. British Diabetic Association, 10 Queen Anne Street, London.

Brodie, M.J. (1990) Management of epilepsy during pregnancy and lactation. *Lancet* **336**(8712): 426–427.

Brudenell, J.M. (1982) Diabetic pregnancy. In Studd, J. (ed.) *Progress in Obstetrics and Gynaecology*, Vol. 2. Edinburgh: Churchill Livingstone.

Brudenell, M. (1989) Diabetic pregnancy. In Turnbull, A. & Chamberlain, G. (eds) *Obstetrics*. London: Churchill Livingstone.

Brumfield, C.G. & Huddleston, J.F. (1984) The management of diabetic ketoacidosis in pregnancy. *Clin. Obstet. Gynaecol.* **27**(i): 50–59.

Burke, B.J., Owens, C.., Pennock, C.A., Turner, G. & Hartog, M. (1985) The management of diabetic pregnancy – inpatient or outpatient? *J. Obstet. Gynaecol.* **6**: 14–18.

Chamberlain, J. (1991) Medical problems in pregnancy. *Br. Med. J.* **302**(6787): 1262–1264.

Crichton, M.A. & Silverton, L.I. (1985) The sweeter side of life: a review of diabetes and its effects on pregnancy. *Midwifery* **1**: 195–206.

Davison, M.M., Katz, A.L. & Linheimer, M.D. (1985) Kidney disease and pregnancy: Obstetric outcome and long term renal prognosis. *Clin. Perinatol.* **12**: 497–519.

Department of Health (1992) *Folic Acid and Neural Tube Defects – Guidelines on Prevention* Circular PL/CMO (92) 18. London: DOH.

deSwiet, M. (1989) Cardiovascular problems in pregnancy. In Turnbull, A. & Chamberlain, G. (eds) *Obstetrics*. London: Churchill Livingstone.

Drugs and Therapeutics Bulletin (1990) *Sodium Valproate and Spina Bifida*, vol. 28:15, pp. 59–60. London: Consumers Association.

Drugs and Therapeutics Bulletin (1994) *Folic Acid to Prevent Neural Tube Defects*, vol. 32:4, pp. 31–32. London: Consumers Association.

Drury, M.I. (1987) Pregnancy in diabetes. *Midwife, Health Visitor & Community Nurse* June: 229–233.

Dunlop, W. & Davison, J.M. (1989) Urinary tract in pregnancy. In Turnbull, A. & Chamberlain, G. (eds) *Obstetrics*. London: Churchill Livingstone.

Editorial (1978) Iron and resistance to infection. *Lancet* **ii**: 325–326.

Essex, N.L. & Pyke, D.A. (1979) Management of maternal diabetes in pregnancy. In Sutherland, H.W. & Stowers, J.M.

(eds) *Carbohydrate Metabolism in Pregnancy and the New-born*, pp. 357–367. Berlin: Springer-Verlag.

Fenton, V., Cavill, I. & Fisher, J. (1977) Iron stores in pregnancy. *Br. J. Haematol.* 37: 145–149.

Gillmer, M. (1983) Diabetes in pregnancy. *Med. Int.* 1(35): 1639–1640.

Green, J.R., Pawson, I.G. & Schumacher, L.B. (1990) Glucose tolerance in pregnancy: ethnic variation and influence of body habitus. *Am. J. Obstet. Gynecol.* 163(1:1): 93–98.

Health Education Authority (1996) *Folic Acid and the Prevention of Neural Tube Defects: Guidance for Health Service Purchasers and Providers.* London: HEA.

Hemminki, E. & Starfield, B. (1978) Routine administration of iron and vitamins during pregnancy: review of controlled clinical trials. *Br. J. Obstet. Gynaecol.* 85: 404–410.

Hinchliff, S. & Montague, S. (1988) *Physiology for Nursing Practice.* London: Baillière Tindall.

Hod, M., Merlob, P. & Friedman, S. (1991) Gestational diabetes mellitus – a survey of perinatal complications in the 1980s. *Diabetes* 4 (Suppl.): 74–78.

Hollingsworth, D.R. (1984) *Pregnancy, Diabetes and Birth: a Management Guide.* London: Williams & Wilkins.

Hunter, D.J.S. (1989) Diabetes in pregnancy. In Chalmers, I., Enkin, M. & Keirse, M.J.N.C. (eds) *Effective Care in Pregnancy and Childbirth.* Oxford: Oxford University Press.

Hunter, D.J.S. & Keirse, M.J.N.C. (1989) Gestational diabetes. In Chalmers, I., Enkin, M. & Keirse, M.J.N.C. (eds) *Effective Care in Pregnancy and Childbirth,* Vol. 1. Oxford: Oxford University Press.

Hytten, F.E. (1976) Metabolic adaptations of pregnancy. In Turnbull, A.C. & Woodford, F.P. (eds) *Prevention of Handicap through Antenatal Care,* pp. 35–39. Amsterdam: Elsevier/North-Holland.

Jacobson, J.D. & Cousins, L. (1989) A population-based study of maternal and perinatal outcome in patients with gestational diabetes. *Am. J. Obstet. Gynecol.* 161(4): 981–986.

Jarrett, R.J. (1993) Gestational diabetes: a non-entity? *Br. Med. J.* 306(6869): 37–38.

Jowett, N.I. & Nichol, S.G. (1987) Diabetic pregnancy. *Midwives Chronicle* February: 33–36.

Kitzmiller, J.L. (1988) Diabetic nephropathy. In Reece, Albert E. & Coustan, D.R. (eds) *Diabetes Mellitus in Pregnancy: Principles and Practice,* pp. 489–510. London: Churchill Livingstone.

Leslie, R.D.G., Pyke, D.A., John, P.N. & White, J.M. (1978) Haemoglobin A₁ in diabetic pregnancy. *Lancet* ii. 958–959.

Mahomed, K. & Hytten, F. (1989) Iron and folate supplementation in pregnancy. In Chalmers, I., Enkin, M. & Keirse, M.J.N.C. (eds) *Effective Care in Pregnancy and Childbirth.* Oxford: Oxford University Press.

Malins, J.M. (1978) Congenital malformations and fetal abnormality in diabetic pregnancy. *J. R. Soc. Med.* 71: 205–207.

Mays, M. (1993) Tuberculosis: a comprehensive review for the certified nurse-midwife. *J. Nurse Midwifery* 38(3): 32–139.

Metcalfe, J. (1984) Dietary control and regular exercise. *Mims Magazine* 1 April: 13–15.

Modell, M. & Modell, B. (1990) Genetic screening for ethnic minorities. *Br. Med. J.* 300(6741): 1702–1704.

Montgomery, E. (1990) Iron levels in pregnancy, physiology or pathology? Assessing the need for supplements. *Midwifery* 6(4): 205–214.

Moore-Giloon, J. (1994) Asthma in pregnancy. *Br. J. Obstet. Gynaecol.* 101(8): 658–660.

Murphy, J., Peters, J., Morris, P., Hayes, T.M. & Pearson, J.F. (1984) Conservative management of pregnancy in diabetic women. *Br. Med. J.* 288: 1203–1205.

Price, J.H., Hadden, D.R., Archer, D.B. & Hartley, J.M.D. (1984) Diabetic retinopathy in pregnancy. *Br. J. Obstet. & Gynaecol.* 91: 11–17.

Puklin, J. (1988) Diabetic retinopathy. In Reece, E.A. & Coustan, D.R. (eds) *Diabetes Mellitus in Pregnancy, Principles and Practice,* pp. 469–488. London: Churchill Livingstone.

Puolakka, J., Jänne, O. & Vihko, R. (1980a) Evaluation by serum ferritin assay of the influence of maternal iron stores on the iron status of newborns and infants. *Acta Obstet. Gynaecol. Scand.* 95 (suppl.): 53–56.

Puolakka, J., Jänne, O., Pakarinen, A. *et al.* (1980b) Serum ferritin as a measure of iron stores during and after normal pregnancy with and without iron supplements. *Acta Obstet. Gynaecol. Scand.* 95 (Suppl.): 43–51.

Reece, Albert E. & Coustan, D.R. (1988) *Diabetes Mellitus in Pregnancy: Principles and Practice.* London: Churchill Livingstone.

Romslo, I., Haram, K., Sagen, N. & Augensen, K. (1983) Iron requirement in normal pregnancy as assessed by serum ferritin, serum transferrin saturation and erythrocyte protoporphyrin determinations. *Br. J. Obstet. Gynaecol.* 90: 101–107.

Salveson, D.R., Brudenell, M.J. & Nicolaides, K.H. (1992) Fetal polycythaemia and thrombocytopaenia in pregnancies complicated by maternal diabetes mellitus. *Am. J. Obstet. Gynecol.* 166(4): 1287–1292.

Schatz, M. (1992) Asthma during pregnancy. *Ann. Allergy* 68(1): 123–133.

Steer, P., Alam, M.A. & Wadsworth, J. (1995) Relation between maternal Hb concentration and birth weight in different ethnic groups. *Br. Med. J.* 6978(25): 489–491.

Stubbs, S.M., Brudenell, J.M., Pyke, D.A., Watkins, P.J., Stubbs, W.A. & Alberti, K.G.M.M. (1980) Management of the pregnant diabetic: home or hospital, with or without glucose meters? *Lancet* i: 1122–1124.

WHO (World Health Organization) (1979) *The Prevalence of Nutritional Anaemia in Developing Countries.* Geneva: WHO.

WHO (1980) Expert Committee on Diabetes Mellitus. *WHO Technical Report* 646: 1–79.

Further Reading

Boore, J.R.P. (1989) Endocrine function. In Hinchliff, S. & Montague, S. (eds) *Physiology for Nursing Practice*. London: Ballière Tindall.

Oakley, C. (1988) A midwife for the woman with diabetes. *Nursing Times* 85(45): 36–38.

Reece, A.E. & Coustan, D.R. (1988) *Diabetes Mellitus in Pregnancy: Principles and Practice*. London: Churchill Livingstone.

Useful Addresses

British Dialietic Association
10 Queen Anne Street
London W1M OBD

Sickle Cell Society
Green Lodge, Barretts Green Road, London NW10 7AP

United Kingdom Thalassaemia Society
107 Nightingale Lane, London N8 7QY

43

Sexually Transmitted Diseases

Vaginal Discharge

Many women report an increase in vaginal discharge during pregnancy known as *leucorrhoea*. In most cases this is due to an excess of cervical mucus and transudate, due to increased vascularity, from the vagina. The discharge is clear or white, and there are no signs of infection. Microscopic examination shows no abnormal organisms and no pus cells; the discharge consists mainly of vaginal epithelial cells and large numbers of Gram-positive bacilli.

MONILIAL INFECTIONS

Commonly the vagina is infected by a yeast-like fungus named *Candida albicans* (Figure 1). This fungus flourishes on a warm, moist mucous surface in an acid environment, particularly in the presence of glucose. It may affect the genitals, skin, gastrointestinal tract and mouth. When the vagina is infected a thick white discharge results, usually associated with severe vulval pruritus, and sometimes with soreness and burning. Clinical examination shows redness of the vulva with white patches of thrush. Microscopic examination of a vaginal cytology smear shows the ovoid spores and long tubes of the fungus. The condition is treated by the administration of antifungal pessaries, tablets or cream containing nystatin, imidazole or triazole. Pessaries containing Nystan 100 000 units are inserted into the vaginal vault every night for two

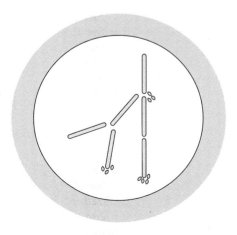

Figure 1   Candida albicans.

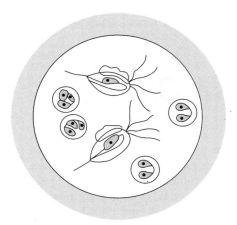

Figure 2   *Trichomonas vaginalis* and pus cells.

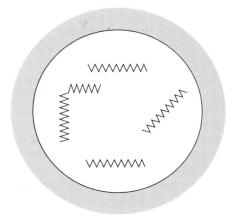

Figure 3   *Treponema pallidum.*

weeks. Clotrimazole (Canesten) vaginal tablets or cream applied for three nights is a good alternative.

TRICHOMONAL INFECTION

A fairly common cause of an abnormal discharge is infection of the vagina by *Trichomonas vaginalis* (Figure 2). This is a flagellated protozoon which can cause severe vulval irritation, dyspareunia and sometimes urinary frequency and dysuria. There is a profuse watery discharge which is offensive. Examination shows a reddened vulva and vagina with small punctuate haemorrhagic areas on the cervix and adjacent tissues. A specimen is obtained from the posterior fornix, added to a drop of isotonic saline, and examined immediately under the microscope. The organism is motile and can be seen moving about in the suspension.

The usual treatment is metronidazole (Flagyl) 400 mg orally twice daily for five days. The woman's partner should be treated at the same time to avoid reinfection. Metronidazole is contraindicated during the first trimester of pregnancy and during lactation. Clotrimazole pessaries and creams are suitable treatments.

SYPHILIS

Syphilis belongs to the family of treponematoses and is caused by *Treponema pallidum* (Figure 3), a spiral microorganism. It is a generalized infection caused by the entry of the organism into the body through mucous membrane or abrasions in the skin, and the spread is via the bloodstream. It is a notifiable disease.

Signs and symptoms

Primary stage   Symptoms appear within 9–90 days of infection; they are usually in the genital tract, but extragenital sites include lip, tongue, mouth, fingers, eyelid, nipple and any part of the skin or mucous membrane.

The primary lesion – the *chancre* – develops at the site of inoculation; it may be at first a raised pimple. This develops into a papula and finally ulcerates. It is most commonly seen on the labia or clitoris, but may occur in the vagina or on the cervix. The lesion is painless but highly infectious. Very soon after infection the organisms penetrate into the lymphatics and the regional lymph nodes become enlarged, firm but painless. Finally they reach the bloodstream where 4–8 weeks after the primary infection antibodies can be detected by serological tests.

Secondary stage   Other symptoms begin to develop about 6–10 weeks after the primary chancre. Symptoms may be so mild that once again they are overlooked and clinical diagnosis is often difficult as syphilis mimics many febrile and skin diseases. There is often a mild pyrexia, headache, sore throat, laryngitis which results in a painless loss of voice and general malaise. Mucous membrane lesions are seen on the lips, cheeks, tongue, pharynx and larynx, nose, vulva, vagina and cervix. These are shallow, painless ulcers with a greyish appearance and are described as 'snail track' ulcers. These lesions are highly infectious. The rash which develops varies in character and degree: the early rash is a faint pink erythema found on the shoulders, chest, back, abdomen and arms. The spots progress to a copper colour and may occur on the trunk, palms, arms, legs, soles, face and genitalia. The constant feature of a syphilitic rash is that it never irritates. In the moist areas such as the vulva and perianal region, flat-topped warts appear (*condylomata lata*); they are very infectious. The hair may fall out in patches (*syphilitic alopecia*) and eye conditions occur, commonly iritis, keratitis and retinitis.

The secondary stage is highly infectious, especially via the mucosal surfaces. As with the primary stage, it may pass unnoticed as the woman may never feel ill, the rash may be missed and other symptoms may not be urgent enough to cause her to seek advice. Occasionally the illness is obvious with a widespread rash, a high pyrexia and all the symptoms of fever and toxaemia.

Tertiary stage   The tertiary stage or late syphilis develops at any time from two years after the initial infection. Only a positive serological test diagnoses syphilis. The first clinical sign may be a tertiary lesion (*gummatous syphilis*) which may form on any part of the body. Cardiovascular syphilis involves blood vessels, particularly the aorta, which is affected by aortitis, an aneurysm, and aortic incompetence. Cerebral and spinal cord vessels may be affected with neurosyphilis developing finally as general paralysis of the insane or tabes dorsalis.

Diagnosis

Diagnosis may be confirmed by demonstrating the presence of *Treponema pallidum* in serum exudate obtained from a chancre using dark ground microscopy.

The following *non-specific serological tests* may be used:

▶ Venereal disease reference laboratory slide test (VDRL).
▶ Rapid plasma reagin (RPR).

A positive reaction may occur in the presence of any treponemal disease (yaws, bejel and pinta). A biological false positive reaction can occur after a viral infection (glandular fever, measles, chickenpox, mumps, herpes simplex and zoster), or following vaccination. Reactive results must be confirmed by a diagnostic *specific test*, such as:

▶ *Treponema pallidum* haemagglutination test (TPHA).

▶ Fluorescent treponemal antibody absorption test (FTA-ABS).

A selection of the non-specific tests are carried out; if these produce a positive reaction the tests are repeated using a specific test.

Congenital syphilis

Congenital syphilis rarely occurs in Britain due to routine screening of all pregnant women although there is now concern about the rising level of syphilis in women and several cases of congenital syphilis have been reported (Nicoll and Moisley, 1994). Prenatal infection is almost 100% when the woman has untreated primary or secondary disease. At birth the baby may appear normal and physically healthy; usually after the first weeks or months the signs of early congenital syphilis appear. These include snuffles due to rhinitis associated with osteitis of the nasal bones; cracks and fissures around the anus, nose or mouth which may heal with radiating scars called *rhagades*; and various skin rashes, including syphilitic pemphigus on the palms and soles.

Late congenital syphilis appears after 2 years of age. The clinical features are similar to adult late disease. The effects can cause a saddle nose, interstitial keratitis, nerve deafness, deformities of long bones and other abnormalities.

Syphilis may cause a late abortion, after 12–16 weeks' gestation, or intrauterine death resulting in a macerated stillbirth; in this case the placenta may be large, pale and heavy.

Prophylaxis and treatment

Routine serological examination should be carried out at the first antenatal visit. A combination of the VDRL test and the TPHA test can confirm syphilis. Sexual contacts and any siblings should also be examined. The usual treatment for early infectious syphilis is 600 000 units of procaine penicillin daily for 10 days. Other stages of syphilis require 900 000 units of procaine penicillin daily for 14–21 days. If the woman is sensitive to penicilllin, erythromycin 500 mg, four times a day for 14–28 days can be given.

The mother can be reassured that prevention of fetal infection is almost 100%, provided treatment is started early in pregnancy, preferably before 16–20 weeks.

If erythromycin is used, or early congenital syphilis

diagnosed, the neonate should be given a course of penicillin.

After treatment has been completed, the woman should be followed up for repeat serological testing and to assess clinical relapse or reinfection.

GONORRHOEA

This is infection of the genital tract by *Neisseria gonorrhoeae* (Figure 4), a bean-shaped intracellular diplococcus. It can infect the immature mucous membrane of the vulva and vagina before puberty. In women it can infect the urethra, cervix, rectum and mouth. Transmission to the fetus at delivery can lead to conjunctivitis in the neonate (*ophthalmia neonatorum*). It is a notifiable disease.

Symptoms and signs

The incubation period is usually 2–5 days. Asymptomatic infection is common in the female, therefore the disease may spread to the Bartholin's glands and fallopian tubes.

In the rare acute case, the woman may complain of a mucopurulent vaginal discharge, dysuria and frequency of micturition and a rectal discharge.

The condition must be differentiated from the commoner monilial vaginitis and trichomonal vaginitis.

The diagnosis is established by culture of a urethral and endocervical smear to identify the characteristic microorganism. The specimen must be plated directly or put into a suitable transport material immediately because the organism is sensitive to heat and drying.

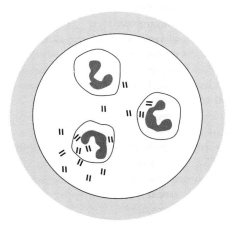

Figure 4   *Neisseria gonorrhoeae* in pus cells.

Treatment

Penicillin (e.g. amoxycillin 2 g) in association with probenecid 1 g as a single dose is sufficient treatment in the majority of cases. For penicillin-resistant gonococci an alternative treatment with cefuroxime 1 g or erythromycin stearate 500 mg twice a day for four days may be necessary.

Sexual partners of the woman should be traced to prevent spread of infection or reinfection.

Gonococcal ophthalmia

If a woman has gonorrhoea the eyes of the fetus may become infected during birth. If untreated, permanent blindness can occur. The signs are profuse purulent discharge occurring within 2–4 days of birth, unilateral or bilateral, and oedema and redness of the eyelid.

Diagnosis is by microscopy and culture of discharge taken from the eye. Saline bathing is performed and the baby nursed to avoid infection of the unaffected eye. Systemic penicillin (e.g. benzyl penicillin) 500 000 units/kg body weight in two divided doses for several days is given.

Ophthalmia neonatorum is highly contagious therefore the mother and baby should occupy a single room in hospital and universal infection control precautions should be adopted.

HERPES GENITALIS

Herpes genitalis is caused by the herpes simplex type II virus and is transmitted by sexual intercourse. Type I virus can cause genital infection but is usually associated with lesions of the face, lips and eyes.

The closely sited vesicles may involve the vulva, vagina, cervix and urethra. The virus can spread to the perianal area, anus and rectum, buttocks and thighs.

Primary herpes presents with painful genital ulcers and inguinal lymphadenopathy occurs. The vulva and the cervix are affected. Fever, malaise, headache, photophobia and viral meningitis can occur. When the urethra and bladder are affected there is severe dysuria and retention of urine is possible.

Reactivation of the virus produces recurrences of the infection which are milder and shorter. The diagnosis must always be confirmed by culture, which can exclude associated infections.

Treatment includes prevention or treatment of secondary infection and analgesics to relieve the pain. Acyclovir 200 mg five times daily for 5–7 days following a first dose of 400 mg can reduce the duration of the primary attack. Recurrent infections may require acyclovir suppressive therapy.

Infection is a potential hazard to the baby during vaginal delivery. If active lesions are detected on the external genitalia, vagina or cervix a Caesarean section should be performed, but only if the membranes have been ruptured for less than four hours.

Neonatal screening should be undertaken following delivery and acyclovir treatment given if necessary. Annual cervical cytology is recommended for all women with this condition.

Genital Warts

Genital warts (condylomata acuminata) are caused by a virus infection. They may affect the introitus and vulva, vagina, cervix, perineum, anus and rectum. The disease can be transmitted by sexual contact so the partner should be screened and treated.

During pregnancy the genital warts may increase in size, but recede again in the puerperium. Treatment is not generally considered during pregnancy unless requested by the woman. Cryotherapy or diathermy may be used but podophyllin should be avoided. Viral shedding is most prevalent during treatment.

An infant or child may develop laryngeal warts due to infection from the mother at delivery, but Caesarean section is only indicated if the warts are extremely large.

Chlamydia trachomatis Infections

The chlamydiae are small, intracellular parasites with features similar to bacteria. They may be the cause of subclinical infections for many years. Chlamydiae may be detected in an endocervical specimen containing epithelial cells, by culture and serological methods.

The incidence of chlamydial infections has increased. In many cases there may be a combined infection of *C. trachomatis* and *N. gonorrhoeae* (Kane, 1984). Women who have any sexually transmitted disease, evidence of pelvic infection, multiple sexual partners, or a partner with non-specific urethritis should be screened for *C. trachomatis*.

Signs and symptoms

Women with chlamydial infections present with a mucopurulent vaginal discharge from the cervix, abdominal pain due to pelvic inflammatory disease, frequency of micturition and dysuria which may have an acute onset.

C. trachomatis is now recognized as a major cause of non-gonococcal cervicitis, salpingitis and pelvic inflammatory disease (Cateral, 1981; Conway *et al.*, 1984). This leads to problems of spontaneous abortion, ectopic pregnancy and infertility.

The newborn infant may develop chlamydial conjunctivitis or severe ophthalmia and a nasopharyngitis or pneumonia. Saline bathing for ocular infection and erythromycin for all infections are used to treat the neonate (Sutherland, 1992).

The mother and her sexual partner must be screened and treated.

Treatment

If there is a risk of pregnancy, a diagnosed pregnancy or breastfeeding occurring the drug of choice is erythromycin 500 mg twice a day for 14 days. The woman's sexual partner should also be examined and treated, if infected.

Viral Hepatitis

There are four forms of viral hepatitis:

1 *Hepatitis A virus* is excreted in faeces and is spread through oral–anal contact.
2 *Hepatitis non-A non-B virus(es)* are transmitted through parenteral and percutaneous routes by blood and blood products. Infection can also occur by transmission from person to person and by sexual contact.
3 *Hepatitis D virus* requires the presence of hepatitis B virus to produce infection.
4 *Hepatitis B virus* is blood-borne and highly infective. The major route of transmission is through sexual contact. Maternal–fetal transmission can occur but is rare.

Signs and symptoms

Acute infection may be subclinical and an unrecognized carrier status may develop. Symptoms of viral hepatitis include fever, headache, malaise, nausea, vomiting, anorexia followed by jaundice. Enlargement of the liver and spleen can occur, with a risk of developing chronic hepatitis or cirrhosis.

Management

Bedrest is advised during acute viral hepatitis and avoidance of alcohol and drugs until liver function tests return to normal. A low-fat, high-protein and high-carbohydrate diet is prescribed.

Intrauterine infection is rare. Acute maternal hepatitis B infection during pregnancy can lead to transmission at birth. Perinatal transmission also occurs from mothers who are chronic carriers. Protection by an immunization programme is offered for the infant. Breastfeeding is recommended for all infants, whether or not they have been immunized.

Human Immunodeficiency Virus (HIV)

The human immunodeficiency virus is a slow-acting retrovirus. The most common carrier is the T helper lymphocyte. Two types of HIV have been recognized: *HIV-1* and *HIV-2*. The virus is contained in blood and body fluids and the main routes of infection are penetrative sexual intercourse, blood transfusion and maternal to fetus or infant.

Serological testing detects the titre of HIV antibodies present. Seroconversion can take 4–12 weeks following infection and a false negative result is obtained during this period.

Signs and symptoms

During seroconversion the majority of people remain asymptomatic. A few people develop malaise, fever, lethargy, sore throat, enlarged lymph glands and sore muscles and joints (Adler, 1987). There are four main diseases caused by HIV:

1 Persistent generalized lymphadenopathy (PGL).
2 AIDS-related complex (ARC).
3 Acquired immune deficiency syndrome (AIDS).
4 Neurological HIV.

Progression from infection to disease varies but half will develop diagnostic criteria within 10 years.

Management

The incidence of HIV in women of childbearing age varies throughout Britain. Anonymous serum screening of antenatal women provides an indication of the present rates. Otherwise antenatal diagnosis is performed on the basis of risk assessment of the mother and with her informed consent or maternal request. In some clinics all women are offered screening for HIV (Chrystie *et al.*, 1995).

A plan of care should be devised in consultation with the woman incorporating obstetric, medical and paediatric services. Counselling should be provided during the antenatal period. Information regarding transmission, maternal prognosis and neonatal infection must be given. The woman may wish to terminate her pregnancy because of her HIV status.

Smoking, alcohol and drug use should be minimized during pregnancy. Referral to specialist agencies may be necessary to achieve abstinence and provide appropriate support. Maintenance of good health and nutrition is important, and any infections should be recognized and treated early. Cervical cytology and screening for other sexually transmitted diseases should be performed.

Routes of maternal transmission of HIV

The three major routes of transmission of HIV during childbirth are:

1 Transplacental.
2 Ingestion or inoculation at birth.
3 Breastfeeding.

Transplacental   Infection can be transmitted to the fetus through the placenta from the maternal circulation. The incidence of vertical transmission is between 15 and 40%. Seroconversion during pregnancy, a rise in HIV-related illness, and a decrease in immune function increase the risk.

Ingestion or inoculation at birth   HIV transmission at birth can occur irrespective of mode of delivery, although Caesarean section may reduce the risk. Artificial rupture of membranes, application of fetal scalp electrode, fetal blood sampling, episiotomy and instrumental delivery appear to increase the risk of infection. Ingestion or inoculation of vaginal fluids or maternal blood is considered responsible. Genital ulceration may be an additional factor.

Breastfeeding The risk of transmission through breastfeeding for women who seroconverted prior to delivery is double, and the risk if the mother is infected postnatally while lactating may be higher. In developed countries where an alternative substitute is available, breastfeeding is not advised.

Neonatal management

All babies are HIV antibody positive at birth but virological and immunological markers can diagnose an infected infant. Some infected infants contract *Pneumocystis carinii* pneumonia in the first few months and die. The prognosis is variable for the remainder therefore routine follow-up is essential. Active and

passive immunization is recommended as the risk of childhood infections outweigh any vaccine risk.

Prevention

Avoidance of high-risk activities such as unprotected sexual intercourse, multiple partners, and intravenous drug-taking can prevent HIV infection.

Reducing the risk of infecting a partner when conception is desired can be achieved by unprotected sexual intercourse occurring only around the time of ovulation. If the partner is HIV positive, reinfection should be avoided as it may accelerate the disease.

Protection of medical staff is based on the use of universal infection control policies whenever providing care. Local policies may indicate additional protective measures for known cases of HIV infection.

References

Adler, M.W. (1987) Development of the epidemic. *Br. Med. J.* **294**: 1083–1085.

Cateral, R.D. (1981) Biological effect of sexual freedom. *Lancet* i: 315–319.

Chrystie, I.L., Wolfe, C.D.A., Kennedy, J. *et al.* (1995) Voluntary named testing for HIV in a community based antenatal clinic: a pilot study. *Br. Med. J.* **311**: 928–931.

Conway, D., Glazener, C.M.A., Caul, E.O. *et al.* (1984) Chlamydial serology in fertile and infertile women. *Lancet* i: 191–193.

Kane, J.L. (1984) *Chlamydia trachomatis* infections and their importance to the gynaecologist. *J. Obstet. Gynaecol.* **4**: 246–254.

Nicoll, A. & Moisley, C. (1994) Antenatal screening for syphilis. *Br. Med. J.* **308**: 1253–1254.

Sutherland, S. (1992) *Chlamydia trachomatis.* In Greenough, A., Osborne, J. & Sutherland, S. (eds) *Congenital, Perinatal and Neonatal Infections*, pp. 35–47. Edinburgh: Churchill Livingstone.

Further Reading

Anonymous (1994) AZT for pregnant women: most physicians say AZT benefits outweigh fears, risks. *AIDS Alert* **9**(4): 53–55.

Batten, L. (1993) Women and HIV/AIDS: a literature review. *Nurs. Plaxis in New Zealand* **8**(2): 4–12.

Blaney, C.L. (1994) Pregnancy and HIV. *Network* **14**(3): 24–26.

Bond, S. & Rhodes, T.Y. (1990) HIV infection and community midwives: knowledge and attitudes. *Midwifery* **6**(2): 86–92.

Brierley, J. (1993) HIV and AIDS in childbirth: are midwives responding to the needs of women? *Midwives Chron.* **106**: 317–325.

Butz, A., Hutton, N. & Larson, E. (1991) Immunoglobulins and growth parameters at birth of infants born to HIV seropositive and seronegative women. *Am, J, Pub. Health* **81**(10): 1323–1326.

Chin, J. (1994) The growing impact of HIV/AIDS pomdemic on children born to HIV-infected women. *Clin. in Perinatol.* **21**(1): 1–14.

Clane, M.J. (1992) The diagnosis and management of maternal and congenital syphilis. *J. Nurs-Mid.* **37**(1): 4–16.

Dinsmoor, M.J. (1994) HIV infection and pregnancy. *Clin. in Perinatol.* **21**(1): 85–94.

Fogel, C.I. (1995) Sexually transmitted diseases. In: *Annual review of women's health*, volume II. *Nat. League for Nurs. Pub.* **2**: 205–219.

Kelley, K.F., Galbraith, M.A. & Vermund, S.H. (1992) Genital human papillomovirus infection in women. *J. Obstet. Gynecol. & Neonatal Nurs.* **21**(6): 503–515.

Killion, C. (1994) Pregnancy: a critical time to target STDs. *Am. J. Nat. Child Nurs.* **19**(3): 156–161.

Kuhn, L., Stein, Z.A., Thomas, P.A. *et al.* (1994) Maternal-infant HIV transmission and circumstances of delivery. *Am. J. Pub. Health* **84**(7): 1110–1115.

Meadows, J., Catalon, J. & Gazzard, B. (1993) HIV antibody testing in the antenatal clinic: the views of consumers. *Midwifery* **9**(2): 63–69.

Nze, K., Sharp, T., Burrows, L. *et al.* (1987) Supporting the mother and infant at risk for AIDS. *Nursing* **17**(11): 44–47.

RCOG (Royal College of Obstetricians and Gynaecologists) (1990) *HIV Infection in Maternity Care and Gynaecology.* London: RCOG.

Squires, K. (1994) HIV infection in women. *J. Women's Health* **3**(5): 383–386.

Walker, C.K. & Sweet, C.L. (1992) Pregnancy and pediatric HIV infection. *Curr. Opin. Infect. Dis.* **5**(2): 201–213.

Weiss, S.H. & Louria, D.B. (1994) Quo vadis: perinatal AIDS issues – 2004. *Clin. in Perinatol.* **21**(1): 179–198.

WHO (World Health Organization) (1990) *AIDS prevention: Guidelines for MCH/FP Programme Managers*, Series I, II & III. Geneva: WHO.

WHO (1995) HIV and AIDS in pregnancy. *Safe Motherhood* **16**: 1 & 4–8.

Williams, A.B. (1990) Reproductive concerns of women at risk for HIV infection. *J. Nurs. Mid.* **35**(5): 292–298.

44

Abnormalities of the Genital Tract (and Female Genital Mutilation)

Approximately 3% of women have a developmental anomaly of the genital tract (Llewellyn Jones, 1990). Pregnancy and labour may also be affected by other conditions such as fibroids or uterine displacements.

Developmental Anomalies

The majority of the female genital tract arises from the Müllerian ducts which form during embryonic life. The ducts fuse and the median septum then breaks down, thus forming a single uterus. Should this process fail, abnormalities such as *double uterus* (with or without a double cervix and vagina), *bicornuate uterus* or *subseptate uterus* will occur (Figure 1). As the Müllerian and Wolffian ducts develop close together in embryonic life, genital tract anomalies may be accompanied by malformations of the kidney and ureter (Tindall, 1987; Rabinerson *et al.*, 1991).

Provided the cervix and vagina are patent the woman is usually fertile: the ovaries are almost always present even if the rest of the genital tract is grossly malformed or absent.

UNICORNUATE UTERUS

This uncommon abnormality arises from failure of development of one of the Müllerian ducts. It is associated with renal tract anomalies on the same side as the

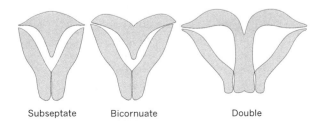

Subseptate   Bicornuate   Double

Figure 1   Uterine malformations.

missing duct. Occasionally a rudimentary or vestigial horn may be present. Pregnancy can be expected to progress normally although breech presentation is common and preterm labour is more likely (Michalas, 1991). Uterine function in labour is usually normal (Tindall, 1987). If the pregnancy develops in a rudimentary horn the outcome is usually spontaneous abortion or occasionally rupture of the rudimentary horn, as the myometrium becomes rapidly stretched. Pre-eclampsia has been reported as a complication of rudimentary horn pregnancy (Emembolu, 1989).

DOUBLE UTERUS (UTERUS DIDELPHIS)

This may be accompanied by a double vagina. As the pregnancy progresses the midwife will notice that the fundus feels unusually wide. Breech presentation is common. As the pregnancy grows the non-pregnant uterus will enlarge under the influence of the pregnancy hormones and may occupy space in the pelvis, thus obstructing labour. Twin pregnancy has been recorded, with a fetus in each half of a double uterus (Kekkonen *et al.*, 1991).

SUBSEPTATE AND BICORNUATE UTERUS

This occurs when complete obliteration of the Müllerian septum fails. A subseptate uterus is outwardly normal but the midwife may recognize a bicornuate uterus which has a wide, heart-shaped fundus. This can be detected on abdominal examination and may even be visible under the abdominal wall in a very slim woman, especially after the third stage of labour. Subseptate and bicornuate uterus are associated with transverse lie and breech presentation, as the abnormal uterine structure hinders the normal process of spontaneous version which occurs between 30 and 34 weeks' gestation. Attempts at external cephalic version of the fetus will be unsuccessful.

The midwife should be aware of any woman with a history of successive malpresentation as this may indicate the presence of a structural abnormality of the uterus. The progress of the first and second stage of labour is usually normal where there is a subseptate or bicornuate uterus. However, retained placenta may occur in the third stage and 50% of women with these types of uterine anomaly require a manual removal of placenta. The incidence of postpartum haemorrhage is also increased (Tindall, 1987).

VAGINAL SEPTUM (Figure 2)

A vaginal septum may be longitudinal or transverse and may be complete or partial. It may be detected on vaginal examination but as the tissue is usually soft and is easily deflected by the examining fingers the diagnosis may be overlooked. A high vaginal septum may prevent cervical dilatation and may obstruct descent of the fetus during labour. Where the breech presents, the fetus may sit astride a longitudinal septum. In the second stage of labour the septum may be palpated or may be visible in front of the advancing presenting part and may require division in order to allow delivery of the fetus (Kelsall, 1992).

ASSOCIATED PROBLEMS

The presence of a uterine malformation is associated with a four-fold increase in the risk of spontaneous abortion and preterm labour (Llewellyn Jones, 1990). The poorly formed myometrium is unable to stretch and develop to accommodate the rapidly growing fetus. Cervical incompetence is common in cases of uterine malformation (Michalas, 1991). The pregnancy will also be unstable and more likely to abort if the placental site is on a septum. Ultrasound scanning during pregnancy will usually reveal the presence of a uterine abnormality. The midwife should inform the doctor so that appropriate care may be planned as there is a higher likelihood of the need for surgical intervention during labour.

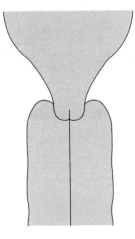

Figure 2   Longitudinal vaginal septum.

Displacements of the Uterus

RETROVERSION OF THE GRAVID UTERUS

Retroversion of the uterus, where the pregnant uterus falls back into the hollow of the sacrum (Figure 3), occurs in at least 10% of women and is normally of little clinical significance. It is not associated with infertility or an increased rate of spontaneous abortion (Llewellyn Jones, 1990). During pregnancy the condition usually resolves spontaneously as the uterus grows, becomes erect and rises into the abdomen around the 12th week.

However, in approximately one in 3000 cases the retroversion fails to resolve and the uterus becomes fixed or incarcerated in the pelvis (Keating *et al.*, 1992). This is more likely to occur where uterine malformation or pelvic adhesions are present (Llewellyn Jones, 1990). By the 14th or 15th week of pregnancy the retroverted pregnant uterus completely fills the pelvis, the cervix is drawn up towards the pelvic brim, the anterior vaginal wall is stretched and so, at the same time, is the urethra. The urethra then becomes narrowed and the mother is unable to pass urine.

Diagnosis

The woman will at first complain of difficulty in micturition and later of complete inability to pass urine, i.e. retention of urine occurs. The bladder becomes more and more distended and, if it is unrelieved, overflow incontinence will occur as small amounts of urine escape.

At this stage the woman will complain of severe abdominal pain. On examination of the abdomen there is a large soft swelling above the pubes. The swelling, which is the bladder, may rise to the level of umbilicus or even above it. The fundus is not palpable at the brim of the pelvis.

Treatment

The woman requires hospital treatment. The bladder is emptied slowly by catheter and is kept empty with a self-retaining catheter draining into a sterile urine collection bag until bladder tone returns. Once the bladder is empty the uterus usually corrects its malposition spontaneously. This may be assisted if the mother lies in the semi-prone or Sims position. The retroversion will not recur, since the uterus is growing steadily and will, in a few days, be too big to fall back into the pelvis. Occasionally spontaneous correction does not occur and then manipulation under anaesthesia is necessary.

Uterine incarceration which persists into the third trimester has been reported but is very rare. In such cases the uterine fundus lies in the pouch of Douglas (Van Winter *et al.*, 1991; Keating *et al.*, 1992).

Dangers

Urinary tract infection is likely due to stasis of urine in the overdistended bladder. The midwife should send a catheter specimen of urine for microscopy and any infection must be treated promptly. In exceptional cases sloughing of the bladder and rupture may occur. The pregnancy is at risk as spontaneous abortion is more likely. Persistent incarceration may cause sacculation of the anterior uterine wall. The pregnancy will then enlarge into the abdomen and this may confuse the diagnosis.

ANTEVERSION OF THE GRAVID UTERUS (PENDULOUS ABDOMEN) (Figure 4)

This unusual condition is commoner in multiparous women whose abdominal muscles have been weakened by repeated pregnancies. Separation of the recti abdominis allows the uterus to fall forward and in extreme cases the fundus may lie below the symphysis pubis. As the uterus becomes heavier the woman will complain of

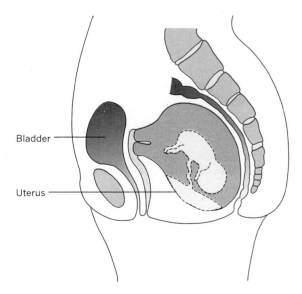

Figure 3   Incarceration of the gravid uterus.

Bladder

Uterus

backache and abdominal pain. The presenting part will not engage and dystocia is likely because the long axis of the uterus is at an angle to the pelvic brim (Llewellyn Jones, 1990). A well-fitting binder or corset will relieve the mother's discomfort and encourage engagement of the presenting part (Llewellyn Jones, 1990). The binder should be worn during labour to facilitate engagement and descent of the fetus. The 'all-fours' delivery position should be avoided.

PROLAPSE OF THE GRAVID UTERUS

Although rarely seen, pregnancy may occur in a partially prolapsed uterus. The condition is much commoner in multiparous women when the uterovaginal supports have become lax and allow the uterus to descend so that the cervix is found at or just behind the vaginal introitus. The condition is most troublesome in the first trimester of pregnancy as the uterus increases in size and weight and the ligaments soften and relax. The doctor may insert a ring pessary to relieve the prolapse. As the uterus grows and becomes an abdominal organ the condition improves. Labour usually proceeds normally and cervical dilatation may

be rapid (Beischer and Mackay, 1986; Llewellyn Jones, 1990; Lewis and Chamberlain, 1990).

Fibromyomata (Fibroids)

Fibroids are clinically apparent in about five per 2000 white women (Lewis and Chamberlain, 1990). They are commoner in older women and in young West Indian and West African women.

On palpation of the uterus one or more smooth rounded swellings may be felt continuous with the wall of the uterus (Figure 5). A large fibroid may be mistaken for a fetal head. In pregnancy, hypertrophy of the myometrial fibres and increased vascularity and oedema cause the fibroid to enlarge and soften. Red degeneration (*necrobiosis*) occurs due to venous obstruction (Lewis and Chamberlain, 1990). These changes often cause pain and local tenderness but surgical intervention is rarely necessary.

The doctor will order analgesic drugs to relieve the pain. Most fibroids are found in the body of the uterus and do not affect the course of labour. Rarely, one may occur in the lower segment beneath the presenting part. This will prevent descent of the fetus into the pelvis and may obstruct labour. A low-lying fibroid may be felt on vaginal examination.

During the third stage of labour postpartum haemorrhage may occur, especially if the placental site overlies a fibroid (Lewis and Chamberlain, 1990).

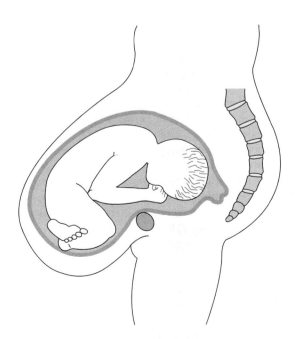

Figure 4   Pendulous abdomen.

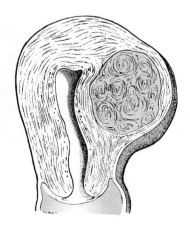

Figure 5   Uterine fibroid

Labour and delivery should take place in hospital in case difficulty should arise. During the puerperium fibroids regress and become smaller as autolysis reduces the myometrial mass.

Ovarian Cyst

An ovarian cyst in association with pregnancy is less common than fibroids, occurring in less than one in 1000 cases. The tumour is malignant in about 10% of women under 30 and the incidence of malignancy rises in older women (Lewis and Chamberlain, 1990).

The cyst may be in the abdomen or in the pelvis and may be discovered on ultrasound scanning or pelvic examination in early pregnancy (Figure 6). It is generally recommended that the cyst should be removed as soon as possible because of the risk of malignancy or torsion (either before or after delivery). Removal before the 12th week carries a risk of miscarriage if the corpus luteum is removed before the placenta is ready to take over the hormonal support of the pregnancy (Lewis and Chamberlain, 1990). If undetected or untreated, an ovarian cyst lying within the pelvic cavity may obstruct labour.

Female Genital Mutilation

The custom of female genital mutilation (female circumcision) is still relatively common among some groups of African women, particularly those from Nigeria, Ethiopia, the Sudan and Egypt. It is a traditional practice among some African Muslims, although there is no Koranic justification for it and it predates the foundation of Islam for it is mentioned in a Greek

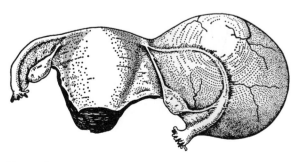

Figure 6 A uterus with a simple serous cyst.

papyrus from around 163 BC (Egwuatu and Agugua, 1981). It is carried out in order to control women's sexuality and to promote chastity.

The operation may be performed at any time from shortly after birth to adolescence (Trevelyn, 1994). There are three main types of female genital mutilation:

▶ Simple excision of the clitoral hood and suturing of the labia majora.
▶ Removal of the clitoris (*clitoridectomy*).
▶ *Infibulation* or *pharaonic circumcision*: This is the most extensive type and is similar to a simple vulvectomy (Jordan, 1994). In this operation the clitoris, labia minora and most of the labia majora are excised and the labial remnants are closed together, leaving a small orifice near the fourchette which allows the escape of urine and menstrual blood.

Female genital mutilation is illegal in the UK and many other countries and is usually carried out in the family's home village by the traditional birth attendant or the older women. Aseptic precautions and anaesthesia are not used. The instrument may be a sharpened piece of metal or glass. Fusion of the labial remnants is encouraged by binding the girl's legs together. Infection and acute urinary retention are common. When healing occurs there may be complete fusion of the labia which requires urgent surgical correction. On marriage, penetrative sexual intercourse may be impossible due to the vulval stenosis and the husband may enlarge his wife's vaginal introitus with a sharp instrument (Thompson, 1989).

Female genital mutilation carries a significant immediate mortality from haemorrhage and sepsis. Lifelong morbidity from urinary infection, pelvic inflammatory disease, endometriosis and renal damage is common. Contraceptive choice is limited by the vulval stenosis and cervical smears are impossible to obtain (Trevelyan, 1994). Psychological trauma and marital disharmony are common (Jordan, 1994).

In pregnancy, urinary tract infection is likely. Progress during labour is hard to assess due to the difficulty in performing a vaginal examination (Trevelyan, 1994). During birth, the second stage of labour may be considerably prolonged because of the rigidity of the scar tissue. This may result in fetal hypoxia and brain damage (Thompson, 1989). The midwife must be prepared to perform an anterior episiotomy, separating the labial remnants. There may be severe damage to the pelvic floor: rupture of the anal sphincter is more likely as the rigidity of the vulval tissue causes undue pressure to be exerted in the posterior part of the birth canal. If the perineum is not meticulously repaired faecal incontinence will result. This would have disastrous consequences for the woman as divorce and social ostracism often follow such problems. The midwife or obstetrician must be careful not to repair the labia in such a way as to restore the infibulated state (Jordan, 1994). This would be illegal, although the midwife may face strong pressure to do so from the woman and her relatives.

Uterine prolapse is not uncommon even following a first baby. If the infant is a girl, the midwife must be aware that the mother may wish to have the child circumcised.

References

Beischer, N. & Mackay, E. (1986) *Obstetrics and the Newborn*. London: Baillière Tindall.

Egwuata, V. & Agugua, N. (1981) Complications of female circumcision in Nigerian Igbos. *Br. J. Obstet. Gynaecol.* **88**: 1090–1093.

Emembolu, J. (1989) Rudimentary horn pregnancy associated with pre-eclampsia. *Int. J. Gynaecol. Obstet.* **30**(4): 367–370.

Jordan, J. (1994) Female genital mutilation (female circumcision). *Br. J. Obstet. Gynaecol.* **101**: 94–95.

Keating, P., Walton, S. & Maouris, P. (1992) Incarceration of a bicornuate retroverted gravid uterus presenting with bilateral ureteric obstruction. *Br. J. Obstet. Gynaecol.* **99**: 345–347.

Kekkonen, R., Nuutila, M. & Laatikainen, T. (1991) Twin pregnancy with a fetus in each half of a uterus didelphys. *Acta Obstet. Gynecol. Scand.* **70**: 373–374.

Kelsall, J. (1992) Unusual delay in the second stage. *A.R.M. Midwifery Matters* 52(Spring): 21, 30.

Lewis, T. & Chamberlain, G. (eds) (1990) *Obstetrics by Ten Teachers*. Sevenoaks: Hodder & Stoughton.

Llewellyn Jones, D. (1990) *Fundamentals of Obstetrics and Gynaecology*, 5th edn, Vol 1: *Obstetrics*. London: Faber & Faber.

Michalas, S. (1991) Outcome of pregnancy in women with uterine malformation: evaluation of 62 cases. *Int. J. Gynecol. Obstet.* **35**: 215–219.

Rabinerson, D., Neri, A. & Yardena, O. (1991) Combined anomalies of the Mullerian and Wolffian Systems. *Acta Obstet. Gynecol. Scand.* **71**: 156–157.

Thompson, J. (1989) Torture by tradition. *Nursing Times* 85(15) 12 April: 16–17.

Tindall, V.R. (1987) *Jeffcoate's Principles of Gynaecology*. London: Butterworths.

Trevelyan, J. (1994) Women's health: discrimination, tradition. *Nursing Times* **90**(15): 49–50.

Van Winter, J., Ogburn, P., Ney, J. & Hetzel, D. (1991) Uterine incarceration during the third trimester: a rare complication of pregnancy. *Mayo Clin. Proc.* **66**: 608–613.

Further Reading

Baker, C., Gilson, G., Vill, M. & Curet, L. (1993) Female circumcision: obstetric issues. *Am. J. Obstet. Gynecol.* **169**(6): 1616–1618.

Higman Davis, J. (1992) Female genital mutilation – a practice that should have vanished. *Midwives Chronicle* February: 33.

Moutos, D., Damewood, M., Schaff, W. & Rock, J. (1992) A comparison of reproductive outcome between women with a unicornuate uterus and women with a didelphic uterus. *Fertil. Steril.* **58**(1): 88–93.

Webb, E. & Hartley, B. (1994) Female genital mutilation: a dilemma in child protection. *Arch. Dis. Childh.* **70**(5): 441–443.

45

Multiple Pregnancy

Currently the incidence of multiple pregnancy is increasing in many countries. This is particularly so in the case of triplets and higher order births and is largely due to improvements in the treatment of infertile couples. The highest reported incidence of twinning is 45 per 1000 maternities in the Yoruba tribe in Nigeria (Nylander, 1967, 1970). Japan, on the other hand, has a rate of only 5.6 per 1000 births (Imaizumi and Inouye, 1984).

In 1989 the twinning rate in the United Kingdom was about 11 per 1000 births and increasing (Registrar General, 1989). Triplet births have more than doubled since 1985. Latest available figures give a rate of 13.16 per 1000 maternities (OPCS London, GRO Scotland and GRO Northern Ireland, 1994) (Table 1). It is possible that the rates of multiple conceptions are much higher than these figures indicate. Early ultrasound scanning of mothers has demonstrated twin fetal sacs in the first trimester of pregnancy but subsequent examinations reveal a singleton pregnancy. This phenomenon is described as the *'vanishing' twin syndrome* (Landy *et al.*, 1986). A further group omitted from the figures are those born before the 24th week of pregnancy. If one infant survives but the other does not, the birth will be registered as a singleton one. It would seem therefore that the incidence of multiple pregnancy may indeed be much higher than the figures suggest (Figure 1).

The implication for maternity and neonatal care of increases in multiple births is of concern. The pregnancies carry high risks for both mother and infants. They put strains on already overstretched neonatal services and are extremely costly (Papiernik, 1991). Perinatal mortality is high, causing great distress for families and stress to the midwifery, nursing and medical staff who care for them (Botting *et al.*, 1987; Bryan, 1991).

Table 1 Incidence of multiple births in the UK, 1994

| | Number of maternities | | | |
	England and Wales	Scotland	N. Ireland	*All UK*
Singletons	650 801	60 429	23 847	734 077
Twins	8 451	778	289	9 518
Triplets	260	16	6	282
Quads and more	8	1	0	9
All multiples	8 719	795	295	9 809
All maternities	659 520	61 224	24 142	744 986
Multiple birth rate per 1000 maternities	13.2	13.0	12.2	13.16

Source: OPCS (London), GRO Scotland and GRO N. Ireland. Crown Copyright.
N.B. Figures include live and stillbirths.

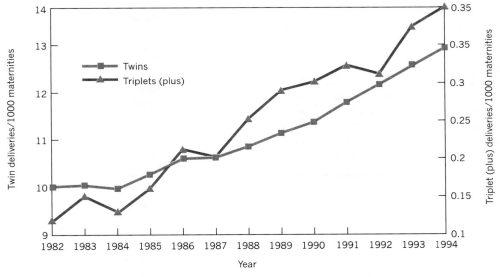

Figure 1 Recent trends in multiple births, England and Wales, 1982–1994. (Reproduced with permission from OPCS, Medical Statistics Division, St. Catherine's House, London.)

Biology of Twinning

At least two types of twins are recognized:

1 *Monozygotic, uniovular* (often described as *identical* or *MZ*) twins are the result of fertilization of a single ovum by one spermatozoon (zygote). Within a few days the embryonic cell mass divides into two identical halves. Each half develops into a single fetus with its own amniotic sac. They usually share a placenta and chorion. Occasionally only one amniotic sac is present. Monozygotic twins are always of the same sex and have the same coloured eyes and blood groups. Conjoined or Siamese twins are rare and result from incomplete division of the blastocyst. There is frequently intrauterine growth retardation of one or both infants. Occasionally one may die in early pregnancy. This fetus becomes flattened and mummified and is known as a *fetus papyraceus*.

2 *Dizygotic, binovular* (also called *fraternal, familial* or *DZ*) twins result from the fertilization of two

ova by two spermatozoa. Two complete, separate fetuses develop in the uterus at the same time, each with their own cord, placenta, chorion and amnion. They may be like sex or boy and girl. They may be as similar or as unalike as any other siblings in a family.

It has been suggested in recent years that a third, very rare type of twinning may exist (Bulmer, 1970; Corney and Robson, 1975). This twinning would be the result of two spermatozoa fertilizing a single ovum which has split. These twins, although monovular, are not monozygotic and diagnosis is difficult.

Aetiology

Monozygotic twinning appears to be constant at 3.5 per 1000 throughout the world. It is the dizygotic twinning rate which varies. Some factors which influence this include:

1   *Maternal age and parity*: Single mothers and those who conceive within three months of marriage are more at risk. It is thought that irregularity of sexual intercourse may account for the high incidence in unwed mothers and very high levels of sexual activity for multiple conception in early marriage (Noble, 1991). Older mothers or those who already have several children are also prone to multiple conception (Bryan, 1992).
2   *Maternal height and weight*: Tall women are more likely to conceive twins than are their smaller counterparts (MacGillivray *et al.*, 1988). Thin, undernourished women are less likely to give birth to twins than those who are of average weight or obese (Campbell *et al.*, 1974).
3   *Fertility*: Mothers expecting twins appear to conceive more easily. Most are pregnant within six months of trying and unplanned pregnancy is common (Spillman, 1992).
4   *Inherited factors*: Most twins inherit dominant rather than recessive genes from their mother. It is suggested that the genotype of the mother rather than that of the father affects the frequency of dizygotic twinning (Linney, 1983).
5   *Treatment of infertility*: Ovulation stimulants are said to account for 10–15% of twin births (Webster and Ellwood, 1985). The introduction of *in vitro* fertilization (IVF), often combined with

drugs, has resulted in many more multiple births, particularly of the higher orders. More recently, the use of gamete intra-fallopian tube transfer (GIFT) has contributed a further increase (Bryan *et al.*, 1991).
6   *Contraceptive use*: It is reasonable to assume that the twinning rate would be rising even more rapidly had not oral contraceptives and other reliable methods of pregnancy prevention been introduced. However, Bracken (1979) reported an increased incidence of twin pregnancy in mothers who conceived soon after discontinuing the use of oral contraceptives.

Diagnosis

Ultrasound examination

It is now common practice in most maternity centres to routinely scan all pregnant women. Some units report nearly 100% detection rates of multiple pregnancies (Patel *et al.*, 1984). As a result it is now very uncommon for multiple pregnancy to remain undiagnosed. When there are triplets or more, the correct number of infants may only be ascertained after several scans (Macfarlane *et al.*, 1990). Ultrasound screening may be carried out as early as six weeks into the pregnancy and most women are aware of the multiple conception by the 18th week (Spillman, 1993a). When the diagnosis is made very early in the pregnancy, there is some doubt as to whether the mother should be told immediately or the news given later when the risk of the 'vanishing twin' syndrome is past (Bryan, 1992). Parents, on the whole, say they would prefer to know.

At whatever stage parents are told, it is essential that whoever shares the news is aware of the effect the revelation may have (Spillman, 1985). Although some mothers and fathers are delighted to know that more than one baby is expected, in many cases there are reactions of shock and disbelief (Spillman, 1986). It is important that an obstetrician or midwife is available to answer questions and give appropriate counselling at this time. It is also helpful if the mother can be put in touch with someone who has twin children who can understand and give reassurance. Equally an introduction to the local Twins Club as soon as possible after the diagnosis will offer access to appropriate literature, advice and support. If there is no club locally, independent membership of the Twins and Multiple Births

Association (TAMBA) may be a helpful alternative (see Useful Addresses).

Although in the United Kingdom, multiple pregnancy is most likely to be diagnosed by the sonographer, there may be situations, particularly in the developing world, where such technology is not available. A skilled midwife can apply other methods of detection.

Inspection

If the mother is sure of the date of her last menstrual period and the uterus looks larger than expected, twins may be the reason. A history of twins in the family would reinforce this suspicion.

Palpation

It much depends on the position of the fetuses in the uterus, how soon in the pregnancy multiples can be confirmed. It is unlikely before 28 weeks of gestation. If *two hard round heads* are felt, the woman has twins. A multiplicity of limbs and excessive fetal movements reported by the mother are also suggestive. A smaller than expected head for the size of the uterus, even if a second head cannot be felt, should also alert the midwife to the possibility that the pregnancy is a multiple one.

Palpation may be difficult, since polyhydramnios is a common complication of a twin pregnancy.

Auscultation

The use of 'Sonicaid' machines in monitoring fetal heartbeats has improved detection of more than one fetal heart rate. If such equipment is not available, two operators should simultaneously listen for at least one minute. If two heartbeats with a variation per minute of ten beats are recorded, almost certainly twin infants are present.

Radiography

The widespread use of ultrasound scanning has resulted in radiography of pregnant women being rarely used. The possible teratogenic effects on the fetus make the use of radiography before the 30th week of pregnancy undesirable.

Antenatal Management

Although the aim, as for all pregnant women, should be continuity of care throughout the pregnancy, this is often difficult to achieve. Broadbent (1985) reported that most of the mothers who expected twins in her study received all their antenatal care in consultant units. When 'shared care' occurred the mother seemed to have a greater rapport with her 'own' doctor and midwife. It would seem that this pattern may be changing. Spillman (1993a) found in a sample of 468 mothers of multiples, that half had received shared care between their general practitioner and attached midwife and the consultant unit. These mothers were happier with their antenatal care arrangements than those who had to travel to the consultant unit for all their antenatal care. However in both groups, many mothers had never previously met the midwives and doctors who were present at the time of delivery of their twins.

The essence of antenatal care should be awareness of possible complications. The aim should be prevention and prompt action should they occur.

It is also important that as well as counselling being offered at the time of diagnosis, parentcraft and relaxation classes should be started earlier in the pregnancy than for a mother expecting one baby. She should be encouraged to stop work at an earlier stage and visits to the delivery suite and neonatal unit should be arranged before the 22nd week of pregnancy.

Midwives should be aware of the enhanced role of fathers of multiples and their co-operation in the mother's care should be sought from the start.

COMPLICATIONS

When the pregnancy is a multiple one, minor disturbances are likely to be exaggerated. *Morning sickness* is often severe and prolonged. *Heartburn* is also often persistent. *Nightmares* are common and increase the risk of sleeplessness, particularly in the third trimester. Increased pressure may cause *oedema* of the ankles and *varicose veins* of the legs and vulva. As the pregnancy progresses, *dyspnoea*, *backache* and *exhaustion* are common.

It is important to encourage the mother to rest adequately in order to lessen the risks of these problems. In the past it was commonplace to admit most mothers expecting twins or more for rest in hospital. However, this has not been proven to be of benefit even for mothers at particular risk of preterm labour (Rydhstrom *et al.*, 1987; Crowther *et al.*, 1989). In France it has been shown that providing more advice and support in the home has resulted in a reduction in pregnancy complications and risk to the infants (Papiernik *et al.*, 1985).

A well-balanced diet should be encouraged. The hospital dietician may be able to offer advice on this aspect.

More serious complications may occur, including the following:

▶ *Pre-eclampsia* is reported to be more frequently found in multiple pregnancies (Bryan, 1992). McMullan *et al.* (1984) found the incidence to be higher in monozygotic than in dizygotic primigravid twin pregnancies.

▶ *Anaemia* is a risk. Two or more fetuses make much greater demands on the mother's stores of iron and folic acid. However, recent research suggests that iron and folic acid supplements prescribed to prevent the development of anaemia are unnecessary in most cases as the condition is transient and resolves. Only mothers with evidence of significant anaemia should be treated (MacGillivray, 1991).

▶ *Polyhydramnios* is more common in multiple pregnancy. This is seen equally in monozygotic and dizygotic twinning (Nylander and MacGillivray, 1975). In cases of feto-fetal transfusion syndrome, polyhydramnios is often a feature. An increase in perinatal mortality associated with polyhydramnios is also reported (Farooqui *et al.*, 1973).

▶ *Preterm labour* is a major risk. Low or very high parity, low maternal age, and monozygosity have been shown to predispose to the onset of early labour (Weekes *et al.*, 1977). The same study showed that cervical cerclage had no effect in reducing the incidence of preterm delivery.

▶ *Antepartum haemorrhage* is significantly increased in multiple pregnancy (MacGillivray and Campbell, 1988). *Placenta praevia* is also more common because of the large placental site encroaching on the lower uterine segment and *placenta abruptio* may occur following rupture of the membranes and subsequent diminution in uterine size, or be associated with pregnancy-induced hypertension.

Intrapartum Care

All mothers expecting a multiple birth should be booked for delivery in a consultant unit. Ideally, in the case of triplets and higher order births this should be a hospital which can offer neonatal intensive care facilities, i.e. a Regional Referral Unit. This avoids the necessity of transferring some or all of the infants postnatally possibly to different hospitals. If the mother lives a long way from such provision, she may be admitted in the third trimester or stay with friends nearby.

COMPLICATIONS

The risk during labour to mother and babies is much greater in multiple pregnancy. As well as preterm delivery other complications are more common.

Although *malpresentations* occur more frequently than with singleton births, in about half of twin pregnancies both babies are cephalic presentations and in three-quarters of cases the first baby presents as a vertex (Campbell and MacGillivray, 1988a). Even when the first baby presents by the breech, it is usual for the second to be cephalic. The lie and presentation of the second twin may change as the first is born. Oblique or transverse lie is uncommon but can be a serious development (Nnatu, 1985). There is a risk of *cord prolapse*, particularly in cases of malpresentation, polyhydramnios and in the interval between the births of the first and second twin.

The length of the first stage of labour is usually similar to that of a singleton birth. However, because of the overstretching of the uterus and abdominal muscles there may be *uterine inertia* in some mothers. The second stage is sometimes prolonged. This may prove dangerous in the case of the second baby as the uterus contracts after the first baby is delivered, the placental site constricts and oxygen supply to the baby may be diminished.

Delay in labour can occur when the second twin delays the descent of the first as in the case of '*locked*' *twins*. This is most likely when the first baby is a breech presentation and the second is cephalic. The head of the second twin is impacted in front of the head of the first, thus preventing further descent.

Following delivery, there is an increased risk of *haemorrhage* from the large placental site. Overstretched uterine muscles may contribute. A degree of *placenta praevia* may have been present and the abdominal muscles are more relaxed.

CARE IN LABOUR

When a mother expecting a multiple birth is admitted in labour, the team which will be present at the delivery should be alerted. As well as midwives and obstetric medical staff, it is desirable that paediatricians are available and that an experienced anaesthetist is in attendance (Bryan, 1992). General and epidural anaesthesia are frequently required and emergency Caesarean section, particularly in the case of the second twin, is not uncommon (Spillman, 1993b). All those in attendance should be introduced to the parents and their presence and role explained. If students and other observers are included, the mother's permission should be sought. Usually there will be no objection providing the father is also present (Spillman, 1987a).

First stage

The first stage of labour is conducted normally. It is important, whenever possible, to encourage the mother to move around in the early stages. This is not advisable if the membranes have ruptured however, because of the risk of cord prolapse. It is also difficult to achieve when continuous monitoring of the infants and contractions is in progress.

Epidural anaesthesia is now commonly offered to mothers giving birth to multiples. It is vital that the anaesthetist is experienced in the procedure. Recent research has shown that when this is not the case, the anaesthesia, even after several attempts, may be ineffective or a spinal tap may result (Spillman, 1993b). When effective, epidural anaesthesia has great advantages. It avoids delay in carrying out manoeuvres such as internal version, forceps delivery, ventouse extraction and emergency Caesarean section. The use of analgesia such as pethidine should be avoided as this may cause respiratory depression, particularly in the case of the second baby who may already be experiencing reduced oxygen levels (Bryan, 1992).

Very often the mother is anxious and may require much reassurance and support throughout labour. Good midwifery care from a sympathetic midwife, where possible one who has been involved in her antenatal care, will do much to alleviate some of her minor discomforts.

Second stage

The obstetrician, anaesthetist and paediatrician should be present together with the midwife when the mother is in the second stage of labour. Continuous monitoring of contractions and both infants' heartbeats should be in progress.

The room where the delivery is to take place should be suitable for the performance of an emergency Caesarean section or in close proximity to an operating theatre. Two sets of resuscitation equipment and incubators should be prepared. The delivery trolley should include the requirements for episiotomy, amniotomy, instrumental delivery and extra cord clamps. Equipment for local and general anaesthesia should be available if epidural anaesthetic is not already established and effective.

The second stage is conducted as usual up to the birth of the first baby. When the labour is preterm, forceps may be used to protect the infant's head during delivery. The cord should be firmly clamped in two places and cut between the clamps. If the maternal side is not secure, the second baby in the case of uniovular twins may suffer exsanguination. When the cord is around the baby's neck and requires cutting before delivery, it is important to check that the cut cord does not belong to the second twin. Very little time is available for delivery of that baby in such a situation. The first infant should be clearly labelled 'Twin 1' or with the parents' chosen name if that is known. The cord should also be labelled Twin 1. The baby should be shown to the mother if the condition is satisfactory or the parents constantly informed of progress if resuscitation is required.

The *lie* of the second baby should now be ascertained by abdominal palpation. If transverse or oblique, this must be corrected to longitudinal. The presentation and fetal heart rate are also checked, as is the mother's blood pressure and pulse rate.

A vaginal examination is then carried out to check the presentation of the second baby. When it has been confirmed that there is no cord presentation, the second sac of membranes is ruptured. Once again a check is made to make sure that the cord has not prolapsed. Normally contractions resume very soon afterwards and the second twin advances rapidly. The delivery is now conducted in the normal way. The interval between the births varies considerably. It has been suggested that 30 minutes should be the maximum time. However Depp *et al.* (1986) advocate applying an electrode to the presenting part of the second twin to monitor the condition and if satisfactory to allow nature to take its course. Campbell and MacGillivray (1988a) conclude that avoidance of undue haste or undue delay would seem to be the safest policy.

If more than two babies are expected and vaginal delivery is chosen, the procedure between each baby is repeated as described.

Third stage

Management may vary in different hospitals. It is usual to give an injection of ergometrine maleate 250–500 μg intravenously or Syntometrine 1 ml intramuscularly with the birth of the anterior shoulder of the last baby. When the uterus is felt to contract, controlled traction is applied to both/all cords at the same time.

Examination of placenta and membranes

This is particularly important following a multiple birth (Bryan, 1992). The midwife must make the usual examination to ensure completeness and detect any deviation from normal. If the babies are of different sex then they must be dizygotic twins and there should be separate placentae and two complete sets of membranes. It should be remembered that the placentae may have fused together and look like one.

When the babies are of the same sex, they may be monozygotic or dizygotic. It used to be thought that there was always a single chorion in the case of monozygotic twins. However, research has revealed that a significant number of dichorionic placentae belong to monozygous twins (Strong and Corney, 1967; Corney, 1975). The latter study failed to find any evidence of monochorionic placentae in dizygotic twins. Thus, if on examination, the midwife identifies only one chorion and a single placenta, the twins are monozygotic. Occasionally a single placenta may divide and cause confusion. It is important that the placentae and membranes are sent for histological examination to confirm the zygosity. This is particularly so if one twin has an abnormality, is stillborn or dies. It is now becoming common practice to take samples of cord blood for zygosity determination (Figure 2).

MANAGEMENT OF COMPLICATIONS

Risks to first and second twins

It is widely accepted that the risk to the second born infant is significantly higher (Campbell and MacGillivray, 1988b; Bryan, 1992). Thompson *et al.* (1983) in a Scottish study report a death rate for first twins of 47.6 per 1000 compared with 64.6 for second twins. Mortality is also higher for boys than girls (Campbell and MacGillivray, 1988b).

During the first stage of labour the presenting part of the first twin is subject to pressure as the cervix dilates. If this is vertex there is a risk of intracranial haemorrhage, particularly if the labour is preterm. During the second stage, forceps may be used to protect the head, or the after-coming head if there is breech presentation.

When the first twin shows signs of fetal distress before the cervix is fully dilated, it may be decided that a Caesarean section should be performed.

If, following the vaginal delivery of twin 1, the second baby is in a transverse or oblique lie, the doctor, or midwife, when no doctor is present, should perform external version to turn the baby to the vertex or breech position. Usually, if this is not possible, an emergency Caesarean section is performed. The alternative of a doctor performing an internal version, grasping a foot and delivering the baby by breech extraction, is seldom carried out nowadays. Such manouvres carry high mortality rates.

Sometimes, after rupturing the membranes of the second twin, there is a delay in the birth and fetal anoxia may occur. A Syntocinon infusion may be administered and contractions re-established.

Forceps delivery or ventouse extraction may be used to expedite the birth although the latter procedure is not recommended if the delivery is very preterm. (Campbell and MacGillivray, 1988a). If there is cord prolapse, the baby must be delivered without delay.

Occasionally the placenta and membranes of the first twin are delivered before the second baby is born. Excessive bleeding may occur from the placental site and the placenta of the second twin may also begin to separate. The second sac of membranes should be ruptured immediately and the baby and placenta delivered as quickly as possible. The uterus should then contract and bleeding be controlled.

Undiagnosed twins

It is unusual nowadays for a multiple pregnancy to remain undiagnosed at the time of delivery. However where ultrasonography is not available or not used routinely for all expectant mothers, this can still occur. Should this be the case, the greatest risk is that ergometrine or Syntometrine may already have been administered. This causes contraction of the uterus which may result in severe anoxia in the second twin, leading to death or precipitate delivery of a possibly brain-damaged infant. Rupture of the uterus is also a risk. The second twin requires immediate delivery. A general anaesthetic may be required and a muscle relaxant given. Caesarean section may be indicated.

It should be appreciated that both parents are likely to be shocked and stressed by this situation (Theroux,

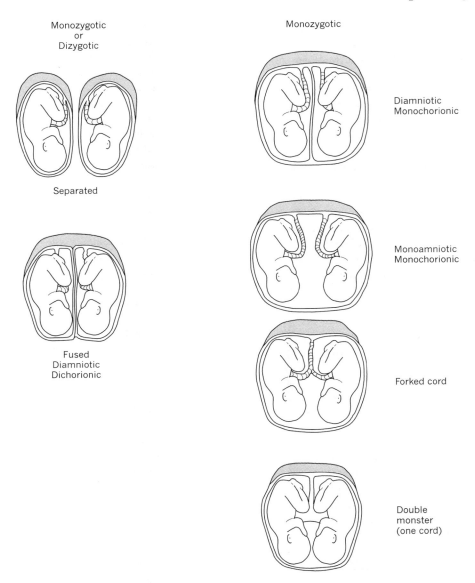

Monozygotic
or
Dizygotic

Separated

Fused
Diamniotic
Dichorionic

Monozygotic

Diamniotic
Monochorionic

Monoamniotic
Monochorionic

Forked cord

Double
monster
(one cord)

Figure 2 Placentation of twins. (Reproduced with permission from Strong and Corney, 1967.)

1989). Suddenly there are two babies to whom they must relate. They may already have formed a bond with the first infant and find it difficult to accept the unexpected baby (Bryan, 1992). Midwives, if aware of the possible problem, can give extra support to allow expression of negative feelings and help acceptance of the new situation.

Locking of twins

This is an extremely rare phenomenon. However, the condition is potentially disastrous and therefore mid-wives should be aware of the possibility, particularly when the labour is preterm and the babies small. Primigravidae are also more at risk (Khunda, 1972).

If locked twins are suspected during the first stage of labour a Caesarean section is performed to prevent obstruction occurring. However, the second stage of labour may be underway before it is realized that, during the breech delivery of the first infant, progress has halted. The descending second baby's head engages in the pelvis ahead of the first twin's head and interlocking of the chins occurs. The first twin will die of asphyxia unless delivered quickly. The mother is anaesthetized without delay and the doctor may attempt to push the head of the second twin out of the way. The first twin can then be delivered followed by the second. Even if Caesarean section is attempted, results are poor. A high fatality rate of the first twin is reported in such cases (Khunda, 1972).

If the doctor's attempt to dislodge the second twin's head is unsuccessful and the first baby has died of asphyxia, it has to be decapitated to allow delivery of the second baby.

Less common types of locking may occur. The fetuses may *collide*, preventing engagement of either. There may be *impaction* when both presenting parts partially engage, and there may be *compaction* when descent cannot take place because both presenting parts are fully engaged. In these situations, Caesarean section should resolve the situation.

Conjoined twins

This rare condition only affects monozygotic twins. With ultrasound scanning, such an abnormality is likely to be detected during the pregnancy. The twins may be joined in various ways and the degree of shared organs and fusion will affect the possibility of successful separation. The babies should be delivered by elective Caesarean section. In developing countries, obstructed labour is a likely outcome and, because of delay in reaching medical assistance, may result in death of the babies and possible rupture of the uterus and death of the mother.

Occasionally in the case of monochorionic twins, *acute feto-fetal transfusion* may occur during labour. Both babies are at great risk. The donor twin suffers severe hypovolaemia and anaemia whilst the recipient is hypervolaemic and then polycythaemic. Both may die of cardiac failure if the condition is not recognized, delivery expedited and urgent treatment given (Bryan, 1992).

When one twin has died before birth, it is preferable, if possible, to deliver the live twin first (Bryan, 1992).

DELIVERY OF TRIPLETS AND HIGHER ORDER BIRTHS

A recent study of triplets and higher order births has revealed that in almost two thirds of cases labour commenced spontaneously. The remainder were induced for a variety of reasons. These included mater-

nal problems, fetal growth retardation and the policy in some units to intervene at what is thought to be an optimum time for survival (Botting *et al.*, 1990).

The most likely method of delivery is by Caesarean section. The higher the order, the more likely this becomes (Pons *et al.*, 1988). However, practices vary greatly between units and some obstetricians favour vaginal delivery in most cases (Thiery *et al.*, 1988). Caesarean sections may be carried out under epidural or general anaesthesia.

Whatever the chosen method of delivery, separate teams of paediatric staff should be available for the resuscitation of each infant. It should be remembered that the large number of people present at such deliveries can be very unnerving for the parents. It is important that explanation is given to them of the need for so many onlookers and participants.

However many infants are involved, the parents should be shown their babies as soon as possible after delivery. They should be allowed to hold those babies who are in a satisfactory condition and the mother can be encouraged to suckle those for whom there is no immediate anxiety.

If it is necessary to transfer some or all of the infants to the neonatal unit, photographs should be taken and brought to the mother as soon as possible. Ideally, the babies should be photographed together so that the realities of the multiple birth are established. However, if this is not possible, the pictures should be clearly labelled with the birth order of the babies.

Postnatal Care

Following delivery, the mother is likely to be very tired. She has probably suffered from a sleep deficit over several months and a more complicated delivery may compound her exhaustion. If she has been delivered by Caesarean section, she is more likely to feel very unwell, have problems with feeding her babies and suffer from postnatal depression (Spillman, 1993b). The lochia in the first few days is often heavier than after a singleton delivery and the mother is more likely to complain of afterpains.

In addition, the mother has two or more babies to whom she must relate and give care. Her anxieties may be increased because her babies are preterm. One, both, or in the case of triplets or more, all, may be nursed in the neonatal unit. In some units, if only one twin or not all of triplets require special care, the well infants may also be admitted to the neonatal unit. The aim is not to separate the babies, and to facilitate parental involvement by not requiring the mother to care for one or more infants in the postnatal ward as well as making regular visits to the neonatal unit to visit and be involved in the care of her sick baby or babies.

Unfortunately, some units are so busy that it is impractical to admit well babies, however psychologically desirable this may be. A compromise may be possible if the postnatal ward is adjacent to the neonatal unit. Nowadays more progressive units have established transitional care wards where small babies can remain with their mothers. Skilled midwives or nurses are available to support, assist and advise and extra warmth and facilities for specialized feeding are available.

Sadly, it is not uncommon for very sick babies to be transferred from the delivery hospital to a Regional Referral Unit where intensive neonatal nursing care can be offered. Sometimes cots are not available in the same hospital for both or all of the babies and separation is inevitable (Bryan, 1992). The distances involved can be great and extremely costly to the parents and the neonatal services (Papiernik, 1991). The mother may remain at the referring hospital whilst her babies are transferred. This situation is traumatic for all the family and may place great strains on the father who has to visit each of the hospitals involved. Midwifery staff must strive to reunite the family as soon as the condition of the babies allows. Regular communication during the separation is vital. The splitting up of the family group is often avoided if the babies are transferred to the Regional Referral Unit *in utero*. Bowman *et al.* (1988) demonstrated that such babies had a better prognosis than those who needed to be transferred after birth.

FEEDING MULTIPLES

Breastfeeding should be encouraged. With support, even mothers of triplets can successfully breastfeed their infants. Help should be available at every feed until the mother feels confident (Bryan, 1992). Mothers who have previously breastfed their children often establish a satisfactory routine for their multiples quickly. Primigravidae may require more sustained help. Some mothers prefer to feed both infants together, thus saving time, others will waken the second to feed immediately after the first and others will feed each baby on demand. There is no one right way

(Spillman, 1987b). The important thing is that the mother should be comfortable. Often the use of a triangular pillow to support the babies is helpful. Many different positions may be chosen. The mother may prefer to feed the babies resting in bed or on a large chair, sofa or beanbag.

If the babies have been born preterm, it may be necessary to establish lactation by expressing milk until the infants are strong enough to suckle. The babies should be feeding well and gaining weight before discharge.

Some mothers choose to wholly or partially bottle-feed their multiples. Partners, family and friends are then able to share in feeding routines. This may lessen the mother's inevitable tiredness.

COMING HOME

The timing of the homecoming should be a joint decision between the parents and the midwifery and paediatric staff. If the babies have been born preterm, the mother may have already been back at home for several days or weeks before her babies can join her. Some parents will prefer to wait until both/all the babies are ready to come home and take them together, whereas others will prefer to settle them at home one at a time. Some units are too busy to keep babies who are fit for discharge until the other twin, triplets or more are well. In such situations, visiting the infant/s still in hospital can be a strain. Criticism of parents who are unable to visit frequently should be avoided. It may be necessary to arrange the re-admission of the mother for a few days before the infants are discharged in order to be sure that she is confident of being able to care for the babies at home.

This transition will be smoother if the mother has adequate help. Often none is offered and extended families and friends struggle to give support and encouragement (Price, 1990). Some general practitioners apply for home help provision for mothers with twins or more whereas others seem unaware that there may be a problem. Midwives are in a position to assess the needs and to approach the social services on the family's behalf.

FAMILY RELATIONSHIPS

A mother may find it difficult to relate to both/all of the babies at the beginning. She is likely to be overtired and become overwhelmed with the enormity of her

FAMILY TYPE	Parents and sibling	Parents, sibling and baby	Parents, sibling and twins	Parents, sibling and triplets
	M ▽ F / S	M ⊠ F / S B	M F / S ⬠ B / B	M F / S ⬡ B / B B
Number in family	3	4	5	6
Number of links per person	2	3	4	5
Total number of links	3	6	10	15
FAMILY LINKS				

Figure 3   Family links.

task. Esther Goshen-Gottstein (1980) found that in the case of twins, mothers spent 35–37% of their time on infant-centred activities compared with the 22–29% needed by mothers of singletons.

A strong preference may develop for one of the babies in the early days. Research has shown that this is usually for the baby who was heavier at birth (Spillman, 1984). The mother should be reassured that this is normal and in time her relationship with the other baby or babies will improve.

There may also be problems with other children in the family, especially toddlers. It is hard enough for a 2-year old child to accept one new baby. When two or more arrive simultaneously there may be real difficulties. What was previously a family of three with three relationships, with the arrival of twins will find the number of links increased to ten and with triplets to 15 (Figure 3) (Rowland, 1991). In an Australian study, 64% of families with young twins reported problems with their older child during the first six months after the twins' birth (Hay *et al.*, 1988).

Partners must be encouraged to play a full part in the care of the children. Marital breakdown is more common when there are twins or higher multiples in the family (Noble, 1990). The parents should be encouraged to find time for their own relationship.

POSTNATAL DEPRESSION

In view of all the possible complications, increased risk of surgical intervention and other stresses involved in

having a multiple birth, it is perhaps not surprising that there is an increased risk of postnatal depression (Powell, 1981; Thorpe *et al.*, 1991; Spillman, 1993b).

The health professionals caring for the mother should recognize the signs that such depression is developing. It is helpful if there is continuity of care by a known midwife and a health visitor who has been introduced to the family *before* the babies are born. A smooth transfer of responsibility can then be achieved. If the babies are still in hospital, it is still important for the mother to receive visits from her midwife and health visitor. Her depression is otherwise likely to be exacerbated and she may become isolated.

BEREAVEMENT

Parents who have a multiple birth are more than three times as likely to experience perinatal loss of their infants than are those who have a singleton baby. Botting *et al.* (1987) found that in the UK, although twins account for less than 2% of births, they are responsible for 9% of perinatal deaths. Preterm birth and its associated complications are responsible for many of the losses.

To lose a baby from a multiple birth poses special problems for the family. They have to grieve for their lost baby or babies, whilst rejoicing in the survival of the other/s. There may be continuing anxiety for the health of the remaining child or children. The loss of the status of being parents of twins, triplets or more is a severe blow. The world may now see them as parents of a singleton infant, twins or triplets, when they continue to think of themselves as parents of twins, triplets or quadruplets (Bryan, 1986; Sainsbury, 1988). It is therefore very important for professionals to include the lost infant or infants in conversations with the family. Remarks such as 'You are lucky to have one healthy baby' or 'it would have been hard work with three' are hurtful and unhelpful.

The parents should be encouraged to make contact with an appropriate self-help group such as the Twins and Multiple Births Association (TAMBA) Bereavement Support Group. Those who have already made contact with their local Twins Club during pregnancy will often find continued support from other families in the club who have experienced similar losses. Clinics for bereaved parents of multiples are held regularly by the Multiple Births Foundation at Queen Charlotte's Hospital in London and in Birmingham and York. TAMBA also have a telephone helpline, called '*Twin-*

line', which is open in the evenings and at weekends when often the statutory services are not available. Midwives should be aware of these services and ensure that bereaved families can make use of them (Spillman, 1993c) (see Useful Addresses).

PLANNING AHEAD

It is important that good family planning advice is offered to the parents following a multiple birth.

Genetic counselling may be needed by those who have lost a baby. Follow-up of survivors should be arranged, especially when the infants are monozygous or have experienced neonatal complications. Midwives who offer optimum support to families who have a multiple birth will find great rewards. The families are always appreciative of those who understand their special needs.

References

Botting, B., Macdonald Davies, I. & Macfarlane, A. (1987) Recent trends in the incidence of multiple births and their mortality. *Arch. Dis. Childh.* **62**: 941–950.

Botting, B., MacFarlane, A.J. & Price, F.V. (1990) *Three Four and More: a Study of Triplet and Higher Order Births.* London: HMSO.

Bowman, E., Doyle, L.W., Murton, L.J., Roy, R.N.D. & Kitchen, W. (1988) Increased mortality of preterm infants transferred between tertiary perinatal centres. *Br. Med. J.* **297**: 1098–1100.

Bracken, M.B. (1979) Oral contraception and twinning: an epidemiological study. *Am. J. Obstet. Gynecol.* **133**: 432–434.

Broadbent, B.A. (1985) Multiple births – womens' needs. *Midwife, Health Visitor & Community Nurse* **21**: 425–430.

Bryan, E.M. (1986) The death of a newborn twin. How can support for the parents be improved? *Acta Genet. Med. Gemellol.* **5**: 115–118.

Bryan, E. (1991) But there should have been two. In Harvey, D. & Bryan, E. (eds) *The Stress of Multiple Births*, pp. 49–55. London: The Multiple Births Foundation.

Bryan, E. (1992) *Twins and Higher Multiple Births: A Guide to their Nature and Nurture.* London: Edward Arnold.

Bryan, E., Higgins, R. & Harvey, D. (1991) Ethical dilemmas. In Harvey, D. & Bryan, E. (eds) *The Stress of Multiple Births*, pp. 35–40. London: Multiple Births Foundation.

Bulmer, M.G. (1970) *The Biology of Twinning in Man.* Oxford: Clarendon Press.

Campbell, D.M. & MacGillivray, I. (1988a) Management of labour and delivery. In MacGillivray, I., Campbell, D.M. & Thompson, B. (eds) *Twinning and Twins*, pp. 143–160. Chichester: John Wiley.

Campbell, D.M. & MacGillivray, I. (1988b) Outcome of twin pregnancies. In MacGillivray, I., Campbell, D.M. & Thompson, B. (eds) *Twinning and Twins*, pp. 179–205. Chichester: John Wiley.

Campbell, D.M., Campbell, A.J. & MacGillivray, I. (1974) Maternal characteristics of women having twin pregnancies. *J. Biosoc. Sci.* **6**: 463–470.

Corney, G. (1975) Placentation. In MacGillivray, I., Nylander, P.P.S. & Corney, G. (eds) *Human Multiple Reproduction*, pp. 40–76. London: W.B. Saunders.

Corney, G. & Robson, E.B. (1975) Types of twinning and determination of zygosity. In MacGillivray, I., Nylander,

P.P.S. & Corney, G. (eds) *Human Multiple Reproduction*, pp. 16–39. London: W.B. Saunders.

Crowther, C.A., Neilson, J.P., Verkuyl, D.A.A., Bannerman, C. & Ashurst, H.M. (1989) Pre-term labour in twin pregnancies, can it be prevented by hospital admission? *Br. J. Obstet. Gynaecol.* **96**: 850–853.

Depp, R., Keith, L. & Sciarri, J. (1986) The mode of delivery in twin pregnancy. Paper given at the Fifth Congress of International Society for Twin Studies. Unpublished. Amsterdam.

Farooqui, M.O., Grossman, J.H. & Shannon, R.A. (1973) A review of twin pregnancy and perinatal mortality. *Obstet. Gynaecol. Survey* **28**: 144–153.

Goshen-Gottstein, E. (1980) The mothers of twins, triplets and quadruplets. *Psychiatry* **43**: 184–204.

Hay, D.A., McIndoe, R. & O'Brian, P.J. (1988) The older sibling of twins. *Aust. J. Early Child.* **13**: 25–28.

Imaizumi, Y. & Inouye, E. (1984) Multiple birth rates in Japan. Further analysis. *Acta Genet. Med. Gemellol.* **33**: 107–114.

Khunda, S. (1972) Locked twins. *Obstet. Gynecol.* **39**: 453–459.

Landy, H.J., Weiner, S., Corson, S.L. *et al.* (1986) The 'vanishing twin': Ultrasonic assessment of fetal disappearance in the first trimester. *Am. J. Obstet. Gynecol.* **155**: 14–19.

Linney, J. (1983) *The Management of Multiple Births.* Chichester: John Wiley.

Macfarlane, A.J., Price, F.V. & Daw, E.G. (1990) Antenatal care. In Botting, B.J., Macfarlane, A.J. & Price, F.V. (eds) *Three Four and More*, pp. 59–79. London: HMSO.

MacGillivray, I. (1991) Obstetrical aspects of multiple births. In Harvey, D. & Bryan, E.M. (eds) *The Stress of Multiple Births*, pp. 11–21. London: The Multiple Births Foundation.

MacGillivray, I. & Campbell, D.M. (1988) Management of twin pregnancies. In MacGillivray, I., Campbell, D.M. & Thompson, B. (eds) *Twinning and Twins*, pp. 111–139. Chichester: John Wiley.

MacGillivray, I., Samphier, M. & Little, J. (1988) Factors affecting twinning. In MacGillivray, I., Campbell, D.M. & Thompson, B. (eds) *Twinning and Twins*, pp. 67–97. Chichester: John Wiley.

McMullan, P.F., Norman, R.J. & Marivate, M. (1984) Pregnancy-induced hypertension in twin pregnancy. *Br. J. Obstet. Gynaecol.* **91**: 240–243.

Nnatu, S. (1985) Presentation in twin pregnancy. *J. Obstet. Gynaecol.* **6**: 35–37.

Noble, E. (1991) *Having Twins.* Boston: Houghton Mifflin.

Nylander, P.P.S. (1967) Twinning in West Africa. *World Med. J.* **14**: 178–180.

Nylander, P.P.S. (1970) Twinning in Nigeria. *Acta Genet. Med. Gemellol.* **19**: 457–464.

Nylander, P.P.S. & MacGillivray, I. (1975) Complications of twin pregnancy. In MacGillivray, I., Nylander, P.P.S. & Corney, G. (eds) *Human Multiple Reproduction*, pp. 137–146. London: W.B. Saunders.

Papiernik, E. (1991) Costs of multiple pregnancies. In Harvey, D. & Bryan, E. (eds) *The Stress of Multiple Births*, pp. 22–34. London: The Multiple Births Foundation.

Papiernik, E., Mussy, M.A., Vial, M. & Richard, A. (1985) A low rate of perinatal deaths for twin births. *Acta Genet. Med. Gemellol.* **34**: 201–206.

Patel, N., Bowie, W., Campbell, D.M. *et al.* (1984) *Scottish Twin Study 1983 Report.* Social Paediatric and Obstetric Research Unit, University of Glasgow & Greater Glasgow Health Board.

Pons, J.C., Mayenga, J.M., Plu, G., Forman, R.G. & Papiernik, E. (1988) Management of triplet pregnancy. *Acta Genet. Med. Gemellol.* **37**: 99–103.

Powell, T. (1981) Symptoms of atypical depression in mothers of twins. Unpublished MSc thesis, University of Surrey.

Price, F.V. (1990) Who helps? In Botting, B.J., Macfarlane, A.J. & Price F.V. (eds) *Three, Four and More: A study of triplet and higher order birth*, pp. 131–150. London: HMSO.

Registrar General (1989) *Birth Statistics.* Series FMI no. 6. Offices of Population Censuses and Surveys. London: HMSO.

Rowland, C. (1991) Family relationships. In Harvey, D. & Bryan, E. (eds) *The Stress of Multiple Births*, pp. 59–67. London: The Multiple Births Foundation.

Rydhstrom, H., Nordenskold, F., Grenert, L. *et al.* (1987) Routine hospital care does not improve prognosis in twin gestation. *Acta Obstet. Gynecol. Scand.* **66**: 361–364.

Sainsbury, M.K. (1988) Grief in multifetal death. *Acta Genet. Med. Gemellol.* **37**: 181–185.

Spillman, J.R. (1984) *The role of birthweight in mother–twin relationships.* Unpublished MSc thesis, Cranfield University.

Spillman, J.R. (1985) 'You have a little bonus my dear': The effect on mothers of the diagnosis of multiple pregnancy. *Br. Med. Ultrasound Soc. Bull.* **39**: 6–9.

Spillman, J.R. (1986) Expecting a multiple birth: some emotional aspects. *Br. J. Nurses Child Health* **10**: 298–299.

Spillman, J.R. (1987a) Emotional aspects of experiencing a multiple birth. *Midwife, Health Visitor and Community Nurse* **23**(2): 54–58.

Spillman, J.R. (1987b) Double exposure – Coping with newborn twins at home. *Midwife, Health Visitor & Community Nurse* **23**(3): 92–94.

Spillman, J.R. (1992) A study of maternity provision in the UK in response to the needs of families who have a multiple birth. *Acta Genet. Med. Gemellol.* **41**: 353–364.

Spillman, J.R. (1993a) Midwives Responding to the needs of multiples. In *Proceedings: 23rd International Congress of Midwives*, Vancouver, Canada, Vol. IV, pp. 1752–1765.

Spillman, J.R. (1993b) Multiple pregnancy – Effects of Caesarean section and epidural anaesthesia on postnatal health. In *Proceedings: 23rd International Congress of Midwives*, Vancouver, Canada, Vol. IV, pp. 1766–1775.

Spillman, J.R. (1993c) Perinatal loss in multiple pregnancy. In *Proceedings: 23rd International Congress of Midwives*, Vancouver, Canada, Vol. IV, pp. 1776–1785.

Strong, S.J. & Corney, G. (1967) *The Placenta in Twin Pregnancy.* Oxford: Pergamon Press.

Theroux, R. (1989) Multiple birth: A unique parenting experience. *J. Perinat. Neonat. Nursing* **3**(1): 35–45.

Thiery, M., Kermans, G. & Derom, R. (1988) Triplet and higher order births. What is the optimal delivery route? *Acta Genet. Med. Gemellol.* **37**: 89–98.

Thompson, B., Pritchard, C. & Corney, G. (1983) Perinatal mortality in twins by zygosity and placentation. Paper given at the 4th Congress of International Society of Twin Studies, London.

Thorpe, K., Golding, J., MacGillivray, I. & Greenwood, R. (1991) Comparison of prevalence of depression in mothers of twins and mothers of singletons. *Br. Med. J.* **302**: 875–878.

Webster, F. & Ellwood, J.M. (1985) A study of the influence of ovulation stimulants and oral contraception on twin births in England. *Acta Genet. Med. Gemellol.* **34**: 105–108.

Weekes, A.R.L., Menzies, D.N. & de Boer, C.H. (1977) The relative efficacy of bed rest, cervical suture and no treatment in the management of twin pregnancy. *Br. J. Obstet. Gynaecol.* **84**: 161–164.

Useful Addresses

Twins and Multiple Births Association (TAMBA)
PO Box 30, Little Sutton, LH66 1TH
Tamba Twinline Co-ordinator
PO Box 30, Little Sutton, LH66 1TH
Twinline tel. 01732 868000

The Multiple Births Foundation (MBF)
Queen Charlottes and Chelsea Hospitals, Goldhawk Road, London W6 0XG

46

The Fetus at Risk

Fetal distress is caused by lack of oxygen (*hypoxia*) *in utero*. In severe cases it causes intracranial damage and may lead to cerebral palsy or occasionally to stillbirth or neonatal death. At birth the baby may be asphyxiated and require urgent resuscitation.

Mechanisms that lead to hypoxia causing brain damage or death are poorly understood, but the main factors are thought to be (Parer and Livingstone, 1990):

▶ Insufficiency of uterine blood flow.
▶ Insufficiency of umbilical blood flow.
▶ Decrease in maternal oxygen content.

The degree and duration of hypoxia and the gestational age and weight of the fetus will influence the outcome (Levene, 1987).

Fetal distress can be either *acute* or *chronic*. One of the aims of good antenatal care is the early identification of women with high risk factors which may lead to chronic or acute fetal distress. More frequent examinations and investigations to monitor the maternal and fetal condition can then be carried out and, if inter-vention is required, it can be offered at the optimum time.

Factors Associated with Chronic Fetal Distress

Social factors
Chronic fetal distress can be related to various social factors:

▶ *Low socio-economic status*: This is associated with increased perinatal morbidity and mortality. Socio-economic status is a reflection not merely of income but also of education, nutrition, physical health and physique.
▶ *Maternal age*: Young teenagers and older mothers over 35 years are associated with high risk.
▶ *Smoking*: This contributes to fetal distress since nico-tine causes vasoconstriction, leading to decreased uterine blood flow whilst carbon monoxide reduces

the transport of oxygen. The perinatal mortality rate is increased (Butler *et al.*, 1972).

▶ *Maternal drug misuse*: Drug misuse in pregnancy is associated with many complications, including intrauterine growth retardation, hypoxia and preterm labour, all of which increase the risk of perinatal death (Thornton *et al.*, 1990; Robins *et al.*, 1993; Siney, 1995).

▶ *Poor obstetric history*: Previous abortions, preterm labour or stillbirth are all associated with a significantly higher fetal loss in the current pregnancy.

Maternal disease

Conditions in the mother that raise the risk of chronic fetal distress can be divided into those that affect the maternal circulatory system and thus cause insufficiency of uterine blood flow, such as:

▶ pregnancy-induced hypertension;
▶ chronic hypertension;
▶ diabetes; and
▶ chronic renal disease;

and those that cause a decrease in maternal arterial oxygen, such as:

▶ sickle cell disease;
▶ severe anaemia, 9 g/dl or below;
▶ pulmonary disease;
▶ cardiac disease;
▶ epilepsy, if not well controlled; and
▶ severe maternal infections.

In these conditions the danger is that maternal acidosis will lead to fetal acidosis and hence to fetal distress.

Placental conditions

Conditions such as placental insufficiency, postmaturity and antepartum haemorrhage may all result in a reduced oxygen supply to the fetus.

Fetal conditions

Certain congenital malformations, intrauterine infections and rhesus incompatibility all carry the risk of intrauterine hypoxia. The risk is also increased in multiple pregnancy.

Intrapartum risk factors

During labour, the following factors are associated with increased risk of fetal distress:

▶ Malpresentations, e.g. breech.
▶ Midcavity forceps delivery.
▶ Caesarean section.
▶ Excessive sedation or analgesia.
▶ Anaesthetic complications, e.g. hypotension or hypoxia.
▶ Prolonged or precipitate labour (Blackburn and Loper, 1992).

Intrauterine Growth Retardation

Chronic, slowly progressive hypoxia produces characteristic changes that can be detected. Growth will slow in a specific way reflecting redistributed blood flow producing a fetus with asymmetrical growth retardation (Jacobs and Phibbs, 1989). Blood flow is increased to the brain, adrenals and heart and decreased to the lungs, gut, liver and spleen. With continued hypoxia fetal organs begin to fail, the placenta ages rapidly and renal blood flow falls, resulting in decreased amniotic fluid. Central nervous system anoxia leads to decreased fetal and respiratory movements and tone, and lack of fetal heart rate variability evident on a cardiotocograph (CTG). Prior to death, myocardial depression and fetal heart rate decelerations occur (Jacobs and Phibbs, 1989). These parameters form the basis of the biophysical profile performed antenatally to assess fetal well-being.

Acute Causes of Fetal Distress

Uterine conditions

Hypertonic uterine contractions are abnormally long and strong and the uterus has a high resting tone which may seriously effect the uteroplacental circulation between contractions, thereby resulting in fetal hypoxia.

Compression of the umbilical cord

Compression of the umbilical cord will interfere with the blood circulation of the fetus and result in hypoxia. The cord may be compressed following 'prolapse', when there is a true knot, or if it is entangled around the fetus.

Placental conditions

Placental separation, as occurs in abruptio placentae, is associated with a high fetal loss.

Depression of the respiratory centre

Respiratory depression in the newborn as a result of analgesics given to the mother in labour and birth injury may cause hypoxia.

Detection of Fetal Compromise Antenatally

Antenatally the important aspects of risk must be updated at every visit, including risks to both mother and fetus. For example, at eight weeks the maternal history is taken to identify specific risk factors. At 34 weeks it is important to assess adequate fetal growth and at term ensure normal fetal movements (Jacobs and Phibbs, 1989). The identification of a predisposition to fetal compromise should initiate appropriate investigations to confirm a diagnosis and future management of the condition can then be planned.

Investigations

Investigations used to detect antenatal fetal compromise include the following:

1 *Ultrasound scan* to assess fetal growth.
2 *Biophysical profile*: A physical examination of the fetus using an ultrasound scan. Parameters measured in this evaluation include:

> ▶ fetal breathing movements;
> ▶ fetal movements;
> ▶ fetal tone;
> ▶ amniotic fluid index;
> ▶ non-stress test (Tucker, 1992).

3 *Non-stress test*: External cardiotocograph (CTG) is performed antenatally. Criteria that should be met include two or more fetal heart rate (FHR) accelerations of at least 15 beats per minute lasting at least 15 seconds in a 20-minute period.
4 *Doppler studies* (see Chapter 21).

Signs of Fetal Distress in Labour

Fetal heart

The fetal heart should be monitored continuously by a cardiotocograph when there is a suspicion or a high risk of fetal distress developing so that early signs may be detected and prompt and appropriate action taken.

The signs of fetal distress are the following:

1 A baseline *tachycardia* above 160 bpm or a baseline *bradycardia* below 120 bpm (Gauge and Henderson, 1992; Miller, 1993).
2 *Early decelerations*: When the drop in heart rate is more than 15 bpm and occurs with a contraction. The deceleration image is mirrored by the contraction and not usually considered to be serious (Evans, 1992).
3 *Variable decelerations*: A common pattern which can sometimes be difficult to define. It can be an early or late drop in fetal heart rate and may not be uniform in shape or occur with contractions (Evans, 1992). The association with fetal acidosis increases with the depth and duration of decelerations and with the presence of other fetal heart rate abnormalities (Bradley, 1991).
4 *Late decelerations*: A drop in the fetal heart rate which shows the lowest level of deceleration lagging behind the highest peak of the uterine contraction (Evans, 1992). Late decelerations arise due to a decrease in uterine blood flow and, in turn, oxygen transfer during a contraction is reduced. There is a significant decrease in fetal cerebral oxygenation (Aldrich *et al.*, 1995). If such a pattern occurs with other fetal heart rate abnormalities this pattern *must* be treated as a serious threat to fetal well-being.
5 *Lack of fetal heartbeat variability*: This may be due to severe or chronic hypoxia where the fetal autonomic nervous system is unable to respond to stress (Gauge and Henderson, 1992).
6 Meconium stained liquor.

Meconium

The passage of meconium occurs in approximately 20% of all deliveries and aspiration occurs in 1–3% of all liveborn infants (Gregory *et al.*, 1974; Katz and Bowes, 1992; Rossi *et al.*, 1989, cited in McNiven *et al.*, 1994). The likely cause of this is thought to be anal sphincter relaxation in response to bowel hypoxia as a result of blood being shunted to vital organs (McNiven et al., 1994). Research has found meconium staining of the amniotic fluid to be associated with an increased risk of neonatal death and morbidity (Fujikura and Kilonsky, 1975; Hobel, 1971).

The presence of thick meconium staining of the amniotic fluid in early labour should alert the midwife to the potential risk of fetal distress and mandates vigilant surveillance of fetal well-being. The available evidence suggests that thin or light meconium confers a similar prognosis to clear fluid (Holtzman et al., 1989).

Management of Labour

The management depends on the woman's medical and obstetric history, the pregnancy history to date and the presence of risk factors. Other considerations include the stage of labour and the degree of hypoxia. The fetal heart should be monitored continuously *only* when there is a high risk of fetal distress developing so that early signs can be detected and appropriate action taken.

FIRST STAGE

The doctor is informed immediately of any signs of fetal distress. Measures to improve placental perfusion are instituted such as a change to a lateral position; hypotension should be corrected and Syntocinon, if in progress, should be discontinued and replaced by Hartmann's solution to keep the vein open. An abdominal palpation and vaginal examination should be performed to assess progress and, if the membranes are still intact, artificial rupture of the membranes should be performed to enable the colour of the liquor to be visualized. During this time contemporaneous records must be kept (UKCC, 1993). The doctor may perform a fetal blood sample (see Chapter 29) if auscultation or electronic fetal heart recordings indicate a fetal heart rate abnormality. A pH between 7.35 and 7.25 is indicative of fetal well-being. A pH of 7.24 is considered pre-acidotic and a pH of less than 7.20 is indicative of fetal distress (Miller, 1993). Grant (1993) claims that better fetal and maternal outcome is evident if fetal blood sampling is employed with fetal heart rate monitoring.

Subsequent management will depend on the findings of the examinations and investigations described.

In severe cases of fetal distress, delivery must be expedited and an immediate Caesarean section becomes necessary. In less severe cases the doctor may decide to observe the fetal condition closely by continuous monitoring of the fetal heart, observation of amniotic fluid for the presence of meconium and repeating the fetal blood sampling. Delivery will be expedited if there is any deterioration in the fetal condition.

SECOND STAGE

When fetal distress occurs in the second stage, if the head is well enough advanced an episiotomy may be performed to hasten delivery. Otherwise a doctor will perform an instrumental delivery and occasionally a Caesarean section may be necessary. Resuscitation equipment must be prepared and a paediatrician called in readiness to receive an asphyxiated baby.

Intrauterine Fetal Death

The fetus may, at any stage of pregnancy, die *in utero*. Intrauterine fetal death before the 24th week of pregnancy would lead to an abortion, whereas after the 24th week the baby would be stillborn.

Causes

Death may be caused by any of the factors previously outlined that are known to cause acute or chronic fetal distress. The risk of fetal death is known to decline as gestation advances and increases in extremes of reproductive age, lower socio-economic groups, smokers and high parous women (Albers and Savitz, 1991). The most common causes of late fetal death are intrauterine growth retardation, placental complications, severe maternal disease or congenital malformations (Brans et al., 1984; Buckell, 1985, cited in Haglund et al., 1993). However, in over half of all stillbirths no cause is found (Healy, 1993).

Signs

Suggestive signs are the absence of fetal movements reported by the mother and the midwife's inability to auscultate fetal heart sounds. Before proceeding any further it is essential to confirm the diagnosis of fetal death. For more than 50 years X-ray was the principal means of establishing a diagnosis (Pitkin, 1987), the most reliable sign being the presence of gas in major blood vessels and the heart which appears within 1–2 days of death. This is known as *Roberts' sign* (Lewis and Chamberlain, 1990). A later sign is overlapping of the cranial bones known as *Spalding's sign*, caused by disintegration of the brain and subsequent collapse of the cranial bones. Ultrasound imaging has now become the 'gold standard' for diagnosis of fetal death. However, Pitkin (1987) claims that this procedure is liable to observer error and death should therefore be confirmed by two independent experts.

Management

At least 75% of women start labour spontaneously within two weeks of fetal death and most of the others will deliver within a further two weeks (Pitkin, 1987). If spontaneous delivery does not occur within 3–4 weeks the risk of disseminated intravascular coagulation increases. This occurs because thromboplastin is released into the circulation from the dead fetal tissue and triggers off the blood clotting mechanism. This results in a gradual decline in the serum fibrinogen level and the platelet count. To diagnose this condition a clotting profile is performed on all women who present with an intrauterine death and it is repeated once or twice weekly until the woman delivers. Heparin is the treatment for disseminated intravascular coagulation, but is discontinued at the onset of labour and fresh blood is cross-matched because of the risk of haemorrhage (see Chapter 40).

When the baby dies before the onset of labour, unless there is some risk to the mother in waiting extra time, the timing of induction should be in accordance with her wishes (Dyer, 1992). If a decision is made to medically induce labour this may be achieved by the use of prostaglandins and oxytocin. Once labour is induced it should be brought to a speedy conclusion, especially once the membranes have ruptured, because of the risk of anaerobic uterine infection from the growth of bacteria in dead fetal tissue (Lewis and Chamberlain, 1990). Llewellyn-Jones (1994) claims that by using any of the above methods, 50% of women will expel the fetus in 12 hours and 90% in 24 hours.

Active management of the third stage of labour is recommended because of the risk of postpartum haemorrhage due to coagulation failure.

Maceration starts when the fetus has been dead for 12–24 hours and is caused by aseptic autolysis. When the fetus is macerated at birth the epidermis peels leaving the red dermis exposed; the tissues are soft and the skull bones loose and overlapping.

References

Albers, L.L. & Savitz, D.A. (1991) Hospital setting and fetal death during labour among women at low risk. *Am. J. Obstet. Gynecol.* **164**(3): 868–873.

Aldrich, C.J., D'Antona, D. & Spencer, J.A. (1995) Late fetal heart deceleration and changes in cerebral oxygenation during the first stage of labour. *Br. J. Obstet. Gynaecol.* **102**(1): 9–13.

Blackburn, S.T. & Loper, D.L. (1992) *Maternal, Fetal and Neonatal Physiology: A Clinical Perspective.* Philadelphia: W.B. Saunders Co.

Bradley, R. (1991) Intrapartum fetal monitoring. *Maternal & Child Health* November: 351–357.

Brans, Y.W., Escobedo, M.B., Hayaski, R.H. *et al.* (1984) Perinatal mortality in a large perinatal centre: five-year review of 31,000 births. *Am. J. Obstet. Gynecol.* **148**: 284–289.

Buckell, E.W.C. (1985) Wessex perinatal mortality survey 1982. *Br. J. Obstet. Gynaecol.* **92**: 550–558.

Butler, N.R., Goldstein, H. & Ross, E.M. (1972) Cigarette smoking in pregnancy; its influence on both weight and perinatal mortality. *Br. Med. J.* **2**: 127–130.

Dyer, M. (1992) Stillborn – Still precious. *MIDIRS Midwifery Digest* **2**(2): 341–344.

Evans, S. (1992) The value of cardiotocograph monitoring in midwifery. *Midwives Chronicle* January: 4–10.

Fujikura, T. & Kilonsky, B. (1975) The significance of meconium staining. *Am. J. Obstet. Gynecol.* **121**: 45–50.

Gauge, S.M. & Henderson, C. (1992) *CTG Made Easy.* Edinburgh: Churchill Livingstone.

Grant, A.M. (1993) Fetal blood sampling as adjunct to heart monitoring. In Enkin, M.W., Keirse, M.J.N.C., Renfrew, M.J. & Neilson, J.P. (eds) *Pregnancy and Childbirth Module.* Cochrane Database of Systematic Reviews: Review no. 07018. 30 July 1992. Oxford: Update Software.

Gregory, G., Gooding, C., Phibbs, R. & Tooley, W. (1974) Meconium aspiration in infants: a prospective study. *J. Pediat.* **85**: 848–852.

Haglund, B., Cnattingiust, S. & Nordstrom, M-L. (1993) Social differences in late fetal death and infant mortality in Sweden 1985–1986. *Paediat. Perinatal Epidemiol.* **7**: 33–44.

Healy, P. (1993) Who knows why? *Nursing Times* **8**(39): 40–41.

Hobel, C.J. (1971) Intrapartum clinical assessment of fetal distress. *Am. J. Obstet. Gynecol.* **110**: 336–342.

Holtzman, R.B., Banzhaz, W.C., Silver, R.K. & Hageman, J.R. (1989) Perinatal management of meconium staining of the amniotic fluid. *Clin. Perinatol.* **16**(4): 825–838.

Jacobs, M.M. & Phibbs, R.H. (1989) Prevention, recognition

and treatment of perinatal asphyxia. *Clin. Perinatol.* **16**(4): 785–807.

Katz, V. & Bowes, W. (1992) Meconium aspiration syndrome: reflections on a murky subject. *Am. J. Obstet. Gynecol.* **166**: 171–183.

Levene, M.I. (1987) Neonatal neurology. In *Current Reviews in Perinatology*, Vol. 3. Edinburgh: Churchill Livingstone.

Lewis, TLT. & Chamberlain, G.V.P. (1990) *Obstetrics by Ten Teachers*, 15th edn. London: Edward Arnold.

Llewellyn-Jones, D. (1994) *Fundamentals of Obstetrics & Gynaecology*, 6th edn. London: Mosby.

McNiven, P., Roch, B. & Wall, J. (1994) Meconium stained amniotic fluid. *Modern Midwife* **4**(7): 17–20.

Miller, S. (1993) Continuous Assessment. *Nursing Times* **89**(23): 48–49.

Parer, J.T. & Livingstone, E.G. (1990) What is fetal distress? *Am. J. Obstet. Gynecol.* **162**(6): 1421–1427.

Pitkin, R.M. (1987) Fetal death: diagnosis and management. *Am. J. Obstet. Gynecol.* **157**(3): 582–589.

Robins, L.N., Mills, J.L., Krulewitch, C. & Allen, A.H. (1993) Effects of in utero exposure to street drugs. *Am. J. Public Health* **83** (Suppl.): 6–32.

Rossi, E., Philipson, E., Williams, T. & Kalham, S. (1989) Meconium aspiration syndrome: intrapartum and neonatal attributes. *Am. J. Obstet. Gynecol.* **161**(5): 1106–1110.

Siney, C. (ed.) (1995) *The Pregnant Drug Addict*. Hale: Books for Midwives Press.

Thornton, L., Clune, M., Maguire, R., Griffin, E. & O'Connor, J. (1990) Narcotic addiction: the expectant mother and her baby. *Ir. Med. J.* **83**(4): 139–142.

Tucker, S.M. (1992) *Pocket Guide to Fetal Monitoring*. St. Louis: Mosby Year Book.

UKCC (UK Central Council for Nursing, Midwifery and Health Visiting) (1993) *Midwives' Rules*. London: UKCC.

47

Preterm Labour

Labour is defined as preterm when it occurs before the end of the 37th week of pregnancy. Babies are described in terms of either birthweight or gestational age. Infants delivered less than 37 completed weeks from the first day of the last menstrual period are referred to as *preterm*, irrespective of weight, while infants weighing less than 2500 g are classified as of *low birthweight*. Many babies, of course, are both preterm and of low birthweight.

Recent advances in neonatal care have resulted in the survival of very small and immature infants and these definitions have been further developed to embrace this category: *very low birthweight infants* (VLBW) are defined as those weighing less than 1500 g at birth and *extremely low birthweight infants* (ELBW) as less than 1000 g at birth (Halliday, 1992).

It is important to differentiate between the low birthweight preterm infant and the baby whose birthweight is low because of intrauterine growth retardation as each group has different needs and problems after birth.

The incidence of preterm delivery as a proportion of all births ranges from 6 to 10% in developed countries and this has changed little over the past 20 years. Rates of preterm delivery increase with increasing gestational age, up to 37 weeks, with less than a quarter occurring before 32 weeks (Griffin, 1993). Preterm birth is directly responsible for 75–90% of all neonatal deaths not due to lethal congenital malformations and is a major cause of both short- and long-term neonatal morbidity (Amon, 1992).

Aetiology

Preterm birth may occur as a result of any of the following situations:

▶ *Elective preterm delivery*: This may be undertaken as a result of severe pre-eclampsia, maternal renal disease or severe intrauterine growth retardation. This group of infants has the best outcome and the lowest handicap rate.
▶ *Premature rupture of the membranes*: This is an antecedent in about 20% of cases of preterm birth.
▶ *Complicated emergency delivery*: The complications

include placental abruption, eclampsia, rhesus iso-immunization, maternal infection or prolapsed cord. This group accounts for about 25% of preterm births.

▶ *Uncomplicated spontaneous preterm labour of unknown cause*: This is the largest group, accounting for up to 40% of preterm births.

These latter two groups tend to have the poorest outcome in terms of survival and handicap (Halliday, 1992).

RISK FACTORS

A number of risk factors have been associated with preterm labour and these may be related to maternal or fetal circumstances. It is important to remember that many of these factors are not causative agents but only markers which may indicate the woman who is at increased risk of preterm labour. (Abrams *et al.*, 1989; Drife, 1989; Alger and Crenshaw, 1989; Main, 1988; Ledger, 1989; Amon, 1992; Roberts *et al.*, 1990; Chamberlain, 1991; Hay *et al.*, 1994; Hedegaard *et al.*, 1993).

Biological/medical factors

▶ Age less than 15 or more than 35 years.
▶ Low body weight (less than 50 kg at conception).
▶ History of hypertension, renal disease or diabetes mellitus.
▶ Generalized infections, especially viral.

Reproductive history

▶ History of previous preterm birth. If the woman has had more than two previous preterm deliveries her risk of preterm birth is 70% for the current pregnancy.
▶ Bleeding in previous pregnancy.
▶ Uterine abnormality: 35% of women with cervical incompetence will deliver preterm and 19% of women with a bicornuate, unicornuate or didelphic uterus will deliver before 37 weeks' gestation.

Current pregnancy

▶ Failure to gain weight adequately.
▶ Bleeding.
▶ Retained intrauterine contraceptive device.
▶ Abdominal surgery.
▶ Infections, especially pyelonephritis.

▶ Genital tract infection, especially non-specific vaginitis, bacterial vaginosis, *Chlamydia* and group B haemolytic *Streptococcus*. This latter organism is carried by 5% of women and is associated with preterm prelabour rupture of the membranes. Amnionitis resulting from genital tract infection may stimulate the local release of prostaglandin and this may cause labour to begin.
▶ Multiple pregnancy: 46% deliver preterm.
▶ Polyhydramnios.
▶ Fetal malformation.
▶ Rhesus disease.
▶ Fetal death.

Socio-economic

▶ Poverty and social deprivation: preterm labour is commoner in women from lower socio-economic groups.
▶ Marital status: preterm labour is commoner in unmarried women.
▶ Employment which involves hard physical work.

Psychological

▶ Psychological distress is associated with preterm delivery.

Cultural/behavioural

▶ Cigarette, alcohol or drug use.
▶ Short inter-pregnancy interval.
▶ Late antenatal booking.
▶ Poor attendance for antenatal care.

Prediction and Prevention of Preterm Labour

Several methods have been used to try to identify women at risk of preterm labour. However, prediction is difficult and may not be effective in preventing preterm birth. Formal *risk-scoring systems* have been used, based on the factors described above. This method has relatively poor predictive value, especially for primigravid women and a low score may induce a false sense of security (Keirse, 1989; Halliday, 1992). Home *monitoring of uterine activity* has also been used but appears to have no effect on the rate of preterm birth (Iams *et al.*, 1987).

Regular pelvic examination will reveal signs of cervical changes which may herald the onset of labour. However this procedure may of itself introduce infection and has a low predictive value for women at risk of preterm birth (Halliday, 1992; Buekens *et al.*, 1994). Ultrasonographic measurement of *cervical length* may predict the likelihood of preterm labour (Andersen *et al.*, 1990). This is, however, a time-consuming technique if applied to a large section of the pregnant population and may therefore be impracticable.

The discovery of a relationship between high levels of *fetal fibronectin* in cervical and vaginal secretions and the onset of preterm labour has led to the development of a bedside test (Lockwood *et al.*, 1991; Mast Diagnostics Ltd, 1993). Fetal fibronectin is a component of the extracellular matrix. It is secreted by the anchoring trophoblastic villi. If preterm labour is imminent there is separation of maternal and fetal tissue at the choriodecidual junction, leading to leakage of fibronectin. The test has a sensitivity of 79.4% and a specificity of 82.7%. There is, however, a false positive rate of 17% (Creasy, 1991). The test should be carried out every two weeks from 24 weeks' gestation and cannot be used in the presence of vaginal bleeding or rupture of the membranes as both blood and amniotic fluid contain fibronectin. The value of the test may therefore be limited.

Fetal breathing movements cease before preterm labour commences and this is a reliable indicator of imminent preterm delivery (Castle and Turnbull, 1983; Besinger *et al.*, 1987). However the time and resources required to screen large populations of at-risk women make this unattractive as a screening procedure (Halliday, 1992).

Prevention of preterm birth is dependent upon preventing uterine activity and/or cervical dilatation. *Bedrest* has been advocated as a preventative measure but has been shown to be ineffective (Papiernik, 1984). Increased *antenatal care* and *education* about preterm labour may reduce the incidence of birth before 34 weeks' gestation (Papiernik *et al.*, 1985). *Progestogens* and *ethanol* are no longer used. *Antibiotic therapy* has been shown to delay the onset of preterm labour in some cases (Norman *et al.*, 1994). Recent work on the use of *glyceryl trinitrate (GTN)* skin patches indicate that this is an effective method of suppressing preterm labour (Lees *et al.*, 1994).

Cervical cerclage may be helpful where there is a recognized cervical weakness such as may follow previous second trimester abortion or cone biopsy. The technique involves the insertion of a strong, non-absorbable suture such as Mersilene tape around the cervix at the level of the internal os. This keeps the cervical canal closed. The procedure is carried out under general anaesthesia. The suture is removed at 39 weeks' gestation or when labour commences.

The role of *social support* in preventing preterm birth has been examined and does not appear to have any influence on physical outcomes, although it may improve psychological well-being (Spencer *et al.* 1989; Mamelle *et al.*, 1989; Bryce *et al.*, 1988; Oakley, 1989).

Preterm Prelabour Rupture of the Membranes

Spontaneous rupture of the membranes before 37 weeks' gestation and before labour commences is termed preterm prelabour rupture. The cause may be unclear but it is associated with cervical incompetence and genital tract infection, especially group B haemolytic *Streptococcus*. Labour may commence soon afterwards but if it does not occur for some days the uterine cavity and the fetus may be colonized by bacteria. This increases the risks to the fetus. There is also the danger of prolapse of the umbilical cord (Lewis and Chamberlain, 1990).

If preterm rupture of the membranes occurs at home the midwife must contact the doctor and arrange for the woman to be admitted to a hospital with a neonatal unit. Most women with preterm prelabour rupture of membranes will deliver within a week (Keirse *et al.*, 1989a). On admission to hospital the midwife should assess the maternal and fetal condition, noting any uterine activity. A speculum examination is carried out to visualize the cervix. A pool of amniotic fluid may be seen in the posterior fornix. A cervical swab is taken and sent for microscopy and culture. Digital vaginal examination should be avoided in order to reduce the risk of ascending infection.

The doctor may prescribe the steroid dexamethasone 12 mg intramuscularly. Two doses are given, 12 hours apart, to accelerate surfactant production in the fetal lungs and reduce the risk of respiratory distress syndrome (*hyaline membrane disease*) at birth. This drug is effective after 24 hours and for up to seven days. It is of most benefit between 24 and 32 weeks' gestation. Although its efficacy has been questioned, a number of randomized controlled trials have indicated its value in promoting fetal lung maturity and many authorities recommend its use (Crowley, 1989; Keirse *et al.*, 1989a; Creasy, 1989; Llewellyn-Jones, 1990; Amon, 1992; Halliday, 1992).

Prophylactic tocolytic drugs are not normally used as they appear to have little value in this situation (Keirse *et al.*, 1989a).

The woman's temperature and pulse should be recorded at least twice daily as chorio-amnionitis occurs in at least 20% of cases of preterm rupture of the membranes. Blood may be taken for serum screening for C-reactive protein. This is a globulin of hepatic origin which rises in the acute phase of any infection. Consecutive values of more than 20 mg/l indicate infection (Drife, 1989). However, its value as an early indicator of intrauterine infection has been questioned (Keirse *et al.*, 1989a). If there is clear evidence of infection or vaginal colonization with pathogenic bacteria the doctor will prescribe antibiotic therapy. Prophylactic antiobiotic therapy in the absence of colonization may be ineffective in preventing maternal, fetal or neonatal infection (Keirse *et al.*, 1989a).

The midwife should monitor the fetal condition and observe the state of the liquor which drains from the vagina. Abnormal maternal signs such as pyrexia, tachycardia, uterine tenderness or offensive liquor or fetal signs such as abnormal fetal heart patterns or alterations in fetal activity should be reported to the doctor. The midwife must be alert for any signs of bleeding as placental abruption may follow preterm prelabour rupture of the membranes, due to the reduction in liquor volume (Keirse *et al.*, 1989a).

If the membranes have been ruptured for more than three weeks the fetal lungs may fail to develop properly due to the reduced liquor volume. This is a particular problem if rupture of the membranes occurs before 24 weeks' gestation. In these circumstances the outlook for the fetus is poor (Steer, 1991).

Management of Preterm Labour and Delivery

Preterm labour may be difficult to recognize but documented cervical changes, cervical effacement of 80% or cervical dilatation of 2 cm or more are accepted as diagnostic (Creasy, 1989). The midwife should be aware of the likelihood of preterm labour in any woman who complains of:

▶ increased painless contractions;
▶ menstrual-like cramps;
▶ backache;
▶ pelvic pressure; or
▶ increased vaginal discharge (Iams *et al.* 1990, 1994).

If labour begins at home the midwife must contact the doctor and arrange for the woman to be admitted to a hospital with a neonatal unit. On admission to hospital the mother should be made comfortable and the fetus should be continuously monitored. The midwife and the doctor should discuss the plans for the management of labour with the couple. The neonatal unit should be informed and a member of the neonatal unit staff should visit the parents to discuss the proposed management of the baby at delivery.

If the gestation is 35 weeks or more labour will probably be allowed to continue as most babies of this age make good progress if given appropriate care after birth. Below 35 weeks the doctor may prescribe a *tocolytic drug* if both mother and fetus are in good condition, with no signs of current vaginal bleeding or rupture of the membranes.

TOCOLYTIC DRUGS

The group of drugs most commonly used are the *beta-adrenergic agonists* such as ritodrine hydrochloride (Yutopar), salbutamol (Ventolin, Salbuvent) and terbutaline (Bricanyl). These compounds stimulate the beta-receptors of the autonomic nervous system and thus relax smooth muscle.

Ritodrine hydrochloride is administered by intravenous infusion, commencing at 50 μg/min and gradually increasing to 300–350 μg/min or until uterine contractions are suppressed, provided the maternal pulse does not exceed 140 beats per minute (RCOG, 1994). The infusion is continued for 12–48 hours after cessation of contractions and then oral therapy, 10 mg six hourly is prescribed for four weeks or until the mother reaches 37 weeks' gestation, whichever is the sooner. Leveno *et al.* (1986) found in their study that although ritodrine treatment significantly delayed delivery for 24 hours or less, it did not significantly modify the ultimate perinatal consequences of preterm labour. As ritodrine crosses the placenta a fetal tachycardia will develop.

Salbutamol is another beta-receptor stimulant drug which reduces uterine activity. The dose is usually 10 μg/min by intravenous infusion but may be increased up to 45 μg/min if required to suppress uterine contractions, providing the maternal pulse rate does not exceed 140 beats per minute. The infusion is maintained until contractions are controlled and then oral salbutamol 4 mg four times daily is prescribed.

Terbutaline is administered by intravenous infusion, commencing at 10 μg/min, increasing to 25 μg/min, until uterine activity ceases. The oral dose thereafter is 5 mg eight hourly.

Maternal side-effects of these beta-adrenergic drugs include nausea, flushing, tremors, hypotension and palpitations. More serious effects are cardiac arrhythmias, myocardial ischaemia and pulmonary oedema which may develop in up to 5% of women treated with beta-adrenergic agonists. It is thought that the drugs stimulate the renin–aldosterone system and promote increased secretion of antidiuretic hormone, thus leading to fluid retention. In the lungs they may also increase the permeability of the alveolar–capillary barrier (Watson and Morgan, 1989; Milos *et al.*, 1988). Pulmonary oedema is more likely to occur in multiple pregnancies (Keirse *et al.*, 1989b). Symptoms include retrosternal chest pain, cough and dyspnoea. Other signs of fluid retention will be present such as a positive fluid balance and haemodilution with a decrease in haematocrit. Chest X-ray will confirm the diagnosis. The midwife should inform the doctor of any woman complaining of chest pain or dyspnoea whilst being treated with these drugs. The oedema disperses once the treatment is stopped.

Prostaglandin synthesis inhibitors such as indomethacin may be used to arrest preterm labour. Prostaglandin endoperoxide synthase converts free arachidonic acid to prostaglandin, which induces changes in the cervical collagen and facilitates cervical dilatation. Indomethacin acts by inhibiting production of this enzyme. Maternal side-effects include nausea, vomiting, diarrhoea, dizziness and headaches. Long-term use may cause fetal effects such as premature closure of the ductus arteriosus, right-sided heart failure and fetal death. Fetal exposure to this drug may be associated with an increased incidence of necrotizing enterocolitis in low birthweight infants (Major *et al.*, 1994). Contraindications are maternal infection, bleeding disorders, renal disease or peptic ulcers (Alger and Crenshaw, 1989; Keirse *et al.*, 1989b; Higby *et al.*, 1993).

Calcium channel blockers such as nifedipine may be used. These are drugs which inhibit muscle contraction by interfering with the movement of calcium ions across the plasma membrane (Marieb, 1992). However, they may not prolong gestation for more than 48 hours (Higby *et al.*, 1993). Research is currently being carried out into the potential for potassium channel openers as tocolytics.

Dexamethasone may be given as described earlier to accelerate fetal production of surfactant.

In all cases where drugs are used to suppress uterine activity, the maternal and fetal condition must be closely observed. Continuous monitoring of uterine contractions should be carried out and recordings of maternal pulse and blood pressure made every 15 minutes. A strict record of fluid balance is essential. Four hourly blood glucose (e.g. by BM Stix) is recommended (RCOG, 1994). Continuous external monitoring of the fetal heart is preferable to intermittent recordings every 15 minutes. Side-effects of the drugs must also be recorded. If the dilatation of the os uteri reaches 4 cm or more or the membranes rupture it is unlikely that the attempt to prevent labour progressing will be successful.

LABOUR AND DELIVERY

If the labour progresses despite attempts to control it, the midwife must inform both an obstetrician and a paediatrician. Continuous monitoring of the uterine contractions and fetal heart are carried out and all tocolytic drugs are stopped. Fetal distress due to cord compression may occur, particularly if the membranes have ruptured before the onset of labour. Amnioinfusion has been used to reduce cord compression following oligohydramnios but insufficient work has been done to allow evaluation of the risks and benefits of this technique (Keirse *et al.*, 1989a). Care must be exercised in the choice and timing of drugs given for pain relief. Epidural anaesthesia or the inhalation of nitrous oxide and oxygen are the preferred methods of pain relief as they have no adverse effect on the fetus. Analgesic drugs, especially morphine and its derivatives, should be given as sparingly as possible and avoided altogether within 3–4 hours of delivery, as they may severely depress the fetal respiratory centre.

Both an obstetrician and paediatrician should be present at delivery. Because of the poor ossification of the fetal skull and therefore the risk of intracranial injury, an elective episiotomy will be made to shorten the perineal phase of the second stage, followed by a very well-controlled normal delivery or forceps may be applied to protect the head during birth. Some obstetricians prefer to deliver the very immature infant by Caesarean section, especially if the presentation is breech, in order to reduce the risk of birth trauma and asphyxia (Alger and Crenshaw, 1989). A 30 second delay in clamping the umbilical cord, with the baby held 20 cm below the introitus, will increase the packed cell volume. This may assist the infant's progress after birth and reduce morbidity (Kinmond *et al.*, 1993).

The paediatrician will resuscitate the baby should it be necessary. Some authorities recommend that the child should be given an injection of phytomenadione (Konakion) 0.5–1 mg to lessen any risk of haemor-rhage. When the mother has seen and held her baby he is transferred to the neonatal unit.

Preterm delivery is extremely stressful for the parents. The birth of the baby often comes as a shock and they will be psychologically unprepared for his/her arrival. Any feelings of joy are quickly submerged by fears for the child's health and both parents need time to discuss the event and its implications with their professional attendants. The financial burden may be considerable if the infant is transferred to another hospital and the parents have to travel long distances to visit. In addition to this there may be the needs of older children to consider and the midwife should not underestimate the stress which preterm birth causes to all the family.

References

Abrams, B., Newman, V., Key, T. & Parker, J. (1989) Maternal weight gain and preterm delivery. *Obstet. Gynecol.* **74**(4): 577–583.

Alger, L. & Crenshaw, M. (1989) Preterm labour and delivery of the preterm infant. In Turnbull, A. & Chamberlain, G. (eds) *Obstetrics.* Edinburgh: Churchill Livingstone.

Amon, E. (1992) Premature labour. In Reece, E., Hobbins, J., Mahoney, M. & Petrie, R. (eds) *Medicine of the Fetus and Mother.* Philadelphia: J.B. Lippincott.

Andersen, H., Nugent, C., Wanty, S. & Hayashi, R. (1990) Prediction of risk for preterm delivery by ultrasonographic measurement of cervical length. *Am. J. Obstet. Gynecol.* **163**(3): 859–867.

Besinger, R., Compton, A. & Hayashi, R. (1987) The presence or absence of fetal breathing movements as a predictor of outcome in preterm labour. *Am. J. Obstet. Gynecol.* **157**: 753–757.

Bryce, R., Stanley, F. & Enkin, M. (1988) The role of social support in the prevention of preterm birth. *Birth* **15**(1): 19–22.

Buekens, P., Alexander, S., Boutsen, M., Blondel, B., Kaminski, M. & Reid, M. (1994) Randomised controlled trial of routine cervical examinations in pregnancy. European Community Collaborative Study Group on Prenatal Screening. *Lancet* **344**(8926): 841–844.

Castle, B. & Turnbull, A. (1983) The presence or absence of fetal breathing movements predicts the outcome of preterm labour. *Lancet* **ii**(8348): 471–472.

Chamberlain, G. (1991) ABC of antenatal care: preterm labour. *Br. Med. J.* **303** (6 July): 44–48.

Creasy, R. (1989) Preterm labour and delivery. In Creasy, R. & Resnik, R. (eds) *Maternal–Fetal Medicine: Principle and Practice*, 2nd edition. London: W.B. Saunders.

Creasy, R. (1991) Preventing preterm birth. *N. Engl. J. Med.* **325**: 727–729.

Crowley, P. (1989) Promoting pulmonary maturity. In Chalmers, I., Enkin, M. & Keirse, M. (eds) *Effective Care in Pregnancy and Childbirth.* Oxford: Oxford University Press.

Drife, J. (1989) Infection and preterm birth. *Br. J. Obstet. Gynaecol.* **96**(10): 1128–1132.

Griffin, J. (1993) *Born Too Soon.* Office of Health Economics, 12 Whitehall, London.

Halliday, H. (1992) Prematurity. In Calder, A. & Dunlop, W. (eds) *High Risk Pregnancy.* Oxford: Butterworth Heinemann.

Hay, P., Lamont, R., Taylor-Robinson, D., Morgan, D., Ison, C. & Pearson, J. (1994) Abnormal bacterial colonisation of the genital tract and subsequent preterm delivery and late miscarriage. *Br. Med. J.* **308**(29 January): 295–298.

Hedegaard, M., Henriksen, T., Sabroe, S. & Secher, W. (1993) Psychological distress in pregnancy and preterm delivery. *Br. Med. J.* **307** (24 July): 234–239.

Higby, K., Xenakis, E. & Pauerstein, C. (1993) Do tocolytic agents stop preterm labour? A critical and comprehensive review of efficacy and safety. *Am. J. Obstet. Gynecol.* **168**(4): 1247–1259.

Iams, J., Johnson, F., O'Shaughnessy, R. & West, L. (1987) A prospective random trial of home uterine activity monitoring in pregnancies at increased risk of preterm labour. *Am. J. Obstet. Gynecol.* **157**: 638–643.

Iams, J., Stilson, R., Johnson, F., Williams, R. & Rice, R. (1990) Symptoms that precede preterm labour and preterm premature rupture of the membranes. *Am. J. Obstet. Gynecol.* **162**(2): 486–490.

Iams, J., Johnson, F. & Parker, M. (1994) A prospective evaluation of the signs and symptoms of preterm labour. *Obstet. Gynecol.* **84**(2): 227–230.

Keirse, M. (1989) An evaluation of formal risk scoring for preterm birth. *Am. J. Perinatol.* **6**(2): 226–233.

Keirse, M., Ohlsson, A., Treffers, P. & Kanhai, H. (1989a) Prelabour rupture of the membranes preterm. In Chalmers, I., Enkin, M. & Keirse, M. (eds) *Effective Care in Pregnancy and Childbirth.* Oxford: Oxford University Press.

Keirse, M., Grant, A. & King, J. (1989b) Preterm labour. In Chalmers, I., Enkin, M. & Keirse, M. (eds) *Effective Care in Pregnancy and Childbirth.* Oxford: Oxford University Press.

Kinmond, S., Aitchison, T., Holland, B., Jones, J., Turner, T. & Wardrop, C. (1993) Umbilical cord clamping and preterm infants: a randomised trial. *Br. Med. J.* 306 (16 January): 172–175.

Ledger, W. (1989) Infection and premature labor. *Am. J. Perinatol.* 6(2): 234–236.

Lees, C., Campbell, S., Jauniaux, E. *et al.* (1994) Arrest of preterm labour and prolongation of gestation with glyceryl trinitrate, a nitric oxide donor. *Lancet* 343(8909): 1325–1326.

Leveno, K., Guzick, D., Hankins, G., Klein, V., Young, B. & Williams, M. (1986) Single centre randomized trial of ritodine hydrochloride for preterm labour *Lancet* i: 1293–1296.

Lewis, T. & Chamberlain, G. (1990) *Obstetrics by Ten Teachers.* London: Edward Arnold.

Llewellyn-Jones, D. (1990) *Fundamentals of Obstetrics and Gynaecology*, Vol. 1, *Obstetrics* 5th edn. London: Faber & Faber.

Lockwood, C., Senyei, A., Dishe, M. *et al.* (1991) Fetal fibronectin in cervical and vaginal secretions as a predictor of preterm delivery. *N. Engl. J. Med.* 325(10): 669–674.

Main, D. (1988) The epidemiology of preterm birth. *Clin. Obstet. Gynecol.* 31(3): 521–532.

Major, C., Lewis, D., Harding, J., Porto, M. & Garite, T. (1994) Tocolysis with indomethacin increases the incidence of necrotising enterocolitis in the low birth weight neonate. *Am. J. Obstet. Gynecol.* 170(1, 1): 102–106.

Mamelle, N., Bertucat, I. & Munoz, F. (1989) Pregnant women at work: rest periods prevent preterm birth? *Paediat. Perinatal Epidemiol.* 3(1): 19–28.

Marieb, E. (1992) *Human Anatomy and Physiology.* Wokingham: Benjamin/Cummings.

Mast Diagnostics UK Ltd (1993) Fetal fibronectin membrane assay kit. Mast Diagnostics Ltd., Bootle, Merseyside.

Milos, M., Aberle, D., Parkinson, B., Batra, P. & Brown, K. (1988) Maternal pulmonary edema complicating beta-adrenergic therapy of preterm labor. *Am. J. Roentgenol.* 151: 917–918.

Norman, K., Pattinson, R., de Souza, J., de Jong, P., Moller, G. & Kirsten, G. (1994) Ampicillin and metronidazole treatment in preterm labour: a multi-centre, randomised controlled trial. *Br. J. Obstet. Gynaecol.* 101(5): 404–408.

Oakley, A. (1989) Can social support influence pregnancy outcome? *Br. J. Obstet. Gynaecol.* 96(3): 260–262.

Papiernik, E. (1984) Proposals for a programmed prevention policy of preterm birth. *Clin. Obstet. Gynecol.* 27: 614–635.

Papiernik, E., Bouyer, J. & Dreyfus, J. (1985) Risk factors for preterm births and results of a prevention policy. The Haguenau Perinatal Study 1971–1982. In Beard, R. & Sharp, F. (eds) *Preterm Labour and its Consequences. Proceedings of the Thirteenth Study Group of the Royal College of Obstetricians and Gynaecologists*, pp. 15–20. London: RCOG.

Roberts, W., Morrison, J., Hamer, C. & Wiser, W. (1990) The incidence of preterm labor and specific risk factors. *Obstet. Gynecol.* 76(1 Suppl.): 855–895.

Royal College of Obstetricians and Gynaecologists (RCOG). (1994) *Guidelines No. 1 – For the Use of Ritodrine.* April, 1994. London: RCOG.

Spencer, B., Thomas, H. & Morris, J. (1989) A randomised controlled trial of the provision of a social support service during pregnancy: The South Manchester Family Worker Project. *Br. J. Obstet. Gynaecol.* 96(3): 281–288.

Steer, P. (1991) Obstetrics for paediatricians: premature labour. *Arch. Dis. Childh.* 66: 1167–1170.

Watson, N. & Morgan, B. (1989) Pulmonary oedema and salbutamol in preterm labour. *Br. J. Obstet. Gynaecol.* 96(12): 1445–1448.

Further Reading

Kuperminic, M., Lessing, J., Yaron, Y. & Peyser, M. (1993) Nifedepine versus ritodrine for suppression of preterm labour. *Br. J. Obstet. Gynaecol.* 100(12): 1090–1094.

McKenzie, H., Donnet, M., Howie, P., Patel, W. & Benvie, D. (1994) Risk of preterm delivery in pregnant women with group B streptococcal urinary infectious or urinary antibodies to group B streptococcal and *E. coli* antigens. *Br. J. Obstet. Gynaecol.* 101: 107–113.

Mercer, B., Crocker, L., Boe, N. & Sibai, B. (1993) Induction versus expectant management in premature rupture of the membranes with mature amniotic fluid at 32–36 weeks: A randomized trial. *Am. J. Obstet. Gynecol.* 169(4): 775–782.

Narahara, H. & Johnston, J. (1993) Smoking and preterm labor: effect of a cigarette smoke extract on the secretion of platelet-activating factor acetyl-hydrolase by human decidual macrophages. *Am. J. Obstet. Gynecol.* 169(5): 1321–1326.

Nelson, L., Anderson, R., O'Shea, T. & Swain, M. (1994) Expectant management of preterm premature rupture of the membranes. *Am. J. Obstet. Gynecol.* 171(2): 350–356.

Romero, R., Sibai, B., Caritis, S. *et al.* (1993) Antibiotic treatment of preterm labor with intact membranes: A multi-center randomized double-blinded, placebo–controlled trial. *Am. J. Obstet. Gynecol.* 169(4): 764–774.

48

Induction of Labour and Post-Term Pregnancy

Induction of Labour

> Decisions to bring pregnancy to an end prior to the spontaneous onset of labour constitute one of the most fundamental ways of intervening in the 'natural history' of pregnancy and childbirth.
>
> (Chalmers and Keirse, 1989: 981)

Induction of labour may be described as the deliberate attempt to pre-empt the spontaneous onset of labour by artificial means. Rates of induction vary considerably between maternity units, but a rate of 17% in England and Wales in 1990 was reported by Lamont (1990), in comparison to a rate of 41% in the mid-1970s (DHSS, 1976).

This decline is due in part to an understanding of the adverse effects of unjustified induction, but it was widespread public criticism by the media in the early 1970s which led to a re-examination of the issue among those providing care for pregnant women.

Most of the indications for induction relate to concern about fetal compromise and are thus clear-cut, but there are other circumstances where the decision is less clear as to whether induction confers benefit or harm. In these situations careful assessment of each individual woman and fetus is needed to select those in whom the risk of continuing the pregnancy is greater than the potential risk of intervention.

MATERNAL INDICATIONS

Post-term pregnancy

Induction of labour may be offered to women with pregnancies over 41 weeks' gestation. This will be considered in more detail later in the chapter.

Hypertension

Hypertensive disorders are one of the principal indications for induction and timely intervention may become necessary to avoid serious maternal morbidity (see Chapter 41).

Other medical conditions

In renal and heart disease where there is concern about the effects of the pregnancy continuing, induction may be indicated (see Chapter 42). Elective delivery at 36–38 weeks' gestation was for many years the classical management for women with diabetes, based on one study which suggested that the stillbirth rate rose above the neonatal death rate after 36 weeks' gestation (Peel and Oakley, 1949, cited in Hunter, 1989). However, it is now felt that there is no valid reason to terminate an otherwise uncomplicated pregnancy in a diabetic woman before term (Hunter, 1989).

Pre-labour spontaneous rupture of the membranes

By definition, this condition occurs before the onset of regular uterine contractions and may occur before 37 weeks when it is referred to as *pre-labour rupture of the membranes preterm* or at 37 weeks or after when it is known as *pre-labour rupture at term*. With the former, the two main risks include preterm delivery and infectious morbidity in the neonate and the woman due to ascending intrauterine infection. Pre-labour rupture at term results in 70% of these women delivering within 24 hours and almost 90% within 48 hours (Grant and Keirse, 1989). The main concerns are related to maternal and neonatal infection and an increased risk of Caesarean section. In a large prospective study of 5041 women with pre-labour rupture of the membranes at term, Hannah *et al.* (1996) randomized women into four groups: induction of labour with intravenous oxytocin; induction of labour with vaginal prostaglandin E_2 gel; or expectant management for up to four days with labour induced by either intravenous oxytocin or vaginal prostaglandin E_2 gel if complications developed. Interestingly, the rates of neonatal infection and Caesarean section were not significantly different among the groups. Clinical chorioamnionitis was less likely to develop in the women in the induction-with-oxytocin group than in those in the expectant management (oxytocin) group as was postpartum fever. In addition, women viewed induction of labour more positively than expectant management.

Placental abruption

In moderate and severe placental abruption once maternal resuscitation has taken place and if the fetus is alive, a decision has to be made about delivery, taking into consideration the estimated maturity of the fetus. This is usually by Caesarean section, but inducing labour and augmenting with oxytocin in conjunction with careful continuous fetal monitoring may result in a 50% decrease in the Caesarean section rate, without a significant increase in perinatal mortality (Hurd *et al.*, 1983).

Maternal request

Induction may be requested by women for social or psychological reasons, for example, difficulties may arise in arranging social support, or women may become depressed about pregnancies which continue longer than expected. In these circumstances induction is usually only performed at term.

Poor obstetric history

A previous stillbirth may be an indication for induction of labour at term.

Unstable lie

Induction may be offered to women at term with an unstable lie once underlying abnormalities such as placenta praevia have been excluded. The lie is corrected to longitudinal by external version followed by induction of labour. However, the risk of cord prolapse may lead the obstetrician to decide on Caesarean section as the safest option.

FETAL INDICATIONS

Fetal compromise

Induction is indicated if there is evidence of diminished fetal well-being caused by placental insufficiency and characterized by intrauterine growth retardation, abnormally reduced fetal movements or abnormal fetal umbilical blood flow detected by Doppler ultrasound. However, if the fetus is severely compromised, Caesarean section will be performed.

Fetal death

It is wrong to assume that all women want the most rapid method of delivery when their baby has died *in utero*. There are no real benefits or hazards for induction compared with waiting for spontaneous labour and the decision should be left to the woman. Although there is a possible increase in the risk of blood coagulation disorders with awaiting spontaneous labour, this is usually when the death has been caused by placental abruption (Keirse and Kanhai, 1989).

Rhesus iso-immunization

Induction of labour is the usual management for established iso-immunization if the fetus is sufficiently mature, before it is too severely affected to be effectively treated by therapy after birth (Gravenhorst, 1989).

Severe congenital abnormalities

Labour may be induced to terminate the pregnancy if the fetus has a lethal abnormality or a defect likely to result in major handicap. Other circumstances may be when the baby would benefit from early surgery.

CONTRAINDICATIONS

Placenta praevia

Even with marginal placenta praevia there is almost no indication for vaginal delivery when the fetus has reached a viable age because of the risks of maternal and fetal haemorrhage, cord accidents and malpresentations (Fraser and Watson, 1989).

Cephalopelvic disproportion

Proven cephalopelvic disproportion may be a contraindication for induction of labour. This is usually only diagnosed following a previous Caesarean section for disproportion and if the fetus in the current pregnancy is of an equivalent or greater weight. However, in the literature successful vaginal delivery occurs over 50% of the time following a Caesarean section for disproportion (Enkin, 1989).

Oblique or transverse lie

These are absolute contraindications because of the risk of cord prolapse and of obstruction.

Severe fetal compromise

In this situation the fetus is unlikely to tolerate the stress of labour or even a minor degree of hypoxia and Caesarean section is the safest option.

TIMING OF INDUCTION

Induction is usually timed for when it will be most successful, that is, near to the onset of spontaneous labour. But there are situations when it will be necessary to intervene before term and both birthweight of the fetus estimated by ultrasound and gestational age are important factors in predicting future problems in the neonatal period. Amniocentesis may be performed to measure the lecithin–sphingomyelin ratio, in order to estimate fetal pulmonary maturity, and corticosteroids should be prescribed for the woman to promote this and thereby reduce the risk of mortality, respiratory distress syndrome and intraventricular haemorrhage in preterm infants (Crowley, 1996).

METHODS

Cervical ripening

The success of induction and subsequent length of labour is primarily determined by the state of the cervix at the time of induction. An 'unripe' cervix fails to dilate adequately and this results in high failure rates of induction, characterized by long and exhausting labours, an increased incidence of Caesarean section and other complications. These include pyrexia and intrauterine infection following amniotomy, and uterine hyperstimulation and drug-induced side-effects with the use of high-dosage oxytocics (Keirse and van Oppen, 1989).

Prior to induction the state of the cervix is assessed using a score based on that originally proposed by Bishop (1964). Five qualities are rated:

- ▶ cervical dilatation;
- ▶ cervical consistency;
- ▶ length of the cervix; and
- ▶ position of the cervix;
- ▶ station of the presenting part (see Table 1).

When the total score is six or over the cervix is said to be favourable.

Prostaglandins Following the introduction of prostaglandins for the induction of labour it was found that smaller doses produced marked softening of the cervix. The use of prostaglandins for cervical ripening have

Table 1 Modified Bishop's scoring system

Features for assessment	Score			
	0	1	2	3
Dilatation of cervix (cm)	closed	1–2	3–4	5+
Consistency of cervix	firm	medium	soft	–
Length of cervix (cm)	3	2	1	0
Position of cervix	posterior	mid	anterior	–
Station in cm above (−) ischial spines	−3	−2	−1	0

since been extensively studied and, in an overview of all the controlled comparisons, Keirse (1992a) summarizes that they are more likely than either placebo or no treatment to start labour and to avoid the need for formal induction with oxytocin. Keirse also comments that prostaglandins markedly reduce the likelihood of not being delivered within 12 hours from the start of induction, decrease the incidence of an interval from induction to delivery in excess of 24 hours and increase the chances of a spontaneous vaginal delivery.

Prostaglandin E_2 (PGE_2) is most commonly used and evidence suggests that it is superior to other forms such as $PGF_{2\alpha}$ because of the lower dosage needed (Keirse and van Oppen, 1989). Oral administration of prostaglandins requires repeated doses over a long period of time to effect cervical ripening and may be associated with unpleasant maternal gastrointestinal side-effects. Of the other routes, vaginal, endocervical and extra-amniotic, evidence does not show that one is clinically superior to the others and therefore the most appropriate route is the one causing least discomfort for the woman (Keirse and van Oppen, 1989).

Higher doses of prostaglandins are used to induce labour after fetal death which may lead to the woman experiencing nausea, diarrhoea and vomiting. However, natural prostaglandins have been structurally modified to produce prostaglandin analogues which, although not suitable for induction of labour with a live fetus, may produce less distressing side-effects for the woman.

Other methods   Only *oestrogens* and particularly oestradiol have been studied with any consistency and, although they are known to ripen the cervix, other outcomes are unclear, for example, whether they increase the likelihood of delivery within a reasonable time interval after induction (Keirse and van Oppen, 1989).

Oxytocin is a poor ripening agent because of the very few oxytocin receptors in the cervix and may be unpleasant for the woman. *Mechanical devices* such as laminaria tents introduced into the cervix or extra-amniotic space, *relaxin* and *breast stimulation* do not appear to be useful approaches to ripening the cervix and are not recommended when there is an obvious need to induce labour (Keirse and van Oppen, 1989).

Risks of cervical ripening   As cervical ripening is the first step to inducing labour, it should not be

attempted unless the aim is to bring pregnancy to an end.

Keirse and van Oppen (1989) describe the risks as:

▶ unnecessary and unjustified induction of labour because of the knowledge clinicians have about ripening the cervix;
▶ intrauterine infection caused by mechanical procedures and extra amniotic drug administration;
▶ uterine hypertonus which may lead to Caesarean section during ripening;
▶ fetal heart rate abnormalities – the significance of which are unclear for the baby;
▶ discomfort for the woman.

In the light of current evidence prostaglandins are the approach of choice for ripening the unfavourable cervix.

Sweeping the membranes

Sweeping or stripping the membranes from the lower uterine segment at term has frequently been used to induce labour in the hope that amniotomy or oxytocic drugs may be avoided.

The theory behind this method is that prostaglandin production is increased (Mitchell *et al.*, 1977) which is in direct relationship to the surface area of detachment occurring between the membranes and uterine wall (Keirse *et al.*, 1983).

However, there is a dearth of evidence from controlled trials to evaluate this practice. In the two trials (Weissberg and Spellacy, 1977; McColgin *et al.*, 1990) overviewed by Keirse (1992b), stripping the membranes increased the likelihood of labour within 48 hours and of being delivered within one week, and decreased the likelihood of delivery after 42 weeks. A larger trial (Allott and Palmer, 1993) of 195 women with pregnancies beyond 40-weeks gestation showed that the probability of labour was twice as high at 3-days post-intervention in the group of women allocated to membrane sweeping. In addition, fewer women in this group required induction of labour by other methods (8% compared to 19%).

Amniotomy

Rupturing the membranes

represents one of the most irrevocable interventions in pregnancy . . . (and) constitutes obstetric interference of the most profound nature. More than any other intervention currently used to induce labour, it embodies a firm commitment to delivery.

(Keirse and Chalmers, 1989: 1058)

The most common approach is *low amniotomy* or fore-water rupture as opposed to *high amniotomy* or hind-water rupture which, if used at all, should be reserved for inducing labour in women with polyhydramnios and a firm indication to end the pregnancy (Keirse and Chalmers, 1989).

Amniotomy may successfully be used alone to induce labour but its onset may be unpredictable and occasionally prolonged (Patterson, 1971). It may be used with oxytocic drugs either at the time of membrane rupture or after an interval of a few hours if uterine contractions have not commenced. From evidence from clinical trials (Patterson, 1971; Saleh, 1975, cited in Keirse and Chalmers, 1989) women who receive oxytocics at the time of amniotomy are more likely to be delivered within 12 hours and less likely to have a Caesarean section or forceps delivery than those who do not receive oxytocics. Also, women who receive oxytocin at the time of amniotomy require less analgesia and sustain lower rates of postpartum haemorrhage than those who receive oxytocin at a later time. Less depressed Apgar scores are also found.

The risks of amniotomy include (Keirse and Chambers, 1989):

▶ *Intrauterine infection*: the longer the interval until delivery the greater the risk.
▶ *Early decelerations* of the fetal heart rate: This may be related to cord compression or prolapse.
▶ *Umbilical cord prolapse*: not necessarily at the time of amniotomy but may occur when labour ensues.
▶ *Bleeding* from the cervix, from fetal vessels in the membranes (vasa praevia) or from the placental site in placenta praevia.

Oxytocin

Currently the most widely used method for inducing labour is intravenous infusion of oxytocin (Syntocinon). This is usually administered through an electronic infusion pump which delivers the drug at a regulated rate in a small volume of isotonic solution or through a fully automated closed loop feedback system in which the dose of oxytocin is regulated by the intensity of uterine contractions.

The regime for administration will vary between maternity units (Irons *et al.*, 1993), but one example is 10 units of Syntocinon diluted in 500 ml of 0.9% saline commencing at 4 milliunits per minute and increasing by 4 milliunits per minute every 15 minutes, up to a maximum of 32 milliunits per minute until effective, regular uterine contractions occur. The minimum effective dose of Syntocinon should be used.

The risks of oxytocin administration include:

▶ Water retention and hyponatraemia due to the anti-diuretic effect of oxytocin, particularly at an early stage of pregnancy when large doses are required to stimulate contractions (Hendricks and Brenner, 1964).
▶ Uterine hyperstimulation causing:
  – fetal hypoxia due to compromised circulation through the placenta;
  – uterine rupture.
▶ Neonatal hyperbilirubinaemia – probably due more to the relative immaturity of the baby as a result of ending the pregnancy than to the use of oxytocin (Keirse and Chalmers, 1989).

Prostaglandins

Prostaglandins have been used since the late 1960s for the induction of labour in a variety of different forms and rates of administration. Several studies, reviewed by Keirse (1992c), have compared prostaglandins with placebo treatments and have shown that the failure rate and the proportion of women needing a further attempt at induction were lower in those receiving prostaglandins (Liggins, 1979; MacKenzie *et al.*, 1981), as were the proportion of women who had not delivered vaginally within 12 hours and within 24 hours (Ulmsten *et al.*, 1982). The rates of Caesarean section were lower in the prostaglandin groups (Liggins, 1979), but those of instrumental vaginal delivery were similar. Most of the trials did not observe uterine hyperstimulation and/or hypertonus (Gordon-Wright and Elder, 1979) and the incidence of gastrointestinal side-effects were low. No difference was observed in terms of Apgar scores (Liggins, 1979; Gordon-Wright and Elder, 1979).

The two main prostaglandins – PGE_2 and $PGF_{2\alpha}$ – stimulate uterine contractions and indeed are naturally formed during spontaneous labour but overall, prostaglandin E_2 is preferable, although it may cause venous erythema when administered intravenously, and hyperthermia (Keirse and Chalmers, 1989).

Currently, the most popular mode of administration of PGE_2 is the vaginal route and may include tablets, pessaries and gels. Gel may also be administered into the extra-amniotic space and into the endocervical canal, although this route is more commonly used for ripening the cervix and its merits and hazards for induction of labour compared to other routes is yet to be assessed.

The risks of prostaglandin administration include (Keirse and Chalmers, 1989):

▶ *Gastrointestinal side-effects*, affecting up to 10% of women when given orally.
▶ *Maternal pyrexia* from the effect of prostaglandins on the thermoregulating centres in the brain.
▶ *Unjustified induction of labour* because of the ready availability of prostaglandins.

Keirse (1993) has reviewed the evidence for the use of prostaglandins versus oxytocin and suggests that prostaglandins are likely to reduce the incidence of operative delivery and may increase the likelihood of delivery within 24 hours, possibly because of the greater mobility women have when given prostaglandins vaginally or orally. However, between 5 and 20% of women will experience gastrointestinal side-effects or pyrexia, depending on the routes, type and dosage given. The relative safety of these drugs for the baby has yet to be determined.

Methods to stimulate natural oxytocin and prostaglandin release

Mechanical nipple stimulation induces uterine contractility by the release of oxytocin from the maternal posterior pituitary gland (Salzmann, 1971). The relationship between nipple stimulation and uterine contractility has been used down through the centuries to prevent postpartum haemorrhage by putting the baby to the breast at birth. However, in the last century Merriman (1838, cited in Thiery *et al.*, 1989) advocated nipple stimulation to 'introduce' labour and there have been several more recent reports of clinicians exploring this effect (Salzmann, 1971; Elliot and Flaherty, 1984; Fragner and Miyazaki, 1987). This effect is thought to remain within a physiological range (Lazaro, 1973, cited in Thiery *et al.*, 1989) but some have reported uterine hyperstimulation resulting in profound fetal bradycardia (Viegas *et al.*, 1984).

Secondly there is thought to be a relationship between female orgasm and the release of oxytocin (Goodlin *et al.*, 1971, 1972). Seminal fluid is known to be a concentrated source of prostaglandins and

therefore intercourse may well ripen the cervix or induce labour in some women.

Post-term Pregnancy

Definition

The standard international definition of a post-term, prolonged or post-dates pregnancy endorsed by the World Health Organization (WHO, 1977) and the International Federation of Gynecology and Obstetrics (FIGO, 1982) is 42 completed weeks or more, i.e. 294 days or more.

Incidence

The reported incidence rates for post-term pregnancy range from 4 to 14%, with an average of about 10%, while that of pregnancies beyond 43 weeks range from 2 to 7% (Bakketeig and Bergsjo, 1989). Reporting on Scandinavian data, Bakketeig and Bergsjo (1989) demonstrate a strong association between nulliparous women and the incidence of post-term birth with the risk being 15–20% higher compared with parous women. Interestingly, they also demonstrate a cumulative risk of repeating a post-term birth, for example, for a woman with two previous post-term births her risk of a subsequent one is 39.1%.

Assessment of gestational age

Most pregnancies are dated according to Naegele's rule but women with long or irregular periods may have a longer interval between menstruation and ovulation than is presupposed by this rule. When data are analysed from studies of gestational length using basal body temperature rise to indicate ovulation, the rate of post-term pregnancy is lower (Stewart, 1952; Boyce *et al.*, 1976). Calculation of the expected date of delivery may pose a problem for women with uncertain menstrual dates. Hall *et al.* (1985) found that in Aberdeen 73% of women had certain dates, 20% approximate and 7% uncertain. Recent use of oral contraception may further complicate the picture.

Clinical estimation of gestational age by bimanual palpation of the uterus in early pregnancy or by abdominal palpation is not accurate (Beazley and Underhill, 1970). The date of quickening, when the woman first feels fetal movement, adds little to the assessment because of wide variation (O'Dowd and O'Dowd, 1985). Early ultrasound examination to assess duration of gestation in the first trimester entails measurement of the fetal crown–rump length and is accurate to within five days in 95% of pregnancies (Robinson and Fleming, 1975). Between 13 and 18 weeks, measurement of the biparietal diameter predicts the date of delivery to within two weeks in 89% of pregnancies (Campbell, 1976). Early scans are also associated with a reduction in induction for post-term pregnancy (Bakketeig et al., 1984; Eik-Nes et al., 1984).

Risk of post-term pregnancy – perinatal mortality and morbidity

Since the 1920s, strong evidence has been presented to suggest that post-term pregnancy is associated with a higher risk of perinatal death (Ballantyne and Browne 1922; Butler and Bonham, 1963). However, there is also a higher incidence of congenital malformation in babies born post-term compared with those at term and many studies fail to correct their risk estimates for deaths from these causes (Crowley, 1989) which account for about 25% of the excess mortality (Naeye, 1978). In a retrospective analysis of 62 804 births in Dublin between 1979 and 1986, the corrected perinatal death rate (which excluded lethal malformation) for post-term births was 6.7 per 1000 while for births at term the rate was 4.5 per 1000 (Crowley, 1989). This study showed a higher incidence of intrapartum and neonatal deaths but not of antepartum deaths. The main cause of mortality was asphyxia with meconium-stained amniotic fluid.

When morbidity is considered for babies born post-term there is an association with perinatal asphyxia and the incidence of neonatal convulsions (Minchom et al., 1987) which in turn are associated with meconium-stained amniotic fluid (Curtis et al., 1988).

Thus the increased mortality and morbidity risks of post-term pregnancy appear to increase with the onset of labour and are strongly associated with meconium-staining of the amniotic fluid.

Associated features of post-term pregnancy

Uteroplacental insufficiency　A tenaciously held but mistaken belief is that the placenta ages as pregnancy progresses. However, no morphological features of the term placenta can be considered as a manifestation of ageing (Fox, 1979; Larsen et al., 1995); indeed, fresh villous growth and continuing DNA synthesis have been demonstrated in the placenta at term

(Sands and Dobbing, 1985; Fox, 1978). Yet in some fetuses there is gradual deterioration in placental function and chronic progressive uteroplacental insufficiency has been postulated to be the mechanism of fetal distress and/or death in post-term pregnancies (Miyazaki and Miyazaki, 1981). Interestingly, it has been suggested that a factor may exist which affects either prostaglandin synthesis or prostacyclin production, or both, which may both delay the onset of labour and jeopardize efficient placental exchange mechanisms (Crowley, 1989).

Post-maturity syndrome　Clifford described this syndrome in the neonate in 1954 and attributed it to placental ageing and dysfunction. Gibb's description of its features is outlined in Table 2 (see also Chapter 68).

Knox Ritchie (1992) describes this syndrome as an expression of chronic fetal malnutrition which is not confined to post-term pregnancy. A minority of post-term pregnancies are complicated by this syndrome which is also associated with oligohydramnios (Clement et al., 1987).

Oligohydramnios　In some post-term pregnancies the volume of amniotic fluid diminishes, thereby limiting its cushioning effect on the cord and fetus. The cord may become vulnerable to compression by the fetus during uterine contractions which may lead to an interrupted supply of oxygen and abnormalities in the fetal heart rate, particularly variable decelerations. Meconium-staining of the amniotic fluid is also associated with a decreased volume (Crowley et al., 1984) which in turn may lead to the *meconium aspiration syndrome* in the baby (Katz and Bowes, 1992).

Table 2　Features of the post-maturity syndrome (Gibb, 1985)

Absence of lanugo
Absence of vernix
Abundant scalp hair
Long fingernails
Dry, cracked desquamated skin
Body length increased in relation to body weight
Alert and apprehensive facies
Meconium staining of skin and membranes

Fetal macrosomia Fetal growth continues, though at a reduced rate, after 38 weeks' gestation (Gruenwald, 1967) and babies born at 42 completed weeks have a 21% incidence of weighing over 4000 g compared with a 12% incidence at 40 weeks and a 5% incidence at 38 weeks (Boyd *et al.*, 1983). This increases the risk of shoulder dystocia, brachial and facial palsy and clavicular fracture in the baby and subsequent morbidity to the woman as a result of intervention. Although there may be some increase in rigidity of the cranial vault, there is, however, little evidence to suggest that moulding is reduced due to supposed increased skull ossification in the baby born post-term (Calkins, 1948, cited by Gibb, 1985).

Management of post-term pregnancy

The two alternatives in providing care for women with post-term pregnancy are either some form of assessing fetal well-being or induction of labour. In practice, these may well be offered before the pregnancy is strictly post-term, i.e. 42 completed weeks or more.

Assessing fetal well-being This may take several forms including cardiotocography, measuring amniotic fluid volume and biophysical profile scoring:

▶ *Cardiotocography*, also called non-stress testing in the USA, essentially observes for the presence or absence of accelerations of the fetal heart which are normally present in a healthy non-compromised fetus. The sensitivity of this test is thought to improve by increasing the frequency of testing to two or three times weekly and when measurement of amniotic fluid volume is added (Eden *et al.*, 1982; Phelan *et al.*, 1984; Cario, 1984). However, others have drawn attention to the high false negative rate of non-stress testing (Miyazaki and Miyazaki, 1981), defined as death *in utero* within one week of a reactive trace, and advocate the oxytocin challenge or contraction stress test as a more sensitive indicator of fetal well-being (Freeman *et al.*, 1981; Khouzami *et al.*, 1983).

▶ *Measurement of amniotic fluid volume by ultrasound* is another method of surveillance. Crowley *et al.* (1984) defined reduced amniotic fluid as the absence of a single vertical pool of fluid measuring greater than 3 cm. If this condition was discovered, women were offered induction of labour; women with normal fluid volume were scanned every four days until labour began or the fluid volume became reduced. Those with reduced fluid volume had a statistically significant increase in meconium-staining and growth-retarded babies and were more likely to require Caesarean section for fetal distress.

▶ *Biophysical profile scoring* was first described by Manning *et al.* (1980) and involves scoring five biophysical variables: fetal breathing movements, gross body movements, fetal tone, fetal heart rate reactivity and amniotic fluid volume (Table 3).

The false negative rate for biophysical scoring, defined as death of a structurally normal fetus within seven days of a last normal test, is less than 0.1% (Manning *et al.*, 1987). The scoring system has been specifically applied to post-term pregnancies (Johnson *et al.*, 1986) and, when performed twice weekly, accurately differentiated normal fetuses from those at risk of hypoxia.

However, it is worth noting that although tests of fetal well-being may detect pregnancies in which there is a problem, Crowley (1989) comments that there is less evidence that their use improves the outcome.

Induction of labour This is the second alternative in managing post-term pregnancy. In an overview of the trials of elective induction of labour at 41+ weeks (at 290 days' gestation or later), Crowley (1994) concludes that such a practice reduces the small risk of perinatal death and may slightly reduce the risk of Caesarean section, particularly in units with high rates. There is no evidence that induction of labour at 41+ weeks affects operative vaginal delivery rates, the incidence of fetal heart rate abnormalities during labour or Apgar scores, but it does reduce meconium-staining of amniotic fluid and appears to increase the incidence of neonatal jaundice. Crowley (1989) also comments that to avoid treating women for a 'disease' from which they are not suffering in the first place, early ultrasound scans should be performed on all women in units where induction of labour is offered for pregnancies of 41 weeks' duration or more.

Women's Views on Induction of Labour

Cartwright's study in 1977 sought to examine women's experiences of induction for any indication and found

Table 3 Biophysical profile scoring (Manning *et al.*, 1980)

Variable	Score 2	Score 0
Fetal breathing movements (FBM)	At least one episode of FBM of at least 60 s duration in 30 min	Absent FBM or no episode of at least 60·s duration in 30 min
Gross body movement	At least three discrete movements in 30 min	Two or less discrete movements in 30 min
Fetal tone	Extremities & trunk in flexion. At least one episode of active extension of limb(s) or trunk and return to flexion	Extremities and trunk in extension/partial flexion. Fetal movement not followed by return to flexion. Fetal hand open
Fetal heart rate (FHR) reactivity	At least two episodes of FHR acceleration of > 15 beats/min and of at least 30 s duration associated with fetal movement in 20 min	Less than two episodes of FHR acceleration associated with fetal movement in 40 min
Amniotic fluid (AF) volume	At least one pool of AF that measures at least 1 cm in the vertical axis	Either no AF pools or a pool > 1 cm in the vertical axis

that 78% of those who had their labour induced would prefer not to have the same experience repeated. For post–term pregnancy as an indication for induction, there is a paucity of information on women's views. Roberts and Young (1991) studied the attitudes of 500 pregnant women to a proposal of conservative management, involving twice weekly ultrasound scans and cardiotocography and fetal movement chart monitoring from 42 weeks, compared with induction at 42 weeks. At 37 weeks, despite intensive education, only 45% of women were agreeable to conservative management. The most common reason given for preferring induction was that women 'could not stand the thought of being pregnant for more than 42 weeks'. At 41 weeks' gestation, 122 women remained undelivered and the figure had dropped to 31% requesting conservative management. The study proposed abandoning the term 'expected date of delivery' and informing women at booking that normal pregnancy may well last beyond that date.

Midwifery Care for Women Undergoing Induction of Labour

Psychological care

The decision to pre-empt the spontaneous onset of labour needs to be made in a climate of honest interchange of information, with the benefits and risks of induction explained by the obstetrician and midwife, so that informed consent may be given. It is likely that care given by the same midwife or small team of midwives throughout pregnancy and during induction will help to alleviate any disappointment felt by the woman and her partner at not achieving a spontaneous labour. Involving the woman and her partner in decision-making is also likely to increase their feelings of control over what happens. A plan of care can then be mapped out and documented in the woman's case notes.

Planning for induction

For women with complicated pregnancies and clear indications for induction thought needs to be given to the timing of the procedure. Liaison with the antenatal ward, delivery suite and special care baby unit, if appropriate, to ensure bed availability and adequate staffing should be planned.

The midwife providing care for a woman with a normal pregnancy will need to consider the appropriate time for referral to an obstetrician in the event of the pregnancy becoming post-term.

Induction protocol

Induction protocols will differ from unit to unit. Some maternity units will admit women the night before planned induction, primarily to assess cervical ripeness. One example of a protocol is as follows:

If the Bishop's score is 5 or less an initial dose of 1 mg of prostaglandin E_2 gel is administered intravaginally at 22.00 to nulliparous women or at 06.00 to multiparous women. Depending on the response to the prostaglandin gel a further dose of 2 mg may be given to nulliparous women the following morning.

In many units midwives assess the Bishop's score and administer the prostaglandin gel according to the dose prescribed. Following insertion of the gel the woman remains in bed for an hour to ensure absorption and the midwife will monitor any contractions, the woman's response to them and the fetal heart rate, usually by means of cardiotocograph tracing. If the cervix is ripe, induction may be carried out by means of an amniotomy and an oxytocin infusion, if indicated.

Once labour ensues issues such as the woman's comfort, position, hygiene and requirements for pain relief need to be addressed. The most appropriate form of monitoring the fetal heart rate and uterine contractions also needs to be considered, particularly if intravenous oxytocin is used with its risk of hyperstimulation (Oláh *et al.*, 1993).

Summary points

▶ Induction is a deliberate intervention to pre-empt the spontaneous onset of labour. As such, clear and justifiable indications should exist.

▶ The ripeness of the cervix is the most significant determinant of the success of induction and the subsequent length of labour. Prostaglandins are the approach of choice in ripening the unfavourable cervix.

▶ Methods to induce labour include sweeping the membranes, amniotomy, administering intravenous oxytocin or intravaginal prostaglandin or stimulating these substances naturally.

▶ Post-term pregnancy has an incidence rate of approximately 10%. Women with post-term pregnancies may be offered either assessment of fetal well-being or induction of labour.

▶ The midwife providing care for a woman undergoing induction of labour needs to consider its planning and timing as well as her role in providing psychological and physical care.

References

Allott, H.A. & Palmer, R. (1993) Sweeping the membranes: a valid procedure in stimulating the onset of labour? *Br. J. Obstet. Gynaecol.* 100: 898–903.

Bakketeig, L. & Bergsjo, P. (1989) Post-term pregnancy: Magnitude of the problem. In Chalmers, I., Enkin, M. & Keirse, M.J.N.C. (eds) *Effective Care in Pregnancy and Childbirth*, Vol. 1, 765–775. Oxford: Oxford University Press.

Bakketeig, L.S., Eik-Nes, S.H., Jacobsen, G. *et al.* (1984) Randomised controlled trial of ultrasonographic screening in pregnancy. *Lancet* 2: 207–211.

Ballantyne, J.W. & Browne, F.J. (1992) The problems of postmaturity and prolongation of pregnancy. *J. Obstet. Gynaecol. Br. Empire* 19: 177.

Beazley, J.M. & Underhill, R.A. (1970) Fallacy of the fundal height. *Br. Med. J.* 4: 404–406.

Bishop, E.H. (1964) Pelvic scoring for elective induction. *Obstet. Gynecol.* 24: 266–268.

Boyce, A., Mayaux, M.J. & Schwartz, D. (1976) Classical &

'true' gestational postmaturity. *Am. J. Obstet. Gynecol.* 125: 911–914.

Boyd, M.E., Usher, R.H. & McLean, F.H. (1983) Fetal macrosomia: prediction, risks, proposed management. *Obstet. Gynecol.* 61: 715–722.

Butler, N.R. & Bonham, D.G. (1963) *Perinatal Mortality*. Churchill Livingstone, Edinburgh.

Calkins, L.A. (1948) Postmaturity, Cited in Gibb, D. (1985) Prolonged pregnancy. In Studd, J. (ed) *The Management of Labour*. London: Blackwell Scientific Publications.

Campbell, S. (1976) Fetal growth. In: Beard, R.W. & Nathanielsz, P.W. (eds). *Fetal Physiology & Medicine*. London: Saunders.

Cario, G. (1984) Conservative management of prolonged pregnancy using fetal heart rate monitoring only: a prospective study. *Br. J. Obstet. Gynaecol.* 91: 23–30.

Cartwright, A. (1977) Mothers' experiences of induction. *Br. Med. J.* 2: 745–749.

Chalmers, I. & Keirse, M.J.N.C. (1989) Evaluating elective delivery. In Chalmers, I., Enkin, M. & Keirse, M.J.N.C.

(eds) *Effective Care in Pregnancy & Childbirth*, Vol. 2 pp. 981–987. Oxford: Oxford University Press.

Clement, D., Schifrin, B.S. & Kates, R.B. (1987) Acute oligohydramnios in postdate pregnancy. *Am. J. Obstet Gynecol.* **157**: 884–886.

Clifford, S. (1954) Postmaturity – with placental dysfunction. *J. Paediat.* **44**: 1–13.

Crowley, P. (1989) Post-term pregnancy: induction or surveillance? In: Chalmers, I., Enkin, M. & Keirse, M.J.N.C. (eds) *Effective Care in Pregnancy & Childbirth* Vol. 1, pp. 776–791. Oxford: Oxford University Press.

Crowley, P. (1994) Elective induction of labour at 41+ weeks gestation. In: Keirse, M.J.N.C., Renfrew, M.J., Neilson, J.P. & Crowther, C. (eds) *Pregnancy and Childbirth Module*. In: The Cochrane Pregnancy and Childbirth Database. The Cochrane Collaboration, issue 2, 1995. Oxford: Update Software.

Crowley, P. (1996) Corticosteroids prior to preterm delivery. In: Keirse M.J.N.C., Renfrew, M.J., Neilson, J.P. & Crowther, C. (eds) *Pregnancy and Childbirth Module*. In: The Cochrane Database of Systematic Reviews. Available in The Cochrane Library. London: BMJ Publishing Group.

Crowley, P., O'Herlihy, C. & Boylan, P. (1984) The value of ultrasound measurement of amniotic fluid volume in the management of prolonged pregnancies. *Br. J. Obstet. Gynaecol.* **91**: 444–448.

Curtis, P.D., Mathews, T.G., Clarke, T.A. *et al.* (1988) Neonatal seizures: the Dublin Collaborative Study. *Arch. Dis. Childh.* **63**: 1065–1068.

DHSS (Department of Health and Social Security) (1976) *On the State of the Public Health for the Year 1975*. London: HMSO.

Eden, R.D., Gergely, R.Z., Schifrin, B.S. & Wade, M.A. (1982) Comparison of antepartum testing schemes for the management of postdate pregnancy. *Am. J. Obstet. Gynecol.* **144**: 683–692.

Eik-Nes, S.H., Okland, O., Aure, J.C. & Ulstein, M. (1984) Ultrasound screening in pregnancy: a randomised controlled trial. *Lancet* i: 1347.

Elliot, J.P. & Flaherty, J.F. (1984) The use of breast stimulation to prevent postdate pregnancy. *Am. J. Obstet. Gynecol.* **149**: 628–632.

Enkin, M. (1989) Labour and delivery following previous Caesarean section. In Chalmers, I., Enkin, M. & Keirse, M.J.N.C. (eds) *Effective Care in Pregnancy and Childbirth* Vol. 2, pp. 1196–1215. Oxford: Oxford University Press.

FIGO (1982) *Report of the Committee Following a Workshop in Monitoring and Reporting Perinatal Mortality and Morbidity*. FIGO Standing Committee on Perinatal Mortality. *Int. Fed. Gynaecol. Obstet.* London: Chameleon Press.

Fox, H. (1978) *Pathology of the placenta*. London: W.H. Saunders.

Fox, H. (1979) The placenta as a model for organ ageing. In Beaconsfield, P. & Villee, C. (eds) *Placenta – A neglected experimental animal*. Oxford: Pergamon.

Fragner, N.B. & Miyazaki, F.S. (1987) Intrauterine monitoring of contractions during breast stimulation. *Obstet. Gynecol.* **69**: 767–769.

Fraser, R., Watson, R. (1989) Bleeding during the latter half of pregnancy. In Chalmers, I., Enkin, M. & Keirse,

M.J.N.C. (eds) *Effective Care in Pregnancy and Childbirth*, Vol. 1, pp. 594–611. Oxford: Oxford University Press.

Freeman, R.K., Garite, T.J., Modanlou, H., Dorchester, W., Rommal, C. & Devaney, M. (1981) Postdate pregnancy: utilization of contraction stress testing for primary fetal surveillance. *Am. J. Obstet. Gynecol.* **140**: 128–135.

Gibb, D. (1985) Prolonged pregnancy. In Studd, J. (ed.) *The Management of Labour*. London: Blackwell Scientific Publications.

Goodlin, R.C., Keller, D.W. & Raffin, M. (1971) Orgasm during late pregnancy: possible deleterious effects. *Obstet. Gynecol.* **38**: 916–920.

Goodlin, R.C., Schmidt, W. & Creevy, D.C. (1972) Uterine tension and heart rate during maternal orgasm. *Obstet. Gynecol.* **39**: 125–127.

Gordon-Wright, A.P. & Elder, M.G. (1979) Prostaglandin E_2 tablets used intravaginally for the induction of labour. *Br. J. Obstet. Gynaecol.* **86**: 32–36.

Grant, J. & Keirse, M.J.N.C. (1989) Prelabour rupture of the membranes at term. In Chalmers, I., Enkin, M. & Keirse, M.J.N.C. (eds) *Effective Care in Pregnancy and Childbirth*, Vol. 2, pp. 1112–1126. Oxford: Oxford University Press.

Gravenhorst, J.B. (1989) Rhesus isoimmunisation. In Chalmers, I., Enkin, M. & Keirse, M.J.N.C. (eds) *Effective Care in Pregnancy and Childbirth*, Vol. 1, pp. 565–577. Oxford: Oxford University Press.

Gruenwald, P. (1967) Growth of the human fetus. In McLaren, A. (ed) *Advances in Reproductive Physiology*, Vol. 2, pp. 279–309. London: Logos Press.

Hall, M.H., Carr-Hill, R.A., Fraser, C., Campbell, D. & Samphier, M.I. (1985) The extent and antecedents of uncertain gestation. *Br. J. Obstet. Gynaecol.* **92**: 445–451.

Hannah, M.E., Ohlsson, A., Farine D., *et al.* (1996) Induction of labor compared with expectant management for prelabour rupture of the membranes at term. *New Engl. J. Med.* **334**: 1005–1010.

Hendricks, C.H. & Brenner, W.E. (1964) Patterns of increasing uterine activity in late pregnancy and the development of uterine responsiveness to oxytocin. *Am. J. Obstet. Gynecol.* **90**: 485–492.

Hunter, D.J.S. (1989) Diabetes in pregnancy. In Chalmers, I., Enkin, M. & Keirse, M.J.N.C. (eds) *Effective Care in Pregnancy and Childbirth*, Vol. 1, pp. 578–593. Oxford: Oxford University Press.

Hurd, W.H., Miodovnik, M., Hertzberg, V. & Lavin, J.P. (1983) Selective management of abruptio placentae: a prospective study. *Obstet. Gynecol.* **61**: 467–473.

Irons, D.W., Thornton, S., Davison, J.M., *et al.* (1993) Oxytocin infusion regimens: time for standardisation? *Br. J. Obstet. Gynaecol.* **100**: 786–787.

Johnson, J.M., Harman, L.C., Lange, I.R. & Manning, F.A. (1986) Biophysical profile scoring in the management of the post-term pregnancy: an analysis of 307 patients. *Am. J. Obst. Gynecol.* **154**: 269–273.

Katz, V.L. & Bowes, W.A. (1992) Meconium aspiration syndrome: reflections on a murky subject. *Am. J. Obstet. Gynecol.* **166**: 171–183.

Keirse, M.J.N.C. (1992a) Any prostaglandin/any route for cervical ripening. In: Keirse, M.J.N.C., Renfrew, M.J., Neilson, J.P. & Crowther, C. (eds) *Pregnancy and Childbirth*

Module. In: The Cochrane Pregnancy and Childbirth Database. The Cochrane Collaboration: Issue 2, 1995. Oxford: Update Software.

Keirse, M.J.N.C. (1992b) Stripping/sweeping membranes at term for induction of labour. In: Keirse, M.J.N.C., Renfrew, M.J., Neilson, J.P. & Crowther, C. (eds) *Pregnancy and Childbirth Module.* In: The Cochrane Pregnancy and Childbirth Database. The Cochrane Collaboration; issue 2, 1995. Oxford: Update Software.

Keirse, M.J.N.C. (1992c) Any prostagalandin vs placebo for induction of labour. In: Keirse, M.J.N.C., Renfrew, M.J. Neilson, J.P. & Crowther, C. (eds) *Pregnancy and Childbirth Module.* In: The Cochrane Pregnancy and Childbirth Database. The Cochrane Collaboration; issue 2, 1995. Oxford: Update Software.

Keirse, M.J.N.C. (1993) Any prostaglandin (by any route) vs oxytocin (any route) for induction of labour. In: Keirse, M.J.N.C., Renfrew, M.J., Neilson, J.P. & Crowther, C. (eds) *Pregnancy and Childbirth Module.* In: The Cochrane Pregnancy and Childbirth Database. The Cochrane Collaboration; issue 2, 1995. Oxford: Update Software.

Keirse, M.J.N.C. & Chalmers, I. (1989) Methods for inducing labour. In Chalmers, I., Enkin, M. & Keirse, M.J.N.C. (eds) *Effective Care in Pregnancy and Childbirth,* Vol. 2, pp. 1057–1079. Oxford: Oxford University Press.

Keirse, M.J.N.C. & Kanhai, H.H.H. (1989) Induction of labour after fetal death. In Chalmers, I., Enkin, M. & Keirse, M.J.N.C. (eds) *Effective Care in Pregnancy and Childbirth.* Vol. 2, pp. 1118–1126. Oxford: Oxford University Press.

Keirse, M.J.N.C., Ohlsson, A. Treffers, P.E. & Kanhai, H.H.H. (1989) Prelabour rupture of the membranes preterm. In Chalmers, I., Enkin, M. & Keirse, M.J.N.C. (eds) *Effective Care in Pregnancy,* Vol. 1, pp. 666–693. Oxford: Oxford University Press.

Keirse, M.J.N.C., Thiery, M., Parewijck, W. & Mitchell, M.D. (1983) Chronic stimulation of uterine prostaglandin synthesis during cervical ripening before the onset of labor. *Prostaglandins* 25: 671–682.

Keirse, M.J.N.C. & van Oppen, A.C.C. (1989) Preparing the cervix for induction of labour. In Chalmers, I., Enkin, M. & Keirse, M.J.N.C. (eds) *Effective Care in Pregnancy and Childbirth,* Vol. 2, pp. 988–1056. Oxford: Oxford University Press.

Khouzami, V.A., Johnson, J.W., Daikoku, N.H., Rotmensch, J. & Hernanadez, E. (1983) Comparison of urinary estrogens, contraction stress tests and non-stress tests in the management of post-term pregnancy. *J. Reprod. Med.* 28: 189–194.

Knox Ritchie, J.W. (1992) Obstetrics for the neonatologist. In Roberton, N.R.C. (ed) *Textbook of Neonatology,* 2nd edn. pp. 83–119. London: Churchill Livingstone.

Lamont, R.F. (1990) Induction of labour: oxytocin compared with prostaglandins. *Contemp. Rev. Obstet. Gynaecol.* 2: 16–20.

Larsen, L.G., Clausen, H.V., Anderson, B. *et al.* (1995). A stereologic study of postmature placentas fixed by dual perfusion. *Am. J. Obstet. Gynecol.* 172: 500–507.

Lazaro, J.L. (1973) Induction of labour with the help of suction to the mammary glands cited in Thiery, M.,

Baines, C.J. & Keirse, M.J.N.C. The development of methods of inducing labour. In Chalmers, I., Enkin, M. & Keirse, M.J.N.C. (eds) *Effective Care in Pregnancy and Childbirth,* Vol. 2, pp. 969–980. Oxford: Oxford University Press.

Liggins, G.C. (1979) Controlled trial of induction of labor by vaginal suppositories containing prostaglandin E$_2$. *Prostaglandins,* 18: 167–172.

MacKenzie, I.Z., Bradley, S. & Embrey, M.P. (1981) A simpler approach to labor induction using lipid-based prostaglandin E$_2$ vaginal suppository. *Am. J. Obstet. Gynecol.* 141: 158–162.

Manning, F.A., Platt, L.D. & Sipos, L. (1980) Antepartum fetal evaluation: development of a fetal biophysical profile. *Am. J. Obstet Gynecol.* 136: 787–795.

Manning, F.A., Morrison, I., Harman, C.R., Lange, I.R. & Menticoglou, S. (1987) Fetal assessment based on fetal biophysical profile scoring: experience in 19 221 referred high-risk patients. 11. An analysis of false-negative fetal deaths. *Am. J. Obstet. Gynecol.* 157: 880–884.

McColgin, S.W., Hampton, H.L., McCaul, J.F., Howard, P.R., Andrew, M.E. & Morrison, J.C. (1990) Stripping membranes at term: can it safely reduce the incidence of post-term pregnancies? *Obstet. Gynecol.* 76: 678–680.

Merriman, S. (1838) A synopsis of the various kinds of difficult parturition cited in Thiery, M., Baines, C.J. & Keirse, M.J.N.C. The development of methods for inducing labour. In Chalmers, I., Enkin, M. & Keirse, M.J.N.C. (eds) *Effective Care in Pregnancy and Childbirth,* Vol. 2, pp. 969–980. Oxford: Oxford University Press.

Minchom, P., Niswander, K., Chalmers, I. *et al.* (1987) Antecedents and outcome of very early neonatal seizures in infants born at or after term. *Br. J. Obstet. Gynaecol.* 94: 431–439.

Mitchell, M.D., Klint, A.P.F., Bibby, J., Brunt, J., Anderson, A.B.M. & Turnbull, A.C. (1977) Rapid increases in plasma prostaglandin concentrations after vaginal examination and amniotomy. *Br. Med. J.* 2: 1183–1185.

Miyazaki, F.S., Miyazaki, B.A. (1981) False reactive nonstress tests in post-term pregnancies. *Am. J. Obstet. Gynecol.* 153: 301–306.

Oláh, K.S., Henderson, C., Birkbeck, J. (1993) Assessment of uterine contractions: midwife or monitor? *Br. J. Midwifery,* 1: 111–118.

Naeye, R. (1978) Causes of perinatal mortality excess in prolonged gestations. *Am. J. Epidemiol.* 108: 429–433.

O'Dowd, M.J. & O'Dowd, T.M. (1985) Quickening – a reevaluation. *Br. J. Obstet. Gynaecol.* 92: 1037–1039.

Patterson, W.M. (1971) Amniotomy, with or without simultaneous oxytocin infusion. *J. Obstet. Gynaecol. Br. Commonwealth,* 78: 310–316.

Peel, J. & Oakley, W. (1949) The management of pregnancy in diabetics cited in Hunter, D.J.S. (1989) Diabetes in pregnancy. In Chalmers, I., Enkin, M. & Keirse, M.J.N.C. (eds) *Effective Care in Pregnancy and Childbirth,* Vol. 1, pp. 578–593. Oxford: Oxford University Press.

Phelan, J.P., Platt, L.O., Yeh, S-Y, Trujillo, M. & Paul, R.H. (1984) Continuing role of the non-stress test in the management of postdated pregnancy. *Obstet. Gynecol.* 64: 624–628.

Roberts, L.J. & Young, K.R. (1991) The management of prolonged pregnancy — an analysis of women's attitudes before and after term. *Br. J. Obstet. Gynaecol.* **98**: 1102–1106.

Robinson, H.P. & Fleming, J.E.E. (1975) A critical evaluation of 'crown–rump length' measurements. *Br. J. Obstet. Gynaecol.* **82**: 702–710.

Saleh, Y.Z. (1975) Surgical induction of labour with and without oxytocin infusion. A prospective study cited in Keirse, M.J.N.C. & Chalmers, I. (1989) Methods for inducing labour. In Chalmers, I., Enkin, M. & Keirse, M.J.N.C. (eds) *Effective Care in Pregnancy and Childbirth*, Vol. 2, pp. 1057–1079. Oxford: Oxford University Press.

Salzmann, K.D. (1971) An untapped source of oxytocin. *J. R. Coll. Gen. Pract.* **21**(106): 282–288.

Sands, J. & Dobbing, J. (1985) Continuing growth and development of the third-trimester human placenta. *Placenta*, **6**: 13–22.

Stewart, H.L. (1952) Duration of pregnancy and postmaturity. *J. Am. Med. Assoc.* **148**: 1079–1083.

Ulmsten, U., Wingerup, L., Belfrage, P., Ekman, G. & Wiqvist, N. (1982) Intracervical application of prostaglandin gel for induction of term labour. *Obstet. Gynecol.* **59**: 336–339.

Viegas, O.A.C., Arulkumaran, S. & Ratman, G.S. (1984) Nipple stimulation in late pregnancy causing uterine hyperstimulation and profound bradycardia. *Br. J. Obstet. Gynaecol.* **91**: 364–366.

Weissberg, S.M. & Spellacy, W.N. (1977) Membrane stripping to induce labour. *J. Reprod. Med.* **19**: 125–127.

WHO (World Health Organization) (1977) *Manual of the International Statistical Classification of Diseases, Injuries and Causes of Death. Based on the Recommendations of the Ninth Revision Conference 1975 and Adopted by the 29th World Health Assembly*, Vol. 1. Geneva: WHO.

49

Prolonged Labour and Disordered Uterine Action

In normal labour the uterine contractions are progressively longer, stronger and more frequent and are associated with completion of effacement and progressive dilatation of the os uteri in the first stage and with the steady expulsion of the fetus in the second stage. Unfortunately there is no way to predict the kind of labour progression (in terms of dilatation and descent) that a given contractile pattern will produce, i.e. the quality of contractions can tell little about the course of labour (Friedman, 1981). Abnormal uterine action may be *inefficient* or *overefficient*.

Prolonged Labour

Labour used to be termed 'prolonged' when it exceeded 24 hours (Baird, 1952). Nowadays the generally accepted limit is the 12-hour period espoused by Driscoll *et al.* (1993). The rationale behind such an arbitrary time is the belief that the longer labour continues, the greater the hazard to both mother and fetus. There is no firm agreement, however, about whether the time of onset starts with the latent or active phase of labour.

Dangers to the mother

The mother suffers from anxiety and the pain of prolonged labour; she may become dehydrated, ketotic and tired (Keirse, 1989).

Maternal distress, a condition of mental and physical exhaustion, results. In this condition the temperature, pulse and blood pressure rise, dehydration, oliguria and ketosis develop and may be accompanied by vomiting. Psychologically the woman becomes demoralized and restless and her pain threshold is lowered. With good standards of care this condition should not occur.

Other dangers to the mother include *intrauterine infection*, especially if the membranes rupture early, the risk of a *ruptured uterus* due to obstructed labour caused by undetected cephalopelvic disproportion, though this should not occur with good standards of care, the risk of *operative intervention, anaesthesia* and *postpartum haemorrhage* because the tired uterus cannot contract strongly. How much mental trauma the mother sustains is difficult to assess.

Dangers to the fetus

Intrauterine hypoxia occurs in prolonged labour and causes fetal acidosis, meconium aspiration and may lead to *perinatal death. Cerebral injury* may follow severe hypoxia or excessive moulding or as a result of a difficult assisted vaginal delivery. With prolonged rupture of the membranes the fetus may be born with an *infection* acquired *in utero*. This may lead to neonatal pneumonia.

Causes

The majority of women whose labours are thus prolonged are primigravidae. The birth of the first child alters the birth canal and subsequent deliveries are easier.

The three main causes of prolonged labour are:

1 Inefficient uterine action.
2 Cephalopelvic disproportion.
3 Posterior position of the occiput.

Very rarely the cause is cervical dystocia.

INEFFICIENT UTERINE ACTION

O'Driscoll *et al.* (1993) cite inefficient uterine action as the most common cause of abnormal labour in primigravidae. Without efficient uterine action it is impossible to assess whether vaginal delivery is possible with minor cephalopelvic disproportion or malposition of the fetal head. Before instigating active management, consideration should be given to using non-invasive methods that influence the progress of labour, such as ambulation (Flynn *et al*, 1978; Hemminki and Saarkowski, 1983), psychosocial support (Klaus *et al.*, 1986) and allowing low-risk women to eat and drink in labour (Grant, 1990).

ACTIVE MANAGEMENT OF LABOUR

Active management or augmentation of labour is undertaken when the progress of labour is slow. This approach was first implemented in 1968 in the National Maternity Hospital in Dublin (O'Driscoll *et al.*, 1969). The main considerations are:

1 *Accurate diagnosis of the onset of labour* otherwise

inappropriate management may be instituted. Effacement of the cervix is given greater emphasis than dilatation.

2 *Early use of amniotomy* (artificial rupture of the membranes) once a diagnosis of labour has been accepted (Boylan, 1989).

3 *Early use of relatively high doses of oxytocin* in order to stimulate labour.

4 *Intense psychological support during labour.* A woman has the support of a student midwife/medical student throughout the whole course of labour.

5 *Rigorous peer review.* Staff sit down on a weekly or monthly basis and evaluate the overall standard and quality of care (Boylan, 1989).

Such an approach in this population achieves a high spontaneous vaginal delivery rate and a low number of operative deliveries with equally impressive mortality and morbidity rates. In order to achieve such impressive outcomes, 45% of primigravidae in labour are augmented with oxytocin (O'Driscoll *et al.*, 1993). A recent overview of trials evaluating the outcomes of active management, as described above, concludes that although operative delivery rate is reduced it is the presence of a constant companion for the woman in labour which is the effective ingredient, not the use of amniotomy and oxytocinon (Thornton and Lilford, 1994).

In general, active management of labour is not normally applied to women in labour with twins or malpresentations. Augmentation should be used with extreme caution in multigravidae and women with uterine scars because of the risk of uterine rupture (DOH, 1994).

The use of the partogram to record observations and progress in labour promotes the early diagnosis of slow progress. Referral and appropriate action can therefore be taken at the optimum time.

The partogram

Progress in active management is measured by linear progression of labour along a prescribed time scale. Friedman (1955) was the first to introduce a *curve* of cervical dilatation measured in centimetres plotted against time in hours. This is otherwise known as 'the partogram'. Others have since modified Friedman's graph of cervical dilatation (Philpot and Castle, 1972a,b) with the introduction of *alert* and *action* lines. The *alert* line or *normogram* (Studd, 1973) represents the mean progressive dilatation of normal primigravidae in labour. The *action* line is two hours to the right

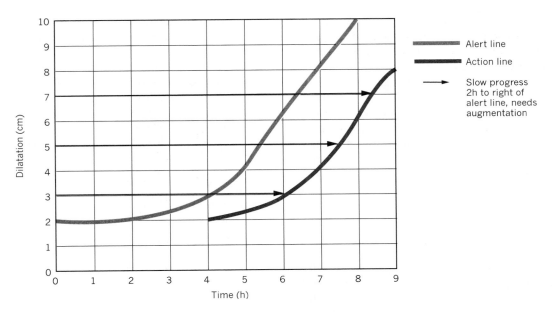

Figure 1   Normogram/partogram of cervimetric progress commencing at 2 cm dilatation. 'Alert' line outlines normal progress. 'Action' line indicates when augmentation should be instituted. (After Studd (1973).)

of the *alert* line and augmentation is instituted at this time (Figure 1).

O'Driscoll *et al.* (1993) adopt a far more aggressive approach, whereby once labour is confirmed cervical dilatation is expected to progress at a rate of 1 cm/h. Augmentation is employed in primigravidae at any deviation to the right of a simple diagonal line drawn at 1 cm/h from the diagnosis of labour.

As part of active management of labour a partogram is used to plot dilatation of the cervix and descent of the head (preferably abdominally). A glance at the partogram will indicate if progress is satisfactory. When progress is slow augmentation in the form of amniotomy and often an intravenous infusion of oxytocin is used to accelerate labour.

It is imperative to distinguish between primigravidae and multigravidae when augmentation is deemed necessary. Prolonged labour rarely occurs in multigravidae, but when it does it is usually due to obstruction. In such cases the injudicious use of oxytocin can result in uterine rupture, an occurrence rarely encountered in primigravidae (O'Driscoll *et al.*, 1993).

Amniotomy

The membranes may be ruptured to accelerate labour. The significant benefits of intact membranes are the maintenance of an even hydrostatic pressure to the whole fetal surface during labour and a reduced likelihood of infection. Fetal hypoxia is less likely because retraction of the placental site and thus impairment of the uteroplacental circulation will not occur (Henderson, 1990). Fetal heart rate abnormalities were less common in the amniotomy group in a study by Barrett *et al.* (1992), but there was no difference in this study between the amniotomy and nonintervention groups in regard to the method of delivery, condition at birth and postpartum pyrexia. The main arguments for amniotomy are to accelerate labour and reveal the presence of meconium (Barrett *et al.*, 1992).

Fraser (1993) reviewed six trials (Wetrich 1970; Stewart *et al.*, 1982; Franks 1990; Fraser *et al.*, 1988; Barrett *et al.*, 1992; Fraser *et al.*, 1991) that examined amniotomy in spontaneous labour. The main conclusion of this meta analysis was that at the present time there is no evidence that one policy of rupturing the membranes or leaving them intact has a clear advantage over the other. Of course the most important views of amniotomy are those of women who experience this intervention. A large trial conducted by the National Childbirth Trust (1989) found that the great majority of women found labour harder to cope with following amniotomy and felt their physiology had been disturbed. Another study (Robson and Kumar, 1980) made the unexpected discovery that maternal affection was more likely to be lacking after delivery if the mother had a forewater amniotomy, experienced a painful, unpleasant labour, and had been given more than 125 mg of pethidine. In this study most mothers had developed affection for their baby within a week of the birth and no further adverse effects were noted.

Before performing amniotomy a clear indication of the need to institute the procedure should be apparent, i.e. if progress is slow, or there is concern regarding fetal well-being. A discussion with the mother regarding the need and the implications should take place and her consent should be obtained. Following amniotomy it may be necessary to augment labour with oxytocin.

Discussion of augmentation with oxytocin

The use of oxytocin in the active management of labour varies from 5% (Bidgood and Steer, 1987) to 45% (O'Driscoll *et al.*, 1993). The proposed benefits of early augmentation with oxytocin are low Caesarean section rate and the correspondingly high spontaneous vaginal delivery rate. (Turner *et al.*, 1986; Lopez-Zeno *et al.*, 1992; O'Driscoll *et al.*, 1993) Disadvantages of this form of augmentation are the increased amount of pain women experience (Hemminki *et al.*, 1985) and the restriction of movement. Keirse (1989) recommends that, while there is a place for oxytocic augmentation in slow labour, other measures such as allowing women to be mobile, and eat and drink should be considered in the first instance, rather than medical intervention. With too narrow a view of normality an increased number of labours would be defined as abnormal and the women concerned may be subjected to unnecessary intervention to treat non-existent dystocia (Crowther *et al.*, 1989).

Haddad and Morris (1985) report that women with a high tendency to anxiety are more likely to require oxytocin to augment uterine contractions. It is thought that high maternal anxiety interferes with normal uterine activity, hence the need for oxytocin. Contractions stimulated by oxytocin tend to be more painful and thus effective analgesia is required. Epidural analgesia is frequently the method of choice.

With active management, few women are in labour longer than 12 hours and, indeed, most have a normal delivery within 8 hours (O'Driscoll and Meagher, 1980). This means that the mother usually has continuous care from one midwife and this is not only reassuring for the woman but also satisfying for the midwife. Occasionally active management fails to accel-

erate the progress of labour sufficiently, or complications such as fetal hypoxia arise, and then an operative delivery is required.

It is most important to make a distinction between primigravidae and multigravidae. Prolonged labour rarely occurs in a multigravida, but when it does it is usually due to obstruction. If the uterus of a multigravid woman in obstructed labour is stimulated, uterine rupture may occur. Therefore oxytocin should be used very sparingly in a multigravida and only after an experienced obstetrician has carefully assessed the labour. On the other hand prolonged labour is common in primigravidae; moreover it is in primigravidae that one is concerned about cephalopelvic disproportion, because the functional capacity of the pelvis is unknown. It is rare for a primigravid uterus to rupture, so oxytocin can be used with confidence, provided it is not given too early, i.e. in the latent phase of labour (Oliah and Neilson, 1994).

MIDWIFERY CARE

The midwife will carefully assess the mother's condition, both physical and mental, and the condition of the fetus by continuous fetal heart monitoring. By abdominal and per vaginam examination she will confirm the presentation and position of the fetus and assess the station of the head, the state of the cervix, the position of the fetus and the degree of caput succedaneum and moulding. The obstetrician will be informed of progress and, because labour is abnormal, takes overall responsibility for the woman's care. He may wish to assess the size and shape of the pelvis and, if more than a minor degree of cephalopelvic disproportion is suspected, operative delivery would be required.

Maternal physical and pyschological wellbeing

The woman and her partner should be cared for and supported by a midwife with whom they have developed a trusting relationship. Good communications are essential to allay unnecessary anxiety and to enable the woman and her partner to understand what is happening and to be involved in all discussions and decisions regarding care.

General midwifery care

The midwife should help the woman find a comfortable position, preferably in an upright position as this often promotes uterine action, and provide support and assistance, as required (Keirse, 1989).

General hygiene measures are necessary both for comfort and to reduce the risks of infection, especially once the membranes have ruptured.

A record of fluid intake and output is made. If there is any likelihood of operative delivery, oral intake will be restricted for women in prolonged labour and drugs, such as ranitidine, may be prescribed to reduce gastric acidity because of the risk of acid aspiration syndrome should an anaesthetic be required. Intravenous fluids will be necessary if oral fluids are restricted.

The woman is given the opportunity to empty her bladder at two-hourly intervals, because a full bladder may reflexly affect uterine contractions and add to the discomfort of labour. Each specimen of urine is tested for ketones and protein. In the event of a woman being unable to empty her bladder, catheterization will be necessary.

Observations

Maternal condition The woman should be assessed holistically, including her impressions about how she is coping with labour, and also how her coping ability may change should augmentation of labour be started.

The temperature, pulse and blood pressure are recorded regularly. A raised temperature is likely to be caused by infection, and a high vaginal swab and a midstream specimen of urine would be obtained for culture and sensitivities. A broad spectrum antibiotic is normally prescribed, which may be given intravenously.

Fluid balance would be noted, especially when labour is being augmented with syntocinon because of its slightly anti-diuretic effect and its loose association with neonatal jaundice (Johnson *et al.*, 1984).

Fetal condition Continuous fetal heart monitoring is usual in prolonged labour and, if indicated by any suspicion of an abnormal fetal heart trace or meconium stained liquor, fetal blood sampling would be carried out to detect a compromised fetus. The amount and colour of the amniotic fluid is observed.

Progress in labour Descent of the fetus is assessed by abdominal examination, the descent of the head being expressed in fifths palpable. The strength, frequency and duration of the uterine contractions are

carefully observed and the midwife also notes the woman's reaction to them. Continuous monitoring of uterine action is usually carried out in prolonged labour.

Examinations per vaginam are made to assess progress, noting in particular cervical dilatation, descent of the head in relation to the ischial spines, the position of the fetus, which is determined by the sutures and fontanelles, and the degree of caput and moulding. Finally the pelvic size is estimated and any abnormality noted. From this examination the cause of prolonged labour may be apparent, for example, malposition or malpresentation, or possibly a contracted pelvis. A decision would then be made about the subsequent management of labour. Provided the maternal and fetal condition are good and there are no contraindications to the use of oxytocin, such as significant cephalopelvic disproportion, labour may be augmented with a syntocinon infusion.

Care with augmentation of labour

Full discussion should take place with the woman and her partner and their informed consent will be obtained for the augmentation of labour. The midwife will also discuss pain relief because the woman will be confined to bed and the strength and frequency of the uterine contractions will be enhanced. She may therefore wish to consider more effective methods of pain relief, such as epidural. Such a decision will be made in conjunction with the woman on a strictly individual basis.

Syntocinon is administered intravenously using an infusion pump and a regime that has been agreed locally. It should be titrated so that contractions occur no more frequently than 4 in 10 minutes. The midwife carefully observes uterine action, ensuring that the uterus relaxes adequately between contractions and that there are no signs of hyperstimulation. As labour progresses the infusion rate may need to be decreased.

Continuous monitoring of the fetal heart and uterine contractions is necessary to detect any signs of fetal distress and signs of hyperstimulation. Careful assessment of progress is made by noting descent of the head per abdomen and by examinations per vaginam at two- to four-hourly intervals.

All other care and observations are as already described for prolonged labour.

After delivery the infusion is continued for one hour

to maintain good uterine action and thereby reduce the risk of postpartum haemorrhage.

Throughout a prolonged and augmented labour the woman and her partner need much support and reassurance. They will particularly appreciate a frequent flow of information about all procedures and the findings of examinations which should be clearly explained. It is most important for the woman's mental health postnatally that she is consulted about all interventions and retains a sense of control.

A debriefing discussion between the woman and the midwife who cared for her in labour should take place at a suitable time, preferably within the first 24 hours after delivery. This can help the woman in coming to terms with the events of her labour and raising her self-esteem.

Prolonged Second Stage of Labour

A survey of midwifery policies in English health districts (Garcia and Garforth, 1989) found that there was a tendency to define a prolonged second stage as one hour in a primigravida and thirty minutes in a multigravida. Thomson (1988) claims that the time restrictions on the second stage have become custom and practice, as opposed to being research based. A large retrospective analysis (Saunders *et al.*, 1992) showed no increase in perinatal mortality or morbidity in second stages lasting up to three hours. Although the frequency of maternal morbidity appears to rise with time, this effect is much less marked in women who deliver spontaneously. Cohen (1977) also found that women who had an operative delivery had an increased incidence of postpartum haemorrhage and infection attributable to the type of delivery, as opposed to the length of second stage.

Causes

Delayed progress may be due to inefficient uterine action, poor maternal effort or loss of bearing down reflex as a result of an epidural block. Other maternal causes of delay in the second stage include a full bladder or rectum, a rigid perineum and, rarely, a contracted pelvic outlet.

Fetal causes of prolonged second stage include a persistent occipitoposterior position, deep transverse arrest, malpresentations, a large baby and a fetal abnormality such as hydrocephaly.

Management

Provided the maternal and fetal condition are satisfactory and progress is evident, limits on the duration of the second stage should be discarded (Sleep *et al.*, 1989). If progress is slow and the woman is able and wishes to adopt an upright position, this should be encouraged because it is thought to direct the presenting part more effectively against the posterior wall of the vagina, stimulating the release of oxytocin (Ferguson's reflex), and thereby enhancing the urge to bear down (Burns, 1992).

Meticulous observations must be made in the second stage, as in the first. The doctor must be informed if there appears to be lack of progress or fetal or maternal distress develops. In this instance an assisted vaginal delivery or occasionally a Caesarean section may be necessary.

Some women experience a sense of failure and become depressed after a prolonged and difficult labour (Cartwright, 1979). The reaction may be exacerbated if the puerperium is complicated by infection. Again a debriefing discussion between the mother and the midwife who attended her in labour should take place within a day or two of delivery, as this can be helpful to the woman.

Overefficient Uterine Action (Precipitate Labour)

Labour is sometimes very rapid with intense frequent contractions and delivery occurs within an hour (Llewellyn-Jones, 1990). This is much more common in the multiparous woman and is usually caused by the minimal resistance of the maternal soft tissues. The first stage of labour has probably occurred almost without pain and only when the head is about to be born does the woman become aware of it. The mother may sustain lacerations of the cervix and perineum and is at risk of postpartum haemorrhage. Fetal complications include hypoxia as a result of intense frequent contractions and intracranial haemorrhage which may occur as a result of rapid descent through the birth canal. Other dangers include injuries sustained as a result of being delivered in an unsuitable place or falling to the ground. Women with a history of precipitate labour are usually admitted to hospital before term.

Tonic Contraction of the Uterus

Tonic contraction of the uterus is a very rare occurrence. It is associated with obstructed labour, when the uterus has been contracting powerfully to overcome the obstruction and eventually one long contraction is maintained. The continuous contraction of the uterus is accompanied by continuous severe pain and rapid deterioriation in the condition of the mother; intrauterine death occurs, since the circulation of blood in the placenta is greatly decreased. Therefore it is important to administer oxygen. The woman must be delivered immediately, usually by Caesarean section, otherwise the uterus may rupture and she may die.

Tetanic uterine action Tetanic uterine action occurs as a result of uterine hyperstimulation. The most common cause is the injudicious use of prostaglandin and syntocinon. If syntocinon is being administered intravenously the infusion should be stopped.

The woman should be encouraged to adopt the left lateral position to enhance uteroplacental blood flow and oxygen should be administered if a fetal bradycardia is present. Medical staff should be informed urgently as delivery may need to be expedited.

Cervical Dystocia

This is a rare condition when there is a structural abnormality of the cervix which may be congenital or acquired. When congenital, the cervix may be fibrous, stenosed or poorly developed. Acquired cervical dystocia may be due to fibrosis and scarring following infection, cautery, surgery, or irradiation. Despite normal uterine contractions, the cervix fails to dilate and feels hard and unyielding. Vaginal delivery is therefore impossible and a Caesarean section is performed.

References

Baird, D. (1952) The cause and prevention of difficult labour. *Am. J. Obstet. Gynecol.* **63**: 1200–1212.

Bidgood, K.A. & Steer, P.J. (1987) A randomized control study of oxytocin augmentation of labour 1. Obstetric outcome. *Br. J. Obstet. Gynaecol.* **94**: 512–517.

Barrett, J.F.R. *et al.* (1992) Randomized trial of amniotomy versus the intention to leave membranes intact until the second stage. *Br. J. Obstet. Gynaecol.* **99**: 5–10.

Boylan, P.C. (1989) Active management of labor: Results in Dublin, Houston, London New Brunswick, Singapore and Valparaiso. *Birth* 16(3): 114–118.

Burns, K.M.L. (1992) The second stage of labour – A battle against tradition. *Midwives Chronicle* **April**: 92–94.

Cartwright, A. (1979) *The Dignity of Labour.* London: Tavistock.

Cohen, W.R. (1977) Influence of the duration of second stage on perinatal outcome and puerperal morbidity. *Obstet. Gynecol.* **48**: 266–269.

Crowther, C., Enkin, M., Keirse, M.J.N.C. & Brown, I. (1989) Monitoring the progress of labour. In: Cholmas, I., Enkin, M. & Keirse, M.J.N.C. (eds). *Effective Care in Pregnancy and Childbirth*, pp. 833–845. Oxford: Oxford University Press.

DOH (Department of Health) (1994) *Report on Confidential Enquiries into Maternal Deaths in the UK 1988–1990.* London: HMSO.

Flynn, A.M., Kelly, K., Hollins, G. & Lynch, P.F. (1978) Ambulation in labour. *Br. Med. J.* **2**: 591–593.

Franks, S.P. (1990) A randomized trial of amniotomy in active labour. *J. Family Pract.* **30**: 49–52.

Fraser, W.D. (1988) *A randomized controlled trial of the effect of amniotomy on labour duration*, MSc thesis. Alberta, Canada: University of Calgary.

Fraser, W.D. (1993) Amniotomy to shorten labour. In: Enkin, M.W., Keirse, M.J.N.C., Renfrew, M.J. & Neilson, J.P. (eds) Pregnancy and Childbirth Module 'Cochrane Database of Systematic Reviews'. Oxford: Update Software.

Fraser, W.D. *et al.* (1991) The Canadian multicentre RCT of early amniotomy *J. Perinat. Med.* **2**.

Friedman, E.A. (1955) Primigravid labor – a graphicostatistical analysis. *Obstet. Gynecol.* **6**: 567–589.

Garcia, J. & Garforth, S. (1989) Labour and delivery routines in English consultant maternity units. *Midwifery* **5**: 155–162.

Grant, J. (1990) Nutrition and hydration in labour. In Alexander, J., Levy, V. & Roch, S. (eds) *Intrapartum Care – A Research Based Approach.* Hampshire: Macmillan Education.

Haddad, P.F. & Morris, N.F. (1985) Anxiety in pregnancy and its relation to use of oxytocin and analgesia in labour. *J. Obstet. Gynaecol.* **6**: 77–81.

Hemminki, E. & Saarikoski, S. (1983) Ambulation and delayed amniotomy in the first stage of labor. *Eur. J. Obstet. Gynecol. Reproduct. Biol.* **15**: 129–139.

Hemminki, E. *et al.* (1985) Ambulation versus oxytocin in protracted labour: a pilot study. *Eur. J. Obstet. Gynecol. Reproduct. Biol.* **20**: 199–208.

Henderson, C. (1990) Artificial rupture of the membranes. In Alexander, J., Levy, V. & Roch, S. (eds) *Intrapartum Care – A research Based Approach.* Hampshire: Macmillan Education.

Johnson, J.D. *et al.* (1984) Oxytocin and neonatal hyperbilirubinaemia; studies of bilirubin production. *Am. J. Dis. Child.* **138**: 1047–1050.

Keirse, M.J.N.C. (1989) Augmentation of labour. In Chalmers, I., Enkin, M. & Keirse, M.J.N.C. (eds) *Effective Care in Pregnancy and Childbirth.* Oxford: Oxford University Press.

Klaus, M.H. *et al.* (1986) Effects of social support during parturition no maternal and infant morbidity. *Br. Med. J.* **293**: 585–587.

Llewellyn-Jones, D. (1990) *Fundamentals of Obstetrics and Gynaecology,* Vol. I *Obstetrics.* London: Faber & Faber.

Lopez-Zeno, J.A. (1992) A controlled trial of a program for the active managment of labor. *New Engl. J. Med.* **326**(7): 450–454.

National Childbirth Trust (1989) *Rupture of the Membranes in Labour: Women's Views.* London: National Childbirth Trust.

O'Driscoll, K. *et al.* (1969) Prevention of prolonged labour. *Br. Med. J.* **2**: 477–480.

O'Driscoll, K. *et al.* (1993) *Active Management of Labour,* 3rd edn. Aylesbury; Mosby Year Book.

O'Driscoll, K. & Meagher, D. (1980) *Active Management of Labour.* Philadelphia: W.B. Saunders.

Oliah, K.S.J. & Neilson, J.P. (1994) Failure to progress in the management of labour. *Br. J. Obstet. Gynecol.* **101**: 1–3.

Philpot, R.H. & Castle, W.M. (1972a) Cervicographs in the management of labour. in the primgravida. 1. The alert line for detecting abnormal labour *J. Obstet. Gynaecol. Br. Commonwealth* **79**: 592–598.

Philpot, R.H. & Castle, W.M. (1972b) Cervicographs in the management of labour in primigravidae. 2. The action line and treatment of abnormal labour. *J. Obstet. Gynaecol. Br. Commonwealth* **79**: 599–602.

Robson, K.M. & Kumar, R. (1980) Delayed onset of maternal affection after childbirth. *Br. J. Psychiat.* **136**: 347–353.

Saunders, N.S.G. *et al.* (1992) Neonatal and maternal morbidity in relation to the length of second stage of labour. *Br. J. Obstet. Gynaecol.* **99**: 381–385.

Sleep, J. *et al.* (1989) Care during the second stage of labour. In Chalmers, I., Enkin, M. & Keirse, M.J.N.C. (eds) *Effective Care in Pregnancy and Childbirth.* Oxford: Oxford University Press.

Stewart, P. *et al.* (1982) Spontaneous labour, when should the membranes be ruptured? *Br. J. Obstet. Gynaecol.* **99**: 5–10.

Studd, J. (1973) Partograms and normograms of cervical dilatation in management of primigravid labour. *Br. Med. J.* **4**: 451–455.

Thomson, A.M. (1988) Management of the woman in normal second stage labour: A review. *Midwifery* **4**(2): 77–85.

Thornton, J.G. & Lilford, R.J. (1994) Active management of labour: current knowledge and research issues. *Br. Med. J.* **309**: 366–369.

Turner, M.J. *et al.* (1986) Active management of labour in primigravidae. *J. Obstet. Gynaecol.* **7**: 79–83.

Wetrich, D.W. (1970) Effect of amniotomy upon labour. *Obstet. Gynecol.* **35**: 800–806.

50

Malpositions of the Fetal Head

An occipitoposterior position is a malposition of the vertex presentation. The occiput occupies a posterior quadrant of the mother's pelvis, whereas the sinciput is directed towards the anterior aspect. It is common, occurring in about 10% of all labours, most of which end normally. It is, however, the commonest cause of prolonged labour and of mechanical difficulties associated with delivery.

Occipitoposterior positions (Figure 1) throw a heavy responsibility on the midwife. Where the labour is progressing satisfactorily she will normally be looking after the mother, either in hospital or at home, and the outcome is likely to be spontaneous rotation to an anterior position followed by a normal vertex delivery. Slow progress, however, should alert the midwife to the possibility of abnormal labour and she must be vigilant to recognize promptly any complications which may arise, and to call for assistance. The midwife caring for the woman in prolonged labour has the exacting task of maintaining a close watch on the progress the mother is making, attending to her physical care and, at the same time, providing the encouragement, reassurance, sympathy and moral support that the woman needs during the course of a tedious and often painful labour.

The chief problem in occipitoposterior positions is that the fetus tends to be in a deflexed attitude, with the anterior fontanelle immediately over the internal os. For this reason it is sometimes called *bregmatic presentation*.

Normally the fetus lies in a round-shouldered attitude, head flexed and chin on chest, forming a compact ovoid shape. The rounded back bulges forward into the mother's abdomen and the flexed head engages easily, fitting into the pelvis as neatly as an egg into an egg cup. In labour it fits the lower uterine segment accurately and presses evenly on the cervix, stimulating good contractions and facilitating dilatation. During birth, the smallest possible diameters stretch the pelvic floor and perineum, while, if moulding occurs, the fetal head is squeezed in the most favourable diameters, so that there is little risk of birth trauma.

In contrast, in the occipitoposterior position, the fetal spine is towards the forward curve of the maternal lumbar spine, so that flexion is easily undone. As the fetal spine straightens, the fetus tends to 'square' his shoulders and raise his chin from his chest, thus adopting an erect or 'military' attitude. This brings the head into a more difficult relationship with the pelvic brim, like an egg put sideways on an egg-cup. It sits

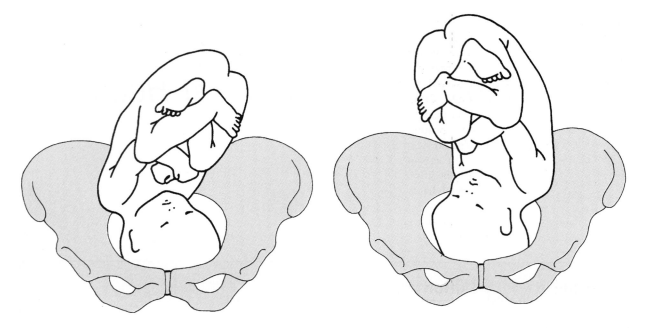

Figure 1   Right and left occipitoposterior positions.

insecurely above the pelvic brim, being slow to engage as larger diameters present. Contractions are not effectively stimulated, descent is delayed, dilatation is uneven and slow, while during birth the larger diameters are liable to cause severe tearing of the vagina and perineum. The fetal head is compressed in unfavourable diameters, with a greater risk of tearing of the tentorium cerebelli and consequent intracranial haemorrhage.

The cause of occipitoposterior position is not satisfactorily explained, though it is often associated with an *android* or *anthropoid* pelvis where the forepelvis is narrow, so that the head has to adjust to enter the pelvic brim. Other causes which have been suggested are a *pendulous abdomen*, *flat sacrum* and *anterior placenta*.

Occipitoposterior Position in Pregnancy

DIAGNOSIS IN PREGNANCY

The diagnosis is made by abdominal examination. On inspection, the abdomen appears flattened, or slightly

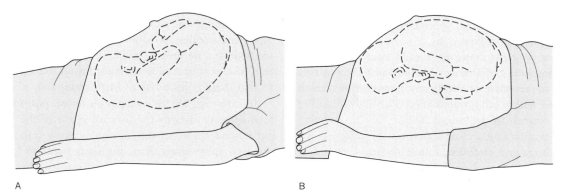

A   B

Figure 2   **A**: Abdominal contour with occipitoposterior position, showing depression at umbilicus. **B**: Rounded abdominal contour with occiptoanterior position.

depressed, below the umbilicus (see Figure 2). On palpation, the fetal head is high. Occipitoposterior position is the commonest cause of a non-engaged head in late pregnancy in a primigravida. If the fetus is almost occipitolateral, the deflexed head may feel large, because the occipitofrontal diameter is palpated, while the fetal back can be palpated out in the flank. If the occiput is markedly posterior, the high head feels small, since it is palpated near the bitemporal diameter; fetal limbs are felt as small knobs on both sides of the uterus and it may be impossible to feel the back (see Figure 3). The fetal heart sounds are often heard just below the umbilicus, while if the heart sounds are audible in one flank, it suggests that the fetal back is directed to that side.

Occipitoposterior Position in Labour

DIAGNOSIS IN LABOUR

The diagnosis may be made by abdominal examination, as described above, though now the head may be flexed and engaged. In this case, a prominence, the sinciput, can be felt above the pubic bone, usually on the left side.

On vaginal examination the findings will depend on the degree of flexion of the fetal head. Palpation of the anterior fontanelle is almost diagnostic of an occipito-

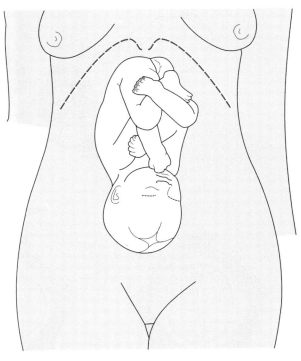

Figure 3   In occipitoposterior positions the anterior shoulder is well out from the midline and fetal limbs are readily palpable. This may cause a mistaken diagnosis of multiple pregnancy. (Reproduced with permission from Beischer and Mackay (1986) *Obstetrics and the Newborn* p. 488. London: Baillière Tindall.)

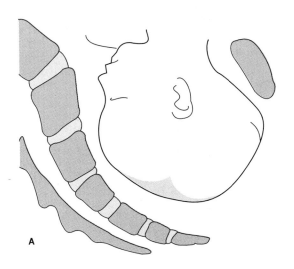

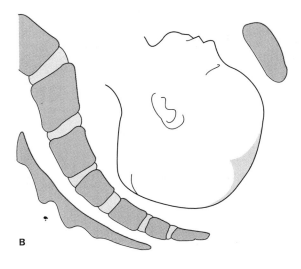

Figure 4   Position of the anterior and posterior fontanelles. **A**: Occipito-anterior; **B**: occipitoposterior.

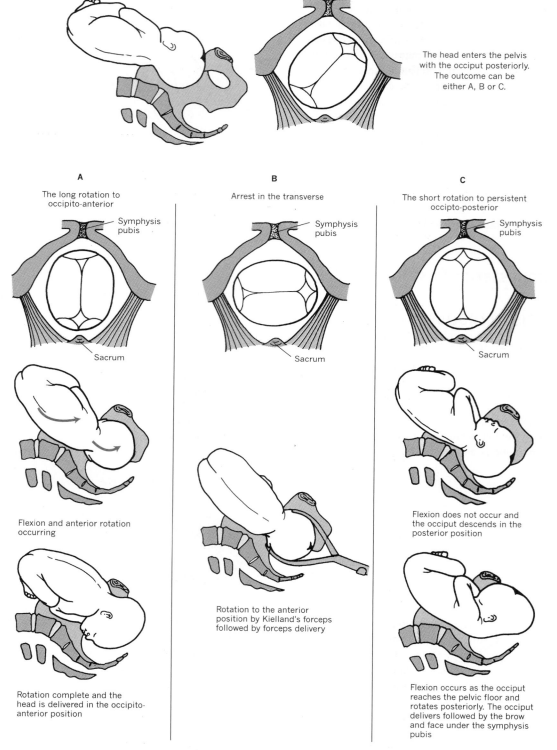

The head enters the pelvis with the occiput posteriorly. The outcome can be either A, B or C.

A

The long rotation to occipito-anterior

Symphysis pubis

Sacrum

Flexion and anterior rotation occurring

Rotation complete and the head is delivered in the occipito-anterior position

B

Arrest in the transverse

Symphysis pubis

Sacrum

Rotation to the anterior position by Kielland's forceps followed by forceps delivery

C

The short rotation to persistent occipto-posterior

Symphysis pubis

Sacrum

Flexion does not occur and the occiput descends in the posterior position

Flexion occurs as the occiput reaches the pelvic floor and rotates posteriorly. The occiput delivers followed by the brow and face under the symphysis pubis

Figure 5 Outcome of an occipitoposterior position. The head enters the pelvis with the occipit posteriorly. The outcome can be **A**, **B** or **C**.

posterior position (Figure 4). When the head is partially or well-flexed the anterior fontanelle is felt towards the front of the pelvis, while occasionally the posterior fontanelle is just within reach at the back. With a deflexed head, the anterior fontanelle is almost central and, unless obscured by the caput, easily recognizable by its size and shape.

PROGRESS IN LABOUR

Head flexed
If the head is flexed, labour will probably be completely normal. The engaging diameter is the suboccipitofrontal (10 cm). The occiput touches the pelvic floor and rotates anteriorly through three eighths of a circle; the baby is born with the occiput anterior (Figure 5A).

Head deflexed
Flexion may often improve, though the deflexed head tends to remain high or to take some time to engage. Labour is slow to become established. Once the head becomes flexed, labour usually speeds up and continues normally, with a long internal rotation and an occipito–anterior birth (Figure 5A).

If the head remains deflexed, however, labour is likely to be prolonged and painful, backache being a prominent characteristic. The sinciput may be the leading part which touches the pelvic floor and rotates anteriorly through one eighth of a circle (45°). This brings the sinciput under the pubic arch and the occiput into the hollow of the sacrum. With good contractions spontaneous delivery ensues. This is called *persistent occipitoposterior position* or *face-to-pubes delivery*; it is often associated with an android pelvis (Figure 5C).

Mechanism of persistent occipitoposterior position
The lie is longitudinal, presentation vertex and attitude deflexed, so that the engaging diameter is the occipito-frontal which measures 11.5 cm. The position may be either right or left occipitoposterior and the presenting part the anterior part of either the right (ROP) or left (LOP) parietal bone.

Descent takes place with deficient flexion and the biparietal diameter of the fetal head is held up on the sacrocotyloid diameter of the maternal pelvis, so that the sinciput becomes the leading part.

When the sinciput meets the resistance of the pelvic floor, it *rotates* forward 45° or one eighth of a circle.

The occiput is delivered over the perineum and the *head is born by flexion*, followed by *extension* to deliver the face from under the symphysis pubis. *Restitution* then takes place when the head rights itself with the shoulders.

Internal rotation of the shoulders occurs when the anterior shoulder reaches the pelvic floor and rotates 45° forward, accompanied by external rotation of the head.

First the anterior shoulder is born under the pubic arch and then the posterior shoulder passes over the perineum. The trunk is born by bending sideways in order to pass through the curve of the birth canal. This is termed *lateral flexion*.

Head high and deflexed
If the head is high and deflexed it may partially extend, so that the *brow presents*. It may also extend completely, resulting in a *face presentation*.

Deep transverse arrest
Deep transverse arrest (Figure 5B) may occur if the head remains deflexed. In this condition the fetal head may attempt a long rotation, but become caught in the transverse diameter of the outlet, between the ischial spines, should they be unduly prominent.

This is suspected if there is delay in the second stage of labour and on examination per vaginam the sagittal suture is found in the transverse diameter of the pelvis with a fontanelle at each end, close to the ischial spines. Rotation of the fetal head to an anterior position and delivery by vacuum extraction or forceps is required.

COMPLICATIONS

1 Prolapse of the cord may occur. As with any ill-fitting presenting part the membranes tend to rupture early and the cord may prolapse.

2 Prolonged labour may occur, which may be associated with a deflexed head, overefficient uterine contractions and a slightly contracted pelvis. The development of either fetal or maternal distress is more likely.

3 Retention of urine is common.

4 Early distension of the perineum and dilatation of the anus can occur while the head is still high. The

woman will feel the need to push before full dilatation of the os uteri has occurred.

5   Operative intervention and anaesthesia are often necessary.

6   The risk of trauma to the mother's soft tissues is increased.

7   Infection is more likely because of early rupture of the membranes, especially if labour is prolonged.

8   Upward moulding of the fetal skull may lead to intracranial damage. The perinatal mortality and morbidity is increased due to hypoxia and birth trauma.

CARE IN LABOUR

First stage

Communications and support   The mother should be fully informed about her progress throughout labour and included in all decisions related to her care. If labour is prolonged, she will particularly appreciate the support, empathy and skill of a caring midwife who works with her to achieve the best possible labour and a good outcome.

Ambulation and position   There is considerable evidence to indicate that an upright position and freedom to move around in labour has beneficial effects on both mother and baby. Several studies have concluded that uterine action is more effective, labour is shorter, there is less need for analgesia and the condition of the fetus in labour and the baby at birth are better (Flynn *et al.*, 1978; Williams *et al.*, 1980; Roberts *et al.*, 1981; Hemminki and Saarikoski, 1983; Roberts, 1989). The midwife should therefore encourage the woman to adopt an upright position and move around as she wishes to promote good progress. This will help to avert the need for augmentation of labour which is commonly required when there is slow progress in labour due to an occipitoposterior position.

Towards the end of the first stage there is often a premature desire to bear down when the fetus is in an occipitoposterior position. To try and stop the woman pushing before the cervix is fully dilated, the adoption of the kneeling position, with the head resting on the forearms may be effective. It relieves pressure on the anterior lip of the cervix (Brayshaw and Wright, 1994: 57). The breathing technique, puff- puff- blow with contractions, may also be helpful because it prevents the diaphragm from fixing and increasing the abdominal pressure, as occurs when pushing takes place.

General comfort and relief of pain   Backache is a common problem for women in labour when the fetus is in an occipitoposterior position. It may be relieved by adopting a position of leaning forward to relieve the weight from the lumbar spine. Examples are sitting astride a chair and leaning forward on to a table or some other form of support, kneeling and leaning forward, as described above, or standing and leaning forward, when the woman can be supported by her partner, or perhaps lean against the wall. Massage of the back in the lumbar/sacral region may also help to relieve the pain. Sometimes relaxing in a warm bath is helpful. A full bladder will add to the woman's discomfort and may also delay progress in labour, so regular emptying of the bladder is necessary. If these measures do not provide adequate relief, the woman may require analgesia and an epidural is usually the most effective method of obtaining good pain relief.

Assessment of progress   The descent of the fetal head, dilatation of the cervix and position of the fetus are carefully monitored to ascertain progress, because prolonged labour is a common problem when the fetus is in an occipitoposterior position. All other observations are carried out as described for normal labour (see Chapter 29). If progress is delayed, augmentation of labour with oxytocic drugs may be required.

Second stage

In about two thirds of occipitoposterior labours long internal rotation to an occipito-anterior position occurs and, in most of these cases, normal delivery follows. In the remaining third, the sinciput is the leading part and the occiput remains persistently posterior. Given good contractions, delivery takes place with the fetal head in the occipitoposterior position, sometimes called face-to-pubes. This method, however, is associated with a higher perinatal morbidity and mortality and maternal morbidity, especially if the baby is large.

In the second stage progress is assessed by the descent of the presenting part. The position adopted by the woman can have a significant effect on her comfort and on progress. The squatting position has the advantage of increasing the sagittal diameter of the pelvic outlet which may be helpful at delivery, as well as raising the intra-abdominal pressure (Russell, 1982;

McKay, 1984; Romond and Baker, 1985). Many women with the fetus in an occipitoposterior position, however, find the kneeling position most comfortable as it helps to relieve the backache which can be a very distressing feature of this labour (Balaskas, 1983). It can also assist the rotation of the fetal head to an anterior position and it reduces the pressure on the perineum and therefore reduces perineal trauma (Grant, 1987). Tears, if any, tend to be labial.

Delivery of the fetus in the occipitoposterior position

Flexion Flexion is maintained as the sinciput emerges from under the symphysis pubis so that a smaller diameter distends the vulval orifice. When the sinciput is delivered as far as the glabella, the occiput passes over the perineum.

Extension Once the occiput is born the midwife moves her hand to grasp the parietal eminences and extends the head until the rest of the face is delivered from under the symphysis pubis.

The rest of the baby is delivered as described for an occipito-anterior position.

Operative deliveries

If descent fails to take place in the second stage of labour, or progress is slow and there is concern about the fetal or maternal condition, an operative delivery is needed to deliver the woman safely of a healthy baby. The situation is discussed with the mother and she is involved in the decision and gives her informed consent for the necessary intevention.

Before attempting an operative delivery the doctor, a senior obstetrician, will make a vaginal examination to determine the station of the head, the position of the fetus, the degree of moulding of the fetal head and the capacity of the pelvis. If there is marked moulding, correction of the lateral or posterior position and asynclitism should precede the application of forceps or the vacuum extractor to reduce the risk of intracranial injury (Vacca and Keirse, 1989).

The vacuum extractor is an effective instrument for achieving rotation of the fetal head and delivery and, in a review of the use of forceps and the vacuum extractor, is considered preferable to forceps (Vacca and Keirse, 1989). The main reasons for this preference are that severe maternal injuries are more likely with the use of forceps and more analgesia is required. Severe perineal trauma may occur in cases of persistent occipitoposterior position, especially when a forceps delivery is performed, even with an episiotomy (Combs et al., 1990; Sultan et al., 1994). According to Sultan et al. (1994), the risk factors associated with third (and fourth)-degree tears are forceps delivery, first vaginal delivery, a large baby weighing over 4 kg and persistent occipitoposterior position. A minimum of two of these factors are present in operative deliveries for occipitoposterior positions. Vaginal and cervical tears may also occur.

If obstetric forceps are used, the fetal head is first rotated to an anterior position, either manually or with Kjelland's forceps, and then a forceps delivery is carried out. In deep transverse arrest, which is a serious cause of delay in the second stage of labour, the treatment is the same: rotation of the fetal head to an anterior position followed by operative delivery.

Occasionally Caesarean section is necessary in cases of occipitoposterior position of the fetal head if complications such as prolapse of the cord and fetal distress occur, or cephalopelvic disproportion is diagnosed.

References

Balaskas, J. (1983) *New Life – The Exercise Book for Childbirth*. London: Sidgwick & Jackson.

Brayshaw, E. & Wright, P. (1994) *Teaching Physical Skills for the Childbearing Year*. Hale: Books for Midwives Press.

Combs, C.A., Robertson, C.A. & Laros, R.J.Jr. (1990) Risk factors for third-degree and fourth-degree lacerations in forceps and vacuum deliveries. *Am. J. Obstet. Gynecol.* **163**(1, Pt. 1): 100–104.

Flynn, A.M., Kelly, J., Hollins, G. & Lynch, P.F. (1978) Ambulation in labour. *Br. Med. J.* **2**: 591–593.

Grant, A. (1987) Reassessing the second stage. *Assoc. Chartered Physiother. Obstet. Gynaecol.* **60**: 26–29.

Hemminki, E. & Saarikoski, S. (1983) Ambulation and delayed amniotomy in the first stage of labour. *Eur. J. Obstet. Gynec. Reprod. Biol.* **15**: 98–139.

McKay, S. (1984) Squatting: an alternate position for the second stage of labor. *Matern. Child Nurs.* **9**: 181–183.

Roberts, J. (1989) Maternal position during the first stage of labour. In Chalmers, I., Enkin, M. & Keirse, M.J.N.C. *Effective Care in Pregnancy and Childbirth*, Vol. 2, pp. 883–892. Oxford: Oxford University Press.

Roberts, J. Malasanos, L. & Mendez-Bauer, C. (1980) Maternal positions in labour: Analysis in relation to comfort and efficiency. March of Dimes Birth Defects Foundation: Original Article Series XVIII: 97–128.

Romond, J.L. & Baker, I.T. (1985) Squatting in childbirth: a new look at an old tradition. *J. Obstet. Gynecol. Neonatal Nurs.* **14**: 406–411.

Russell, J.G. (1982) The rationale of primitive delivery positions. *Br. J. Obstet. Gynaecol.* **87**: 712–715.

Sultan, A.H., Kamm, M.A., Hudson, C.N. & Bartram, C.I. (1994) Third degree obstetric and sphincter tears: risk factors and outcome of primary repair. *Br. Med. J.* **308**: 887–891.

Vacca, A. & Keirse, M.J.N.C. (1989) Instrumental vaginal delivery. Cited in Chalmers, I., Enkin, M. & Keirse, M.J.N.C. *Effective Care in Pregnancy and Childbirth*, Vol. 2, p. 1217. Oxford: Oxford University Press.

Williams, R.M., Thom, M.H. & Studd, J.W.W. (1980) A study of the benefits and acceptability of ambulation in spontaneous labour. *Br. J. Obstet. Gynaecol.* **87**: 122–126.

51

Malpresentations

Any presentation other than the vertex is termed a malpresentation. The malpresentations are therefore *breech*, *face*, *brow* and *shoulder*.

In all malpresentations, as in malpositions, there is an ill-fitting presenting part. This is often associated with early rupture of the membranes due to uneven pressure on the bag of forewaters and there is an increased risk of cord prolapse. An ill-fitting presenting part is also associated with poor uterine action and therefore labour may be prolonged.

Breech Presentation

Breech presentation occurs when the fetal buttocks lie lowermost in the maternal uterus. The lie is longitu-dinal, the denominator is the sacrum and the present-ing diameter is the bitrochanteric, which measures 10 cm.

INCIDENCE

The incidence of breech presentation at the time of delivery is 3–4%. For singleton babies weighing more than 2500 g, the incidence is slightly lower, 2.6–3% (Kauppila, 1975). Spontaneous version occurs with diminishing frequency as pregnancy advances. West-gren *et al.* (1985) found that spontaneous version of the fetus occurred in 57% of pregnancies after 32 weeks, and in 25% after 36 weeks. It is more likely to occur in multigravidae, especially in those who have not had a previous breech presentation, and least likely when there are extended fetal legs or a short umbilical cord.

TYPES OF BREECH PRESENTATION

Four types of breech presentation are described (Figure 1):

1 *Complete or flexed breech*: The fetus sits 'tailor-wise' over the pelvis, the thighs and knees flexed and the feet close to the buttocks. This type is commonest in multigravidae.

2 *Extended breech*: The breech with extended legs is also known as a *frank breech*. The fetal thighs are flexed, but the legs are extended at the knees and lie alongside the trunk, the feet being near the head. This is the commonest type of breech presentation, occurring most frequently in primigravidae towards term, because their firm uterine and abdominal muscles allow only limited fetal movement. The fetus is therefore unable to flex its legs and turn to a cephalic presentation.

3 *Footling presentation*: One or both feet present below the buttocks, with hips and knees extended. This type of breech presentation is more likely to occur when the fetus is preterm, but is relatively rare.

4 *Knee presentation*: One or both knees present below the buttocks, with one or both hips extended and

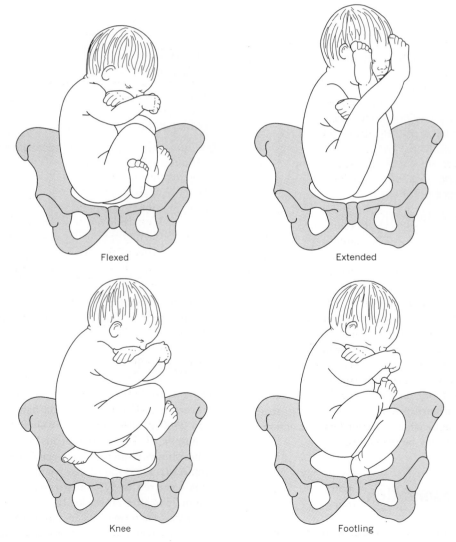

Flexed

Extended

Knee

Footling

Figure 1 Types of breech presentations.

the knees flexed. This is the least common of all types of breech presentation.

CAUSES

One fetus in four will present by the breech at some stage in pregnancy, but by the 34th week most of these fetuses have turned, so that the vertex presents. Thus, if a woman has a preterm labour, it is not surprising to find the breech presenting; indeed preterm infants comprise a quarter of all babies born by the breech.

Many of the probable causes of breech presentation are associated with conditions which either restrict the freedom of the fetus to turn in the uterus, or allow the fetus to change its presentation frequently because of excessive space within the uterus.

Causes which may inhibit freedom of fetal movement and therefore spontaneous version to a cephalic presentation include:

▶ Primigravidae with firm abdominal and uterine muscles, especially when the fetal legs are extended, as described above (Westgren *et al.*, 1985).
▶ Uterine anomalies, such as bicornuate uterus. Previous breech birth may also be associated with a uterine anomaly.
▶ Oligohydramnios, because the reduced volume of amniotic fluid restricts the ability of the fetus to turn in the uterus. The condition may also be associated with fetal anomalies and/or compromise.
▶ Placental location: Placenta praevia may prevent the fetal head from fitting into the lower uterine segment and entering the pelvis. The fetus therefore adopts a breech presentation. A placenta situated in one or other cornua of the uterus reduces the breadth of space in the upper segment.
▶ Uterine fibroids which interfere with fetal activity or are situated in the lower uterine segment.
▶ A contracted pelvis because the fetal head is unable to enter the pelvic brim.
▶ Fetal anomalies which restrict fetal activity or prevent engagement in the pelvis, e.g. hydrocephalus.
▶ Multiple pregnancy because there is usually insufficient space to turn. Twins may present vertex and breech, like a pair of shoes in a box, fitting so closely that spontaneous version is unlikely.

Causes associated with excessive space in the uterus include:

▶ Grande multiparity, because of lax abdominal and uterine muscles.
▶ Polyhydramnios which causes overdistension of the uterus and therefore allows the fetus to be more mobile.

Fetal causes of breech presentation include:

▶ Fetal death.
▶ Decreased fetal activity, often due to a compromised fetus.
▶ Impaired fetal growth, which may be associated with fetal or maternal conditions having an adverse effect on the fetus.
▶ Short umbilical cord which restricts fetal mobility.

DIAGNOSIS

History

A history of a previous breech presentation may be significant, as the cause could be an uterine anomaly. The woman may give a history of discomfort under the ribs due to the presence of the hard fetal head there, or of kicking in the lower pole of the uterus.

Abdominal examination

The diagnosis is made chiefly by abdominal examination. Though inspection reveals nothing unusual, on palpation the presenting part feels firm, but not 'bony' hard, and less rounded than the head. The diagnosis is made by feeling the head, hard, round and ballottable in the fundus of the uterus, and the diagnosis may be very easy and obvious. It is more difficult, however, in a primigravida with firm abdominal muscles, especially if the legs are extended and the breech is deep in the pelvis, because the presentation is nearly out of reach of the midwife's palpating fingers and can be mistaken for the deeply engaged head. The baby's feet, lying under the chin, so immobilize the head that ballottement cannot be elicited. The placenta may lie on the anterior uterine wall and still further obscure the head. The fetal heart sounds, classically 'above the umbilicus' in breech presentation, may well be heard at maximum intensity at the supposedly 'vertex' point: halfway between the anterior superior iliac spine and the umbilicus.

Examination per vaginam

An examination per vaginam may be made to exclude a deeply engaged head. The fetal shoulders, palpated just above the brim of the pelvis when the head is deeply engaged, are sometimes difficult to distinguish from the breech (Chalmers *et al.*, 1989).

The midwife should be aware of these deceptive findings; unless she is certain that the vertex presents from 32 weeks' gestation onwards, she should be cautious and ask a doctor to see the mother.

Ultrasound

The diagnosis may be confirmed by ultrasound. In areas where ultrasound is not available, a radiograph will confirm the presentation. A scan for fetal anomalies should also be done at the time of diagnosis.

Diagnosis on examination per vaginam in labour

In labour the presenting part may be high at first. On examination per vaginam the breech feels soft and irregular and no sutures and fontanelles are palpable. The hard sacrum and the anus will be palpable and it is important to distinguish these from a face presentation. Fresh meconium from the anus on the examining finger is diagnostic of a breech presentation. The genitalia are soft and not easily recognized because they become oedematous. In a flexed breech the feet may be palpable alongside the buttocks. The features of the foot which help to distinguish it from a hand on vaginal examination include shorter digits of more even length, the larger size and limited range of movement of the big toe as compared to the thumb, and the presence of the heel.

RISKS OF BREECH PRESENTATION

Breech presentation places a healthy mother and fetus at increased risk of a complicated vaginal delivery or Caesarean section (Hofmeyr, 1991). The risks of breech presentation for the mother are associated with the increased risks of intervention, including the greater likelihood of Caesarean section. For the fetus, breech presentation and vaginal delivery can be a serious hazard. The perinatal mortality of breech deliveries has been estimated to be four times that of well-flexed cephalic presentations (Rovinsky *et al.*, 1973). Other figures are very variable and range from 0 to 35 per 1000 (Kauppila, 1975). It will be recalled that in vertex delivery the fetal head enters the bony pelvis either before or soon after labour begins. It is gradually compressed, moulds by slow degrees and finally emerges slowly, the pressure being gradually released. Once the head is born, the baby can breathe and,

indeed, sometimes does so before the shoulders emerge.

In a breech delivery, however, the fetal head does not approach the maternal pelvis until after the thorax and arms are born, while less than 10 minutes later the head is born. Until recently it was thought that the traumatic stresses undergone by the after-coming head as it passes swiftly through the birth canal, thereby undergoing rapid compression, with an equally sudden release of pressure as it emerges that puts pressure on the tentorium cerebelli and its contained and adjacent blood vessels, were the major cause of intracranial haemorrhage. Nowadays it is thought that the major cause of intracranial haemorrhage is anoxia.

Placental separation may occur in the second stage of labour and, as the after-coming head enters the pelvis, it inevitably compresses the cord; this lack of oxygen continues and while the fetal head is still in the vagina, the hypoxia can stimulate breathing. As a result liquor, blood and mucus may be inhaled, so that after birth it is difficult or impossible to clear the air passage and initiate normal breathing.

Additional dangers to the baby are fractures, rupture of abdominal organs and damage to muscles and nerves.

The dangers of breech delivery can be summarized thus:

▶ Intra- and extrauterine anoxia.
▶ Intracranial haemorrhage.
▶ Fractures and dislocations.
▶ Damage to muscles and nerves, especially the sternomastoid muscles due to traction, and to the brachial plexus.
▶ Rupture of abdominal organs due to pressure or faulty handling.
▶ Genital oedema and bruising due to caput formation.

The incidence of congenital anomalies is higher in fetuses presenting by the breech (Lauszus *et al.*, 1992), and especially so in those of very low birthweight (Kauppila *et al.*, 1981).

There also appears to be a correlation between breech delivery and children who develop growth hormone deficiency. Goodman *et al.* (1968) noted this association in 11% out of 35 children, and Rona (1976) in 11% out of 140 children. Albertsson-Wikland *et al.* (1990) postulate that the cause could be related to damage to the hypothalamic–pituitary region, but further studies are required to confirm the association and, if proven, to identify the cause.

MANAGEMENT OF PREGNANCY

If the midwife diagnoses, or suspects, a breech presentation at 32–34 weeks, she should refer the mother to an obstetrician. The obstetrician will study the woman's notes, examine her, discuss the situation with her and assess all the information available which may influence the management of the remainder of her pregnancy and her delivery. Attempts may be made to convert the fetus to a cephalic presentation.

Promotion of spontaneous cephalic version

There are many reports of attempts to promote spontaneous cephalic version by encouraging the mother to adopt various positions and exercises. One of the positions advocated is the knee–chest position. In Elkins' study (1982), cited by Chalmers *et al.* (1989), women adopted the knee–chest position for 15 minutes every two hours during the daytime for five days. Spontaneous version and normal vaginal delivery occurred in 65 out of 71 women. It has also been noted that a distended bladder which displaces the breech and the hands and knees position often used by women to assist their descent from the examination couch may promote spontaneous version in some cases (Hofmeyr, 1983).

Another study in which women raised their pelvis, abducted their thighs and carried out relaxed abdominal breathing for between 10 and 60 minutes a day significantly increased the rate of spontaneous version of the fetus to a cephalic presentation (Bung *et al.*, 1987).

Further studies are required to study the effectiveness of the use of the various positions and exercises to promote spontaneous cephalic version.

It is reported that persistent breech presentation after 34 weeks' gestation can be corrected in almost 80% of cases using a Chinese acupuncture technique called *moxibustion*. This involves the application of a moxastick containing the herb *Artemis vulgaris* (mugwort) to the B67 acupuncture point at the base of the little toenails twice a day for five days (Budd, 1992). At present a research study is being carried out to show what effect the moxibustion technique has on mother and fetus which may explain the apparent increase in spontaneous version of breech presentation fetuses with this technique (Simms *et al.*, 1994).

EXTERNAL CEPHALIC VERSION

External cephalic version is manual manipulation of the fetus through the abdominal wall to convert it from a breech to a cephalic presentation. There has always been considerable controversy about the effectiveness and safety of this procedure, especially when performed before 36 weeks. It is not without risk and contraindications include:

► a history of infertility;
► elderly primigravidae;
► cephalopelvic disproportion;
► placenta praevia;
► placental abruption;
► multiple pregnancy;
► hypertension;
► congenital malformations;
► intrauterine fetal death;
► rhesus negative mother, although many obstetricians nowadays do not consider this a contraindication because anti-D immunoglobulin can be given to the mother to prevent iso-immunization;
► uterine scar, although again this is not an absolute contradiction since Flamm *et al.* (1991) reported no serious maternal or fetal complications following attempted external cephalic version on women with lower segment uterine scars.

If Caesarean section is necessary because of complications affecting the pregnancy, it would obviously be unnecessary to attempt external cephalic version. Many obstetricians do not attempt the procedure anyway, preferring to deliver the woman with a breech presentation at term by Caesarean section.

Hofmeyr (1994a) reviewed the policy of planned elective Caesarean section at term for breech presentation (Collea *et al.*, 1978) and found that, although there was some decrease in short-term perinatal morbidity, there was an increase in maternal morbidity. He therefore concludes that there is inadequate evidence to substantiate or refute the effectiveness of Caesarean section for term breech presentation in improving perinatal outcome (Hofmeyr, 1994a).

Complications of external cephalic version include:

► cord entanglement;
► fetal distress;
► premature rupture of the membranes;
► premature separation of the placenta; and
► preterm labour.

Fetal mortality following the procedure is reported to be in the region of 1% (Hofmeyr, 1991). Several studies on external cephalic version before term have shown that it fails to have any effect on the incidence of breech delivery, Caesarean section rates and perinatal outcome (Chalmers *et al.*, 1989). Nowadays there is considerable evidence to support delaying external cephalic version until term (Saling and Muller-Holve, 1975; Hofmeyr, 1990; Mahomed *et al.*, 1991).

As far back as 1975 Saling and Muller-Holve reported that external cephalic version was successful in most pregnancies after 37 weeks' gestation, with the aid of betamimetic drugs such as ritodrine to relax the uterus. Other studies support these findings (Thunedborg *et al.*, 1991; DeRosa and Anderle, 1991; Mahomed *et al.*, 1991). There is also evidence that, in many pregnancies, tocolytic drugs are unnecessary (Hofmeyr, 1983; Robertson *et al.*, 1987). The advantages of delaying external cephalic version until term include the following:

▶ allows more time for spontaneous version to occur;
▶ less reversions to breech presentation;
▶ fetal mortality rate is reduced;
▶ other pregnancy complications which may affect the mode of delivery have become evident;
▶ in the event of complications occurring during the procedure, expediting the delivery of a mature fetus carries less risk;
▶ reduced incidence of breech delivery: Mahomed *et al.* (1991) report that external cephalic version at term using tocolysis reduced the frequency of breech presentation during labour from 83% to 17%;
▶ reduced incidence of Caesarean section: Mahomed *et al.* (1991) report a reduction in Caesarean section rate from 33% to 13%.

Other studies support the findings of a reduced incidence of breech delivery and Caesarean section when external cephalic version is performed at term (Hofmeyr, 1983, 1990, 1991; Brocks *et al.*, 1984; Morrison *et al.*, 1986; Mahomed *et al.*, 1991). Hofmeyr (1994b) reviewed five studies and found that there was a significant reduction in non-cephalic birth and Caesarean section rate when external cephalic version is attempted at term. No additional risks to the fetus have been reported.

The main disadvantage of delaying external cephalic version until term is that the membranes may rupture or labour start before version is attempted.

Procedure for external cephalic version   For this manoeuvre, the mother, her bladder empty, lies flat on a couch, while the midwife chats with her to reassure her and to aid relaxation. A cardiotocogram may be recorded before the procedure, or the fetal heart auscultated with a fetal stethoscope or Sonicaid. Tocolytic drugs may be administered intravenously to promote myometrial relaxation. Talcum powder may be sprinkled on the abdomen.

After disimpacting the breech from the pelvis, the obstetrician applies pressure to both poles of the fetus and rotates it to a cephalic presentation. To achieve this gentle pressure is maintained, moving breech and head, a little at a time, until the head lies over the pelvis and the breech is in the fundus. Usually a forward somersault is promoted, but sometimes it is easier to achieve success with a backward somersault. In some cases the version is so easily achieved that the fetus is turned without the mother realizing it. The fetal heart is auscultated during the manoeuvre and the vulva is exposed for evidence of bleeding or amniotic fluid.

On completion of the manoeuvre the fetal heart may be monitored by cardiotocograph for 30 minutes, or longer if the trace is abnormal, or other complications occur such as uterine contractions, ruptured membranes or bleeding per vaginam. The woman is asked to report any such abnormal findings if they occur later.

Persistent breech presentation

If version is unsuccessful or contraindicated and a breech presentation persists, the doctor will carefully assess the woman and discuss the mode of delivery with her. Vaginal delivery may be attempted in low-risk women after careful assessment which would include the following factors:

▶ Age.
▶ Parity.
▶ Period of gestation.
▶ Past obstetric history.
▶ Progress of present pregnancy.
▶ Size and shape of pelvis.
▶ Condition of the fetus.

Lauszus *et al.* (1992) found in their retrospective study of singleton breech delivery at term that low maternal age, low vaginal parity and high birthweight reduced the vaginal success rate. Roumen and Luyben (1991) agree with these findings. They conclude, however, that 80% of carefully selected women with a breech presentation at term deliver successfully per vaginam and that this should be considered a safe option. Assessment of pelvic size and shape and the size of the fetus in relation to the maternal pelvis is essential before considering vaginal delivery, because the largest part of the fetus, the head, only starts to enter the pelvis once the buttocks are delivered and a diagnosis of cephalopelvic disproportion at that stage could be disastrous. Pelvic size can be assessed clinically on vaginal examination and also by radiograph, an erect lateral pelvimetry giving the anterior–posterior diameters of the brim, cavity and outlet. It also shows the shape of the sacrum, whether it is well-curved or straight.

Wright *et al.* (1992) report on the accuracy of magnetic resonance imaging (MRI) for pelvimetry in assessing the size of the pelvis. One of the advantages is that it shows soft tissue structures as well as bone.

Fetal size is assessed, initially by abdominal examination but ultrasound may also be used to determine size and to screen for anomalies.

Finally, the period of gestation is considered. The practice of most obstetricians caring for a woman with a

breech presentation is to effect delivery between 38 and 40 weeks' gestation, thereby avoiding post-maturity and the problems of a larger fetus with a more ossified skull which does not mould easily. The risks of breech delivery are increased in preterm babies. Kiely (1991) found that the risk of neonatal death was significantly higher for babies weighing between 501 and 1750 g who had been delivered vaginally, than for those delivered by Caesarean section. Similarly the risks for babies with birthweights over 3000 g were increased. A survey conducted by Penn and Steer (1991) on obstetricians' management of the preterm breech found that 76% of them favoured Caesarean section to avoid the increased risks of trauma.

MECHANISMS OF LABOUR

There are six positions in breech presentations. The denominator is the sacrum and its relationship to the maternal pelvis determines the position. The positions are the same as the vertex presentations, substituting the sacrum for the occiput (Figure 2):

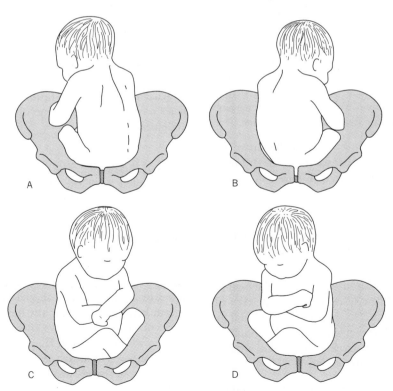

Figure 2 Breech positions. **A**: Left sacro-anterior; **B**: right sacro-anterior; **C**: right sacroposterior; **D**: left sacroposterior.

1 *Left sacro-anterior position* (LSA): The sacrum points to the left iliopectineal eminence and the abdomen and legs are directed towards the right sacroiliac joint. The left buttock is anterior and the bitrochanteric diameter is in the left oblique diameter. The natal cleft is in the right oblique diameter. A caput may form on the left buttock and on the genitals.

2 *Right sacro-anterior position* (RSA): The sacrum points to the right iliopectineal eminence, and the abdomen is directed towards the left sacroiliac joint. The right buttock is anterior.

3 *Left or right sacrolateral* (LSL, RSL): The sacrum is towards the left or right side of the pelvis.

4 *Left or right sacroposterior* (LSP, RSP): The sacrum points to the left or right sacroiliac joint, and the abdomen towards the right or left iliopectineal eminence.

Breech in the left sacro-anterior position
Birth of the buttocks

Descent The breech engages with the bitrochanteric diameter (10 cm) in the left oblique diameter of the pelvic brim and descends into the pelvic cavity.

Internal rotation of the buttocks The anterior buttock reaches the pelvic floor, is rotated forwards through one-eighth of a circle and comes to lie behind the symphysis pubis. The bitrochanteric diameter now lies in the anteroposterior diameter of the outlet.

Lateral flexion of the trunk Lateral flexion of the trunk allows the continued descent of the buttocks along the curve of the birth canal (Figure 3).

Birth of the buttocks The anterior buttock passes under the symphysis pubis and is born followed by the posterior buttock which passes over the perineum.

Birth of the shoulders
Internal rotation of the shoulders With the birth of the buttocks the shoulders descend into the pelvis with the bisacromial diameter (11 cm) in the left oblique diameter of the brim. Internal rotation of the shoulders through one-eighth of a circle brings the anterior shoulder behind the symphysis.

Birth of the shoulders The left (anterior) shoulder and arm escape under the symphysis and the right (posterior) shoulder and arm pass over the perineum.

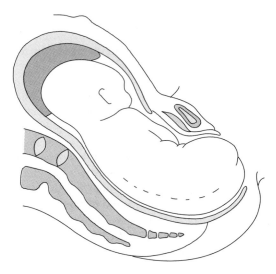

Figure 3 Lateral flexion and birth of the buttocks.

Internal rotation of the head and external rotation of the trunk The flexed head engages with the suboccipitobregmatic (9.5 cm) or suboccipitofrontal diameter (10 cm) lying in the right oblique or transverse diameter of the brim. Internal rotation of the head carries the occiput behind the symphysis. The face now lies in the hollow of the sacrum. External rotation of the buttocks and shoulders is produced by the internal rotation of the head. The back of the baby's head now faces in the same direction as the mother's abdomen.

Birth of the head The chin, face, vertex and occiput are expelled over the perineum by a movement of flexion to complete the delivery.

MANAGEMENT OF LABOUR

The labour is conducted in hospital, under the supervision of an experienced obstetrician, with care being given by a midwife and an anaesthetist and a paediatrician being available for the delivery.

Some obstetricians have attempted external cephalic version with tocolysis in labour, prior to rupture of the membranes. (Hofmeyr, 1983; Ferguson and Dyson, 1985). In the latter small study the success rate was 73%.

If the mother has not gone into spontaneous labour by 40 weeks, labour is usually induced. Some obstetricians recommend induction of labour at 38 weeks, when the fetus will be smaller.

First stage of labour

The first stage differs little from that of normal labour. If the breech is not engaged, as is probable in a flexed breech, there is a risk of early rupture of the membranes and prolapse of the umbilical cord. For this reason some obstetricians prefer the woman to remain in bed. Others consider the physiological advantages of the mother being upright in labour (see Chapter 29) outweigh any possible benefits of her remaining in bed. Where the breech is engaged, the legs are probably extended and the risk of cord prolapse is less, therefore the mother can safely be ambulant. Whether the mother is ambulant or in bed, the moment the membranes rupture, the midwife should make a vaginal examination, primarily to detect prolapse of the cord, though, at the same time, the usual observations are made to assess progress.

Continuous monitoring of the fetal heart should be undertaken where possible, or, if the mother is ambulant, intermittent monitoring, or telemetry. If external cardiotocography is unsatisfactory the electrodes can be applied to the fetal buttocks. Observations on the maternal condition and progress in labour are carried out carefully. In most cases the first stage progresses normally. Sometimes, however, uterine action is hypotonic and labour is augmented with oxytocic drugs.

Epidural anaesthesia is usually advocated for effective pain relief. The breech tends to slip through the cervix before it is fully dilated and this gives the mother a desire to 'push'. The buttocks may then descend easily, but the larger head cannot pass through the incompletely dilated cervix and dangerous delay results. Accordingly the mother must be discouraged from pushing until full dilatation of the cervix has been confirmed by vaginal examination. This problem does not usually arise when the mother has had epidural anaesthesia as she is unaware of the expulsive nature of her contractions.

Disadvantages of epidural analgesia for vaginal breech delivery have been reported. Chadha *et al.* (1992) conducted a large retrospective study on breech presentation in labour and epidural analgesia. They found that the use of epidural was associated with a longer duration of labour, increased need for augmentation with oxytocin and a significantly higher Caesarean section rate in the second stage. A signifi-

cant decrease in the intensity of uterine contractions associated with epidural anaesthesia occurs in both the first and second stages of labour and therefore affects the maternal expulsive effort. As a result there is an increase in the incidence of breech extraction or Caesarean section. Chadha *et al.* (1992) therefore suggest that the use of epidural anaesthesia for vaginal breech delivery is inappropriate. Crawford (1974) also noted that the second stage was longer in women who had epidural anaesthesia, but the incidence of breech extraction was not increased.

It is therefore important for the midwife who is caring for a woman who is having epidural analgesia to ensure that top-ups are carefully timed so that maternal expulsive efforts in the second stage of labour are not adversely affected. In cases where epidural analgesia is not given for breech presentation in labour, when the woman first shows signs of bearing down inhalational analgesia is administered, and breathing patterns which discourage pushing are encouraged, until the second stage is confirmed by vaginal examination (see Chapter 25).

Second stage of labour

It is essential to make a vaginal examination to confirm full dilatation of the os uteri before allowing the mother to push. For the second stage the mother adopts a semi-recumbent, upright or supported squatting position which will aid her expulsive efforts. For the actual delivery the obstetrician usually prefers the woman to be in the lithotomy position. An anaesthetist is present at the delivery in case operative intervention suddenly becomes necessary. A paediatrician waits in readiness to receive the baby who may require resuscitation. An experienced obstetrician prepares to deliver the baby. The midwife prepares the necessary equipment for forceps delivery, and for the reception and resuscitation of the baby, and plays an essential role in supporting the mother and her partner. She also notifies the neonatal unit of the imminent delivery of the baby.

Spontaneous breech delivery The delivery occurs with little assistance from the doctor or midwife. It is more common in multigravidae, or in the small pre-term breech.

Assisted breech delivery The bladder is emptied prior to delivery. When the posterior buttock distends the perineum, the perineum is infiltrated with local anaesthetic (unless the mother has had epidural anaesthetic or a pudendal block) and an episiotomy is performed. The posterior buttock then emerges and the breech advances more quickly. There should be no interference until the baby is born as far as the umbilicus. Then the legs are gently disengaged (unless they have already slipped out). Unless the cord is under tension there is no value in pulling it down.

With the next contraction the shoulder blades appear; the arms, which are normally flexed across the chest, are easily slipped out and the shoulders are born.

Burns–Marshall manoeuvre The baby is now allowed to hang by his own weight for a few moments to facilitate descent and flexion of the head. When the nape of the neck and hairline come into view, showing that the head is now ready to be born (Figure 4), the baby is grasped by his ankles and, using slight traction,

the trunk is carried up in a wide arc over the mother's abdomen (the *Burns–Marshall manoeuvre*). The perineum should then be depressed with the fingers to expose the mouth of the fetus. It is cleared of mucus to allow the fetus to breathe without inhaling the fluid (Cox, 1986). As soon as the nose appears at the vulva the nostrils are cleared. The baby should then be able to breathe freely.

The birth of the head then proceeds very slowly indeed. If it were allowed to 'pop out' quickly the sudden release of pressure could easily give rise to an intracranial haemorrhage. To avoid this danger the obstetrician applies Wrigley's or Neville Barnes obstetric forceps to the after-coming head. This enables him to control exactly the speed with which the head is born. It is brought down until the baby's mouth and nose are accessible so that the air passages can be cleared and oxygen can be given as soon as the baby

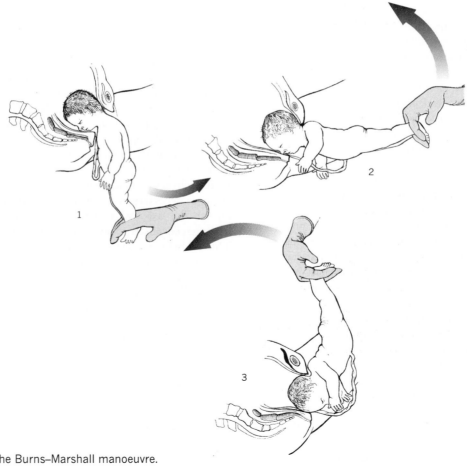

Figure 4   The Burns–Marshall manoeuvre.

gasps. Subsequently the birth of the head proceeds very slowly. An oxytocic drug is given to the mother as the head crowns.

Mauriceau–Smellie–Veit manoeuvre Sometimes the Mauriceau–Smellie–Veit method of delivering the head is used (Figure 5). This method should ensure good control of the head. It may also be used when there is delay in the descent of the head, although more commonly obstetric forceps would be applied. This manoeuvre is a combination of jaw flexion and shoulder traction. It can be used for any breech delivery, but is of particular value when the fetal head is extended and forceps cannot be applied. The obstetrician straddles the baby across his or her left arm, slides three fingers into the vagina, and feels for the baby's mouth; then inserting the middle finger into the mouth and resting the other two, one on each malar bone, the head is flexed. The index and ring fingers of the obstetrician's right hand are hooked over the baby's shoulders, to apply traction, while the middle finger presses on to the occiput to aid flexion. An assistant may apply suprapubic pressure. As gently as possible the baby's head is pulled through the cavity to the outlet, after which the trunk is raised to bring the mouth into view. The air passages are then cleared and the birth of the head completed in the usual way. The midwife can, in an emergency, perform this manoeuvre, though it is not often needed. She does well to remember the rule 'flexion before traction'.

Complications of breech delivery

Delay with extended legs Sometimes in a primigravid woman the legs splint the trunk, limiting the movement of lateral flexion. Usually the contractions are moderate rather than really strong. The obstetrician, with a forefinger in each of the baby's groins, exerts gentle traction, just sufficient to assist the descent of the buttocks. Once the popliteal fossa is seen the legs can be released by gentle pressure outwards behind the knees to abduct and flex the knees.

Extended arms If the baby's arms are not folded across the chest they are likely to be stretched up alongside the head. It is not possible for head and arms to enter the pelvis together, so the arms must come first and then the head. This is best achieved by *Lövset's manoeuvre*, which is shown in Figure 6, with the baby in a right sacrolateral position. The manoeuvre depends on the fact that the posterior shoulder is below the sacral promontory while the anterior shoulder is above the symphysis pubis. The obstetrician, grasping the baby's thighs with thumbs over the sacrum, pulls the baby gently downwards at the same time turning him, back upwards, through a half circle (180°). The former posterior shoulder, now anterior, appears under the symphysis, while the other shoulder has been brought into the pelvic cavity. The baby is then turned back through a half circle and the other arm is released in the same way. This procedure does

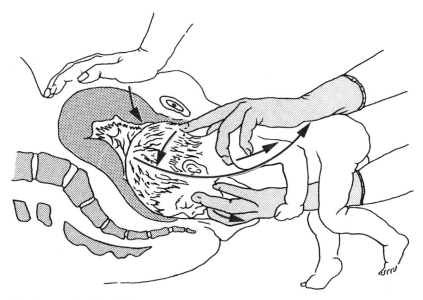

Figure 5 The Mauriceau–Smellie–Veit manoeuvre.

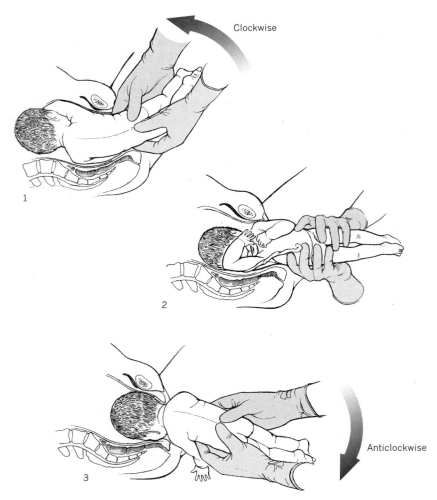

Clockwise

Anticlockwise

Figure 6   Birth of the arms using Lövset's manoeuvre.

not require an anaesthetic, it can be carried out by a midwife and, correctly performed, it is safe and successful, even in cases where the baby has one arm at the back of the neck (*nuchal displacement*).

Extended head   After the birth of the shoulders the baby is allowed to hang from the vagina to facilitate descent and flexion of the head. If the neck and hairline are not visible within a few seconds, the most likely reason is extension of the head. Forceps delivery is then required. Alternatively, the head may be delivered by the Mauriceau–Smellie–Veit manoeuvre, described above. This would be the method of delivery adopted in this situation by the midwife.

Entrapment of the fetal head   This is a most dangerous situation when the breech is expelled, but the head is trapped by the incompletely dilated cervix. The midwife, if faced with this situation, must call for a doctor urgently and try to create a channel for air to reach the fetal airways by placing her fingers or a Sim's speculum in the vagina and holding the maternal tissues away from the baby's nose and mouth. Secretions from the air passages are aspirated. The doctor will try to release the head from the cervix, but mortality and morbidity rates are high. Shushan and Younis (1992) report the use of *McRobert's manoeuvre* to facilitate the release of the fetal head. In this manoeuvre, which is more commonly used for shoulder dystocia, the woman lies on her back and draws her knees up to her chest, thereby lifting her buttocks a little off the bed (see Chapter 52).

Undiagnosed cephalopelvic disproportion

This is a grave emergency. Emergency Caesarean section may be attempted, but abdominal delivery can be difficult and traumatic when the breech is partially delivered vaginally. Symphysiotomy may save the life of the fetus whose head is trapped by disproportion (Klufio and Amoa, 1991).

Breech extraction

This method of delivery is sometimes used for delivery of the second twin. The operation is not without risk and should not be attempted unless there is no cephalopelvic disproportion, the cervix is fully dilated, the mother has a general or epidural anaesthetic and a skilled obstetrician is available. The obstetrician extracts the breech from the birth canal, manipulating the fetus, in contrast to the movements of the fetus produced by uterine contractions when labour is normal. In developed countries there is hardly any place for this manoeuvre.

Undiagnosed breech presentation

Occasionally breech presentation is diagnosed for the first time in labour. When this happens there is often pressure to deliver the woman by Caesarean section because antenatal assessment for vaginal delivery has not been carried out and there are fears of increased perinatal mortality. The relevant history, clinical assessment of the pelvis, X-ray pelvimetry and estimation of fetal size by clinical examination and ultrasound can usually be carried out in labour. A retrospective study, conducted by Nwosu *et al.* (1993), reported that breech presentations diagnosed in labour are more likely to deliver vaginally, with no excess morbidity or mortality. They conclude that there are no grounds for delivering all undiagnosed breech presentations by Caesarean section.

It is possible, for a variety of reasons, for a midwife to be faced with an emergency breech delivery. In community practice, the midwife should make every effort to get the mother into hospital. When labour is not advancing very quickly this is usually possible. Sometimes, however, the mother's labour is progressing rapidly, delivery is imminent and it would be foolhardy to attempt to move her. Such rapid progress could occur only if the uterine contractions were exceptionally strong. If, therefore, this mother is having really good strong contractions, there is every chance that she will have a smooth and easy breech delivery, but even so the midwife should call for skilled medical help as unexpected complications may occur. Meanwhile the midwife's management of the delivery is as described above.

Face Presentation

Face presentation is uncommon, occurring in about one in 500 of all deliveries. The head and spine are fully extended but the limbs are flexed, so that the fetus lies in the uterus in a curious S-shaped attitude, the occiput against its shoulder blades and the face directly over the internal os.

CAUSES

In *primary face presentation*, which is present before the onset of labour, the fetus is often abnormal. In *anencephaly*, which is quite common, there is no vertex to present; in the rarer *fetal goitre*, the head cannot flex; occasionally there is excessive tone in the fetal extensor muscles and he maintains the extended attitude for a few days after birth.

Secondary face presentations develop in labour, often unaccountably. In a deflexed occipitoposterior position the biparietal diameter may have difficulty in passing the sacrocotyloid diameter of the maternal pelvis. The bitemporal diameter descends more quickly, the head extends and the face presents. Where the uterus is tilted sideways (*uterine obliquity*) the force of the uterine contractions may be directed towards the front of the head, so that the head extends as it enters the pelvis. Face presentation is also more likely to occur in a *flat pelvis*, in a *lax uterus*, in *prematurity* and where there is *polyhydramnios* or a *multiple pregnancy*.

DIAGNOSIS

Face presentation is not easily diagnosed in pregnancy. It should be suspected if a deep groove is felt between the fetal head and back. The heart sounds, heard through the anterior chest wall on the side where the limbs are palpated, may seem unusually loud and clear when the position is mento-anterior. In mentoposterior positions the fetal heart sounds are more difficult to hear because the chest is posterior. Ultrasound in pregnancy may by chance disclose an unsuspected face presentation.

In labour the high presenting part may give rise to suspicion. The diagnosis can be made on vaginal examination, when gentle palpation will reveal the orbital ridges and the mouth with the gums. The presence of the gums distinguishes the mouth found in a face presentation from the anus which is located in a breech presentation. Occasionally the fetus will further help the diagnosis by sucking the examining finger. Once a face presentation is diagnosed it is essential to determine the position of the chin, whether it is anterior or posterior. A posterior face presentation, unless it rotates to an anterior position, will lead to obstructed labour. As labour progresses it becomes increasingly difficult to distinguish facial landmarks on examination per vaginam because the face becomes very oedematous. Examinations must be very gentle to avoid trauma to the eyes.

When a midwife diagnoses a face presentation she must inform a doctor. If the chin is lateral or posterior she should stress the urgency of the situation.

MECHANISMS

The lie is longitudinal.

There are six positions in which the face may present (Figure 7). The chin or mentum is the denominator:

1 *Right mentoposterior* (RMP) is an extension of the LOA. The chin points to the right sacroiliac joint.
2 *Left mentoposterior* (LMP) is an extension of an ROA. The chin points to the left sacroiliac joint.
3 *Right mentolateral* (RML) is an extension of an LOL. The chin is directed towards the right side of the pelvis.
4 *Left mentolateral* (LML) is an extension of an ROL. The chin is directed towards the left side of the pelvis.

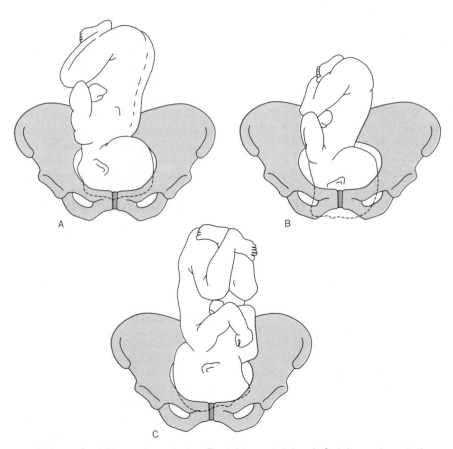

Figure 7   Face presentations. **A**: right mentoposterior; **B**: right mentolateral; **C**: left mento-anterior.

5 *Left mento-anterior* (LMA) is an extension of an ROP. The chin points to the left iliopectineal eminence.

6 *Right mento-anterior* (RMA) is an extension of an LOP. The chin points to the right iliopectineal eminence.

Face presentation develops before the head is engaged in the pelvis. The left mento-anterior position is probably the commonest.

Mento-anterior mechanism

The extended head enters the brim of the pelvis, the face presenting; the chin points to the iliopectineal eminence and the sinciput to the opposite sacroiliac joint. The submentobregmatic diameter (9.5 cm) engages; the face descends into the pelvis; the chin, being the lowest part, meets the resistance of the pelvic floor and is rotated through one-eighth of a circle, to escape under the pubic arch, and the face appears at the vulval outlet (Figure 8). Further uterine contractions drive the vertex and occiput over the perineum and thus, by a movement of flexion, the head is born. Restitution and external rotation take place.

Only if the chin is anterior can face presentation be born spontaneously. There is no mechanism by which the chin can be born when it lies at the back of the pelvis, such as is possible with a vertex presentation in a persistent occipitoposterior position. For the birth of a mentoposterior position the head and chest of the fetus would have to enter the pelvis together. This is impossible and obstructed labour will occur. However, spontaneous rotation of the head from the mentolateral or mentoposterior to the mento-anterior position can

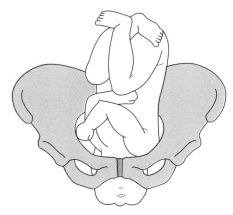

Figure 8 The face at the outlet, the chin passing under the pubic arch.

and occasionally does take place. Spontaneous delivery may then occur.

In a face presentation with the chin to the front, and a normal pelvis and fetus, with good contractions, labour will probably progress normally.

MANAGEMENT

In a mento-anterior position labour often proceeds normally, though, as in any malpresentation, the membranes may rupture early, prolapse of the cord is possible, and labour is sometimes prolonged. In the second stage normal delivery is anticipated, aided by an episiotomy, since, although the submentobregmatic diameter is only 9.5 cm, it is the submentovertical of 11.5 cm which distends the perineum at the time of delivery. If there is delay in the second stage the doctor will apply forceps. If normal delivery occurs, extension is maintained by applying pressure on the sinciput until the chin has escaped under the symphysis pubis; the head is then flexed to allow the vertex and occiput to sweep the perineum.

Mentolateral and mentoposterior positions are much more hazardous. Spontaneous delivery is unlikely, obstructed labour is possible and immediate treatment is thus essential.

The obstetrician may, either manually or with Kielland's forceps, rotate the head to a mento-anterior position and carry out a forceps delivery. In a primigravida, where these manoeuvres are more difficult, a Caesarean section is preferable and, indeed, is usually the treatment of choice for all women these days.

At birth, though the baby is usually in good condition, his eyelids and lips are grossly oedematous, his whole face is congested and bruised and his unsightly appearance could cause his mother considerable alarm and anxiety. Nevertheless, she will want to see him and if she cannot she will be even more anxious. She is therefore told how he looks and at the same time assured that this disfiguring bruising and oedema will subside within a few days; sucking, at first difficult, is usually normal in 48 hours.

Complications which may occur with a face presentation include:

▶ Cord prolapse.
▶ Obstructed labour, because:
  (a) the face does not mould and therefore cannot overcome minor degrees of cephalopelvic disproportion;

(b) a persistent posterior face presentation leads to obstructed labour.

▶ Emergency operative delivery may be necessary.

▶ Severe perineal trauma may occur because, although the presenting diameter, the submentobregmatic, is only 9.5 cm, it is the submentovertical of 11.5 cm which distends the vagina and perineum.

▶ Abnormal moulding of the fetal skull may lead to intracranial haemorrhage.

▶ Facial bruising and oedema.

Brow Presentation

Brow presentation (Figure 9) is less common than face presentation, occurring once in about 2000 labours. The causes are, with the exception of anencephaly, the same as in face presentation.

The head is midway between flexion and extension, with the mentovertical diameter of 13 cm attempting unsuccessfully to enter the 13 cm transverse diameter of the pelvic brim. A small head might enter a large pelvis only to be arrested in the cavity. Brow presentation, undiscovered and untreated, can cause this and obstructed labour could develop.

DIAGNOSIS

On abdominal examination the head is very high and the presenting diameter unusually large. A groove may be felt between the occiput and the back. On vaginal examination the presenting part may be too high to identify. If the brow is within reach, the orbital ridges are felt on one side and the anterior fontanelle on the other. The diagnosis may be confirmed radiographically or by ultrasound.

MANAGEMENT

The midwife must quickly call a doctor if she suspects or diagnoses a brow presentation in labour and a mother in her own home should be immediately taken to hospital. As in all malpresentations, the membranes are likely to rupture early and there is a risk of cord prolapse; thus an examination per vaginam is made as soon as the membranes rupture to detect cord prolapse. If brow presentation is diagnosed early in labour it may convert to a face presentation by becoming fully extended or it may flex to a vertex presentation. If the brow persists, however, and the fetus is a normal size, it will be impossible to deliver vaginally and a Caesarean section will be performed. Rarely are manoeuvres such as manual conversion to face presentation undertaken nowadays. The safest treatment for mother and baby is delivery by Caesarean section.

Oblique and Transverse Lie Leading to Shoulder Presentation

The normal lie of the fetus is longitudinal. Non-longitudinal lie may be transverse or oblique and will, if not corrected, become a shoulder presentation in labour (Figure 10). Shoulder presentation causes obstructed labour and must be prevented.

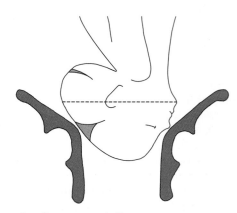

Figure 9   Brow presentation.

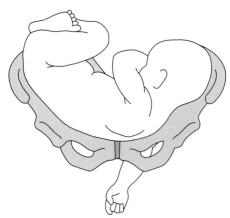

Figure 10   Shoulder presentation with prolapse of one arm.

CAUSES

The commonest cause is *laxity* of the uterine and abdominal muscles. Thus transverse, oblique, or often unstable lie is seen most frequently in women of high parity (grande multiparae).

Of various underlying causes, the most serious is *placenta praevia*. If, therefore, a mother has a persistent oblique lie, even though she has had no bleeding, she may have a placenta praevia. Other contributory factors are *multiple pregnancy, polyhydramnios*, a *uterine abnormality*, a *contracted pelvis* and occasionally a *large uterine fibroid*. An overdistended bladder may displace the presenting part and cause a transient oblique lie.

DIAGNOSIS

A transverse lie is easily diagnosed in pregnancy from the shape of the uterus, which appears too broad, with a bulge on either side of the abdomen, while the fundus is unusually low. Palpation will reveal the fetal head on one side and the breech on the other, but there is *no presenting part* entering the pelvis. An oblique lie may also be suspected by the shape of the uterus on inspection. On palpation the fetal head, or breech, is found in one or other iliac fossa. If a non-longitudinal lie is found after the 32nd week a doctor should be informed.

Ultrasound may be used to confirm the diagnosis and to detect the possible cause.

MANAGEMENT

The doctor may attempt to correct the lie by external version to a longitudinal lie and cephalic presentation. The likelihood of reversion to an oblique or transverse lie is high, however, and consequently some obstetricians do not recommend repeated external cephalic versions before planned delivery, or the onset of labour (Phelan *et al.*, 1986). The risk of leaving external cephalic version to this time is that the membranes may rupture and the cord may prolapse, or labour start, before the lie is corrected.

At each antenatal visit the doctor checks the lie and presentation and auscultates the fetal heart. If ultrasound examination excludes placenta praevia, a vaginal examination may be made to detect any pelvic abnormality such as a contracted pelvis. X-ray pelvimetry may also be required. Ultrasound examination would detect any fetal or uterine abnormality.

As pregnancy advances a non-longitudinal lie tends to revert to longitudinal and stabilize. Phelan *et al.* (1986) found that, after 37 weeks' gestation, a transverse lie persisted in only 17% of pregnancies. Similar findings are reported in other studies (Chalmers *et al.*, 1989).

Phelan *et al.* (1986) recommend that, when the fetal lungs are mature, the mother should be admitted to hospital for external cephalic version which is performed in the delivery area. This may then be followed by induction of labour with oxytocic drugs. The lie is closely monitored and, if necessary, gentle lateral pressure may be applied to the uterus to help maintain a longitudinal lie. Both the fetal heart and uterine contractions are monitored electronically, if possible, and the fetal and maternal condition are carefully observed. Once labour is established and the fetal head enters the pelvis, the membranes may be ruptured. Labour should then progress normally. In cases where the woman has a poor obstetric history, or if complications occur in labour, Caesarean section may be the safest mode of delivery.

If these precautions are not taken, when labour begins the fetal shoulder may be forced down towards the pelvis. The membranes are likely to rupture early and the cord to prolapse, while in addition the fetal arm may also prolapse.

A midwife would recognize shoulder presentation by abdominal examination, as described above, and by vaginal examination, when the shoulder is recognized by feeling the fetal ribs and the hand (to be distinguished from the foot because she can 'shake hands with it'). Vaginal examination is best avoided, however, unless placenta praevia has been excluded.

The midwife should send urgently for a doctor or, in community practice, for the obstetric emergency services. The more advanced the labour, the more difficult it is to correct the lie; after the membranes have ruptured it may be impossible. In such cases, Caesarean section is necessary and it may well be the safest mode of delivery even when the fetus is dead.

A midwife with no doctor at hand may find, after the birth of a first twin, that the second child is lying transversely. Immediate action is necessary and she should correct the lie by external version and rupture the second bag of membranes, thus stabilizing the longitudinal lie and hastening the birth of the child.

Compound Presentation

This term is used to describe a presentation in which a hand or foot lies alongside the head. Very rarely both a hand and a foot come down. It tends to occur when the fetus is small and the pelvis large or when there is any condition preventing the descent of the head into the pelvis. Compound presentation is of real significance only in advanced labour when the membranes have ruptured. Usually the presenting limb will recede as the presenting part descends. Replacement of an arm or leg is hardly ever necessary. Labour usually ends in a normal or a low instrumental delivery.

References

Albertsson-Wikland, K., Niklasson, A. and Karlberg, P. (1990) Birth data for patients who later develop GHD: Preliminary analysis of a national register. *Acta Paediat. Scand. (Suppl.)* **370**: 115–120.

Brocks, V., Philipsen, T. & Secher, N.J. (1984) A randomized trial of external cephalic version with tocolysis in late pregnancy. *Br. J. Obstet. Gynaecol.* **91**: 653–656.

Budd, S. (1992) Traditional Chinese medicine in obstetrics. *Midwives' Chronicle*, **105**(1253): 140–143.

Bung, P., Huch, R. & Huch, A. (1987) Ist die indische wendung eine ertdgreiche Methode zur senkung der Beckenendlagefrequenz? *Geburtsh Frauenheilk* **47**: 202–205.

Chadha, Y.C., Mahmood, T.A., Dick, M.J., Smith, N.C., Campbell, D.M. & Templeton, A. (1992) Breech delivery and epidural analgesia. *Br. J. Obstet. Gynaecol.* **99**: 96–100.

Chalmers, I., Enkin, M. & Keirse, M.J.N.C. (1989) *Effective Care in Pregnancy and Childbirth.* Oxford: Oxford University Press.

Collea, J.V., Robin, S.C., Weghorst, G.R. & Quilligan, E.J. (1978) The randomized management of term frank breech presentation: vaginal delivery versus Caesarean section. *Am. J. Obstet. Gynecol.* **131**: 186–195.

Cox, L.W. (1986) Breech presentation: a review of current practice. *Midwifery* **2**(2): 71–80.

Crawford, J.S. (1974) An appraisal of lumbar epidural blockade in patients with a singleton fetus presenting by the breech. *J. Obstet. Gynaecol. Br. Commonwealth* **81**: 876–872.

DeRosa, J. & Anderle, L.J. (1991) External cephalic version of term singleton breech presentations with tocolysis: a retrospective study in a community hospital. *J. Am. Osteopathic Assoc.* **91**(4): 351–352.

Elkins, V.H. (1982) In Enkin, M. & Chalmers, I. (eds). *Effectiveness and Satisfaction in Antenatal Care*, p. 216. London: Spastics International Medical Publishers.

Ferguson, J.E. & Dyson, D.C. (1985) Intrapartum external cephalic version. *Am. J. Obstet. Gynecol.* **152**: 297–298.

Flamm, B.L., Fried, M.W., Lonky, N.M. & Giles, W.A. (1991) External cephalic version after previous cesarean section. *Am. J. Obstet. Gynecol.* **165**(2): 370–372.

Goodman, H.J., Grumbach, M.M. & Kaplan, S.L. (1968) Growth and growth hormone. *N. Engl. J. Med.* **278**: 58–68.

Hofmeyr, G.J. (1983) Effect of external cephalic version in late pregnancy on breech presentation and caesarean section rate: a controlled trial. *Br. J. Obstet. Gynaecol.* **90**: 392–399.

Hofmeyr, G.J. (1990) External cephalic version at term. In Chalmers, I. (ed.) *Oxford Database of Perinatal Trials*, Version 1.2, Disk Issue 4, Record no. 3087. Oxford: Oxford University Press.

Hofmeyr, G.J. (1991) External cephalic version at term: how high are the stakes? *Br. J. Obstet. Gynaecol.* **98**(1): 1–3.

Hofmeyr, G.J. (1994a). Planned elective Caesarean section for term breech presentation. In Enkin, M.W., Keirse, M.J.N.C., Renfrew, M.J. & Neilson, J.P. (eds) *Pregnancy and Childbirth Module.* Cochrane Database of Systematic Reviews: Review no. 05287. Cochrane Update on Disk, Disk Issue 1. Oxford: Update Software.

Hofmeyr, G.J. (1994b) External cephalic version at term. In Enkin, M.W., Keirse, M.J.N.C., Renfrew, M.J. & Neilson, J.P. (eds) *Pregnancy and Childbirth Module.* Cochrane Database of Systematic Reviews: Review no. 03087. Cochrane Update on Disk, Disk Issue 1. Oxford: Update Software.

Kauppila, O. (1975) The perinatal mortality in breech deliveries and observations on affecting factors; a retrospective study of 2227 cases. *Acta Obstet. Gynecol. Scand. (Suppl)*, **39**: 1–79.

Kauppila, O., Groonos, M., Aro, P. *et al.* (1981) Management of low birth weight delivery: should caesarean section be routine? *Am. J. Obstet. Gynecol.* **57**: 289–294.

Kiely, J.L. (1991) Mode of delivery and neonatal death in 17 587 infants presenting by the breech. *Br. Obstet. Gynaecol.* **98**(9): 898–904.

Klufio, C.A. & Amoa, A.B. (1991) Breech presentation and delivery. *Papua New Guinea Med. J.* **34**(4): 289–295.

Lauszus, F.F., Petersen, A. & Praest, J. (1992) Strategy for delivery in breech presentation. A retrospective study. *Ugeskr. Laeger* **154**(3): 123–126.

Mahomed, K., Seeras, R. & Coulson, R. (1991) External cephalic version at term. A randomized controlled trial using tocolysis. *Br. J. Obstet. Gynaecol.* **98**: 8–13.

Morrison, J.C., Myatt, R.E., Martin, J.N. *et al.* (1986) External cephalic version of the breech presentation under tocolysis. *Am. J. Obstet. Gynecol.* **154**: 900–903.

Nwosu, E.C., Chia, P. & Atlay, R.D. (1993) Undiagnosed breech. *Br. J. Obstet. Gynaecol.* **100**: 531–535.

Penn, Z.J. & Steer, P.J. (1991) How obstetricians manage the problem of preterm delivery with special reference to the preterm breech. *Br. J. Obstet. Gynaecol.* **98**(6): 531–534.

Phelan, J.P., Boucher, M., Mueller, E., McCart, D., Horenstein, J. & Clark, S.L. (1986) The non laboring transverse lie. A management dilemma. *J. Reprod. Med.* **31**: 184–186.

Robertson, A.W., Kopelman, J.N., Read, J.A., Duff, P., Magelssen, D.J. & Dashow, E.E. (1987) External cephalic version at term: is a tocolytic necessary? *Obstet. Gynaecol.* **70**: 896–899.

Rona, R. (1976) An epidemiological and genetic study of idiopathic GHD. Department of Growth and Development, Institute of Child Health, University of London, Unpublished thesis.

Roumen, F.J. & Luyben, A.G. (1991) Safety of term vaginal breech delivery. *Eur. J. Obstet. Gynaecol. Reprod. Biol.* **40**(3): 171–177.

Rovinsky, J.J., Miller, J.A. & Kaplan, S. (1973) Management of breech presentation at term. *Am. J. Obstet. Gynecol.* **115**: 497–513.

Saling, E. & Muller-Holve, W. (1975) External cephalic version under tocolysis. *J. Perinatal Med.* **3**: 115–122.

Shushan, A. & Younis, J.S. (1992) McRoberts manoeuvre for the management of the aftercoming head in breech delivery. *Gynecol. Obstet. Invest.* **34**(3): 188–189.

Simms, C., McHaffie, H., Renfrew, M.J. & Ashurst, H. (1994) *The Midwifery Research Database, MIRIAD.* Hale: Book for Midwives Press, pp. 202–203.

Thunedborg, P., Fischer-Rasmussen, W. & Tollund, L. (1991) The benefit of external cephalic version with tocolysis as a routine in late pregnancy. *Eur. J. Obstet. Gynecol. Reprod. Biol.* **42**(1): 23–27.

Westgren, M., Edvall, H., Nordstrom, E. & Svalenius, E. (1985) Spontaneous cephalic version of breech presentation in the last trimester. *Br. J. Obstet. Gynaecol.* **92**: 19–22.

Wright, A.R., English, P.T., Cameron, H.M. & Wilsdon, J.B. (1992) MR pelvimetry – a practical alternative. *Acta Radiol.* **33**(6): 582–587.

Part Eleven

Obstetric Emergencies and Operative Procedures

52

Shoulder Dystocia

Shoulder dystocia is an obstetric emergency with a potentially catastrophic outcome. It refers to deliveries where manoeuvres other than normal gentle downward traction are needed to complete the delivery of the anterior shoulder (Resnik, 1980). Smeltzer (1986) suggests that shoulder dystocia is caused by a failure of the shoulders to spontaneously traverse the pelvis after the fetal head has been delivered. A sign that shoulder dystocia may have occurred is that the infant's chin burrows into the mother's perineum, and the head looks as though it is trying to return into the vagina. This is caused by reverse traction from the anterior shoulder which is wedged on to the symphysis pubis and the posterior shoulder which has not yet negotiated the pelvic inlet (Figure 1).

Instinct may suggest pulling to deliver the anterior shoulder, but pulling on the infant's head will further impede delivery by wedging the infant's anterior shoulder more firmly on to the symphysis pubis. The midwife must recognize shoulder dystocia and summon obstetric and paediatric help immediately as the out-

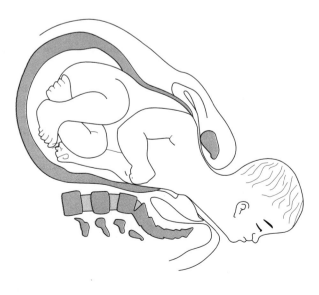

Figure 1 Shoulder dystocia.

come for both mother and infant is potentially very serious. She must then institute proven effective manoeuvres to release the shoulders and complete delivery.

The midwife must also remain calm and in control of the situation, and maintain communication with the mother. The mother may require additional analgesia, or regional or general anaesthesia prior to some of the following manoeuvres. The midwife must therefore also summon an anaesthetist, and meanwhile provide the best level of pain relief possible until such help may arrive. Meanwhile she should not delay in attempting to complete the delivery.

Incidence

It is generally agreed that the incidence of shoulder dystocia is around two per 1000 deliveries (0.2%). The risk rises with increasing birthweight and length of gestation (Hopwood, 1982; Acker *et al.*, 1986; Gross *et al.*, 1987; Al-Najashi *et al.*, 1989; Vermeulen and Brolmann, 1990).

Risk Factors

IDENTIFICATION OF RISK FACTORS

Ideally all potential cases of shoulder dystocia would be identified antenatally and the associated maternal and neonatal morbidity and mortality could then be prevented. At present midwives and doctors can do no more than anticipate the problem by identifying those factors which give a strong index of suspicion.

The antenatal booking history should alert the midwife to certain risk factors:

▶ *Maternal age*: The definition of advanced maternal age is over 35 years. O'Leary (1992: 13) suggests that the significance of advanced maternal age in this context is its relationship to increased birthweight and therefore shoulder dystocia.

▶ *Maternal obesity*: The most frequently occurring factor associated with shoulder dystocia is maternal obesity (maternal weight at delivery over 90 kg) (Sack, 1969; Modanlou *et al.*, 1982; Boyd *et al.*, 1983; Acker *et al.*, 1986; Spellacy *et al.*, 1985).

▶ *Maternal birthweight*: It has been demonstrated by Klebanoff *et al.* (1985), that a mother's own birthweight has a strong influence upon her infant's birthweight. The study looked at 1335 women and concluded that maternal birthweight was an accurate predictor of macrosomia (birthweight over 4000 g). The results of this study were verified by a larger study (16 320 mothers, 17 092 infants) undertaken by Seidman *et al.* (1988). O'Leary (1992) suggests that on the strength of these studies the mother's birthweight should be recorded at the antenatal booking to help to predict macrosomia and thus prevent some cases of shoulder dystocia.

▶ *Maternal diabetes and gestational diabetes*: Spellacy *et al.* (1985) studied the data from 33 545 deliveries and concluded that women with either insulin-dependent or gestational diabetes are more likely to deliver a macrosomic infant and are therefore at a higher risk of a delivery complicated by shoulder dystocia.

▶ *Pelvic abnormality*: Those women who have a platypelloid type of pelvis have an increased risk of developing shoulder dystocia (O'Leary, 1992: 65).

▶ *Fetal size*: The risk of shoulder dystocia increases with birthweight. Infants of non-diabetic mothers who have birthweights of 4000–4449 g have a 10% risk of shoulder dystocia, while infants of the same weight born to diabetic mothers have a 31% risk of developing shoulder dystocia (Acker *et al.*, 1985; Spellacy *et al.*, 1985).

Use of ultrasound to predict the macrosomic infant

Ultrasonic estimation of fetal weight is widely used as it is objective and can be reproduced (Combs *et al.*, 1993). However, Chaun *et al.* (1992) suggest that ultrasonic diagnosis of the large infant is generally no more accurate than clinical estimation. Ultrasonic estimation of fetal weight is currently used along with clinical judgement to assess the safest method of delivery, especially for the post-mature, macrosomic fetus.

Prediction of impending shoulder dystocia

In some cases the first hint of trouble the midwife may experience during a delivery is the slow extension of the baby's head and then the chin remaining tight against the mother's perineum (Coates, 1995). In spite of current technology, shoulder dystocia usually occurs unexpectedly (Al-Najashi *et al.*, 1989). It is therefore important that the midwife has a sound knowledge of the manoeuvres that may be used to complete the delivery in the shortest time possible, thus ensuring the best outcome for the mother and her infant.

Manoeuvres for Management of Shoulder Dystocia

McROBERTS' MANOEUVRE

This manoeuvre was described by Gonik *et al.* (1983) for the relief of shoulder dystocia. It is named after William A. McRoberts Jr MD who taught the method in Houston, Texas. The manoeuvre (Figure 2) requires the woman to lie on her back and to be assisted into an exaggerated knee–chest position. Once the woman is in this position then the midwife should be able to proceed with a normal delivery of the shoulders. Smeltzer (1986) suggests that the manoeuvre:

1 rotates the symphysis pubis superiorly by approximately 8 cm;
2 elevates the anterior shoulder;
3 pushes the posterior shoulder over the sacrum;
4 flexes the fetal spine;
5 straightens maternal lordosis;
6 opens the pelvic inlet to its maximum;
7 brings the inlet perpendicular to the maximum expulsive force;
8 removes weight-bearing forces from the sacrum; and
9 removes the sacral promontory as a point of obstruction (Figures 3 and 4).

Maternal and fetal models were used by Gonik *et al.* (1989) to assess the forces used to extract the fetal shoulders. The McRoberts' manoeuvre was compared

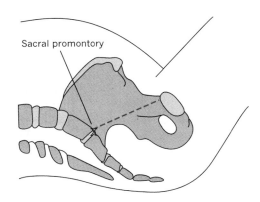

Figure 3   Diagram to show brim of pelvis in dorsal position.

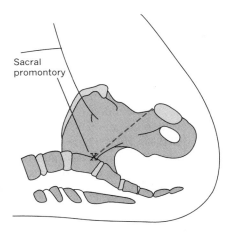

Figure 4   Diagram to show brim of pelvis in McRoberts' position.

with the lithotomy position and consistently required less force to remove the shoulders.

Gonik *et al.* (1983), Smeltzer (1986), Mashburn (1988), O'Leary and Leonetti (1990) advocate the use of the McRoberts' manoeuvre as a first step if shoulder dystocia is diagnosed, and suggest that if the manoeuvre is unsuccessful at the first attempt to try it a second time before attempting other manoeuvres.

WOODS' MANOEUVRE AND RUBIN MANOEUVRE

Woods' manoeuvre

The laws of physics were applied by Woods (1943) to overcome the problem of shoulder dystocia. Using a

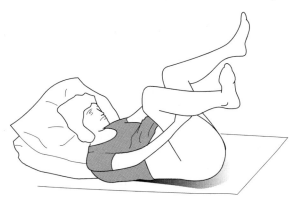

Figure 2   McRoberts' position.

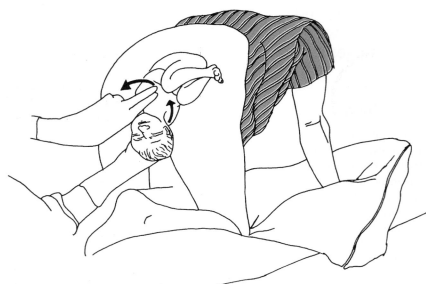

Figure 5 Woods' manoeuvre with mother in all-fours position.

wooden manikin he demonstrated that after the head has been delivered, the shoulders of the baby 'resemble a longitudinal section of a screw engaged in three threads' (Woods, 1943: 797). These 'threads' are the sacral promontory, the symphysis pubis and the coccyx. As a screw offers the greatest resistance to its release by pull, Woods points out that pulling on the baby's head or neck would be inappropriate as it contravenes the laws of physics.

To undertake the Woods' or the Rubin manoeuvre, the midwife should assist the woman into the lithotomy position with her buttocks well over the edge of the bed so that there is no restriction to the sacrum or coccyx during the manoeuvre. If this is not possible, then the McRoberts' manoeuvre detailed earlier should be used. Even if this has failed to deliver the baby, it still provides a useful position for undertaking further manoeuvres. Alternatively, the woman could be assisted into an all-fours position. These positions remove restrictions to the sacrum and coccyx which are present when the mother is in the dorsal or semi-recumbent positions. Positioning the mother as described will facilitate manoeuvres to rotate the fetal shoulders off the symphysis pubis and complete the delivery.

The method Woods used to relieve shoulder dystocia involves applying one hand to the mother's abdomen, putting firm but gentle pressure on to the fetal buttocks, and inserting two fingers of the other hand into the vagina, locating the anterior surface of the posterior shoulder (clavicle). The shoulder is then rotated through 180° in the direction of the fetal back (Figure 5). This rotation may disimpact the anterior shoulder and enable the posterior shoulder to enter the pelvic brim. The posterior shoulder, now anterior following the rotation, may be delivered by normal downward traction and the delivery completed.

Rubin manoeuvre

Rubin (1964) emphasized the importance of having both of the infant's shoulders adducted and presented measurements to demonstrate that in this position the circumference of the baby's body is less than if the shoulders were abducted. (Abduction would result from the use of the Woods' manoeuvre.) To achieve the Rubin manoeuvre a hand must be inserted into the vagina as far as is necessary to locate a shoulder. Then, working from behind the fetus, push the shoulders into the oblique diameter. Once the shoulders are in the oblique diameter and free of the symphysis pubis, then delivery can be completed (Figure 6).

O'Leary (1992) suggests that both the Woods' and Rubin manoeuvres may be more successful if they are used in conjunction with gentle but firm suprapubic pressure in the direction that facilitates the vaginal rotation (Figure 7).

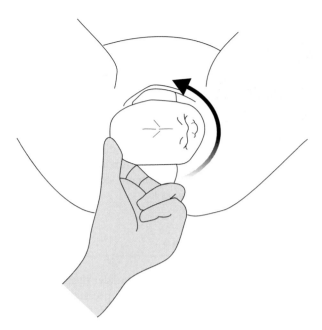

Figure 6   Rubin manoeuvre. The posterior shoulder is rotated anteriorly; the shoulders are adducted.

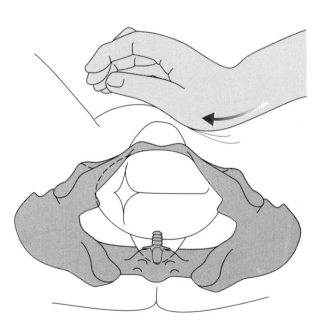

Figure 7   Diagram to illustrate correct use of and direction of suprapubic pressure when the fetal back is on the mother's right.

DELIVERY OF THE POSTERIOR ARM

Schwartz and McClelland Dixon (1958) advocate this manoeuvre to relieve shoulder dystocia as they found it caused less fetal injury when compared with traction and pressure (50 cases). The technique is to insert a hand into the vagina along the curve of the sacrum and locate the posterior arm or hand. The fetal arm should then be swept over the chest and delivered (Figure 8). If this manoeuvre fails once the posterior arm has been delivered, rotate the fetus using either the Woods' or Rubin manoeuvre so that the shoulder and arm that have been delivered are rotated to the anterior position, thus unlocking the obstruction.

ZAVANELLI MANOEUVRE

The Zavanelli manoeuvre is a revolutionary concept (Sandberg, 1985). Unlike the other manoeuvres described it reverses the mechanism of delivery. Cephalic replacement is then followed by a Caesarean section.

To carry out the manoeuvre the obstetrician would return the fetal head to the pre-restitution position of either direct occipito-anterior or direct occipito-posterior position. The head is then manually flexed and returned to the vagina with remarkable ease (Sandberg, 1988) (Figure 9). Delivery is then completed by Caesarean section.

The role of the midwife in such circumstances would be to support the mother, monitor and record the condition of both the mother and the fetus, and ensure that all the personnel necessary are available to deal with this obstetric emergency.

O'Leary (1992) states that this technique of cephalic replacement was developed in anticipation of the undeliverable shoulder in 1976. Sandberg (1985: 482) suggests that the Zavanelli manoeuvre ' . . . must occupy the bottom priority until its virtue and applicability . . . can be confirmed'. O'Leary (1992) reviewed all the data available for the cases where the Zavanelli manoeuvre had been used. The obstetricians who had used the manoeuvre described it as easy, simple or gratifying. The outcome for the infant was good. Apgar scores at one minute were low but normal at 5 and 10 minutes. Antibiotics were used prophylactically in all cases. One woman had undergone a hysterectomy at delivery for a ruptured uterine constriction ring. All the mothers made an uneventful post-operative recovery.

Those infants who had been followed up for two years were all found to be normal.

Other Procedures

CLEIDOTOMY

Deliberate fracture of the clavicle has also been considered by some authors to be necessary to accomplish delivery. This is a difficult procedure especially in a large, mature fetus. O'Leary (1992: 78) points out that although clavicular fracture is often mentioned 'its use has never been substantiated.' In the past, cutting of the clavicle has also been advocated but is considered to be dangerous and potentially mutilating for both mother and fetus.

EPISIOTOMY

Shoulder dystocia is a bony dystocia and as such is not greatly affected by soft tissue. However, all the authors mentioned thus far have recommended the use of an episiotomy to try to prevent any further injury to the mother's pelvic floor and perineum during any direct manipulation of the fetus.

Maternal Outcome

Maternal deaths associated with shoulder dystocia have been caused by the use of fundal pressure causing *uterine rupture* (Seigworth, 1966), and from *haemorrhage* during delivery or immediately postpartum (O'Leary, 1992: 155).

Benedetti and Gabbe (1978) described maternal morbidity from shoulder dystocia as considerable: in their study 68% of cases had an estimated blood loss of more than 1000 ml. Others have recorded extensive *vaginal, cervical and perineal lacerations*, uterine rupture and *vaginal haematoma* as a sequelae to shoulder dystocia (Hopwood, 1982; Gross *et al.*, 1987).

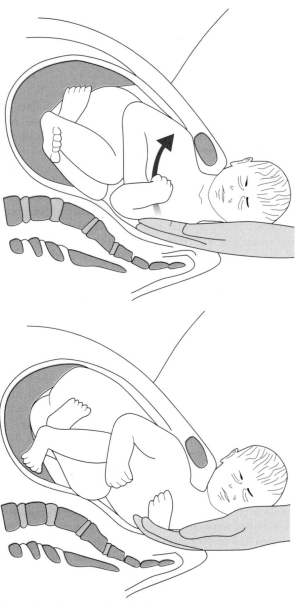

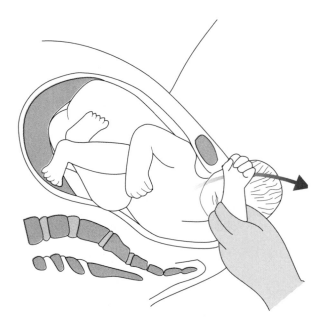

Figure 8   Delivery of posterior arm.

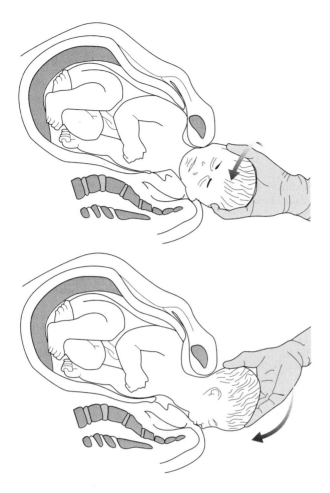

Figure 9   Zavanelli manoeuvre.

It would be wise to anticipate postpartum haemorrhage if shoulder dystocia is encountered, and to examine the cervix, vagina and labia very carefully following delivery to diagnose any lacerations (see Chapter 56).

Fetal Outcome

The most obvious and immediate consequence of a delivery complicated by shoulder dystocia is *birth asphyxia*. *Meconium aspiration* is also frequently associated with these deliveries (Gordon *et al.*, 1973; Benedetti and Gabbe, 1978; Boyd *et al.*, 1983). Meconium may not have been seen prior to the second stage of labour. However, the asphyxia caused by the delay in completion of the delivery is likely to cause the fetus to expel meconium prior to delivery. Midwives should therefore prepare for the reception of an asphyxiated baby, and call for a paediatrician to attend the delivery.

The most commonly reported injury following delivery complicated by shoulder dystocia is *Erb's palsy*. Fundal pressure together with traction provide the worst outcome for *brachial plexus injury* (Gross *et al.*, 1987). Infants experiencing shoulder dystocia are known to have serious immediate and long-term morbidity. It is therefore essential that the midwife summons a person skilled in advanced neonatal resuscitation as soon as shoulder dystocia is suspected, and prepares for resuscitation of the infant after delivery (see Chapter 69).

References

Acker, D.B., Sachs, B.P. & Friedman, E.A. (1985) Risk factors for shoulder dystocia. *Obstet. Gynecol.* **66**(6): 762–768.

Acker, D.B., Sachs, B.P. & Friedman, E.A. (1986) Risk factors for shoulder dystocia in the average weight infant. *Obstet. Gynecol.* **67**(5): 614–618.

Al–Najashi, S., Al–Suleiman, S.A., El–Yahia, A., Raman, M.S. & Raman, J. (1989) Shoulder dystocia – A study of 56 cases. *Aust. New Zealand J. Obstet. Gynaecol.* **29**(2): 129–131.

Boyd, M.E., Usher, R.H. & McLean, F.H. (1983) Fetal macrosomia, prediction risks and proposed management. *Am. J. Obstet. Gynecol.* **61**(6): 715–722.

Benedetti, T.J. & Gabbe, S.G. (1978) Shoulder dystocia a complication of fetal macrosomia and prolonged second stage of labour with mid pelvic operative delivery. *Obstet. Gynecol.* **52**(5): 526–529.

Chaun, S.P., Lutton, P.M., Bailey, K.J., Guerrieri, J.P. & Morrison, J.C. (1992) Intrapartum clinical, sonographic, and parous patients' estimates of newborn birth weight. *Obstet. Gynecol.* **79**: 956–958.

Coates, T.H. (1995) Shoulder dystocia. In Alexander, J., Levy, V. & Roch, S. (eds) *Midwifery Practice*, Vol. 5. London: Macmillan.

Combs, A.C., Singh, N.B. & Khoury, J.S. (1993) Elective induction versus spontaneous labour after sonographic diagnosis of fetal macrosomia. *Obstet. Gynecol.* **81**: 492–496.

Gordon, M., Rich, H., Deutschberger, J. & Green, M. (1973) Immediate and long term outcome of obstetric birth trauma. *Am. J. Obstet. Gynecol.* **117**: 51–56.

Gonik, B., Allen Stringer, C. & Held, B. (1983) An alternate maneuver for management of shoulder dystocia. *Am. J. Obstet. Gynecol.* **117**: 882–883.

Gonik, B., Allen, R. & Sorab, J. (1989) Objective evaluation of the shoulder dystocia phenomenon: Effect of maternal pelvic orientation on force reduction. *Obstet. Gynecol.* **74**(1): 44–48.

Gross, S.J., Shime, J. & Forrine, D. (1987) Shoulder dystocia: Predictors and outcome. A five year review. *Am. J. Obstet. Gynecol.* **56**(2): 336–344.

Hopwood, H.G. (1982) Shoulder dystocia: Fifteen years experience in a community hospital. *Am. J. Obstet. Gynecol.* **29**(2): 162–166.

Klebanoff, M.A., Mills, J.L. & Berendes, H.W. (1985) Mother's birthweight as a predictor of macrosomia. *Am. J. Obstet. Gynecol.* **153**: 253–256.

Mashburn, J. (1988) Identification and management of shoulder dystocia. *J. Nurse Midwifery* **33**(5): 225–231.

Modanlou, H.D., Komatsu, G., Dorchester, W., Freeman, R.K. & Bosu, S.K. (1982) Large-for-gestational-age neonates: Anthropometric reasons for shoulder dystocia. *Obstet. Gynecol.* **60**(4): 417–423.

O'Leary, J.A. (ed.) (1992) *Shoulder Dystocia and Birth Injury: Prevention and Treatment*. New York: McGraw-Hill.

O'Leary, J.A. & Leonetti, H.B. (1990) Shoulder dystocia: prevention and treatment. *Am. J. Obstet. Gynecol.* **162**: 5–9.

Resnik, R. (1980) Management of shoulder girdle dystocia. *Clin. Obstet. Gynecol.* **23**(2): 559–564.

Rubin, A. (1964) Management of shoulder dystocia. *J. Am. Med. Assoc.* **189**: 835.

Sack, R.A. (1969) The large infant. *Am. J. Obstet. Gynecol.* **104**: 195–203.

Sandberg, E.C. (1985) The Zavanelli maneuver: A potentially revolutionary method for the resolution of shoulder dystocia. *Am. J. Obstet. Gynecol.* **152**(4): 479–484.

Sandberg, E.C. (1988) The Zavanelli maneuver extended: Progression of a revolutionary concept. *J. Obstet. Gynecol.* **158**(6): 1347–1353.

Schwartz, B.C. & McClelland Dixon, D. (1958) Shoulder dystocia. *Obstet. Gynecol.* **11**: 468–471.

Seidman, D.S., Ever-Hadani, P., Stevenson, D.K., Slater, P.E., Harlap, S. & Gale, R. (1988) Birth order and birth weight re-examined. *Obstet. Gynecol.* **72**(2): 158–162.

Seigworth, G.R. (1966) Shoulder dystocia a review of five years experience. *Obstet. Gynecol.* **28**: 764–767.

Smeltzer, J.S. (1986) Prevention and management of shoulder dystocia. *Clin. Obstet. Gynecol.* **29**(2): 299–308.

Spellacy, W.N., Miller, S., Winegar, A. & Peterson, P.Q. (1985) Macrosomia, maternal characteristics and infant complications. *Obstet. Gynecol.* **66**(2): 158–161.

Vermeulen, G.M. & Brolmann, H.A. (1990) Shoulder dystocia: a retrospective study. *Ned. Tijdschr. Geneeskd* **134**(23): 1134–1138.

Woods, C.E. (1943) A principle of physics as applicable to shoulder delivery. *Am. J. Obstet. Gynecol.* **45**: 796–805.

53

Presentation and Prolapse of the Umbilical Cord

In approximately one in 300 births the umbilical cord descends below the presenting part (Lewis and Chamberlain, 1990). The vessels in the cord may become occluded by pressure from the descending presenting part. Such a profound hypoxic insult will result in irreversible brain damage, stillbirth or neonatal death.

Presentation of the cord occurs when a loop of cord lies below the presenting part of the fetus, the membranes being intact. When the membranes rupture the cord is said to be *prolapsed*. Occult cord presentation occurs when a loop of cord lies alongside, rather than in front of, the presenting part (Lewis and Chamberlain, 1990). This will not be felt on vaginal examination but may be the cause of unexplained fetal distress in labour, characterized in the early stages by deep early decelerations of the fetal heart. When confronted with a case of unexplained fetal distress the midwife should consider the possibility of cord compression.

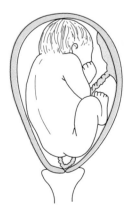

Figure 1   Cord presentation.

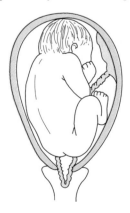

Figure 2   Cord prolapse.

Causes

Presentation and prolapse of the umbilical cord may occur in any situation which results in a poorly fitting presenting part: under normal circumstances the well-flexed fetal head enters the pelvis in late pregnancy or in early labour and thus prevents descent of the cord. An unusually *long umbilical cord* may also constitute a risk for this condition. Cord presentation and prolapse is common in *malpresentations* such as *shoulder presentation* (1 in 5) and *breech presentation* (1 in 22) especially a flexed or footling breech: the available space around the fetal legs in the lower pole of the uterus favours descent of the cord (Llewellyn Jones, 1990).

Preterm fetuses are at increased risk because there is a higher incidence of malpresentation, especially before 34 weeks' gestation, due to the relatively large quantity of amniotic fluid compared to fetal size, which permits increased mobility of the fetus. The small and immature parts of the preterm fetus do not fit into the lower pole of the uterus as snugly as those of the term fetus and this adds to the risk.

Malpositions such as *occipitoposterior positions*, where the presenting part tends to remain high, may also favour cord presentation and prolapse. *Polyhydramnios* encourages fetal mobility and often results in a high presenting part. When the membranes rupture the gush of amniotic fluid may bring down the cord. Similarly, the cord may prolapse during *artificial rupture of the membranes* if the presenting part is ill-fitting or high. The fetal heart should always be auscultated before and after artificial rupture of the membranes and if any unexplained fetal distress occurs after this procedure the possibility of cord compression should be considered.

Multiple births are associated with cord presentation and prolapse as malpresentation is not unusual. The second fetus in a twin delivery may take advantage of the extra available space in the uterus and turn to become a malpresentation after the birth of the first child. This predisposes to cord presentation and the person conducting the delivery must be mindful of this when rupturing the second amniotic sac.

Multiparous women are at increased risk because their relatively lax abdominal musculature favours non-engagement of the fetal head until labour begins. *Malformation or contracture of the pelvis* and *cephalo-pelvic disproportion* are associated with a high presenting part and therefore constitute a risk for cord presentation and prolapse, as do conditions such as *fibroids* or *placenta praevia* because they occupy space in the pelvis and prevent the fetal head from becoming engaged. The midwife should remember that *obstetric manipulations* such as *external cephalic version* of the fetus may also promote cord presentation (Llewellyn Jones, 1990).

Diagnosis

Cord presentation may be diagnosed in pregnancy by ultrasound scanning (Pelosi, 1990). In 1985 Lange *et al.* demonstrated the reliability of this method in a study of 1471 high-risk women. In nine of these women cord presentation was suggested on ultrasound examination and this was later confirmed in eight of the nine. There were no cases of cord prolapse among the remaining women whose cord position was normal on ultrasonography. These authors suggest that women with a malpresentation or a poorly fitting presenting part at term should have an ultrasound scan to exclude cord presentation in order to identify fetuses at risk and so plan the appropriate place and mode of delivery.

Vaginal examination may occasionally reveal a cord presentation, the soft, irregular, rope-like cord being palpated through the fetal membranes. Pulsation will be evident and will be synchronous with the fetal heart. If the presenting part is very high the cord may float away from the examining fingers. Pulsation felt in the vaginal fornices which are caused by the uterine arteries will be synchronous with the maternal pulse – the midwife should auscultate the fetal heart and take the maternal pulse if she is unsure of the source of the pulsation. If a cord presentation is suspected the midwife must keep the membranes intact and should attempt to reduce any cord compression by placing the mother in an exaggerated Sims' position with the hips and buttocks elevated by a wedge or pillows. Medical assistance should be called at once and the midwife should stay with the woman. By elevating the maternal pelvis the umbilical cord may be encouraged to move but if cord presentation persists the fetus will be delivered by Caesarean section.

When the membranes rupture it is essential to auscultate the fetal heart and to make a vaginal examination in order to diagnose cord prolapse. The risk of cord prolapse should be borne in mind whenever there is a high head, malpresentation or malposition, poly-hydramnios or multiple pregnancy. The prolapsed cord may be palpated in the cervical canal or in the vagina or may be visible at the vulva. The midwife should quickly assess cervical dilatation and the descent of the presenting part as management of this condition depends upon the stage of labour.

Dangers

The fetus is at risk of having its oxygen supply cut off when the cord is compressed between the presenting part and the maternal pelvis. In addition, cooling, drying or handling of the cord will cause the umbilical vessels to go into spasm. The prognosis for the fetus depends on where the mother is when the emergency occurs. If she is in hospital where delivery can be immediately effected, the perinatal mortality may be 15–20%, whereas in isolated centres or at home it may be more than 50% (Beischer and Mackay, 1986). The outcome for the fetus may be worse where the presentation is cephalic as the hard head is more likely to compress the cord than the breech or the shoulder (Lewis and Chamberlain, 1990).

The dangers for the mother are those associated with operative delivery and anaesthesia and include the risk of Mendelson's syndrome, haemorrhage and sepsis. The midwife should remember that, unless sensitively handled, the psychological trauma inflicted by the emergency and the need for a rapid and often operative delivery may cause distress and may affect the woman's ability to form a nurturing relationship with the child.

Management of Cord Prolapse

The management will depend upon the stage of labour and whether the fetus is alive or dead. If there are no pulsations in the cord and the fetal heart is not heard then the fetus is dead. This may be confirmed on ultrasound scan if a portable scanner is readily available. Once fetal death has been confirmed labour is allowed to proceed without further intervention and will culminate in the normal delivery of a stillborn infant. If the fetus is known or suspected to be alive the treatment is immediate delivery. The midwife must

attempt to keep the fetus in good condition until delivery is effected.

First stage

Medical assistance is summoned urgently. Meanwhile, the midwife must attempt to relieve pressure on the cord by moving the woman into the knee–chest position or the exaggerated Sims' position. The foot of the bed is elevated if possible. In addition, the midwife should introduce two fingers into the vagina and push up the presenting part during contractions to further relieve cord compression. If the cord is protruding from the vulva the midwife should replace it gently within the vagina in order to prevent spasm of the umbilical vessels.

Should this emergency arise while labour is being induced the midwife should stop the Syntocinon infusion. Oxygen may be administered by facemask at a rate of 4 l/min. Maternal oxygen therapy has been shown to increase Po_2 levels in the hypoxic fetus. It does not appear to cause constriction in the placental bed (McClure and James, 1960; Nicolaides et al., 1987; Battaglia and Hobbins, 1992). However this treatment can only be of benefit if there is still some feto-placental circulation; the midwife must therefore make every effort to ensure that cord compression is relieved and the feto-placental circulation maintained.

Manual replacement of the umbilical cord within the uterine cavity (funic reduction) has been shown to have some success in selected parous women (Barrett, 1991). However the midwife should not attempt this manoeuvre as successful replacement is unlikely and handling the cord will exacerbate fetal hypoxia. The doctor may commence an intravenous infusion of a tocolytic drug such as ritodrine (Yutopar) to arrest uterine contractions. The use of tocolytic infusions combined with filling the maternal urinary bladder with 500–700 ml of sterile normal saline to elevate the presenting part has been successful in maintaining good fetal condition while preparations are made for delivery by Caesarean section (Katz et al., 1988).

Second stage

If the cervix is fully dilated and there is no evidence of cephalopelvic disproportion or malpresentation, an immediate forceps delivery is performed. Late in second stage the midwife should make an episiotomy and encourage the woman's expulsive efforts in order to effect a quick delivery. Caesarean section may be the preferred mode of delivery even in second stage if there is evidence of malpresentation which would require correction or if the presentation is breech with the buttocks high in the pelvis.

The midwife should remember that the woman and her partner are likely to be confused and frightened by the sudden nature of the emergency and the speed with which delivery is effected. Careful explanations should be given as soon as the midwife is aware of the possibility of cord presentation or prolapse. Even if the outcome is good the feelings of powerlessness engendered by the situation may cause the couple to feel resentful or angry. The midwife should ensure that she makes the opportunity for time to discuss the events with them and reflect on their reactions and feelings.

References

Barrett, J.M. (1991) Funic reduction for the management of umbilical cord prolapse. *Am. J. Obstet. Gynecol.* **165**(3): 654–657.

Battaglia, F. & Hobbins, J. (1992) Fetal–placental perfusion and transfer of nutrients. In Reece, E., Hobbins, J., Mahoney, M. & Petrie, R. (eds) *Medicine of the Fetus and Mother.* Philadelphia: J.B. Lippincott.

Beischer, N. & Mackay, E. (1986) *Obstetrics and the Newborn.* London: Baillière Tindall.

Katz, Z., Shohan, Z., Lancet, M., Blickstein, I., Mogilner, B. & Zalel, Y. (1988). Management of labor with umbilical cord prolapse: A 5 year study. *Obstet. Gynecol.* **72**(2): 278–281.

Lange, I.R., Manning, F.A., Morrison, I., Chamberlain, P.F. & Harman, C.R. (1985) Cord prolapse: is antenatal diagnosis possible? *Am. J. Obstet. Gynecol.* **151**: 1083–1085.

Lewis, T.L.T. & Chamberlain, G.V.P. (1990). *Obstetrics by Ten Teachers, 15th edn.* Sevenoaks: Hodder & Stoughton.

Llewellyn Jones, D. (1990) *Fundamentals of Obstetrics and Gynaecology,* Vol. 1: *Obstetrics,* 5th Edn. London: Faber & Faber.

McClure, J. & James, B. (1960) Oxygen administration to the mother and its relation to blood oxygen in the newborn infant. *Am. J. Obstet.* **80**: 554–557.

Nicolaides, K., Bradley, R., Soothill, P., Campbell, S., Bilardo, C. & Gibb, D. (1987) Maternal oxygen therapy for intrauterine growth retardation. *Lancet* 25 April (8539): 942–945.

Pelosi, M.A. (1990) Antepartum ultrasonic diagnosis of cord presentation. *Am. J. Obstet. Gynecol.* **162**(2): 599–601.

Further Reading

Critchlow, C., Leet, T., Benedetti, T. & Daling, J. (1994) Risk factors and infant outcomes associated with umbilical cord prolapse: a population-based case-control study among births in Washington State. *Am. J. Obstet. Gynecol.* **170**(2): 613–618.

Griese, M. & Prickett, S. (1993) Nursing management of umbilical cord prolapse. *J. Obstet. Gynecol. Neonatal Nursing* **22**(4): 311–315.

Manning, F., Menticoglou, S. & Harman, C. (1989) Fetal assessment by biophysical methods: ultrasound. In Turnbull, A. & Chamberlain, G. (eds) *Obstetrics.* London: Churchill Livingstone.

54

Cephalopelvic Disproportion, Obstructed Labour and Uterine Rupture

Cephalopelvic Disproportion

Cephalopelvic disproportion is failure of the fetal head to descend through the pelvis in the presence of efficient uterine contractions and moulding of the head. It is caused by a misfit between the fetal head and the maternal pelvis, because the presenting diameter of the fetal head is larger than the diameters of the maternal pelvis through which it has to pass. Malpresentations, malpositions, pelvic tumours and fetal abnormalities which prevent the head descending through the pelvis are viewed as constituting *obstruction* rather than causes of cephalopelvic disproportion.

The head is the largest part of the fetus and if it has passed through the brim of the pelvis the rest of the fetus should pass through without difficulty. The probability is that the cavity and outlet are also of adequate dimensions to accommodate the passage of a normal fetus. However, in practice cephalopelvic disproportion can take place at the cavity or outlet of the pelvis too. The reader is reminded of the different types of pelves and how these may influence the way the fetal head negotiates its passage through the bony canal (see Chapter 2).

During the last 2 or 3 weeks of pregnancy it will sometimes be found that the head is not engaged and, in some cases, cannot be made to engage. Reasons for non-engagement of the fetal head have been discussed in Chapter 19. In about 50% of primigravidae the fetal head engages between 38 and 42 weeks (Weekes and Flynn, 1975). The most common reason for non-engagement is an occipitoposterior position of the fetal head, because of the larger presenting diameter of the deflexed head, the occipitofrontal diameter of which is 11.5 cm. In labour, however, the head usually flexes, and descends into the pelvis.

Diagnosis

The possibility of disproportion should be considered if there is a history of:

▶ medical conditions such as rickets or osteomalacia

which could adversely affect the size and shape of the pelvis;

▶ spinal deformities such as scoliosis;

▶ pelvic fractures or injuries which may have altered the normal shape and dimensions of the pelvis;

▶ obstetric complications such as previous prolonged labour, difficult delivery, Caesarean section or perinatal death.

On examination of the woman the possibility of cephalopelvic disproportion should be considered if:

▶ the woman is of short stature, less than 1.52 m; or

▶ the fetus seems unduly large.

It used to be thought that size of feet was a useful guide to the size of the pelvis and so it was common practice to ask pregnant women for their shoe size. Mahmood *et al.* (1988), however, found that maternal shoe size was not a useful parameter for predicting cephalopelvic disproportion. Maternal height is considered a more useful guide; nevertheless they found that 80% of women who were less than 1.60 m tall delivered vaginally.

The possibility that disproportion is present is much greater in a primigravida than in a multigravida with a history of previous normal deliveries, but it can never be ruled out since the size of the fetus may have been smaller in previous pregnancies. It is difficult to assess the size of the fetus accurately by palpation, but with experience it is possible to determine whether the fetus is unduly large for the duration of pregnancy. As ultrasound technology and expertise become increasingly more sophisticated, more accurate estimation of fetal size is possible. Technology, however, is no substitute for the expert midwifery skills required to obtain an accurate medical and obstetric history from the woman, or for midwives developing the clinical expertise to assess fetal and pelvic size and interpret the idiosyncratic combinations of all the above findings and take appropriate action.

If the head is not engaged by the 38th week of pregnancy in a primigravida, the mother is normally referred to an obstetrician for an opinion, chiefly to exclude the possibility of cephalopelvic disproportion. Head-fitting tests (see Chapter 19) or pelvic assessment may be performed, although opinion varies regarding their value.

When clinical examination reveals no evidence of pelvic contraction or cephalopelvic disproportion, no further action is taken and a vaginal delivery is antici-pated. If there is a suspicion of cephalopelvic dispro-portion, however, X-ray pelvimetry may be required, particularly in the circumstances described below.

X-Ray pelvimetry   X-Ray pelvimetry is indicated for:

▶ any primigravida with the fetal head not engaged at term in whom clinical examination suggests pelvic contraction;

▶ a primigravida with a breech presentation, if external version has failed or is contraindicated, and vaginal delivery is being considered; or

▶ any multipara with a history of difficult labour, for example, failure to progress in labour, prolonged labour and operative delivery. In these cases it is preferable to perform a radiological assessment of the pelvis in the puerperium, rather than in a subsequent pregnancy, because of the risks of radia-tion to the fetus.

An erect lateral X-ray pelvimetry will reveal the size and shape of the pelvis and also the relationship of the fetal head to the brim. Details of the size and shape of the pelvis seen on X-ray pelvimetry are as follows:

▶ General shape of the pelvis.

▶ Shape of the sacrum.

▶ Inclination between the sacrum and the pelvic brim.

▶ Anteroposterior diameter of the brim, cavity and outlet.

▶ Width of the sacro-sciatic notch.

▶ Depth of the pelvis.

An erect lateral X-ray of the pelvis may be supplemen-ted by an anteroposterior view showing the transverse diameter of the brim and the bispinous diameter.

The sole influence that pelvic radiological assess-ment plays in deciding whether a trial labour should take place in cases of minor cephalopelvic dispropor-tion has been debated for some time (Hogston, 1989; Thubisi *et al.*, 1993). Except where gross contraction is suspected, Lavin *et al.* (1982) conclude that pelvimetry has limited value in predicting the likelihood of vaginal delivery. Evaluation of the progress of labour is con-sidered a far more accurate indicator of cephalopelvic disproportion (Rosen & Dickinson, 1990).

As an alternative to X-ray pelvimetry, Moore *et al.* (1992) conducted a small study which highlighted the benefits of magnetic resonance imaging (MRI) pelvi-metry as giving more accurate measurements of the pelvic outlet, without the dangers of ionizing radiation or other biological hazards to the mother or fetus.

Further studies are required to evaluate this development.

Management

From these examinations and investigations the obstetrician is able to place the mother into one of three categories:

1 No disproportion is present and spontaneous labour and vaginal delivery can be awaited.
2 There is definite disproportion, either because the pelvis is small or abnormal in shape or because the fetus is unusually large. Vaginal delivery is out of the question and Caesarean section is necessary.
3 There is a slight degree of disproportion which may well be overcome successfully in labour. Provided there are no other complications, the woman is admitted to hospital for trial labour. Careful monitoring and surveillance of both mother and fetus are conducted and the facilities and personnel required for any emergency intervention are readily available.

Dangers

If cephalopelvic disproportion is not detected it will lead to obstructed labour which may result in a ruptured uterus and in maternal and fetal death.

Trial Labour

Trial labour is an ordinary labour conducted in hospital with the special object of ascertaining if the contractions of labour will flex and mould the fetal head sufficiently to make it engage and descend through the pelvis when there is a minor degree of cephalopelvic disproportion. If the head engages labour is likely to continue normally. The purpose is to give maximum opportunity for the woman to benefit from a vaginal delivery within the parameters of fetal and maternal safety. A successful trial labour prevents unnecessary operative intervention and the associated risks of increased morbidity and mortality, including psychological problems. It also influences the management of future labours, in that if the woman delivers safely vaginally, this is likely to be the pattern in the future.

Nowadays it is considered that all primigravidae with a non-engaged head are undergoing a trial labour and, with careful selection in the antenatal period and

an upright position in labour, or the active management of labour which ensures effective uterine action, most deliver normally.

Conditions necessary in labour when a minor degree of cephalopelvic disproportion is suspected

The presentation must be *cephalic*. A trial labour is never carried out in breech presentations. There should be no *major* degree of cephalopelvic disproportion. The woman should be *young* and *healthy* with a good medical and obstetric history. There should be *no complications* of pregnancy such as hypertension or antepartum haemorrhage and the pregnancy must not be postmature, otherwise the fetal head will not mould satisfactorily. A condition necessary in the past was that there should be *no uterine scar*, but there is now increasing evidence to suggest that it is safe to conduct a trial labour with a transverse lower segment uterine scar, provided there is careful management and monitoring in labour. The probability is that there will be a successful vaginal delivery with minimal risks of morbidity associated with scar dehiscence or uterine rupture (Flamm *et al.*, 1994). The midwife caring for a woman in labour with a uterine scar will be constantly on the alert for the signs and symptoms of impending rupture of the uterus which are described later in this chapter.

Management

Labour will take place in a major obstetric unit where there are both the facilities and the personnel available for electronic monitoring and any interventions which may be required to achieve a safe outcome to the labour for both mother and baby. Although midwifery care is given as in normal labour, the obstetrician will be the lead professional in a trial labour. The midwife may find that the couple require a high level of support and need to be kept very well-informed of progress, or the lack of it, and be involved in all decisions related to their care. Good preparation of the woman and her partner before the onset of labour is essential to gain their understanding of the situation and their co-operation in labour.

During labour the mother is encouraged to be ambulant because an upright position promotes flexion and descent of the head, cervical dilatation and the maintenance of contractions (Enkin *et al.*, 1993).

Continuous monitoring of the fetal heart and uterine contractions is preferable to intermittent recordings and may be carried out by telemetry if the mother is ambulant. Progress is assessed by:

1 the efficiency of the uterine contractions;
2 abdominal palpation to determine descent of the fetal head;
3 vaginal examination to note descent of the head, effacement of the cervix and dilatation of the os uteri. The obstetrician may wish to make all vaginal examinations.

All observations and findings of examinations are plotted on a partogram. This facilitates rapid recognition of any delay in cervical dilatation and descent of the head and indicates when action should be taken to aid progress. Cervical dilatation of less than 1 cm per hour over a two-hour period is regarded as delayed progress (O'Driscoll and Meagher, 1986).

If progress is found to be slow due to inefficient uterine action, active management of labour may be undertaken, after the mother has been carefully assessed by an obstetrician. Oxytocic drugs are used to overcome active phase arrest which is unrelated to cephalopelvic disproportion (Handa and Laros, 1993). Otherwise a diagnosis of cephalopelvic disproportion may be made in cases when the real problem is inefficient uterine action. The use of oxytocin in trial labour may be viewed as controversial because of the risk of uterine rupture. Several studies, however, support its use, provided electronic cardiotocography is carried out and facilities for the management of any emergencies are readily available (Farmer *et al.*, 1991; Leung *et al.*, 1993). In the study conducted by Leung *et al.* (1993), it was found that the increase in the incidence of ruptured uterus was caused by the overuse of Syntocinon. It should be stressed that active management would never be undertaken if more than a minor degree of cephalopelvic disproportion was suspected. Selective and judicious use of oxytocin is necessary when it is used to improve uterine efficiency in cases of minor cephalopelvic disproportion.

Conditions necessary for the use of oxytocin in a trial labour can be summarized thus:

▶ expert midwifery care to monitor uterine activity both by abdominal palpation and by skilled interpretation of the cardiotocography trace;
▶ continuous electronic cardiotocography;
▶ close surveillance of fetal and maternal well-being;
▶ avoidance of hyperstimulation of uterine activity by

oxytocin and, in the absence of significant progress, a limited period of use.

If hyperstimulation occurs, the oxytocin is immediately stopped and the obstetrician informed. If progress in labour does not improve with the use of oxytocin for a limited period, Caesarean section is indicated (Barton *et al.*, 1992).

It is never possible to forecast exactly how labour will progress, as so many factors are uncertain. However, if the uterine contractions are effective, the fetal head moulds, the pelvic joints relax and the maternal and fetal condition remains satisfactory, vaginal delivery is likely.

If contractions are ineffective, no 'trial' is possible. Oxytocic drugs may therefore be used to augment labour, as described above. If with effective contractions the head fails to engage, a Caesarean section will be performed. Similarly, if fetal distress should arise, the trial is abandoned as immediate operative delivery will be necessary. Studies by Ollendorff *et al.* (1988) and Flamm *et al.* (1994) show a 60–70% success rate for vaginal delivery following previous Caesarean section for cephalopelvic disproportion, or failure to progress in labour. In these studies the incidence of morbidity in the mothers was no higher than that found in women undergoing trial labour following previous Ceasarean section for non-recurrent conditions. This leaves open to question how absolute are the diagnoses of cephalopelvic disproportion?

Engelkes and van Roosmalen (1992) suggest that *symphysiotomy* is worthy of consideration in the management of cephalopelvic disproportion in selected cases. Such cases may include the following:

▶ to facilitate a ventouse extraction when the os uteri is fully dilated. Forceps delivery is contraindicated following a symphysiotomy because of the risk of injury to the bladder and to the thinned lower segment of the uterus;
▶ when operative intervention is best avoided, perhaps due to lack of facilities, particular hazards or cultural preferences;
▶ in cases of entrapment of the after-coming head of the breech (Menticoglou, 1990).

According to Engelkes and van Roosmalen (1992), symphysiotomy is associated with minimal morbidity in expert hands and so is another form of management to be considered in cases of cephalopelvic disproportion. It is rarely carried out in the UK because Caesarean section is considered safe and would appear to be more culturally acceptable. (See Chapter 55 for more on symphysiotomy.)

Obstructed Labour

Obstructed labour will occur in any case in which there is an insuperable barrier to the passage of the fetus through the birth canal, in spite of good uterine contractions.

Causes

Obstructed labour may occur in the following circumstances:

- ▶ if the maternal pelvis is grossly contracted, probably due to rickets, osteomalacia or severe injury;
- ▶ if the available space in the pelvis is occupied by a large tumour, e.g. a fibroid or an ovarian cyst;
- ▶ if the fetus is unusually large or abnormal with a condition such as hydrocephalus;
- ▶ if malpositions or malpresentations such as shoulder, brow and persistent mentoposterior face presentations occur or an impacted breech;
- ▶ if cephalopelvic disproportion is unrecognized.

It is important to distinguish clearly between *delay in labour*, known as *active phase arrest*, when progress is slow, probably because the uterine contractions are not sufficiently strong, but delivery is possible, and *obstruction*, when there is no progress in spite of good uterine contractions, because delivery is mechanically impossible.

Signs and symptoms

Obstructed labour should be suspected if there is little or no progress in labour, including no descent of the fetus, despite good uterine contractions. On examination the presenting part remains high and the cervix dilates slowly and is described as hanging like an 'empty sleeve' because the presenting part remains high and is therefore not well applied to it. The membranes often rupture early and so there is a risk of prolapsed cord. Recognition of the condition at this stage will prevent serious complications.

If the condition is allowed to continue the contractions become longer, stronger and more frequent in an effort to overcome the obstruction, until eventually tonic contractions occur. Uterine exhaustion may occur, especially in primigravidae, when the contractions cease for a while and then restart with renewed vigour. The mother is in severe and continuous pain, greatly distressed and looks very anxious and ill. The temperature is raised, the pulse is rapid; she may be vomiting and showing signs of dehydration. When the abdomen is inspected the uterus appears closely moulded around the fetus, the liquor amnii having drained away. On palpation the presentation remains high and the uterus is continuously hard instead of contracting intermittently. In advanced obstructed labour an oblique ridge may actually be seen running across the abdomen. This is *Bandl's retraction ring*, which denotes a marked difference in thickness between the tonically retracted upper uterine segment and the dangerously thinned lower segment, which is now in imminent danger of rupturing. The continuous retraction soon cuts off the fetal oxygen supply; hence at this stage the fetal heart sounds are no longer heard because the fetus is dead. The woman herself is in grave danger of dying from exhaustion or from rupture of the uterus. On vaginal examination the vagina may feel hot and dry and the presenting part remains high. A large caput succedaneum will be present and, if the presentation is cephalic, there will be excessive moulding. Urinary output is reduced and the woman may sustain a vesicovaginal fistula due to injury caused by prolonged pressure on the bladder.

Morbidity and mortality associated with obstructed labour

Morbidity and mortality associated with obstructed labour are greatly increased in cases where the condition is not recognized at an early stage, and where there is delay in referral and perhaps inadequate facilities and trained personnel to cope with such an emergency. According to Ozumba and Uchegbu (1991), it is mainly a problem in certain well-defined geographical regions in Africa and the Indian subcontinent. One of the initiatives of the World Health Organization, in its campaign to halve the number of maternal deaths in the world by the year 2000, is the introduction of the partogram for use in developing countries by all those who attend women in labour, including traditional birth attendants (WHO, 1994). This should enable those who are trained to use the partogram to recognize delay in labour at an early stage and initiate early referral. Where there is provision for good ante- and intranatal care by well-qualified professionals, obstructed labour should not occur.

Management

Prevention   By good antenatal care and close observation in early labour, the causes of obstructed labour can be recognized and treatment instituted before obstruction occurs (Kwast, 1992). Thus, an ovarian cyst is removed during pregnancy, a Caesarean section is planned in late pregnancy for conditions such as cephalopelvic disproportion, a transverse lie is corrected at the onset of labour, or earlier, and safe delivery is achieved. If obstruction occurs later in labour, for instance, when the fetal head extends to a brow presentation or to a posterior face presentation, immediate Caesarean section is performed. In the second stage of labour early recognition of deep transverse arrest is essential so that the woman can be safely delivered with forceps once the fetal head has been rotated.

A midwife called to a mother at home and finding her in obstructed labour should immediately notify an emergency obstetric team and arrange for ambulance paramedics to transfer the woman to hospital. She may give the woman an injection of pethidine hydrochloride to relieve her pain, blood is taken for cross-matching and an intravenous infusion of Hartmann's solution will be set up before the woman is transferred to hospital. Nothing by mouth is given as the woman will need to be prepared for anaesthesia and careful observations of the maternal and fetal condition are made and recorded.

In hospital the treatment is immediate Caesarean section to deliver the fetus, whether alive or dead. Once the baby is delivered the obstetrician will closely examine the uterus for signs of rupture.

There is rarely a place in modern obstetrics for destructive operations such as craniotomy and cleidotomy in cases of obstructed labour because of the risk of trauma to the overstretched and thinned lower uterine segment, and to other parts of the birth canal. There is also the profound psychological trauma to the parents to be considered when such procedures are undertaken. Gupta and Chitra (1994), however, suggest that there remains a limited place for destructive operations in developing countries in carefully selected cases which present late with obstructed labour, an intrauterine death and advanced intrauterine sepsis.

Uterine Rupture

Rupture of the uterus is a serious obstetric emergency which can result in fetal and/or maternal death. In the *Report on Confidential Enquiries into Maternal Deaths in the United Kingdom 1991–1993* (DOH, 1996), four cases of ruptured uterus are reported. Three of them were spontaneous ruptures, one through a lower segment Caesarean section scar and two in association with a severe abruptio placentae. The fourth death was due to traumatic uterine rupture following a failed vacuum extraction and forceps delivery.

The true incidence of ruptured uterus is difficult to determine from the medical literature because authors have different interpretations of what constitutes a ruptured uterus. Some only include a complete rupture whereas others do not distinguish between complete and incomplete ruptures. The incidence of ruptured uterus is higher in parts of the world where ante- and intranatal care are deficient and obstructed labour is a more frequent occurrence (Rachagan *et al.*, 1991). According to Duncan's (1991) estimation it occurs ten times more often in developing than in developed countries. Grace *et al.* (1993), however, dispute these figures and postulate that while the incidence of uterine rupture is decreasing in developing countries due to improvements in antenatal care, the incidence in developed countries may actually be on the increase due to a rising number of vaginal deliveries following Caesarean section and the increased use of oxytocin to augment labour.

Causes

In modern obstetric practice the misuse of oxytocic drugs is more often responsible for uterine rupture than instruments or intrauterine manipulations, or complications such as obstructed labour (Grace *et al.*, 1993).

Scar rupture   The cause may be previous uterine surgery, usually a Caesarean section. A classical scar (that is a longitudinal scar in the body of the uterus) is particularly likely to rupture (O'Connor and Gaughan, 1993). The most likely time for rupture to occur is in late pregnancy or in labour. Because of the high risk of uterine rupture following a classical uterine incision, an elective Caesarean section is usually planned in a subsequent pregnancy at about 38 weeks' gestation.

The incidence of uterine rupture following a lower

segment Caesarean section is 0.82% (Leung *et al.*, 1993). In these cases the rupture is more likely to occur when the woman is in labour (Mahomed, 1987).

Other causes of scarring of the uterus include surgery for conditions such as evacuation of the uterus, fibroids and some investigations, for example hysteroscopy. During these procedures trauma or perforation which is not always recognized may lead to a scarred uterus which results in rupture, usually at the fundus, in a subsequent pregnancy (Howe, 1993).

Traumatic rupture   Traumatic rupture is caused by:

▶ the use of instruments;
▶ intrauterine manipulations; and
▶ the misuse of oxytocic drugs.

Because of the increased maternal and fetal morbidity and mortality associated with high or mid-cavity forceps deliveries, Caesarean section is now considered a preferable mode of delivery. Similarly, intrauterine manipulations to correct unstable lie or malpresentation, such as a shoulder presentation, are considered hazardous procedures for both mother and fetus because of the high risk of uterine rupture. The risks are increased when manipulations are attempted in cases of prolonged or obstructed labour, because of the excessive thinning of the lower uterine segment, and also when the integrity of the uterus is suspect, as in grande multigravidae and when there is scarring.

Great care must be exercised in the use of oxytocic drugs for inducing or augmenting labour, especially in multiparous women because hypertonic contractions are more easily stimulated. There is also an increased risk of uterine rupture in those with an intrauterine fetal death if high levels of oxytocic drugs are administered because the effects on the fetus do not have to be considered. A cervical tear may extend into the lower uterine segment and cause serious haemorrhage because of the poor retraction there.

Spontaneous rupture   This may occur as a result of very strong uterine contractions (not induced or augmented by the use of oxytocic drugs). The cause of spontaneous rupture is not always clear. It may occur due to unrecognized trauma to the uterus which occurred in a previous pregnancy. Another cause is obstructed labour which results in tonic uterine contractions; this will lead to a ruptured uterus if the condition is not diagnosed and delivery effected quickly. In this case the rupture is usually in the lower

uterine segment. Abruptio placentae increases the risk of uterine rupture, because of disruption and distension of the uterine wall (Golan *et al.*, 1980; DOH, 1994). The risk is further increased when oxytocic drugs are used to stimulate uterine action. Although spontaneous rupture of the primigravid uterus is rare, several authors cite examples of this occurrence (Golan *et al.*, 1980; Guirgis and Kettle, 1989; Churchill and Bloomfield, 1992).

Types of uterine rupture

Complete or true rupture   This involves the full thickness of the uterine wall and pelvic peritoneum. Flamm (1985) describes it as a sudden, acute event associated with pain and blood loss and a raised maternal and fetal morbidity. It is most commonly associated with spontaneous or traumatic rupture of an unscarred uterus.

Incomplete rupture   This involves the myometrium but not the pelvic peritoneum which remains intact. It may also be called *occult* or *silent rupture*, or sometimes *dehiscence* or *uterine window*. Incomplete rupture is more frequently associated with a previous lower segment Caesarean section scar and tends to present with less violent and dramatic signs and symptoms, possibly due to the avascular nature of the scar tissue (O'Connor and Gaughan, 1993).

Sites of uterine rupture

The unscarred uterus   Between 60 and 70% of uterine ruptures are reported to occur in the unscarred uterus (Elkins *et al.*, 1985; Eden *et al.*, 1986), and longitudinal tears appear to be more common in these cases. Many cases in the literature describe a cervical tear which extends longitudinally into the lower uterine segment, either anteriorly or posteriorly (Golan *et al.*, 1980). It may further extend into the vascular upper uterine segment, thereby increasing morbidity and mortality (Mahomed, 1987). In some cases a rupture may occur in the upper uterine segment only. Ruptures in the unscarred uterus are usually complete and therefore associated with higher maternal and fetal morbidity and mortality rates.

The scarred uterus   In these cases the rupture is usually through the scar. The risk of scar rupture in a subsequent pregnancy following a longitudinal incision in the upper uterine segment (i.e. a classical Caesarean section) is estimated to be 2% (Golan *et* al., 1980). In a pregnancy following a previous lower segment Caesarean section the risk of rupture is 0.82% (Leung *et al.*, 1993).

Although the rupture usually follows the line of the scar, there are cases documented when this does not happen, for example transverse rupture into the posterior lower uterine segment, or vertical lower segment ruptures (Golan *et al.*, 1980).

Signs and symptoms

Complete rupture of the uterus often presents as an acute event with dramatic maternal collapse. The mother usually complains of severe and constant abdominal pain, followed by a marked reduction or cessation of uterine contractions, and vaginal bleeding. The fetus may be palpated in the abdomen separate from the uterus and fetal distress followed by intrauterine death is usual.

An incomplete rupture is far less dramatic. It may be called a silent rupture as the onset of signs and symptoms is gradual and it is often difficult to diagnose. Sometimes it is diagnosed after delivery or at Caesarean section (O'Connor and Gaughan, 1993), especially in cases where there are no signs and symptoms before delivery (Rachagan et al., 1991; Guirgis and Kettle, 1989). The mother may complain of constant abdominal pain and her contractions slow or cease. Although abdominal pain and/or scar tenderness are regarded as classical signs, Rachagan *et al.* (1991) found that these symptoms presented in only 35.3% of cases. A rise in maternal pulse rate and the cessation of fetal heart sounds were identified by Rachagan *et al.* (1991) as the most common clinical features of impending rupture. Vaginal bleeding may also occur. There is a gradual deteriorioration in the mother's condition. If the rupture is diagnosed early and delivery is expedited, the fetus might survive.

Management

The initial management will depend on the maternal and fetal condition. If the mother is in a state of shock she is urgently resuscitated and prepared for immediate surgery, either Caesarean section or, if the rupture is suspected after delivery, laparotomy. A blood transfusion will be necessary for severe haemorrhage and/or shock. Once the baby is delivered and the obstetrician has identified the type, location and extent of the rupture, the appropriate treatment can be instituted. The surgical options are:

▶ simple repair of the rupture: this is the treatment of choice whenever possible according to O'Connor and Gaughan (1993);
▶ uterine and internal hypogastric artery ligation to control haemorrhage; and
▶ hysterectomy; the uterus should always be sent for histological examination (DOH, 1994).

Aftercare

It is essential that mothers and their partners who have experienced such traumatic complications in childbirth receive adequate support and a clear explanation of the events from their obstetrician and midwife during the postnatal period. Some mothers suffer long-term psychological problems after a traumatic birth experience (Raphael-Leff, 1991; Kitzinger, 1992). Menage (1993) likens it to post-traumatic stress disorder. The opportunity to debrief and the provision of good support from midwife, doctor and family may help to prevent these additional problems. On occasions the midwife will realize that the mother needs specialist help which is beyond her capabilities and referral for appropriate professional counselling or treatment may be required. Midwives themselves may also need the opportunity to debrief after caring for a woman who has experienced such traumatic complications in childbirth. Reflecting on the events with colleagues not only helps the midwife to learn from her experience (Palmer *et al.*, 1994), but also helps her to work through her own feelings and obtain support.

References

Barton, D.P.J., Robson, M.S., Turner, M.J. & Stronge, J.M. (1992) Prolonged spontaneous labour in primigravidae whose labour was actively managed: results of an audit. *J. Obstet. Gynaecol.* **12**(5): 304–308.

Churchill, D. & Bloomfield, P.I. (1992) Uterine rupture in the primigravida. *J. Obstet. Gynaecol.* **12**(5): 314.

DOH (Department of Health) (1996) *Report on Confidential Enquiries into Maternal Deaths in the United Kingdom 1991–93.* London: HMSO.

Duncan, S. (1991) Rupture of the uterus in pregnancy or labour. *Africa Health* **13**(3): 21–22.

Eden, R.D., Parker, R.T. & Gall, S.A. (1986) Rupture of the

pregnant uterus: A 53 year review. *Obstet. Gynecol.* **68**(5): 671–674.

Elkins, T., Onwuka, E., Stovall, T., Hagood, M. & Osborn, D. (1985) Uterine rupture in Nigeria. *J. Reprod. Med.* **30**(3): 195–199.

Engelkes, E. & van Roosmalen, J. (1992) The value of symphysiotomy compared with caesarian section in cases of obstructed labour. *Social Sci. Med.* **35**(6): 789–793.

Enkin, M.W., Keirse, M.J.N.C., Renfrew, M.J. & Neilson, J.P. (1993) Upright versus recumbent position during first stage of labour. In *Pregnancy and Childbirth Module.* Cochrane Database of Systematic Reviews: Review no. 03334. Cochrane Updates on Disk. Oxford: Update Software.

Farmer, R.M., Kirschbaum, T., Potter, D., Strong, T.H. & Medearis, A.L. (1991) Uterine rupture during trial of labour after previous caesarean section. *Am. J. Obstet. Gynecol.* **165**(4, Part 1): 996–1001.

Flamm, B.L. (1985) Vaginal birth after caesarean section: controversies old and new. *Clin. Obstet. Gynecol.* **28**(4): 735–744.

Flamm, B.L., Goings, J.R., Liu, Y. & Wolde-Tsadik, G. (1994) Elective repeat caesarean delivery versus trial of labour: a prospective multi-centre study. *Obstet. Gynecol.* **83**(6): 927–932.

Grace, D., Lavery, G. & Loughran, P.G. (1993) Acute uterine rupture and its sequalae. *Int. J. Obstet. Anaesth.* **2**: 41–44.

Golan, A., Sandbank, O. & Rubin, A. (1980) Rupture of the pregnant uterus. *Obstet. Gynecol.* **56**(5): 549–554.

Guirgis, R.R. & Kettle, M.J. (1989) Uterine rupture in a primigravid patient. *J. Obstet. Gynaecol.* **9**(3): 214–215.

Gupta, U. & Chitra, R. (1994) Destructive operations still have a place in developing countries. *Int. J. Gynaecol. Obstet.* **44**(1): 15–19.

Handa, V.L. & Laros, R.K. (1993) Active phase arrest in labour: predictors of cesarean delivery in a nulliparous population. *Obstet. Gynecol.* **81**(5, Part 1): 758–763.

Hogston, P. (1989) Should we abandon x-ray pelvimetry? *Br. J. Clin. Pract.* **43**(2): 71–73.

Howe, R.S. (1993) Third-trimester uterine rupture following hysteroscopic uterine perforation. *Obstet. Gynecol.* **81**(5, part 2): 827–829.

Kitzinger, S. (1992) Birth and violence against women. In Roberts, H. (ed.) *Women's Health Matters.* London: Routledge.

Kwast, B.E. (1992) Obstructed labour: its contribution to maternal mortality. *Midwifery* **8**: 3–7.

Lavin, J.P., Stephens, R.J., Miodovnik, M. & Barden, T.P. (1982) Vaginal deliveries in patients with a prior cesarean section. *Obstet. Gynecol.* **59**(2): 135–148.

Leung, A.S., Farmer, R.M., Leung, E.K., Medearis, A.L. & Paul, R.H. (1993) Risk factors associated with uterine rup-

ture during trial of labour after cesarean delivery: A case-study control. *Am. J. Obstet. Gynecol.* **168**(5): 1358–1363.

Mahmood, T.A., Campbell, D.M. & Wilson, A.W. (1988) Maternal height, shoe size, and outcome of labour in white primigravidae: a prospective anthropometric study. *Br. Med. J.* **297**(6647): 515–516.

Mahomed, K. (1987) A five year review of rupture of the pregnant uterus in Harare, Zimbabwe. *J. Obstet. Gynecol.* **7**: 192–196.

Menage, J. (1993) Post traumatic stress disorder in women who have undergone obstetric and/or gynaecological procedures. *J. Reprod. Infant Psychol.* **11**(4): 221–228.

Menticoglou, S.M. (1990) Symphysiotomy for the trapped aftercoming parts of the breech: A review of the literature and a plea for its use. *Aust. New Zealand J. Obstet. Gynaecol.* **30**(1): 1–9.

Moore, N.R., Dickenson, D.R.M. & Gillmer, M.D. (1992) Royal College of Radiologists Annual Meeting – Abstract. *Clin. Radiol.* **46**: 414.

O'Connor, R.A. & Gaughan, B. (1993) Rupture of the gravid uterus and its management. *J. Obstet. Gynecol.* **13**: 29–33.

O'Driscoll, K. & Meagher, D. (1986) *Active Management of Labour.* 2nd edn. Eastbourne: Saunders.

Ollendorff, D.A., Goldberg, J.M., Minogue, J.P. & Socol, M.L. (1988) Vaginal birth after cesarean section for arrest of labour: Is success determined by maximum dilatation during the prior labour? *Am. J. Obstet. Gynecol.* **159**(3): 636–639.

Ozumba, B.C. & Uchegbu, H. (1991) Incidence and management of obstructed labour in Eastern Nigeria. *Aust. New Zealand J. Obstet. Gynaecol.* **31**(3): 213–216.

Palmer, A., Burns, S. & Bulman, C. (1994) *Reflective Practice in Nursing: The Growth of the Professional Practitioner.* Oxford: Blackwell Scientific.

Rachagan, S.P., Raman, S., Balasundram, G. & Balakrishnan, S. (1991) Rupture of the uterus – a 21 year review. *Aust. New Zealand J. Obstet. Gynaecol.* **31**(1): 37–40.

Raphael-Leff, J. (1991) *Psychological Processes of Childbearing.* London: Chapman & Hall.

Rosen, M.G. & Dickinson, J.C. (1990) Vaginal birth after caesarean. *Obstet. Gynecol.* **76**(5, Part 1): 865–868.

Thubisi, M., Ebrahim, A., Moodley, J. & Shwini, P.M. (1993) Vaginal delivery after previous caesarean section: Is x-ray pelvimetry necessary? *Br. J. Obstet. Gynaecol.* **100**: 421–424.

Weekes, A.R.L. & Flynn, M.J. (1975) Engagement of the fetal head and its relationship to the duration of gestation and time of onset of labour. *Br. J. Obstet. Gynaecol.* **82**: 7–11.

WHO (World Health Organization) (1994) *Partograph Reduces Complications of Labour and Childbirth*, 7 June. Geneva: WHO.

55

Anaesthesia and Operative Procedures in Obstetrics

General Anaesthesia

Pharmacological preparations are used to bring about induced reversible analgesia, a state of unconsciousness and muscle relaxation to enable surgical procedures to be performed. In obstetric anaesthesia the safety of both the mother and the fetus have to be considered. It is usually managed by the use of induction agents which may be barbiturates (e.g. thiopentone) or benzodiazepines (e.g. diazepam or midazolam) to induce maternal unconsciousness rapidly with the minimum of side-effects, whilst avoiding at the same time, direct or indirect fetal depression (Capogna and Celleno, 1993).

Anaesthesia is maintained by low concentrations of inhalational anaesthetic agents such as nitrous oxide (mixed with a high percentage of oxygen) combined with volatile agents such as halothane (Fluothane) or enflurane (Ethrane) which enhances anaesthetic depth, improves uterine blood flow by reducing circulating

catecholamines in response to noxious stimuli and improves fetal acid–base status (Capogna and Celleno, 1993). This method is considered to provide adequate depth of anaesthesia during the interval between induction of the anaesthetic and delivery, at the same time reducing maternal awareness (Capogna and Celleno, 1993). Muscle relaxation is brought about by depolarizing relaxants, e.g. suxamethonium (Scoline), or non-depolarizing agents, e.g. pancuronium (Pavulon).

Obstetric anaesthesia is fraught with difficulties and a recent report by the Department of Health indicates a need for vigilance in the care of the woman in pregnancy and childbirth undergoing general anaesthesia, especially when this is carried out in an emergency (DOH, 1996). The problems of obstetric anaesthesia may include raised maternal intragastric pressure, acidity of gastric contents, aortocaval occlusion if the supine position is employed, the adverse effect on the fetus of the drugs used, or of maternal hypoxia or

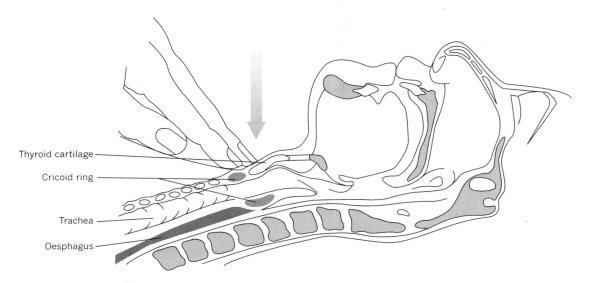

Thyroid cartilage

Cricoid ring

Trachea

Oesophagus

Figure 1   The technique of cricoid pressure (Sellick's manoeuvre). The oesophagus is compressed and occluded between the cricoid ring of the trachea and the bodies of the cervical vertebrae. Pressure is applied as soon as the patient loses consciousness and is maintained until the trachea is intubated with a cuffed endotracheal tube. (Reproduced with permission from Reeder, S.J. *et al.* (1983) *Maternity Nursing*, 15th edn, p. 515. Philadelphia: Lippincott.)

hypotension, placental insufficiency or intrapartum fetal hypoxia. These problems are exacerbated in the case of preterm infants.

Obstetric anaesthesia requires prevention of acid aspiration syndrome and neonatal respiratory depression, avoidance of hypoxia, hypotension, uterine atony and maternal hyperventilation, maintenance of utero-placental blood flow, adequate relaxation, and avoidance of intraoperative awareness throughout the procedure by avoiding a light plane of anaesthesia (Moir and Thorburn, 1986).

ACID ASPIRATION SYNDROME (MENDELSON'S SYNDROME)

Acid aspiration syndrome is a serious and potentially life-threatening syndrome which arises from the inhalation of acid gastric contents when laryngeal reflexes are absent, as in general anaesthesia. It was first described by Mendelson in 1946. It gives rise to *adult respiratory distress syndrome* (ARDS) due to aspiration pneumonitis and presents as acute bronchospasm, dyspnoea, cyanosis, tachycardia and wheezing. The pregnant woman is at risk due to delayed gastric emptying arising from gastric hypotonia, altered position of the stomach and pressure of the enlarged

uterus, gastric hypersecretion in labour and decreased lower oesophageal tone due to progesterone secretion (Moir and Thorburn, 1986).

Prevention is the significant feature and a number of measures are employed to prevent the occurrence of acid aspiration syndrome. These include the administration of antacid preparations such as sodium citrate 30 ml given orally 30 minutes prior to the induction of the anaesthetic, and rotating the woman to and fro to allow adequate mixing in the stomach (Ostheimer, 1992). Histamine-2 (H_2)-receptor antagonists, such as ranitidine 150 mg may be given, usually prior to surgery. It is recommended that it is administered to all women suffering from pre-eclampsia due to the high incidence of mortalities from acid aspiration syndrome in this group of women (DOH, 1994). Metoclopramide may be given by intramuscular injection as it increases lower oesophageal sphincter pressure, shortens gastric emptying and is an anti-emetic.

The question of nutrition or fasting in labour is controversial (Johnson *et al.*, 1989). Swift (1991) and Ludka (1993) recommend policies allowing ingestion of food and fluids in labour to avoid the detrimental effects of fasting on both the mother and the fetus. Ludka (1993) reports no increase in maternal mortality or detrimental outcomes for mother or infant in normal labour. A policy of 'nil by mouth' still prevails in many units for all women, due to the perceived risk of acid aspiration syndrome in the event of general anaesthesia (Johnson *et al.*, 1989). However, a more liberal approach allowing low-fat, low pH drinks and foods, e.g. yoghurt drinks etc., appears to be under consideration. After administration of analgesia, such as pethidine, water only or ice is recommended (Newton, personal communication, 1993).

The increased use of epidural and spinal blocks for operative delivery has reduced the need for general anaesthesia and hence the risk of acid aspiration syndrome. The use of large-bore stomach tubes to empty the stomach, and/or an emetic such as apomorphine are not usually recommended, as emptying of the stomach is not guaranteed (Moir and Thorburn, 1986). 'Crash induction' to reduce the risk of inhalation of gastric contents in an emergency situation is effective.

Sellick's manoeuvre (cricoid pressure) during the passage of an endotracheal tube is essential in all cases to protect the airway from regurgitated stomach contents (Figure 1). The cricoid cartilage is compressed between the finger and thumb towards the cervical spine to occlude the oesophagus (Bevis, 1985). The assistant, who may be the midwife, maintains the pressure until the endotracheal tube is in place. Intubation in the pregnant woman may be difficult due to the posture of the neck in pregnancy or laryngeal oedema in cases of pregnancy-induced hypertension. A strict protocol to follow in the case of 'failed or difficult induction' is mandatory to prevent fatalities and it is recommended that administration of obstetric anaesthesia should only be performed by an experienced anaesthetist (Moir and Thorburn, 1986; DOH, 1994, 1996).

When surgery is completed oxygen is given, inhalational agents are discontinued, muscle relaxation by non-depolarizing agents is reversed using prostigmine and atropine. Extubation involves removal of the endotracheal tube when reflexes have returned, suction is carried out and the operating table is tilted head down. Vigilance at this stage is important as the woman may not be fully conscious and inhalation of gastric contents may still occur. The woman is placed on her side to maintain an airway, assist drainage of secretions and prevent airway obstruction by the tongue.

In the immediate post-operative recovery period temperature, pulse, blood pressure, respirations, colour, state of consciousness, vaginal loss, wound dressing, catheter and wound drainage are observed, as appropriate. Infusion of intravenous fluids is monitored and recorded on the anaesthetic sheet. An analgesic may be administered for pain relief. The anaesthetist will give permission for the woman to be discharged to the care of the ward staff once he or she is satisfied about her post-operative condition. Instructions and details of the surgery and anaesthetic are recorded in the notes and given to the receiving midwife.

Spinal (Subarachnoid) Analgesia

Spinal analgesia involves introduction of a local anaesthetic into the subarachnoid space through an interspace between L2 and L5 to avoid the spinal cord which usually extends to L1, by piercing the dura and adherent arachnoid mater using a small-gauge spinal needle. This reduces the risk of postural headache which occurs more frequently in pregnant women (incidence 6%) and is thought to be multifactorial. Factors include decreased intravascular fluid volume due to blood loss, vomiting in labour and changes in pressure in the epidural space due to resolution of epidural venous engorgement after delivery which affect the regeneration and pressure of cerebrospinal fluid. The position adopted is the left or right lateral, similar to a lumbar puncture position. For Caesarean section it is recommended that the right lateral position be used to avoid pooling of the anaesthetic on the left side of the dural sac which may result in inadequate block on the woman's right side (Ostheimer, 1992).

The blood pressure is taken and recorded in the supine and lateral position before the block is initiated and is monitored frequently. The fetal heart rate is electronically monitored. Spinal analgesia has a rapid onset, is effective and quicker to perform than epidural, uses a small dosage of hyperbaric spinal anaesthetic (heavy bupivacaine 0.5% in glucose solution) so the risk of toxicity is reduced and, as it is a single-shot procedure, there is no risk of catheter breakage. It is not without disadvantages:

▶ it is not continuous;
▶ it commonly gives rise to hypotension;
▶ control of spread of the local anaesthetic is not possible; and
▶ it may give rise to headaches (Moir and Thorburn, 1986).

Preparation, care and contraindications are similar to those for epidural analgesia. It is being used increasingly in conjunction with spinal opiates for operative delivery, and manual removal of the placenta and membranes.

Operative Procedures in Obstetrics

FORCEPS DELIVERY

Forceps delivery involves the use of a specially designed instrument, an obstetric forcep, which is used to expedite delivery of the infant. The use of forceps as an aid to vaginal delivery has been known since their invention by the Chamberlen family in the 1600s (Pearson, 1981).

Since the introduction of forceps many attempts have been made to improve the efficacy and safety of the instrument for specific obstetrical situations, and the shortcomings of current forceps design is acknowledged (Hibbard and McKenna, 1990). The basic instrument consists of a blade, shank, handle and pelvic and cephalic curves. In addition there may be a locking or traction device. Particular variants of the instrument are usually named after the person who was responsible for the design (Figure 2).

Forceps may be used in two ways:

1. to exert traction without rotation (non-rotational), e.g. Simpson, Neville Barnes or Haig Ferguson; or
2. to correct malposition, e.g. occipitoposterior, by rotation prior to traction (rotational), e.g. Kielland's.

The function dictates the shape and size of the instrument. The operation may be performed at the pelvic outlet or mid-pelvic level. Forceps are correctly applied to the sides of the fetal head when the blades are located symmetrically between the orbits and the ears, reaching from the parietal eminences to the malar area and cheeks (Vacca and Kierse, 1989). Forceps delivery occurs in 5–15% of cases and is more common in primigravidae (83%) (Johanson *et al.*, 1993a).

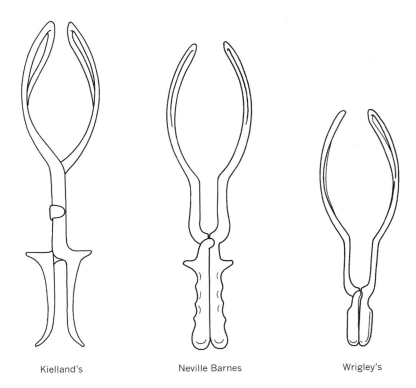

Kielland's   Neville Barnes   Wrigley's

Figure 2   Obstetric forceps.

Indications

The main indications for forceps delivery are:

1 Delay in the second stage of labour, the most frequent causes are:

   ▶ poor uterine contractions;
   ▶ deep transverse arrest of the head;
   ▶ persistent occipitoposterior position.

2 Fetal or maternal distress.
3 To spare the mother muscular effort as is necessary in severe pre-eclampsia, hypertension, heart disease and tuberculosis.
4 To protect the infant, as in the birth of a preterm baby, or in breech delivery with forceps applied to the after-coming head.

Contraindications   (Dennen, 1994)

▶ Unengaged head.
▶ Malpresentation (face/brow).
▶ Inability to define position.
▶ Head above level of ischial spines.
▶ Fetal macrosomia (>4–4.5 kg estimated weight, especially in maternal diabetes).
▶ Inexperience/lack of training.
▶ Fetal death with postmortem changes.

Prerequisites for forceps delivery

The following conditions must be present for forceps delivery to proceed:

1 The os uteri must be fully dilated.
2 The bladder must be empty.
3 The membranes ruptured.
4 No cephalopelvic disproportion.
5 Uterine contractions satisfactory.
6 The head engaged and no obstruction below the head.
7 The position, station and moulding of the fetal head known.
8 Adequate analgesia/anaesthesia available.
9 An episiotomy performed (usually).
10 Attention given to the comfort, dignity, morale and co-operation of the mother.
11 The operator familiar with and experienced in the use of the chosen instrument.
12 Full explanation of the procedure and rationale given to the woman and her partner.
13 A paediatrician should be in attendance for the delivery (where possible).
14 Neonatal resuscitation equipment available and checked.

Analgesia

Pudendal nerve block and perineal infiltration may be used, either alone or in combination. Epidural or spinal analgesia may be used for rotational forceps delivery (see Chapter 32). Very occasionally a general anaesthetic is required (Johanson *et al.*, 1993b).

Preparation of the mother

Every effort should be made to facilitate understanding by the mother and her partner of the indications for the intervention and they should be given all the information they require. The mother is placed in the lithotomy position. It is the midwife's responsibility to position the mother correctly. Both legs must be flexed simultaneously on to the abdomen and the feet moved to the outer sides of the supports and placed in the leg rests or stirrups to avoid sacroiliac strain. To prevent obstruction of venous return and possible thrombosis by pressure, care is taken to ensure the legs are fully abducted. Once the mother is correctly positioned, the foot part of the bed is lowered and the mother's buttocks lifted to the edge of the bed. The operator can now proceed.

Following delivery the baby should be observed for forceps marks, abrasions or signs of cerebral irritation.

Trial forceps delivery

In situations where there is doubt as to whether the instrumental delivery will be successful, the procedure is performed in an operating theatre so that Caesarean section may be undertaken without delay. Failed forceps delivery, followed by Caesarean section, is most common with Kielland's delivery (Johanson *et al.*, 1993b).

Complications

Maternal morbidity This may be *physical* and *psychological*, *short* or *long term*. Significant *perineal* and *vaginal trauma* may be caused, including *third-degree tears*. Occasionally the *cervix* and *lower segment of the uterus* may be damaged if the forceps delivery is attempted before full dilatation of the os uteri is achieved and such lacerations may cause *serious postpartum haemorrhage* and *shock*. There may be *bladder problems* including retention of urine, possibly due to bruising and oedema of the urethra and bladder neck,

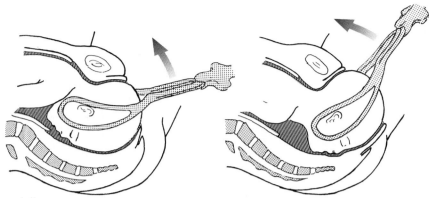

Figure 3   Forceps delivery.

which may require urinary catheterization with continuous bladder drainage during the early days of the puerperium. *Perineal pain* due to bruising, oedema and episiotomy may be present and *dyspareunia* may occur later. The *psychological effects* of forceps delivery may include fear and anxiety in relation to subsequent pregnancy, and feelings of inadequacy and disappointment (Johanson *et al.*, 1993a).

Fetal morbidity   This is reported to be more severe with rotational forceps deliveries (Johanson *et al.*, 1993b). A *cephalhaematoma* may develop due to friction between the fetal head and pelvis or forceps blade. *Facial palsy*, which is usually temporary, may occur due to the forceps blade compressing the facial nerve which runs anteriorly to the ear. Rarely, *intracranial haemorrhage* may occur if the forceps blades are incorrectly applied, or excessive traction is used. *Facial or scalp abrasions* or *marks* are common. *Bruising* of the scalp may cause *neonatal jaundice*. The mother should be reassured, and be given an explanation in the event of any of these problems occurring. The occurrence of unexplained *convulsions* appears to be restricted to the use of Kielland's forceps, and Johanson *et al.* (1993b) suggest more research is needed to provide more evidence on the long- and short-term consequences. However, forceps delivery is the commonest method of operative delivery in the UK and, in expert hands, serious complications are rare (Figure 3).

VACUUM EXTRACTION

Vacuum extraction is a method of instrumental delivery which involves the use of a vacuum device as a traction instrument to assist delivery. The technique was developed from early work by Young in 1705, Simpson in 1905 and others (Carter, 1990). The modern version was developed by Malmström in the 1950s and has since been modified by others (Vacca, 1992) (Figure 4).

The vacuum extractor or ventouse consists of a cup made of metal or soft material such as silicone rubber, a traction device and a vacuum system which provides negative pressure by which the cup is attached to the fetal scalp. The apparatus may be used to expedite delivery in cases of prolonged labour, usually in the second stage. It may be used in the first stage, but there are conflicting opinions about the merits of this (Carter, 1990; Vacca, 1992). Local or regional anaesthesia is employed.

Factors affecting vacuum extraction

The success of vacuum extraction may be affected by various factors (Vacca, 1992):

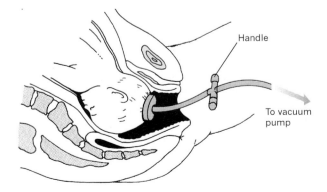

Handle

To vacuum pump

Figure 4   Vacuum extraction.

▶ Expertise of the operator.
▶ Accurate diagnosis of fetal position and station.
▶ Well-being of the fetus.
▶ Recognition of cephalopelvic disproportion.
▶ Uterine action.
▶ Cervical dilatation.
▶ Progress in the first stage of labour.
▶ Duration of the second stage.
▶ Degree of moulding of the fetal head.
▶ Good working order of the equipment.
▶ Correct application of the cups selected.

Indications

Indications for vacuum extraction are similar to those for forceps delivery in the second stage of labour, as already described, with the following additions (Carter, 1990):

▶ Prolapse of the umbilical cord when the os uteri is more than 7 cm dilated.
▶ Delivery of the second twin.
▶ Borderline cephalopelvic disproportion.
▶ Following symphysiotomy (van Roosmalen, 1991).

Contraindications

Contraindications in addition to those for forceps are (Vacca, 1992):

▶ Malpresentations, e.g. face, brow, breech.
▶ Abnormal lie, e.g. transverse, oblique.
▶ Unco-operative woman.
▶ Suspected fetal coagulopathy.
▶ Preterm labour at less than 36 weeks' gestation.
▶ Any significant reduction in maternal expulsive effort, e.g. general anaesthetic.
▶ Poor uterine action.
▶ Cervix not fully dilated (controversial subject, conflicting opinions).

If used to accelerate dilatation of the os uteri late in the first stage, Vacca and Kierse (1989) highlight the need for caution, applying this technique only when prompt delivery is mandatory and when it is likely that the cervix will recede.

Equipment and procedure

The original instrument consisted of a rounded metal cup of various sizes with a chain and traction handle attached and a suction pump. The cups are made in three sizes, 40, 50 and 60 mm in diameter, and the largest size which can be slipped through the cervix is used. A number of modifications to the apparatus have been made, including soft cups made of silastic (Silastic), silicone rubber (Silc), plastic (Mityvac) and malleable polyethelyne plastic (CMI) and anterior and posterior cups designed by Bird and O'Neil (Vacca, 1992) (Figure 5).

Preparation of the mother is as for forceps delivery. The cup is applied to the fetal head and, using suction, a vacuum is created applying a negative pressure of 0.2 kg/cm. The cup is checked for position and to exclude any entrapment of maternal tissue, and the vacuum is increased either in stages or rapidly to a maximum of 0.8 kg/cm. The artificial 'caput', is drawn into the cup, which is thus firmly fixed (Figure 4). Traction is then applied to coincide with the uterine contractions and maternal expulsive effort. Once the delivery is completed the vacuum is released and the cup is detached. If used in the first stage of labour, the head is pulled down on to the slowly dilating cervix, in an effort to stimulate stronger contractions. Although the vacuum extractor was perceived to be slower than forceps delivery, evidence suggests the time is similar for both instruments (Vacca, 1992).

Neonatal morbidity

This is reported to be reduced with the use of soft cups and there is little evidence of any long-term ill-effects, but further research is needed to establish the long-term outcomes (Johanson *et al.*, 1993b).

Asphyxia   After any instrumental vaginal delivery the baby may suffer hypoxia, have lower Apgar scores and need appropriate resuscitation.

Chignon, scalp marking and abrasion   The large caput succedaneum, described from its shape as a 'chignon', gives the baby a bizarre appearance. It subsides quickly, becoming a circular bruised area which clears more slowly. Abrasions of the scalp may occur in a minority of cases; these are more common in difficult procedures due to inadvertent detachment of the cup and prolonged traction. Parental reassurance and daily inspection of the lesion is important (Figure 5).

Neonatal jaundice   Mild neonatal jaundice has been reported for which no specific cause is given and which does not usually require phototherapy treatment. It may be due to reabsorption of haemoglobin associated with bruising (O'Grady, 1988).

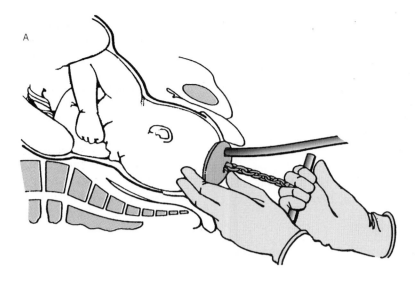

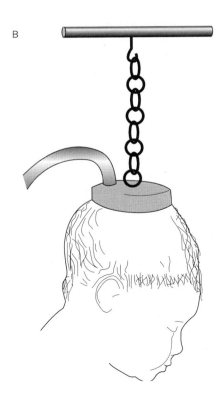

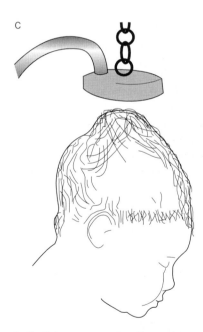

Figure 5   **A**: Outlet vacuum extraction using *Dreifingergriff* (three-finger grip) traction with a metal cup vacuum extractor (Bird's modification). **B**: Correct mid-occipital application of a rigid cup vacuum extractor. **C**: Chignon produced by a rigid cup vacuum extractor. (Reproduced with permission from O'Grady, J.P. (1988) *Modern Instrumental Delivery*, p. 178. Baltimore: Williams and Wilkins.)

Cephalhaematoma, subgaleal haemorrhage Cephalhaematoma is more likely after vacuum extraction than after forceps delivery. The most serious complication to occur is that of subgaleal haemorrhage (subaponeurotic). This potentially life-threatening condition is reported to have increased since the introduction of the vacuum extractor. The incidence varies but is reported to be in the region of 1–3.8%.

Retinal haemorrhage This is more common in vacuum than forceps deliveries but it has no residual effect and is transitory (Vacca, 1992).

Perinatal mortality

Use of the vacuum extractor has been responsible for some mortalities in the past, but in current practice this is rare and not attributed specifically to the vacuum extractor (Vacca, 1992).

Maternal morbidity

Maternal trauma, both physical and psychological, is less severe after vacuum extraction than after forceps delivery (Johanson et al., 1993b). The mother can take an active part by bearing down and this may contribute to her emotional fulfilment. However, women are likely to be concerned about the appearance of the infant due to the presence of the 'chignon'. A positive attitude towards the infant by the midwife and other health care professionals is an important factor in helping parents to accept the appearance of the infant.

The vacuum extractor is a useful instrument in the selection available for operative delivery, reducing maternal injury, requiring less analgesia and hence diminished anaesthetic risk, and with a higher vaginal delivery rate than for forceps delivery. It is recommended that the vacuum extractor is the first choice as the method for instrumental delivery (RCOG, 1993). Use appears to be based on tradition and varies between countries and obstetricians (Vacca, 1992).

CAESAREAN SECTION

Caesarean section is a surgical procedure which may be performed under general, epidural or spinal anaesthesia or, rarely, local infiltration, in which the fetus, placenta and membranes are delivered through an incision in the abdominal wall and in the uterus, usually after the 28th week of pregnancy. If performed to terminate the pregnancy before the 24th week it is referred to as a hysterotomy, but this procedure is rarely performed now (Plauche et al., 1992).

Incidence

The incidence of Caesarean section births in Britain increased in 1993 to 14.6%, a rise from 13% in 1992 (Francome et al., 1993). There is considerable variation in the Caesarean section rate between maternity units in the UK. A survey based on a sample of 90 000 births in Britain in 1993 revealed that, of the 85 hospitals in the sample, only one had a Caesarean rate below 10%, whereas in some others the rate was approaching 20%. In Holland in 1993 the Caesarean rate was 8%. The increasing Caesarean section rate in the UK is attributed by doctors to a variety of reasons, including delivery of preterm infants now likely to survive with good neonatal care, and improved safety due to better anaesthesia. Avoidance of litigation and individual obstetrician's preferences in their practice are also major factors (Savage and Francome, 1993).

Caesarean sections are increasingly being performed under epidural rather than general anaesthetic. This removes the risk associated with general anaesthetic and enables the mother to see and hold her baby at birth. In some cases the partner is invited to be present too so that he can support the mother and share in the experience of his baby's birth (DHSS, 1986).

Indications

Indications for Caesarean section include the following:

► Hypertensive disorders, e.g. pre-eclampsia and eclampsia.
► Fetal distress.
► Failure or delay to progress in labour.
► Malpresentations such as breech, brow or shoulder presentations, but a breech presentation may be delivered vaginally if there is no suspected cephalo-pelvic disproportion or other complications.
► Prolapse of the umbilical cord in the first stage of labour.
► Antepartum haemorrhage, due to abruption or placenta praevia.
► Cephalopelvic disproportion.
► Severe intrauterine growth retardation.
► Severe rhesus iso-immunization.
► Multiple pregnancy, usually only if there are additional complications which substantially increase the risks to mother or babies.
► Peri- and post-mortem delivery, where appropriate.

▶ Active herpes genitalis.
▶ Previous vaginal reconstruction surgery.
▶ Pelvic tumours, e.g. cervical myomas (fibroids).
▶ Fetal macrosomia (high birthweight).
▶ Fetal abnormality, e.g. hydrocephalus, gastroschisis.
▶ High risk factors which may include:
  – Bad obstetric history – this may include previous Caesarean section, but this is not necessarily an indication for a repeat section.
  – Previous neonatal death.
  – Maternal age, e.g. elderly primigravida.
  – History of infertility.

The *Reports on Confidential Enquiries into Maternal Deaths in the United Kingdom 1988–1990* and *1991–1993* indicate that the majority of Caesarean sections are performed for *hypertensive disorders of pregnancy*, *antepartum haemorrhage* or *fetal distress* (DOH, 1994, 1996). The overall mortality rate for this procedure in the UK is reported to be 0.33 per 1000 Caesarean sections, the main immediate causes being pulmonary embolism, hypertensive disease and haemorrhage. Maternal deaths following Caesarean section account for 48.8% of all direct deaths reported in the recent *Confidential Enquiry* (DOH, 1996). It is important to note that when a Caesarean section is performed in the interest of the fetus, it may increase the risk to the mother (Hillan, 1991a).

Types of Caesarean section

Elective   The election to deliver by Caesarean section is usually made in the antenatal period when it becomes apparent that vaginal delivery is inadvisable.

Emergency (planned and unplanned)   Emergency Caesarean section is performed when the fetus or mother are in a life-threatening situation, either in the antenatal or intranatal period. A planned emergency Caesarean section is one in which appropriate preparatory procedures have been followed. An unplanned emergency Caesarean section is defined as one where the need for the operation overrides strict adherence to normal preparatory measures (DOH, 1991).

Pre-surgical preparation

The woman is seen by an anaesthetist who explains the anaesthetic procedure and establishes fitness for anaesthesia. Following explanation of the surgical procedure, written consent is obtained using the appropriate form (NHSME/DOH, 1990). A sample of venous blood is collected for full blood count, haemoglobin level and cross-matching; two units of blood are usually ordered. The abdominal and pubic areas are shaved, the bowel may be emptied by the use of an enema or suppositories, and the woman has a shower or bath to ensure skin cleanliness. Prophylactic measures are taken against Mendelson's syndrome (acid pneumonitis) (see earlier in this chapter). The urinary bladder is emptied and kept empty during the procedure by catheter, inserted just prior to the operation. The fetal heart is checked immediately prior to the commencement of the operation.

If the procedure is to be performed under epidural or spinal anaesthesia, the cannula or needle is inserted, appropriate analgesia is obtained, the anaesthetist ensuring that the blockade is effective before allowing the operation to proceed. All necessary precautions and monitoring of the fetal and maternal condition apply. To minimize the risk of supine hypotensive syndrome, the operating table is tilted laterally, or the woman is wedged at a lateral tilt until the infant is delivered. A foot cushion is usually employed to elevate the legs from the table to avoid venous stasis in the calf muscles; other means, e.g. anti-embolic stockings, may be used to avoid the risk of venous thrombosis.

Pre-surgery checklist   Compliance with a checklist, setting out all the elements of care which are the responsibility of the midwife in preparing the mother for surgery, ensuring that necessary equipment is available, and that final checks on mother and fetus are carried out, facilitates high standards of care.

Requirements   The operating theatre is checked for completeness and working order of equipment prior to commencement of the operation. Attention is given to the environment regarding health and safety regulations. Staff should be conversant with theatre technique and the management of peri- and post-operative care and have an annual update in cardiopulmonary resuscitation technique. All staff should be familiar with and able to perform Sellick's manoeuvre (cricoid pressure) for the prevention of acid aspiration during the induction of the anaesthetic (see Figure 1) (Power, 1987). A paediatrician should be present for the delivery.

The following equipment should be available:

► Resuscitation equipment and an incubator for the baby.

► Anaesthetic trolley and/or equipment for epidural or spinal anaesthesia.

► Cardiac monitors and blood pressure equipment for monitoring maternal condition.

► Intravenous fluids for infusion and anaesthetic drugs.

► General laparotomy or LSCS instrument pack.

► Obstetric forceps (usually Wrigley's).

► Oxytocic drugs, e.g. Syntometrine, for injection into the uterine muscle or intravenously, and broad-spectrum antibiotics, e.g. penicillin, for prevention of post-operative morbidity (Enkin *et al.*, 1989).

Anaesthesia

Many Caesarean sections are performed under *epidural* or *spinal*, rather than *general anaesthesia*. This removes the risks associated with general anaesthesia (DOH, 1991) and enables the mother to see and hold her baby at birth. It is reported that this method is superior in facilitating the mother/baby relationship. The partner may be present, so that he can be supportive to the mother and share in the experience of the birth (Hillan, 1991b). Recent evidence suggests this makes for a more satisfying experience for both the woman and her partner, and for the health care professionals involved. After considerations of safety, the preference of the mother regarding the type of anaesthesia should be paramount (Pearson and Rees, 1989).

Operative procedure

The incision in the abdominal wall may be *vertical, paramedian* or *midline suprapubic*, or the *transverse* (Pfannensteil or Cohen) incision (Pearson and Rees, 1989). The popular *Pfannensteil incision* is more acceptable because of the cosmetic appearance of the scar (Pearson and Rees, 1989). The *Cohen incision* does not separate the fascia from the muscle and the peritoneum is incised transversely as opposed to vertically as in the Pfannensteil.

The incision in the uterus, as distinct from that in the abdominal wall described above, may be performed in two ways as follows:

Lower segment Caesarean section (LSCS)   This involves a transverse incision in the lower uterine segment. This is the method of choice and is used widely because it is regarded as a safe procedure since the uterus is less likely to rupture in subsequent pregnancies (incidence 0.5%) (Creighton *et al.*, 1991).

Classical upper segment Caesarean section   This involves a longitudinal incision in the upper uterine segment and is rarely performed due to the higher risk of scar rupture in a subsequent pregnancy (incidence 2.2%). It may be used in the case of a major degree of placenta praevia, cervical carcinoma, lower segment uterine myomas, or for the delivery of preterm infants prior to the 28th week when the lower uterine segment has not fully formed. A modified classical incision (*De Lee*), in which the vertical incision is not carried up on to the fundus, is reported to decrease the risk of subsequent rupture (Creighton *et al.*, 1991).

Post-operative care

Post-operative care starts as soon as the operation is completed and, after an assessment of the care required, a plan is made to meet the needs of the individual woman and her baby.

Immediate post-operative care   The mother is transferred to the post-operative recovery room where her condition is closely observed and monitored. Observations include the following:

► Pulse rate.

► Blood pressure.

► Respiratory rate.

► Colour.

► State of consciousness, following a general anaesthetic.

► Airway.

► Oxygen administration, as per instructions.

► Vaginal blood loss.

► Wound for bleeding and, if inserted, drainage from wound drains.

► Intravenous therapy.

► Degree of sensation, following epidural or spinal analgesia.

► Pain relief.

► Urinary output.

Baby   If the mother is conscious and the baby appears well at birth he or she may be given to the mother immediately. Otherwise the baby is received by a midwife and any necessary resuscitative measures are carried out by a paediatrician or anaesthetist in the theatre. Once the baby's condition is satisfactory he or she is transferred to a warm nursery. A preterm or ill baby will be admitted to the neonatal unit for special or intensive care. The parents will naturally be very anxious if their baby requires such care and should be encouraged to visit as often as possible.

Accurate and contemporaneous records are made of all observations and treatments. When the mother is conscious and the anaesthetist is satisfied with her post-operative condition, she is transferred to the postnatal ward. The midwife responsible for the care of mother and baby will give a detailed handover report to the ward midwife. This report will include the condition of the mother and the baby at birth, and the care and any treatment given before transfer to the ward or, in the case of a sick or preterm baby, to the neonatal ward. This information is important to enable all staff involved with the mother and baby in the early postnatal period to give appropriate care and support.

Subsequent postnatal care   The physical and psychological condition of the mother is monitored frequently for the first 24–48 hours, then according to individual needs. Pain relief will be required, unless the mother has an epidural or spinal anaesthesia in progress. Initially pain relief is usually administered in the form of intramuscular opiates, e.g. morphia or diclofenac 100 mg (Voltarol), but later suppositories or oral analgesics will be given, as required, within prescribed limits.

Oral fluids are offered soon after the operation and a light diet started when the woman feels ready to eat, unless the surgeon requests that food is withheld until bowel sounds are heard, usually about the third post-operative day. Intravenous fluids are then maintained until bowel sounds are heard and the woman has started to eat. The urinary catheter is removed once the maternal condition is satisfactory, but the urinary output is monitored until the woman is passing adequate amounts of urine spontaneously.

Early ambulation and active and passive leg exercises are taught to prevent deep vein thrombosis. Deep breathing and coughing are also encouraged, especially after a general anaesthetic.

Personal hygiene is an important part of postnatal care and the woman will be shown how to use the bidet and will require assistance with showers until she can manage safely alone.

Many women require a mild aperient such as magnesium hydroxide, usually on the second post-operative day and, if flatulence and constipation persist, may need suppositories such as bisacodyl the following day.

Wound care includes inspection and, if a drain is present, it is shortened and removed according to the doctor's instructions. If clips or non-absorbable skin sutures have been used, they too will be removed at a time directed by the surgeon, usually about the fifth post-operative day. Strict attention must be paid to the prevention of infection by appropriate infection-control procedures, according to local policy.

The haemoglobin is estimated, usually on the third postnatal day, and anaemia treated if diagnosed. In severe cases a blood transfusion may be necessary.

Breast care is as for any woman during the postnatal period, although lactation may take a little longer to become established.

The mother with a painful abdominal wound may require help in finding a comfortable position in which to breastfeed her baby. The midwife can suggest that she tries lying on her side in bed with her baby alongside her, or sitting in a chair with her baby supported on a pillow, perhaps with his trunk and feet under her arm when feeding, rather than lying across her abdomen. Although early contact and involvement in the care of her baby is encouraged, a Caesarean section is a major abdominal operation and the mother will require more help and support during the first few post-operative days, and again when she is transferred home.

Most women following Caesarean section are transferred home on the fifth or sixth post-operative day to the care of their midwife in the community and their general practitioner. Contraception will be discussed before discharge and advice given, if required, about the provision of services and appropriate methods.

Following Caesarean section, the six-week postnatal examination is usually conducted by the obstetrician at the hospital.

Psychological effects of Caesarean section

The psychological effects of Caesarean section have been the subject of recent research (Hillan, 1991b). Some mothers experience a sense of loss or failure because they have been unable to deliver their baby vaginally. The mother also has to recover from the effects of major surgery and, at the same time, learn to care for her new baby. It therefore takes more time to recover physically and emotionally from a Caesarean section and extra support is needed.

Trowell (1986) found that women who had been delivered by Caesarean section remembered the birth as a bad experience, expressed doubts about their ability to care for their baby and were depressed and overanxious. One year later these feelings were still present. Similar findings were found in an earlier American study (Murat and Mercer, 1981). Women with supportive families and friends usually cope, but those with social problems who lack a close, supportive relationship appear to be in particular need of more help and support. In some parts of the UK self-help groups have developed to provide the extra help and support which many of these women need.

Complications

A number of complications may occur during or following Caesarean section. They include physical and psychological problems and may be immediate or of a long-term nature.

Haemorrhage The amount of blood lost during the operation varies. It may be excessive and the mother will then require a blood transfusion. A very serious complication is the unsuspected continuation of intra-peritoneal bleeding after the operation. The midwife must record the pulse and blood pressure regularly after the operation. If the pulse rises or the blood pressure begins to fall, if there is excessive vaginal bleeding, or if recovery of consciousness is delayed, a doctor should be notified immediately.

Anaesthetic complications General anaesthetics in obstetric patients are a hazardous procedure and must be carried out by senior anaesthetists. One of the complications which may occur is acid aspiration syndrome, a life-threatening condition which should not occur if adequate precautions are taken (see earlier in this chapter). Other problems which may occur include drug sensitivity, hypoxia and hypotension.

Complications associated with epidural and spinal anaesthesia include hypotension, dural tap causing severe spinal headache, toxic reaction to drugs, total spinal anaesthesia and infection.

Infection Symptoms vary according to the virulence of the infection. A mild uterine infection presents on about the third postnatal day with a raised temperature and pulse rate, subinvolution of the uterus and profuse red, offensive lochia. If untreated it may cause perito-

nitis and the danger signs, for which the midwife should be constantly on the alert, include a rising pulse rate, pyrexia, vomiting, abdominal pain and distension. *Paralytic ileus* frequently accompanies peritonitis and is recognized by an inability to pass flatus or have the bowels open because the bowel has become paralysed. This is a very serious complication. Antibiotic drugs are given to overcome the infection. Because the absorption of fluids and nutrients from the paralysed intestinal tract is disrupted, fluids, electrolytes and glucose are given intravenously until the condition is resolved. Aspiration of the stomach with a Ryle's tube is necessary until the paralytic ileus recovers and the mother is able to take fluids by mouth without vomiting.

Pulmonary embolism There is always a possibility of pulmonary embolism whenever a laparotomy has been performed. Collapse and even sudden death may occur from this serious complication, often between the 10th and 14th post-operative day. Exercises, leg movements and early ambulation have helped to reduce the incidence of this complication.

Urinary tract problems Retention of urine may be a transient postnatal problem, but more serious problems which are rare now in the Western world include damage to the bladder or ureters which can result in incontinence.

Long-term problems These include *abdominal adhesions* which may lead to intestinal obstruction, and *defective uterine scar* which may cause concern in a subsequent pregnancy because of the risk of rupture (Hillan, 1991a). *Psychological problems* may also be a long-term problem.

Risks of Caesarean section to the fetus

Low Apgar scores and relative fetal acidosis may occur, due to maternal cardiovascular changes, especially with spinal anaesthesia. Later respiratory distress syndrome may develop, the incidence being four times greater in babies delivered by elective Caesarean section than in those who are delivered vaginally (see Chapter 69).

Very occasionally the baby may have scalpel lacerations or, even more rarely, sustain fractures if the delivery is difficult.

Trial of scar – vaginal birth after Caesarean section

Vaginal birth after Caesarean section (VBAC) is successful in about 50% of cases, and depends largely upon whether the indication for the previous Caesarean section is likely to recur (Francome *et al.*, 1993). Consumer awareness has been raised in the media and by a support group which publishes and disseminates information about the number of women who successfully deliver vaginally following a previous Caesarean section (Francome *et al.*, 1993).

It is recommended that women who have had a Caesarean section should have the next labour conducted by an obstetrician in hospital. From 34 weeks onwards there is always a slight risk that the uterine scar will rupture, therefore the woman must be asked to report any tenderness over the scar and contact the hospital at the first sign of the onset of labour. In labour, termed a trial of scar, meticulous observations of maternal and fetal condition are made, including noting any tenderness or pain over the Caesarean scar. Epidural anaesthesia is not now contraindicated for trial of scar but, if used, the woman would be unaware of any uterine tenderness and therefore the midwife must be extremely vigilant in observing signs of impending uterine rupture. The use of oxytocic drugs to induce or augment labour may be contraindicated because of the risk of uterine rupture. If used, great caution must be exercised by restricting the dose of the oxytocic drug to the absolute minimum and by close observation of uterine action and maternal and fetal condition. The oxytocic drug should be stopped immediately if uterine action becomes hypertonic and the midwife should inform the obstetrician. Following delivery the doctor makes an examination per vaginam to explore the lower uterine segment to determine the integrity of the scar.

Legal and ethical issues

A competent woman can refuse medical treatment, including consent to Caesarean section. In a recent case, however, the woman's decision not to have a Caesarean section was overruled by a court. This case, and indeed others, raises many legal and ethical issues relating to human rights which affect the practice of midwives (Hewson, 1992).

There is concern about the high increase in the rate of Caesarean section births, many being performed for fear of litigation (Francome *et al.*, 1993). Recent evidence suggests that personal support in labour by a midwife reduces the need for Caesarean section (Butler *et al.*, 1993). More midwifery-led care in the future therefore may reduce the number of Caesarean births.

Sterilization may be recommended following the third LSCS, as the risks associated with this operative delivery increase.

SYMPHYSIOTOMY

Symphysiotomy is the incision of the fibrocartilage of the symphysis pubis through part, but not all, of its thickness (Figure 6). The procedure follows that described by Crichton and Seedat (1963) and Gebbie (1982). It is performed in labour and enlarges the transverse measurements of the pelvis. This facilitates the process of birth in cases of cephalopelvic disproportion with a live fetus (van Roosmalen, 1991). Symphysiotomy is not performed when fetal death has occurred. Occasionally it may be carried out following a failed vacuum extraction in the second stage of labour, or for the after-coming head in a breech delivery (Yasmin and O'Sullivan, 1992).

According to Gebbie (1982), three criteria should be satisfied before carrying out this procedure:

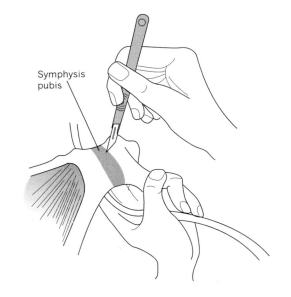

Symphysis pubis

Figure 6   Protection of the urethra by the left hand during the procedure of symphysiotomy. (Reproduced with permission from van Roosmalen, J. (1991) In Studd, J. (ed) *Progress in Obstetrics and Gynaecology*, vol. 9, p. 158. Edinburgh: Churchill Livingstone.)

1 one third or more of the fetal head should have entered the pelvic brim;
2 the fetal head should not be felt prominent in front of the symphysis pubis; and
3 cervical dilatation should be more than 7 cm in a primigravida.

Before carrying out this procedure it is essential that a self-retaining catheter is passed to empty the bladder. Following symphysiotomy the vacuum extractor may be used to hasten delivery. The use of obstetric forceps is contraindicated because of the risk of vesico–vaginal fistula (van Roosmalen, 1991).

Symphysiotomy is rarely carried out in the UK but is more commonly employed in the management of disproportion in countries where the risks of Caesarean section are particularly high and, in some places, culturally unacceptable (van Roosmalen, 1991). A great advantage of symphysiotomy is that the pelvis remains permanently enlarged, so that subsequent deliveries should be easier. Repeat symphysiotomy is not undertaken in subsequent births which need operative intervention, however, because of fibrotic scarring of the symphysis pubis.

After delivery, broad strapping is applied around the pelvis and the legs may be bound together. The mother is nursed on her side. Occasionally the bladder or urethra is injured during symphysiotomy, so after delivery the self-retaining catheter remains *in situ* for 3 or 4 days and the urinary output is carefully observed. The more serious complication of vesico–vaginal fistula is more likely to result from obstructed labour than symphysiotomy (van Roosmalen, 1991).

VERSION

Version is the practice of turning the fetus *in utero* to obtain a more favourable lie or presentation. Three kinds of version are described: *external version*, usually during the antenatal period but sometimes in labour before the rupture of the membranes; *internal version*; and, rarely, *bipolar version* when the woman is in labour. External cephalic version (Figure 7) is undertaken by many obstetricians in the UK, but it is considered safer to deliver the mother by Caesarean section rather than to attempt internal and bipolar versions.

External cephalic version

External cephalic version is manipulation of the fetus through the abdominal wall to turn it to a cephalic

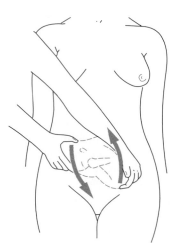

Figure 7 External cephalic version.

presentation. Gentle pressure is exerted by the obstetrician on each pole of the fetus simultaneously to turn it by a traditional forwards, or newer backflip, method to a cephalic presentation (Clay *et al.*, 1993) (Figure 8).

Indications External cephalic version is indicated:

1 To convert a breech to a cephalic presentation when there are no other complications, thereby reducing the incidence of breech presentation in labour with its associated risks. If successful, it also reduces the Caesarean section rate and perinatal mortality and morbidity associated with vaginal breech delivery (Yasmin and O'Sullivan, 1992) (see Chapter 51).
2 To correct a transverse lie, usually in a multigravida. The fetus is usually easily turned, but often reverts to a transverse lie. If the lie continues to be unstable the mother is admitted to hospital so that the lie can be corrected at the onset of labour.
3 To correct a transverse lie in a second twin. If the midwife is responsible for the mother, she should correct the lie and then rupture the membranes (see Chapter 45).

External cephalic version has been known since the time of Hippocrates. It was widely performed prior to the 1970s, usually between 30 and 40 weeks' gestation, but then declined in popularity (Hofmeyr, 1991). Now it is being performed more frequently again and increasingly at term (Hofmeyr, 1989). This is because the safety of the procedure has been improved with the use of ultrasound scanning, fetal heart monitoring and

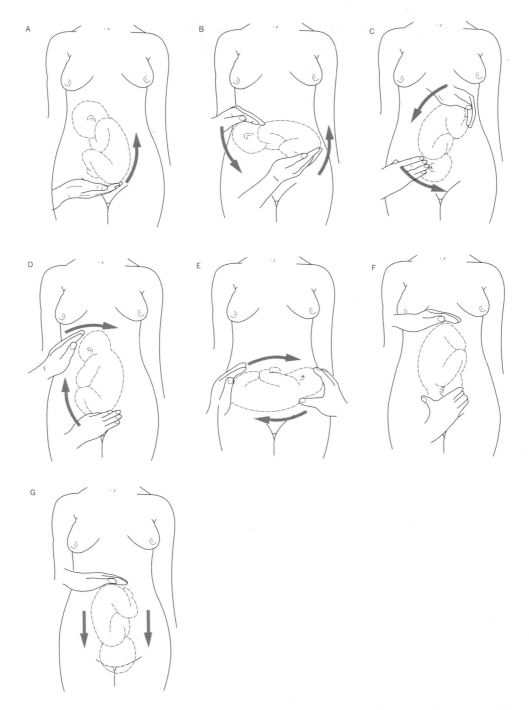

Figure 8   External cephalic version. **A**: Palpation and mobilization of the breech. **B**: Manual forward rotation using both hands, one to push the breech and the other to guide the vertex. **C**: Completion of forward roll. **D**: Backward flip using both hands. **E**: Quarter turn accomplished. Continue to push breech upwards and vertex downward. **F**: Completion of external version. **G**: Gently push the breech downwards to direct vertex into pelvis. (Reproduced with permission from Clay *et al.*, 1993, p. 77S.)

tocolytic drugs. These drugs are myometrial muscle relaxants and reduce the risk of feto-maternal haemorrhage (Clay *et al.*, 1993). General anaesthesia is rarely used nowadays because it is thought to increase the risks of the procedure, probably because there is a tendency to use more force when there is no maternal resistance.

Preparation Before performing the version, informed consent is obtained from the woman, after discussing with her the advantages and potential risks of the procedure. Immediately before the procedure the woman is asked to empty her bladder and she then lies in a supine or dorsal position and is encouraged to relax (Clay *et al.*, 1993).

For success it is recommended that the following criteria are met:

- singleton fetus in the third trimester;
- a reactive fetal monitoring trace performed immediately prior to the external cephalic version;
- an adequate amount of liquor amnii.

Engagement of the presenting part, estimated fetal weight of greater than 4000 g, and occipitoposterior positions are thought to militate against the success of external cephalic version.

Following the procedure the fetal heart is monitored and the woman is encouraged to rest. She is advised to report any vaginal bleeding, loss of amniotic fluid or uterine contractions. Rhesus-negative women have a Kleihauer test carried out and are given anti-D immunoglobulin because of the risk of feto-maternal haemorrhage and subsequent iso-immunization.

Contraindications *Absolute contraindications* (Clay *et al.*, 1993) include the following:

- Multiple pregnancy, due to risk of cord accident, e.g. entanglement.
- Severe intrauterine growth retardation, due to compromised fetus.
- Severe oligohydramnios, also associated with a compromised fetus and rarely successful.
- Fetal abnormality, also often associated with a compromised fetus.
- Any contraindications to a vaginal delivery.
- Significant third trimester bleeding, because there is a risk of causing further placental separation and haemorrhage, and a compromised fetus.

- Rhesus iso-immunization, due to the risk of feto-maternal haemorrhage.
- Nuchal cord, because of the risk of fetal distress.

Relative contraindications (Clay *et al.*, 1993) include the following:

- Uterine abnormality, e.g. bicornuate uterus, because a successful outome is more difficult to achieve.
- Maternal illness (e.g. cardiac disease, hypertension, diabetes mellitus, thyroid disease), because tocolytic drugs may be contraindicated.

Complications These are reported to be rare and include:

- Transient bradycardia or abnormal fetal heart rate, which recovers spontaneously on cessation of the procedure and repositioning of the woman.
- Placental abruption.
- Premature rupture of the membranes.
- Cord complications, e.g. entanglement or knot.
- Onset of labour.
- Feto-maternal haemorrhage.
- Negative psychological effects on the mother if the version fails.

It is recommended that external cephalic version is carried out in maternity units with all the facilities necessary to deal with any complications which may arise.

Internal podalic version

This manoeuvre is performed when the woman is in labour and the os is fully dilated (podalic is from the Greek *podos* = foot) provided there is no cephalopelvic disproportion.

Indications Internal podalic version is indicated:

1 To convert a malpresentation which it is not possible to deliver as such to a presentation which is more easily delivered, for example a shoulder to a breech in circumstances when Caesarean section cannot be performed.
2 To deliver the second of twins when the shoulder presents. Nowadays this is the only indication for this procedure (Beischer and Mackay, 1986).

Procedure With the mother under a general or spinal anaesthetic, a hand is inserted into the vagina and uterus and, by manipulation on the abdomen with one hand and by internal manipulation with the other, a foot is grasped and drawn down, so that the presentation is converted to a breech. Unless great care is taken during this procedure, the uterus may rupture, especially when labour has been prolonged and the lower segment is overstretched. There is also a risk of injury to the fetus.

Bipolar podalic version

This is a somewhat similar procedure, performed early in labour, with only two fingers in the uterus and the other hand on the abdomen. The presentation is converted to a breech and then the membranes are ruptured and a foot is brought down through the cervix to ensure that the lie remains longitudinal. Since this manoeuvre is carried out in early labour before the cervix is sufficiently dilated to admit the hand, there is usually opportunity to transfer the woman to hospital for Caesarean section, so this difficult manoeuvre is no longer attempted.

CERVICAL CERCLAGE

Cervical cerclage is a surgical intervention performed usually under general anaesthetic in the second trimester of pregnancy, whereby a suture is placed around the cervix to prevent it from dilating where there is cervical incompetence (Figure 9). The aim of the procedure is to prolong pregnancy and thus improve the fetal and neonatal outcome (Grant, 1989). 'Cervical incompetence', a term first used by Gream in 1865, is a condition where there is laxity of the cervix which causes the cervical os to dilate very easily (Jackson

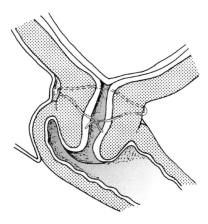

Figure 9   Cervical cerclage.

and Garite, 1992). It may be the cause of mid-trimester miscarriage, or preterm labour and delivery.

Causes

Cervical incompetence may be congenital, for example uterine abnormality, or it may be caused by intrauterine exposure to diethylstilboestrol, or it may be the result of previous cervical surgery, for example, excessive dilatation for curettage, cone biopsy, Manchester repair or cervical amputation. Other causes include hormonal and biochemical influences (Jackson and Garite, 1992).

Diagnosis

The diagnosis is usually made on *previous obstetric history* (Grant, 1989). Typically the history is one of successive mid-trimester abortions, characterized by rupture of the membranes in the absence of painful uterine contractions and a short, relatively painless labour with a live fetus (Ware Branch, 1986).

It may also be diagnosed by *serial vaginal examinations* to assess the dilatation of the cervix.

Ultrasound scans show changes in the length of the cervix, with the internal os more than 3 cm dilated and funnelling of the membranes.

Recent evidence indicates that cervical cerclage should be offered to women who have had two previous mid-trimester abortions or preterm labours, and that it is beneficial in these cases despite the risks associated with increased medical intervention and infection.

Techniques

Cervical cerclage may be performed by the technique described by Shirodkar (1960), or McDonald (1957), the latter being simpler and more commonly used now because the bladder is not dissected from the uterus, and the knot of the purse-string suture is more easily accessible for removal (MRC/RCOG, 1993). A recent study indicates that the McDonald procedure may be safely performed under pudendal nerve block, but research work continues (McCulloch *et al.*, 1993). Very occasionally a transabdominal technique is used for women with a cervical defect (Jackson and Garite, 1992).

Procedure

A non-absorbable suture of either mersilene tape, nylon or heavy silk is inserted into the cervix, rather like the purse-string suture in an appendicectomy. This holds the cervix closed and therefore prevents spontaneous abortion. The suture is removed just before term, or earlier if labour commences.

The treatment is successful in many cases, but is not without risk and involves at least two hospital admissions and a general anaesthetic for insertion of the suture. Obstetric interventions such as induction of labour, use of oral betamimetics and Caesarean section may be necessary and there is a higher risk of puerperal sepsis (MRC/RCOG, 1993).

Contraindications

Contraindications to cervical cerclage include:

▶ Significant uterine contractions.
▶ Ruptured membranes.
▶ Proven or suspected intrauterine infection.
▶ Uterine bleeding.
▶ Fetal abnormality (Ware Branch, 1986).

Complications

Complications that may occur following cervical cerclage include:

▶ Cervical laceration.
▶ Premature rupture of the membranes.
▶ Stimulation of myometrial activity.
▶ Sepsis.
▶ Endotoxic shock.
▶ Cervical dystocia or cervical stenosis.
▶ Vesico-vaginal fistula.
▶ Uterine rupture.
▶ Anaesthetic complications.
▶ Maternal death (Grant, 1989).

EMBRYOTOMY

Embryotomy is a destructive procedure whereby the fetus is destroyed to facilitate vaginal delivery. It may take the form of craniotomy, when the head is perforated to facilitate delivery, e.g. in cases of hydrocephalus, cleidotomy when the clavicles are severed to allow delivery of impacted shoulders, and decapitation as in the case of locked twins. It may be necessary when Caesarean section cannot be safely performed, usually in cases of cephalopelvic disproportion or major fetal malformations (Myerscough, 1982).

References

Beischer, N.A. & Mackay, E.V. (1986) *Obstetrics and the Newborn*. London: Baillière Tindall.

Bevis, R. (1985) *Anaesthesia in Midwifery*. London: Ballière Tindall.

Butler, J., Abrahams, B., Parker, J., Roberts, J.M. & Laros, R.K. (1993) Supportive nurse-midwife care is associated with a reduced incidence of caesarean section. *Am. J. Obstet. Gynecol.* **168**(3): 1403–1407.

Capogna, G. & Celleno, D. (1993) The effects of anaesthetic agents on the newborn. In Reynolds, F. (ed.) *Effects on the Baby of Maternal Analgesia and Anaesthesia*. London: W.B. Saunders.

Carter, J. (1990) The vacuum extractor. In Studd, J.W.W. (ed.) *Progress in Obstetrics and Gynaecology*. Vol. 8, pp. 107–126. Edinburgh: Churchill Livingstone.

Clay, L.S., Criss, K. & Jackson, U.C. (1993) External cephalic version. *J. Nurse Midwifery* **38**(2) (Suppl.): 72S–79S.

Clayburn, P.A. & Rosen, M. (1993) The effects of opioid and inhalation analgesia on the newborn. In Reynolds, F. (ed.) *Effects on the Baby of Maternal Analgesia and Anaesthesia*. London: W.B. Saunders.

Crichton, D. & Seedat, E.K. (1963) The technique of symphysiotomy. *South Afr. Med. J.* **37**: 227–231.

Crichton, S.M., Pierce, J.M. & Stanton, S.L. (1991) Complications of Caesarean section. In Studd, J.W.W. (ed.) *Progress in Obstetrics and Gynaecology*, Vol. 9. Edinburgh: Churchill Livingstone.

Dennen, P.C. (1994) Forceps delivery. In James, D.K., Steer, P.J., Weiner, C.P. *et al.* (eds) *High Risk Pregnancy*. London: WB Saunders.

DHSS (1986) *Report on Confidential Enquiries into Maternal Deaths in England and Wales, 1979–1981*. London: HMSO.

DOH (Department of Health) (1991) *Report on Confidential Enquiries into Maternal Deaths in the UK, 1985–1987*. London: HMSO.

DOH (1994) *Report on Confidential Enquiries into Maternal Deaths in the UK, 1988–1990*. London: HMSO.

DOH (1996) *Report on Confidential Enquiries into Maternal Deaths in the UK, 1991–93*. London: HMSO.

Enkin, M., Enkin, E., Chalmers, I. & Hemminki, E. (1989) Prophylactic antibiotics in association with caesarean section. In Chalmers, I., Enkin, M. & Keirse, M.J.N.C. (eds) *Effective Care in Pregnancy and Childbirth*. Oxford: Oxford University Press.

Francome, C., Savage, W., Churchill, H. & Lewison, H. (1993) *Caesarean Birth in Britain*. London: Middlesex University Press, NCT.

Gebbie, D.A.M. (1982) Symphysiotomy. *Clin. Obstet. Gynaecol.* **9**: 663–683.

Grant, A. (1989) Cervical cerclage. In Chalmers I., Enkin, M. & Keirsen, M.J.N.C. (eds) *Effective Care in Pregnancy and Childbirth*. Oxford: Oxford University Press.

Hewson, B. (1992) When 'no' means 'yes'. *The Law Societies Gazette* **45**(9): 2.

Hibbard, B.M. & McKenna, D.M. (1990) The obstetric forceps – are we using the appropriate tools? *Br. J. Obstet. Gynaecol.* 97: 374–380.

Hillan, E. (1991a) Caesarean section: maternal risks. *Nursing Standard* 5(48): 26–29.

Hillan, E. (1991b) Caesarean section: Psychosocial effects. *Nursing Standard* 5(50): 30–33.

Hillan, E. (1991c) Caesarean section: Perinatal risks. *Nursing Standard* 5(49:) 37–39.

Hofmeyr, G.J. (1989) Breech presentation and abnormal lie in pregnancy. In Chalmers, I., Enkin, M. & Keirse, M.J.N.C. (eds) *Effective Care in Pregnancy and Childbirth*. Oxford: Oxford University Press.

Hofmeyr, G.J. (1991) External cephalic version at term: how high are the stakes? (Commentaries) *Br. J. Obstet. Gynaecol.* 98: 1–3.

Jackson, D.J. & Garite, T.J. (1992) Surgical correction of uterine abnormalities. In Plauche, W.C., Morrison, J.C. & O'Sullivan, M.J. (eds) *Surgical Obstetrics*. Philadelphia: W.B. Saunders.

Johanson, R.B., Wilkinson, P., Bastible, A., Ryan, S., Murphy, H. & O'Brien, S. (1993a) Health after childbirth: a comparison of normal and assisted vaginal delivery. *Midwifery* 9: 161–168.

Johanson, R.B., Rice, C., Doyle, M. *et al.* (1993b) A randomised prospective study comparing the new vacuum extractor policy with forceps delivery. *Br. J. Obstet. Gynaecol.* 100: 530–534.

Johnson, C., Kierse, M.J.N.C., Enkin, M. & Chalmers, I. (1989) Nutrition and hydration in labour. In Chalmers, I., Enkin, M. & Keirse, M.J.N.C. (eds) *Effective Care in Pregnancy and Childbirth*. Oxford: Oxford University Press.

Ludka, L.M. (1993) Eating and drinking in labour: a literature review. *J. Nurse-Midwifery* 38(4): 199–207.

McCulloch, B., Bergen, S., Pielet, B., Kellet, J. & Elrad, H. (1993) McDonald suture under pudendal nerve block. *Am. J. Obstet. Gynaecol.* 168(2): 499–502.

McDonald, I.A. (1957) Suture of the cervix for inevitable miscarriage. *J. Obstet. Gynaecol. of Br. Empire* 64: 346–350.

McDonald, I.A. (1980) Cervical cerclage. *Clin. Obstet. Gynaecol.* 7: 461–479.

Mendelson, C.L. (1946) The aspiration of stomach contents into the lungs during obstetric anaesthesia. *Am. J. Obstet. Gynecol.* 52: 191–205.

Moir, D. & Thorburn, J. (1986) *Obstetric Anaesthesia and Analgesia*, 3rd edn. London: Baillière Tindall.

Myerscough, P.R. (1982) Reductive embryotomy. In Myerscough, P.R. (ed.) *Munro Kerr's Operative Obstetrics*, 10th edn. London: Baillière Tindall.

MRC/RCOG (1993) Final report of the Medical Research Council, Royal College of Obstetricians and Gynaecologists Multiple Randomised Trial of Cervical Cerclage. *Br. J. Obstet. Gynaecol.* 100: 516–523.

Murat, J.S. & Mercer, R.T. (1981) The caesarean experience: implications for nursing. *Birth Defects Original Article Series* 17: 129–152.

NHSME/DOH (1990) *A Guide to Informed Consent for Examination or Treatment*. London: NHSME/DOH.

O'Grady, J.P. (1988) *Modern Instrumental Delivery*. Baltimore: Williams & Wilkins.

Ostheimer, G.W. (1992) *Manual of Obstetric Anaesthesia*. New York: Churchill Livingstone.

Pearson, J.F. (1981) A short history of the obstetric forceps. *Maternal Child Health* May: 198–204.

Pearson, J. & Rees, G. (1989) Technique of caesarean section. In Chalmers, I., Enkin, M. & Keirse, M.J.N.C. (eds) *Effective Care in Pregnancy and Childbirth*, Vol. 2. Oxford: Oxford University Press.

Plauche, W.C. (1992) Vacuum extraction. In Plauche, W.C., Morrison, J.C. & O'Sullivan, M.J. (eds) *Surgical Obstetrics*. Philadelphia: W.B. Saunders.

Plauche, W.C., Morrison, J.C. & O'Sullivan, M.J. (1992) *Surgical Obstetrics*. Philadelphia: W.B. Saunders.

Power, K.J. (1987) The prevention of acid aspiration (Mendelson's syndrome). A contribution to reduced maternal mortality. *Midwifery* 3: 143–148.

RCOG (Royal College of Obstetricians and Gynaecologists) (1993) *Effective Procedures in Obstetrics*. Manchester: Medical Audit Unit (RCOG).

Savage, W. & Francome, C. (1993) British caesarean section rates: have we reached a plateau? *Br. J. Obstet. Gynaecol.* 100: 493–496.

Shirodkar, V.N. (1960) Habitual abortion in the second trimester. In: Shirodkar, V.N. (ed.) *Contributions to Obstetrics and Gynaecology*. Edinburgh: Livingstone.

Swift, L. (1991) Labour and fasting. *Nursing Times* 87(48): 64–65.

Trowell, J. (1986) Emotional effects of a caesarean. *Nursing Times* 28 May: 64.

Vacca, A. (1992) *Handbook of Vacuum Extraction in Obstetric Practice*. London: Edward Arnold.

Vacca, A. & Keirse, M.J.N.C. (1989) Instrumental vaginal delivery. In Chalmers, I., Enkin, M. & Keirse, M.J.N.C. (eds) *Effective Care in Pregnancy and Childbirth*, Vol. 2, pp. 1217–1233. Oxford: Oxford University Press.

van Roosmalen, J. (1991) Symphysiotomy – a re-appraisal for the developing world. In Studd, J.W.W. (ed.) *Progress in Obstetrics and Gynaecology*, Vol. 9, pp. 149–161. Edinburgh: Churchill Livingstone.

Ware Branch, D. (1986) Operations for cervical incompetence. *Clin. Obstet. Gynaecol.* 29(2): 240–254.

Yasmin, S. & O'Sullivan, M.J. (1992) Assisted breech extraction. In Plauche, W.C., Morrison, J.C. & O'Sullivan, M.J. (eds) *Surgical Obstetrics*. Philadelphia: W.B. Saunders.

Further Reading

AIMS (1991) VBAC: The right to a normal birth. *AIMS J* 4: 3.

Barth, W.H. (1990) Emergent cerclage. *Surg. Gynecol. Obstet.* **170**: 323–326.

Bronham, D.R. (1988) Caesarean section and post operative care. *Update* August: 262–268.

Donald, W.L. & Barton, J.J. (1990) Ultrasonography and external cephalic version at term. *Am. J. Obstet. Gynecol.* **162**: 1542–1547.

Frazer, M. (1987) 'So great a cruelty' – historical aspects of caesarean section. *Midwifery* **3**: 72–74.

Hanns, W. (1990) The efficacy of external version and its impact on the breech experience. *Am. J. Obstet. Gynecol.* **162**(60): 1459–1464.

Lilford, R.J., Van Coeverden de Groot, H.A., Moore, P.J. &

Bingham, P. (1990) The relative risks of caesarean section and vaginal delivery: a detailed analysis to exclude the effects of medical disorders and other acute pre-existing physiological disturbances. *Br. J. Obstet. Gynaecol.* **97**: 883–892.

Macdonald, A.G. (1985) The gastric acid problem. In Atkinson, R.S. & Adams, A.P. (eds) *Recent Advances in Anaesthesia and Analgesia*, Vol. 15, pp. 107–132.

Mahomed, K., Seeras, R. & Coulson, R. (1991) External cephalic version at term. A randomised trial using tocolysis. *Br. J. Obstet. Gynaecol.* **98**: 8–13.

Seidman, D.S., Laor, A. & Gale, R. (1991) Long term effects of vacuum extraction and forceps delivery. *Lancet* **337**: 1583–1585.

56

Complications of the Third Stage of Labour

Postpartum Haemorrhage

Postpartum haemorrhage is, to the midwife, the most serious of all the complications of midwifery. It may happen without warning after any delivery and, as there is a placental circulation of approximately 600 ml/min at term, the mother can lose blood with alarming rapidity (Zahn and Yeomans, 1990). Postpartum haemorrhage is still a significant cause of maternal mortality and morbidity in the United Kingdom (DOH, 1994). Often there is no doctor present and in this situation the prompt and intelligent action of the midwife may spare the mother dangerous blood loss and perhaps even save her life. It is therefore essential that the midwife has a thorough understanding of this subject.

Definition

Postpartum haemorrhage is defined as excessive bleeding from the genital tract occurring any time from the birth of the child to the end of the puerperium. *Primary haemorrhage* refers to the first 24 hours. This condition complicates approximately 6% of all deliveries (including Caesarean sections). Haemorrhage occurring after 24 hours and before the end of the puerperium, that is, the sixth postnatal week, is called *secondary* or *puerperal haemorrhage*. This is much less common, occurring in fewer than 1% of all deliveries (Consumers Association, 1992). Postpartum haemorrhage is further classified according to its source. Most commonly the bleeding is from the placental site and results from poor tone of the uterine muscle; hence it is sometimes called *atonic haemorrhage*. Less frequently, excessive bleeding occurs from a laceration of some part of the genital tract, when it is termed *traumatic haemorrhage*.

The word 'excessive' requires careful interpretation. Traditionally a loss of 500 ml or more at delivery is regarded as a postpartum haemorrhage. Later in the puerperium lesser amounts would be classified as excessive.

But blood lost at the end of labour is extremely difficult to measure. It stains sheets, towels and gowns; it mixes with liquor; it trickles to the floor and is mopped up; it clots and the clot is conscientiously collected and measured in a jug, but it is not always appreciated that the 360 ml clot is only the solid part of more than 600 ml of blood. These estimates are at best approximate and often unreliable. Underestimation of blood loss is the commonest error and the haemorrhage may be underestimated by 30–50% (Levy and Moore, 1985; Levy, 1990; Combs *et al.*, 1991). This is especially likely to occur when a large volume of blood has been lost.

However the exact amount lost is less important than the effect on the mother of the blood loss. In this context 'excessive' means *any amount*, however small, which adversely affects the mother.

Postpartum haemorrhage (PPH) unqualified, means primary haemorrhage from the placental site, this being the commonest and most dangerous type. Traumatic and secondary postpartum haemorrhage are described specifically by these names.

PRIMARY POSTPARTUM HAEMORRHAGE FROM THE PLACENTAL SITE

Causes

The immediate cause is failure of the uterus to contract and retract adequately. If the many uterine blood vessels are not squeezed or ligated by compression from the muscle fibres surrounding them, blood loss can be rapid and dangerous.

It is not possible to predict accurately that any particular woman will have a postpartum haemorrhage, but the risk is increased in certain circumstances. These are as follows:

▶ A *history* of previous postpartum haemorrhage or retained placenta. This may recur.
▶ *High parity*: Women who have had three or more children may be at increased risk because with each pregnancy more fibrous tissue replaces muscle fibres in the uterus and therefore contraction and retraction is less efficient. However not all studies have shown an increased risk for grande multiparae (Combs *et al.*, 1991).
▶ *Multiple pregnancy, polyhydramnios and fetal macrosomia*: In these circumstances the overdistended uterus may not retract well. Also, in multiple preg-

nancy there is a larger placental site from which bleeding may occur.
▶ *Anaemia*: An anaemic woman is less able to withstand haemorrhage and she may collapse after even a small loss.
▶ *Antepartum haemorrhage*: A woman who has suffered either placenta praevia or abruptio placentae may subsequently have a postpartum haemorrhage. In the case of placenta praevia this is because the retractile ability of the lower uterine segment is deficient and therefore control of bleeding from the placental site is poor. A Couvelaire uterus may occur in severe, concealed placental abruption and the damaged muscle fibres fail to contract and retract effectively to control haemorrhage. The midwife should remember that a woman who has had an antepartum haemorrhage may be somewhat anaemic and this further increases the threat from postpartum haemorrhage.
▶ *Prolonged labour*: If contractions have been weak or uncoordinated in the first and second stages of labour this may be expected to continue in the third stage and the uterus will fail to contract and retract effectively. Occasionally prolonged labour due to mechanical difficulty may lead to uterine exhaustion, atony and thus postpartum haemorrhage.
▶ *Pre-eclampsia*: This association may be a reflection of the fact that these women are more likely to have induced labours and an operative delivery. Also, some drugs used to prevent seizures may contribute to uterine atony.
▶ *General anaesthesia*: Uterine atony may occur if anaesthesia is prolonged. It is especially likely if halogenated anaesthetic agents are used.
▶ *Fibroids*: The presence of uterine fibroids may interfere with efficient retraction.
▶ *Mismanagement of the third stage of labour*: Massaging, squeezing or otherwise 'fiddling' with the uterus can disrupt the rhythm of myometrial activity, causing only partial separation of the placenta.
▶ *Retained placenta*: Unless the uterus is empty it cannot retract completely so that a partially separated retained placenta (whether or not the result of mismanagement) or retained blood clot can themselves diminish the contractions and worsen bleeding.
▶ *Tocolytic drugs*: Drugs given to suppress uterine activity in preterm labour may cause atony in the

third stage should labour progress. This will contribute to postpartum haemorrhage.

▶ *Induced or augmented labours*: The uterine inefficiency which necessitates the use of oxytocics may contribute to postpartum haemorrhage.

▶ *Inversion of the uterus*: Any degree of uterine inversion will interfere with efficient contraction and retraction and will precipitate postpartum haemorrhage.

▶ *Infection*: Chorioamnionitis is associated with primary postpartum haemorrhage.

The midwife must remember that postpartum haemorrhage may occur as a complication of otherwise completely normal labours when even the most careful retrospective assessment fails to explain it (Zahn and Yeomans, 1990; Lewis and Chamberlain, 1990; Combs *et al.*, 1991; ACOG Technical Bulletin Number 143, 1990).

The foregoing account deals only with postpartum haemorrhage resulting from inadequate contraction and retraction of the uterus. In some cases a steady oozing of blood persists even though the uterus is well contracted and the blood remains liquid. This condition may be caused by *disseminated intravascular coagulation* (DIC) which uses up the supplies of circulating fibrinogen and other blood clotting factors and leads to a blood coagulation disorder. Disseminated intravascular coagulation may complicate concealed abruptio placentae, amniotic fluid embolus, severe pre-eclampsia and eclampsia and may follow prolonged retention in the uterus of a dead fetus.

As the condition worsens, blood levels of fibrin degradation products (FDPs) rise. These are toxic to the myometrium and will interfere with efficient uterine contraction and retraction, thus exacerbating the haemorrhage.

At *every* delivery the midwife should note whether the blood is clotting and whether the clot is firm or friable. Absent or unstable clot formation is an indication of coagulopathy: this must be treated promptly and the midwife should call a doctor without delay. If DIC is allowed to progress the condition will become uncontrollable and maternal death will ensue.

Medical disorders such as idiopathic thrombocytopenia and inherited coagulopathies such as Von Willebrand's disease also increase the risk of primary postpartum haemorrhage (Sipes and Weiner, 1992).

Prophylaxis

Prevention of postpartum haemorrhage begins at the initial booking interview when the midwife will identify those women at higher risk. Any woman whose history suggests that postpartum haemorrhage may occur should be booked for delivery in hospital where special arrangements are made, first to minimize bleeding and secondly, if it does occur, to institute immediate treatment. Conditions such as anaemia will be detected and anaemic women should be treated with iron and folic acid supplements. In severe cases intramuscular iron or even blood transfusion may be required to raise the haemoglobin level above 11 g/dl before delivery.

During labour careful management will reduce the likelihood of postpartum haemorrhage for those women at risk. When labour starts an intravenous cannula is inserted and a blood sample is taken: the haemoglobin level is estimated and the blood group confirmed. The serum is saved: this speeds up the process of cross-matching donor blood should it become necessary. The midwife will monitor the progress of labour; it is important to avoid dehydration and exhaustion and the doctor should be informed if there are any signs of prolonged labour. A Syntocinon infusion may be required and this should be maintained for at least one hour after the end of the third stage of labour. The bladder should also be kept empty.

Correct management of the third stage of labour is crucial. Syntometrine 1 ml (containing ergometrine maleate 500 µg and Syntocinon 5 units) is given by intramuscular injection with the crowning of the head or with the birth of the anterior shoulder. Ergometrine maleate 500 µg should be available for intravenous injection if required. Umbilical vein oxytocin has been used in an attempt to shorten the third stage of labour and reduce blood loss. The diffusion of oxytocin from the villous vessels of the placenta into the intervillous space triggers local myometrial contractions, resulting in separation of the placenta. Oxytocin 10–20 units in 20 ml of normal saline is injected into the umbilical vein immediately after clamping the cord. However, there is contradictory evidence as to the effectiveness of this technique and it is not normally used (Young *et al.*, 1988; Reddy and Carey, 1989; Porter *et al.*, 1991). The placenta is delivered by controlled cord traction.

The midwife should discuss the management of the third stage of labour with the woman, preferably before the onset of labour. Some women would prefer not to have Syntometrine but physiological management is considered unsafe for the woman at risk of postpartum haemorrhage.

Treatment

Before delivery of the placenta   While, at the first opportunity, the midwife must send an urgent message for medical help, she must stay with the mother and treat her while awaiting the doctor. In the community or in a hospital without immediate medical aid the midwife would herself send a message to call for emergency obstetric help. This may be the emergency obstetric unit from the consultant unit or a paramedic team from the Ambulance Service. The midwife should always be aware of what assistance is available in the area. In the case of postpartum haemorrhage at home a blood transfusion should be started and the placenta removed if possible before transferring the woman to hospital (Lewis and Chamberlain, 1990).

When haemorrhage is first noted the midwife must quickly determine the likely cause by locating the fundus and assessing the degree of uterine contraction. In primary postpartum haemorrhage due to uterine atony the fundus will feel soft and flaccid. The first consideration is to make the uterus contract. The quickest way to do this is by massaging the uterus. The midwife should therefore take the following actions:

1   'Rub up' a contraction by massaging the uterus, when, within a few minutes, it will become hard.
2   Give an oxytocic drug, either an intramuscular injection of Syntrometrine 1 ml which will make the uterus contract within 2.5 minutes or an intravenous injection of either Syntometrine 1 ml or ergometrine maleate 500 μg which will act in 45 seconds. The midwife should not, on her own authority, administer more than two 500 μg doses of ergometrine maleate as this drug may cause severe peripheral vasoconstriction and a sharp rise in blood pressure (Lewis and Chamberlain, 1990).
3   Attempt to deliver the placenta when the uterus contracts.
4   If this fails, pass a catheter to empty the bladder and, having ensured again that the uterus is well-contracted, attempt once again to deliver the placenta by controlled cord traction.
5   If the placenta is still unable to be delivered, prepare for the doctor to perform a manual removal of

the placenta and membranes under general anaesthesia or under epidural anaesthesia if this is in progress. Before this procedure is carried out it is essential to set up an intravenous infusion, if not already in progress, and to take blood for cross-matching.

When dealing with a case of postpartum haemorrhage the midwife should not elevate the foot of the bed as this would encourage blood to pool within the uterine cavity and would hinder uterine contraction and retraction. Instead the mother's legs may be elevated on pillows, taking care to avoid undue pressure on the calves which would predispose to venous thrombosis.

After delivery of the placenta   Massage of the uterus to stimulate a contraction and expel any blood clot and the administration of an intravenous injection of ergometrine maleate 500 μg or an intramuscular injection of Syntometrine 1 ml are usually sufficient to control the bleeding. A catheter is passed to empty the bladder if bleeding persists.

The placenta and membranes are examined to ensure that they are complete. If the placenta is incomplete an exploration and evacuation of the uterus is carried out by the doctor under general or epidural anaesthesia.

If bleeding continues bimanual compression of the uterus may be performed.

External bimanual compression   The left hand dips down as far as possible behind the uterus; the right hand is pressed flat on the abdominal wall; the uterus is compressed and, at the same time, pulled upwards in the abdomen. The bleeding area is thus compressed while the pulling up of the uterus straightens the kinked uterine veins and, by allowing free drainage from them, relieves the congestion and decreases the bleeding.

Internal bimanual compression   (Figure 1) This may be carried out when the mother is anaesthetized if bleeding persists after a manual removal of the placenta and membranes or following evacuation of the uterus. The right hand is introduced into the vagina, closed to form a fist, and pushed up in the direction of the anterior vaginal formix. The left hand, on the abdominal wall, dips down behind the uterus and pulls it forwards and towards the symphysis. The two hands are pressed firmly together, thus

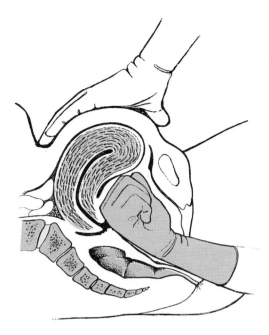

Figure 1   Internal bimanual compression of the uterus.

compressing the uterus and therefore the placental site. The pressure is maintained until the uterus contracts and remains retracted.

Once bleeding is controlled uterine contraction is maintained by an intravenous infusion of Hartmann's solution to which oxytocin is added. The usual dose is 20–40 units of Syntocinon in 500 ml of Hartmann's solution. The concentration of the drug and the rate of infusion are determined by the obstetrician. Blood transfusion may be required. If the bleeding persists or recurs the doctor may decide to carry out an exploration of the genital tract under general anaesthesia.

In cases of massive obstetric haemorrhage a senior obstetrician and the duty anaesthetic registrar must be called. The anaesthetist will be responsible for managing fluid replacement. Two large-bore intravenous cannulae and a central venous pressure line are inserted. Blood samples are taken for clotting studies. At least six units of cross-matched blood are requested; plasma expanders such as Gelofusine, Haemaccel or Hespan may be used. The use of dextran should be avoided as it may interfere with typing and cross-matching of blood and can also prolong bleeding times if the correct dose is exceeded (Royle and Walsh, 1992; DOH, 1994). All maternity units should keep at least two units of emergency group O rhesus negative blood

in the blood fridge and this may be used while awaiting cross-matched supplies. The blood should be passed through a warming coil and infused as rapidly as possible using a compression cuff. Martin's pumps should not be used as they do not provide a sufficiently rapid infusion rate (Seeley, 1989; DOH, 1994).

If the uterus remains flaccid in spite of conventional oxytocics the doctor may order Hemabate (Carboprost) 250 µg. This is given as a deep intramuscular injection and may be repeated at 90-minute intervals. An intravenous infusion of prostaglandin E_2 (PGE_2), 5 mg in 500 ml of normal saline may be used. This is given at an initial rate of 40 drops per minute. Continuous intrauterine irrigation with small doses of PGE_2 has also been successful in controlling severe postpartum haemorrhage (Sarkar and Mamo, 1990; Peyser and Kupferminc, 1990). In very severe cases of haemorrhage a laparotomy will be performed and, if measures such as the injection of oxytocic drugs directly into the uterus and direct compression of the aorta fail to stop the bleeding, internal iliac ligation will be necessary. The obstetrician will make every attempt to conserve the uterus but if the internal iliac ligation fails to control the bleeding hysterectomy is now the only way to save the mother (Ratnam and Rauff, 1989).

Observations

The amount of blood loss is measured and assessed and, once bleeding is controlled, the total loss is estimated. The greater the blood loss the more difficult it is to estimate it accurately. Haswell (1981) found that estimates of blood loss over 500 ml were only about half the true amount. Brant (1967) also found that estimates become more inaccurate the higher the loss.

A fluid balance chart is maintained to record the fluid intake and urinary output. A self-retaining catheter is inserted, attached to a urometer, and urine output is measured and recorded hourly. Central venous pressure should be measured when it is necessary to give large volumes of fluid intravenously in order to avoid overtransfusion. The mother's general condition is assessed and her pulse and blood pressure are recorded every 15 minutes until her condition is satisfactory.

It is important to palpate the fundus repeatedly to ensure that it remains well-contracted and to observe the lochia.

The best treatment for hypovolaemic shock is to replace the circulating blood volume, but other measures such as elevating the woman's legs, sedation and giving oxygen are also employed. All wet bed linen is removed and the mother is kept dry and comfortable.

If it is noted that the blood does not clot or the clotting studies indicate incipient coagulation failure the haematologist should be called. Fresh blood is usually the best treatment as this will contain platelets and coagulation factors V (pro-accelerin) and VIII (anti-haemophilic factor). Fresh frozen plasma also contains factors V and VIII as well as fibrinogen (factor I).

TRAUMATIC POSTPARTUM HAEMORRHAGE

A woman may sustain severe blood loss from a laceration of some part of the genital tract. Occasionally this arises from a perineal tear or episiotomy, while lacerations including the labia or clitoris often bleed freely. Deep lacerations of the vaginal walls, cervix and, exceptionally, lower uterine segment will produce severe haemorrhage. This is much more likely to complicate a difficult, instrumental delivery than a normal one for which the midwife would be taking responsibility, though it sometimes follows a very rapid labour. Uterine rupture may also occur in obstructed labour or if a scar ruptures.

Superficial bleeding points are easily seen and treated by direct pressure. A laceration of the cervix is suspected if the bleeding begins the moment the child is born and continues steadily though the uterus is well-contracted. It may be temporarily controlled by digital pressure or by the application of a sponge or arterial pressure forceps. The doctor is summoned and the laceration is sutured. Tears of the upper part of the vagina, the cervix or the uterus are sutured under general or epidural anaesthesia. In cases of severe haemorrhage from a ruptured uterus, it may be necessary to perform a hysterectomy.

For secondary postpartum haemorrhage, see Chapter 5.

FOLLOWING POSTPARTUM HAEMORRHAGE

Following postpartum haemorrhage the mother is liable to suffer from chronic iron-deficiency anaemia unless adequate treatment is instituted during the puerperium. She is more likely to develop puerperal sepsis and lactation is often poor. In cases of severe and prolonged shock the woman may develop anuria due to tubular necrosis. Another serious complication is anterior pituitary necrosis. If the mother survives she will suffer from Sheehan's syndrome.

The midwife should make the opportunity to discuss the events which have occurred with the parents. They will both wish to know the reason for the haemorrhage and whether it is likely to happen again. The partner, in particular, is very vulnerable in the emergency situation and is likely to have been very frightened. The sudden nature of the emergency often means that explanations given at the time are brief, hurried and poorly assimilated by the couple. The midwife should give them time to ask questions and can advise them about the likely management of future deliveries. The woman should avoid another pregnancy until she has completely recovered.

Postpartum haemorrhage is still a cause of maternal death in the UK, although with improving social conditions, including better nutrition and better obstetric care the number of deaths attributed to this cause is decreasing.

Subsequent pregnancies

All mothers who have had a postpartum haemorrhage should be booked for subsequent deliveries in hospital under the care of an obstetrician. An intravenous cannula is sited when labour begins and Syntometrine 1 ml or ergometrine 500 µg are administered by injection with the crowning of the head or the birth of the anterior shoulder to reduce the risk of a further postpartum haemorrhage.

Prolonged Third Stage

With active management of the third stage of labour, the placenta and membranes are normally expelled within 10 minutes of the birth of the baby (Spencer, 1962; Lewis and Chamberlain, 1990). The third stage is considered prolonged when the time exceeds 30 minutes, though the midwife should summon the doctor after 20 minutes or earlier if there is excessive bleeding or if she is in any way concerned about the mother's condition. With physiological management of the third stage a longer time may be allowed, up to one hour, provided the maternal condition is good, with no signs of undue bleeding.

The retained placenta may be partially or completely separated but trapped in the cervix or lower uterine segment, so bleeding will occur from the placental site. If the retained placenta is completely adherent to the uterine wall there can be no bleeding from the placental site.

Causes

Causes of a prolonged third stage include the following (Beischer and Mackay, 1986; Zahn and Yeomans 1990; Romero *et al.*, 1990; Lewis and Chamberlain, 1990; Combs and Laros, 1991; Legro *et al.*, 1994; Jaffe *et al.*, 1994):

▶ *Uterine inertia*: The atonic uterus fails to contract and retract sufficiently to facilitate placental separation. This may follow prolonged, or (occasionally) very rapid, labour.
▶ *Full bladder*: The bladder occupies space in the pelvis and impedes efficient uterine contraction and retraction.
▶ *Mismanagement of the third stage*: 'Fiddling' with the uterus may induce weak, dysrhythmic uterine contractions which only partially separate the placenta. A similar result will occur if controlled cord traction is attempted before the Syntometrine has taken effect.
▶ *Constriction ring*: This is a localized spasm of uterine muscle just above the lower segment which prevents the descent of the placenta.
▶ *Uterine abnormality*: Retained placenta is more likely if the uterus is bicornuate or subseptate.
▶ *Preterm birth*: This is particularly likely at very early gestations and where preterm labour is induced for medical reasons.
▶ *Morbid adherence of the placenta*: This is more likely to occur in women with a history of uterine curettage, previous Caesarean section and placenta praevia. There may be a relationship between abnormally adherent placenta and fetal sex, the fetus being significantly less likely to be male (Khong *et al.*, 1991). In some cases there is a history of elevated maternal serum alpha-fetoprotein levels in the second trimester (Kupferminic *et al.*, 1993).

There are three types of abnormally *adherent placenta*:

1 *Placenta accreta*: The decidua basalis is deficient and the chorionic villi are attached to the myometrium.

2 *Placenta increta*: The villi deeply invade the myometrium.
3 *Placenta percreta*: The villi have penetrated the myometrium as far as the serous coat of the uterus. This is very rare.

The area of adherence may be focal, partial or total. Cases of focal or partial adhesion may be successfully treated by manual removal of the placenta, possibly followed by blunt curettage. Attempts to remove a placenta percreta are likely to result in uterine perforation and haemorrhage. The obstetrician may carry out a hysterectomy or may leave the placenta *in situ* to be reabsorbed. In the latter situation methotrexate has been used to achieve destruction of the trophoblastic tissue and thus accelerate reabsorption. However, use of this drug is not successful in all cases.

Management

The dangers of haemorrhage and shock are increased when the placenta is retained. An attempt is made to deliver the placenta and membranes following catheterization to empty the bladder, and, if this fails, the woman is prepared for manual removal of the placenta and membranes under a general anaesthetic. First, however, blood is taken for cross-matching and an intravenous infusion is commenced because there is a risk of severe haemorrhage occurring during the procedure.

The woman is anaesthetized and put into the lithotomy position. Strict aseptic precautions are essential; the vulva is cleaned with antiseptic solution and chlorhexidine (Hibitane) obstetric cream 1% is used for lubrication of the tissues. Special sterile elbow length gloves are sometimes worn during this procedure. The obstetrician forms the right hand into a cone shape and inserts it into the vagina. With the left hand on the abdomen (a sterile towel intervening) he or she steadies the uterus from above. It is helpful if an assistant holds the cord taut. The cord is followed up to its placental insertion and the separated area or the edge of the placenta is located. With a gentle sawing motion the remainder of the placenta is stripped off the uterine wall. The obstetrician removes the placenta and then explores the uterine cavity to ensure that no placental fragments have been missed (Figure 2).

Occasionally, the presence of a constriction ring makes removal of the placenta difficult. Relaxation can be achieved by the administration of anaesthetic agents such as fluothane or cyclopropane. Inhalation of

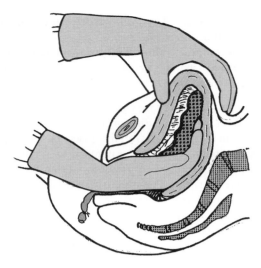

Figure 2   Manual removal of the placenta.

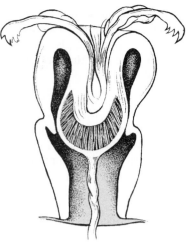

Figure 3   Inversion of the gravid uterus.

amyl nitrite will also achieve relaxation of a constriction ring but this drug is rarely used now.

Following manual removal uterine contraction is achieved by intravenous Syntometrine or ergometrine maleate 500 μg. An intravenous infusion of Hartmann's solution with Syntocinon is commenced. The dose and rate of administration is prescribed by the doctor: 20 units of Syntocinon in 500 ml of infusion solution is the usual amount. This will maintain uterine contraction. If bleeding recurs or continues bimanual compression may be required. Antibiotics are given as manual removal of the placenta is a highly invasive procedure and there is a risk of puerperal sepsis.

If the placenta is retained in community practice the midwife should call for emergency obstetric help without delay. An intravenous infusion is commenced at home and blood is taken for cross-matching. If attempts to deliver the placenta fail, the mother should be transferred to hospital for a manual removal of placenta and membranes under general anaesthesia. Usually it is possible to deliver the placenta and membranes at home before transferring the woman to hospital.

Acute Inversion of the Uterus

This is a rare but most serious complication of the third stage of labour. The uterus is partly or completely turned inside out (Figure 3). In partial inversion the fundus is turned inside out but does not pass through the cervix. In more severe cases the fundus protrudes through the cervix and lies in the vagina. Once inversion has begun, it may continue until the uterus is completely inverted and appears outside the vulva.

Causes

Inversion of the uterus may be due to various causes, including the following:

▶ *Mismanagement of the third stage of labour*: This is the commonest cause of uterine inversion and results either from pressure on the fundus or from traction on the cord when the uterus is relaxed. It is particularly likely to occur when the placenta is situated in the uterine fundus.
▶ *Short cord.*
▶ *Manual removal of placenta*: Inversion of the uterus may occur if the operator's hand is quickly withdrawn from the uterus while the other hand is still applying some degree of fundal pressure.
▶ *Precipitate delivery*: Especially if the woman is in an upright position.
▶ *Spontaneous inversion*: Occasionally spontaneous inversion occurs and the cause is unknown. It may result from uterine atony and a sudden increase in the intra-abdominal pressure such as occurs when coughing, sneezing or a straining effort.

Dangers

The condition is associated with profound shock and possibly haemorrhage, if the placenta has partly or wholly separated from the uterus. If the mother survives she may suffer from anuria and Sheehan's syndrome as a result of shock and the risk of puerperal sepsis is high.

Diagnosis

Minor degrees of uterine inversion may not be recognized if there is only a slight indentation of the fundus. The woman may complain of pain and the lochia is likely to be heavy. This type of inversion usually corrects itself spontaneously (Ratnam and Rauff, 1989).

If the inversion is more serious the woman will complain of pain and on palpation of the abdomen a hollow will be felt in the fundus of the uterus. Haemorrhage will occur if the placenta has separated.

If there is a complete inversion, the uterus will not be palpable in the abdomen and the inverted fundus will be visible at the vulva. If the uterus cannot be palpated in the abdomen or seen at the vulva, a vaginal examination should be made as it is likely to be in the vagina. The woman will complain of severe lower abdominal pain and may report a sensation of prolapse or 'something coming down'. Haemorrhage and neurogenic shock due to traction on the infundibulopelvic and round ligaments will follow (Ratnam and Rauff, 1989; Zahn and Yeomans, 1990).

Management

Where possible the uterus should be replaced immediately as maternal shock will increase and may become irreversible. Replacement is easier if it is carried out at once, before the uterus has had time to become congested. If immediate replacement is not possible and the uterus is outside the vulva, it should be gently replaced inside the vagina, if possible. The foot of the bed should be raised in order to reduce traction on the infundibulopelvic ligaments and to alleviate shock. An intravenous infusion is commenced: plasma expanders such as Gelofusine or Haemaccel may be given. Blood is taken for cross-matching as blood transfusion will be required. The woman is also given an injection of morphine 15 mg intramuscularly. If the placenta is still attached to the inner uterine wall the midwife must make no attempt to detach it as torrential haemorrhage may result.

Once shock is treated the uterus must be replaced without any delay. The mother is anaesthetized and the uterus is replaced either manually or by the hydrostatic method. By manual manipulation the part of the uterus which inverted last, that is the lower segment, is replaced first and the fundus last. The other hand should be placed on the abdomen to give counterpressure, otherwise the uterus may be pushed up too high.

Some obstetricians prefer the hydrostatic method as described by O'Sullivan (1945). Opinion varies as to whether the placenta should be removed just prior to replacement of the uterus: removal of the placenta reduces the mass which must be replaced but may precipitate haemorrhage. The woman is anaesthetized and put in the lithotomy position. The obstetrician replaces the uterus in the vagina. Warm normal saline is then infused into the vagina via a douche nozzle from a container suspended approximately 1 m above the uterus. At least 2–3 litres of fluid will be required. The tube or nozzle is held in the vagina and the introitus sealed around the forearm by the other hand. The pressure exerted by the fluid distends the vagina and effects the replacement of the uterus, often within 5–10 minutes. If these procedures fail, laparotomy may be necessary (Ratnam and Rauff, 1989; Momani and Hassan, 1989).

Following replacement of the uterus an intravenous injection of ergometrine maleate 250–500 µg is given to ensure that the uterus contracts and bleeding is controlled. Further treatment for shock may then be required. The woman should be seen by the obstetrician six weeks after delivery in order to exclude chronic uterine inversion. The midwife should encourage the woman to carry out her postnatal exercises; referral to an obstetric physiotherapist may be helpful if the abdominal and pelvic floor muscle tone is particularly poor. A woman who has suffered an acute inversion of the uterus should be referred to a doctor and booked for delivery in hospital if she becomes pregnant again.

Shock

Shock is a condition in which the circulation cannot meet the metabolic requirements of the cells (Seeley, 1989). The blood pressure falls and tissue perfusion is reduced (Campbell, 1993). Irreversible organ damage may result. Shock is usually classified according to its cause (Dildy and Cotton, 1992; Campbell, 1993):

▶ *Cardiogenic shock*: This is reduced cardiac output due to heart failure. In midwifery it may occur as a result of pulmonary embolism, congenital cardiac defects, acquired valvular disease or severe anaemia.
▶ *Hypovolaemic shock*: This occurs when the circulat-

ing blood volume is too low to meet tissue requirements. It is associated with severe obstetric haemorrhage, such as antepartum or postpartum haemorrhage, ruptured ectopic pregnancy and genital tract trauma. It may follow coagulopathy such as that associated with amniotic fluid embolism.

▶ *Neurogenic shock*: This occurs as a result of an insult to the central nervous system. It is associated with uterine inversion, regional anaesthesia and aspiration of gastric contents.

▶ *Toxic shock* (septic shock, bacterial shock): This occurs as a result of a severe generalized infection. This topic will be considered separately.

▶ *Anaphylactic shock*: This may occur as a result of an adverse drug reaction.

The effects of shock may be exacerbated by pain, dehydration and exhaustion.

The term 'obstetric shock' has been used to describe collapse. This rather catch-all term, which generally signifies hypovolaemic shock, should no longer be used.

Signs of deterioration

The midwife should be alert for changes in the condition of any woman in her care. The following signs indicate deepening shock which will affect all the body organs and systems:

1 *Pulse*: A pulse rate of over 90 is not normal. As it continues to rise the volume grows weaker until the rapid thready pulse of severe haemorrhage is noted.
2 *Blood pressure*: Though the mother is losing blood, for some time the compensatory mechanisms in her body will keep her blood pressure at a normal level. Peripheral, splanchnic and renal vasoconstriction ensure that vital organs such as the heart and brain continue to be perfused. If the systolic pressure falls below 100 mmHg there is cause for anxiety. Readings of 90 and 80 mmHg indicate seriously deepening shock.
3 *Increasing pallor of the skin*: The skin is covered with a cold sweat. The lips are bluish and the mucous membranes blanched.
4 *Temperature*: This falls to a subnormal level.
5 *Respiration*: Breathing becomes deep and sighing. The mother is sometimes restless and may complain of thirst, nausea or faintness. She may lose consciousness.

The midwife should call a doctor at the first sign of a rising pulse rate and if, in addition, the mother's blood pressure begins to fall, she should call for emergency obstetric help at once.

Whether the cause is clearly postpartum haemorrhage or whether some less obvious condition is present is immaterial. In either case the mother is in urgent need of resuscitative treatment.

Treatment

The principles underlying treatment are as follows (Dildy and Cotton, 1992):

1 *Administration of fluid*: Two large-bore intravenous cannulae are sited. Blood is taken and cross-matching requested: at least six units of donor blood will be required. In the meantime, the circulation can be maintained by plasma expanders such as Gelofusine, Haemaccel or Hespan.
2 *Other means of maintaining the circulation*: Inotropic drugs such as dopamine increase myocardial contractility and may be effective. Vasopressor agents such as noradrenaline may also be required; this type of drug is used with caution as pulmonary and renal vasoconstriction may occur. The midwife should be aware that any inotropic or vasopressor substance used in the treatment of a pregnant woman will have an effect on uteroplacental perfusion and may therefore further compromise the fetus.

In an emergency situation raising the woman's legs may assist in maintaining the core circulation.
3 *Monitoring*: A central venous pressure line is inserted to monitor maternal responses to fluid therapy. The heart rate should be monitored continuously by electrocardiograph (ECG) if possible and a pulse oximeter applied. The doctor will take blood for estimation of plasma gases, haemoglobin, clotting studies, urea and electrolytes. The patency of the airway must be monitored and the woman's position should be adjusted so as to allow adequate ventilation and lung expansion. The midwife must watch carefully for any signs of cyanosis. Frequent records of pulse, blood pressure, respiratory rate, blood loss, urine output and level of consciousness are maintained.
4 *Pain relief and rest*: An intramuscular injection of morphine may be given to relieve pain and allay anxiety. The mother should be kept as quiet and undisturbed as possible.
5 *Oxygen*: Especially if air hunger is noticeable the

mother benefits from inhalation of oxygen. It is administered by nasal prongs or facemask at an initial rate of 6 l/min. The rate may be adjusted according to the results of blood gas estimation or pulse oximetry.

6 *Avoiding warmth*: The cold, pale skin is evidence that the body's compensatory mechanism is at work. The superficial capillaries and arterioles are constricted and blood is being diverted to the parts of the body where the need is greatest; that is the heart and brain. To warm the skin until it is flushed may well undo this important compensatory mechanism and even deepen the shock to an irreversible degree.

BACTERIAL SHOCK

This is cardiovascular collapse due to septicaemia. The causative organisms are commonly the Gram-negative anaerobes, particularly the Enterobacteriaceae. *Escherichia coli*, *Klebsiella*, *Serratia* and *Clostridium welchii* may all cause septic shock. Occasionally Gram-positive aerobic organisms such as Staphylococci and Streptococci may be implicated. Endotoxins released by organisms such as *Escherichia coli* or *Clostridium welchii* enter the bloodstream and cause intense vasoconstriction of the post-capillary vessels. Blood therefore collects in the capillary bed rather than returning to the heart, the cardiac output is reduced and peripheral failure ensues. This results in tissue destruction, especially to the kidneys.

Together with vasoconstriction there is disseminated intravascular coagulation. The woman will have a high fever with rigors. Tachycardia, tachypnoea and oliguria are present. The skin is usually hot and dry. Adult respiratory distress syndrome may develop and this, in combination with generalized sepsis, has a mortality of over 80% (Pearlman and Faro, 1990). Bacterial shock may follow puerperal uterine infection, septic abortion, intra-amniotic infection and urinary tract infection.

Management

The woman is isolated. A midstream specimen of urine, high vaginal swab and blood cultures are sent for bacterial investigation. Serum electrolytes and blood urea are measured and screening tests for clotting disorders performed.

Treatment includes blood transfusion if required, measurement of central venous pressure as a guide to

cardiac output, the administration of intravenous antibiotics, correction of acidosis and an accurate assessment of urinary output. Steroids may be given to decrease peripheral resistance and improve pulmonary circulation. Any infected products of conception must be removed from the uterus. The midwife should pay attention to the woman's personal hygiene and general comfort.

Amniotic Fluid Embolism

Amniotic fluid embolism occurs when amniotic fluid is forced into the maternal circulation via the uterine sinuses of the placental bed. It may occur at or close to term, during labour or immediately after delivery. The diagnosis is usually made post-mortem when fetal squames and lanugo are found in the lungs. The mortality rate associated with this condition is very high: approaching 80%. It may occur in older, multiparous women and where labour has been tumultuous or hypertonic. This includes cases where oxytocic drugs have been used to induce or accelerate labour. However, amniotic fluid embolism has occurred during elective Caesarean section (DOH, 1994). It may also complicate multiple pregnancy or follow polyhydramnios.

In all these cases the intra-amniotic pressure is increased and when the membranes rupture, either spontaneously or artificially, amniotic fluid may be forced into the maternal circulation (DOH, 1994). In 40% of cases, fetal death occurs before clinical signs of amniotic fluid embolus occur and placental abruption is found in 50% of cases (Chatelain and Quirk, 1990).

Symptoms may occur gradually or be sudden in onset. They include cyanosis, chest pain, dyspnoea, bloodstained frothy sputum, convulsions and collapse (Lewis and Chamberlain, 1990; Davies and Harrison, 1992). As amniotic fluid is rich in thromboplastins, disseminated intravascular coagulation may be expected to develop and if the woman survives the initial embolus she may subsequently die from coagulation failure. As amniotic fluid depresses myometrial activity, the uterus may become atonic and this will compound the haemorrhage due to coagulopathy (Clark, 1990).

When amniotic fluid embolism occurs the midwife must call for medical assistance at once and should commence cardiopulmonary resuscitation. High concentrations of oxygen should be administered. An intravenous infusion and a central venous pressure line are inserted. The woman may be intubated and mechanically ventilated. Delivery is effected by Caesarean section as quickly as possible: the aim here is not simply to salvage the fetus but also because adequate and effective resuscitation of the mother is better achieved when the uterus is empty.

Although uncommon, amniotic fluid embolus is often fatal and the midwife must remember that care of the partner forms a large part of her role in this situation.

References

ACOG Technical Bulletin No. 143 (1990) Diagnosis and management of postpartum haemorrhage. *Int. J. Gynecol. Obstet* **36**: 159–163.

Beischer, N. & Mackay, E. (1986) *Obstetrics and the Newborn*. London: Baillière Tindall.

Brant, H. (1967) Precise estimation of postpartum haemorrhage: difficulties and importance. *Br. Med. J.* **1**: 389–400.

Campbell, J. (1993) Making sense of shock. *Nursing Times* **89**(5): 34–36.

Chatelain, S. & Quirk, G. (1990) Amniotic and thromboembolism. *Clin. Obstet. Gynecol.* **33**(3): 473–481.

Clark, S. (1990) New concepts of amniotic fluid embolism: a review. *Obstet. Gynecol. Survey* **45**(6): 360–368.

Combs, C. & Laros, R. (1991) Prolonged third stage of labour: morbidity and risk factors. *Obstet. Gynecol.* **77**(6): 863–867.

Combs, C., Murphy, E. & Laros, R. (1991) Factors associated with postpartum haemorrhage with vaginal birth. *Obstet. Gynecol.* **77**(1): 69–76.

Consumers Association (1992) The management of postpartum haemorrhage. *Drug Ther. Bull.* **30**(23): 89–92.

Davies, M. & Harrison, J. (1992) Amniotic fluid embolism: maternal mortality revisited. *Br. J. Hosp. Med.* **47**(10): 775–776.

Dildy, G. & Cotton, D. (1992) Trauma, shock and critical care obstetrics. In Reece, E., Hobbins, J., Mahony, M. & Petrie, R. (eds) *Medicine of the Fetus and Mother*. Philadelphia: J.B. Lippincott.

DOH (Department of Health) (1994) *Report on Confidential Enquiries into Maternal Deaths in the United Kingdom 1988–1990*. London: HMSO.

Haswell, J. (1981) Measured blood loss at delivery. *J. Indiana State Med. Assoc.* **74**(1): 34–36.

Jaffe, R., DuBeshter, B., Sherer, D., Thompson, E. & Woods, J. (1994) Failure of methotrexate treatment for term placenta. *Am. J. Obstet. Gynecol.* **171**(2): 558–559.

Khong, T., Healy, D. & McCloud, P. (1991) Pregnancies complicated by abnormally adherent placenta and sex ratio at birth. *Br. Med. J.* **320** (16th March): 625–626.

Kupferminic, M., Tamura, R., Wigton, T., Glassenberg, R. & Socol, M. (1993) Placental accreta is associated with elevated maternal serum alpha-fetoprotein. *Obstet. Gynecol.* **82**(2): 266–269.

Legro, R., Price, F., Hill, L. & Caritis, S. (1994) Nonsurgical management of placental percreta: a case report. *Obstet. Gynecol.* **83**(5, Part 2): 847–849.

Levy, V. (1990) The midwife's management of the third stage of labour. In Alexander, J., Levy, V. & Roch, S. (eds) *Midwifery Practice: Intrapartum Care – a research-based approach*. London: MacMillan.

Levy, V. & Moore, J. (1985) The midwife's management of the third stage of labour. *Nursing Times* **1**(5): 47–50.

Lewis, T. & Chamberlain, G. (1990) *Obstetrics by Ten Teachers*. Sevenoaks: Hodder & Stoughton.

Momani, A. & Hassan, A. (1989) Treatment of puerperal uterine inversion by a hydrostatic method; reports of five cases. *Eur. J. Obstet. Gynecol. Reprod. Biol.* **32**: 281–285.

O'Sullivan, J.V. (1945) Acute inversion of the uterus. *Br. Med. J.* **2**: 282–283.

Pearlman, M. & Faro, S. (1990) Obstetric septic shock: a pathophysiological basis for management. *Clin. Obstet. Gynecol.* **33**(3): 482–492.

Peyser, M. & Kupferminic, M. (1990) Management of severe postpartum haemorrhage by intra-uterine irrigation with prostaglandin E_2. *Am. J. Obstet. Gynecol.* **162**(3): 694–697.

Porter, K., O'Brien, W., Collins, M., Givens, P., Knuppel, R. & Bruskivage, L. (1991) A randomised comparison of umbilical vein and intravenous oxytocin during the puerperium. *Obstet. Gynecol.* **78**(2): 254–256.

Ratnam, S. & Rauff, M. (1989) Postpartum haemorrhage and abnormalities of the third stage of labour. In Turnbull, A. & Chamberlain, G. (eds) *Obstetrics*. London: Churchill Livingstone.

Reddy, V. & Carey, J. (1989) Effect of umbilical vein oxytocin on puerperal blood loss and length of the third stage of labor. *Am. J. Obstet. Gynecol.* **160**(1): 206–208.

Romero, R., Hsu, Y.C., Athanassiadis, A. *et al.* (1990) Preterm delivery: a risk factor for retained placenta. *Am. J. Obstet. Gynecol.* **163**(3): 823–825.

Royle, J. & Walsh, M. (1992) *Watson's Medical–Surgical Nursing Related Physiology* London: Baillière Tindall.

Sarkar, P. & Mamo, J. (1990) Successful control of atonic primary post-partum haemorrhage and prevention of hysterectomy using I.V. prostaglandin E_2. *Br. J. Clin. Pract.* **44**(11): 756–757.

Seeley, H. (1989) Massive blood loss in obstetrics. In Turnbull, A. & Chamberlain, G. (eds) *Obstetrics*. London: Churchill Livingstone.

Sipes, S. & Weiner, C. (1992) Coagulation disorders in pregnancy. In Reece, E., Hobbins, J. Mahony, M. & Petrie, R. (eds) *Medicine of the Fetus and Mother*. Philadelphia: J. B. Lippincott.

Spencer, P. (1962) Controlled cord traction in the management of the third stage of labour. *Br. Med. J.* 1: 1728–1832.

Young, S., Martelly, P., Greb, L., Considine, G. and Coustan, D. (1988) The effect of intra-umbilical oxytocin on the third stage of labour. *Obstet. Gynecol.* 71(5): 736–738.

Zahn, C. & Yeomans, E. (1990) Postpartum haemorrhage: placental accreta, uterine inversion and puerperal hematomas. *Clin. Obstet. Gynecol.* 33(3): 422–431.

Further Reading

Bakri, Y., Sundi, T., Mansi, M. & Jaroudi, K. (1993) Placenta percreta with bladder invasion: report of three cases. *Am. J. Perinatol.* 10(6): 468–470.

Fava, S. & Galizia, A. (1993) Amniotic fluid embolism. *Br. J. Obstet. Gynaecol.* 100(11): 1049–1050.

Gibb, D., Soothill, P. & Ward, K. (1994) Conservative management of placenta accreta. *Br. J. Obstet. Gynaecol.* 101(1): 79–80.

Khang, T. Y. & Khang, T. K. (1993) Delayed postpartum haemorrhage: a morphologic study of causes and their relation to other pregnancy disorders. *Obstet. Gynecol.* 82(1): 17–22.

Llewellyn-Jones, D. (1990) *Fundamentals of Obstetrics and Gynaecology* Vol. 1, *Obstetrics*. London: Faber & Faber.

Maher, J., Wenstrom, K., Hauth, J. & Meis, P. (1994) Amniotic fluid embolism after saline amnioinfusion: two cases and review of the literature. *Obstet. Gynecol.* 83(5, 2): 851–854.

Robson, S., Boys, R., Hunter, S. & Dunlop, W. (1989) Maternal hemodynamics after normal delivery and delivery complicated by post-partum haemorrhage. *Obstet. Gynecol.* 74(2): 234–239.

Part Twelve

Complications of the Puerperium

57

Complications of the Puerperium

During the puerperium many women experience considerable discomfort. Whilst this is generally minor, on occasion serious disorders such as infection, thromboembolism or haemorrhage can occur. Such complications will invariably prolong hospital stay, delay postnatal recovery and may lessen the mother's enjoyment of her new baby. Infection can adversely affect subsequent fertility (Hibbard, 1988) whilst other disorders such as stress incontinence can result in long-term health problems after childbirth (MacArthur *et al.*, 1991; Glazener *et al.*, 1993).

An important role of the midwife is to monitor the physical and mental health of the mother throughout the puerperium. Any deviation from normal must be reported to a doctor for further investigation and treatment in accordance with the *Midwives' Rules* (UKCC, 1993).

Discomforts

After-pains
After-pains occur during the first 2–3 days of the puerperium and are caused by the myometrial contraction of the uterus. They are more common in the multipara than the primipara. The pains are accentuated during breastfeeding because suckling stimulates the release of oxytocin from the posterior pituitary and this causes the uterus to contract. A mild analgesic such as paracetamol is usually effective.

Soreness of the perineum
Most women experience some perineal discomfort or pain postnatally, particularly following episiotomy (Greenshields and Hulme, 1993). Perineal pain is also reported to be greater in women who have epidural

anaesthesia during labour. Infiltrating the perineum prior to suturing, even when the epidural is still providing adequate anaesthesia, prevents overtight suturing and has been shown to reduce this discomfort (Khan and Lilford, 1987).

The mother needs sympathetic understanding of her perineal discomfort. Clear and specific instructions on perineal hygiene should be given and only therapies that are of proven benefit should be recommended for the treatment of sore perinea. The application of cooling agents such as crushed ice, witch hazel or tap water may provide short-term relief and locally applied anaesthetics such as aqueous 5% lignocaine spray or gel can be of benefit (Grant and Sleep, 1989). Paracetamol is usually effective in controlling mild pain.

The effectiveness of oral proteolytic enzymes and locally applied physiotherapies as treatments for sore perinea has yet to be clearly established (Grant and Sleep, 1989).

Haemorrhoids

After the second stage of labour, haemorrhoids may become prolapsed and extremely painful so that analgesia is required. Local treatment may include the application of an anaesthetic cream (Anusol) or an ice pack. The haemorrhoids can be digitally replaced when any oedema has subsided. Constipation should be avoided so a high-residue diet is encouraged. A stool-softening agent such as liquid paraffin may be required.

Breast engorgement

Breast engorgement is a generic term for both vascular and milk engorgement of the breast.

After the placenta has been delivered, prolactin levels rise and milk synthesis begins. Blood supply to the breasts is increased, causing vascular engorgement. The mother experiences a sensation of increased warmth and fullness of the breasts and she may feel uncomfortable.

Milk, once produced, is stored in the alveoli. If it is not adequately removed, the stored volume increases and the capacity of the alveoli may be exceeded. The alveoli become distended, the breasts increasingly uncomfortable and eventually milk production is suppressed. This milk engorgement continues until the volume of milk produced is downregulated to that removed by the baby.

Milk engorgement is preventable by the early initia-

tion of unrestricted feeding. Correct positioning of the baby will ensure that milk is removed effectively at each feed. If the breast is over-full, expressing a small amount of milk prior to feeding will soften the breast to enable attachment.

Sore nipples

Nipple trauma is sustained when the baby is incorrectly positioned at the breast. It is caused by friction of the nipple against the hard palate.

Various ointments and sprays have been evaluated to prevent sore nipples but none has been found to be effective (Inch and Renfrew, 1989).

Different treatment regimes for sore nipples have been compared (Nicholson, 1985). Correctly repositioning the baby at the breast, the use of a nipple shield and resting the breast and expressing the milk have been found equally effective in promoting nipple healing. However, nipple shields may be unacceptable to some mothers and both nipple shields and the use of a breast pump can reduce milk yield (Woolridge et al., 1980; Howie et al., 1980).

Skilled help and advice should be given to the mother from the first feed onwards to ensure that she is able to position her baby correctly at the breast. This is the single most important factor in both the prevention and treatment of sore nipples.

Puerperal Infection

Any bacterial infection of the genital tract occurring after delivery is referred to as a puerperal infection.

Prior to the introduction of antibiotics in 1936, puerperal sepsis ranked first amongst the causes of maternal mortality. Although this is no longer the case, genital tract infection remains one of the most common and serious complications of the puerperium (Cunningham et al., 1993). Thromboembolic disorders can also be associated with infection and are the leading cause of maternal death (DOH, 1996).

Infections of the urinary tract, the breast and surgical incision sites can result in widespread maternal morbidity.

The midwife must notify a doctor if the newly delivered mother develops any signs and symptoms of infection. *Generalized signs* comprise an elevated temperature, rigors, tachycardia and malaise. *Localized signs* such as a subinvoluted and tender uterus, a red and painful segment of the breast or dysuria will usually indicate the site of infection.

Careful diagnosis is essential in view of the fact that a transient rise in temperature can be a normal feature of the puerperium and reflects the physiological changes taking place within both the uterus and the breast as lactation is initiated (Hibbard, 1988).

It is also possible for a woman to develop a pyrexial illness in the early puerperium which is unconnected with her confinement. The treatment of any intercurrent infection is the same as in any other circumstances. Isolation and disinfection are of vital importance in order to protect other mothers and babies.

Disorders of the Genital Tract

INFECTION

Women are at increased risk of infection postpartum because the placental site is a large unhealed vascular area, providing the warmth, darkness and moisture in which many bacteria thrive. Lacerations in any part of the genital tract can also become infected. This includes episiotomy wounds and tears of the perineal body, vaginal walls and cervix. Infection of Caesarean section wound sites can also occur.

Infecting organisms and their source

Infecting organisms originate from one of two sources:

1   *Endogenous bacteria* are those normally present in the body and are responsible for the majority of puerperal infections (Cunningham *et al.*, 1993). Examples are *Streptococcus faecalis* and *Clostridium welchii* which are usually present in the vagina and *Escherichia coli* which inhabit the bowel. Infection will normally only occur when there is tissue damage or cross-contamination as these bacteria ascend the genital tract.

2   *Exogenous bacteria* originate from a source other than the mother and are responsible for the more severe, although less common, puerperal infections (Hibbard, 1988). Attendants on the mother with colds and sore throats can disperse organisms such as the virulent group A beta-haemolytic streptococci by droplet infection, as can asymptomatic carriers. *Chlamydia trachomatis* has recently been implicated as a cause of uterine infection (Berenson *et al.*, 1990). Staphylococci, in particular *Staphylo-*

coccus aureus, are commonly responsible for wound infections.

Factors predisposing to infection

Poor nutrition can impair cell immunity and reduce resistance to infection. Iron deficiency anaemia is also generally thought to increase the risk of infection although there is conflicting evidence as to the benefit of iron therapy in this respect (Cook and Lynch, 1986).

A protracted labour, prolonged rupture of membranes, frequent vaginal examinations and a traumatic delivery all predispose to puerperal infection, but the single most important risk factor is Caesarean section (Cunningham *et al.*, 1993). Retained fragments of placenta are also an ideal culture medium for the growth of microorganisms.

Clinical features

These vary according to the nature and virulence of the organism and the natural defence mechanisms of the mother (Simpson *et al.*, 1988).

Localized uterine infection (*endometritis*) typically presents around the third postpartum day with a rise in temperature to 39°C and a corresponding tachycardia. Headache and rigors may also be present. This is accompanied by a bulky, tender uterus and profuse red lochia which, in anaerobic and coliform infections, has an offensive smell.

Management

The mother should be isolated and the doctor inquires about her symptoms, reviews her labour and examines her. Swabs are taken from high in the vagina and any wound sites. These, and a midstream urine specimen, are sent to the laboratory to identify the causative organism and ascertain its sensitivity to antibiotic drugs. A full blood count will be taken to determine the systemic response to the infecting organism. Blood cultures may also be required if there is a swinging pyrexia. Antibiotic therapy is commenced immediately; usually with a combination of drugs to combat both Gram-positive and Gram-negative organisms (Howie, 1995a). The antibiotic regime may need changing when the culture results are known.

If the infection is severe the mother will feel very unwell. She should be nursed in a side-ward with access to her own toilet and bidet (if she is able to get up). Her temperature and pulse rate should be measured and recorded four-hourly and antipyretics given as necessary. Fluid intake should be maintained at a level appropriate to the degree of fever and intravenous fluids may be required to achieve this. A record of fluid balance should be kept.

The baby should remain with the mother in case it is an asymptomatic carrier of the infection (Simpson *et al.*, 1988). Help with feeding and caring for the baby will be required during the acute phase of the infection, at which time lactation may temporarily diminish.

Spread of infection

With very virulent organisms, or if the mother's resistance is impaired, the infection can extend beyond the uterus to the pelvic cellular tissue, the pelvic peritoneum or along the fallopian tubes to the ovaries. Thrombophlebitis of the uterine veins can transport infected clots to other organs.

Septicaemia can be caused by bacteria such as *Clostridium welchii*. The mother will be extremely ill with a swinging temperature, rigors, vomiting and sometimes anaemia and jaundice. Antibiotic treatment must be started as soon as possible because the mother's condition can deteriorate rapidly.

In the *Report on Confidential Enquiries into Maternal Deaths in the United Kingdom (1991–93)*, there were 15 deaths associated with genital tract sepsis (DOH, 1996). This is a a similar number to that of the previous report covering the years 1988–1990.

RETAINED PRODUCTS OF CONCEPTION

Small fragments of membrane or placenta may be retained in the uterine cavity following delivery and are known as retained products of conception. The placenta and membranes are examined following delivery and if the placenta is thought to be incomplete a digital exploration and evacuation of the uterine cavity under general anaesthetic will be carried out. If the membranes are incomplete a record of this is made in the case notes. In most instances the membrane is expelled spontaneously within a few days.

SUBINVOLUTION

The uterus involutes progressively during the first week of the puerperium and is no longer palpable above the symphysis pubis by about the 10th postpartum day. Within 6–8 weeks of delivery it will approximate to its pre-pregnant size and position. Delay in this process is known as subinvolution and may be caused by a full bladder or rectum, retained products of conception, infection or fibroids. If no specific cause can be found and, providing the lochia are normal, this condition may be of no significance.

The rate of uterine involution does not appear to be directly affected by parity or the method of infant feeding (Rodeck and Newton, 1976; VanRees *et al.*, 1981). However, birthweight has been positively correlated with uterine size in the puerperium (Lavery and Shaw, 1989). As birthweight generally increases with successive pregnancies, this may account for the observed delay in involution in grande multiparous women and following a multiple pregnancy.

Management

Constipation and overdistension of the bladder should be avoided. Careful management of the third stage of labour will reduce the risk of retained products of conception.

SECONDARY POSTPARTUM HAEMORRHAGE

A profuse haemorrhage occurring after the first 24 hours of the puerperium is known as a secondary postpartum haemorrhage. In most cases this is due to a portion of placenta being retained in the uterus, but may also be caused by a blood clot or fibroid preventing contraction of the uterus. It is also commonly associated with infection.

The haemorrhage usually occurs within 7–14 days of delivery but can be later. Often it is preceded by heavy red lochia which may be offensive, subinvolution and, if secondary to infection, a low-grade pyrexia and tachycardia.

Management

The uterus is massaged, if palpable, to cause it to contract. Any clots are expelled and the midwife ensures that the bladder is empty. If the bleeding is severe, an intravenous injection of ergometrine maleate 250–500 μg or an intramuscular injection of Syntometrine 1 ml is given to contract the uterus and control haemorrhage. Medical aid must be summoned. An intravenous infusion is commenced and blood is cross-matched in case transfusion is required. Evacuation of the uterus under general anaesthesia and antibiotic therapy may be necessary. If the haemorrhage occurs at home, arrangements should be made to transfer the mother to hospital. Depending upon the severity of the bleeding and local arrangements, this may be by the paramedic ambulance service. If the haemorrhage is less severe it can be managed at home with oral ergometrine and antibiotics.

Disorders of the Urinary Tract

URINARY TRACT INFECTION

Urinary tract infection occurs in approximately 12% of women postpartum (Barnick and Cardozo, 1990). The physiological changes in the urinary tract which occur during pregnancy take about six weeks to resolve so the potential for infection following delivery remains. Women who experienced urinary tract infections antenatally or those with asymptomatic bacteriuria are particularly susceptible to a recurrence of infection, as are those who required catheterization during labour. In the puerperium, perineal lacerations and sutures can make micturition painful and predispose to retention of urine. Similarly, a lax abdominal wall or epidural analgesia during labour may cause the mother to be unaware that her bladder is distended. Retention of urine predisposes to infection. The organism commonly responsible is *Escherichia coli*.

Diagnosis

Cystitis presents with urinary frequency, dysuria and a slight rise in temperature. In pyelonephritis the condition is more severe, with pain radiating from the loin to the groin, pyrexia, rigors and vomiting. The woman feels very unwell. The urine is opalescent, acid in reaction, smells offensive and on microscopic examination pus cells are evident. A midstream specimen of urine is obtained to identify the causative organism.

Treatment

The mother is urged to drink at least 3000 ml daily. If she is vomiting, adequate hydration is maintained with intravenous fluids. Both fluid intake and urinary output should be monitored. Analgesia and antipyretics are given as necessary.

A broad-spectrum antibiotic is commenced immediately. This may be changed when the infecting organism has been identified. After the course of antibiotics has been completed a repeat specimen of urine is sent for investigation to ensure that treatment has been effective.

Following the six-week postnatal examination, frequent or recurrent urinary tract infections will be investigated by intravenous pyelography and cystoscopy.

URINARY INCONTINENCE

Retention with overflow

Trauma to the bladder and urethra during delivery, epidural analgesia and fear of micturition due to a painful perineum can all predispose to retention of urine. If this remains undetected, urine will eventually leak from the overdistended bladder. This form of incontinence is referred to as retention with overflow. The uterus is displaced upwards or to one side and the bladder is palpable abdominally, despite the frequent passage of urine. An indwelling catheter is placed in the bladder and left on continuous drainage for 48 hours. Following catheter removal urinary output is carefully measured. If retention of urine persists, suprapubic catheterization is required until the volume of residual urine falls below 100 ml on two successive occasions (Cardozo, 1995).

Stress incontinence

Stress incontinence is the involuntary loss of urine from the bladder on exertion or sudden movement.

The major cause of stress incontinence following delivery is incompetence of the urinary sphincter mechanism (Cardozo, 1995). This can be damaged or weakened during labour either by direct injury to the nerve supply or stretching of the supporting structures at the bladder neck. The severity of this injury can be related to the length of the second stage of labour, instrumental delivery and multiparity (Swash, 1988). Pelvic floor exercises to improve the tone of the sphincter mechanism are of limited value if the incontinence is caused by nerve injury. Most of the damage to these nerves recovers spontaneously within three months of childbirth (Swash, 1988).

Vesico-vaginal fistula

Rarely, a vesico-vaginal fistula develops between the bladder or urethra and vagina as a result of damage sustained during labour. This may be caused by devitalization of the tissue at the base of the bladder due to prolonged pressure of the fetal head against the back of the symphysis pubis. Sloughing of the devitalized area takes 8–12 days to complete, following which the mother becomes incontinent of urine.

A vesico-vaginal fistula may also be caused by direct trauma to the bladder during a difficult instrumental delivery. In this case incontinence occurs almost immediately. Initial treatment is antibiotic therapy and continuous bladder drainage for 2–3 weeks to encourage the fistula to close spontaneously. If this treatment fails operative repair is necessary.

Close surveillance during labour should prevent the development of this complication.

Breast Disorders

BREAST INFECTION

Mastitis

Mastitis can be either non-infective or infective. *Non-infective mastitis* occurs when the milk flow from one segment of the breast is obstructed. This may be caused locally by a blocked duct, compression from tight clothing or pressure from holding the breast too tightly when feeding. Any extraneous factors preventing drainage of the breast, such as poor positioning or a restrictive feeding regime, can have the same effect.

The alveoli become overdistended with milk and may be felt as a lump in the breast. If the pressure is not relieved, milk substances are forced out into the adjacent tissue, activating the mother's immune system. The affected segment of the breast is painful and appears red and swollen. The mother complains of flu-like symptoms; her temperature and pulse rate are raised and rigors are common. If this condition is not resolved progression to infective mastitis is likely.

Infective mastitis is caused when bacteria enter the breast, commonly through a crack in the nipple. The causative organism is usually *Staphylococcus aureus* originating from the baby's pharynx. If left untreated, this can develop into a breast abscess.

Management

Correct positioning of the baby at the breast and unrestricted feeding will help prevent the development of mastitis. Factors predisposing to localized obstruction should be avoided.

The mother should continue to breastfeed. Manual or mechanical expression after a feed will ensure the breasts are completely emptied. Analgesia suitable for breastfeeding women should be given as required. Whilst she is feeling unwell, the mother is likely to require both emotional support and practical assistance in caring for her baby.

A differential diagnosis between *infective* and *non-infective mastitis* can be obtained from leucocyte and bacterial counts on a specimen of breast milk (Thomsen *et al.*, 1984). Antibiotic therapy is commenced if the mastitis fails to resolve with good feeding technique and expression or where infective mastitis is confirmed.

Breast abscess

Bacteria entering the breast, commonly through a crack in the nipple, can cause infection in either the superficial cellular or deeper connective tissue. If untreated, this can progress to the formation of a breast abscess. In addition to the signs and symptoms of mastitis, there will be a fluctuant swelling under the reddened area and there may be pitting oedema of the overlying skin. Surgical incision and drainage of the abscess or local aspiration (Dixon, 1988) will be required. Breastfeeding can continue on the affected side of the site if the incision permits. If not, feeding should continue on the unaffected breast until the incision has healed.

Thromboembolic Disorders

SUPERFICIAL THROMBOPHLEBITIS

Thrombophlebitis is caused by the formation of a clot in a superficial varicosed vein as a result of stasis and the hypercoaguable state of pregnancy and the puerperium. Varicose veins commonly occur during pregnancy because of increased venous pressure in the legs and the action of progesterone. Anaemia is also a predisposing factor to thrombophlebitis. A red, inflamed and tender area appears over the vein which feels firm on palpation from the clot lying within it. There is usually a slight increase in the temperature and pulse rate.

Management

The mother is encouraged to mobilize wearing correctly fitting anti-thromboembolic stockings. When sitting, the leg is elevated and exercises are performed. Local warmth-inducing applications such as a kaolin poultice or glycerine and ichthammol paste may provide additional comfort. The inflammation usually subsides within a few days. Whilst the clot remains in a superficial vein there is no immediate hazard to the mother but she is closely observed for signs of deep vein thrombosis.

DEEP VEIN THROMBOSIS

This is a less common but more serious condition. A clot has formed in the deep calf, femoral or iliac veins and there is a risk that fragments will become detached causing a pulmonary embolus. Risk factors for the development of thrombosis and thromboembolism are increasing maternal age, obesity, operative delivery, immobilization and a previous history of thromboembolism (DOH, 1994). It is also associated with the administration of oestrogens; thus these drugs are no longer prescribed for the suppression of lactation.

The clinical features of deep vein thrombosis are variable (Cunningham *et al.*, 1993). There may be a slight rise in the temperature and pulse rate. The woman may complain of calf pain. Oedema and changes in leg colour and temperature can also be present (Leclerc and Hirsh, 1988). Alternatively, the woman may be asymptomatic; the first sign of thromboembolic disease being a pulmonary embolism. High-risk women should therefore be observed vigilantly.

Management

Early ambulation decreases the frequency of deep vein thrombosis in the puerperium. Where suspected, diagnosis should be confirmed by real-time ultrasound, ascending phlebography or isotope venography (Howie, 1995b) because of the non-specific nature of clinical signs. A positive diagnosis has implications for subsequent contraception and future pregnancies. The oestrogen-containing contraceptive pill is contraindicated where there is a history of deep vein thrombosis and prophylactic anticoagulation will be required in a subsequent pregnancy.

Anticoagulant therapy is commenced to prevent further clotting and to reduce the risk of pulmonary embolism.

A typical regime is a bolus dose of 5000–10 000 IU intravenous heparin followed by 1000–1600 IU/hour in saline, administered via an infusion pump (Howie, 1995b). The total dose of heparin should not exceed 40 000 units in any given 24-hour period. Treatment is continued until the acute signs have resolved.

Whilst the woman remains in bed, the foot of the bed is elevated and the weight of the bedclothes removed from the leg by a cradle. Analgesics are given as required. Careful observation for bleeding is necessary; in particular the colour and amount of the lochia should be noted. Protamine sulphate is the antidote to heparin and should be available to reverse the effects, if excessive bleeding occurs. When signs and symptoms have completely abated mobilization can recommence with the leg well supported.

Anticoagulant therapy should continue for six weeks until the risk of recurrent thrombosis has passed (Bonnar, 1981). Treatment is maintained either by self-administered subcutaneous low-dose heparin or the oral anticoagulant warfarin. The dose of warfarin is calculated by regular measurement of the prothrombin time (which is prolonged to 1.5–2.0 times the control value) at an outpatient clinic. Breastfeeding is not contraindicated with either heparin or warfarin therapy.

PULMONARY EMBOLISM

A pulmonary embolism occurs when a clot has become detached from the leg vein, is carried along the inferior vena cava and into the pulmonary artery. Small clots passing into the lung cause pulmonary infarction. If the artery is completely blocked death occurs rapidly. The most recent *Report on Confidential Enquiries into Maternal Deaths in the United Kingdom 1991–1993* (DOH, 1996) details 30 deaths from pulmonary embolism, 17 of which occurred postpartum.

Major pulmonary emboli present with acute chest pain due to ischaemia of the lungs, dyspnoea, cyanosis, haemoptysis, pyrexia and collapse. This may be preceded by warning signs of a slight, unexplained rise in temperature and respiratory rate, an unproductive cough, transitory dyspnoea or chest pain.

Suspected pulmonary embolism should be investigated and the diagnosis confirmed by chest X-ray, a ventilation/perfusion scan of the lungs or pulmonary angiography.

Management

Medical aid is summoned urgently. The mother is sat upright and given oxygen to assist breathing. Vital signs are measured at 15-minute intervals. If resuscitation is required external cardiac massage and artificial ventilation are commenced. The doctor will start anticoagulation therapy with intravenous heparin and a strong analgesic such as morphine will be given to provide pain relief.

If the woman survives, anticoagulation therapy will continue and a thrombolytic drug such as streptokinase may be prescribed to accelerate the breakdown of the existing clot. An embolectomy may be required if this management is unsuccessful.

Emergencies of the Puerperium

Any medical or surgical emergency may occur in the puerperium. Women with pre-existing pulmonary disease are at increased risk of developing pneumonia postpartum. Avoiding heavy sedation and maintaining good hydration will help to prevent this. The early puerperium is also particularly hazardous for women with heart disease or when pregnancy has been com-plicated by severe pre-eclampsia. Eclampsia occurs postpartum in approximately 25% of reported cases (Novy, 1994). An eclamptic fit is most likely within 48 hours of delivery but can occur up to 10 days later.

Surgical problems are more common following operative delivery or adjunctive surgery such as ster-ilization. The increased vascularity of pelvic tissues predisposes to post-operative bleeding.

Post-anaesthetic complications such as hypotension, airway obstruction, laryngospasm or the aspiration of vomit can occur and require emergency treatment. Observation of the pulse, blood pressure and respira-tory rate should be made at 15-minute intervals for at least one hour following operative delivery and there-after until they remain stable. Medical aid must be summoned urgently if a deterioration in the woman's condition is noted or resuscitative measures are required.

References

Barnick, C.G.W. & Cardozo, L.D. (1990) The lower urinary tract in pregnancy, labour and the puerperium. In Studd, J.W.W. (ed.) *Progress in Obstetrics and Gynaecology*, Vol. 9. Edinburgh: Churchill Livingstone.

Berenson, A.B., Hammill, H.A., Martens, M.G. *et al.* (1990) Bacteriologic findings of post-cesarean endometritis in ado-lescents. *Obstet. Gynecol.* 75(4): 627–629.

Bonnar, J. (1981) Venous thromboembolism and pregnancy. In Wood, S.M. & Beeley, L. (eds) *Clinics in Obstetrics and Gynaecology*, Vol. 8, Part 2, p. 455. London: W.B. Saunders.

Cardozo, L.D. (1995) Urinary tract disorders in pregnancy. In Whitfield, C.R. (ed.) *Dewhurst's Textbook of Obstetrics and Gynaecology for Postgraduates*, 5th edn. Oxford: Blackwell Science.

Cook, J. D. & Lynch, S.R. (1986) The liabilities of iron deficiency. *Blood* 68(4): 803–809.

Cunningham, F.G., MacDonald, P.C., Gant, N.F. *et al.* (1993) *Williams Obstetrics*, 19th edn. London: Prentice-Hall.

Dixon, J.M. (1988) Repeated aspiration of breast abscess in lactating women. *Br. Med. J.* 297: 1517–1518.

DOH (Department of Health) (1994) *Report on Confidential Enquiries into Maternal Deaths in the United Kingdom 1988–1990*. London: HMSO.

DOH (1996) *Report on Confidential Enquiries into Maternal Deaths in the United Kingdom 1991–93*. London: HMSO.

Glazener, C., Abdalla, M., Russell, I. & Templeton, A. (1993) Postnatal care: a survey of patients' experiences. *Br. J. Midwifery* 1(2): 67–74.

Grant, A. & Sleep, J. (1989) Relief of perineal pain and discomfort after childbirth. In Chalmers, I., Enkin, M. & Keirse, M.J.N.C. (eds) *Effective Care in Pregnancy and Childbirth*. Oxford: Oxford University Press.

Greenshields, W. & Hulme, H. (1993) *The Perineum in Child-birth. A Survey Conducted by the National Childbirth Trust*. London: National Childbirth Trust.

Hibbard, B. (1988) *Principles of Obstetrics*. London: Butter-worths.

Howie, P.W., McNeilly, A.S., McArdle, T. *et al.* (1980) The relationship between suckling induced prolactin response and lactogenesis. *J. Clin. Endocrinol. Metab.* 50: 670–673.

Howie, P.W. (1995a) The puerperium and its complications. In Whitfield, C.R. (ed.) *Dewhurst's Textbook of Obstetrics and Gynaecology for Postgraduates*, 5th edn. Oxford: Blackwell Scientific.

Howie, P.W. (1995b) Coagulation and fibrinolytic systems and their disorders in obstetrics and gynaecology. In Whitfield, C.R. (ed.) *Dewhurst's Textbook of Obstetrics and Gynaecology for Postgraduates*, 5th edn. Oxford: Blackwell Scientific.

Inch, S. & Renfrew, M.J. (1989) Common breastfeeding problems. In Chalmers, I., Enkin, M. & Keirse, M.J.N.C. (eds) *Effective Care in Pregnancy and Childbirth*. Oxford: Oxford University Press.

Khan, G.Q. & Lilford, R.J. (1987) Wound pain may be reduced by prior infiltration of the episiotomy site after delivery under epidural anaesthesia. *Br. J. Obstet. Gynae-col.* 94(4): 341–344.

Lavery, J.P. & Shaw, L.A. (1989) Sonography of the puerperal uterus. *J. Ultrasound Med.* 8: 481–486.

Leclerc, J.R. & Hirsh, J. (1988) Venous thromboembolic disorders. In Burrow, G.N. & Ferris, T.F. (eds) *Medical Complications During Pregnancy*, 3rd edn. Philadelphia: W.B. Saunders.

MacArthur, C., Lewis, M. & Knox, E.G. (1991) *Health after Childbirth*. London: HMSO.

Nicholson, W. (1985) Cracked nipples in breastfeeding

mothers – a randomised trial of three methods of management. *Newsletter Nursing Mothers Aust.* **21**(4): 7–10.

Novy, M. (1994) The normal puerperium. In DeCherney, A.H. & Pernoll, M.L. (eds) *Current Obstetric and Gynaecologic Diagnosis and Treatment*, 8th edn. London: Prentice-Hall.

Rodeck, C.H. & Newton, J.R. (1976) Study of the uterine cavity by ultrasound in the early puerperium. *Br. J. Obstet. Gynaecol.* **83**: 795–801.

Simpson, M.L., Gaziano, E.P., Lupo, V.R. & Petersen, P.K. (1988) Bacterial infections during pregnancy. In Burrow, G.N. & Ferris, T.F. (eds) *Medical Complications During Pregnancy*, 3rd edn. Philadelphia: W.B. Saunders.

Swash, M. (1988) Childbirth and incontinence. *Midwifery* **4**: 13–18.

Thomsen, A.C., Espersen, T. & Maigaard, S. (1984) Course and treatment of milk stasis, non-infectious inflammation of the breast and infectious mastitis in nursing women. *Am. J. Obstet. Gynecol.* **149**(5): 492–495.

UKCC (UK Central Council for Nursing, Midwifery and Health Visiting) (1993) *Midwives' Rules*. London: UKCC.

VanRees, D., Berstine, R.L. & Crawford, W. (1981) Involution of the postpartum uterus: an ultrasonic study. *J. Clin. Ultrasound* **9**: 55–57.

Woolridge, M., Baum, D. & Drewett, R.F. (1980) Effect of a traditional and of a new nipple shield on sucking patterns and milk flow. *Early Human Devel.* **4**(4): 357–364.

58

Psychiatric Disorders Associated with Childbirth

There is an increased risk of mental illness associated with childbirth, mostly in the postpartum period, but problems may also be present before or during pregnancy. Many of the factors associated with postnatal mental illness, such as lack of a confiding relationship and support, marital tension, socio-economic problems and a previous psychiatric history, are present before and during pregnancy (O'Hara and Zekowski, 1988; Romito, 1989) and so depression may occur both in pregnancy and the postpartum period (Green and Murray, 1994; Clement et al., 1994; Watson et al., 1984). The incidence of mental illness in the first trimester of pregnancy is thought to be as high as 15%. Only about 5% of these women will have suffered from previous episodes of mental illness. In the second and third trimesters of pregnancy the incidence of new episodes of mental illness is less, only about 5%.

Minor Mental Illness in Pregnancy

The majority of episodes of new mental illness during pregnancy are minor conditions or neuroses. The commonest condition is the depressive neurosis with anxiety, but phobic anxiety states and obsessional compulsive disorders may also occur. In most cases these neurotic mental illnesses resolve by the second trimester of pregnancy and there seems to be no added risk of these women developing postnatal depression.

The outlook is different for those women who begin their pregnancies with chronic neurotic conditions. Their illness is likely to continue throughout pregnancy and may be exacerbated during the puerperium.

MINOR MENTAL ILLNESS IN THE FIRST TRIMESTER

Minor mental illness is more likely to occur in the first trimester of pregnancy in women who have marked neurotic traits in the pre-morbid personality. It also tends to occur in women who have a history of neurotic disorders and in those with social problems such as marital tension. Other predisposing factors include a history of previous abortion and the possibility of the present pregnancy being terminated.

Care

The majority of these illnesses resolve spontaneously by the second trimester of pregnancy. The woman will require support, counselling, reassurance and information which is communicated in a caring, intelligible way. Rarely are psychotropic drugs necessary or prescribed at this stage of pregnancy. Instead therapy to help the woman relax and reduce her anxiety may be employed and seems to be effective. Midwives may be involved in counselling and supporting these women and teaching them relaxation techniques. Sometimes a social worker is also required to help tackle social problems which may be the cause of the problem.

MINOR MENTAL ILLNESS LATER IN PREGNANCY

The onset of minor mental illness later in pregnancy, usually during the third trimester, is less common than in the first trimester. When it occurs at this stage in pregnancy, however, the risk of the woman developing postnatal depression is increased (Oates, 1989; Clement et al., 1994). The midwife therefore has an important role to play in the detection of such illness so that the mother can be given appropriate counselling, support and therapy.

Social support in pregnancy can have a beneficial effect on women with obstetric and social problems (Hodnett, 1994a, b), and strategies to diagnose depression and the institution of appropriate psychological interventions to treat the condition in pregnancy may prevent it becoming a long-term postnatal problem. Clement (1995) suggests the use of the Edinburgh Postnatal Depression Scale for the detection of depression in pregnancy for high-risk groups, followed by 'listening visits' in pregnancy and continued in the postpartum period. 'Listening' intervention for women with postnatal depression has been shown to be effective (Holden et al., 1989) and the introduction of psychological screening and 'listening' therapy for selected women in pregnancy may be equally beneficial. The risk of postnatal depression may therefore be reduced.

Major Mental Illness in Pregnancy

Major mental illnesses include manic depression, severe depression and schizophrenia. The risk of a woman developing a new episode of one of these conditions in pregnancy is lower than at other times in her life. When women with a history of major mental illness become pregnant, there is no particular increase in the risk of a relapse during pregnancy if they are well stabilized and their illness is in remission.

Although the risk of major mental illness is reduced in pregnancy, it is greatly increased in the first three months after delivery.

Care

Preconception and antenatal care Women who have had single episodes of major mental illness in the past but who have been well for some time are usually advised by their psychiatrist to stop their medication before conception and throughout their pregnancy. There is no substantial risk of relapse during pregnancy. However, there is a markedly increased risk of their developing a puerperal psychosis during the first three months after delivery (Cox, 1986).

The problem is more complex in the woman who has had several episodes of major mental illness. If the psychiatrist feels that there is a substantial risk of relapse if the woman's medications are withdrawn, then this risk has to be weighed against that of the drugs having a teratogenic effect on the fetus.

It may be possible to adjust the drugs to minimize any possible adverse effect on the fetus. For instance the woman suffering from schizophrenia and schizophrenia-like conditions will probably be maintained on low-dose phenothiazines together with antiparkinsonian agents such as benzhexol. The low-dose phenothiazines may be continued during pregnancy, if necessary, but it is often possible to withdraw the antiparkinsonian agent for the first 12–16 weeks of pregnancy at least. Similarly the drugs used to treat affective illnesses such as manic depressive illness, mania and severe depressive illness may also be adjusted before and during pregnancy. Lithium is probably teratogenic in the first trimester and may also be hazardous in the last trimester when it can affect the fetal thyroid, cause infantile diabetes insipidus and produce hypotonia and cyanosis at birth. It should therefore be withdrawn before conception and throughout pregnancy. Again, antiparkinsonian agents would be withdrawn during the first trimester but other drugs such as phenothiazines and butyro-phenones may be continued in low doses during pregnancy, if necessary. Women with a history of major depressive illness who are considered to have a substantial risk of a relapse may take conventional tricyclic antidepressants such as amitriptyline, imipramine and dothiepin during pregnancy. The newer drugs should be avoided however as their long-term effects are unknown. The dose of tricyclics may have to be reduced in the third trimester and the drug gradually withdrawn before delivery because of adverse effects on the newborn. These include irritability, jitteriness and convulsions. The drugs may be recommenced immediately after delivery.

Puerperal Mental Disorders

As many as 16% of mothers will develop mental illness in the puerperium, and in most cases this will be a new episode of a major mental illness. The risk of becoming mentally ill during the puerperium is therefore greater than at other times in the woman's reproductive life. In 1992 the World Health Organization included puerperal mental disorders in their International Classification of Diseases (Table 1).

Mild and severe mental and behavioural disorders which may occur in the puerperium are included in this chapter. These include postnatal depression, minor mental illness such as neurosis and puerperal psychosis.

POSTNATAL DEPRESSION

Postnatal depression is a non-psychotic depressive disorder of variable severity which occurs in the first year after childbirth. It occurs in 10–15% of women (Cox *et al.*, 1982; Kumar and Robson, 1984), and in about half of these depression starts in the first two weeks after delivery. In many cases it is not detected by professionals, and only a few women seek or receive the medical help which is available. Although the majority of women recover spontaneously from postnatal depression in time, in a significant number of cases the illness becomes chronic and may persist for the first year or more after the birth of the child (Taylor *et al.*, 1994). Longstanding untreated depressive illness is distressing not only for the mother, but also for her partner and her children. It may result in marital problems, or exacerbate existing problems, and have an adverse effect on the children's intellectual and emotional development (Uddenberg and Englesson, 1978; Coghill *et al.*, 1986). Early diagnosis and effective treatment is therefore important for the health of the whole family.

Some researchers have questioned whether postnatal depression is any different from depression which may occur at other times in a woman's life. A controlled study by Cox *et al.* (1993) compared depression in parturient and non-parturient women, and found a marked increase in the onset of depression in parturient women within one month of delivery. He therefore concluded that postnatal depression is a direct consequence of the physical and psychological stresses of childbirth. Others consider postnatal

Table 1 ICD-10 classifications of puerperal disorders

F53	**Mental and behavioural disorders associated with the puerperium, not elsewhere classified**
	This classification should be used only for mental disorders associated with the puerperium (commencing within 6 weeks of delivery) that do not meet the criteria for disorders classified elsewhere in this book, either *because insufficient information is available*, or because it is considered that *special additional clinical features are present which make classification elsewhere inappropriate*. It will usually be possible to classify mental disorders associated with the puerperium by using two other codes: the first is from elsewhere in chapter V (F) and indicates the specific type of mental disorder (usually affective (F30–F39)), and the second is 099.3 (mental diseases and diseases of the nervous system complicating the puerperium) of ICD-10.
F53.0	***Mild*** **mental and behavioural disorders associated with the puerperium not elsewhere classified**
	Includes: postnatal depression NOS
	postpartum depression NOS
F53.1	***Severe*** **mental and behavioural disorders associated with the puerperium, not elsewhere classified**
	Includes: puerperal psychosis NOS
F53.8	**Other mental and behavioural disorders associated with the puerperium, not elsewhere classified**
F53.9	**Puerperal mental disorder, unspecified**

Source: Reproduced by permission of WHO, from *The ICD-10 Classification of Mental and Behavioural Disorders: Clinical Descriptions and Diagnostic Guidelines.* Geneva, World Health Organization, 1992.

depression unique because it follows childbirth and has atypical signs and symptoms (Pitt, 1968; Dalton, 1980).

Aetiology

It is difficult to identify the cause because, despite marked differences in society over the last century, there has been little change in the incidence of major mental illness associated with childbirth. Similarly the incidence of minor mental illness related to childbirth has remained much the same over the last two decades. The cause is therefore unlikely to be a particular change in society or obstetric practice. Rather it is probably multifactorial and a combination of biological, psychological and social factors.

Biological reasons include genetic make-up, gynaecological and obstetric problems (Stein *et al.*, 1989), parity and maternal age, the hormonal changes which occur in the early puerperium and the appearance and behaviour of the baby. Psychological factors may include the woman's early relationship with her parents, personality development, acceptance of her sexuality and the ability to accept dependence (Cox, 1986). Women who display anxious or obsessional traits in their personality, or appear too controlled and compliant have a greater risk of developing postnatal depression. The previous psychiatric history of the woman (and her family) has been found to be a risk factor in many cases (Wolkind *et al.*, 1988). Women who have a severe episode of the postnatal blues may develop depression and therefore need close observation to detect the possible onset.

Social factors include a wide range of conditions and situations which include:

▶ Stressful life events such as family and housing problems (Paykel *et al.*, 1980).
▶ Poor social support (Stein *et al.*, 1989).
▶ Unsupportive partner (Playfair and Gowers, 1981).
▶ Low socio-economic status (Stein *et al.*, 1989).
▶ Tiredness, loneliness and not being able to cope (Levy and Kline, 1994).

Diagnosis

Midwives have a major role in recognizing women at high risk of developing postnatal depression, and of detecting the early signs of this distressing condition. It is sometimes difficult at first to distinguish between the tiredness and emotional instability which are common features of the puerperium, and the onset of a depressive illness. Careful assessment of the woman's emotional state is an essential part of the midwife's role in postnatal care. To achieve this the midwife must encourage the woman to express her feelings and anxieties, not only about her baby but also about herself, and listen carefully both to what she says and to what she may not be able to express openly. Many women are embarrassed by what they see as their inability to cope and are sometimes reticent about admitting it. An empathic, non-directive, empowering approach by the midwife can enable the mother to voice her anxieties and true feelings. If depression is suspected help can then be offered.

Women at risk of postnatal depression have already been discussed and will require particularly close observation in the postnatal period. Possible signs and symptoms of the condition are tearfulness, despondency, feelings of inadequacy and inability to cope, anxiety and a ruminative worry, often about the baby, and guilt about their perceived poor mothering skills, yet the baby is usually well cared for and thriving. Sleep disturbance is a common symptom and may be early morning waking or difficulty in getting off to sleep. Because so many postnatal women are disturbed at night by their baby, this symptom is often missed. During the day the mother will feel constantly tired and will often go to bed to rest and avoid the company of others.

Profound and consistent lowering of the mood, depressive ideation, slowing of psychomotor functions and biological symptoms such as early morning waking are features of severe depression. Another symptom is 'anomie', which is a painful feeling of inability to experience love or pleasure. These mothers often feel that they do not or cannot love their babies, but their baby is obviously lovingly handled and cared for by the mother. This dissonance between the mother's comments and behaviour is an important diagnostic point and one which the midwife, if still in attendance, should recognize.

The Edinburgh Postnatal Depression Scale has been developed for the diagnosis of postnatal depression (Cox and Holden, 1994) (see Tables 2 and 3). It is a simple, self-rating, 10-item scale which was designed to be used at about six weeks postpartum. It can also be used at other times, including the antenatal period for high-risk women (Clement, 1995). Scores for individual items range from 0 to 3 according to severity and the total score for all items is added together. Women who score 12 or more on the scale are likely to be suffering from depressive illness. Refer-

Table 2   Edinburgh Postnatal Depression Scale

Today's date . . . .   Baby's age . . . .   Baby's date of birth . . . .
Birth weight . . . .   Triplets/twins/single . . . .   Male/female . . . .
Mother's age . . . .   Number of other children: 0 1 2 3 4 5 5+

HOW ARE YOU FEELING?

As you have recently had a baby, we would like to know how you are feeling now. Please <u>underline</u> the answer which comes closest to how you have felt in the past 7 days, not just how you feel today.
Here is an example, already completed:

> I have felt happy:
>   Yes, most of the time   No, not very often
>   <u>Yes, some of the time</u>   No, not at all

This would mean: 'I have felt happy some of the time' during the past week. Please complete the other questions in the same way.

IN THE PAST SEVEN DAYS

1. I have been able to laugh and see the funny side of things:
   As much as I always could
   Not quite so much now
   Definitely not so much now
   Not at all
2. I have looked forward with enjoyment to things:
   As much as I ever did
   Rather less than I used to
   Definitely less than I used to
   Hardly at all
3. I have blamed myself unnecessarily when things went wrong:
   Yes, most of the time
   Yes, some of the time
   Not very often
   No, never
4. I have felt worried and anxious for no very good reason:
   No, not at all
   Hardly ever
   Yes, sometimes
   Yes, very often
5. I have felt scared or panicky for no very good reason:
   Yes, quite a lot
   Yes, sometimes
   No, not much
   No, not at all

6. Things have been getting on top of me:
   Yes, most of the time I haven't been able to cope at all
   Yes, sometimes I haven't been coping as well as usual
   No, most of the time I have coped quite well
   No, I have been coping as well as ever
7. I have been so unhappy that I have had difficulty sleeping:
   Yes, most of the time
   Yes, sometimes
   Not very often
   No, not at all
8. I have felt sad or miserable:
   Yes, most of the time
   Yes quite often
   Not very often
   No, not at all
9. I have been so unhappy that I have been crying
   Yes, most of the time
   Yes, quite often
   Only occasionally
   No, never
10. The thought of harming myself has occurred to me:
   Yes, quite often
   Sometimes
   Hardly ever
   Never

Edinburgh Postnatal Depression Scale: Scoring Sheet

1. I have been able to laugh and see the funny side of things:
   As much as I always could — 0
   Not quite so much now — 1
   Definitely not so much now — 2
   Not at all — 3
2. I have looked forward with enjoyment to things:
   As much as I ever did — 0
   Rather less than I used to — 1
   Definitely less than I used to — 2
   Hardly at all — 3
3. I have blamed myself unnecessarily when things go wrong:
   Yes, most of the time — 3
   Yes, some of the time — 2
   Not very often — 1
   No, never — 0
4. I have felt worried and anxious for no very good reason:
   No, not at all — 0
   Hardly, ever — 1
   Yes, sometimes — 2
   Yes, very often — 3
5. I have felt scared or panicky for no very good reason:
   Yes, quite a lot — 3
   Yes, sometimes — 2
   No, not much — 1
   No, not at all — 0

6. Things have been getting on top of me:
   Yes, most of the time I haven't been able to cope at all — 3
   Yes, sometimes I haven't been coping as well as usual — 2
   No, most of the time I have coped quite well — 1
   No, I have been coping as well as ever — 0
7. I have been so unhappy that I have had difficulty sleeping:
   Yes, most of the time — 3
   Yes, sometimes — 2
   Not very often — 1
   No, not at all — 0
8. I have felt sad or miserable:
   Yes, most of the time — 3
   Yes, quite often — 2
   Not very often — 1
   No, not at all — 0
9. I have been so unhappy that I have been crying:
   Yes, most of the time — 3
   Yes, quite often — 2
   Only occasionally — 1
   No, never — 0
10. The thought of harming myself has occurred to me:
   Yes, quite often — 3
   Sometimes — 2
   Hardly ever — 1
   Never — 0

Source: Cox, J. and Holden, J. (eds) (1994) *Perinatal Psychiatry*, pp. 139–143. Reproduced with permission from Gaskell and Royal College of Psychiatrists, London.

Table 3 EPDS record sheet

Health professional . . . .   District . . . .

Name	Baby's D.O.B.	5–8 wk EPDS		10–14 wk EPDS		20–26 wk EPDS		Counselling support		Referred?
		Date	Score	Date	Score	Date	Score	Start	End	Date

Source: Cox, J. and Holden, J. (eds) (1994) *Perinatal Psychiatry*, pp. 139–143. Reproduced with permission from Gaskell and Royal College of Psychiatrists, London.

ral for further assessment and treatment should then be offered.

Management

Postnatal depression may be treated by counselling, cognitive therapy or medication. Non-directive counselling has proved to be a very useful method of managing postnatal depression in many cases. It is a 'person-centred' approach which enables the client to talk through their feelings freely in a nurturing, non-judgemental atmosphere. The counsellor does not interfere, only listens and conveys interest and warmth, thereby enabling the clients to come to know themselves better and find their own solutions to their problems (Holden *et al.*, 1989). Clement (1995) recommends the introduction and auditing of this form of counselling for women in pregnancy who are depressed.

Postnatal support groups may be very helpful to women who feel isolated and lonely after childbirth and may offer the support which a woman needs from those who are experiencing similar problems. The Association for Postnatal Illness and the National Childbirth Trust provide peer support and information about postnatal depression. In some cases support groups are linked to health care workers who can identify those who are in need of treatment, or a review of their treatment.

Antidepressant drugs may be required for the treatment of some mothers suffering from postnatal depression. These include amitriptyline and tetracyclic drugs such as mianserin, both of which must be given in adequate dosages to be effective. Once a satisfactory response has been achieved they are continued for a further 3–4 months at least. Good supervision and support are also required. Referral to a psychiatrist is necessary if the woman fails to respond to antidepressant drugs, or has suicidal tendencies.

Mothers with severe depressive illness should be admitted to a psychiatric unit, preferably a special mother and baby unit with their baby. Treatment with ECT may be required, together with antidepressant drugs which should be continued for six months. Most mothers with postnatal depression respond very well to treatment, usually within 4–6 weeks.

Prognosis

Mothers who have suffered from severe depressive illness following childbirth have a one in five increased risk of recurrence following the birth of another child.

MINOR MENTAL ILLNESS

Minor mental illness, or neurosis, is used to describe a very common group of conditions in which the signs and symptoms vary only in intensity from those which are a normal human reaction to stress. The symptoms of emotional turbulence, anxiety and unhappiness tend to predominate and can be very distressing and disabling. There is not usually any impairment in the mother's perception of reality. The commonest condition is that of *depressive neurosis*, also known as reactive depression. *Anxiety states, panic disorder* and *phobic anxiety states* are also fairly common, whereas *obsessional compulsive illness* is much rarer. The incidence of these conditions is probably the same as in non-puerperal women.

Aetiology

Some women are particularly likely to develop puerperal neurosis due to personality problems, social problems and recent major life events.

Signs and symptoms

Although these illnesses may start within the first few weeks after delivery, they rarely present until three months or so after delivery. The neurotic illness often focuses on perceived problems concerning the baby.

Management

Support groups where mothers can share their problems can be very helpful. They may help to reduce the guilt and a feeling of alienation which many of these mothers experience. A social worker may be able to help with social problems. Medication is not the first line of treatment but when required the benzodiazepines are usually prescribed for these minor depressive and anxiety states.

PUERPERAL PSYCHOSIS

The term 'puerperal psychosis' is used to describe a group of illnesses which occur following childbirth and are characterized by delusions, hallucinations and impaired perception of reality. The majority of puerperal psychoses are affective (manic or depressive) conditions. A minority are schizophrenia-like conditions. True, chronic schizophrenia arising for the first time in the puerperium is very uncommon.

The incidence of puerperal psychosis is 2–3 per 1000 live births (Cox, 1986).

Signs and symptoms

The onset of the mania and schizophrenia-like illnesses and about a third of the depressive psychoses is abrupt and occurs between the 3rd and 14th postnatal day (Kendell *et al.*, 1987). In most cases therefore the midwife is attending the mother when the illness develops. The mother looks physically unwell and is in a state of perplexity, confusion, fear and distress. She is restless, suffers from insomnia and may also be disorientated about time and place. Insomnia is one of the most important symptoms and any woman who has a sleep disturbance not explained by a crying baby, noise, or other legitimate reasons should be closely observed by the midwife.

Nineteenth-century French psychiatrists described this initial phase of puerperal psychosis as the '*delirée triste*'. At this stage it is difficult to make a specific psychiatric diagnosis. The mental state then changes rapidly with the emergence of prominent delusions, hallucinations and disturbances of behaviour. These symptoms are generally very severe in women suffering from puerperal psychosis; more severe than in non-puerperal patients suffering from a major mental illness. The symptoms often focus on the baby or the recent delivery. The mother may have delusions that the baby has died, or that something dreadful is going to happen to it. Women with puerperal psychosis are also more likely to be manic than non-puerperal patients with manic depressive illness.

Within a few days of the onset of the symptoms it is usually possible to recognize whether the illness is affective (manic or depressive) or a schizophrenia-like condition.

Aetiology

It is now thought that biological factors, including genetic factors, are likely to be as important, or perhaps even more important, than possible psychosocial and obstetric factors (Cox and Holden, 1994). A family or personal history of affective psychosis is therefore a major risk factor and should always be elicited when the history is taken in early pregnancy. The risk for a woman with a previous history of affective psychosis is estimated to be as high as 1 in 3 and 1 in 2 (Kendell *et al.*, 1987; Wieck *et al.*, 1991). Cox and Holden (1994) recommend that a woman with a personal history of affective psychosis should be referred to a specialist psychiatrist during her pregnancy. Prophylactic treatment, started usually soon after delivery, can then be considered.

Another recent explanation for the development of puerperal psychosis is the major change which occurs in the levels of the steroid hormones at this time, especially the drop in oestrogen (Wieck, 1989). It is thought that high-risk patients develop a hypersensitivity of the central D_2 receptors and that this may be related to the effect of the drop in the oestrogen level on the dopamine system. Another theory is that the condition is related to the fall in progesterone level which occurs after delivery (Dalton, 1985).

A recent study found the development of the maternity blues was associated with high antenatal progesterone concentrations, low postnatal progesterone concentrations, and a steep fall in concentration after delivery (Harris *et al.*, 1994). A severe episode of the blues in the postnatal period may lead to depression, and therefore the researchers suggest that it may be possible to reduce the problem of the blues by treating mothers with progesterone. Further studies are required to test the effects of treatment with progesterone on the severity of the blues.

Psychosocial and obstetric factors are also thought to be possible causes of puerperal psychosis. Those who appear to be at higher risk include:

▶ primiparae who have had major obstetric problems, including Caesarean section;
▶ those from the higher socio-economic groups;
▶ those who are older than average at the birth of their first child, are married, and have a relatively long interval from marriage to the birth of their first child; and
▶ those who have had a major life event shortly before or after the birth of their child.

Severe episodes of the blues may lead to postnatal depression and untreated depression may develop into a major depressive psychosis (Cox, 1986).

Management

These women are profoundly disturbed and require admission to hospital together with their babies, where possible. Psychiatric units with specialized mother and baby sections where such mothers can be skilfully nursed and treated should be available (Oates, 1994), but according to Prettyman and Friedman (1991), fewer than half the health districts in the United Kingdom have facilities for admitting the mother with her baby. Separation from the baby is inadvisable since it invariably causes an increase in the symptoms, including delusions that the baby is dead or will come to serious harm. The presence of the baby in hospital with the mother aids her treatment, thereby shortening her hospital stay and, in the longer term, improves the mother–baby relationship.

The immediate priority is to *sedate* the mother sufficiently to reduce symptoms, yet allow for adequate hydration and nutrition. If the mother is in a postnatal ward when puerperal psychosis first presents, she may be sedated there for about 48 hours and closely observed. In a significant minority of cases the illness will resolve quickly and admission to a psychiatric unit will then be unnecessary. This is particularly likely if a psychotic episode arises following a Caesarean section. The majority of mothers, however, will eventually require admission to a psychiatric unit. Adequate sedation is usually achieved with the phenothiazines or butyrophenones. These drugs also reduce perplexity and fear. A dose of 50 mg of chlorpromazine may be given three times a day, plus 75 or 100 mg at night because the mental state is often worse then. After a few days when a diagnosis of affective or schizophrenia-like illness can be made, the appropriate treatment can be instigated. *Electroconvulsive therapy* (ECT) may be required for mania and schizophrenia-like conditions if they do not respond to medication with 3–7 days. In the case of the early onset of depressive illness, ECT may be the treatment of choice as soon as a diagnosis is made. The tricyclic antidepressants take 10–14 days before they take effect and thus are not appropriate as first-line treatment for severely disturbed, depressive psychotic patients.

Prognosis

The short- and long-term prognosis is good following puerperal psychosis, despite the initial severity of the illness. Manic patients usually respond to treatment within two weeks, often in a few days. Most of the severe depressive puerperal psychoses will resolve within 6–8 weeks. By six months after the onset of the illness most mothers will have made a full recovery. Only a few have a more protracted recovery. There is a danger of relapse occurring, however, particularly in the early weeks after delivery, so the phenothiazines may be continued for some weeks, or until the baby is three months old. One in five of the women who have had a puerperal psychosis will be at risk of developing a further episode of mental illness following the birth of their next child (Cox, 1986). The illness is likely to follow a similar pattern and will have the same prognosis. The risks are lower for those who developed a psychosis following a Caesarean section or a major life event. Nearly one-third of all women who suffer from puerperal psychosis will develop a manic depressive illness not related to childbearing at a later stage in life. It therefore seems that women who are susceptible to manic depressive illness are especially vulnerable in the puerperium.

Table 4 Drugs and breastfeeding

Tricyclic antidepressants	Safe in full dosage
Chlorpromazine ⎫	
Trifluoperazine ⎬ phenothiazines	Safe in moderate dosage
Haloperidol ⎭	
Benzodiazepines/alcohol	Best avoided
Lithium	Dangerous

Drugs and Breastfeeding

Psychotropic drugs are invariably prescribed for women who develop severe mental illness following childbirth. It is when the mother is breastfeeding that particular care must be taken to ensure that drugs are prescribed which are not only effective for the mother but also safe for the baby (see Table 4). The continuation of breastfeeding is often very important to the mother and, indeed, should be encouraged as it will aid the recovery of her self-esteem and promote her relationship with her baby. Discontinuing breastfeeding only adds to the burden of guilt the mother often feels later. The tricyclic antidepressants appear to be safe in full dosage for breastfeeding mothers. The phenothiazines are also probably safe in moderate dosages, although the baby should be closely observed and breastfeeding may have to be suspended if the baby becomes too drowsy and does not feed well. In this case the breast milk must be expressed and discarded. It is important to try and maintain lactation by regular expression of the breasts until it is considered safe for the baby to resume breastfeeding. Lithium is not considered a safe drug to give to breastfeeding women. With close consultation and co-operation between the professionals caring for the woman it is usually possible to enable the mother to maintain her lactation and breastfeed successfully in due course.

References

Clement, S. (1995) 'Listening visits' in pregnancy: a strategy for preventing postnatal depression? *Midwifery* 11: 75–80.

Clement, S., Sikorski, J., Wilson, J. *et al.* (1994) Unpublished data. Antenatal Care Project, Dept of General Practice, United Medical and Dental School of Guy's and St. Thomas's Hospital, London.

Coghill, S.R., Caplan, H.L., Alexandra, H., Robson, K.M. & Kumar, R. (1986) Impact of maternal postnatal depression on cognitive development of young children. *Br. Med. J.* 292: 1165–1167.

Cox, J. (1986) *Postnatal Depression. A Guide for Health Professionals.* Edinburgh: Churchill Livingstone.

Cox, J., Holden, J.M. & Sagovsky, R. (1987) Detection of postnatal depression: development of the 10-item Edinburgh Depression Scale. *Br. J. Psychiat.* 150: 782–786.

Cox, J. & Holden, J. (eds) (1994) *Perinatal Psychiatry.* London: Gaskell.

Cox, J.L., Connor, Y. & Kendell, R.E. (1982) Prospective study of the psychiatric disorders of childbearing women. *Br. J. Psychiat.* 140: 111–117.

Cox, J., Murray, D. & Chapman, G. (1993) A controlled study of the onset, duration and prevalence of postnatal depression. *Br. J. Psychiat.* 150: 27–31.

Dalton, K. (1980) *Depression after Childbirth.* Oxford: Oxford University Press.

Dalton, K. (1985) Progesterone prophylaxis used successfully in postnatal depression. *Practitioner* 229: 507–508.

Green, J.M. & Murray, D. (1994) The use of the Edinburgh Postnatal Depression Scale in research to explore the relationship between antenatal and postnatal dysphoria. In Cox, J.L. & Holden, J.M. (eds) *Perinatal Psychiatry: Use and Misuse of the Edinburgh Postnatal Depression Scale.* London: Gaskell.

Harris, B., Lovett, L., Newcombe, R.G., Read, G.F., Walker, R. & Riad-Fahmy, D. (1994) Maternity blues and major endocrine changes: Cardiff puerperal mood and hormone study 11. *Br. Med. J.* 308: 949–953.

Hodnett, E.D. (1994a) Support from caregivers during at-risk pregnancy. In Enkin, M.W., Keirse, M.J.N.C., Renfrew, M.J. & Neilson, J.P. (eds) *Pregnancy and Childbirth Module.* Cochrane Database of Systematic Reviews: Review no. 04169. Disk Issue 1. Oxford: Update Software.

Hodnett, E.D. (1994b) Support from caregivers for socially disadvantaged mothers. In Enkin, M.W., Keirse, M.J.N.C., Renfrew, M.J. & Neilson, J.P. (eds) *Pregnancy and Childbirth Module.* Cochrane Database of Systemic Reviews. Review no. 07674. Disk Issue 1. Oxford: Update Software.

Holden, J., Sagovsky, R. & Cox, J.L. (1989) Counselling in a general practice setting: a controlled study of health visitor intervention in the treatment of postnatal depression. *Br. Med. J.* 298: 223–226.

Kendell, R.E., Chalmers, L. & Platz, C. (1987) The epidemiology of puerperal psychoses. *Br. J. Psychiat.* **151**: 662–673.

Kumar, R. & Robson, K. (1984) A prospective study of emotional disorders in childbearing women. *Br. J. Psychiat.* **144**: 35–47.

Levy, V. & Kline, P. (1994) Perinatal depression: a factor analysis. *Br. J. Midwifery* **2**(4): 154–159.

Oates, M.R. (1989) Management of major mental illness in pregnancy and the puerperium. In Oates, M.R. (ed.) *Psychological Aspects of Obstetrics and Gynaecology. Clinical Obstetrics and Gynaecology*, Vol. 3, pp. 839–856. London: Baillière Tindall.

Oates, M.R. (1994) Postnatal mental illness: organisation and function of services. In Cox, J. & Holden, J. *Perinatal Psychiatry*, pp. 18–19. London: Gaskell.

O'Hara, M.W. & Zekowski, E.M. (1988) Postpartum depression: a comprehensive review. In Kumar, R. & Brockington, I.F. (eds) *Motherhood and Mental Illness*. London: John Wright.

Paykel, E.S., Emms, E.M., Fletcher, J. & Rassaby, E.S. (1980) Life events and social support in puerperal depression. *Br. J. Psychiat.* **136**: 339–346.

Pitt, B. (1968) Atypical depression following childbirth. *Br. J. Psychiat.* **114**: 1325–1335.

Playfair, H.R. & Gowers, J.I. (1981) Depression following childbirth – a search for predictive signs. *J. R. Coll. Gen. Pract.* **31**: 201–208.

Prettyman, R.J. & Friedman, T. (1991) Care of women with puerperal psychiatric disorders in England and Wales. *Br. Med. J.* **302**: 1345–1346.

Romito, P. (1989) Unhappiness after childbirth. In Chalmers, I., Enkin, M. & Keirse, M.J.N.C. (eds) *Effective Care in Pregnancy and Childbirth*. Oxford: Oxford University Press.

Stein, A., Cooper, P.J. & Campbell, E.A. (1989) Social adversity and perinatal complications: their relation to postnatal depression. *Br. Med. J.* **171**: 1073–1074.

Taylor, A., Adams, D. & Glover, V. (1994) Postnatal depression: identification, risk factors and effects. *Br. J. Midwifery* **2**: 253–257.

Uddenberg, N. & Englesson, X. (1978) Prognosis of postpartum mental disturbances. *Acta Psychiat. Scand.* **58**(3): 201–212.

Watson, J.P., Elliot, S.A., Rugg, A.J. & Brough, D.A. (1984) Psychiatric disorder in pregnancy and the first postnatal year. *Br. J. Psychiat.* **144**: 453–462.

WHO (World Health Organization) (1992) *The ICD-10 Classification of Mental and Behavioural Disorders*. Geneva: WHO.

Wieck, J.P. (1989) Endocrine aspects of postnatal depression. In *Psychological Aspects of Obstetrics and Gynaecology, Clinical Obstetrics and Gynaecology*, Vol. 3, Part 4, pp. 857–877. London: Baillière Tindall.

Wieck, A., Kumar, R., Hirst, A.D. *et al.* (1991) Increased sensitivity of dopamine receptors and recurrences of affective psychoses after childbirth. *Br. Med. J.* **303**: 613–616.

Wolkind, S., Zajicek-Coleman, E. & Ghodsian, M. (1988) Continuities in maternal depression. *Int. J. Family Psychol.* **1**:167–181.

Part Thirteen

Sexuality and Fertility

59

Sexuality and Childbearing

Sexuality

Sexuality is the state or quality of being sexual and is distinct from gender classification which is, according to Cucchiari (Ortner and Whitehead, 1981), the 'symbolic or meaning system that consists of two complementary yet exclusive categories into which all human beings are placed'. Gender in effect describes socially constructed behavioural attributes. Sexuality is also distinct from sex which can mean the biological basis of gender determination, i.e. the characteristics associated with the sex chromosomes, or commonly, the act of coitus. Sexuality is a modern concept that encompasses the whole person. It is concerned with sexual orientation, desires, expressiveness, innate feelings, sexual instincts and identity at every stage of the lifespan. This being so, the childbearing year is no exception, and in fact sexuality impinges on the process for the women, their partners and their carers to an extent which is not always recognized.

Sexual Response Pattern

Sexual arousal was first studied scientifically as a physiological process by Masters and Johnson (1966) in what have become classical laboratory studies. It can be triggered off in a great many ways and by a variety of stimuli, both physical and psychological (Haeberle, 1983). Although all the senses can be involved in the arousal process, the sense of touch is probably the one most often involved. Masters and Johnson (1966) described the human sexual response pattern as a cycle having four phases: excitement, plateau, orgasm and resolution, the first and last being the longest.

THE MALE RESPONSE

The primary sign of male excitement is the erection of the penis. As he is stimulated the spongelike structures in the corpora cavernosa and the corpus spongiosum fill with blood and cause the penis to rise and stiffen (penile tumescence). Simultaneously the dartos muscle of the scrotum and the spermatic cord contracts, causing the testes to be drawn up towards the body. As the excitement increases there is a rise in the heart rate and blood pressure and in fair-skinned men there may appear a flush or red rash over the lower abdomen, the shoulders, the neck and the face. The nipples also undergo a change and they become erect (Walton, 1994).

Following full erection, the penis may undergo slightly more vasocongestion (the plateau phase) and Cowper's glands may secrete a drop or two of fluid containing spermatozoa. As the myotonia and nervous tension increase there is a sudden release followed by a series of involuntary contractions aided by thrusting movements from the pelvis. This is the orgasm which also causes involuntary, rhythmic contractions of the internal organs. During the orgasmic phase about 3 ml of semen is forced out in quick spurts through the urethral orifice. Breathing becomes very rapid and the heart and blood pressure rise even further than before. Orgasm and ejaculation usually but not necessarily occur together. Following orgasm comes the fourth and final phase of the cycle, the resolution phase, during which the penis and the rest of the body, e.g. the blood pressure returns to the unexcited state.

Accompanying the physiological resolution is a period of subjective calm of variable length during which the man is incapable of having another orgasm. This refractory period is thought to be a peculiarly male phenomenon because women are capable of being multi-orgasmic in a short period of time (Masters and Johnson, 1966).

THE FEMALE RESPONSE

In females the first obvious sign of sexual stimulation is wetness of the vagina. Blood vessels (the vestibular bulbs) are linked to the clitoris and as it is stimulated they become engorged with blood. Lymph is transuded across the vaginal walls and the whole of the vagina is lubricated and it increases in length and in width at the inner end. The clitoris itself undergoes tumescence similarly to the penis but unlike the penis does not undergo erection. The shaft of the clitoris enlarges to lie in closer apposition to the underlying tissue and retracts further under the prepuce. The labia minora darken and increase in size whilst the labia majora flatten out and expose the vaginal orifice (more so in a parous woman).

During this phase the breasts become engorged and swollen and the nipples become erect. Most women exhibit the sexual flush which reaches its peak during the plateau period and resolves abruptly during resolution.

When the excitement has reached a high just prior to orgasm the clitoris retracts under the prepuce (the *plateau period*). The outer third of the vagina contracts and Bartholin's glands secrete a few drops of fluid. Hyperventilation occurs, and the heart rate and the blood pressure increase. Just prior to orgasm there is an increase in muscle tension throughout the body. As the orgasm takes place contractions start in the outer third of the vagina (the *orgasmic platform*). Involuntary spasms occur in the anal sphincter and the uterus also starts to contract beginning at the fundus and ending in the lower segment (Walton, 1994). Pregnancy increases sensitivity to the effects of orgasm, particularly in the last two trimesters.

Rapid decongestion of the areolar tissue occurs immediately afterwards and is external evidence that orgasm has been reached. Multi-orgasmic women have orgasm after orgasm, but after the final orgasm the sex organs return to their unexcited state.

Pregnancy

THE FIRST TRIMESTER

One of the most common worries in pregnancy is whether to have sex or not. However, it does not usually constitute too much of a problem in early pregnancy until it is confirmed. Then women may react in one of two ways: They may either feel liberated and extremely libidinous, or they may find that their sexual desire is reduced. The pelvic congestion may have the effect of increasing desire and, for some women, it enables them to experience orgasm for the first time. For others, there is a fear of harming the fetus and an associated avoidance of orgasm.

Physiological problems

The breasts of a nulliparous woman undergo an increase in size of approximately 25% in the plateau period of sexual activity and by the end of the first trimester have undergone a similar increase in size (Masters and Johnson, 1966). So when there is sexual activity in pregnancy, the resultant 50% increase does cause some women to complain of discomfort.

Backache can occur after coitus but, although not usually of any great significance, it can be upsetting and worrying. Some women also complain of a slight ache after intercourse in the midline over the pubic area. This could be due to either an orgasmic response in the uterus itself, or tension on the round ligaments as the uterus takes on a more upright and rounded shape.

Libido

Early pregnancy is a time when women feel very tired and so desire may decrease. Some women may associate sex with a desire for pregnancy and now do not feel the need to indulge. Or they may dislike sexual intercourse for any of a number of reasons. It may be a longstanding sexual problem such as pain or psychological reasons or the partner may not be a skilful lover and the woman may use the pregnancy as an excuse to reduce the chance of disappointment. Or she may simply be worried and frightened, particularly if there is a history of infertility or miscarriage. She or her partner may worry that they will harm the fetus in some way. Although research has been limited there is no evidence (Behrman *et al.*, 1989) to suggest that it is a significant factor in miscarriage.

Male worries

Male partners may also worry that they may do some harm to the fetus and a small number worry that the fetus will damage them. If a man worries that he may be hurting his partner, or damaging his unborn baby, then it may be quite difficult for him to gain and maintain an erection. It is easier to keep it in perspective and have less anxiety if the couple are well informed. So midwives should give information about sex in pregnancy in as factual and objective way as all other advice in pregnancy is given.

There may be social, religious or cultural factors which may make a couple abstain from sex in pregnancy. However, there are generally no physical reasons to abstain unless there is a history of infection, bleeding or previous early miscarriage, in which case the couple should seek advice from their general practitioner.

Being pregnant is not all sexually negative because for many couples it is the best time of all. The fear of pregnancy has gone so there is no need to use contraception. Pelvic congestion and an increase in oestrogen and progesterone results in increased lubrication of the vagina and the woman may experience a heightened response and the man may feel very sensitive, proud and protective.

THE SECOND TRIMESTER

In the second trimester the woman's shape is noticeably changing and how the couple react to the changes depends very much on their attitudes to body shape in general and to the pregnancy. Some women are really proud of their increasing size whilst others feel that they have become fat. Likewise with men, some adore the look of pregnant women and others simply do not. It is all a matter of individual taste, socialization and religious and cultural upbringing.

The second trimester is mainly one of heightened sexual awareness and eroticism. For most women the minor disorders of pregnancy have ceased, they no longer feel quite so tired and they may have finished working. They no longer need to fear miscarriage and yet they are not so large as to be uncomfortable. The leucorrhoea of pregnancy ensures lubrication and ease of penetration. The venous congestion of pregnancy results in a heightened manifestation of all aspects of the sexual act so that the area becomes congested, the orgasm is heightened and the vaginal lumen becomes smaller, thus gripping the penis tighter. There is also a tendency for the uterus to contract but these contractions do not seem to be harmful. On the contrary they are of the Braxton Hicks type and perfuse the uterus with blood.

THE THIRD TRIMESTER

There is a sharp decrease in sexual activity in the third trimester (Kenny, 1976). This is due to many factors, but in the main is associated with the discomforts of late pregnancy (Walton, 1994). There may also be medical conditions in some women that mitigate against increased sexual activity, e.g. diabetes mellitus with its accompanying and irritating monilial infections. Some women report an overall lack of interest in sex, and an overwhelming preoccupation with the unborn baby and the forthcoming labour. This is particularly so as the estimated date of confinement draws near or is passed. There is also the worry that intercourse will bring on a preterm labour or injure the fetus. It can also be very frightening if there is spotting of blood after intercourse, which is quite likely in late pregnancy due to the friability of the extremely engorged cervical mucosa.

The man may also be quite worried about causing damage to the baby and find that his desire is reduced because of it.

There are several factors which combine at the end of pregnancy to start labour off, e.g. increased size, reduction in oxytocinase and increase in prostaglandins and oxytocin (see Chapter 28). Sexual intercourse in itself is not usually sufficient to do so, but at the end of pregnancy semen, which contains prostaglandins, may bathe the cervix and facilitate the action of the oxytocin from the pituitary glands. The uterus may contract during orgasm and this may facilitate the onset of labour, but not if the other factors are absent. So, sex in late pregnancy is unlikely to start preterm labour. It is highly unlikely that the fetus will be endangered by such activity, although in a compromised pregnancy uterine contractions in themselves may cause a deceleration in the fetal heart rate. Sexual intercourse should be avoided if there is bleeding or ruptured membranes.

PRACTICES IN PREGNANCY

Lack of knowlege about safe practices in pregnancy may make couples very anxious. They usually fear for the baby or worry about possible infection. It is not enough to tell them to be careful. Most people do not know what that means and so make up their own rules as they go along.

In the main there are only two practices that should not be undertaken:

1 *Blowing of air into the vagina*: Cunnilingus in itself is not harmful if it is restricted to oral stimulation of the clitoris and external genitalia. It is unlikely to cause damage because the operculum will prevent air entering the uterus, but it must be stressed that forceful blowing of air into the vagina may be highly dangerous.
2 *Insertion of foreign bodies into the vagina*: There is the physical danger of piercing the vaginal walls, or damaging the cervical os, and there is a risk of altering the pH balance of the vaginal walls and causing infection.

Fellatio (oral stimulation of the male genitalia) is not considered dangerous (except with other high-risk factors present, e.g. HIV) because, even though semen contains prostaglandins, they will be destroyed by the stomach acid.

Some positions in pregnancy can be uncomfortable, but the missionary position can actually cause problems. The inferior vena cava will be compressed by the gravid uterus when the woman lies on her back. Venous return is impeded and this will be compounded if the woman has the weight of her partner on her as well. It is probably better in late pregnancy to make use of woman-on-top positions, i.e. either sitting on her partner's knee or straddling him whilst he lies on his back. These have the advantage of enabling the woman to control the depth of penetration. Rear entry positions with the woman either kneeling or lying in the spoon position may also be better at this time (Walton, 1994).

Sexual intercourse does not necessarily mean penetrative sex. There are other ways for couples who do not want to do it, or have been advised against it for some reason. These include masturbation (self and mutual), oral sex, deep massage or simply kissing and cuddling. There is no right or wrong way unless one of the couple is not happy with the proposed practices.

The fears about infection are very often unfounded. There is little chance of infection except where there are ruptured membranes, or where there is a pre-existing infection in one of the couple which can be transmitted sexually, e.g. *Trichomonas vaginalis* or gonorrhoea.

The professional should always remember that some women are pregnant as a result of incest or rape within or without marriage, or they may be an adult survivor of sexual abuse, or they may be in an abusive situation. This will give rise to fears, anxieties, disempowerment, or at least ambiguous feelings towards sex in pregnancy, and which may continue afterwards. They will need a great deal of support and possibly expert counselling or practical help.

Labour

Childbirth is not often considered a sexual and erotic event but it is sexuality expressed through the body. It is the endpoint of a process that began with the sexual act. Physiologically it is very similar, it is genital focused and is a time of intense emotional responses. It is strange that this is not recognized, if only by the couple themselves, but perhaps it is, but not acknowledged.

The beginning of labour is different for everyone but there are shared similarities, one of which is a feeling of excitement and anticipation. When this is shared each becomes very exhilarated and, when a young couple are in a state of excitement and shared animation, this is arousal. It does not necessarily mean they are about to have sexual intercourse, but they might, and perhaps in this case they should. However, most couples are unlikely to do so unless all is well, they are at home and they know that no harm will be done. This is assuming that sexual arousal is expressed as coitus.

During labour the woman needs to be reassured that she is coping well and is in control. She will be helped by a confident partner who gives her all the physical and emotional support possible. An important aspect of care in labour is pain relief. Pain sets up a vicious circle whereby emotional and physical distress causes more painful contractions, a longer labour and a lowering of the pain threshold. If the woman is helped to manage the pain, the brain releases endorphins and the contractions are perceived as less painful and labour becomes easier.

There are two main ways to do this, either by pharmacological methods or by non-pharmacological methods which stimulate the gate response to pain (Melzack and Wall, 1965). One of the objectives of the non-pharmacological process is to induce a sense of well-being and confidence and a reduction in stress and tension. This is done by having present people in whom the woman has confidence, and by relaxation techniques, warm baths, aromatherapy, massage and transcutaneous electrical nerve stimulation (see Chapters 22 and 32). Some writers (Kitzinger, 1983; Flint, 1986) have drawn attention to the need for a cherishing approach to women in labour, and the need for privacy. With privacy the couple will be able to become more intimate and communicative. If the couple are able to lock the door, given comfortable surroundings and encouraged to hug, kiss and caress each other, it could have an extremely beneficial effect on the woman in labour.

During the earlier part of the first stage the couple could lie on the bed and perhaps have a sleep together, or the partner could massage the woman. As labour progresses many women complain of pains down their inner thighs and over the symphysis pubis. These could be alleviated to some extent by their partner stroking the inside of the thigh and over the mons veneris. This could be seen as so overtly sexual that they would be totally inhibited without privacy, but it could be beneficial in so many ways and may prove to

be another and effective method of pain relief. Oiling of the perineum is thought to help the perineum to stretch and reduce the incidence of trauma, but the supporting evidence to date is not conclusive (Avery and Burkett, 1986; Mynaugh, 1991). It is, however (according to anecdotal reports), very relaxing, particularly if it is performed by the partner, but again privacy is essential.

Stimulation of the nipples causes a rush of oxytocin from the posterior pituitary gland which makes the uterus contract. It could be performed by the partner as part of the process of labour (Dunham et al., 1991).

As the first stage of labour progresses it becomes physiologically similar to the sexual arousal process in many ways. The woman's blood pressure and her pulse rate may rise slightly. Contractions become more frequent and more intense. There is a feeling of mounting anticipation within the room and, for most women, it is a time to withdraw into herself. Outside events become no more than an unwelcome distraction.

Many women find the practices carried out in labour to be embarrassing, frightening and disturbing. These include vaginal and speculum examinations and having to be exposed. Not only is pain a factor here, but there are more subtle feelings of being powerless and vulnerable. Women who are sexual abuse survivors feel this even more keenly (Kitzinger, 1992; Grant, 1992; Draucker, 1992).

During labour the cervix dilates and is taken up until it is fully dilated and the second stage begins. The fetal head descends and comes down through the vagina, giving a feeling of movement and pressure in the rectum and on the perineum. This feeling is met with different reactions. Some women feel relief and push well. For others the feeling of fullness is hard to bear. Dependent on the individual, the feelings engendered may be pain and distress, or anticipation and excitement.

After the birth of the baby the mood is in some ways similar to that following orgasm. Both parents may be tired, but whilst normally after orgasm the woman will sleep, in this case she probably will not.

The long-term effect on sexuality of the practices and procedures carried out in labour have not been researched well, but there is enough in the literature to give some idea. The obstetric interventions fall into two categories. There are those like vaginal examinations that are considered merely to be uncomfortable and embarrassing, and there are those such as forceps deliveries that are considered traumatic. Most of the research (e.g. Ross, 1986) in this field concentrates on the physical long-term effects, rather than those of sexuality. However there are signs that this may be changing. Some midwives (Flint, 1986; Sleep and Grant, 1987; Wright, 1994) have pointed to factors which affect sexuality, e.g. throbbing and aching of the clitoris following delivery, and dyspareunia up to three months postnatally.

The Postnatal Period

The postnatal period in all countries has long been associated with taboos and restrictions on sexuality and this is no less true of the West. Much of the advice that is given forbids the resumption of sexual relationships in this period. There seem to be three main reasons for this: Mainly it seems to be due to a perceived threat of *infection*, i.e. the introduction of organisms into the vagina by the penis, but there is very little supporting evidence for this. Another reason is the *danger to the reproductive organs and unhealed sutures* and again, unless there is very inconsiderate, rough behaviour, this is not supported by the evidence. The third, and probably the most significant, is a *cultural prohibition*. Blood, and particularly the blood of childbirth, has long been seen as polluting and dangerous and, to counteract this pollution a number of religious and cultural restraints have arisen.

Sexuality can be expressed in many ways in the postnatal period, with or without coitus. Kissing, cuddling, and being held close are very significant. The important thing is to feel loved and supported at this time. For many couples the return to a harmonious sex life following the birth of the baby is unproblematic. However, this is not true of everyone because there may be several factors that intervene. These include ritual, physical, emotional, social and contextual factors.

Ritual factors

This is a time when the might of society is powerfully focused on the woman's body. The rituals of the institution act as the 'gaze' of the institution (Foucault, 1973). These rituals, which include procedures such as the postnatal examinations and the visits by the community midwife as well as religious customs, temper sexual activity.

Physical factors

Physical factors which mitigate against sexual activity include vaginal slackness, bruising and tenderness, sutures and scar tissue from Caesarean section, episiotomy or laceration, haemorrhoids, lacerations of the fine mucosa around the clitoris and the labia minora, monilial infections, sore nipples and high prolactin levels. Problems with one or more of these can affect the libido.

Emotional factors

There may be problems (new or existing) with regard to body image. It may be that the couple's sex life was not satisfactory before pregnancy and problems are longstanding and unresolved. New factors such as striae gravidarum can cause distress and compound poor body image. This may lead to anxiety which in itself can lead to disinterest or frigidity.

There may be feelings of resentment and anger on both sides due to the pain of labour, or to the presence (or death) of the baby, which can lead to problems within the relationship unless they are resolved. Sexual problems may be linked with postnatal depression and one in ten women referred to psychiatric clinics postnatally suffer from sexual dysfunction (Hesford and Bhanji, 1986). Or they may be as a result of male anxiety and feelings of inadequacy resulting from the delivery.

Social factors

Caring for a new baby is a very demanding and tiring occupation which in itself can lead to a loss of desire. If this is coupled with adverse social factors such as poor housing, lack of money, and poor family support, then it can lead to exhaustion and depression and low libido.

Contextual factors

Some couples have little or no privacy. They may share accommodation or they may have toddlers and young children who demand their attention at all times of the day and night. There may be teenagers at home whose presence is an inhibiting factor. Then of course there is the baby. Many couples feel worn out in the early weeks because of the demands of the baby and this is more so if the baby is fractious. Some sleep apart at this time in order for one or the other to have some sleep. It is a good idea if couples are encouraged to actively make time and space for themselves at this time.

Breastfeeding

Breastfeeding does not usually affect sexual activity. High levels of prolactin may counteract the effects of oestrogen, but does not usually cause dryness of the vagina. If it does a water-based lubricating gel can be advised. The orgasmic effect causes the milk to flow and some couples find this enhances their lovemaking, whilst others find it off putting. It is a matter of individual preference.

Breastfeeding is very satisfying for many women and they have a very special relationship with the baby at this time. Contrary to some myths it is not erotic, even though there are physical similarities in that the uterus is caused to contract by the action of the oxytocin produced.

Contraception

Anxiety is a major cause of sexual problems and one anxiety that fertile couples face is the prospect of pregnancy. This being so it is extremely important that they have an acceptable and effective method of contraception. The midwife or the general practitioner will give advice in the postnatal period and the general practitioner may provide ongoing family planning services. If not, the couple will be referred to the nearest family planning clinic. Alternatively the address of the nearest clinic can be found in the telephone book.

References

Avery, M.D. & Burkett, B.A. (1986) Effect of perineal massage on the incidence of episiotomy and perineal laceration in a nurse-midwifery service. *J. Nurse Midwifery* **31**: 128–134.

Behrman, S.J., Kistner, R.W. & Patton, G.W. (1989) *Progress in Infertility*, 3rd edn. Boston: Little Brown & Co.

Dunham, C., Myers, F., Barnden, N. *et al.* (1991) *Mamatoto. A Celebration of Birth*. London: Virago Press.

Draucker, C.B. (1992) *Counselling Survivors of Child Sexual Abuse*. London: Sage Publications.

Flint, C. (1986) *Sensitive Midwifery*. Guildford: Heinemann.

Foucault, M. (1973) *The Birth of the Clinic: An Archaeology of Medical Perception*. New York: Pantheon Books.

Grant, L.J. (1992) Effects of child sexual abuse: issues for obstetric caregivers. *Birth* **19**: 220–221.

Haeberle, E.J. (1983) *The Sex Atlas*. London: Sheldon Press.

Hesford, A. & Bhanji, S. (1986) Sexual dysfunction in women. *Nursing Times* 2 April: 49–51.

Kenny, J.A. (1976) Sexual attitudes and behaviour patterns during and following pregnancy. *Arch. Sexual Behaviour* **5**: 539–551.

Kitzinger, J.V. (1992) Counteracting not re-enacting, the violation of women's bodies: the challenge for perinatal caregivers. *Birth* **19**: 219–220.

Kitzinger, S. (1983) *Women's Experience of Sex*. London: Dorling Kindersley.

Masters, W. & Johnson, V. (1966) *Human Sexual Response*. London: J & A Churchill.

Melzack, R. & Wall, P.D. (1965) Pain mechanisms: a new theory. *Science* **150**: 971.

Mynaugh, P.A. (1991) A randomised study of two methods of teaching perineal massage: effect on practice rates, episiotomy rates, and lacerations. *Birth* **18**: 153–159.

Ortner, S.B. & Whitehead, H. (1981) *Sexual Meanings. The Construction of Gender and Sexuality*. Cambridge: Cambridge Press.

Ross, C. (1986) Let it rip? The healing of the perineum following spontaneous vaginal delivery. In *Research and the Midwife, Conference Proceedings, Glasgow*. Manchester: Department of Nursing Studies, Manchester University.

Sleep, J. & Grant, A. (1987) Pelvic floor exercises in postnatal care. *Midwifery* **3**(4): 158–64.

Walton, I. (1994) *Sexuality and Motherhood*. Hale: Books for Midwives Press.

Wright, A. (1994) Perineal pain after childbirth. *Midwives' Chronicle and Nursing Notes* **107**(1272): 22–23.

60

Family Planning

Family planning involves more than just the use of contraceptive techniques. However, the midwife must have a knowledge of these techniques if she is to offer a mother sound advice. During pregnancy and in particular in the early puerperium many women are receptive to advice and help; this should never be forced upon them, but because some are reticent about such matters, opportunities should be created for discussion.

In April 1974 the family planning service in the UK became the responsibility of the then Area Health Authorities and since then both services and supplies have been provided free under the National Health Service. A couple requiring family planning advice and supplies may go either to their general practitioner or to a community or hospital family planning clinic. In some areas there is also a domiciliary service for selected clients who for some reason do not attend the clinics.

The Family Planning Association still provides a service in many parts of the UK but charges are made.

Under-16-year-old girls may obtain contraceptive advice and services from any general practitioner or clinic without parental consent, secure of confidentiality. In these cases the doctor has a duty to try to persuade the girl to inform her parents. If this is not acceptable the doctor can still advise and prescribe contraceptives for her provided she is considered mature enough to understand fully the situation and risks involved.

The Role of the Midwife

Midwives recognize the importance of choice for mothers and their families, choices in place of birth, receiving continuity of care, and in spacing their families to suit their individual needs. Although primarily involved with mothers when the pregnancy is already established, midwives have a responsibility in providing information about contraception and safer sex.

Many women conceive their first child unintentionally and, while this may result in a wanted child, it is not always possible to adapt well to unplanned parenthood. The physical risks and emotional toll of pregnancies which occur at inopportune times are serious and may have long-term consequences for the whole family.

Every mother should be able to obtain help and support from her midwife, discussing her individual needs and those of her partner at some time during her pregnancy, childbirth or postpartum care. It is a vulnerable time for mothers and a sensitive midwife will be able to offer the information and education tailored to meet each family's needs at appropriate times during their care.

An appreciation of the emotional lability of mothers in the postpartum period, coupled with the physiological changes occurring after delivery, will be required if the information and management of this aspect of the midwives' care is to be handled effectively.

Religion and cultural beliefs also require some understanding. It is important that both partners have an opportunity to discuss these things in privacy, so that they may also express anxieties about resuming intercourse, if these exist, and obtain a clear understanding of how best to avoid further pregnancies until they are prepared for them. Partners may also need to talk through birth incidents and express their feelings about their experiences.

If the couple have used contraception previously and planned the pregnancy satisfactorily, then they may wish to resume the same method. If, however, the pregnancy was the result of contraceptive failure, then alternative methods may need to be discussed. The midwife should give information about the range of methods available, but being careful not to impose their beliefs, since the choice of method must be acceptable to the couple and they make the final decision.

The return of ovulation following delivery varies individually, but research suggests that the earliest possible ovulation occurs 21 days postpartum (Gray *et al.* 1987). It is therefore advisable to commence protection at this time. Mothers who breastfeed their babies on demand are likely to suppress ovulation for a longer time. Exactly how long will depend on the suckling of the baby at frequent intervals and include at least two full feeds during the night (McNeilly and Howie, 1982). Babies who vary in their feeding requirements and occasionally sleep through the night will not stimulate enough prolactin to provide control of ovulation.

The return of menstruation, when it occurs, indicates retrospective return of ovulation 14 days before.

It is therefore important that the mother understands that printed information on packets of hormonal contraceptives does not relate to postpartum situations, which need to be commenced independently of menstruation.

Mothers who sleep with their babies alongside them and who encourage demand feeding 24 hours a day over several years will have natural spacing of infants. Some cultural taboos include abstinence of intercourse during breastfeeding. There is considerable evidence that mothers and babies benefit physically and emotionally if they have two or three years together before the next sibling takes over the nest.

Male Contraception

Resuming relationships

The effects of witnessing a delivery, particularly of a beloved partner, is a highly emotional experience and may result in tension or guilt for the man if the mother has painful stitches, or is generally less than well after delivery; occasionally partners require time to discuss their anxieties, and may appreciate a sympathetic professional ear. Having a third party who is known to both will often assist them in talking frankly about their experiences and allowing them to express their feelings and fears. The man may feel rejected when the baby is establishing a relationship with its mother. Expecting effective use of a condom from a partner who is overwrought and disturbed by his recent involvement in the delivery is likely to produce serious difficulties and may put him off using a condom for a long time. It is well for the midwife to realize that women have far better opportunities than men for obtaining professional and friendly advice on these intimate and delicate matters, so it is important that she takes the time to provide good opportunities for counselling. Relationships may flounder for want of a little helpful support.

BARRIER METHODS

Condom or sheath

The condom or sheath is probably the most widely used contraception in the first few months after childbearing and is almost universally popular. As a barrier method, it not only provides protection against conception but is also effective in preventing the transmission of sexually transmitted diseases.

In the UK, condoms can be obtained free from family planning clinics or purchased at chemists, via slot machines, at petrol stations and through many other retail outlets. A recent study investigated the distribution of condoms through general practitioners and concluded that there were many opportunities but that staff training and the development of clear policies are required (Jewitt, 1993).

A wide variety of condoms are available and individual preference will determine choice, although the presence of the kitemark indicates that safety standards have been met. Some condoms are already lubricated with spermicide; these are more comfortable and slightly more effective than those without spermicide.

The correct use of a condom is important to maximize its effectiveness and it is essential that every midwife should know how to demonstrate the application of a condom using a model. The teat-ended condoms are designed to provide space for the ejaculate and air should be expelled from this or from the tip of a rounded condom before it is rolled up the erect penis. When the penis is withdrawn or becomes flaccid, the condom should be removed and disposed of. It is worth a glance to ensure that it is still intact; accidents do occur when sheaths split, even though they are thoroughly tested during manufacture. In the event of damage, it would be advisable to seek advice from a general practitioner, family planning nurse or midwife regarding the need for emergency contraception.

The use of condoms alongside other methods of contraception is now widely advocated to guard against the spread of HIV and other sexually transmitted diseases (Grieco, 1987; Goldsmith, 1987). The regular use of condoms must be encouraged and the attitudes of health care professionals in this matter are of great importance in influencing the attitude of the public. A variety of coloured and flavoured condoms are available which attract public attention and increase wider usage.

Safety   The condom is 97% effective if it is always used properly (Filshie and Guillebaud, 1989). One study indicated a pregnancy rate of 0.7% in women of 35 years and over, and 3.6% in women between 25 and 34 years of age (Filshie and Guillebaud, 1989). The addition of a spermicide may increase protection from pregnancy and certainly from sexually transmitted diseases. The use of condoms has been found to prevent the transmission of AIDS-associated retrovirus (Conant *et al.*, 1986). It is therefore considered a safe, convenient and highly successful method.

OTHER METHODS

Coitus interruptus

This is a method which is used by a large number of couples at some stage in their relationship. It depends on the man withdrawing his penis from the vagina before ejaculation takes place and thus requires control. This may be acceptable to some couples but may cause considerable frustration and stress in others.

Because of the risk of leakage of seminal fluid before withdrawal, coitus interruptus is not considered a very safe method. As there is no effective information about numbers of couples using this method regularly, it is impossible to assess its efficacy with any certainty. It may be worth providing information on other methods in case a safer method is equally acceptable.

Female Contraception

Resuming relationships

Women vary in their approach to resuming marital relations after childbirth and also in their ability to express how they feel. It is common for newly delivered mothers to feel extremely tired and also guilty about their refusal to have intercourse. There is a need for emotional support as well as for practical assistance; sometimes the partner is fully occupied and does not always appreciate the whirlwind of emotions associated with the adaptation to motherhood. In addition there may be a fear of pain if there has been damage to the perineum, or a fear of another pregnancy, in addition to a generally low libido.

The level of emotional tension often makes it difficult for either parent to discuss the topic easily. A midwife who is a trusted professional is in an ideal position to introduce the subject and allow both parents an opportunity to say how they feel, to ask questions and to resolve any misunderstandings. This type of support by an understanding midwife will make a great contribution to the future stability of the relationship.

PHYSIOLOGICAL METHODS

For some people this is the only acceptable method of contraception. The 'safe period' refers to the time during the menstrual cycle when conception is less likely to take place. It is known that ovulation occurs 14 days before the onset of the next menstrual period and that fertilization is possible up to five days before and two days afterwards. Allowing an extra day either end, intercourse should be avoided for these 10 or 11 days during the cycle. Theoretically this is very easy, but in practice to determine the exact time of ovulation takes time and patience, particularly during the post-partum period.

The physiological return of ovulation following childbirth is difficult to assess and the variability of its return makes this method very unreliable in the first few months after delivery. The importance of spacing babies and of women having recovered from childbirth both physically and emotionally before starting to cope with another pregnancy is a significant factor in a mother's life. Relying on trying to determine the 'safe period' will be difficult and may result in pregnancy.

Various methods have been developed to allow the 'safe period' to be worked out. These include:

▶ The temperature method.
▶ The Billings or mucus method.
▶ The calendar method.
▶ Combination of methods.

Temperature method The temperature rises about 0.3°C (1°F) at the time of ovulation and remains at this higher level during the latter half of the menstrual cycle due to the action of progesterone. The woman is taught to take her temperature each morning at the same time, before getting out of bed, and when it has been raised for 72 hours and there is no other likely cause, it is considered to be due to ovulation.

If the mother is breastfeeding, many months may go by before ovulation occurs and there are many reasons too why there may be erratic temperature patterns, such as variability in breastfeeding and minor infections. These will cause confusion and it may take several months of observation to resume the identification of ovulation.

Billings or mucus method Three or four days before ovulation occurs the cervical mucus increases in amount and becomes thinner in consistency to allow the spermatozoa to pass through the cervix more easily. The woman and her partner can be taught to recognize these changes in cervical mucus which precede ovulation so that they can avoid intercourse at that time. It is wise to use the mucus method in conjunction with the temperature method and then the couple know when it is safe to resume intercourse.

Although these changes in the cervical mucus are usually very easy to recognize, they will be changed for some weeks after childbirth while the cervix returns to the non-pregnant state. The lochia usually stop after 2–3 weeks, but occasionally there is some discharge for several weeks and again breastfeeding usually delays the return of ovulation. The woman will therefore need to check daily for good *Spinbarkeit* mucus (that is, a thin, watery consistency with marked stretchability in its threads).

Billings *et al.* (1972) first described these cervical mucus symptoms associated with ovulation. Since then the World Health Organization has conducted a major study which has confirmed the potential effectiveness of mucus symptom observations as a means of family planning (WHO, 1981a,b, 1983, 1984, 1987). A large natural family planning study in India showed that with effective teaching and high motivation the failure rate is very low, equal to that of the combined contraceptive pill, 0.2 pregnancies per 100 women users yearly (Ghosh *et al.*, 1982). According to the WHO (1981a,b) 93% of women can identify the symptoms associated with ovulation and therefore it is a very useful method which confers considerable power to couples to control their fertility (Ryder, 1993).

Calendar method This useful but traditional method is fraught with problems after childbirth. The interruption of menstruation for nine months of pregnancy may result in a different pattern of periods when they resume. Until six months of menstruation have passed, this method will provide poor guidelines for the prediction of ovulation. Mothers using the safe period should be encouraged to use a combination of methods to assess their ovulatory cycle.

Some electronic monitors are said to provide good information regarding ovulation and, when there is sufficient evidence of reliability, they may greatly assist mothers who wish to use this natural method.

To predict the 'safe period' a record of the first day of each menstrual period is kept for at least six months, preferably a year. If periods are absolutely regular the time of ovulation is fairly easy to predict, but in most women the length of the menstrual cycle and time of ovulation vary from month to month and thus they have to work out their 'safe period'. Calculation of probable ovulation is determined each month by deducting 18 days from the number of days in the shortest cycle and 11 days from the number of days in the longest cycle of the preceding six months.

Allowing at least 48 hours for ovum life and at least three days for sperm survival, although it is thought that in some cases this may extend up to seven days. It is essential that ovulation is predicted as accurately as possible. Conception is possible, therefore, between days 7 and 20, and less likely before day 7. The safest time in the cycle is 48 hours after ovulation has taken place, so assessing the time of the individual's ovulation each month is critical for a satisfactory outcome.

As it will take some time following delivery to obtain a history of menstrual patterns it is worth educating an interested couple so that they can use additional precautions when necessary.

Combination of methods   Many women use a combination of methods. The *mucothermal* method is a combination of recording the temperature and detecting changes in the cervical mucus. The *symptothermal* method combines recording the temperature together with changes in the cervical mucus and any other symptoms of ovulation such as slight lower abdominal pain known as *Mittelschmerz* (Figure 1).

The disadvantages of these methods are that they are particularly unreliable when there are considerable menstrual irregularities and illness or emotional upset which may alter the cycle. They are also unreliable during lactation and the menopause.

BARRIER METHODS

Occlusive caps

These devices (Figure 2) cover the cervix and mechanically obstruct the entrance of spermatozoa. Initially they must be fitted by a doctor, midwife or nurse, who has been trained in family planning. Caps are checked for fit at intervals, especially after childbirth or loss of weight.

All caps are made in a variety of sizes and must be

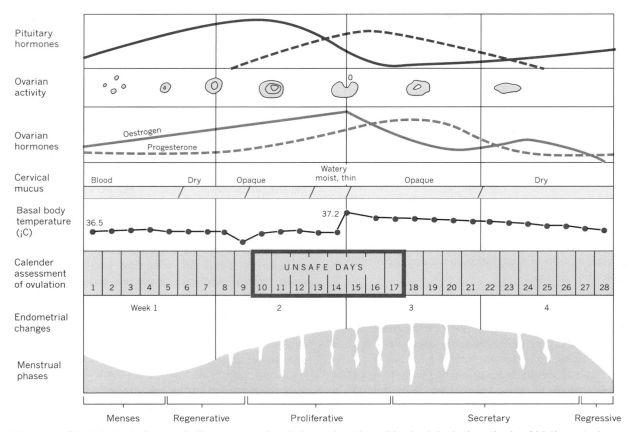

Figure 1   Physiological changes in the menstrual cycle in conjunction with physiological methods of birth control. (Reproduced with permission from Cowper and Young, 1989, p. 103.)

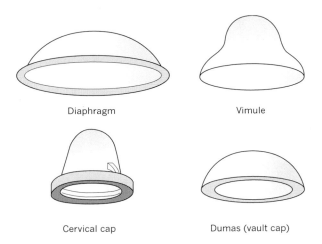

Diaphragm

Vimule

Cervical cap

Dumas (vault cap)

Figure 2 Examples of female barrier methods. (Reproduced with permission from Cowper and Young, 1989, p. 78.)

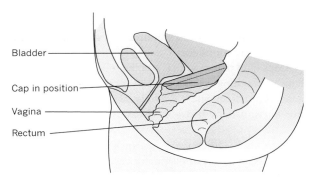

Bladder

Cap in position

Vagina

Rectum

Figure 3 Diaphragm cap in position. (Reproduced with permission from Cowper and Young, 1989, p. 79.)

fitted individually. The woman is taught how to insert the cap, how to check that it is in position, how to remove it and how to care for it. She is sent home with written instructions and a practice cap and is asked to return a week later with the cap in position. She is warned not to rely on the cap as an adequate contraceptive during this time.

At the next visit the doctor, midwife or nurse is able to check the fit and to test the woman's ability to insert the cap in the correct position. Nervousness at the first visit often causes a tense muscle reaction in the vagina so a large enough cap may not be given. At this visit a new cap is supplied together with a spermicidal cream. A choice of contraceptive jelly, cream or foam should be available. The woman is seen at regular intervals and a new cap supplied as necessary.

The use of occlusive caps demands a high level of motivation and confidence by the woman. With correct and conscientious use the rate of pregnancy can be as low as two per 100 woman years (Spencer, 1986).

The diaphragm or Dutch cap This is one of the oldest methods of female contraception and has changed very little in design. A postnatal mother who wishes to use a diaphragm will require careful fitting and assessment at more frequent intervals than usual.

The shallow rubber cap has a circular spring around its perimeter; this may be of flat metal, or a round spring allowing the cap to be compressed and inserted into the vagina rather like a tampon. Some caps have an arcing spring enabling them to be inserted under a protruding cervix. It is necessary to fit the cap so that it rests in the posterior fornix of the vagina posteriorly and on the suprapubic ridge anteriorly (Figure 3). The caps come in graduated sizes from 60 mm to 95 mm and are therefore individually fitted so that the anterior wall of the vagina and cervix are covered by a cap which remains comfortably and firmly in place.

A woman who has used a cap before will require a larger size after delivery and this size will need adjustment as the vaginal muscle tone improves. A cap which is too large protrudes and causes discomfort, or may produce extra pressure, giving rise to urethritis-type discomfort. Too small a cap will move around and will not provide protection. A well-fitting cap is unobtrusive and will not be noticed during intercourse.

It is necessary to allow a mother a few days to practise inserting and removing the cap to ensure she is happy with the use of it. Spermicide is necessary in conjunction with the cap to provide acceptable safety levels. A 5 cm strip of spermicide cream or jelly should be applied on the upper surface before the cap is inserted. This can be done at any convenient time. A further application of spermicide can be inserted with an introducer before intercourse – jelly, cream or foam can be used and is quickly applied. The cap should remain *in situ* for six hours after intercourse and is then removed at a convenient time and washed, rinsed and dried.

A mother should be reassessed for size at 1–2 monthly intervals after childbirth until her muscles have returned to normal. A cap may then be prescribed for a year and, unless there is weight loss or gain of more than 3 kg (7 lb), she will not require further assessment. Teaching a mother to insert and remove a cap takes a few minutes and some supervision before she is confident.

Caps and spermicides can be obtained free from family planning clinics or on prescription through general practice, where a family planning trained practice nurse usually provides this care.

Other caps   Other types of cap less commonly used may be very useful in particular cases. They all rely on suction to remain in place. The use of spermicide on both surfaces and the removal after six hours remain a consistent feature of use. No spermicide should be placed on the rim, or suction will be adversely affected.

Vault caps These are also graduated in several sizes and are thicker rubber than a diaphragm without a spring rim. The cap sits in the fornices of the vagina covering the cervix and remains in position by suction. The benefit of vault caps is that they can be used when the vaginal muscle tone is poor and will not support a diaphragm. They are a little more difficult to insert and require long fingers and some dexterity to remove.

The cervical cap This is designed in several sizes to fit over the cervix. It may be a good cap for women who have a straight-sided cervix. They are small, quite thick rubber, but neat and popular with a small minority (Figure 4).

The vimule This combination of vault and cervical cap has a powerful suction capability and is used to cover the cervix which is small, irregular or partially amputated. It is rarely used but may be the most appropriate cap for a small number of women.

Spermicide   The use of spermicide with caps is important, the efficacy of the method relies on it and this can be applied when the cap is introduced, and should be reapplied without removing the cap if intercourse occurs after three hours, by placing a couple of spermicide pessaries in the vagina. Spermicide foam is a valuable form of protection as, unlike other methods, it does not melt but remains stable at the top of the vagina for up to four hours. Mothers complaining about 'stickiness and mess' may find the whole concept of barrier methods much more acceptable with foam.

Female condoms

These plastic tubular condoms are inserted with the

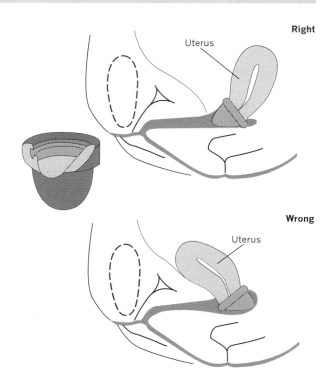

Figure 4   Cervical cap in position.

use of a plastic ring and line the vagina. A soft but firm plastic ring at the entrance covers the genitalia and needs to be steadied in position during intercourse. Spermicide is advised, and it provides useful lubrication. This condom provides protection both from pregnancy and from sexually transmitted diseases but, like all methods, it requires practice. The condoms are available from chemists and are not available on the NHS, although they should be available in all clinics dealing with contraception for teaching purposes. In a study to test the reliability of the female condom, there was a 15% failure rate (Agnew, 1992).

SPERMICIDAL AGENTS

There are a variety of chemical substances that kill or inactivate spermatozoa. They are incorporated into jellies, creams, pessaries, aerosol foams and rice paper. Directions for use vary and should be followed carefully to obtain maximum safety. To insure that spermicides are used effectively it is worthwhile taking time to introduce the spectrum of available types and encourage the mother to select a spermicide with an acceptable taste and smell. It is often small factors like this which make for better compliance.

Most spermicides are used in conjunction with barrier methods and thus enhance their safety. Infrequently foams or pessaries may be used on their own where fertility is already low to reduce the risk of pregnancy; for women with average fertility spermicides alone would result in a high proportion of unplanned pregnancies.

INTRAUTERINE CONTRACEPTIVE DEVICES

The history of intrauterine contraceptive devices (IUCDs), which have been used all over the world since Biblical times, makes a fascinating study. Nowadays IUCDs (Figures 5 and 6) are small plastic devices which are placed in the uterine cavity by means of a special introducer. All have copper or silver threads added which increases the efficiency of the device.

They act by reducing the permeability of cervical mucus to sperm and by making the endometrium hypotrophic. The copper has a spermicidal effect and therefore is hostile to sperm. It is also thought that the device causes some reduction in tubular contraction, thereby reducing the speed of the ovum along the fallopian tube and there is some evidence of infrequent ovulation while the device is *in situ*.

There may also be an increased production of prostaglandins in the uterus which increases uterine activity and causes the expulsion of the fertilized ovum. The IUCD may be expelled, especially around the time of menstruation, within the first six months following insertion.

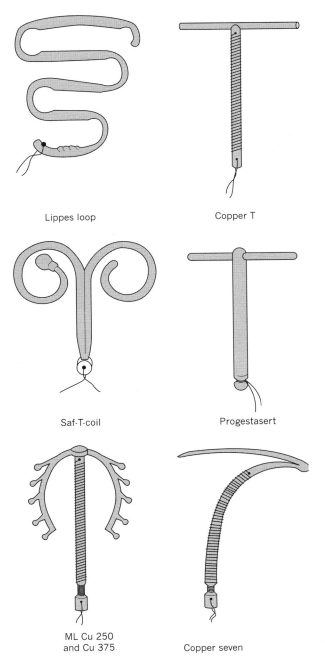

Lippes loop Copper T

Saf-T-coil Progestasert

ML Cu 250 and Cu 375 Copper seven

Figure 5 Intrauterine devices. (Reproduced with permission from Cowper and Young, 1989, p. 89.)

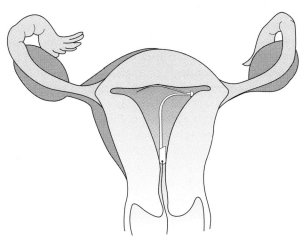

Figure 6 Intrauterine device (copper seven) in position. (Reproduced with permission from Cowper and Young, 1989, p. 96.)

Contraindications to the use of an IUCD include pelvic disease, submucus fibroids, cervicitis, menorrhagia and suspected malignancy.

The introduction of an IUCD following delivery is generally delayed until six weeks postpartum when involution of the uterus is likely to be complete. If it is inserted before involution is complete it will not remain in the optimum position and is more likely to be expelled. Particular care is required after Caesarean section to ensure that the wound has fully healed. In some cases a device is inserted at the time of termination of pregnancy if requested by the woman.

When inserting an IUCD after delivery, the cervix is still soft and the walls of the uterus may be friable, so the doctor inserting the device needs to be experienced in the technique, as perforation of the uterus could occur. In general, the devices are introduced easily and quite quickly, although some dysmenorrhoea-type pain may be experienced for an hour or two after insertion. Threads from the stem of the device can be felt at the top of the vagina, enabling the woman to check that the device remains in position.

A variety of types are now available. All have copper or copper and silver thread on the stem.

The new Levonorgestrel IUCD Mirena is now available, and statistically is more effective than sterilization. The bore of this device is a little wider than traditional devices because of the progestogen reservoir in the stem. The use of a paracervical block or a suitable oral relaxant prior to insertion is advantageous. The proximity of the progestogen to the endometrium reduces its thickness, so that after an initial few weeks of erratic bleeding episodes the blood loss diminishes, and amenorrhoea is not uncommon. The progestogen also causes a physiological mucus plug to form in the cervix which safeguards the uterus from infection. At present the Mirena needs changing every three years. Product research indicates a rapid return to ovulation following removal.

The third generation IUCDs currently are:

▶ Ortho-Gyne T200, duration of effectiveness five years;
▶ Novagard/Nova T200, duration of effectiveness five years;
▶ Multiload CU250, duration of effectiveness seven years;
▶ Ortho Gyne T380 slimline, duration of effectiveness seven years;
▶ Multiload CU375, duration of effectiveness eight years.

An IUCD may be inserted at any time in the month and should be inserted at the convenience of the client. It is necessary to ensure that the woman is not pregnant before the device is introduced. Careful questioning, examination and discussion should reveal a possible pregnancy which is unlikely to be dislodged with the insertion of the device, although there is a slightly raised risk of a mid-trimester miscarriage if a coil is in the uterus. The devices remain *in situ* for 3–8 years and require only minimal supervision following insertion. They have an excellent record in preventing pregnancy and are generally trouble-free, requiring no action prior to intercourse. Reported pregnancy rate with the use of the intrauterine contraceptive device is 1.4 per 100 woman years; Pearl Index (Ryder, 1993). (Pearl Index is the number of pregnancies per 100 woman years.) In a few cases, menstruation is prolonged by a couple of days when an IUCD is *in situ*. A few people with dysmenorrhoea may find the pain is worsened by the introduction of a device. Women with recurrent infection in the reproductive tract would be wise to use another method. While the device does not introduce infection, any infection which may occur is likely to be more difficult to treat.

Follow up The follow-up visits for women with intrauterine contraceptive devices are generally arranged between 3–6 weeks after insertion and then at six months and thereafter annually, until the device requires removal and changing. The woman is advised to check the threads each month after a period. The technical ability and attitude of the doctor fitting the device, and that of the staff supporting and teaching the method, have been demonstrated to be more important for the success of this method than the type of device used (Snowden, 1975). It is extremely important that women receive calm, friendly support during the insertion. If pregnancy does occur when the device is *in situ*, removal is advised, providing the device can be easily dislodged by traction on the threads.

Emergency IUCD contraception In the event of unprotected intercourse having occurred, an intrauterine contraceptive device may be fitted up to five days after the probable day of ovulation in that cycle. The presence of an IUCD in the uterus will probably prevent a fertilized ovum from embedding.

Removal of an IUCD   Unless pregnancy is planned no device shoud be removed between day 7 and day 21 of the menstrual cycle unless there has been no sexual intercourse for seven days or if barrier methods have been used.

HORMONAL CONTRACEPTION

Oral contraception

There are an estimated 60 million women taking oral contraceptives in the world (Cowper and Young, 1989). These may be the *combined pill*, which contains both oestrogen and progesterone, or the *progestogen-only pill*.

Improvements in the manufacture of synthetic progesterones mean that a new generation of pill has become available. This third generation of combined pills came under media attack regarding safety and provoked concern amongst both users and professionals. The economic and political interest in banning newer and, therefore, more expensive drugs provoked cynicism amongst professionals.

All women who are prescribed the pill should be prepared for media scares and be ready to seek sensible advice if they are concerned about their pills, and to avoid a panic reaction which may result in unwanted pregnancies. It is worth noting that the third-generation pills in question are twice as safe as having a baby (Bulletin from the Margaret Pyke Centre, January 1996).

The Family Planning Association recommends that in the event of a woman missing a pill, additional precautions should be taken for seven days. This advice applies to both combined oestrogen and progesterone pills and the progestogen-only pill (FPA, 1993).

Combined pill   The combined oestrogen and progesterone pill contains between 30 and 50 µg of oestrogen and varying amounts of progesterone. It acts by inhibiting ovulation by suppressing the production of gonadotrophins from the anterior pituitary gland. It also alters the consistency of the cervical mucus, making it impenetrable to sperm, reduces the motility of the uterine tubes so that the sperm have difficulty in passing along the tube, and causes a change in the endometrium making it unsuitable for implantation.

The latter three back-up mechanisms are due to the action of progesterone.

The timing of administration of the combined pill is important, for if the follicle begins to ripen ovulation will occur. For complete efficiency the course should begin on the fifth day after the commencement of the last menstrual period and continue for 21 days. This is followed by seven days without tablets, during which time withdrawal bleeding occurs. It is imperative that the instructions given with the various products are carefully followed as there are slight variations in the number of days tablets are taken. When taken correctly the combined oral contraceptive pill is virtually 100% reliable. The reported pregnancy rate is 0.18 per 100 woman years (Ryder, 1993).

Major contraindications include thromboembolic disorders, breast neoplasia, liver disease and focal migraine. In diabetes mellitus stability may be affected and it may be necessary to adjust treatment. Other relative contraindications include hypertension, heart disease, epilepsy and obesity. A family history of venous or arterial disease in close family under 45 years of age must also be considered serious risk.

Oral contraceptives have certain side-effects which include weight gain, nausea, breast heaviness, headaches, depression and loss of libido. Some of these may diminish in time.

Most doctors now recommend that women review the options available before taking the combined oral contraceptive pill, especially if they smoke and are overweight, as there is an increased risk of thromboembolic disease, myocardial infarction and cerebral vascular accident. Other methods of contraception should then be employed.

After delivery, the mother who is not breastfeeding may start the combined pill 21 days postpartum. The regime of 21 days of pills followed by seven pill-free days is followed. The oestrogen content of the pill is inclined to reduce lactation and is also passed to the baby in the breast milk so the combined contraceptive pill containing both oestrogen and progesterone is not recommended for breastfeeding mothers.

Progestogen-only pill   Progestogen is an effective method of contraception postpartum and is satisfactory for breastfeeding mothers. The progestogen does not affect the lactation and any small quantity passing through the milk is not a problem for babies. The mother commences at 21 days after delivery and takes the tablets continuously from packet to packet without a break. There may be some delay in menstruation, but it will be a 'proper' period when it arrives. Mothers should be advised that progestogen does cause erratic bleeding patterns, but this usually settles after a few months and the periods may gradually disappear. This is a sign of suppression of ovulation and a reassuring sign of good contraceptive cover.

Progestogen acts by causing cervical mucus to form a natural plug in the cervix and prevents the sperm entering the uterus, and also reduces the motility of the uterine tubes. In some cases, the progestogen also causes suppression of ovulation. The reported pregnancy rate with the progestogen–only pill is 1.2 per 100 woman years (Ryder, 1993).

Emergency contraception (oral)   The risk of pregnancy arising from an episode of unprotected intercourse can be reduced substantially if the woman receives a specially prepared combined oral preparation of two tablets of 50 mg of oestrogen followed by a further two, 12 hours later. This should be commenced within 72 hours of intercourse. This information should be widely known, publicized and given as general information to the public, who as yet are largely ignorant of the service and as a result, fail to obtain appropriate help in time. Although the midwife may not need to recommend this method of contraception very often in a direct way with her mothers, it is an important part of health education in the community, especially in schools and colleges.

Injectable contraceptives

Depo-Provera   Progesterone may be given intramuscularly and will last for 3–6 months, according to the dose. Depo-Provera 150 mg is most commonly used and may be repeated at three-monthly intervals. It acts by making the cervical mucus impenetrable to sperm, causes changes in the endometrium and may lead to irregular bleeding or amenorrhoea. It is suitable for women who have been given rubella vaccination, for those awaiting sterilization or whose partners have had a vasectomy, or for poorly motivated women who need to limit the size of their family.

Depo-Provera can usually be commenced at six weeks postpartum provided the woman has not had unprotected intercourse. It is not given before six weeks because it may provoke bleeding and, at a time when secondary postpartum haemorrhage may occur, could make diagnosis of pathology difficult and cause

unnecessary blood loss at a vulnerable time for the mother.

Noristerat   Norethisterone oenanthate 200 mg may be given intramuscularly every eight weeks. The high level of progesterone suppresses ovulation and there are few side-effects. The main disadvantage is amenorrhoea, which may occur after two injections of progestogens.

Implants

Norplant   Norplant is the commonest contraceptive implant used at present in the UK. Six small silastic tubes containing progestogen (Levonorgestrel) are inserted superficially under the skin of the upper arm using a minor surgical technique and local anaesthetic. The progestogen is absorbed at a steady rate of approximately 80 µg per day for the first week, slowly reducing to 34 µg over six months. It is recommended that Norplant should be replaced every five years. This regime produces a highly effective care-free protection. The efficacy is slightly affected if the woman's weight is over 70 kg; very heavy women have less effective cover. The implant should not be arranged before six weeks postpartum and may be delayed until lactation has ceased. Menstrual irregularities in the first three months do occur, but a gradual improvement can be expected thereafter and amenorrhoea after the first year is not unknown. Studies have shown a first year pregnancy rate with implanted levonorgestrel of 0.2%, rising to a maximum of 1.6% in the fourth year, and a five year cumulative rate of 3.9% (Mascarenhas, 1994). The preliminary results from a study show that the tolerance of contraceptive implants (Norplant and Implanon) is improved by good counselling for women.

Care of women receiving hormonal contraceptives

Before hormonal contraceptives are prescribed a detailed family, medical, obstetric and menstrual history is obtained and the medical examination includes weight, blood pressure, urine analysis, examination of the breasts and examination per vaginam. A cervical smear is taken and repeated at regular intervals. The blood pressure and weight should be checked at every visit to the family planning clinic. The woman is also asked to fill in a small record card which has a place to indicate the date, whether a tablet was taken, if spotting occurred and when bleeding occurs; this is seen by the doctor or nurse at each visit.

Sterilization

Tubal ligation, laparoscopic sterilization or the application of potentially removable clips to the uterine tubes are methods of sterilization which may be performed in the woman (Figure 7). These methods should be considered permanent. In the male, ligation of the deferent ducts is considered a permanent method of sterilization.

Before carrying out sterilization it is essential that the couple are carefully counselled. The psychosocial aspects of the decision as well as the physical factors concerned with the procedure should be considered.

Some couples like time to reflect on the matter before making a final decision. The emotionally stable couple usually accept sterilization without regret, but those of a neurotic disposition may use the operation to rationalize disturbances that arise later in life.

Female sterilization is best carried out at about 6 or 8 weeks after delivery. The success rate is higher at that time than in the earlier postnatal period and by that time any problems affecting the baby which could influence the couple's decision are usually evident.

Most women will agree to use some other reliable form of contraception until the operation can be arranged. If the operation is delayed, perhaps due to long waiting lists, then intramuscular progestogen may be selected as the most appropriate contraceptive.

About 1% of those who are sterilized request reversal at a later date. The commonest reasons are related to a change in marital status, sudden infant death, the death of an older child and the desire for more children (Buckley, 1986). The success rate for reversal is low, so these methods should be considered permanent.

Vasectomy

This is ligation of both deferent ducts (vas deferens) (Figure 8). In some cases the male partner chooses to be sterilized as it is a safer procedure than tubal ligation. It can be done as an outpatient procedure under local anaesthetic. Again skilled counselling is essential before a final decision is made. The man should understand that sexual desire and activity are not affected by the operation. Men are capable of fathering a child well into old age and the couple may wish to take this into consideration. A couple should appreciate that sterilization will reduce the woman's likely reproductive years by 5–8 years approximately, whereas for a man it could be about 40 years.

Both partners also need to be sure that there are no specific reasons why one or other may require surgery in the near future, for example a woman with fibroids may require a hysterectomy.

Ligation of the deferent ducts prevents the sperm reaching the seminal vesicles and ejaculatory duct. As spermatozoa may survive in the ducts for some time, the couple should continue to take contraceptive precautions until two semen specimens without sperm are produced. This can take up to three months.

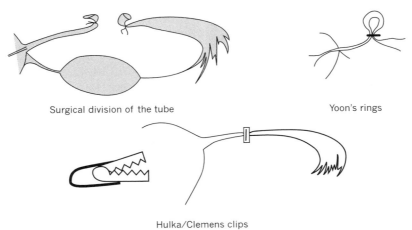

Surgical division of the tube

Yoon's rings

Hulka/Clemens clips

Figure 7 Sterilization methods. (Reproduced with permission from Cowper and Young, 1989, p. 109.)

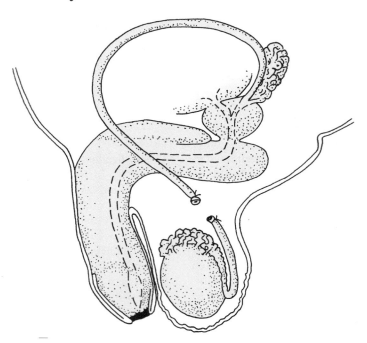

Figure 8   Ligation of the vas deferens.

There has been some concern about increased risks of testicular cancer after vasectomy, but a recent study concludes that there is no increased risk (Møller *et al.*, 1994).

References

Agnew, T. (1992) Women in charge. *Nursing Times* 88(39): 21.

Andersson, K. *et al.* (1994) Levonorgestrel releasing system and copper releasing IUD (Nova 1) over a period of 5 years – a randomized trial. Department of Obstetrics and Gynaecology, Gotenberg, Sweden.

Billings, E.L., Billings, J.J., Brown, J.B. & Burger, H.G. (1972) Symptoms and hormonal changes accompanying ovulation. *Lancet* i: 282–284.

Bounds, W. & Guillebaud, J. (1984) Effectiveness and acceptability of the Collatex sponge ('Today') and the diaphragm. *Br. J. Family Planning* 10: 69.

Buckley, D. (1986) Modern trends in sterilization. *J. Obstet. Gynaecol.* 6(Suppl.2): 5116–5118.

Conant, M., Hardy, D., Sernatinger, J. *et al.* (1986) Condoms prevent transmission of AIDS associated retrovirus. *J. Am. Med. Assoc.* 255: 1706.

Cowper, A. & Young, C. (1989) *Family Planning. Fundamentals for Health Professionals.* London: Chapman & Hall.

Filshie, M. & Guillebaud, J. (1989) *Contraception Science and Practice.* Oxford: Heinemann.

FPA (Family Planning Association) (1993) New POP guidelines announced. *Family Planning Today* Second Quarter: 1.

Ghosh, A.F., Saha, S. & Chattergee, G. (1982) Sympothermia vis a vis fertility control. *J. Obstet. Gynaecol. India.* 32: 443–447.

Goldsmith, M.F. (1987) Sex in the age of AIDS calls for condom sense. *J. Am. Med. Assoc.* 257(17): 2261–2264.

Gray, R.H., Campbell, O.M., Zacur, H.A., Labbok, M.H. & MacRae, S.L. (1987) Postpartum return of ovarian activity in non breastfeeding women monitored by urinary essays. *J. Clin. Endocrinol. Metab.* 64: 645–650.

Grieco, A. (1987) Cutting the risks for STD. *Med. Aspects Human Sexuality* March: 70–84.

Jewitt, C. (1993) Distributing condoms through general practice. *Family Planning Today* Second Quarter: 6.

Mascarenhas, L. (1994) Long acting methods of contraception. *Br. Med. J.* 308: 991–992.

McNeilly, A. & Howsie, P. (1982) *Clin. Endocrinol.* 17: 323–332.

Møller, H. *et al.* (1994) Risk of testicular cancer after vasectomy: a cohort of 73 000 men. *Br. Med. J.* 309(6)950: 295–299.

Notes and News (1984) The man's role in contraception. *Lancet* i: 1194.

Ryder, R.E.J. (1993) 'Natural family planning': effective birth control supported by the Catholic Church. *Br. Med. J.* 307(6906): 723–726.

Snowden, R. (1975) Attitudes of staff versus outcome of IUCDs. Personal communication, University of Exeter.

Spencer, B. (1986) If the cap fits . . . *Nursing Times* January: 22–24.

WHO (World Heath Organization) (1981a) A prospective multicentre trial of the ovulation method of natural family planning. I The teaching phase. *Fertil. Steril.* **36**: 152–158.

WHO (1981b) A prospective multicentre trial of the ovulation method of natural family planning. II The effectiveness phase. *Fertil. Steril.* **36**: 591–598.

WHO (1983) A prospective multicentre trial of the ovulation method of natural family planning. III Characteristics of the menstrual cycle and of the fertile phase. *Fertil. Steril.* **40**: 773–778.

WHO (1984) A prospective multicentre trial of the ovulation method of natural family planning. IV The outcome of pregnancy. *Fertil. Steril.* **41**: 593–598.

WHO (1987) A prospective multicentre trial of the ovulation method of natural family planning. V Psychosexual aspects. *Fertil. Steril.* **47**: 765–772

61

Infertility and Assisted Conception

Couples are classified as infertile or subfertile if pregnancy has not occurred after one year of regular, unprotected intercourse (that is no contraception has been used). On average, a normally fertile couple aged in their twenties, who are having sexual intercourse three or four times a week, have a 1 in 4 chance of conceiving each month. Most couples will have achieved a pregnancy within a year.

Infertility can occur in anyone regardless of class, race or social background. It is estimated that up to 1 in 10 couples may experience fertility problems in the Western world. This may increase to as high as 1 in 6 if those with secondary infertility are included, that is after a pregnancy has occurred, whether or not it resulted in a birth.

Infertility is often thought to be a female problem, which seems to be more socially acceptable, but in fact a third of all cases have causes that are primarily male, a third primarily female and the rest have both male and female problems.

Causes of Infertility

The causes of infertility can simply be divided into three groups:

1 Female problems.
2 Male problems.
3 Problems as a couple.

Female problems

The woman may not be ovulating, that is producing and releasing ova. She may ovulate but irregularly or infrequently, reducing the number of chances she has to become pregnant over a given period of time, or making the timing of intercourse around her most fertile time very difficult.

As women get older they become less fertile (Boukje van Noord-Zaadstra *et al.*, 1991), pregnancy may take longer to occur, the chance of miscarriage is increased, and there is a sharp rise in the risk of fetal abnormality. There are several reasons for this:

Viability of eggs   A woman's eggs are already *in situ* when she is born (Tan and Jacobs, 1991). They remain in her body virtually unchanged until they are released as part of a menstrual cycle. Therefore an ovum released this month is as old as the woman herself, so a woman of 40 years old, is ovulating 40-year-old eggs. The eggs that are produced by older women may be of poorer quality, they may not be released regularly and may not fertilize easily; this situation is not echoed in the male. Sperm are produced all the time from puberty onwards. They take about three months to mature, so men tend to stay fertile longer. The sperm do not age and there is little decline in fertility until men are in their sixties.

Damaged fallopian tubes   A woman may have damaged fallopian tubes, which may hinder or block the eggs and sperm meeting and thus prevent fertilization. If fertilization does happen, the fertilized egg may be unable to continue its journey to the uterus and embeds itself into the tube. This situation will lead to an ectopic pregnancy, which as the conceptus grows will eventually rupture the tube causing haemorrhage. Without surgical intervention this may lead to death. Even if it is diagnosed early, and surgical intervention planned, the most likely result will be salpingectomy, or removal of all, or part of the affected fallopian tube. This of course may further compromise the woman's fertility (Winston, 1994).

Abnormal uterus   The woman may have an abnormality in the uterus which may inhibit implantation or cause it to occur in an abnormal site, for example fibroids or a structural abnormality such as bicornuate uterus or dividing septum (Jones, 1981).

Endometriosis   Endometriosis, which can cause painful periods, is not thought to be significant unless severe enough to cause tubal damage (Booker, 1988) or cause cysts on the ovaries, called endometriomas.

Male problems

The man may not be producing any sperm, not enough or too many abnormal sperm. If the sperm produced are not motile they will also be incapable of natural fertilization.

The characteristics of a normal semen sample are as follows (WHO, 1994):

Volume	2–4 ml
Liquefaction	Complete in 30 minutes
Count	20 million/ml or more
Motility	40% (progressing forward)
Morphology	30% or more normal forms (ovals).

It must be remembered that semen analysis results vary greatly from sample to sample and so results from just one should not be seen as conclusive. A low volume may indicate that the sample was not complete, but if this persists it may indicate an obstruction of the ejaculatory ducts or the congenital absence of the seminal vesicles. A sample should be produced for assessment no less than 36 hours and no more than 72 hours since the last ejaculation. If the sample contains less than 10 million sperm/ml this is described as oligospermia. This does not necessarily mean the man is sterile, but that his fertility is compromised (Sharpe and Irvine, 1994).

Azoospermia   If no sperm are seen in two samples, the man is described as *azoospermic*, therefore fertilization cannot take place. Further investigation is needed to establish if this situation is unchangeable. Complete testicular failure, as indicated by a high follicle-stimulating hormone (FSH) and a normal or low testosterone level is not treatable, whereas azoospermia with a normal FSH and testosterone level may indicate the need for a testicular biopsy to identify if any spermatogenesis is occurring, and therefore a blockage is likely (Hirsch, 1992).

Sperm abnormalities   Human semen samples usually contain up to 30% sperm abnormalities. These may occur in the head, midpiece or tail of the sperm, but appear to have little effect on the potency of the sample. If, however, there are more than 60% abnormal sperm, this is likely to be significant and will indicate a fertility problem.

Sperm motility   Motility of sperm is expressed as the percentage of sperm that are moving in a sample. It is important that at least 50% of them are moving progressively forward, if not it is unlikely that fertilization will occur.

Impotence   The male partner may be impotent, or unable to maintain an erection, making intercourse impossible. The causes for this may be either organic, e.g. diabetes mellitus, hyperprolactinaemia or previous surgery, or it may be psychological. Treating this condition needs expertise and sensitivity and the man should be referred appropriately. Premature ejaculation, a condition where the man is unable to deposit his ejaculate into his partner's vagina, or retrograde ejaculation where the semen is passed into his bladder at orgasm, will also prevent pregnancy occurring.

Damaged tubes   The tubes leading from the testes to the urethra may have been damaged by an injury that has occurred in the past. The damage could be genetic, but most commonly has been caused by infection or deliberately by vasectomy.

Varicocele   In about 10% of men a condition exists called varicocele (Baker *et al.*, 1985). This is a collection of tortuous and dilated veins (rather like varicose veins), which can be detected as a soft swelling above the testicles. The extra blood flowing around the testicles in these enlarged vessels is generally thought to raise the temperature in the testes (which are placed outside the body to keep cool) and this may affect sperm production. Much debate goes on to try to establish how true this is and if surgical correction of this problem has any benefit.

Problems as a couple

Around the time of ovulation the cervical mucus changes its appearance and consistency. It becomes clear and extremely stretchy and many women can identify this time of their cycle purely by this change (Clubb and Knight, 1992). When examined under a microscope the mucus cells arrange themselves into fern-like shapes, and the stretchiness of the Spinbarkeit cells will allow the sample to be pulled to over 30 cm long.

After intercourse, some of the sperm swim through the mucus to the uterus, whilst others remain in the cervix for up to 24 hours. These can be examined using the post–coital test (PCT). The woman attends hospital 6–10 hours after making love and a mucus sample is collected. This is examined under a microscope and the behaviour of any sperm present is noted (Brinsden and Rainsbury, 1992). If sperm are not seen at all, when a normal semen sample has been seen before, then perhaps there has been a coital dysfunction, or if all the sperm are immotile this may suggest an incompatibility, or the presence of sperm antibodies. The PCT has now fallen very much out of favour due to its intrusiveness and its unreliability, and because it is extremely difficult to schedule its performance at an appropriate time.

Antibodies are substances produced by the body's defence mechanism to protect it against foreign bodies, in order to avoid infection. Occasionally some women produce antibodies to their partners' sperm and this may be another cause of infertility (Thompson and Heasley, 1992). This is not a clear-cut diagnosis, however, as antibodies have been found in normally fertile women.

Most commonly the factors affecting a couple's chance of conceiving may be of a more practical nature. The couple may not be making love regularly and this could be due simply to pressure of work making them too tired, shiftwork allowing little opportunity, or working away from home. They may have little privacy if they share accommodation with others, or perhaps they have other children. After several months or years of trying they may simply have given up, as once 'making babies' becomes more important than 'making love' the pleasurable aspects may be forgotten and the time spent together seen as a chore that can build resentment and anger into a relationship.

More serious psychosexual problems can be identified when a couple wish to have a baby, for example non-consummation or vaginismus, and these may need to be resolved before conception can occur. Occasionally a couple may need some very basic information about sex and how pregnancy occurs which may be all that is needed for them to achieve a pregnancy, but it is very important that they retain their dignity and do not feel belittled by their lack of knowledge.

Very commonly no cause of the couple's infertility can be identified. This is described as *unexplained infertility* and, while some may be reassured that no problem has been found, others find the uncertainty unbearable and their distress and anxiety can soar.

Investigations

When a couple are referred for investigation they will need to undergo a few basic tests in order for a diagnosis to be identified as quickly as possible. These tests can be easily arranged by the general practitioner or referring doctor and should include the following:

(A) *Female blood tests*

1 *Luteinizing and follicle-stimulating hormones (LH/FSH)*: Blood for these tests needs to be taken within the first five days of the menstrual cycle. If the woman is amenorrhoeic the test can be taken at any time.

2 *Prolactin and thyroid-stimulating hormone*: These tests only need to be undertaken if the woman's menstrual cycles are more than 42 days long. They can be undertaken at any time.

3 *Thalassaemia and sickle cell*: These tests need to be undertaken for any woman who comes from outside Northern Europe; if either proves to be positive her partner needs to be tested wherever he comes from. These tests can be taken at any time.

4 *Rubella*: This test needs to be done if the woman's rubella status is not known. It can be taken at any time.

5 *Haemoglobin*: This needs to be checked if the woman has a history of menorrhagia or dietary restriction.

6 *Luteal phase progesterone*: This needs to be done to assess if ovulation has occurred. The blood needs to be taken seven days after ovulation and so will vary which day of the cycle it falls on, depending on the length of the cycle. Ovulation is best identified by using an ovulation kit but can be calculated by calendar if the cycles are regular. The blood sample can be taken seven days before the next period is expected, but if the result is low and menstruation delayed, this may need to be repeated.

(B) *Cervical smear*

Take if due for routine screening.

(C) *Male semen test*

This test is best arranged at the hospital to which the man will be referred, as clinics interpret the results their own way, and this will reduce the risk of misinterpretation. The sample should be collected in a sterile container, and the client should be advised to abstain from intercourse for 36–48 hours prior to the test.

By requesting the general practitioners to do the initial tests, the time taken for this will be substantially reduced. It also gives the clients the opportunity to talk to their doctor about their problem, to gain basic preconception advice and to be better prepared to attend the specialist clinic (Lilford, 1992).

FIRST VISIT TO SPECIALIST CLINIC

Prior to attending the clinic the couple may be asked to fill out quite a lengthy questionnaire about their previous medical, reproductive and sexual history. This may seem unnecessary as they will have to go over this at the first visit, but it is important as it gives the couple some idea of the questions they will be asked. By completing it at home they have time to remember details and consider their replies in privacy as they may have situations in their past that they do not want their partners to know about. They may feel under pressure to disclose them if awkward questions are sprung on them unexpectedly in an interview situation. This could be very distressing for the partner and may result in lasting damage to their relationship.

The first interview may be scheduled to coincide with an *ultrasound scan* which needs to be performed in the first five days of a menstrual cycle. This scan will show the uterus and ovaries and any structural abnormalities can be identified. It is performed at the beginning of the cycle when there is least activity in the ovaries, and cysts can easily be identified.

The scan of the uterus may show congenital abnormality, for example a bicornuate uterus or dividing septum. Very occasionally a forgotten intrauterine contraceptive device may be identified, which may of course prevent pregnancy occurring! The scan will not show tubal patency. Ideally the nurse performing the scan will be able to continue the interview and go through the questionnaire with the couple. The continuation of care is important as a relationship of trust and security will help the couple discuss issues that may be very painful as well as personal to them. The nurse is also able to use any information gained whilst scanning the woman in the interview.

Preconception advice can be reinforced to the couple now; advice about smoking, drinking, the use of social drugs and dietary advice may need to be given. Smoking is well known to be harmful for the fetus, it is also known to increase the risk of miscarriage and cot death, but few men know that it can also have a detrimental effect on their sperms' potency (Miller, 1992). So men with a less than optimal semen analysis could be well advised to give up smoking. Advice on a sensible, well-balanced diet and general advice on healthy living could also be included as all women should be advised to be as healthy as possible prior to commencing pregnancy. All women are now routinely advised to take folic acid supplements for up to 12 weeks prior to conception in order to reduce the risk of fetal abnormalities, e.g. spina bifida (DOH, 1994).

By the time the couple have arrived in the clinic their relationship may already have been adversely affected by their fertility problem, and many welcome the opportunity to talk about this (Hirsch, 1989). It would be unwise, however, to attempt a full counselling situation here as it is not appropriate, but advice as to how it could be arranged if necessary should be offered. It is often a relief for the problem to be aired at this point however and it is reassuring to know that others also cry, argue or ignore the problem, and this is a normal way for couples to cope.

The couple's sexual relationship may also have suffered during the time they have been trying for a pregnancy and this too may need to be discussed openly. This may be the first time that they have been able to put how they feel about it into words and this may be very difficult for them, but if handled sensitively, talking can bring a great sense of relief, realizing that this may only be temporary and is very common to other couples experiencing the same problems.

Written information describing the treatments that will be available to them and their chances of success can also be given to prepare the couple for their next hospital appointment with the specialist doctor.

FURTHER INVESTIGATION

After the initial investigations have been completed there are two more questions to be answered:

▶ What is the tubal status of the woman?
▶ Can the eggs and sperm achieve fertilization together?

To discover if the woman's fallopian tubes are damaged or blocked they can be examined either by a *hysterosalpingogram* (HSG) or *laparoscopy*. An HSG is an X-ray examination, during which dye is passed through the cervix, uterus and fallopian tubes. If the dye is seen to pass easily into the pelvic cavity then the tubes are clear. If there is a blockage and the dye does not pass through, this may indicate either a blockage which would prevent sperm ever meeting the egg, or a spasm of the tube which is causing a temporary problem.

A laparoscopy is slightly more complicated as it is usually performed under a general anaesthetic, which has its own risk factors. Two small incisions are made into the abdomen, one below the umbilicus and the other just below the pelvic hairline. Through the first gas is pumped to inflate the abdominal cavity and a small telescope passed in through the same incision to visualize the pelvic organs to see if there are any structural abnormalities or damage done by previous infection or endometriosis. Often both of these tests are performed as one gives information about the inside of the reproductive tract and the other information about the outside. In larger centres where assisted conception is available, neither test may be performed, as regardless of their results the next step may be *in vitro* fertilization treatment (IVF).

In order to assess if the sperm are capable of fertilizing eggs, IVF needs to be performed so that their behaviour can be observed. If fertilization occurs then the fertilized eggs will be returned to the body.

Treatment

Treatments for subfertility are being developed all the time, but those most commonly available include the following:

▶ Ovulation induction.
▶ Tubal surgery.
▶ *In vitro* fertilization.
▶ Assisted conception.
▶ Ovum donation.
▶ Surrogacy.
▶ Intracytoplasmic sperm injection.
▶ Surgical retrieval of sperm.
▶ Donor insemination.

OVULATION INDUCTION

In order to decide how to treat anovulation (that is, when no ovulation occurs) it is necessary to diagnose why it is happening.

The most common causes of amenorrhoea (no periods for over six months) are

1   Polycystic ovaries.
2   Hypothalamic hypopituitarism.
3   Hyperprolactinaemia.
4   Premature ovarian failure (premature menopause).

Polycystic ovaries (PCO)

Polycystic ovaries are the commonest pathological cause of anovulation and menstrual dysfunction (McLure *et al.*, 1991). It is estimated by Franks *et al.* (1985) that it may affect up to 75% of women with infertility due to ovulation disorders. It can be diagnosed by ultrasound, the ovaries are generally larger than normal with many tiny cysts covering the surface. Polycystic ovary syndrome can also have the following symptoms:

▶ *Menstrual disturbance*, periods that are either very infrequent – oligomenorrhoea, completely absent – amenorrhoea, or occasionally too frequent.
▶ *Acne*, extra *body hair* or *greasy skin* (usually caused by too much testosterone).
▶ *Obesity*.

There is a familial tendency for polycystic ovaries, and often the woman's mother, sisters or daughters may have the same symptoms.

Many of the women with polycystic ovaries will be overweight and the first course of action should be to encourage them to lose weight as treatment of the condition is easier if weight is within normal limits.

The simplest treatment is clomiphene citrate which can be taken in 50 mg (Glasier, 1992) tablet form for five days at the beginning of each cycle and will stimulate the follicles to grow. It acts on both the hypothalamus and the pituitary gland to induce ovulation by stimulating the pituitary to produce more follicle-stimulating and luteinizing hormone.

This is often given as a first treatment, but should, ideally, also be monitored by ultrasound as occasionally the ovaries can be overstimulated resulting in multiple pregnancy and hyperstimulation. Although the simplest of treatments to take, the results are very favourable, with 70–75% achieving ovulation. About 5% of the pregnancies of women taking clomiphene result in twins (Tan and Jacobs, 1991). If this treatment fails, hMG may be used.

Other drugs which are occasionally used for ovulation induction are tamoxifen, cyclofenil and epimestrol, which are also taken orally and work in a similar way.

Hypothalamic hypopituitarism

In this condition the pituitary gland does not secrete enough follicle-stimulating and luteinizing hormones to stimulate the ovary to ripen and release the ova. Diagnosis can be made if low levels of these hormones

are detected. The most common cause is usually subnutrition, which results in the menstrual cycle stopping when the woman's weight drops. This could be caused by food shortage, but is more often seen as a result of severe dieting or in women with eating disorders such as anorexia nervosa. The most obvious treatment is to regain normal weight.

If the cause of the low levels of FSH and LH is a result of pituitary failure, then these hormones can be replaced by injections of human menopausal gonadotrophin (hMG). This is collected from the urine of post-menopausal women and is available in several virtually identical preparations. It works by stimulating the growth of follicles in the ovaries (Winston, 1994). This method of treatment requires careful monitoring by ultrasound as there is a significant risk that the woman will overrespond and this could result in ovarian hyperstimulation, which could be extremely dangerous to the patient if left untreated. (This treatment can, however, be used to overstimulate the ovaries deliberately, to produce several eggs if they are to be collected in order to be used in assisted conception techniques such as IVF.) Women who conceive when taking drugs to stimulate ovulation have an increased chance of a multiple pregnancy. Tan and Jacobs (1991) estimate that this could be as high as 25%, mainly twin pregnancies, but also triplets or higher order. Often the couple are not warned that this is a possibility and although twins are frequently described as an 'ideal outcome' for infertile couples, the reality of the physical, financial and emotional implications are often underestimated and the difficulties of coping with triplets even greater (Botting *et al.*, 1990; Harvey and Bryan, 1991).

Hyperprolactinaemia

Prolactin is a hormone that is secreted by the pituitary gland and its release is predominantly regulated by the hypothalamus. It is secreted in large amounts in pregnancy and prevents menstruation occurring by suppressing the release of FSH and LH.

If high levels of prolactin are produced in a nonpregnant woman it results in amenorrhoea. A common symptom of this condition is galactorrhoea, that is the presence of milk in the breasts that either leaks spontaneously or can be expressed when squeezed. The best-known treatment for this condition is the drug bromocriptine, which can be taken in tablet form. It usually reduces the prolactin level to normal in a few weeks, the menstrual cycle returns to normal and the chances of conceiving will then be equal to those of any normal woman.

Premature menopause

A menopause is defined as premature if it occurs before the age of 40 years. This affects 1% of the female population. It can be diagnosed by detecting the presence of high levels of FSH and LH with a low oestradiol level. Another name for this condition is premature ovarian failure. It has been reported in women in their twenties and nothing can be done to treat it. Ova cannot be produced so pregnancy could only be achieved by the woman accepting a donor egg from another woman (see Ovum donation).

TUBAL SURGERY

Tubal damage is generally caused by pelvic infection such as pelvic inflammatory disease, resulting in varying degrees of tubal damage or obstruction. Tubal disease is thought to be responsible for 30–40% of the cases of female infertility (Margara, 1992). Tubal surgery has been performed using high-magnification microscopes since 1959. It requires not only high-quality equipment but also a highly skilled operator. There is some degree of argument about how useful microsurgery is in improving pregnancy rates, and whether the increased risk of ectopic pregnancy is justified, but it is now well-established and is a routine procedure for tubal infertility (Winston, 1994).

Tubal surgery may also be used to reverse tubal sterilization but pregnancy rates vary according to the site of the occlusion and how much tube has been left.

IN VITRO FERTILIZATION

In vitro fertilization (IVF) was originally developed to bypass blocked fallopian tubes but is now used for the treatment of various other causes of infertility, such as:

▶ Unexplained infertility.
▶ Male factor infertility.
▶ Failed donor insemination.
▶ Cervical hostility.
▶ Failed ovulation induction.

The chances of achieving a pregnancy from IVF are, on average, 1:5 per cycle, rising to 1:3 if two or more good embryos are replaced (Tan *et al.*, 1992).

The basic principle involves stimulating the woman to develop several eggs, which are then removed from her ovaries, fertilized outside the body using sperm from either her partner or a donor and then transferring one or more of the fertilized eggs (or embryos) into her uterus. Returning the embryos into the uterus is called *embryo transfer* (ET).

The first stage of the process is to downregulate the ovaries using a course of buserelin administered either by subcutaneous injection or nasally. The buserelin works as a luteinizing hormone releasing hormone analogue which desensitizes the pituitary gland and prevents it from releasing FSH and LH, thus ensuring that the stimulation is controlled. Once desensitization has occurred daily injections of hMGs are given to stimulate the ovaries. The progress of the follicles is monitored by ultrasound scanning until the leading ones measure 16 mm in diameter. At this stage an injection of a hormone called human chorionic gonadotrophin (hCG) is given to cause the final maturation of the eggs.

The next day the eggs are collected under ultrasonic vision per vaginam, or occasionally by laparoscope. Some centres are able to give women a choice of either a general anaesthetic or intravenous sedation and analgesia for this procedure.

The eggs are then placed with the prepared sperm sample and the dish is placed in the incubator overnight.

The next morning the sample will be examined to see if fertilization has taken place. If it has the egg is now called a pre-embryo and remains in the laboratory until 36 hours after the egg collection. It will then have developed enough to be replaced in the uterus.

Generally no more than two embryos should be replaced at any time as more would raise the risk of a multiple pregnancy. The number of replaced embryos may be increased to three only in exceptional circumstances, for example if the woman is over 40 years old. The couple then have to wait for 14 days to see if implantation occurs and a pregnancy develops. This is obviously a very difficult time and although the couple is well aware that the chances of success are very low, the feeling of despair and hurt when the treatment fails is always acute.

ASSISTED CONCEPTION

Other methods of assisted conception are based on the same principles but differ by the site in which the gametes are placed and at what stage of their development they are returned.

- ▶ *GIFT* (gamete intrafallopian transfer) – eggs and sperm are placed into the woman's fallopian tubes.
- ▶ *DIPI* (direct intraperitoneal insemination) – sperm are injected into the pouch of Douglas at the expected time of ovulation.
- ▶ *POST* (peritoneal oocyte and sperm transfer – both eggs and sperm are injected into the pouch of Douglas close to the opening of the fallopian tubes.
- ▶ *ZIFT* (zygote intrafallopian tube transfer).
- ▶ *PROST* (pronuclear stage tubal transfer).
  In ZIFT and PROST fertilized eggs are transferred into the fallopian tubes 18 hours afer insemination.
- ▶ *TET* (tubal embryo transfer).
- ▶ *TEST* (tubal embryo stage transfer).
  In TET and TEST fertilized eggs are transferred into the fallopian tubes when the pre-embryo has developed into more cells.
- ▶ *DOT* (direct oocyte transfer) – the eggs are transferred into the uterus before fertilization has taken place but when the sperm are clustered around it.

OVUM DONATION

When a woman is unable to produce ova, either because she is menopausal, because her ovaries have been removed surgically or because she is infertile due to chemotherapy, she may still be able to experience pregnancy and childbirth by accepting a donor egg. If she is a carrier of a genetic disorder that could be passed on to her child she may also prefer to use a donor. Donor eggs are collected from healthy volunteers who have had their own children already. Generally they are altruistic and donate solely to help others. Occasionally women undergoing IVF may be asked if they would consider donating any spare eggs they have.

This treatment must be very carefully considered before being commenced and counselling, information giving and support, are essential for both partners. Donors are usually anonymous but occasionally known donors may be used. Although this has some advantages, in that the donor is well-known to the recipient (perhaps a sister or cousin) this may lead to problems in the future with relationships between donor, baby and mother not clearly defined. Donors are all tested for human immunodeficiency virus (HIV) and so they too must be carefully counselled and

support offered. To produce enough eggs the donor is stimulated with hMG and the eggs are collected in the same way as in IVF, which at best is uncomfortable, or at worst, painful. A general anaesthetic may be used, but this of course also has risks involved. At the same time the recipient's menstrual cycle is synchronized to that of the donor so that the eggs, after fertilization with the sperm of the recipient's partner, can be transferred at an appropriate time of her cycle.

Some women opt to use donated embryos, which have their genetic material donated from both male and female donors. Because of the great advances made in embryo cryopreservation, embryos that are available can be frozen until the recipient is ready to use them, thus allowing her greater flexibility in choosing how to space her family.

SURROGACY

Surrogacy is an option for women who have no suitable uterus of their own. They may have suffered a hysterectomy, have an abnormality that makes carrying a pregnancy to term impossible, or they may have suffered multiple miscarriages with no identifiable cause.

The gametes used may come from the commissioning parents (HOST surrogacy, where the surrogate acts solely as an incubator). The surrogate may provide her eggs and be inseminated by the commissioning father's sperm or donor sperm, either directly or by IVF.

This situation is obviously very risky to all involved as conceiving, pregnancy and giving birth are all major events and the emotions involved in these may force people to change their minds or regret the promises they made. Before any treatment can occur all parties involved must undergo counselling and be absolutely certain that they are all happy with the arrangements, approval must then be gained from the treatment centre's ethical committee. Payment, except for expenses, is illegal in the UK.

INTRACYTOPLASMIC SPERM INJECTION

In vitro fertilization has been used increasingly to treat couples with mild to moderately impaired sperm quality, as it has been recognized that a relatively small number of spermatozoa are required for fertilization *in vitro* to occur. A further step to help treat couples with very low numbers of sperm or very few normal sperm is currently being introduced into many clinics in the UK. This is intracytoplasmic sperm injection

(ICSI) in which micromanipulation techniques are used to place a sperm inside the egg itself by injection. This then promotes fertilization of the ovum. Many children have already been conceived by this method and it has been heralded as an important breakthrough in the treatment of male infertility.

SURGICAL RETRIEVAL OF SPERM

About 50% of infertile men who have no sperm identified in their samples (azoospermia) have normal testes but the passageways through which the sperm have to pass are obstructed. The three common causes of this are:

1　The vas deferens was not formed and so is said to be congenitally absent.
2　A past infection has caused a blockage in the epididymis near the testes.
3　The client has had a vasectomy in the past and attempts to reverse it by reconstructing the vas deferens have failed.

Using a delicate surgical technique known as microsurgical epididymal sperm aspiration (MESA), sperm are recovered from the epididymis close to the testes using an operating microscope. These sperm can then be used to fertilize the eggs of his partner collected as part of an IVF treatment cycle.

Sperm can also be retrieved from the vas (vas aspiration) which can again be used for IVF.

DONOR INSEMINATION

For some men, however, there is still no treatment available that will help to cure their sterility as they do not produce any sperm. Also some men with an hereditary condition may choose not to use their own genetic material. For all these men their only option to have a family is to use a donor. This option is acceptable to some but not to others and careful counselling and support must be given to the couple before treatment is commenced.

The donors are usually anonymous, and traditionally are often students who use their 'expenses' to supplement their grants. New semen banks have been opened that encourage donors to give their semen altruistically and tend to be used by men who have had their family and wish to allow others to have the experience. All donors have to undergo a careful screening process, to ensure that they have no transfer-

able genetic condition, that they are free from infection and that they understand the implications of donating their semen.

Treatment is, of course, given totally to the client's partner, either simply by intracervical or intrauterine insemination, or by using other assisted conception techniques.

Human Fertilisation and Embryology Authority

The Human Fertilisation and Embryology Authority was set up in 1991 to replace the Interim Licensing Authority, in order to act as a body to maintain standards and issue licences to all fertility centres in the UK wishing to provide either *in vitro* fertilization or donor insemination treatment. The Human Fertilisation and Embryology Act 1990 ensured that couples seeking such treatments would be able to do so confidentially, with permission being needed from them before the clinic could disclose any information about them to any other party. Rules to limit the number of embryos replaced in *in vitro* fertilization cycles have drastically reduced the number of higher order births (i.e. quadruplets or quintruplets). All clinics are required to consider the needs/rights of the unborn child, and they are obliged to take this into consideration before they agree to commence treatment.

Conclusions

As can be seen, infertility is a complex problem that can affect a couple's relationship in many ways. Not only do they have to deal with their own feelings about the problem but also those of their partner. The experience of infertility can damage what was a good relationship and guilt, anger and fear can often result. Couples feel isolated and unhappy before they arrive at the clinic and then they may have to face long waiting lists and limited availability of treatment in the NHS which may lead to frustration and helplessness. All clinics must have open access to counsellors who are specially experienced in dealing with these problems. Counselling should not be viewed as a service only needed by the inadequate but should be promoted as an extra support that can be used to help the individual to find methods to cope with their unique experience.

Much of the treatment and care of clients is carried out directly by nurses and midwives, giving an opportunity for continuity of care which is satisfying for the nurse or midwife and reassuring for the client. Many treatments seem complicated or risky, the chances of success low and the waiting times interminable, but with confidence in the clinic personnel and personal strength many couples succeed in their wish to start a family. For those not so lucky, the nurse or midwife can play a crucial role in supporting the couple through difficult times, helping them to come to terms with their situation and to make new plans with dignity and confidence.

References

Baker, H.G.W., Burger, H.G., de Kresner, D.M., Hudson, B., Rennie, G.C. & Straffon, W.G.E. (1985) Testicular vein ligation and fertility in men with varicoceles. *Br. Med. J.* **291**: 1678–1680.

Booker, M. (1988) Endometriosis. *Br. J. Hospital Med.* May: 440–445.

Botting, B.J., Price, F.V. & Macfarlane, A.J. (1990) *Three, Four and More: A Study of Triplet and Higher Order Births*. London: HMSO.

Boukje van Noord-Zaadstra, M., Caspar, W.N., Looman, Hans *et al.* (1991) Delaying childbearing: effect of age and outcome of pregnancy. *Br. Med. J.* **302**: 1361–1365.

Brinsden, P.R. & Rainsbury, P. (1992) *A Textbook of In Vitro Fertilisation and Assisted Reproduction*. Carnforth, Lancs: The Parthenon Publishing Group.

Clubb, E. & Knight, J. (1992) *Fertility, a Comprehensive Guide to Natural Family Planning*. Newton Abbott: David & Charles.

DOH (Department of Health) (1994) Pregnancy, folic acid and you (leaflet). London: DOH.

Franks, S., Adams, J., Mason, H. & Polson, D. (1985) Ovulatory disorders in women with polycystic ovary syndrome. *Clin. Obstet. Gynecol.* **12**: 605–632.

Glasier, A. (1992) Ovarian function and ovulation induction. In Shaw, R., Soutter, P. & Stanton, S. (eds) *Gynaecology*. Edinburgh & London: Churchill Livingstone.

Harvey, D. & Bryan, E.M. (1991) *The Stress of Multiple Births*. London: Multiple Births Foundation.

Hirsch, A. (1989) The effect of infertility on marriage and self-concept. *J. Obstet. Gynaecol. Neonatal Nurs.* January/February: 13–20.

Hirsch, A. (1992) The investigation and treatment of infertile men. In Brinsden, P.R. & Rainsbury, P. (eds) *A Textbook of In Vitro Fertilisation and Assisted Reproduction*, Ch. 2. Carnforth, Lancs: The Parthenon Publishing Group.

Jones (1981) Obstetrical significance of female anomalies. *Obstet. Gynecol.* **10**: 1039–1043.

Lilford, R. (1992) How general practitioners can help subfertile couples. *Br. Med. J.* **305**: 1376.

Margara, R.A. (1992) Tubal disease. In Shaw, R., Soutter, P. & Stanton, S. (eds) *Gynaecology*. Edinburgh & London: Churchill Livingstone.

McLure, N., Healy, O.L., Kovacs, G.T., McDonald, J., McQuinn, B. & Burger, W.G. (1991) Ovulation induction in polycystic ovarian syndrome. In Teoh, Eng-Soon, Shan Ratman, S. & Macnaughton, M. (eds) *Fertility, Sterility and Contraception*. Carnforth, Lancs: The Parthenon Publishing Group.

Miller, S. (1992) Warning: smoking may damage your sperm. *New Scientist* 17 October: 13–14.

Sharpe, R.M. & Stewart Irvine, D. (1994) What makes a man infertile? *MRC News* Spring: 32–35.

Thompson, W. & Heasley, R.N. (1992) Investigation of the infertile couple. In Shaw, R., Soutter, P. & Stanton, S. (eds) *Gynaecology*. Edinburgh & London: Churchill Livingstone.

Tan, S.L. & Jacobs, H.S. (1991) *Infertility; Your Questions Answered*. Singapore: McGraw-Hill.

Tan, S.L., Royston, P., Campbell, S. *et al.* (1992) Cumulative conception and livebirth rates after in-vitro fertilisation. *Lancet* **339**: 1390–1394.

WHO (World Health Organization) (1994) *World Health Organization Laboratory Manual for the Examination of Human Semen and Semen–Cervical Mucus Interaction*. Cambridge: Cambridge University Press.

Winston, R. (1994) *Infertility, a Sympathetic Approach*. London: Optima.

Further Reading

Cotton, K. (1992) *Second Time Around*. Herts: Dornoch Press.

Davis, H. & Fallowfield, L. (1991) *Counselling and Communication in Health Care*. Chichester: John Wiley & Sons.

Johnson, M. & Everitt, B. (1988) *Essential Reproduction*. Oxford: Blackwell Scientific.

Mason, M.-C. (1993) *Male Infertility – Men Talking*. London & New York: Routledge.

Snowden, R. & Snowden, E. (1993) *The Gift of a Child, A Guide to Donor Insemination*. Exeter: University of Exeter Press.

62

The Menopause

The term 'menopause' refers specifically to the end of menstruation, a normal physiological event, which occurs at an average age of 51 years – an age which has changed very little this century. The menopause can only be diagnosed retrospectively after a year with no menstrual bleeding.

The term 'climacteric' or perimenopause refers to the transitional phase during which ovarian function ceases. This commonly spans five years on each side of the menopause.

The problems associated with the climacteric are currently assuming greater importance because of the steady increase in female life expectancy due to improved health care. At the beginning of this century many women did not live long enough to reach the menopause but nowadays, in developed countries, the average female life expectancy is approximately 80 years. Consequently women can expect to spend over one third of their lives in a postmenopausal oestrogen-deficient state. In England and Wales it is estimated that menopausal women constitute 20% of the entire population (OPCS, 1991).

Statisticians have predicted there will be a 50% increase in the number of women over 85 years old during the next 30 years, which will inevitably place increasing demands on health care resources in the future.

Social Influences at the Menopause

Western society's attitude to the ageing woman has tended to be negative (Greer, 1992) and many women approach the menopause with anxiety and fear. They may be concerned about a marital relationship which is failing or they may be jealous of their partner's success which means that he spends more time at the office and has less time at home. Unemployment and redundancy are common and women may resent having their partner at home before he was due to retire. Libido which has been declining over the years may become non-existent with the onset of the menopause.

Children can be an additional source of worry: they may have left home for the first time and the mother can feel very unneeded and alone now that a main purpose in her life has gone. She may be anxious that they are not working hard enough, or mixing with friends who will be a bad influence now that she can no longer keep a watchful eye on them.

Parents become elderly and sick and demand more time and energy than the woman can afford to give. Women often end up caring for their elderly parents or parents-in-law which can cause even more friction in a relationship already trying to survive with difficulties.

A woman may also realize that the ambitions and aspirations of her younger days have little chance of becoming a reality and she has to re-evaluate many aspects of her life and her hopes for the future. The 'change' not only includes physical changes but also encompasses social, psychological and relationship factors.

Physiology of the Menopause

Ovarian function declines during the climacteric years and the ovaries eventually fail when they run out of primordial follicles. Initially this results in increasing failure of ovulation, together with an associated rise in pituitary gonadotrophins in an attempt to stimulate ovarian follicular growth. Despite this, ovarian hormone production progressively declines, resulting in symptoms that are commonly associated with low oestrogen levels, such as flushes, sweats, vaginal dryness and depression.

The menstrual cycle during the climacteric can be erratic with many women experiencing an 18–21-day cycle with heavy bleeding. This may lengthen to periods occurring every 2–3 months, before they eventually stop.

PREMATURE MENOPAUSE

Premature menopause occurs in 1% of women under the age of 40 years. In additon to the typical clinical features, the diagnosis must be confirmed by raised follicle-stimulating hormone (FSH) levels on two or more separate occasions. All the long-term effects of the menopause commence at a much earlier age and therefore these women have an increased risk of osteoporosis and ischaemic heart disease and are in particular need of long-term hormone replacement therapy. This must be given in an adequate dose to protect the bones from osteoporosis.

Many women postpone starting a family until their thirties and the tragedy of a premature menopause for them is the unexpected loss of fertility. These women need a great deal of counselling to enable them to come to terms with their infertility, although more fertility clinics are now offering the possibility of ovum donation which has an average pregnancy rate of 30% (Abdalla *et al.* 1990).

Resistant ovary syndrome is a rare condition that is clinically indistinguishable from premature menopause, but it may spontaneously recover with an unexpected return of fertility. It is important for women with premature ovarian failure to realize that there is a possibility of pregnancy, although this will be very remote.

Other causes of premature menopause are the following:

▶ *Surgical*: If both ovaries are removed then obviously ovarian function ceases immediately. However, even if the ovaries have been conserved during hysterectomy they fail sooner than would have been expected without surgery (Siddle *et al.*, 1987).
▶ *Radiotherapy and chemotherapy*: An increasing number of women are being rendered menopausal at an early age through radiotherapy and chemotherapy. These are administered to treat a wide range of malignant diseases with a primary outside the pelvis, in which the ovary is a well-recognized site for metastatic disease.

Symptoms and Effects of the Menopause

Short-term effects

Vasomotor symptoms Hot flushes and night sweats are the most characteristic manifestations of the menopause. About 70% of women will experience these symptoms; they cause acute physical distress in 50% and persist for more than five years in 25% (Studd *et al.* 1977). Vasomotor symptoms are most severe in the 1–2 years preceding the menopause and can also include palpitations, headaches, giddiness, insomnia and faintness.

Urogenital symptoms Oestrogen maintains healthy vaginal epithelium and consequently vaginal dryness and atrophy are frequent menopausal problems.

Dyspareunia is common and is often associated with discharge, infection and vaginal bleeding leading to a secondary loss of libido.

Similar atrophy can affect the lower urethra, resulting in a high incidence of urinary symptoms such as frequency, urgency and dysuria.

Psychological symptoms A broad spectrum of psychological symptoms are common in menopausal women. Depression, irritability, loss of confidence, poor memory, difficulty in concentration, primary loss of libido, loss of energy and panic attacks are found to peak in women aged 45–55 years. These symptoms may not be caused by the menopause alone and may be a result of the 'empty nest' syndrome when the children have left home or are causing problems and the marriage may be unsatisfactory.

Skin After the menopause there is a generalized loss of collagen from skin, muscle and bone. This results in thin, dry, flaky skin, brittle nails, dry hair and generalized musculoskeletal aches and pains.

Long-term effects

Osteoporosis Bone density gradually declines in both sexes after the third decade, but in women this loss accelerates substantially after the menopause. Women lose 50% of their total skeleton by the age of 70 years, whereas men lose only 25% by the age of 90 years. Osteoporosis costs the National Health Service an enormous sum of money every year for fracture management and results in:

▶ pain;
▶ fractures (vertebral, hip, wrist);
▶ deformity (kyphosis or dowager's hump); and
▶ loss of height.

Ideally all climacteric women should be screened for osteoporosis by means of a bone density scan, as the knowledge of a low bone density may persuade a woman to seek the most effective treatment before she suffers any fractures.

Oestrogen replacement therapy is the treatment of choice and even in low doses has been shown to prevent further loss of bone density. If HRT is given for five years it reduces the lifetime risk of a hip fracture by 50%. Oestrogen implants are the most potent form of oestrogen administration and have been shown to increase vertebral bone density 8.4% in one year (Studd *et al.* 1990).

Cardiovascular disease Mortality from ischaemic heart disease substantially increases in women after the menopause. Studies have shown that hormone replacement therapy significantly reduces the risk of cardiovascular disease by at least 40% (Stampfer and Colditz, 1991), and the risk of stroke by about 20% (Paganini-Hill *et al.*, 1988). The prevention of cardiovascular symptoms and deaths is probably the strongest reason why HRT should be used, even in women considered to be at 'high risk'. Therefore the presence of angina, previous myocardial infarction, hypertension, smoking and a family history of ischaemic heart disease should be regarded as a positive indication for HRT rather than a contraindication.

Alzheimer's disease New research appears to indicate that HRT could lower the risk or slow the progression of Alzheimer's disease. Larger and longer trials are urgently needed (Paganini-Hill, 1996).

Hormone Replacement Therapy (HRT)

Patient demand for hormone replacement therapy has increased steadily over the past decade, but despite the irrefutable evidence that it improves the quality of life and reduces premature morbidity from osteoporosis and cardiovascular disease, the use of HRT remains very low with only about 10% of women aged 50–60 years on HRT.

With all types of oestrogen replacement therapy it is established practice to give cyclical progestogen for 10–13 days every month to women who have a uterus. This prevents the development of endometrial hyperplasia and has proved effective in removing the risk of endometrial carcinoma which had previously been associated wtih unopposed oestrogen therapy (Paterson *et al.* 1980).

Oestrogen is administered in the UK in four different ways:

▶ Oral.
▶ Transdermal.
▶ Subcutaneous.
▶ Vaginal.

Oral HRT

There are many different formulations of oral therapy and oestrogen and progestogen may be prescribed separately or as a combined preparation. In women with a uterus a combined preparation will offer convenience and guarantee compliance with the progesterone phase but at the expense of flexibility.

Advantages of oral HRT

▶ Familiar.
▶ Flexible.
▶ Inexpensive.
▶ Easily discontinued.

Disadvantages of oral HRT

▶ Poor compliance.
▶ Nausea.
▶ Bolus effect.
▶ First-pass hepatic effect.
▶ Reverse of premenopausal oestradiol:oestrone ratio.

Transdermal HRT

Transdermal HRT can be with either patches or gel. Patches need to be changed every 3–4 days, or new 7-day patches are now available, in order for the hormones to pass readily into the skin. The first type of patch that was available was a thin multilayered patch, but newer single-membrane patches are now available which are cosmetically more pleasing and have reduced adhesion problems and skin irritations.

Some patches are available combined with progestogen, but usually this is prescribed separately in pill form which gives greater flexibility and variability with doses.

Gel containing a measured amount of oestrogen is rubbed into the skin daily. Although this type of HRT is relatively new in the UK it has been widely used in France and other European countries for many years.

Advantages of transdermal HRT

▶ Flexible.
▶ Easily discontinued.
▶ Controlled oestradiol release.
▶ Avoid first-pass hepatic effect.
▶ Premenopausal oestradiol:oestrone ratio.
▶ No effect on clotting factors or lipid metabolism.

Disadvantages of transdermal HRT

▶ Skin reactions.
▶ Adhesion problems.
▶ Unsightly.
▶ Can make a 'crackling' noise.
▶ Expensive.

Subcutaneous implants

Implant therapy is the only method of HRT that can elevate oestrogen levels back to the higher physiological level of the premenopausal range. Such levels may be important in some women in order to obtain maximal remedial treatment of osteoporosis and to obtain relief from psychological symptoms. Testosterone may also be added to an oestrogen implant which is an effective treatment for postmenopausal primary loss of libido. Progestogen cannot be given as an implant so must be prescribed separately as pills in those women who have a uterus.

Advantages of subcutaneous implants

▶ Compliance.
▶ Controlled release.
▶ Convenient and cheap.
▶ Avoid first-pass hepatic effect.
▶ Premenopausal oestradiol:oestrone ratio.
▶ Greater dose range.
▶ Testosterone implant can be added.
▶ Increases bone density.

Disadvantages of subcutaneous implants

▶ Minor surgical procedure.
▶ Occasional rejection of pellet.
▶ Difficult to remove.
▶ Prolonged duration of action.
▶ May need to have periods 1–2 years after the last implant.
▶ Supraphysiological levels of oestradiol.

Vaginal oestrogen

Local vaginal oestrogen in ring, cream, pessary or tablet form is suitable for women who solely complain of vaginal symptoms and do not wish to experience bleeding or take systemic HRT. It is important to monitor the dose since systemic absorption can occur, resulting in unopposed oestrogen with its potentially deleterious effect on the endometrium.

Livial Tibolone (Livial) is an oral preparation and is a synthetic steroid with weak oestrogenic, progestogenic and androgenic properties. It relieves menopausal symptoms and prevents postmenopausal bone loss but is only suitable for postmenopausal women who have had at least a year of amenorrhoea. The advantage of Livial is that it offers the prospect of bleed-free HRT, but whilst this is true for most women, approximately 15% experience irregular spotting and bleeding.

It is important to prescribe the right preparation of HRT for the right patient and to discuss the reasons for this choice with the woman who must feel happy with the form of HRT that is chosen for her.

CONTRAINDICATIONS TO HRT

There are very few absolute contraindications to HRT, and many of those listed in the data information sheets enclosed with HRT preparations are not relevant as the information is extrapolated from data on the oral contraceptive pill. Hypertension, hyperlipidaemia and previous myocardial infarction, as previously mentioned, are positive indications that HRT should be used as cardiovascular disease is substantially reduced in those high-risk women on HRT.

The main contraindication is recent *endometrial or breast cancer*, and these women need help with finding alternative therapies to help them during the climacteric. In those women who have severe menopausal symptoms with a very poor quality of life it may be reasonable to offer help with low-dose HRT provided they are adequately counselled, as recent uncontrolled reports suggest that the prognosis for breast and endometrial cancer may be better if the patients are subsequently given oestrogens.

Undiagnosed genital tract bleeding needs investigation before HRT is commenced.

Pregnancy is an absolute contraindication and a suspected pregnancy should be excluded before starting HRT.

Otosclerosis is a rare ear problem causing deafness and is said to worsen with HRT, however there is no good evidence for this.

SIDE-EFFECTS OF HRT

Side-effects of HRT can be broken down into two main groups:

▶ those associated with the oestrogen component; and
▶ those associated with the progestogen component.

Side-effects of oestrogen
These include:

▶ nausea;
▶ breast tenderness;
▶ leg cramps; and
▶ weight gain.

It is important that women are informed that they may experience some of these symptoms initially, and reassured that such symptoms are transient and will usually settle after 2 or 3 months. Unfortunately women often interpret these side-effects to mean that HRT does not suit them and will discontinue therapy without taking medical advice.

Side-effects of progestogen
Progestogenic side-effects can be divided into two categories – *premenstrual syndrome (PMS)-like effects* and the *withdrawal bleed* – and it is undoubtedly this element of HRT that is a major factor in the low number of women starting HRT and the large number of women who discontinue therapy within one year.

Many of these problems can be resolved by good counselling before commencing HRT about the importance of progestogen in preventing endometrial hyperplasia and warning of possible side-effects.

Management of progestogenic symptoms involves changing the type of progestogen, reduction in dosage and shortening the course. As research continues into HRT, new formulations have become available for women who are at least one year postmenopausal which should avoid the need for a regular bleed. The number of different HRT preparations has increased dramatically recently in attempts to find the 'perfect' HRT with minimal side-effects.

COMMON ANXIETIES AND MISCONCEPTIONS ABOUT HRT

Over the years the menopause and hormone replacement therapy have come to be surrounded by so many myths and superstitions that many women approach their middle age with trepidation and are reluctant to seek medical help for fear of 'interfering with nature'.

Some common misconceptions voiced by women include the following:

▶ *HRT restores fertility*: Some women associate the return of menstruation which occurs with HRT, with a return to fertility. This is not the case.

▶ *Contraceptive pill was contraindicated*: Women may think that if they were not allowed the contraceptive pill for any reason then they will certainly be denied HRT. Explanation is needed that HRT uses *natural* oestrogens, whilst the combined pill uses *synthetic* oestrogens and the usual dose of oestrogen used in HRT is approximately one sixth of that commonly used in the pill.

▶ *Weight gain*: HRT does not cause true weight gain – overeating does!

▶ *Fear of breast cancer*: Statistics and studies give conflicting information about the true incidence of breast cancer whilst on HRT. Overall it seems that HRT taken for longer than ten years slightly increases the risk of developing breast cancer *but* this is balanced by a corresponding reduction in mortality. The explanation of this paradox is unknown but the effect of HRT on breast cancer is probably neutral.

▶ *Fear of thrombosis*: There is no increased risk of thromboembolism with the natural oestrogens used in HRT, and the risk of cardiovascular disease is substantially reduced in women using HRT.

Non-hormonal Help at the Menopause

Women should be encouraged throughout their lives to adopt a healthy lifestyle and this is as important during the menopause as it was during pregnancy and lactation.

There are four main areas of health education and lifestyle advice that should be addressed and the appropriate advice given. This advice is very similar to that which is given during antenatal care:

▶ Regular exercise, preferably weight bearing.
▶ Balanced diet, rich in calcium.
▶ Stop smoking.
▶ Decrease alcohol intake.

Those women who are at risk of osteoporosis, or already have established osteoporosis, should be advised that oestrogen is the only completely effective method of treatment and will prevent further bone loss. *Calcium supplements* are of limited benefit for women who have a well-balanced diet, but may be beneficial for those at particular risk of dietary deficiency, e.g. vegans and those with lactose intolerance.

Other preparations that may be considered for the treatment of osteoporosis when HRT is contraindicated include:

▶ Bisphosphonates.
▶ Calcitonin.
▶ Sodium fluoride.
▶ Vitamin D.

Treatment for the relief of menopausal symptoms without using HRT can include *clonidine* for hot flushes, *antidepressants* or *tranquillizers* for mood changes and depression and *vaginal lubricants* for vaginal dryness and dyspareunia. The benefits of all of these treatments are limited but they may make menopausal symptoms more bearable in some women.

Contraception

It is always important at any stage in life that adequate contraception is used if a pregnancy is not planned. This is especially vital in the perimenopausal woman as maternal morbidity and mortality are increased, and certain chromosomal abnormalities of the fetus are more common in this age group. An unplanned pregnancy in the older woman can be devastating and may result in great psychological trauma.

During the climacteric it is difficult to assess how fertile a woman is, but it is accepted that fertility declines with age and that ovulation occurs less frequently after the age of 40 years. The fertility of a woman at 40 years is said to be reduced to about half of what it was at the age of 25 years, with a further decline after 45 years, but there are few statistics to substantiate this evidence. Although anovulatory cycles increase with age, ovulation and conception can occur right up to the menopause and diagnosis of the menopause can only be made retrospectively. The commonly accepted recommendation is that contraception should be continued for two years if the last menstrual period was when a woman is aged under 50 years, and for one year if the last menstrual period occurred over the age of 50 years.

There is no single 'best' method of contraception for the perimenopausal woman and time needs to be spent giving advice on all the methods available and their suitability. Due to the decline in her fertility a method which may have been unacceptable to her when she was younger due to a higher failure rate, may now be a suitable option.

Sterilization   Both male and female sterilization are suitable.

Combined oral contraception   It is now possible for a woman with no risk factors to stay on the combined pill until she reaches the menopause. It is particularly important that those women are carefully assessed and are healthy, non-smoking, normotensive and with no risk factors for thrombosis or heart disease. However use of the combined pill will mask some climacteric symptoms, and it is not suitable for use in conjunction with HRT.

Progestogen-only pill   This may be used up to the menopause, and can be used concurrently with standard cyclical combined oestrogen/progestogen HRT preparations. In theory this would provide adequate contraception but there are no data to support this.

Depot progestogens   These are not an ideal method for this age group due to irregular vaginal bleeding. Amenorrhoea is a well-known consequence of depot progestogens and cannot be assumed to be due to the menopause.

Intrauterine contraceptive device (IUCD)   This method is suitable for the older woman whether or not she is using HRT. It is not appropriate in women with fibroids or menorrhagia and all IUCDs should be removed one year after the menopause due to the possibility of cervical stenosis.

The new levonorgestrel-releasing intrauterine system (IUS) marketed under the name 'Mirena' will be especially useful for women in this age group as not only is it contraceptive, but it also reduces blood loss due to the direct effect of the progestogen on the endometrium. In the woman who is already established on HRT it will provide continuous low-dose progestogen, thereby protecting the endometrium and hopefully avoiding the necessity of a regular bleed.

Barrier methods   Male and female barrier methods are both reliable and appropriate for this age group, and may also be used in conjunction with HRT. The contraceptive sponge is undervalued and would be suitable for the perimenopausal woman.

Spermicides   These can provide additional lubrication in women in whom vaginal dryness is a problem, but the use of spermicides alone can only be recommended for use after the age of 50 years and for the year following the menopause.

'Natural' family planning   This method tends to be unreliable for the older woman due to irregular menstruation and erratic ovulation.

Modern HRT preparations do not suppress ovulation in the perimenopausal woman and are not contraceptive. It is vitally important that women who are still menstruating before they commence HRT are advised to also use an effective method of contraception in addition to their HRT.

Conclusion

The menopause is a natural event that is not without risks to women's health. Women need to be given accurate information about what is happening to their bodies and impartial advice about hormone replacement therapy, enabling them to make informed choices about whether or not to start therapy. The use of HRT and its follow-up involves essentially fit, healthy, normal women and specialist menopause clinics are increasingly being set up in general practice and in family planning clinics to cater for their needs. Midwives, nurses and doctors need to have a broad knowledge of the menopause, HRT and contraceptive issues so that they can accurately advise perimenopausal women in their care.

References

Abdalla, H.I., Baber, R., Kirkland, A., Leonard, T., Power, M. & Studd, J.W.W. (1990) A report on 100 cycles of oocyte donation; factors affecting the outcome. *Human Reprod.* 5(8): 1018–1022.

Greer, G. (1992) *The Change*. London: Penguin.

OPCS (Office of Population Censuses and Survey) (1991) *Mortality Statistics Cause 1990*, Series DH2, No. 17. London: HMSO.

Paganini-Hill, A. (1996) Oestrogen replacement therapy and Alzheimer's disease. *Br. J. Obstet. Gynaecol.* 103(13): 80–86.

Paganini-Hill, A., Ross, R.K. & Henderson, B.E. (1988)

Postmenopausal oestrogen treatment and stroke: a prospective study. *Br. Med. J.* 297: 519–522.

Paterson, M.E.L., Wade-Evans, T., Sturdee, D., Thom, M. & Studd, J. (1980) Endometrial disease after treatment with oestrogens and progestogens in the climacteric. *Br. Med. J.* 280: 822–824.

Siddle, N., Sarrel, P. & Whitehead, M. (1987) The effect of hysterectomy on the age of ovarian failure: identification of a subgroup of women with premature loss of ovarian function and literature review. *Fertil. Steril.* 47(1): 94–100.

Stampfer, M.J. & Colditz, G.A. (1991) Estrogen replacement therapy and coronary heart disease; a quantitative assessment of the epidemiological evidence. *Prevent. Med.* 20: 47–63.

Studd, J.W.W., Chakravati, S. & Oram, D. (1977) The climacteric and the menopause. In Greenblatt, R. & Studd, J.W.W. (eds) *Clinics in Obstetrics and Gynaecology*, Vol 4, Part 1, pp. 3–29. London: W.B. Saunders.

Studd, J.W.W., Savvas, M., Watson, N. *et al.* (1990) The relationship between plasma oestradiol and the increase in bone density in post-menopausal women after treatment with subcutaneous hormone implants. *Am. J. Obstet. Gynecol.* 163: 1474–1479.

Further Reading

Cooper, W. (1988) *No Change.* 3rd edn. London: Arrow Books.

Smith, R. & Studd, J.W.W. (1993) *The Menopause and Hormone Replacement Therapy.* London: Martin Dunitz.

Whitehead, M. & Godfree, V. (1992) *Hormone Replacement Therapy, Your Questions Answered.* Edinburgh: Churchill Livingstone.

Useful Addresses

British Menopause Society 83 High Street, Marlow, Buckinghamshire SL7 1AB Tel. 01628 890199

The Amarant Trust 80 Lambeth Road, London SE1 7PW Tel. 0171 401 3855

National Osteoporosis Society PO Box 10, Barton Meade House, Radstock, Bath BA3 3YB Tel. 01761 432472 Helpline: 01761 431594

Part Fourteen

The Newborn Baby

63

Physiology and Care of the Newborn

The satisfactory transition from fetus to newborn infant is the greatest hazard the baby has to overcome. It necessitates a very rapid change from the warmth and shelter of the uterus to the cold uncertain world outside. Survival depends on the baby's ability to make this transition. Major physiological adjustments are therefore necessary at birth and continue within the next few days and weeks. These include the establishment of respirations, changes in the cardiovascular system and the blood, the regulation of body temperature, digestion and absorption of food and the development of a resistance to infection. A basic understanding of the physiological changes happening at birth is necessary as a background to the steps needed to care for the newborn baby.

Outline of Physiological Changes at Birth

RESPIRATION

In uterine life the fetus obtains oxygen and excretes carbon dioxide via the placenta. Although the lungs are not used for gaseous exchange, the healthy fetus makes breathing movements for 80% of the time *in utero* to exercise the muscles of respiration. The lungs contain fluid, some of which is expelled when the chest is compressed during a vaginal delivery. At birth, when the cord is clamped and cut, it is vital that respirations are quickly established to enable the baby to obtain oxygen and excrete carbon dioxide via the lungs. The whole respiratory system must be intact and the airways clear to enable this gaseous exchange to take place.

A high negative intrathoracic pressure of as much as 30–40 cm of water may be required initially to inflate the lungs at birth. Subsequently the negative pressure required for breathing is much smaller, only about 5 cm of water. This is because of the presence of a phospholipid called *surfactant* which is present in the lung fluid. It has the property of reducing surface tension in the alveoli and thus prevents them collapsing completely once they have been inflated. Less pressure is therefore required to re-inflate the alveoli after each breath (see Chapter 26).

The first breath is thought to be triggered by stimuli to the *respiratory centre* in the medulla. At birth, when the cord is clamped, there is a relative reduction of oxygen and an accumulation of carbon dioxide in the baby's blood. This stimulates the respiratory centre and initiates respiration. A severe or prolonged oxygen lack, together with very high levels of carbon dioxide, will depress, rather than stimulate, the respiratory centre. Sensory stimuli such as touch, the impact of cool air on the skin, light and noise are also thought to activate the respiratory centre.

Initially the baby's respiratory rate is about 50 per minute but settles to about 40 per minute soon after birth. Respirations in the newborn are irregular, mainly abdominal and interspersed with short periods of apnoea, which are not severe enough to cause a change in colour.

CARDIOVASCULAR SYSTEM

When the umbilical cord is clamped and cut at birth, major circulatory changes take place to divert the blood to the lungs rather than to the placenta for oxygenation. As the baby takes his first breath and the lungs expand, more blood flows through the pulmonary arteries to the lungs, rather than into the ductus arteriosus which bypasses the lungs. The *ductus arteriosus* therefore contracts and gradually closes. The increased volume of blood from the lungs returns to the heart, thereby increasing the pressure in the left atrium. This assists in closing the flap-like valve, the *foramen ovale*, between the two atria. The flow of blood from the right to the left atria through the foramen ovale therefore ceases. The vessels which in intrauterine life carried deoxygenated blood to the placenta, the *hypogastric arteries*, and those which conveyed oxygenated blood from the placenta to the fetus, namely the

umbilical vein and the *ductus venosus*, also close and in time become ligaments.

These circulatory changes are not completed once and for all immediately after birth, but take place over a period of hours or even days. Respiratory and cardiac disorders accompanied by hypoxia and acidosis may delay, or even reverse, the circulatory changes in the heart and lungs.

Changes in the blood

At birth the baby has a high haemoglobin of about 17 g/dl and much of the haemoglobin is of the fetal type, HbF. This high concentration of HbF is required *in utero* to increase the oxygen-carrying capacity of the blood, since oxygenated blood from the placenta is soon mixed with deoxygenated blood from the lower part of the fetus. The overall oxygen saturation of the fetal blood is therefore reduced. After birth, when this problem no longer exists, the high number of red blood cells is not required, so haemolysis of excess red blood cells takes place. This may result in physiological jaundice of the newborn within 2–3 days of birth. By the age of about three months the haemoglobin has fallen to about 12 g/dl. The conversion of fetal haemoglobin to adult haemoglobin (HbA) starts *in utero* and is completed during the first year or two of life.

At birth the prothrombin level is low due to lack of vitamin K. Vitamin K is required as a cofactor for the activation of several clotting proteins in the blood. A deficiency of vitamin K may result in spontaneous bleeding in the newborn between the third and sixth day of life. The administration of vitamin K can rapidly correct such a clotting problem. By the fifth or sixth day, milk feeding is usually established and the bacteria necessary for the synthesis of vitamin K are present in the intestine (see Chapter 72).

TEMPERATURE CONTROL

After birth the newborn has to adjust to a lower environmental temperature and one which is liable to change. The heat-regulating mechanism in the newborn is inefficient and the baby may sustain a significant drop in body temperature unless great care is taken to avoid chilling. Heat is lost from the skin by radiation, convection, evaporation and conduction. This can be reduced if the baby is born into a warm environment of 21–24°C, dried carefully and wrapped warmly. The newborn cannot shiver and increase heat production by this method. Stores of brown fat are present in the baby at birth, however, and can be utilized for heat production when required. Brown fat is stored between the shoulder blades, behind the sternum, in the neck and around the kidneys and suprarenal glands. An adequate intake of food is also essential for heat production. If the baby's temperature falls, more energy contained in the diet will have to be used for the production of heat rather than for growth and the consumption of oxygen will be increased. Every effort therefore must be made to avoid unnecessary heat loss in the newborn (see Chapter 66).

GASTROINTESTINAL TRACT

In utero the fetus obtains all the nutrients required in a predigested form from the maternal blood via the placenta. After birth the baby has to suck, swallow, digest, absorb and excrete for himself. All the digestive enzymes required are present in the baby at term and the process of digestion is similar to that of the adult, except that it mostly takes place in the small intestine. Breast milk is more easily digested than cows' milk.

Meconium is a soft, greenish-black viscid substance which has gradually accumulated in the intestine from about the 16th week of intrauterine life. It consists of mucus, epithelial cells, swallowed amniotic fluid, fatty acids and bile pigments. Meconium is passed for about two days after birth, the first stool being passed within the first 24 hours. As the baby takes food the residue mixes with the remaining meconium and the stool changes to a greenish-brown colour, the 'changing stool'. The passage of meconium indicates that the lower bowel is patent, whereas the passage of a changing stool indicates that the whole gastrointestinal tract is patent. By the fourth or fifth day the stools become yellow. The breastfed baby passes soft, bright yellow, inoffensive stools whereas the baby who is artificially fed passes paler, more formed stools with a slightly offensive odour. The breastfed baby may pass stools as often as five or more times a day when the mother's milk comes in between the fourth and fifth day after delivery. After 3 or 4 weeks, however, when breastfeeding is fully established, the baby may only pass one soft yellow stool every 2 or 3 days, as there are few waste products from breast milk. The artificially fed baby passes stools more regularly when feeding is established and has a tendency to be constipated.

RENAL SYSTEM

The fetus passes urine into the amniotic fluid during pregnancy. At term the kidneys are relatively immature, the renal cortex being more immature than the medulla. The glomerular filtration rate is reduced and the ability to concentrate urine is deficient. Relatively large amounts of fluid are required to excrete solids. If the baby becomes dehydrated the excretion of solids such as urea and sodium chloride is further impaired.

The baby should pass urine within 24 hours of delivery. Initially urinary output is about 20–30 ml per day, rising to 100–200 ml daily by the end of the first week as fluid intake increases. The urine has a low specific gravity.

PROTECTION AGAINST INFECTION

In utero the fetus is protected from infection by the intact amniotic sac and the barrier mechanism of the placenta, although certain microorganisms do cross the placenta and infect the fetus. During the last trimester of pregnancy there is a transplacental transfer of IgG from the mother to the fetus. This gives the baby protection against the infectious diseases to which the mother has antibodies. These antibodies give the baby a passive immunity for about six months.

The newborn baby has no immunity to the common organisms, however, and thus when exposed to them for the first time at birth is highly susceptible to infection. Soon after birth the baby becomes colonized by microorganisms, staphylococci on the umbilicus and skin, *Escherichia coli* in the lower gut and streptococci in the upper respiratory tract. Early and frequent contact with the mother encourages colonization by her bacteria. Clinical infection occurs when the poorly developed defence mechanisms of the baby are overwhelmed by the number and virulence of the organisms. Every effort must therefore be made to protect the baby from infection. Breastfeeding encourages specific bacteria to multiply in the bowel and the acid conditions that result from this may help to prevent the overgrowth of potential pathogens. It therefore provides the baby with some protection from infection.

CENTRAL NERVOUS SYSTEM

The newborn baby has very poor motor development compared with other mammals but highly developed sensations (sight, hearing, taste, smell), hence the importance of picking babies up, talking to them and stroking them to stimulate them and evoke response.

Care of the Newborn Baby at Birth

The healthy fetus has been in a warm, safe and stable environment where all needs have been catered for without any effort. The physical effects of labour and birth are carefully monitored and action can be taken to relieve most problems which arise, but the psychological effects of this traumatic event are not well understood. At birth the baby should therefore be handled gently by the midwife, and be given to the mother where the baby will feel secure and comforted in her arms.

Establishment of respiration (see Chapter 69)

The first consideration is the establishment of respiration and for this the air passages must be clear. The fetus has been living surrounded by liquor amnii, making slight movements with the respiratory muscles ('practising' breathing, as it were) and some liquor thus enters the upper respiratory tract (Kelnar et al., 1995). There may, in addition, be other material, such as mucus, a little blood or vernix and possibly meconium in the liquor and thus in the air passages.

Accordingly, when the baby's head emerges the midwife should gently wipe the nostrils and mouth clear of mucus; when he is born, she places him in a head-down position to help the liquor to trickle out of the air passages. By now he may be crying vigorously or the midwife may need to gently clear the pharynx of more tenacious mucus, using a soft mucus extractor. Vigorous suction must be avoided as it induces laryngospasm and apnoea (Rosen and Roberton, 1984) and is no greater stimulus to breathing than brief, gentle suction.

As soon as respiration begins, the baby's colour, hitherto rather bluish, changes quickly to rosy pink. Sometimes the peripheral circulation is a little uneven, and the baby's skin may be mottled or the hands and feet bluish, but this is not usually important.

Apgar score

At one minute after birth the Apgar score (Table 1) is assessed. This is a method of assessing the baby's condition by observing five vital signs:

1   Respiratory effort.
2   Heart rate.
3   Colour.
4   Muscle tone.
5   Response to stimuli.

For each vital sign the baby is given 2, 1 or 0 points and the points are then totalled. An Apgar score of 8–10 indicates that the baby is in good condition at birth. A score of 4–7 indicates a moderate birth asphyxia and a score of 1–3 severe birth asphyxia. Urgent resuscitative measures are then necessary. The Apgar score is reassessed five minutes after birth and repeated at five-minute intervals in cases of asphyxia when the baby is being resuscitated. Most healthy babies have an Apgar score of 9 at birth, one point being lost for colour because the extremities often remain a blue colour for some hours after birth due to poor peripheral circulation.

Mother and baby relationship

The relationship between mother and baby begins long before birth and may be affected by a range of factors, including the woman's experience of pregnancy. Oakley (1987) believes that the relationship begins before conception and reflects the way the woman herself was mothered. The mother's apparent reaction to her baby

Table 1   The Apgar score

Sign*	Score		
	0	1	2
Heart rate	Absent	Slow (below 100)	Fast (above 100)
Respiratory effort	Absent	Slow Irregular	Good Crying
Muscle tone	Limp	Some flexion of extremities	Active
Reflex irritability (stimulation of foot or oropharynx)	No response	Grimace	Cry, cough
Colour	Blue Pale	Body pink Extremities blue	Completely pink

*The first two, heart rate and respiratory effort, are the most important.

at birth will vary greatly according to her culture, experience, expectations and the environment, and will also be affected by her physical and emotional well-being at the time.

In some cultures the mother will wish to have immediate and close social contact with her baby from the moment of birth, whereas in others the woman may prefer to have her baby cleaned and perhaps wrapped before he is presented to her. Discussion with the mother before labour and delivery will elicit her feelings and wishes, but these may change when the baby actually arrives and so the midwife needs to be flexible to adapt to the mother's reactions at the time.

It is common practice to deliver the baby on to the mother's abdomen if she is in a semi-recumbent position, or otherwise into her arms as far as the length of the cord will allow, where she has physical contact with her baby from the moment of birth. When the cord is clamped and cut and provided respirations are established, the mother should be given her baby to cuddle immediately. Usually this is a very joyous and emotional moment for both parents.

Mothers tend to go through a sequence in their early contact with their new baby. First she just looks at her baby, making eye-to-eye contact as she holds him in an en face position. It is known that newborn babies can focus at a distance of 20–25 cm (Schaffer, 1971) and therefore the baby can see the mother when held closely in her arms. Next, using her fingertips, she explores and often massages hands, fingers and toes, then gathers the baby to her and finally places her whole hand on his body (Klaus et al., 1972, 1975; Klaus and Kennell, 1982). The father, too, is usually involved in this early contact with his child and should also be given the opportunity to cuddle him.

There is evidence that early and unhurried contact between the mother and baby during the first hour after birth significantly affects maternal emotional well-being when measured at six weeks after delivery (Ball, 1994). It also gives mother, father and their baby the opportunity to start getting to know one another and, as this is thought to be a sensitive period for human attachment (this period may last for about three days) and the baby is usually awake at this time, the social interaction between them at this early stage promotes attachment (Klaus and Kennell, 1976).

The baby is offered the breast if the mother wishes to breastfeed and at first may just lick the nipple but in due course usually sucks well. This early sucking not only promotes mother/baby attachment, but also has a positive effect on maternal emotional well-being. It also stimulates the breasts to secrete milk and research has shown that mothers who breastfeed their babies soon after delivery breastfeed for longer (Salariya et al., 1978). Other advantages of this early breastfeed are that the baby is usually alert and sucks well, which is most encouraging for the mother, and the baby has a good feed of colostrum which has a high protein and low fat content. It also contains antibodies which give the baby some protection against infection. In addition, as the baby sucks oxytocin is released from the posterior pituitary gland to aid contraction of the uterus.

Mothers who plan to feed artificially should also be given the opportunity to offer their baby a feed soon after delivery. When the baby is cuddled in the mother's arms for a feed the en face position is achieved and feeding gives pleasure to both mother and baby (Ball, 1984).

The midwife should be aware that some mothers are disappointed in their baby at birth. Others may not want to touch and cuddle their child until he has been washed and made presentable. In these instances the midwife's role is to promote bonding by gently encouraging the mother to touch and hold her baby. The baby can be wiped clean to make him more acceptable. Positive helpful comments should be made to the mother about her baby. Careless remarks such as 'he's rather a scraggy little thing' can do much harm in that they may make the mother feel a failure and even ashamed of her baby. Instead she should be encouraged to feel that she has achieved a marvellous feat by giving birth to such a lovely baby.

The midwife should ensure that all mothers have the opportunity for early, prolonged and intimate contact with their baby soon after birth, preferably in the first hour. Only when the medical condition of the mother or baby mitigate against it should it be delayed. Then arrangements will need to be made for the mother to see and touch her baby at the earliest opportunity. This early contact establishes the foundation for a good mother–child relationship and less feeding and behavioural problems are likely to occur later.

Warmth (see Chapter 66)

It is important that the baby is kept warm at birth. He has been accustomed to a constant intrauterine temperature of 37.7°C and is born into a much cooler atmosphere of 21–24°C. At birth he should be gently dried to prevent evaporation from his wet skin, and then given to his mother who will keep him warm. Warm wrappers are placed over the baby and if necessary an overhead heater may be used whilst he is in his mother's arms. Later he is wrapped warmly and placed in a preheated cot under a heat lamp. Unnecessary exposure should be avoided. Within an hour of birth the baby's axillary temperature is taken using a low-reading thermometer.

Umbilical cord

The umbilical cord is usually clamped (Figure 1) and cut immediately after birth. Two pairs of artery forceps are used, one being placed 7.5 cm and the other 12.5 cm from the umbilicus. The cord is then cut between the clamps with blunt-ended scissors, the end being covered with a sterile gauze dressing. Great care must be taken to avoid the introduction of infection. It is also essential to ensure that the clamp is secure, otherwise the cord may bleed. A blood loss of 30 ml from a baby is equivalent to 600 ml in an adult.

A haemostat will then be applied to the cord 2.5 cm from the umbilicus. The haemostat may be a plastic or metal clamp, an elastic band or nylon tape ligature. The excess cord is then cut off and the stump is wiped dry with a sterile swab. The practice of applying antiseptic solution or spray has largely been abandoned since such treatment has been found to delay separation of the cord (Lawrence, 1982; Barr, 1984; Rush *et al.*, 1989).

Identification of the baby

In hospital it is important to label the baby with the mother's name, hospital number, date of birth and sex as soon as possible after delivery. Various types of identification are used and the midwife should carefully follow the policy of her employing authority. The important principles are that the form of identification used should be checked by the mother, applied soon after birth and certainly before mother and baby are separated, and should be secure and reliable. The midwife will check each day that the labels are still on the baby. There should be a clear written policy to follow if labels become detached from the baby for any reason during the time he is in hospital. A cot card is also completed and attached to the baby's cot.

Birthweight and measurements

The baby is weighed within an hour or so of birth, his weight being checked by a second midwife. His length is measured from crown to heel and is usually 50–52 cm at term. Length measurements are difficult to perform accurately without a measuring device such as a rollametre or neonatometer. If this is not available, a tape measure is usually used and there should be a clear protocol which is carefully followed to improve the accuracy of this method of measurement. The baby is measured lying on his side initially on a flat surface before he is clothed. The starting point on the baby's head may be the upper border of the posterior fontanelle because it is easy to identify and therefore more consistent measurements are achieved. The tape measure is then applied down the baby's back before he is rolled over to the dorsal position, making sure that the starting position is still correct and that the tape measure is taut. The legs are then straightened and the length of the baby is measured from the upper

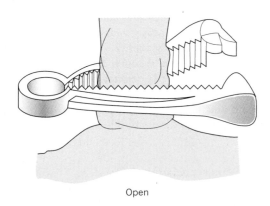
Open

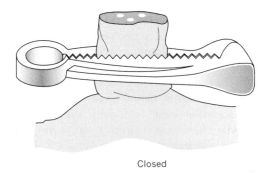
Closed

Figure 1   A cord clamp.

border of the posterior fontanelle to the heel, with the feet at a 90° angle to the tape measure (Burn, 1995).

Finally the occipitofrontal head circumference is measured and should be approximately 35 cm. All these measurements are recorded in the notes.

Examination of the newborn

Whilst the baby is exposed, the midwife carries out a detailed examination in the presence of the parents and takes his temperature. The midwife may now be responsible for the full medical examination of the baby, provided that she has been trained in the procedure (UKCC, 1993; DOH, 1993). During the examination the midwife explains what she is doing and involves the parents as much as possible in the procedure. Questions are answered and appropriate health education given. The midwife will already have noted that the baby is healthy and, on cursory observation, normally developed. The baby is unwrapped and examined gently in a warm, well-lit room.

General observations   The term baby is breathing regularly; he is pink and plump with abundant subcutaneous fat and a smooth skin. Vernix caseosa, a white greasy substance, is found only in the skin creases of mature babies, but may also cover the trunk of those who are preterm. It is secreted by the fetal sebaceous glands and protects the skin from its watery environment *in utero*. Postmature babies have lost this protective covering and thus tend to have a dry peeling skin. The baby has a variable amount of hair and blue-grey eyes which may later change their colour. Lanugo is fine body hair and is mainly a feature of the preterm baby, but some is often still present on mature babies. The baby's movements and muscle tone are noted. Though his limbs move actively he tends to keep them flexed.

The examination is then carried out in a systematic manner, starting from the head and finishing at the feet.

Head   The size and shape of the baby's head are observed. There may be a caput succedaneum (see Chapter 74) and sometimes the shape of the head has been distorted by moulding. The midwife observes the skull formation, the width of the sutures and the size and tension of the fontanelles. A third fontanelle palpated between the anterior and posterior fontanelles may be associated with Down's syndrome.

Face   The features are observed for normality. Unusual features may be associated with abnormal conditions such as Down's syndrome. The eyes and ears are observed, noting the development and symmetry. Low-set ears (i.e. ears which are significantly lower than the level of the outer canthus of the eye) are associated with a number of syndromes. Similarly, accessory skin tags and auricles may be associated with abnormality, usually of the renal tract. Small pink, flame-shaped marks called *capillary naevi* may be seen on the upper eyelids, the midline of the forehead, the upper lip and the nape of the neck. They are common and unimportant since they always fade over a period of months. Capillary naevi found elsewhere may not fade and can be quite extensive (port wine stain). Haemorrhages under the conjunctiva are bright red and look alarming but they, too, soon disappear. The eyes should be checked for the presence of congenital cataracts and the presence of a slant, epicanthic folds and white flecks in the iris (*Brushfield's spots*) would also be noted because they may be signs of Down's syndrome.

Babies have wandering eye movements during the early weeks of life, but can focus on a distance of 20–25 cm. Tears are rarely produced with crying until the baby is about a month old. During this time the baby is particularly liable to develop eye infections. Many babies have tiny white spots called *milia* over the nose. They are caused by blocked sebaceous glands. It would be difficult to overlook a cleft lip, but the mouth should be examined, the hard palate being felt with a finger and the soft palate inspected. Small, white spots, called *Epstein's pearls*, may be seen at the junction of the hard and soft palate. *Tongue-tie*, in which the frenulum appears to anchor the tongue to the floor of the mouth restricting free movement, often causes the mother anxiety. She may be reassured about this, since it rarely causes a problem. Rarely the baby is born with one or two teeth. They tend to become loose, however, and therefore are usually extracted. Facial palsy occasionally occurs after an instrumental delivery and this would be noted.

Neck   Any webbing, a short neck and a large fold of skin on the back of the neck would be noted because these characteristics may be associated with chromosomal abnormalities. Any swelling would also be detected. If it is caused by a sternomastoid tumour it is usually 2–3 weeks before it becomes evident. The clavicles are examined for fractures.

Chest   Next the midwife inspects the chest, noting the baby's respirations and any asymmetry. The development and position of the nipples are noted and the chest is palpated for the apex beat. If the midwife is responsible for the full medical examination she will listen to the heart and lungs. A stethoscope is used to listen to the air entry on both sides of the chest which should be equal. The heart is auscultated, listening for both first and second heart sounds. Any abnormalities such as heart murmurs would be referred to a doctor. Many disappear, but others such as a murmur associated with a ventricular septal defect may present later. During the examination of the heart the midwife will note any cyanosis and feel the peripheral pulses. Absence of the femoral pulses may be associated with coarctation of the aorta (Rose, 1994).

Abdomen   The state of the cord and any abdominal swelling is noted. Palpation of the abdomen will reveal any abnormal swelling. The liver edge should be noted and is normally 2 cm below the costal margin. Both kidneys can normally be palpated but the spleen should not be felt.

External genitalia   In baby boys the penis is inspected and the position of the urethral orifice noted. No attempt is made to retract the foreskin from the glans as it is adherent and separates spontaneously during the early years of life. Both testes should be present in the scrotum. The presence of inguinal hernias would be noted. In baby girls the labia are gently separated to observe the presence of the urethral and vaginal orifices. A thick white discharge is often present at birth.

Back   The baby's back is inspected and a finger run down the spine will reveal any unevenness. A baby of Asian or Black ancestry may have a Mongolian blue spot, like a bruise, over the sacral area. The presence of a sacrococcygeal dimple and sometimes a patch of hairiness may be associated with a blind sinus. Finally the presence and position of the anus is noted. Only when the baby passes meconium can it be considered patent.

Limbs and hips   The limbs are examined for normal and equal length and observed for normal movement. Examination of the hips is described next but in practice it may be left to the end of the examination because it usually causes the baby to cry. *Ortolani's and*

Barlow's tests (Ortolani, 1937; Barlow, 1968) are carried out for the diagnosis of congenital dislocation of the hips. The baby lies on his back and the examiner gently grasps each leg with knees and hips flexed. The middle fingers of the examiner's hands are placed over the greater trochanters and the thumbs on the inner aspect of the thighs. The thighs are then fully abducted. The dislocated femoral head may clunk back into the acetabulum during this manoeuvre (*Ortolani's sign*). Alternatively the dislocated femoral head may fail to reduce and the thighs cannot then be fully abducted, staying at about 45° to the horizontal. This is an important sign of a dislocated hip which will be present even when there is no clunk or feeling of instability. Barlow's test is performed by holding the baby's legs in the same way and then, with the hips abducted to 45°, the examiner applies upward and inward pressure with the middle finger of each hand in turn. A clunk will be felt if the head of the femur slips back into the acetabulum. Finally the examiner applies downward and outward pressure with the thumbs and in some cases the femoral head slips backwards out of the acetabulum again. The doctor will be consulted if a clunk or feeling of instability is present, or if the hips fail to abduct fully.

The feet and ankles are next carefully inspected. Mild degrees of talipes are sometimes noted and, like any other abnormality, must be recorded and reported to the doctor. Finally the fingers and toes should be counted and any webbing noted. It is surprisingly easy to overlook extra digits, but they may be associated with a syndrome and therefore further investigations may be required.

Neurological examination

Throughout the above physical examination the midwife will observe the baby's movements, tone and reflexes. Any asymmetry will be noted, recorded and reported. Certain stimuli evoke specific responses which give some indication of normal neuromuscular development. Some of the responses depend on the gestational age of the baby and on the baby's state of alertness at the time of the examination. The following primitive neonatal reflexes and tendon reflexes are carried out. Some are omitted because performing them does not provide extra information (Dubowitz and Dubowitz, 1981).

Rooting reflex   With the head in the midline position the corner of the mouth is stroked. This causes the baby to open his mouth and turn to the side stimulated. This reflex is most easily elicited when the baby is awake and hungry, and can be used when attaching the baby to the breast. It may be absent in a baby who is lethargic.

Sucking reflex   A clean finger or teat is placed in the baby's mouth and the baby responds by sucking. The strength and rhythmicity of the suck can therefore be determined. This reflex is affected by many factors, including the timing of the last feed, the sleep state of the baby, gestational age and sedatives given to the mother (Berger, 1989). Weak sucking in a term baby may be associated with neurological problems.

Moro reflex   The Moro reflex is elicited by startling the baby. He is supported in the supine position on the hand and forearm of the examiner. When the baby is relaxed the head is suddenly allowed to drop back a few centimetres. The reflex consists of rapidly flinging out the arms with hands open, though the fingers often remain curved; this is followed by slow adduction of the arms as in an embrace. The most common cause of an absent or depressed Moro reflex is a generalized disturbance of the central nervous system (Berger, 1989). If the reflex is asymmetrical it may be associated with an *Erb's palsy.*

Palmar grasp reflex   Pressure on the palm of the hand elicits the grasp reflex which is very strong in the healthy term infant. A weak or absent reflex is likely to be associated with a generalized disturbance of the central nervous system.

Tendon reflexes   The knee and sometimes the ankle jerks are the easiest to elicit in the newborn baby. The correct sized reflex hammer should be used and the degree and symmetry of the response should be noted.

Although the foregoing account of the examination seems long, a careful methodological examination to detect the presence of any abnormalities is essential and does not take much time. Most babies are normal and the parents can be reassured that their baby appears healthy and no abnormalities have been detected. If any abnormalities are suspected or detected, the parents are gently and sensitively informed of the signs which are giving rise to concern. The midwife should try not to cause undue alarm at this stage, but explain that she would like a paedia-

trician to see the baby and then make arrangements for referral as soon as possible.

Following this examination the baby is gently cleansed and warmly dressed and wrapped. Later, provided his temperature is normal, he may be bathed.

Vitamin K

In many parts of the UK the baby is given vitamin K with the first feed, provided the mother gives her consent. It is given as a prophylactic measure to reduce the risk of haemorrhagic disease in the newborn which appears to be increasing in frequency and has a poor prognosis. Since the publication of two studies which reported an increased risk of childhood cancer in babies who had been given vitamin K (Golding *et al.*, 1992; Draper and Stiller, 1992), there has been controversy about the administration of this drug to the newborn. The risk appears to be linked to injections of vitamin K rather than to administration by the oral route.

Not all paediatricians accept the findings of these trials (Hull, 1992) and further controlled trials are required to clarify the issue. Meanwhile, it is recommended that the drug is administered by the oral route and 0.5 mg is given after the first feed and two further doses of 0.5 mg are given to breastfed babies at the age of 1 and 6 weeks (Kelnar *et al.*, 1995). Only when administration by the oral route is not possible is an intramuscular or intravenous injection prescribed by a paediatrician (Report of the Expert Committee, 1992). The midwife must record the administration of the drug in the usual way (UKCC, 1994).

Records

Before transferring the mother and baby to a postnatal ward the case notes are completed, including a record of whether the baby has passed urine and meconium. Finally the birth notification form is completed in readiness to send within 36 hours to the appropriate medical officer (UKCC, 1994).

The First Few Days

OBSERVATIONS

Behaviour

At first the baby does not distinguish night from day, sleeping, waking, crying, feeding and sleeping again throughout the 24 hours, but sleeping most of the time. By the time he is 4 or 5 weeks old he is usually sleeping longer at night and is more wakeful in the day time; up to this time and beyond he usually requires night feeds (Matsuoka *et al.*, 1991). The fairly organized circadian sleep and wakefulness rhythm develops around 16 weeks of age (Matsuoka *et al.*, 1991).

His principal needs are for food and fluid, sleep, warmth, security and love. His mode of expression is crying and it is in this way that he signals his needs.

Mother–baby attachment

After the time of prolonged contact at birth, mother and baby should be kept together as much as possible during the early neonatal period when they are getting to know one another and mothering skills are developing. Rooming-in, where the baby's cot remains beside the mother's bed, is therefore recommended (Maternity Services Advisory Committee, 1985). Restricted contact between mother and baby in the early postnatal period is associated with less affectionate maternal behaviour and maternal feelings of incompetence and lack of confidence (Thomson and Westreich, 1989). Maternal/infant attachment, established from birth, is strengthened by handling, so the mother is encouraged to care for her baby soon after birth. Unrestricted access allows her freedom to respond to her baby whenever he is awake. The father, too, should be involved in his child's care and progress, otherwise he may feel neglected and become jealous of the close relationship developing between mother and baby.

Three stages have been described in the maternal–infant attachment process. The first is when the mother and baby first become acquainted and involves early physical contact. The next is the care-taking relationship when the mother learns to care for her baby, to feed, change, wash and bath him. The final stage is called *identity*, when the child is incorporated into the family. To reach this final stage mother and baby grow to know and love each other as they interact. The newborn may initiate interaction by crying. The mother responds by rocking the cot or picking him up and cuddling him. This is the expression of a normal mother's instinct to tend and protect her child and it should be encouraged rather than repressed. The baby stops crying when he is picked up and becomes alert and responsive, so the mother should be encouraged to talk and establish eye-to-eye contact with him. In turn the baby gazes at his mother and

responds; thus mother–baby interaction is sychronized and attachment develops. Even a very young baby shows preference for stimuli such as the human face, voice and touch and soon learns to recognize his mother.

In some situations mother and child have to be separated due to maternal illness or the need for special and intensive care of the newborn, and most mothers are likely to overcome any adverse effects of this separation (Thomson and Westreich, 1989). Some consider that the degree to which a mother perceives separation as having an adverse effect on her mothering ability may be related to the outcome (Richards, 1978; Ross, 1980). It is possible that women of low socio-economic status who have low social support may be more adversely affected by restricted contact with their baby than their more affluent counterparts (Thomson and Westreich, 1989). This was demonstrated in a study by Anisfeld and Lipper (1983) and highlights the benefits to women with low social support and their babies when they have early and prolonged contact soon after birth. Those with high levels of social support of course also benefit, but usually form close attachments to their babies whether or not they have early contact.

Some mothers are worried because they do not feel a maternal instinct or that they really love their baby during the early days of motherhood. These feelings are not at all uncommon at this time, though few women actually express them openly. They need reassurance that their feelings are quite normal and that, as they learn to know their baby and he them, they will gradually fall in love with him.

It is important to promote attachment between mother and child because the quality of this early relationship can influence the ability of the child to form good relationships in later life.

Daily observations and care

Colour   The well-marked, pink colour noted at birth is evidence that the haemoglobin value of the blood is unusually high, 17 g/dl being normal at birth. This extra haemoglobin was needed before birth, when the oxygen supply was relatively poor, but is now more than sufficient. The baby therefore destroys old erythrocytes in greater quantity than he manufactures new ones, and his colour becomes gradually somewhat paler. If his liver function is not sufficiently mature to deal immediately with the released bilirubin, he may show slight, transient jaundice. If, however, the baby is more than slightly jaundiced, or if he is pale and cyanotic, a doctor should be consulted as the baby may be ill.

Weight   A baby may lose up to 10% of his birthweight during the first three days after birth. During this time he takes little food, but passes meconium and loses fluid in passing urine, and from the skin and in respiration. Once he is taking more food he gains weight, reaching or passing his birthweight by about the tenth day. Subsequently he gains approximately 200 g per week.

Muscle tone   The baby is active and vigorous, kicking energetically, though when he lies quietly he is usually in a flexed attitude, as he was before birth. He should not be kept too tightly tucked up, but rather given freedom to move.

Temperature   The baby's axillary temperature may be recorded daily using a low-reading thermometer. It should not fall below 36.6°C.

The environmental temperature should be 21°C both day and night.

Respirations   The respiratory rate is about 40 per minute. Respirations continue to be irregular.

Stools   A record is made of the number and character of all stools passed.

Urinary output   Similarly a record is made of the number of wet napkins in each 24-hour period. The odour and colour of the urine is also noted. Occasionally a red stain is found on the napkin due to urates colouring the urine.

Skin   The skin is observed daily for soreness, rashes and septic spots. The midwife should make every effort to avoid trauma to the child's skin or, indeed, to any superficial tissues. Accordingly the vernix is allowed to remain on his skin, since it will help to protect the skin surface. He may be cleansed with an antiseptic cream rather than immersed in water. Cleaning procedures in general are kept to a minimum, but whether or not the child is bathed, the skin, especially the creases, should be inspected daily. The face and hands are washed each day and the buttocks and groins in particular need gentle cleansing each time the napkin is changed. A barrier cream should then be applied to prevent soreness. If the buttocks are not regularly and carefully cleaned, bacteria on the skin convert urea from the urine to ammonia and the buttocks become sore due to an ammoniacal burn.

Umbilical cord   A good handwashing technique is essential before attending to the cord, otherwise there may be a spread of *Staphylococcus aureus* which can be highly dangerous. The umbilical cord is inspected daily by the midwife for signs of infection and separation. It separates by a process of dry gangrene usually between the fifth and seventh day. The mother should be taught to place the cord outside the napkin to promote drying and prevent soiling. If the cord is soiled by a dirty napkin it should be cleaned with water only and dried with cottonwool swabs.

The application of spirit and powder or antiseptic sprays was shown to delay separation of the cord as far back as the early 1980s (Magowan *et al.*, 1980; Lawrence, 1982; Barr, 1984). In these studies, cords not treated or treated only with an antibacterial powder separated by the seventh day and there was no increase in infection. A larger, more recent study confirms the findings that there is no increase in infection when the umbilical cord is not treated with alcohol wipes and hexachlorophene powder (Dignan, 1994). In this study the cords in the untreated group were cleaned with water only, if it was necessary, and the only difference was that the cords took a little longer to separate in this group. In both groups the cord took longer to separate in male babies because the umbilical area is more likely to be moistened by urine. In another study the researcher assessed the effect of the different methods of treatment of the umbilical cord on the work of midwives, and distinguished between cord separation and cord stump healing. This was because in some cases although the cord had separated, the umbilical stump remained moist, sticky or infected and therefore more home visits were required by the community midwife. The findings concluded that although cord separation time is shorter with the use of antiseptic powder (Sterzac), the use of this powder is associated with a longer time to heal (Mugford *et al.*, 1986). The granulation tissue (stump) is treated by the application of copper sulphate.

Eyes   Usually the eyelids are wiped with sterile swabs at birth; after this the baby's eyes are inspected every day. If clean they are left alone.

Mouth   The mouth is similarly inspected; if it remains clean no treatment is necessary. The same applies to the ears.

Nose   The nostrils are also inspected and, if clean, left alone. If there is any mucus or other material visible the surface only is wiped, wool swabs and water being used. On no account should twists of wool be inserted into the nares.

By these means the baby's skin, eyes, ears, nose and mouth are kept clean but protected from injury and thus from infection.

INFECTION

Because the newborn infant has little resistance to microorganisms, he is highly susceptible to infection. The organisms to which he most commonly succumbs are the staphylococci, streptococci, *Escherichia coli*, *Pseudomonas aeruginosa* and the *Proteus* group. An apparently mild infection can rapidly become a serious condition in the newborn, so every effort must be made to protect him from infection.

There are three main factors concerned in avoiding infection:

1   Keep the baby's skin in a healthy condition and intact, so that if bacteria should be deposited upon him there is no portal of entry whereby they could invade the tissues.
2   Limit the bacteria in the baby's surroundings.
3   Adopt a barrier-nursing technique to avoid cross-infection.

Sources of infection
The infant may be infected in a number of ways:

▶ *Attendants*: The nose, throat or skin of those dealing with the baby may harbour dangerous organisms (staphylococci and streptococci). This includes not only the midwife and doctor but the parents themselves.
▶ *Hands and clothing*: Infection may be carried to the infant by the hands or clothing of the attendant. Again, the midwife, doctor or parent may be responsible. The hands may carry infection from one baby to another or convey skin infection or gastrointestinal infection from the attendant to the baby.
▶ *Dust*: The air and dust in maternity wards and

nurseries contain many bacteria, one of which, the staphylococcus, is most liable to cause infection.
▶ *Fomites*: Infection may be spread by unsterilized instruments, bowls and dressings. Clothing and napkins may be the source. Before the era of pre-packed feeds and disposable bottles and teats in hospitals, inadequately sterilized bottles and teats were a source of infection. This may still be the case in the home.
▶ *Cross-infection*: The close proximity of a number of babies in a nursery or ward makes the spread of infection from one baby to another extremely easy. If one baby should become infected the infection may spread to others and become an epidemic. It will be spread by the methods already mentioned, namely by the attendant's hands, by the use of communal equipment and through the air and dust.

Prevention of infection
The midwife should always have in mind the possible sources of infection:

▶ *Infection from the attendant*: No person with a cold, sore throat, boil or indeed any other infection should attend a newborn baby.
▶ *Hands and clothing*: Facilities for washing the hands must be available both after personal toilet and in the nursery and wards. Preferably disposable hand towels should be used. The hands must be washed before and after attending each baby. Antiseptic hand cream, applied to the hands after washing, is valuable.
▶ *Dust*: The ward and nursery should be adequately ventilated. Cleaning must be thorough but it should be done in such a way that dust is not scattered around the room. Floors are cleaned using vacuum cleaners with filters which prevent bacteria passing out of the machine into the air. Damp dusting is advisable. Babies are taken out of the ward or nursery during cleaning. Cots, trollies and tables can be wiped over with dilute antiseptic.
▶ *Fomites*: All instruments and bowls used for the care of the baby should be sterilized. Dressings must be sterile. Clean linen and napkins in adequate quantities must be available at all times for the baby. The midwife should give the mother every encouragement to establish and maintain breastfeeding. If she is unsuccessful, or prefers artificial feeding, she must be taught that scrupulous attention is

required to clean and sterilize feeding bottles and teats.

▶ *Cross-infection*: Rooming-in, whereby the baby is nursed beside his mother's bed, is the usual practice nowadays. This not only aids the bonding process, but also reduces the risk of cross-infection. Overcrowding in wards and nurseries should be avoided. The greater the number of babies and the more crowded, the greater the risk of cross-infection. Individual equipment for bathing and changing should be provided, disposable articles being used whenever possible. Prepacked artificial feeds and disposable bottles and teats help to reduce the risk of infection in babies who are not being breastfed. Any baby suspected of infection should be isolated from other babies.

The main routine care of the baby involves changing the napkins, washing or bathing, and feeding. There is no evidence that routine medicated baby bathing reduces staphylococcal skin colonization and therefore infection (Rush *et al.*, 1989). The baby should therefore be bathed in plain water. Soiled linen and napkins should be handled as little as possible, placed in containers and removed from the environment. Whilst the baby is being bathed, care must be taken to prevent abrasions of the skin which might allow entry of bacteria. Great care must also be taken of the eyes and cord, the other two places liable to infection.

Careful handwashing should never be neglected before and after touching the baby on each occasion as this is one of the most effective ways of preventing the spread of infection.

SCREENING TESTS

Various tests and examinations may be carried out in the early neonatal period to detect the presence of specific abnormal conditions. The effects of many conditions may be ameliorated by early diagnosis and treatment. Thus, some inborn errors of metabolism may be managed with diet and/or drugs. The traditional criteria for deciding what conditions to screen for are as follows:

1 The incidence of the disease must not be vanishingly small.
2 The consequences of failure to diagnose the condition until it declares itself clinically must be serious and costly.

3 Effective treatment must be available only if it is commenced before the onset of symptoms.
4 A satisfactory screening test must be available; it must be simple, cheap, specific (few false positives) and sensitive (few false negatives).

Tests for the diagnosis of phenylketonuria
Guthrie test   The Guthrie test for the detection of phenylketonuria is carried out between the 6th and 14th day, by which time the baby should be well-established on milk feeds (see Chapter 72). It must be deferred if the baby is receiving antibiotics at the time when the bacterial inhibition test is used because the antibiotics will destroy *Bacillus subtilis* and a false result is thus likely. Nowadays the specific fluorometric method is more commonly used.

A level of 4 mg/100 ml (240 μmol/l) or more is considered positive for phenylketonuria and further investigations would then be carried out. If the diagnosis is confirmed the instigation of early treatment can prevent brain damage leading to severe mental retardation.

Test for the diagnosis of hypothyroidism
The baby is also screened for hypothyroidism by measuring the level of thyroxine or thyroid-stimulating hormone (TSH) in the blood which is taken for the Guthrie test. Further investigations of thyroid function will be required if the test result is abnormal. If the condition is confirmed, early treatment with thyroxine will prevent mental handicap and promote normal growth (Kelnar *et al.*, 1995).

Tests for the detection of cystic fibrosis
Immunoreactive trypsin (IRT) test   The immunoreactive trypsin test on blood obtained from a heel prick is the most reliable test which is available at the moment for the detection of cystic fibrosis. A positive result would be followed by a sweat test to confirm the diagnosis. Early diagnosis of cystic fibrosis improves the prognosis.

It is now possible to carry out the antenatal diagnosis of cystic fibrosis in many cases, but there is no antenatal screening test available.

Tests for the diagnosis of congenital dislocation of the hip
Ortolani's and Barlow's tests   These tests (see earlier in this chapter) are carried out on all babies at birth

to diagnose congenital dislocation of the hips. Ultrasound examination of the hips to confirm the diagnosis of congenital dislocation is now possible (Berman and Klenerman, 1986). It may also be carried out on high-risk babies, for instance when there is a family history or following breech delivery (Curro and Bianchi, 1989). When ultrasound is used Berman and Klenerman (1986) found that dislocation was detected in a small number of clinically normal hips. Also unnecessary splinting of normal hips was avoided.

Tests for hearing

Auditory response cradle   The auditory response cradle is used in some hospitals to screen all infants for deafness. A set of headphones is used to play noises to the baby and a computer analyses his movements in response to the sounds. The examination is brief, simple and accurate. The value of such a test is that children with hearing impairments can be given extra help at an early age to develop speech. Further hearing tests are carried out during the next few months and at eight months all babies should be tested.

Other tests

At the same time as the six-day blood spot is screened for phenylketonuria and hypothyroidism, it can also be screened for antibodies to rubella, of both the IgG and IgM classes. This test could be important since the absence of IgG directed against rubella indicates that the mother is not immune and should be vaccinated, while the presence of specific IgM demonstrates that congenital infection has occurred.

Screening for other diseases is largely restricted to particular population groups, as with sickle cell disease and thalassaemia. Other diseases are too rare, have no suitable remedy, or often cause the damage before the results of a screening test would be available.

THE PROGRESS OF THE BABY

Weight   The normal baby has doubled his birthweight by the 5th–6th month. He gains about 100 g weekly from the fifth month onwards and trebles his birthweight by the end of his first year.

Measurements   The average length of a newborn baby is 50–52 cm. At six months he measures 60 cm and at the end of his first year he measures about 70 cm.

The circumferences of the head and chest at birth are almost the same: 30–35 cm; sometimes the chest is slightly smaller. At six months the head and chest are about 40 cm and at the end of the first year about 45 cm.

Teeth   The two lower central incisors usually erupt at about the 6th or 7th month; after a few weeks the two upper central incisors appear, followed by the two lateral incisors in the upper jaw. Occasionally the lower lateral incisors come through before the first birthday, so at the end of the first year the average baby has six or eight teeth. This is the usual order in which the first teeth appear, but there are wide variations even in normal babies. The first tooth may appear as late as the tenth month and teeth may then not come through in the above order.

A healthy baby suffers little inconvenience from teething; one who is not well may suffer some disturbance, especially if the digestive or respiratory tract is affected.

Behaviour   For the first two months, the baby often sleeps for the greater part of the 24 hours. His cry should be lusty, but crying should not be excessive. At six weeks he should begin to smile and at three months take note of his surroundings. At six months the baby should be sitting up but still needing support; at 9–10 months crawling; and starting to walk at about a year.

It must be emphasized that these 'milestones' are only approximate and that many perfectly normal babies show wide variations from this pattern.

FOLLOW-UP OF THE BABY

The care of the baby is transferred from the midwife to the health visitor between the 10th and 28th day after birth. The health visitor usually visits the mother and baby at home on or around the 11th day. She discusses problems with the mother, gives advice on topics such as childcare and family planning and encourages the mother to take her baby to the child health clinic or to her general practitioner regularly to be weighed, to have vaccinations and to allow regular developmental assessments to be carried out. The general practitioner is responsible for general medical care, but some babies with medical problems are also followed up by a paediatrician.

Minor Disorders of the Newborn

Skin rashes (non-infective)

Erythema toxicum   Also called urticaria neonatorum, this is a blotchy red rash with pinhead papules which commonly occurs during the first week of life. It is not an infective condition and disappears within a day or two. No treatment is required.

Heat rashes   These commonly occur and are recognized as reddened areas, often in the skin folds with hard pinpoint centres. The rash quickly disappears when the baby cools down.

Miliaria or sweat rash   This is due to obstruction of the sweat glands and is seen in babies who become overheated. Fewer cot blankets, less clothing and more fresh air may help. The skin may be dabbed with calamine lotion or sprinkled lightly with a sterile dusting powder.

Chafing or intertrigo

This is caused by friction between two skin surfaces and is usually seen in the groin or axilla and in the folds of the neck. It indicates that the child's skin has not been adequately dried after being washed or bathed. The energetic removal of vernix caseosa may also be the cause. After a bath, the folds in the skin should be dried by a dabbing movement with a soft towel. Where chafing has occurred, drying and a very light dusting with an antiseptic powder will heal the lesion.

Sore buttocks

Redness and excoriation may be produced around the anus and buttocks by frequent loose stools. This is more likely to occur in babies who are artificially fed than in those being breastfed. Causes include infrequent changing of the napkin, poor hygiene, loose frequent stools, incorrect laundering of napkins, diet (for instance the addition of extra sugar to feeds) and infection such as candidiasis.

This condition is very painful and great care is needed in its treatment. The buttocks should be washed with swabs of absorbent wool and well dried with a gentle dabbing. If soap is used it must be pure and non-irritating. Treatment includes finding the cause, high standards of hygiene and exposing the buttocks to the air.

An Anglepoise lamp may be used in conjunction with exposure of the sore area. The lamp should be arranged 33 cm away from the buttocks in such a position that if it is knocked or falls it avoids the baby. This method not only dries the area but also provides warmth for the baby. The midwife should remember that the buttocks are a large area and when they are exposed heat is lost and the baby's temperature may fall. To prevent this the cot should be placed somewhere warm, away from draughts. If sore buttocks last for more than a day or two, medical advice should be sought. Preterm babies are very prone to sore buttocks. Feeding must be investigated, as the feed may not suit the baby. Thrush infection often causes sore buttocks and the mouth should therefore be examined carefully, especially if the buttocks remain persistently red. Candidal infections are treated with oral and local application of nystatin. A barrier cream such as zinc and castor oil is applied to the buttocks when the soreness has improved and the baby is dressed in a napkin.

Napkin rash (ammoniacal dermatitis)

This is usually confined to the area covered by the napkin, but the heels, legs and back may also be affected. The skin may be reddened or become wrinkled and shiny. In more severe cases vesicles or pustules may form or the skin may become raw and moist. The skin is affected over the convexities, the flexures usually escaping. The condition is produced by prolonged skin contact with napkins soaked in urine and faeces. The urea in urine is rapidly converted to ammonia by bacteria present in the faeces. The ammonia is an irritant to the skin. A napkin rash is therefore usually an ammoniacal dermatitis. The development of a napkin rash should be prevented by frequent changing of napkins. The buttocks should be cleansed before applying a clean napkin which has been thoroughly washed and boiled to remove ammonia and destroy bacteria. A zinc and castor oil cream may be applied to protect the skin. If a napkin rash has occurred it may be cured by using these preventive measures but the rash may heal more quickly if the buttocks are not covered by the napkin but left completely exposed to the air. The child lies on his side on the napkin, the trunk and legs adequately covered, in a warm room or in the open air if the weather is fine.

Infection skin rashes

These may occur when there are pustules, pemphigus neonatorum (see Chapter 73), candidiasis, rubella, toxoplasmosis, cytomegalovirus infection or syphilis.

Breast engorgement

The breasts may become engorged in both male and female infants on about the third day of life. After the baby is separated from its mother at birth, its serum oestrogen levels fall and this stimulates the breasts to secrete milk. No treatment is required as the condition will subside spontaneously. Squeezing the breasts and trying to express the so-called 'witch's milk' may result in infection.

Pseudo-menstruation

Oestrogen withdrawal may also lead to pseudo-menstruation in baby girls. A blood-stained vaginal discharge is present on about the third day. No treatment is required.

Constipation

Constipation most commonly occurs in babies who are artifically fed. Extra water may be given. Breastfed babies may not pass a stool for 2 or 3 days once feeding is established but this is quite normal providing the stools are the usual soft, yellow consistency.

Vomiting

The baby may swallow liquor amnii, blood, mucus or other foreign material shortly before birth. If, after birth, he vomits watery fluid or mucus, possibly streaked with blood, it is usually of no importance. A thriving baby taking large feeds may regurgitate a little milk. This effortless possetting after feeds is also unimportant. Vomiting other than this may well be abnormal and is associated with the following more serious conditions.

1 *Feeding errors* which include both overfeeding and underfeeding, feeding too quickly, swallowing excessive air and feeds which are too concentrated.
2 *Infection* of either the alimentary tract or elsewhere.
3 *Intracranial injury*, most commonly in preterm babies.
4 *Congenital malformations* of the alimentary tract. Oesophageal atresia with or without tracheo-oesophageal fistula presents with excessive dribbling or vomiting of frothy mucus. Vomiting of bile-stained fluid is due to intestinal obstruction which may be atresia, stenosis or volvulus of the small intestine, meconium ileus or Hirschsprung's disease of the large intestine. Vomiting due to pyloric stenosis is projectile and occurs later, usually after the tenth day.

5 *Haemorrhagic disease* often presents with haematemesis. Blood-stained vomit may also be due to blood swallowed at delivery or from a cracked nipple.
6 *Metabolic disorders* such as hypoglycaemia and galactosaemia.

Observations on the vomit include its colour, amount, frequency, timing in relation to feeds and whether or not it is projectile. The general condition of the baby is assessed and feeding carefully supervised. The baby may be screened for infection and further investigations are carried out to detect congenital abnormalities or metabolic disorders, if necessary.

No feeds are given and the doctor is summoned if the baby is dribbling excessive mucus at birth or if the vomit is bile-stained.

Failure to thrive

Causes　*Errors in the proportion or quantity of feeds.* Errors and underfeeding can arise if dried milk is measured in teaspoonfuls instead of by the measure provided and if the water is also incorrectly measured.

Excessive dosage of vitamin D combined with artificial feeding on unmodified cows' milk, which contains three to four times more calcium than breast milk, can be followed by an excess of calcium in the blood. The baby may suffer from constipation, vomiting and failure to gain weight. Vitamin D 500–1500 units daily is sufficient to prevent rickets.

Infection Acute infection of the gastrointestinal or respiratory tract will usually be associated with obvious illness requiring immediate treatment, but in urinary tract infection the clinical picture is much less clear-cut. It may be suspected if the child fails to thrive.

A thrush infection of the mouth may cause the baby to refuse to feed properly.

Constitutional disease Congenital abnormalities, for example malformation of the heart, may be associated with failure to thrive. Some abnormalities such as those of the urinary tract may be revealed only by special investigations. Iron-deficiency anaemia is particularly common in preterm infants and may be a cause of failure to thrive; it can be readily remedied by iron therapy. Diseases such as cystic fibrosis and galactosaemia may be responsible for failure to thrive. Coeliac disease begins after weaning and is due to intolerance of gluten; it can be cured by a correct diet.

Failure in mother–child attachment This may be the cause of failure to thrive, thus should be considered. Child abuse may occur in these cases.

Signs Signs of failure to thrive may include some of the following:

▶ Pale or grey colour, or jaundice.
▶ Reluctance to feed.
▶ Failure to gain weight or loss of weight.
▶ Vomiting.
▶ Constipation or frequent loose stools.
▶ A crying, fretful baby, or a lethargic, drowsy infant.

In addition, other signs specific to certain conditions may be apparent.

Management Any signs of infection or abnormal behaviour of the infant should be detected by the midwife when she makes her daily examination of the newborn. At that time she also discusses feeding with the mother and, if concerned about the infant failing to thrive, will observe the mother feeding her baby. It is also important to check that artificial feeds are being made up correctly. Jones and Belsey (1978) found that many serious errors are made by parents when making up feeds.

If the cause of failure to thrive appears to be more than a simple feeding problem, the midwife will refer the baby to a doctor.

The doctor carries out a full physical examination and usually requests investigations to screen the baby for infection. Antibiotics would be prescribed for any infection detected. If congenital conditions are suspected the appropriate investigations are performed. Treatment, if possible, is instigated for any abnormal condition diagnosed.

The mother's behaviour and attitude to her baby are noted. Any problems in managing the baby are discussed and extra support and supervision from the midwife or health visitor may be required. An over-anxious mother may have an adverse effect on her baby in that the infant senses her anxiety and may respond by being tense and fretful. Reassurance and support are required to relieve anxiety and build up the mother's confidence in her ability to give good care to her child.

Occasionally child abuse is suspected and then the child must be admitted to hospital.

Signs that a child is thriving

Appearance The skin is warm and the colour good, the muscles feel firm and the skin elastic. Eyes and hair are bright. The fontanelle begins to close and is closed by the time the child is 18 months old. Teeth begin to appear from 5–8 months onwards. The expression is intelligent.

Behaviour The cry is lusty but not prolonged; the baby is vigorous, takes food eagerly, sleeps well and is generally contented. The child begins to sit up at about six months, to crawl at about 8–10 months and to take his first steps at about a year.

Digestion There is no apparent discomfort after feeds and no vomiting. The urine is normal; the stools are normal in number and colour and cause no soreness of the buttocks.

Weight There is a gradual gain in weight and, although it may be more in the first few weeks, an average weekly gain of 150–200 g is maintained.

References

Anisfeld, E. & Lipper, E. (1983) Early contact, social support and mother–infant bonding. *Pediatrics* **72**: 79–83.

Ball, J.A. (1994) *Reactions to Motherhood*. Hale: Books for Midwives Press.

Barlow, T.G. (1968) Congenital dislocation of the hip. *Nursing Times* **64**(29): 967–968.

Barr, R.J. (1984) The umbilical cord: to treat or not to treat? *Midwives' Chronicle* July: 224–226.

Berger, H. (1989) Clinical examination of the newborn. In Chalmers, I., Enkin, M. & Keirse, M.J.N.C. (eds) *Effective Care in Pregnancy and Childbirth*, p. 1413. Oxford: Oxford University Press.

Berman, L. & Klenerman, L. (1986) Ultrasound screening for hip abnormalities: preliminary findings in 1001 neonates. *Br. Med. J.* **293**: 719–722.

Burn, J. (1995) A study to assess the reliability of measurements and measuring techniques of newborn babies. Unpublished MSc dissertation, University of Surrey.

Curro, V. & Bianchi, A. (1989) Clicking hips: a risk factor for congenital hip dislocation. *Lancet* 17 June: 1393.

Dignan, K. (1994) Is cord care really necessary? *Br. J. Midwifery* **2**(2): 121–125.

DOH (Department of Health) (1993) *Changing Childbirth*, Report of the Expert Committee. London: HMSO.

Draper, G.H. & Stiller, C.A. (1992) Intramuscular vitamin K and childhood cancer. *Br. Med. J.* **305**: 709.

Dubowitz, L. & Dubowitz, V. (1981) The neurological assessment of the preterm and fullterm infant. In *Clinics in Developmental Medicine*. London: Heinemann.

Golding, J., Birmingham, K., Greenwood, R. *et al.* (1992) Childhood cancer, intramuscular vitamin K and pethidine given during labour. *Br. Med. J.* **305**: 341–346.

Hull, D. (1992) Vitamin K and childhood cancer. The risk of haemorrhagic disease is certain: that of childhood cancer is not. *Br. Med. J.* **305**: 326–327.

Jones, R. & Belsey, E. (1978) Common mistakes in infant feeding. Survey of a London Borough. *Br. Med. J.* **2**: 112–114.

Kelnar, J.H., Harvey, D. & Simpson, C. (1995) *The Sick Newborn Baby*. London: Baillière Tindall.

Klaus, M.H. & Kennell, J.H. (1976) *Maternal–Infant Bonding*. St. Louis: C.V. Mosby.

Klaus, M.H. & Kennell, J.H. (1982) *Parent–Infant Bonding*. St. Louis: C.V. Mosby.

Klaus, M.H., Jerauld, R., Kreger, N.C., McAlpine, W., Steffa, M. & Kennell, J.H. (1972) Maternal attachment: importance of the first post-partum days. *New Engl. J. Med.* **286**: 460–463.

Klaus, M.H., Trause, M.A. & Kennell, J.H. (1975) Does human maternal behaviour after delivery show a characteristic pattern? In: Porter, E. & O'Connor, M. (eds) *Parent–Infant Interaction*. Ciba Foundation Symposium No. 33. Amsterdam: Associated Scientific Publishers.

Lawrence, C.R. (1982) Effect of two different methods of umbilical cord care on its separation time. *Midwives' Chronicle Nursing Notes* June: 204–205.

Magowan, M., Andrews, A. & Pinder, B. (1980) The effect of an antibiotic spray on the umbilical cord separation times. *Nursing Times* 16 October: 1841.

Maternity Services Advisory Committee (1985) Third Report, *Maternity Care in Action*, Part III. London: HMSO.

Matsuoka, M., Segawa, M. & Higurashi, M. (1991) The development of sleep and wakefulness cycle in early infancy and its relationship to feeding habits. *Tohoku J. Exp. Med.* **165**: 147–154.

Mugford, M., Somchiwong, M. & Waterhouse, I. (1986) Treatment of umbilical cords: a randomised controlled trial to assess the effect of treatment on the work of midwives. *Midwifery* 2(4): 177–186.

Oakley, A. (1987) Mother love – do midwives help or hinder? *Lancet* i: 379.

Ortolani, M. (1937) Un segno poco noto e sua importanza pe la diagnosi; precoce di prelussazione congenita dell'anca. *Pediatria* **45**: 129–136.

Report of the Expert Committee (1992) *Vitamin K Prophylaxis in Infancy*. London: British Paediatric Association.

Richards, M.P.M. (1978) Possible effect of early separation on later development. In Brimblecombe, F.S.W., Richards, M.P.M. & Roberton, N.R.C. (eds) *Early Separation and Special Care Nurseries*. Clinics in Developmental Medicine. London: SIMP/Heinemann Medical Books.

Rose, S.J. (1994) Physical examination of the full-term baby. *Br. J. Midwifery* 2(5): 209–213.

Rosen, M. & Roberton, N.R.C. (1984) Resuscitation of the newborn. *Midwives' Chronicle* May: 142–148.

Ross, G.S. (1980) Parental responses to infants in intensive care: a separation issue re-evaluation. *Clin. Perinatol.* **7**: 47–61.

Rush, J., Chalmers, I. & Enkin, M. (1989) Care of the new mother and baby. In Chalmers, I., Enkin, M. & Keirse, M.J.N.C. (eds) *Effective Care in Pregnancy and Childbirth*, p. 1334. Oxford: Oxford University Press.

Salariya, E.M. Easton, P.M. & Cater, J.I. (1978) Duration of breast feeding after early initiation and frequent feeding. *Lancet* ii: 1141–1143.

Schaffer, H.R. (1971) *The Growth of Sociability*. Harmondsworth: Penguin Books.

Thomson, M. & Westreich, R. (1989) Restriction of mother–infant contact in the immediate postnatal period. In Chalmers, I., Enkin, M. & Keirse, M.J.N.C. (eds) *Effective Care in Pregnancy and Childbirth*, p. 1324. Oxford: Oxford University Press.

UKCC (UK Central Council for Nursing, Midwifery and Health Visiting) (1993) *Midwives' Rules*. London: UKCC.

UKCC (1994) *The Midwife's Code of Practice*. London: UKCC.

64

Breastfeeding

Breastfeeding is recognized worldwide as being the optimal method of feeding for the human baby. As well as important benefits for babies there are also advantages for mothers.

Advantages of Breastfeeding for the Baby

Breast milk is an ideal form of nutrition, containing all that the baby needs and with a greater propensity for digestion and absorption of constituents than artificial formulae. In a controversial study (Lucas *et al.*, 1992), it was found that preterm babies who received mother's milk in the early weeks (even by nasogastric tube) had a significantly higher intelligence quotient at the age of $7\frac{1}{2}$–8 years, than those who did not. A dose–response relationship was reported and the hypothesis made that breast milk constituents promote brain growth and maturation.

Unlike artificial formulae, breast milk contains living cells and other substances which help to protect the baby from infection. This factor probably accounts for the fact that the incidence of sudden infant death syndrome is lower in breastfed infants, though Gilbert *et al.* (1995) argue that bottle feeding is not a significant independent risk factor. Coeliac disease and Crohn's disease are also reduced and recent research suggests that exclusive breastfeeding with delayed exposure to artificial formula based on cows' milk can significantly reduce the risk of diabetes mellitus in children (Karjalainen *et al.*, 1992). The act of breastfeeding can provide intimate closeness for mother and baby as well as mutual pleasure and interaction which promotes the mother–baby relationship. As research continues it has become increasingly clear that breast milk is much more than just a form of nutrition.

PREVENTION OF INFECTION

During the early months after birth, babies are at increased risk of infection due to immature immune systems. Every pathogen which challenges the mother stimulates the production of specific antibodies and these are present in breast milk. They protect the infant by binding pathogens (e.g. bacteria, viruses, parasites, etc.) and preventing their attachment to mucosal membrane. Secretory IgA antibodies which are specific against rubella, rotavirus, *Giardia lamblia*, *Escherichia coli*, *Shigella* and *Salmonella* have been found in human milk. In this way passive immunity can be transferred from mother to infant. IgA is present in colostrum and breast milk up to a year. IgG and IgM are also present but at lower levels. The baby's own defence system against infection is stimulated by factors contained in breast milk and the production of secretory IgA is known to be enhanced in the urinary tract, saliva and nasal secretions.

Factors other than antibodies provide protection from infection. Lactoferrin, a protein which binds iron in breast milk for improved absorption, thereby deprives pathogenic bacteria (e.g. *E. coli*) of iron necessary for growth. Some oligosaccharides in human milk inhibit bacterial attachment to respiratory and urinary tract epithelium (Coppa *et al.*, 1990). Lysozyme, an enzyme which is bacteriolytic against Gram-positive bacteria and possibly some viruses, is found at higher levels in breast milk than in milk of most other species and is about 3000 times that of cows' milk (Lonnerdal, 1985). The high lactose content and presence of bifidus factor facilitate the growth of lactobacilli which metabolize lactose to lactic acid. Proliferation of pathogens like *Candida albicans*, *E. coli* and parasites is prevented by the more acid stool which results, thus protecting the infant against gastrointestinal disease. Cellular immunity is also transferred from mother to baby via breast milk, mainly in the form of macrophages, though neutrophils, T and B lymphocytes are also present. In the first ten days colostrum and breast milk contain more leucocytes than blood. Concentrations decrease in mature milk but increasing milk volume intakes by the baby compensate for this.

The immune components of human milk provide an antigen avoidance system that decreases the severity of infections for breastfed babies (Goldman, 1993). Pisacane *et al.* (1995) suggest that as a result of milder inflammatory responses to infection, their immune system is programmed to last several years and those children who breastfeed for longer than three months are less likely than controls to develop acute appendicitis.

Constituents of Breast Milk

Mature breast milk varies in its composition from one mother to another. It also varies in the same mother, between breasts, between feeds, over the course of lactation and even during a feed.

Protein

Human milk contains less than one third the amount of protein contained in cows' milk. As a result breastfed infants have a lower solute load than artificially fed infants, due to lower blood urea and amino acid levels (Walker, 1993). The whey protein *alpha-lactalbumin* is the main protein and it is easier to digest and more nutritive than cows' milk protein which is mainly caseinogen. In breast milk the casein:whey ratio is 30:70 whereas in artificial formulae it ranges from 18:82 to 60:40 (WHO, 1991). When breast milk casein is digested, peptides are released which are thought to stimulate the baby's immune system (Ebrahim, 1990).

Taurine, a free amino acid is present in high levels in breast milk (5 mg per 100 ml as compared with 0.3 mg per 100 ml in cows' milk). It is necessary for the conjugation of bile salts and hence fat absorption in the first week of life until glycine takes over this function. Taurine is also necessary for the myelination of the central nervous system and is added to artificial formulae in the UK (Walker, 1993) in quantities similar to those is mature breast milk.

Carbohydrates

Lactose is the main carbohydrate in human milk and is present in much higher levels than in cows' milk. It helps to promote the growth of *Lactobacillus bifidus* in the intestine and leads to the increased acidity of the stools. This resulting fall in stool pH helps to stabilize calcium salts for easier absorption and also facilitates iron absorption. Another carbohydrate known as *bifidus factor*, which is not found in cows' milk, also encourages the growth of lactobacilli.

Breast milk also contains free glucose, galactose and about 25 other oligosaccharides. The latter are found in substantial amounts in the urine of breastfed infants during the first month of life and it is thought that they may have a protective effect against urinary tract infection (Coppa *et al.*, 1990).

Fats

After birth, fats become an important energy source for the baby. The lipids found in breast milk are more readily digested and absorbed than most other types of fats. *Arachidonic acid* (AA) and *docosahexaenoic acid* (DHA) are long-chain fatty acids which are consistent components of breast milk (Crawford, 1993). They are particularly important for the development of membrane-rich systems such as the brain, neural and vascular tissue. Prostaglandin synthesis is dependent on the availability of AA and another fatty acid called *linoleic acid*. Human milk is a rich source of these, being four times higher than cows' milk (WHO, 1991). Prostaglandins enhance digestion and maturation of intestinal cells, which helps in protection from infection.

Fetal stores of long-chain fatty acids can provide an important energy buffer for the newborn, who has immature enzyme systems for synthesis of these lipids. However, the quality of these stores depends on maternal nutrition, placental development and gestational age at birth and some newborns may be deficient. Deficits of AA and DHA have been found in both term and preterm babies who have been formula fed (Farquharson *et al.*, 1992). Artificial milk powders have been supplemented with vegetable oils to increase the linoleic content, the precursor fatty acid to AA, which in excess amounts may inhibit the conversion of alpha-linolenic to DHA.

Crawford (1993) argues that such supplementation is inadequate as human milk is animal fat and not vegetable and that the conversion of precursors linoleic acid and α-linolenic acid to AA and DHA respectively is not as effective as supposed. He recommends the supplementation of term and preterm artificial formulae with AA and DHA, using human milk as a guide to their composition. One babymilk company now adds substances which contain AA and DHA and it is hoped that others will follow suit. Lucas *et al.* (1992) have postulated that the accumulation of long-chain lipids such as DHA in the developing brain and retina may account for the higher IQ in children who have been breastfed. Pisacane and colleagues (1994) found an association between prolonged breastfeeding and a decreased risk of multiple sclerosis. They suggest that there may be defective membrane formation in the brain, due to lower amounts of unsaturated fatty acids in formula-fed babies, which allows easier entry of an infective agent to accelerate myelin degradation.

Breast milk is also rich in *free fatty acids* which are an important energy source for the baby. Fat digestion is significantly improved in breastfed babies as the enzyme lipase is another constituent (lipase is destroyed by heating expressed breast milk). Human milk is rich in cholesterol and after three months, the exclusively breastfed infant's serum cholesterol is significantly higher than in those who are receiving artificial formulae (Jooste *et al.*, 1991). The importance of this is not understood. Early exposure may affect adult handling of this important lipid as regards cardiovascular disease but this has not been proven. Fat content is significantly increased in the hindmilk of a feed and is usually in higher concentrations in late morning and early afternoon.

Mineral salts

Mineral salts total only about 0.2% in breast milk compared to about 0.7% in cows' milk. This means that the kidneys of breastfed babies have a lower solute load presented to them. Healthy babies can usually cope with the higher solute of artificial formulae, provided feeds are correctly reconstituted and they do not become dehydrated. Hypernatraemia (raised serum sodium) can result otherwise, which can lead to irreversible brain damage. A long-term effect of high solute load in the early months is a predisposition to hypertension in later life.

Calcium is more readily absorbed as breastfed babies' stools are more acid and its ratio to phosphorus is 2:1. Although calcium content is high in cows' milk it is less well absorbed due to the higher phosphorus content and higher pH of the stools in artificially fed babies. Hypocalcaemia can result in neonatal tetany and convulsions (Walker, 1993) and may be associated with an increased incidence of dental caries in early childhood.

Up to 70% of breast milk *iron* is absorbed due to the lower stool pH in breastfed babies and the presence of lactoferrin which binds iron. Cows' milk is a poor iron source and artificial formulae have to be fortified with iron as well as ferrous sulphate and ascorbic acid to aid its absorption. *Zinc* is present in small but sufficient amounts and is more readily absorbed than from breast milk substitutes. Dietary *lead* intake is much lower in breastfed infants. Excess lead impairs neurological development. *Trace elements* like copper, cobalt and selenium are generally at optimal levels and higher than cows' milk.

Vitamins

Vitamin concentrations are almost always adequate for infant needs though they can vary with maternal intake. It is therefore essential that the mother's diet contains a good supply of all vitamins.

Vitamin A concentrations are higher in human than in cows' milk and vitamin A deficiency has been shown to be substantially reduced in breastfed babies in developing countries (Mahalanibis, 1991). *Vitamin K* is higher in colostrum and early milk than in later milk but by then babies would normally be synthesizing their own vitamin K. Being fat-soluble it is present in hindmilk mostly. It is important that infants are not deprived of colostrum or hindmilk, as a deficiency of vitamin K can lead to haemorrhagic disease. *Vitamin D* is present in small amounts in breast milk but babies do not become deficient unless the mother's intake of vitamin D is low and she and her baby have inadequate exposure to sunlight. Vitamin D deficiency is especially common in Asian women.

Enzymes

At least 70 enzymes have been identified in breast milk and the role of most of these is not known. Some are bacteriolytic (e.g. lysozyme), and some actively digest fats (i.e. lipase), and starches (i.e. amylase). The activity of amylase is considerably higher in human and especially in preterm milk, than in cows' milk and is thought to compensate for low salivary and pancreative amylase activity in the newborn period (Lonnerdal, 1985).

Hormones

A large number of hormones and hormone-releasing factors are present in human milk. These include prolactin, oxytocin, prostaglandins, insulin, thyroid-stimulating hormone and thyroxine, to name but a few. Growth hormones are also present of which the most potent is epidermal growth factor which is important for gut development and maturation. Endocrine responses differ between breastfed and artificially fed infants and there are significant differences in the secretion of insulin, enteroglucagon and other hormones (Ebrahim, 1990).

Colostrum

Colostrum is a yellowish fluid which is secreted by the breasts from about the 16th week of pregnancy. It is a high-density, low-volume feed which requires little digestion and is readily absorbed into the baby's bloodstream. It differs from mature milk in that it contains less lactose, fat and water-soluble vitamins but is richer in protein, some minerals and fat-soluble vitamins, in particular vitamins A and K. Colostrum has been referred to as 'nature's prescription as well as nature's food' (WHO, 1991). This is because it is rich in anti-infective properties such as IgA, lactoferrin, lysozymes and leucocytes. It evolves into mature milk between 3 and 14 days.

Allergy

Atopic disease is a common health problem that is on the increase; the major cause is genetic. If one or both parents have a history of asthma, eczema, etc., then the baby will also be at risk of allergy. Environmental factors can also be responsible for atopy and up to 10% of affected children have healthy non-atopic parents (Saarinen and Kajosaari, 1995). Newborn babies may have either inherited sensitivities to certain food antigens, e.g. cows' milk protein, and/or become sensitized during early infancy. The immune system of the baby is physiologically immature as is the gut mucosa, both of which may allow high macromolecule absorption of foreign proteins. Breast milk is thought to help protect against allergy in two ways. First by promoting the natural maturation of the intestinal mucosal barrier and secretory immune system and secondly, it contains IgA antibodies, which can prevent the contact of food antigens with the mucosal lining of the infant's gut and prevent their systemic absorption. A small study has found that a lack of IgA in maternal milk permits the development of allergy symptons, which may explain why not all exclusively breastfed babies are protected against atopic disease (Machtinger and Moss, 1986).

It has been suggested that the mother of a hypersensitive child should avoid allergens such as cows' milk when she is breastfeeding and breastfeed exclusively for 4–6 months (Ebrahim, 1988). Some research has shown that early feeding with cows' milk formula has no significant effect on the incidence of atopic disease in children up to the age of fourteen years who have been breastfed (Gustafsson *et al.*, 1992). However, Saarinen and Kajosaari (1995) have found that breastfeeding for six months or more achieves the greatest benefit in reducing substantial atopy at the age of 17 years. It appears to be beneficial in reducing both food and respiratory allergy even if feeding is sustained for longer than one month. A significant difference in the rate of atopy (65% *vs* 42%) and substantial atopy (54% *vs* 8%) was found between those who received no breast milk or were breastfed for less than one month and those who had prolonged breastfeeding (>6 months) (Saarinen and Kajosaari, 1995). The differences were significant irrespective of positive or negative heredity, which demonstrates that breastfeeding offers protection to all and not only to those at risk.

Advantages for the Mother who Breastfeeds

The mother's metabolism is more efficient during lactation so that her food intake is more effectively utilized. Fat stores laid down in pregnancy can also be metabolized so she is more likely to return to her pregravid weight. Women who breastfeed have a lower incidence of breast and ovarian carcinoma and, as more recently suggested, have a higher resistance to urinary tract infection (UK National Case Control Study Group, 1993; Coppa *et al.*, 1990). In the mother who is fully breastfeeding, prolactin levels can be high enough to suppress ovulation, so that return to full menstruation is delayed. This effect permits the mother to recover her iron stores, which enhances her immune and nutritional status and general health. The lactational amenorrhoea method (LAM) is a form of natural birth control available to women who are fully or almost fully breastfeeding and amenorrhoeic (Norman, 1995). Finally, mothers who breastfeed generally derive great emotional and physical satisfaction from it and a very close interdependent relationship develops between mother and child. Not only is the baby dependent on the mother for food, but she depends on him for comfort and relief at feed times when her breasts are full.

Contraindications

A few women find the idea of breastfeeding repulsive and are unlikely to succeed even if persuaded to try. Those with severe debilitating or infective conditions such as tuberculosis should not breastfeed. Human immunodeficiency virus can be transmitted to the baby via breast milk and affected mothers need to be aware of this risk. Breast milk may be important in preventing intercurrent infections which could accelerate HIV-related disease in already infected or exposed infants, but more research is needed to demonstrate if this is so.

Since most drugs taken by the mother pass in her milk to the baby, breastfeeding is contraindicated when drugs which may be harmful to the baby are prescribed, e.g. antithyroid or cytotoxic drugs. Babies with galactosaemia or lactose intolerance cannot be fed on either human or other milk containing lactose. Breast milk can be combined with special formulae in the treatment of maple-syrup urine disease and phenylketonuria, provided in the latter case serum phenylalanine levels are monitored. Certain congenital abnormalities such as cleft lip and palate and Pierre-Robin syndrome make breastfeeding difficult if not impossible.

With the very preterm or ill baby, breastfeeding may not be possible at first. However, these babies in particular need breast milk and the mother may feel that she is making a positive contribution to her baby's care if she expresses her milk for his feeds until he can go to the breast. Preterm babies who are exclusively formula fed are 6–10 times more likely to develop necrotizing enterocolitis than those fed breast milk alone and three times more than those fed formula and breast milk (Lucas and Cole, 1990).

Choice of Infant Feeding Method

Most women have decided on their method of feeding before the baby is born. Women are influenced in their choice by various factors. In 1990, a survey showed that the most common reason given by women who chose to breastfeed was that it was best for baby (OPCS, 1992). Another important reason given was that it was more convenient, as they did not have to make up feeds etc. Convenience was also seen to be a reason for women who chose to bottle feed, as other people could feed the baby. For women having a second or subsequent child, their previous method exerts a strong influence on their choice of feeding, with few mothers who had successfully breastfed previous babies choosing to bottle feed and vice versa. Social class is another determinant and women from social class I are much more likely to choose breastfeeding (89%) than women from social class V (47%) (OPCS, 1992). Nevertheless, attendance at antenatal classes was associated with a higher likelihood of intending to breastfeed for manual and non-manual classes.

The mother's level of education is also highly associated with the likelihood of her breastfeeding. Among women having their first child who left full-time education after the age of 19, 93% chose to breastfeed compared to 57% of women who left school at 16 or less (OPCS, 1992). This may account in part for social class differences, but one small Scottish study has shown that a major reason for working-class primiparae not choosing to breastfeed was that it was socially unacceptable and embarrassing (McIntosh, 1985). This in turn reflects the attitude that breasts are often perceived as sexual objects in Western society as opposed to their primary function of nurturing the infant. Breastfeeding in public places is frowned upon by some sectors in society and it is rare to see it portrayed by the media except perhaps in the context of Third World poverty (Entwistle, 1991). For these reasons some women may be discouraged from breastfeeding at all though it is possible to feed in a public place and be discreet about it. Women are also influenced by family and friends in their choice of feeding. If their mothers breastfed them, they are more likely to breastfeed.

Partners also have a major influence, depending on their attitudes to breastfeeding and level of support they are able to give. Some men find their partner's breastfeeding attractive whereas others find it off-putting or feel jealous that the baby has usurped 'their' domain. In an American study it was found that fathers who preferred bottle feeding were more likely to have negative attitudes about breastfeeding, e.g. it would interfere with sex, it spoils the shape of the breasts, etc. Fathers who supported breastfeeding were more aware of the benefits to the baby of breast milk and respected women who fed their baby this way (Freed et al., 1992). Attitudes of friends, whether they be negative or positive to breastfeeding, also influence the woman's choice. Older women tend to breastfeed more than younger women. In a study of the attitudes of Liverpool teenagers to breastfeeding, it was found that many regarded bottle feeding as more convenient and fashionable (Gregg, 1989). Women who smoke are less likely to breastfeed than non-smokers and this is true for almost every social class; mothers on maternity leave are more likely than all others to breastfeed (OPCS, 1992), which suggests that returning to work does not influence women against choosing breastfeeding. Finally, breastfeeding has become a 'green' issue for women concerned with energy conservation.

THE ROLE OF THE MIDWIFE

The role of the midwife is to ensure that women and their families are aware of the many important benefits of breastfeeding and hazards of artificial feeding (Walker, 1993). She should also discuss any relevant contraindications for individual women so that choice of infant feeding method is informed. It follows that the midwife must ensure that she keeps up-to-date with important research related to infant feeding in order to fulfil this role accordingly. Certain practices without any scientific basis were advocated by midwives in the past and were counterproductive to successful breastfeeding, such as restricting sucking time on the breast, the need to offer both breasts at a single feed and the giving of complements (Fisher, 1985). Some of these practices still persist today with the results that women get conflicting advice and do not succeed in breastfeeding (Garforth and Garcia, 1989). The support offered to women to initiate and establish breastfeeding is a vital aspect of health promotion for the child and mother and midwives must give it the commitment required. Good interpersonal skills and sensitivity to parents' attitudes are also required, so that adequate information is given yet is not perceived as overzealous promotion of breastfeeding. Mothers should feel comfortable and supported with their choice of infant feeding, so that their relationship with the baby is enhanced.

Midwives' attitudes to breastfeeding vary enormously (Garforth and Garcia, 1989). Some see breastfeeding support as integral to their role, whilst others treat it as a low priority or even omit it. These variations may reflect midwives' knowledge, skill and/or belief in breastfeeding. Some may be reluctant to promote it for fear of making bottle-feeding mothers feel guilty, thus demonstrating a paternalistic attitude (Walker, 1993). However, breastfeeding is a health issue and should be treated as such. Health professionals need to be aware of negative attitudes and beware of discouraging women who wish to breastfeed by word or action. Midwives are the professionals who are most in contact with mothers in the early days of breastfeeding and they have an important role in its promotion and support.

Management of Breastfeeding

Ideally the baby should breastfeed in the first hour after delivery, as at this time the baby is particularly receptive and exhibiting a strong rooting reflex. A successful first feed can have a positive effect on the mother's confidence and research has shown that undisturbed contact between mother and baby until the first feed is accomplished has a positive effect on the duration and success of breastfeeding (Salariya *et al.*, 1978; Righart and Alade, 1990). The midwife should therefore encourage and support the mother who wishes to breastfeed following delivery and facilitate this undisturbed contact as much as possible. Widström and colleagues (1987) describe how babies make spontaneous sucking and rooting movements after 15 minutes of comparative inactivity following delivery. When lain in the prone position between mothers' breasts, infants spontaneously find the nipple and start to suckle by 55 minutes on average. When pethidine is given to women towards the end of the first stage of labour, it can adversely affect early contact and initiation of breastfeeding (Rajan, 1994). Additional support of such mothers is needed, or better still an alternative to pethidine.

The mother should feed her baby in whatever position she finds most comfortable. This may be lying on her side, sitting upright well-supported by pillows in a comfortable chair or any other position which the mother and the midwife can devise. The baby's body should be close to the mother's body with his head and shoulders facing her breast and his mouth at the same level as her nipple. To achieve this position the baby may be supported on a pillow on the mother's lap, or alongside her on the bed.

The correct positioning of the baby on the breast is one of the most important factors for successful breastfeeding and the midwife must ensure that the mother is able to achieve this. The baby needs to be alert and rooting for the breast. The rooting reflex is stimulated by the smell of his mother's milk and by stroking the baby's cheek with the nipple if necessary. When he opens his mouth widely, the baby should be guided gently towards the breast so that his lower lip and gum are directed below the base of the nipple. The mother will not be able to see this point of contact but to achieve it the breast can be tilted up slightly as the baby's head is brought towards the breast. When this relationship is achieved, the breast can be almost 'folded down' into the baby's mouth (Woolridge, 1986a). In this way he is able to grasp both the nipple and the areola and apply pressure with his tongue to the underlying ducts. During this manoeuvre the mother can support her breast underneath so that the flat of her hand is against her ribs and her thumb encircles the breast but does not impinge on the nipple, as this may interfere with correct attachment. Once the baby is attached, support of the breast should be relaxed so as not to put undue pressure on the ducts and inhibit milk flow. The baby's head should be slightly extended so that his nostrils are clear of the breast and there is no need to press the breast away from his nose (Figures 1 and 2).

When properly fixed on the breast, the baby's mouth should be wide open with his lower lip curled back and below the base of the nipple (Figure 1). When feeding, the baby's jaw action extends back to his ears with little movement seen in the cheeks. The nipple, with surrounding and underlying breast tissue, is drawn out into a teat by the baby's sucking. This teat is about three times as long as the nipple at rest; it extends as far back as the junction between the hard and soft palate; its shape is dictated by the internal structures of the baby's mouth (Figure 2). The milk is then stripped from the ampullae and propelled towards the back of the baby's mouth by peristaltic waves along the surface of the tongue (Woolridge, 1986a). If the

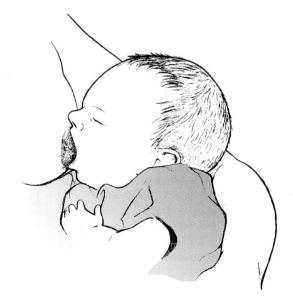

Figure 1 The correct position for breastfeeding.

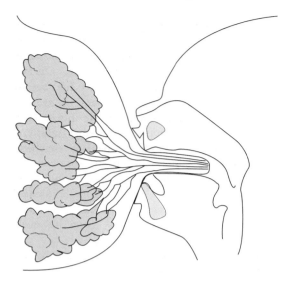

Figure 2 Breast tissue formed into a teat in the baby's mouth.

baby is not correctly fixed, the mother must gently remove him from the breast, by applying firm pressure with a finger on his chin to break the vacuum and then try again. Otherwise the baby obtains insufficient milk and becomes fretful and frustrated and the mother is likely to develop sore nipples. Some babies fix quickly and easily at the breast whereas others take a little time to fix properly. The midwife should be available to give guidance and support to the mother until she can confidently manage alone.

The baby will take rest periods at intervals during a feed which is quite normal. There is no need to stimulate the baby to suck constantly. It is important, however, to ensure that the areola does not slip out of the baby's mouth when he is resting, leaving only the nipple for him to suck, since this is a common cause of sore nipples. The mother should be encouraged to allow the baby to finish feeding at the first breast before offering the second so that he obtains the calorific hindmilk. It may be that he only wants to feed at one breast at an individual feed and the mother should be reassured that this is quite acceptable. The other breast can be offered at the next feed so that milk production is stimulated in both breasts. When the baby receives mostly foremilk through not being allowed to finish feeding at the first breast, he will not be satisfied for long and will require frequent feeding (Woolridge and Fisher, 1988).

BABY-LED FEEDING

The healthy breastfed baby is fed whenever he is hungry and feeds are baby-led or on demand rather than at scheduled times. The intervals between feeds can range from 1 to 8 hours (RCM, 1988) and healthy babies need not be woken up for feeds or frequency and length of feeds restricted. When the baby is allowed to regulate the frequency of feeds himself, he is awake and ready for his feed and therefore is more likely to suck vigorously than a sleepy baby who is woken for feeds at scheduled times. As a result the baby thrives and the mother is encouraged to continue with breastfeeding for longer. Milk engorgement of the breasts on the 3rd or 4th day is unlikely to occur if the baby is feeding frequently at this time.

The main disadvantage of baby-led feeding is that the mother may become overtired. In the early weeks she needs to make sure that she has some rest and sleep during the day at a time when the baby is sleeping, as she will almost certainly be disturbed at night as well as feeding frequently during the day. Nevertheless, she may sit or lie down to breastfeed. The act of feeding can be very relaxing and unlike women who bottle feed, she has no preparation of feeds, sterilization of equipment, etc. to do.

The mother may find it difficult to plan her time, as she does not know exactly when the baby will require feeding. Initially she should reduce activities such as housework to a minimum to avoid exhaustion and concentrate her energies on her baby, partner and any other children in the family. Involvement of her partner in the care of the baby and other children and his taking responsibility for household chores will allow her more opportunity to rest.

At times the baby's feeds may coincide with her own meals. She needs a nutritious diet in order to breastfeed successfully and to maintain her own health, so it is important that arrangements are made to ensure that her dietary needs are met. In due course feeding tends to settle down into a pattern and the mother will then have the freedom to plan the day ahead.

The Problems of Breastfeeding

INSUFFICIENT MILK

The most common reason given by mothers for stopping breastfeeding is insufficient milk (OPCS, 1992).

Very few women are in fact unable to produce enough milk for their baby if breastfeeding is managed properly. Mismanagement occurs when the frequency and duration of feeds is restricted or the baby is not positioned correctly on the breast. Sore nipples and engorgement then arise which further exacerbate the problem. The baby is not satisfied and becomes fretful which can affect the mother's confidence in her ability to breastfeed. She may then consider giving additional fluids which will further jeopardize her chances of establishing successful breastfeeding. This cycle of events could be avoided if the midwife teaches the mother from the beginning that the milk supply is related to demand and how to ensure that the baby is positioned properly. She also needs support and encouragement to help promote confidence in her ability to breastfeed.

If the mother appears to have insufficient milk the midwife should encourage her to put the baby to the breast more frequently and for longer periods. This extra stimulus will increase the milk supply within the next day or two. She must allow the baby to finish feeding at the first breast, so that he can obtain the calorific and satisfying hindmilk. Otherwise, when there is enforced change from the first to the second breast, the baby receives mostly low-fat foremilk and will soon appear hungry again. This practice is also thought to explain colic, wind and loose bowel movements (Woolridge and Fisher, 1988). The midwife can reassure the mother that the baby is getting enough milk from her breast by drawing her attention to how satisfied he is after a feed, or to the fact that he is gaining weight, having frequent wet nappies, etc.

Complementary feeds are those given in addition to breastfeeds; *supplementary feeds* are those given instead of a breastfeed. Both of these should be avoided as many studies have shown that their use is strongly associated with early cessation of breastfeeding (RCM, 1988; OPCS, 1992). They exacerbate the problem of insufficient milk by reducing breast stimulation and can seriously undermine the mother's confidence. Exclusively breastfed babies do not require water supplements even in hot humid weather (Sachdev *et al.*, 1991). Babies can become accustomed to feeding from bottles which may lead to difficulties when trying to position them properly at the breast. This nipple confusion can compound the problem of inadequate drainage of milk from the breast and may result in lactation mastitis (Dahlen, 1993). Another important consideration is that giving cows' milk based formula could interfere with the development of the baby's immune system and cause an allergic reaction in sensitive babies (Walker, 1993). The midwife should inform the mother of the implications of giving complements or supplements and try to restore her confidence in her ability to breastfeed through encouragement and support.

There is often a temporary reduction in milk supply when the mother becomes more active. At this time the midwife should advise her to have adequate rest and a good diet and to try to relax. Many mothers give up breastfeeding by six weeks for reasons of insufficient milk. This may be because of a lack of understanding of the supply-on-demand theory at times when the baby needs more milk perhaps because of a growth spurt. It may also be that by this time the breasts feel softer and smaller, as the let-down reflex becomes conditioned and lactation has settled down.

SORE OR CRACKED NIPPLES

The nipples may feel tender during the first few days of breastfeeding but the discomfort then normally subsides. If the nipples become sore, feeds should be supervised to check that the baby is correctly positioned at the breast. This is a particular risk for women with non-protractile or inverted nipples. When the baby has insufficient breast tissue presented to him, an adequate teat cannot be formed. Frictional trauma and suction lesions can result as the baby tries to retain the teat in his mouth and strip milk from it (Woolridge, 1986b). The remedy is to reposition the baby at the breast so that he has adequate breast tissue in his mouth. Some mothers are inclined to depress the breast away from the baby's nose so that the nostrils are clear. This practice alters the position of the nipple in the baby's mouth and can result in sore nipples. It may be that the baby is being held too closely into the breast so that the nostils are occluded. The mother should allow the baby's head to extend a little when on the breast so that his nose only slightly indents the breast and he can breathe easily. The incidence of sore nipples is not affected by the duration of the feed and there is no rationale for limiting sucking time at the breast so long as the baby is properly positioned. Resting and expressing the breasts can produce nipple healing but stimulation of lactation is not as effective as with direct suckling.

If the nipple is badly cracked, it may be too painful for the mother to continue feeding on the affected side. She can be advised to feed on the unaffected side and gently hand express from the affected side. This expressed milk can then be given to the baby by bottle, cup or spoon. When the crack has healed sufficiently, feeding can be resumed on the affected side. Some mothers may prefer to use a nipple shield. These can reduce stimulation for lactation and reduce milk transfer to the baby, especially with the traditional rubber type, and should be used for the minimum of time if at all. There is no scientific evidence that nipple creams, sprays, etc. will prevent sore nipples or treat the condition once developed.

Non-protractile and *inverted nipples* can become more protracted with successful breastfeeding but initially these mothers will need more support and help with positioning. The mother may need to change the position in which she feeds the baby to achieve good attachment. It has been shown that the use of breast shells during pregnancy for the treatment of these conditions may reduce the chances of success-ful breastfeeding (Alexander *et al.*, 1992). The multi-centre randomized controlled Main trial (Main Trial Collaborative Group, 1994) has investigated the effects of breast shells and Hoffman's exercises on pregnant women with inverted and non-protractile nipples. Hoffman's exercises were intended to stretch and free the nipple by manipulation so that it became more prominent. However, the Main trial has found no basis for recommending either Hoffman's exercises or the use of breast shells and rejects the need for routine breast examination in pregnancy for this purpose.

ENGORGEMENT OF THE BREASTS

Vascular engorgement may occur in the first 2–4 days after delivery due to increased blood supply to the breasts required for milk production. Placental oestro-gen levels in the mother's blood have fallen sufficiently by this time so the action of prolactin is not inhibited. The mother may experience pain and tenderness in the breasts which are flushed, tense and hot to the touch. Her temperature and pulse may be slightly raised. As milk production follows the increased blood supply, milk engorgement can occur if it is not efficiently removed from the breast by the baby. This can occur when the baby is incorrectly positioned, not allowed to feed on demand day and night, or because he is made to feed from both breasts at each feed. The breast becomes hard, knotty and painful as the alveoli are distended with milk. If this condition is not resolved quickly, milk production can be suppressed.

The mother will probably require analgesia and should be advised to keep the breasts well supported between feeds. The midwife should try to discover the reason for the problem and advise accordingly. She may need to help the mother position the baby properly on the breast as it is difficult when the breast is tense and hard. It may be necessary to express a little milk before feeds to enable the baby to fix more easily. The breast should feel softer and more comfortable following a good feed by the baby.

BLOCKED DUCTS

Occasionally one of the milk ducts becomes blocked due to pressure from tight clothing or because of incorrect positioning or rough handling during a feed. It is recognized by a reddened tender area which overlies a swelling and can be termed *non-infective mastitis*. If the obstruction is not relieved, this condi-tion can develop into infective mastitis due to stasis of milk.

The midwife should advise the mother to continue feeding frequently, particularly from the affected side. As well as ensuring good positioning, she should show her how to gently massage the affected area downwards towards the nipple during and after a feed to help clear the obstruction in the duct. She may also need to advise about not wearing tight clothing and gentle handling of the breasts. Excess milk should be expressed after feeds as it has been shown to signifi-cantly decrease the duration of symptoms and improve outcome (Thomsen *et al.*, 1984).

Conclusion

A source of skilled help and support to call upon when problems arise is necessary for all breastfeeding mothers; initially the midwife is available and then the health visitor. In many areas breastfeeding support groups have been established and provide a very valu-able service. They are usually composed of mothers who are, or have previously, breastfed and may be led by a midwife or health visitor, or by a member of a voluntary organization such as the National Childbirth Trust or La Leche League. It is becoming more com-mon for maternity units to employ an experienced midwife as infant feeding advisor. She can monitor levels of successful breastfeeding and address local practices which are counterproductive such as giving conflicting advice. This should not mean, however, that other midwives neglect the art of giving consistent sound advice and support to the breastfeeding mother when required.

The trend away from breastfeeding is concerning and unacceptable in the light of overwhelming evidence of breast milk superiority as an infant feeding method. The World Health Organization and UNICEF have launched a worldwide Baby Friendly Hospital Initiative, to help reverse this trend. It is designed to encourage hospitals and other health care facilities to examine their practices and redefine what steps they are taking to assist successful breastfeeding. Exclusive breastfeeding from birth should be protected, promoted and supported and the initiative gives health care facilities guidelines to assess their achievement of the Ten Steps required for Baby Friendly designation. Health professionals need to continue and improve their efforts to increase general awareness and communicate to parents the importance of breast milk to the health and well-being of their children and future generations.

References

Alexander, J.M., Grant, A.M. & Campbell, M.J. (1992) Randomised controlled trial of breast shells and Hoffman's exercises for inverted and non-protractile nipples. *Br. Med. J.* **304**: 1030–1032.

Coppa, G.V., Gabriella, O., Giorgi, P. *et al.* (1990) Preliminary study of breastfeeding and bacterial adhesion to uroepithelial cells. *Lancet* **335**: 569–571.

Crawford, M.A. (1993) The role of essential fatty acids in neural development: implications for perinatal nutrition. *Am. J. Clin. Nutr.* **57** (Suppl.): 703S–710S.

Dahlen, H. (1993) Lactation mastitis. *Nursing Times* **89**: 36, 38–40.

Ebrahim, G.J. (1988) The place of breast feeding in modern paediatrics. *Maternal Child Health* October: 278–280.

Ebrahim, G.J. (1990) The scientific contribution of breast feeding research. *Maternal Child Health* March: 92–93.

Entwistle, F. (1991) Breastfeeding. The most natural function. *Nursing Times* **87**: 18, 24–26.

Farquharson, J., Cochburn, F., Ainslie Patrick, W., Jamieson, E.C. & Logan, R.W. (1992) Infant cerebral cortex phospholipid fatty-acid composition and diet. *Lancet* **340**: 810–813.

Fisher, C. (1985) How did we go wrong with breast feeding? *Midwifery* **1**: 48–51.

Freed, G., Fraley, K. & Schanler, R. (1992) Attitudes of expectant fathers regarding breast feeding. *Pediatrics* **90**: 224–227.

Garforth, S. & Garcia, J. (1989) Breast feeding policies in practice – no wonder they get confused. *Midwifery* **5**: 75–83.

Gilbert, R.E., Wigfield, R.E., Fleming, P.J. *et al.* (1995) Bottle feeding and the sudden infant death syndrome. *Br. Med. J.* **310**: 88–90.

Goldman, A.S. (1993) The immune system of human milk: antimicrobial, anti-inflammatory and immunomodulating properties. *Pediat. Infect. Dis. J.* **12**: 664.

Gregg, J.E.M. (1989) Attitudes of teenagers in Liverpool to breast feeding. *Br. Med. J.* **299**: 147–148.

Gustafsson, D., Lowhagen, T. & Anderson, K. (1992) Risk of developing atopic disease after early feeding with cows' milk based formula. *Arch. Dis. Childhood* **67**: 1008–1010.

Jooste, P.L., Rossouw, L.J., Steenkamp, H.J. *et al.* (1991) Effect of breast feeding on the plasma cholesterol and growth of infants. *J. Pediat. Gastroenterol. Nutr.* **13**: 139–142.

Karjalainen, J., Martin, J., Knip, M. *et al.* (1992) A bovine albumin peptide as a possible trigger of insulin-dependent diabetes mellitus. *New Engl. J. Med.* **327**(5): 302–307.

Lonnerdal, B. (1985) Biochemistry and physiological function of human milk proteins. *Am. J. Clin. Nutr.* **42**: 1299–1377.

Lucas, A. & Cole, T.J. (1990) Breast milk and neonatal necrotising enterocolitis. *Lancet* **336**: 1519–1523.

Lucas, A., Morley, R., Cole, T.J. *et al.* (1992) Breast milk and subsequent intelligence quotient in children born preterm. *Lancet* **339**: 261–264.

Machtinger, S. & Moss, R. (1986) Cow's milk allergy in breast-fed infants: The role of allergen and maternal secretory IgA antibody. *J. Allergy Clin. Immunol.* **77**: 341–347.

Mahalanabis, D. (1991) Breast feeding and vitamin A deficiency among children in a diarrhoea treatment centre in Bangladesh: a case-control study. *Br. Med. J.* **303**: 493–496.

Main Trial Collaborative Group (1994) Preparing for breast feeding: treatment of inverted and non-protractile nipples in pregnancy. *Midwifery* (December) **10**: 200–213.

McIntosh, J. (1985) Barriers to breast feeding: Choice of feeding method in a sample of working class primiparae. *Midwifery* **1**: 213–224.

Norman, C. (1995) Does nature know best? Background and mechanism of natural family planning. *Midwives* **108**: 1, 85–88.

OPCS (Office of Population Censuses and Surveys) (1992) *Infant Feeding 1990*. London: HMSO.

Pisacane, A., Impagliazzo, N., Russo, M. *et al.* (1994) Breast feeding and multiple sclerosis. *Br. Med. J.* **308**: 1411–1412.

Pisacane, A., de Luca, U., Impagliazzo, N. *et al.* (1995) Breast feeding and acute appendicitis. *Br. Med. J.* **310**: 836–837.

Rajan, L. (1994) The impact of obstetric procedures and analgesia/anaesthesia during labour and delivery on breast feeding. *Midwifery* **10**: 87–103.

RCM (Royal College of Midwives) (1988) *Successful Breast Feeding. A Practical Guide for Midwives (and others supporting breast feeding mothers)*. London: RCM.

Righart, L. & Alade, M.O. (1990) Effect of delivery room

routines on success of first breast feed. *Lancet* **336**: 1105–1107.

Saarinen, U.M. & Kajosaari, M. (1995) Breast feeding as prophylaxis against atopic disease: prospective follow-up study until 17 years old. *Lancet* **346**(8982): 1065–1069.

Sachdev, H.P.S., Krishna, J., Puri, R.K. *et al.* (1991) Water supplementation in exclusively breast-fed infants during summer in the tropics. *Lancet* **337**: 929–933.

Salariya, E.M., Easton, P.M. & Cater, J.I. (1978) Duration of breast feeding after early initiation and frequent feeding. *Lancet* **ii**: 1141–1143.

Thomsen, A.C., Espersen, T. & Maigaard, S. (1984) Course and treatment of milk stasis, noninfectious inflammation of the breast and infectious mastitis in nursing women. *Am. J. Obstet. Gynecol.* **149**: 492–495.

UK National Case Control Study Group (1993) Breast feeding and risk of breast cancer in young women. *Br. Med. J.* **307**: 17–20.

Walker, M. (1993) A fresh look at the risks of artificial infant feeding. *J. Human Lactation* **9**(2): 97–107.

WHO (World Health Organization) (1991) Lactation. In Akre, J. (ed.) *Infant Feeding. The Physiological Basis*. Geneva: WHO.

Widström, A.M., Ransjo-Arvidson, A.B., Christensson, K. *et al.* (1987) Gastric suction in healthy newborn babies. *Acta Paediat. Scand.* **76**: 566–572.

Woolridge, M.W. (1986a) The anatomy of infant sucking. *Midwifery* **2**: 164.

Woolridge, M.W. (1986b) Aetiology of sore nipples. *Midwifery* **2**: 172–176.

Woolridge, M.W. & Fisher, C. (1988) Colic, 'overfeeding', and symptoms of lactose malabsorption in the breast-fed baby: a possible artifact of feed management? *Lancet* **ii**: 382–384.

Further Reading

Palmer, G. (1988) *The Politics of Breast Feeding*. London: Pandora.

Renfrew, M., Fisher, C. & Arms, S. (1990) *Best Feeding. Getting Breast Feeding Right for You*. Berkeley, CA: Celestial Arts.

Riordan, J. & Auerbach, K.G. (1993) *Breast Feeding and Human Lactation*. London: Jones & Bartlett.

65

Artificial Feeding

Although breastfeeding is recommended as best for both mother and child (see Chapter 64), for many women artificial feeding is the method of choice, often because of the social and cultural factors discussed in Chapter 64. In a few cases, breastfeeding is contra-indicated and the mother is advised to feed her baby artificially for medical reasons (see Chapter 64).

Some mothers choose to bottle feed their baby from birth whilst others attempt to breastfeed at first but discontinue after a few days or weeks. Of the 63% who start breastfeeding, 38% have stopped by six weeks (White *et al.*, 1992). Consequently there is a large group of mothers who artificially feed their babies for a variety of reasons. These include social and cultural factors, physical or temperamental problems and, in the case of those who attempt to breastfeed but discontinue, lack of confidence in their ability to breast-feed successfully and, possibly, mismanagement of feeding (MacIntyre, 1982; Fisher, 1984; Dix, 1991; RCM, 1991).

The mother should at no stage be given the impression that artificial feeding is equivalent to breastfeeding (RCM, 1991). Human milk is superior for the newborn infant; milk substitutes, however, play a necessary role in infant nutrition (Goedhart and Bindels, 1994). Ultimately, the mother must be allowed to make her own decision (RCM, 1991) and midwives should ensure that those mothers who choose to bottle feed their infants do so safely.

The Baby's Requirements

When considering any diet, the following factors must be evaluated and taken into account:

1 Energy requirements.
2 Fluid requirements.
3 Balance of ingredients.

Energy requirements
The average baby will thrive satisfactorily on an intake of 440 kJ per kilogram of body weight per day. Breast milk or infant formula contains approximately 90 kJ

per 30 ml. Thus a baby weighing 3.5 kg will require 1540 kJ in 24 hours, i.e. approximately 525 ml of milk.

It should be emphasized that this is only a guide and the baby will take as much as is required at each feed in order to satisfy his needs. The amount may vary considerably from one feed to another but this should not be a cause for concern if the baby appears well and is gaining weight.

Fluid requirements

In order to keep a healthy baby hydrated, he needs to drink about 150–165 ml of fluid per kilogram of body weight per day. Thus a 3.5 kg baby requires approximately 525–575 ml per day. This indicates that when infant formula is given, both energy and fluid requirements are met. Babies have a wide range of appetites, however, and it must be understood that the figures quoted are only guidelines.

Balance of ingredients

Human milk is balanced to suit the needs of the baby just as cows' milk is balanced to meet the needs of the calf. If the latter is used for a baby it must be modified.

The report *Present-day Practice in Infant Feeding* (DHSS, 1988) pointed out the dangers of giving unmodified milk to babies under 12 months of age. Modified milks are those in which all the constituents have been adjusted to resemble human milk as closely as possible. Much of the casein is removed and replaced by whey milk protein which contains a higher percentage of lactalbumen. Some of the milk fat is removed and replaced by vegetable fat. Lactose is added to increase the energy value.

Statutory Instrument (1995) stipulates that the constituents of infant formula must be as shown in Table 1. It is also stipulated that the concentration of vitamins added to artificial milk should be as near to that of human milk as possible, although in human milk the levels vary since they are influenced by the mother's diet. Similarly the concentration of minerals in artificial milk should resemble that of human milk. This can only be achieved with minerals such as sodium by the process of demineralization, whereby the mineral content of cows' milk is reduced. The risk of conditions such as hypernatraemia and neonatal tetany are then reduced.

Human milk contains about 76 µg/100 ml iron whereas cows' milk contains only about 50 µg/100 ml. Breastfed babies also absorb and utilize iron more

Table 1 Comparison of the composition of reconstituted infant formulae and mature human milk (per 100 ml)

		Infant formula	Mean values for mature human milk
Energy	(kJ)	250–315	293
	(kcal)	60–75	70
Protein	(g)	1.2–1.95	1.3
Carbohydrate	(g)	4.6–9.1	7
Fat	(g)	2.1–4.2	4.2
Vitamins			
A	(µg)	39–117	60
D	(µg)	0.65–1.63	0.01
E	(µg)	>0.33	0.35
K	(µg)	2.6	0.21
Thiamin	(µg)	265	16
Riboflavin	(µg)	39	30
Niacin	(µg)	163	620
B6	(µg)	22.8	6
B12	(µg)	0.07	0.01
Total folate	(µg)	2.6	5.0
C	(mg)	5.2	3.8
Minerals			
Sodium	(mg)	13–39	15
Potassium	(mg)	39–94	60
Chloride	(mg)	32.5–81	43
Calcium	(mg)	19.5	35
Iron	(µg)	325–975	76

Source: Adapted from DOH (1994) p. 55 and Statutory Instrument 77 (1995).

efficiently than those fed on cows' milk. It is therefore necessary to add iron to cows' milk which is modified for infant feeding.

Types of Infant Formulae

Infant formulas are artificial feeds which are manufactured to take the place of human milk in providing a sole source of nutrition for the young infant (White *et al.*, 1992: 48). The essential composition of these formulae was set down as a Parliamentary Statute, or law, which came into force in March 1995 (Statutory Instrument 77, 1995).

The majority of infant formula brands can be divided into two groups: those which are *whey dominant* and those which are *casein dominant*. When whey is the dominant protein the whey:casein ratio is closer to human milk. Casein dominant formulae have a whey:casein ratio closer to cows' milk and are therefore not as comparable to breast milk (White *et al.*, 1992).

Examples of infant formulae available in the UK for infant feeding are given below:

Whey-dominant formulae	*Casein-dominant formulae*
SMA Gold	SMA White
Farleys First Milk	Farley's Second Milk
Cow and Gate Premium	Cow and Gate Plus
Milupa Aptamil	Milupa Milumil
Boots Formula 1	Boots Formula 2

Some manufacturers claim that casein-dominant formula is more satisfying for the baby than whey-dominant formula. White *et al.* (1992) suggests that, although there is no firm evidence to show that this formula is more suitable, parents may well be influenced by such claims.

Soya milk formulae

Some soya-based milk substitutes conform to the compositional guidelines (DHSS, 1988; Statutory Instrument, 1995). They have been approved for prescription in the National Health Service for established forms of milk intolerance (DHSS, 1988). Soya-based formulae of entirely plant origin are acceptable to vegans. Some 2–3% of infants are fed on soya-based formula (White *et al.*, 1992).

Follow-on milks

Follow-on milks may be used by some parents to provide the drink element of a more diversified diet in an infant of more than six months of age (DOH, 1994; Statutory Instrument, 1995).

Ready-to-feed formulae

Some formula milks are available in a liquid or ready-to-feed format. The liquid formula just requires decanting into a sterile feeding bottle. Although more costly than the powdered formula, the mother may find ready-made formula useful, for example, if she is travelling with her baby.

Preparation of Feeds

All parents should be shown how to prepare artificial feeds and how to clean and sterilize the utensils. Ideally they should then practise, under supervision, until proficient. Jones and Belsey (1978) give details of the many serious errors which are made by those making up infant feeds. They include using the wrong scoop for the brand of milk, over- or underfilling the scoop, adding too little or too much water and adding sugar or cereals to the feed. These mistakes are more common in parents with more than one child than first-time parents and occur in all social classes. Hence it is not safe to assume that multiparae or those in the higher social groups will make up feeds accurately. All parents need careful teaching and supervision.

Equipment required

To prepare for bottle feeding the following equipment is needed:

1 Wide-necked upright polypropylene bottles, three or better still six: these are easy to clean and the feed can be made up in the bottles, so that the risk of contamination is reduced.
2 Bottle caps, teats and teat covers.
3 Plastic spatula for levelling dried milk powder.
4 Bottle brush.
5 Salt.
6 Sterilizing equipment.

It is best if a special area in the kitchen is used for preparing the baby's feeds. It should be thoroughly cleaned before the feeds are made up. The hands are washed and all articles required for preparing the feeds are collected. The lid is then removed from the sterilizing unit and the packet of milk opened. After washing the hands again, the bottles, teats, teat covers and a spatula are removed from the sterilizing unit and may be rinsed with cool, boiled water. The milk is then reconstituted, carefully following the directions on the packet.

Usually the correct amount of cool, boiled water is poured into the bottle. Next the milk powder is accurately measured in the scoop provided and added to the water. It is particularly important to follow the manufacturer's instructions about the amount of milk in each scoop. Extra milk powder makes the feeds too concentrated and may cause hypernatraemia; too little powder used in making up feeds may lead to malnourishment. Finally the cap is fitted to the bottle and it is then shaken to mix the feed. Most mothers make up sufficient feeds for 24 hours and store them in the refrigerator.

Management of Feeding

Parents usually enjoy giving their babies a bottle feed soon after birth. Babies have a very good sucking reflex within the hour or so of birth so usually suck very well at this time. This early feed can therefore be a very satisfying experience for both parents and baby.

Demand feeding

Subsequently, like the breastfed infant, the baby should be fed on demand. This means the baby is offered a milk feed whenever he wakes up and appears hungry rather than at scheduled times. In addition the baby is free to take the amount of milk he requires at each feed. On the first day or two after birth the baby may take only small feeds but his requirements increase daily until by the third or fourth day he is fully feeding. Even so the amount of milk the baby takes may vary from feed to feed and the mother should be dissuaded from trying to encourage the baby to empty the bottle each time. A normal, healthy baby is the best judge of how much he requires to satisfy his hunger. In a hot environment he may just be thirsty and cooled, boiled water can be offered between milk feeds.

Feeding Technique

Feeds which have been stored in the refrigerator should be warmed to room temperature or above, up to about 33°C. After washing the hands, the teat is put carefully on the bottle and then covered with a sterile cover until the baby is ready to feed.

Preparation of the baby is as for those who are breastfed. The parent should find a comfortable position and be prepared to relax and enjoy this time with their baby. The temperature of the feed is checked by sprinkling a few drops of milk from the bottle on to the inner aspect of the arm. Then, cradling the baby in the arms and holding him close to the body, the baby is offered the teat. The bottle should be tilted to ensure that the teat and neck of the bottle are filled with milk, otherwise the baby will suck in air.

The baby may require 'winding' once or twice during the feed and again at the end. It is not unusual for the baby to posset a little curdled milk when bringing up wind. Most babies complete their feed in about 15 minutes.

If the feed seems to be progressing slowly, yet the baby is sucking well, the cause must be sought. The teat could be under rather than over the baby's tongue, or the teat hole may be too small or it could be blocked. The correct sized hole should provide a steady drip of milk. A gentle shake of the bottle on to the hand will show whether the teat is blocked and if so it must be changed. It is important that artificial feeding, like breastfeeding, should be an unhurried, relaxed experience when the baby feels secure and loved. In due course the demand-fed infant tends to settle into a fairly regular regimen.

Sterilization of Feeding Utensils

Any milk left in the bottle at the end of the feed should be discarded. The bottle, teat and cover are rinsed in cold running water and then thoroughly washed with a bottle brush in a bowl of warm soapy water. If salt is used to clean the teat then all traces should be rinsed off and then the teat washed in warm soapy water. All the equipment is then thoroughly rinsed before being sterilized.

Sterilization methods

There are various methods of sterilizing feeding utensils available nowadays.

Chemical sterilization   There are several different brands of sterilizer available, or the mother may use any large plastic or glass container in which all the feeding equipment can be submerged. Sodium hypochlorite in the form of tablets, liquid or crystals is then made into a solution with cold water according to manufacturer's instructions. The clean feeding equipment is then immersed in the solution for the recommended length of time. Once the equipment is sterile, cool boiled water may be used to rinse before feeding. A new batch of solution has to be made up every 24 hours.

Boiling   A large pan can be set aside for the purpose of sterilizing equipment. The feeding equipment is washed in the usual way, then boiled for 10 minutes in the pan. The clean equipment is left, covered, in the pan until required.

Microwave sterilization   A microwave bottle sterilizer is needed, but a microwave alone is not enough to sterilize feeding equipment. The manufacturer's instructions must be followed. It takes, on average, seven minutes to sterilize equipment using this method.

Electrical steam sterilizer   Steam sterilizes enough bottles and teats for four feeds in about five minutes.

Vitamins

The Department of Health (1991) states that a baby who is being breastfed from a well-nourished mother and a child who is being fed on one of the modified infant formulae to which vitamins have been added should be receiving an adequate supply of vitamins without further supplementation. Infants who should receive vitamin supplementation include those of low birthweight. The standard dose of children's vitamin drops is five drops daily and each dose contains vitamin A 200 µg, vitamin C 20 mg and vitamin D 7 µg. Vitamin drops are started from 4 weeks of age and continued until weaning. The health visitor advises the parents on the time to discontinue giving vitamin drops to their infant. The drops may be obtained from Child Health Clinics at a minimal cost and are free to families receiving Income Support.

Expectant mothers and children under 5 in families receiving Income Support are entitled to receive milk free of charge. This may be taken as 900 g of specified brands of infant formula or liquid cows' milk. Families in receipt of family credit may purchase Welfare milk at reduced rates (DOH, 1994).

Weaning

Mixed feeding should not be started until the baby is 4–6 months old and no later than six months of age (DOH, 1994). Normal growth and development continue when the baby is fed on milk alone up to and indeed beyond six months of age. When solids are introduced the rule about gradual changes still applies and at first only small quantities of fruit, vegetable or gluten-free cereal are offered. The baby's likes and dislikes will soon become evident.

Good weaning practices contribute to dental health. The use of a cup or beaker should be encouraged from six months to optimize dental health (DOH, 1994). Fruit juices should never be fed from a bottle as this constitutes a risk to dental health (DOH, 1994).

As the baby takes more mixed food, so breast and bottle feeds are gradually replaced by the meals he takes. He may enjoy a drink of well-diluted orange juice when he wakes in the morning and he will probably take a breast or bottle feed last thing at night. Most babies like to continue this late feed for several months after they are taking ordinary meals.

International Code of Marketing of Breast Milk Substitutes

In May 1981, the World Health Assembly approved an International Code of Marketing of Breast Milk Substitutes (WHO, 1981). Its purpose is to protect breastfeeding and to help control the marketing of products for the artificial feeding of infants. Of particular concern is the reduction of breastfeeding, especially in developing countries where mortality rates are particularly high for artificially fed infants. The code is not restricted to developing countries, however, but is expected to be adopted by all nations. Its implementation depends on agreements between manufacturers and governments, backed by legislation if necessary. Many violations of the code have been reported.

In the UK the Food Manufacturers' Federation (FMF), now the Food and Drink Federation, in conjunction with the Ministry of Agriculture and the Department of Health have drawn up what appears to be a modified and weakened version of the international code (Food Manufacturers' Federation, 1983; *Lancet*, 1986). This was published in 1983 and is an attempt to regulate the way in which baby milk companies market and promote products for the artificial feeding of infants in the UK. In addition, a DHSS circular was published in 1983 which should be used in conjunction with the FMF code (DHSS, 1983). This circular lays down the responsibilities of professionals in relation to the code.

Recently a strict new code banning the advertising of baby milks has been adopted by the European Parliament. This was backed up by Statutory Instrument 77 (1995) and makes illegal all promotion of baby milks through health professionals. Thus manufacturers are not allowed to give packs of milk powder to doctors, midwives or health visitors for free distribution to mothers.

Midwives should be aware of the content of these codes, the health circular, and Statute otherwise they may inadvertently encourage violations.

References

Dix, D.N. (1991) Why women decide not to breastfeed. *Birth* 18(4): 222–225.

DHSS Health Services Dept (1983) *International Code of Marketing of Breast Milk Substitutes*, HC (83) 13. London: DHSS.

DHSS (Department of Health and Social Security) (1988) *Present Day Practice in Infant Feeding*. Report on Health and Social Subjects No. 32. Third Report. London: HMSO.

DOH (Department of Health) (1991) *Dietary Reference Values for Food Energy and Nutrients for the United Kingdom*. Report on Health and Social Subjects No. 41. London: HMSO.

DOH (1994) *Weaning and the Weaning Diet*. Report on Health and Social Subjects No. 45. London: HMSO.

Fisher, C. (1984) The initiation of breast feeding. *Midwives' Chronicle and Nursing Notes* February: 39–41.

Food Manufacturers' Federation (1983) *Code of Practice for the Marketing of Infant Formulae in the United Kingdom and Schedule for a Code Monitoring Committee*. London: Food Manufacturers' Federation.

Goedhart, A.C. & Bindels, J.C. (1994) The composition of human milk as a model for the design of infant formulas: Recent findings and possible applications. *Nutr. Res. Rev.* 7: 1–23.

Jones, R. & Belsey, E. (1978) Common mistakes in infant feeding. Survey of a London borough. *Br. Med. J.* 2: 112–114.

Lancet (1986) Infant feeding today. *Lancet* i: 17–18.

MacIntyre, S. (1982) Rhetoric and reality: mothers' breast feeding intentions and experiences. *Research and the Midwife, Conference Proceedings*, pp. 39–62.

RCM (Royal College of Midwives) (1991) *Successful Breastfeeding*, 2nd edn. Edinburgh: Churchill Livingstone.

Statutory Instruments No. 77 (1995). *Food. The Infant Formula and Follow-on Formula Regulations*. London: HMSO.

White, A., Freeth, S. & O'Brian, M. for the Office of Population Censuses and Surveys (1992) *Infant Feeding 1990*. London: HMSO.

WHO (World Health Organization) (1981) *International Code of Marketing of Breast Milk Substitues*. Geneva: WHO.

Further Reading

Commission of the European Communities (1991) Directive on infant formulae and follow-on formulae. 91/321/EEC. *Official J. Eur. Community* L175: 35–49.

WHO/UNICEF (1989) *Protecting, Promoting and Supporting Breastfeeding: the Special Role of the Maternity Services*. Geneva: World Health Organization.

66

Thermoregulation and the Neonate

No newborn baby can afford the effects of cold stress. Those least able to tolerate hypothermia include pre-term and/or growth-retarded babies and ill babies. Maintenance of an optimal thermal environment is a vital part of neonatal care and studies have shown that environmental temperatures influence growth and survival of the neonate.

Taking into consideration the short history of neonatal care itself, the maintenance of a stable neutral thermal environment has only recently begun to be recognized.

Historical Background

WRAPPING AND SWADDLING

It was recorded in the Bible and some ancient Greek texts that as soon as the baby was born it was cleansed by rubbing salt into its skin and then wrapped in swaddling clothes. The custom of using salt on the baby's skin was later discontinued because it was found to cause skin irritation, although it remained popular in some parts of England as late as the eighteenth century. A Dr Buchan advised midwives that, following the birth, it was better to wash the baby in warm water (Dick, 1987). A midwife of that time, Mrs Sharpe, washed healthy babies in wine, though she preferred to use warm water if the child showed signs of weakness. Afterwards she would rub the skin with acorn oil prior to swaddling. It is of interest to note that both wine and salt have mild antiseptic properties which would help to protect babies exposed to the unhygienic practices of their times, and the acorn oil would have helped to insulate the baby's skin against the cold (Dick, 1987).

After cleansing, babies would be wrapped in swaddling clothes. In some parts of the world, such as Sparta, Greece and in the Scottish Highlands, swaddling was not used because it was believed that babies should be exposed to severe hardening practices such as being carried naked, even in the winter. This was considered a way of ensuring that only the fittest and strongest individuals survived.

Swaddling was used primarily to counteract the limb deformities resulting from rickets caused by malnutrition. It involved wrapping cloth around the baby in a bandage-like fashion, often so tight that the skin became excoriated, the compressed flesh became gangrenous and the circulation was affected (Dick, 1987). By the end of the eighteenth century the practice of swaddling babies had become unfashionable in England and America, though it continued in France and Germany until the nineteenth century.

Modified swaddling, that is, wrapping the baby in a tight bundle, is still practised today in many countries and cultures, though the rationale for it has changed as nutrition has improved and the focus has moved to the need to keep the baby warm and comfortable. Whether the baby is more comfortable in restraining folds of cloth is debatable and, as can be seen, owes more to the history above than to reasoned judgement.

More recently, comparisons have been made between the progress and well-being of sick neonates clothed and warmly wrapped, and those nursed naked in incubators. It was found that the most effective means of maintaining the temperature and reducing energy loss was to dress the baby and nurse him in an incubator (Sinclair, 1992: 44). This reduces heat loss by hindering excessive movement by the baby and thus conserves energy, whilst preventing heat loss via conduction and radiation.

TEMPERATURE CONTROL

By 1870 it was recognized that temperature played a part in the survival of babies, although the methods used to keep babies warm were sometimes less than satisfactory. One method involved placing the baby into a pot stuffed with poultry feathers placed near a fire. Several factors, such as the inflammable nature of the feathers and the proximity of the open fire, proved rather hazardous and resulted in many babies being burned (Dick, 1987). Another equally dangerous method was to place the cot by the fireside at night. The use of sheepskin or other animal skins was one of the more successful developments and the use of artificial and real sheepskins continues to be an effective means of keeping the neonate warm and comfortable today (Dick, 1987).

In 1878 the first incubator was developed in Paris, by obstetrician Etienne Stephen Tarnier. This was designed with the help of a zoo keeper and it is interesting to note that, at that time, the incubated babies were put 'on show' as exhibits for the entertainment of the general public. The object of the exercise was thus more to provide exhibits than to help the babies survive and indeed few babies did survive.

An understanding of the thermal requirements of the high-risk baby was slow to develop. Pierre Budin, with the help of E.S. Tarnier, was the first neonatologist to show the clinical importance of the thermal environment. In 1907, in his pioneering book *The Nursing*, he emphasized the need for temperature control after noting the increased survival rate for babies nursed in temperatures between 36 and 37°C. He recommended an air temperature of 30°C for the small (1 kg), fully clothed baby. These observations were not fully understood or developed until the latter 50 years of this century.

Blackfan and Yaylou between 1926 and 1933 showed that babies weighing 1360–2270 g nursed in high humidity and air temperature of 25°C were being maintained in a suitable environment (Dick, 1987). This practice became the basis of care. Significant but unstudied changes were made in the baby's thermal environment during the next 29 years. At one point the humidity was increased to the point that it was impossible to see the babies in the incubators!

In the 1940s in a bid to improve observation, the baby was nursed naked without increasing the incubator temperature. The importance of incubator temperature and humidity was finally resolved by W.A. Silverman in 1957. He noted a striking difference in survival rates with an increase in incubator temperature alone.

In the late 1950s Dr June Hill found that in 20% oxygen, oxygen consumption and rectal temperature varied with the environmental temperature. She noted a set of thermal conditions at which heat production (measured as oxygen consumption) was minimal, yet core temperature was within the normal range; this is known as the '*neutral thermal environment*'. She also showed that by reducing the environmental temperature, oxygen consumption would not increase if the environmental temperature was lowered beyond a certain limit, and also that a baby given less oxygen (12%) would fail to maintain an adequate core temperature.

This work and others, demonstrated that the human baby is a *homeotherm* (Greek: *homoios* = 'similar', *therme* = 'heat'), that is, the human organism can maintain its core body temperature within narrow limits in spite of large variations in environmental temperature (Dunn *et al.*, 1994: 238). In contrast, animals such as the turtle are *poikilothermic* (Greek: *poikilos* = 'variable', *therme* = 'heat'). Their body temperature will vary widely in response to environmental change. These observations became the basis of our understanding of temperature control today (Klaus and Fanaroff, 1979).

Physiology of Thermoregulation

The human body is equipped with a complex sensory system capable of detecting whether the temperature has risen or fallen. Information from temperature receptors, distributed widely in many parts of the body, is transmitted to the *hypothalamus*, where autonomic responses are co-ordinated, and to the *cerebral cortex*, where behavioural responses are co-ordinated.

Thus when the body temperature rises, the typical human autonomic response is peripheral vasodilatation and sweating to cool the skin, whilst the behavioural response is to seek a cooler environment and take some clothes off. These responses either reduce heat load or increase the heat loss. On the other hand, when body temperature falls, the typical responses are peripheral vasoconstriction and shivering and for the individual to seek warmth and put on more clothing. All these responses reduce heat loss or increase internal heat production. In either case the responses act to prevent or reverse the temperature changes that initiate them.

The outcome of normal thermoregulatory function is that over a wide range of ambient temperatures, body core temperature is controlled at a relatively stable level – generally between 36.5 and 37°C. The ambient temperature range over which normal body temperature is achieved with minimal activation of metabolic and evaporative processes, is called the *thermoneutral zone*. For a naked adult, this zone is between approximately 27°C and 33°C. Deviations of body temperature may take three forms:

1 Heat gain can exceed heat loss despite the compensation reactions and body temperature will rise and hyperthermia occurs.
2 Heat loss can exceed heat gain and body temperature will fall and hypothermia occurs.
3 The control mechanisms may break down and

temperature will rise or fall according to the environmental factors. If the rectal temperature rises above 40°C or falls lower than 35°C, there is increasing malfunction and risk of tissue damage and ultimately death.

THERMOREGULATION IN THE FETUS

The placenta is a very effective heat exchanger for the fetus who can rely totally on the mother for thermoregulation. Fetal body temperature is generally about 0.6°C above maternal body temperature.

During pregnancy, the heat generated by the mother increases by 30–35% and thus the woman can be expected to have a temperature of 37.5°C during pregnancy. This response is due to the effect of progesterone on metabolism and basal metabolic rate (BMR). This leads to the perception of the mother being more tolerant of a cool environment and having an intolerance of heat.

In the maternal system, there is an increase of 4–7 times the cutaneous bloodflow and activity of sweat glands (Tucker Blackburn and Lee Loper, 1992: 678).

Fetal temperature is inevitably tightly linked to the maternal temperature regulation and therefore cannot be controlled by the fetus autonomously. This has been referred to as the *heat clamp*. The fetal temperature is usually 37.6–37.8°C (Polin and Fox, 1992: 477; Tucker Blackburn and Lee Loper, 1992: 678–679).

The placental role in thermoregulation is influenced by:

▶ Fetal and placental metabolic activity.
▶ Thermal diffusion capacity of heat exchange within the placenta.
▶ Rates of blood flow in the placental and intervillous spaces (Adamsons, 1966).

It is also thought that some of the fetally generated heat is dissipated into the amniotic fluid via the umbilical cord (Morishima *et al.*, 1977). The heat generated by fetal metabolism is therefore dispersed by the amniotic fluid or the placenta to maternal blood in the intervillous spaces. Transfer of heat is facilitated by the maternal–fetal gradient, which is significant when the mother is exposed to changes in temperature, either during exercise or illness or through environmental factors such as taking a sauna (Cohen, 1987; Smith *et al.*, 1988). In these cases the gradient may be reversed or reduced, which can lead to the fetal temperature rising. Changes in fetal temperature will, however, tend to follow at a slower pace than maternal changes due to the insulatory effects of the amniotic fluid (Tucker Blackburn and Lee Loper, 1992: 679).

THERMOREGULATION IN THE NEONATE

Thermoregulation is a critical physiological function in the neonate and is closely linked to the baby's survival and health status. As has been described, during fetal life thermoregulation of the neonate is balanced by the feto-maternal unit. However, birth precipitates the baby into a harsh and cold environment in which the neonate must make major physiological adaptations and changes, including thermoregulatory independence. The newborn baby has the additional problem of not being as efficient in his ability to thermoregulate as the adult. Since the ability to generate heat depends on body mass, and heat loss to the environment on the surface area, the fact that a neonate has a surface area-to-mass ratio about three times higher than that of an adult will lead to difficulty in maintaining his temperature in a cold environment.

Babies with a low body mass are even more at risk. Although a full-term baby has a control over peripheral vascular circulation equal to that of an adult, the autonomic thermoregulatory responses are not fully developed. The healthy baby can increase basal heat production by 2.5 times in response to cold within 1–2 days of birth, though this is less so in the first 24 hours. Rarely able to shiver, the increased heat comes from the noradrenergic lipolysis of the brown fat deposits characteristic of the neonate, and activation of specially adapted mitochondria in the brown fat to produce heat. Sweating in the first few days of life is localized mainly to the skin of the head. Such sweat mechanisms that are active at birth develop late in gestation, so that the baby born three weeks before term sweats very little and if born more than eight weeks before term will not sweat at all.

Mortality rises in small babies if they are kept in an environment as little as 1°C below their neutral temperature. Hypothermia in babies tends to result in metabolic acidosis, hypoglycaemia, and an increased risk of kernicterus. Many babies whose body temperatures fall below 27–32°C will not survive.

The most usual thermal hazard facing a newborn baby is that of hypothermia. However, hyperthermia can also occur and, in extreme cases, can cause death within the first 24 hours after birth.

The significance of the internal and external gradients

The *internal gradient* is the transfer of heat from within the body to its surface. This process relies on an effective and extensive blood flow of capillaries and venous plexi. Further it is influenced by tissue insulation provided by subcutaneous fat and the convective movement of heat through the blood. This process is under sympathetic control and results in changes in the skin blood flow by vasoconstriction and vasodilatation.

Heat loss through this gradient is increased in the neonate because there is a thinner layer of subcutaneous fat and a larger surface-to-volume ratio than in the adult. The surface-to-volume ratio is only 16% in neonates but 35% in adults (Tucker Blackburn and Lee Loper, 1992: 680).

The *external gradient* refers to the heat loss from the neonate's body surface area to the environment. The rate of heat loss is directly proportional to the difference between skin temperature and the environment.

Heat transfer by the external gradient is increased in the neonate because of an increased surface area and an increased thermal transfer coefficient. Therefore, the neonate maintains his temperature by means of the external gradient, i.e. the temperature changes of the skin, whereas the adult uses the internal gradient to control temperature changes. This is especially significant for the preterm baby in which the control and effects of changes in the environment temperature are more profound.

The external and internal gradient are interdependent.

Heat loss

As a rule babies are treated as homeotherms who attempt to maintain their body temperature within a comparatively narrow range. They respond to heat loss by generating more heat. Four routes of heat loss are recognized (Hammarlund and Sedin, 1986):

1   *Evaporation*: Heat loss occurs when water evaporates from the skin and respiratory tract. Evaporative heat loss is highest immediately following delivery and after a bath.
2   *Convection*: Heat is lost to moving air or fluid around the neonate. The amount of heat lost depends on the difference between the skin and air or fluid temperature, the amount of body surface exposed to the environment, and the speed of air or fluid movement.

3 *Radiation*: The neonate will radiate heat from his surface to surrounding colder solid objects such as cold windows or incubator walls. This is the predominant mode of heat loss after the first week of life in babies born before 28 weeks and in all other babies throughout the neonatal period.
4 *Conduction*: Babies conduct heat to cold objects they come into contact with such as a cold mattress, scales and radiograph plates.

Other significant heat loss factors Another form of losing heat is by *insensible water loss* (i.e. water lost through the skin, urine, faeces and respiratory tract that cannot be seen). This water loss is increased in both preterm and low birthweight babies (Rutter, 1985). Increased insensible water loss occurs in these babies because of the large ratio of surface area to body mass, the small amount of subcutaneous fat, the immature structure of their epidermal skin layer and their increased body water content. Preterm and low birthweight babies are at risk from heat loss in environments where insensible water loss is increased. This is because 0.58 kcal of heat is lost with each gram of water lost through evaporation (Hammarlund and Sedin, 1986).

Basal metabolic rate

Measurement of body temperature alone is of limited value in assessing the probable metabolic state of a baby. A neonate with a specific body temperature will become hypermetabolic if the environmental temperature drops below the skin temperature. This causes a rate of heat loss exceeding the rate of heat generated by the baby's basal metabolic activity. Even with a low body temperature, however, if the environment temperature is rising, or is close enough to the skin temperature to limit heat loss to a rate not exceeding the rate of basal heat production, a baby will not become hypermetabolic. High body temperatures also activate distress mechanisms that require an increase in metabolic work (Polk, 1988).

Heat production in the neonate

Heat production is a result of metabolic processes that generate energy by oxidative metabolism of glucose, fats and proteins. The organs that generate the greatest energy are the brain, heart and liver. To maintain a constant body temperature, heat loss from the surface of the body must equal heat gain.

This stability involves heat production by metabolic processes, and is noticeable when the baby is exposed to cold stress when heat production is by physical or chemical mechanisms. In the baby, though the hypothalamus will receive stimuli from other areas of the body, the most sensitive receptors are contained within the *trigeminal area*. This is the most sensitive part of the face and, when exposed to cold, is thought to result in the physiological cascade of *non-shivering thermogenesis* (Baldino and Geller, 1982).

The *physical mechanisms* include involuntary reactions such as shivering, and voluntary reactions in the form of muscular activity, for example, crying, restlessness and hyperactivity. These responses can be affected by anaesthetics, damage to the brain, or drugs, such as muscle relaxants or sedatives.

Chemical or non-shivering thermogenesis is the process by which the neonate generates heat through an increase in the metabolic rate and through brown adipose tissue (BAT) metabolism. This process can be utilized by adults and neonates, but in the adult the metabolic rate can be increased by about 10–15%, whereas the neonate can increase metabolic rate by up to 100% (Guyton, 1979).

Thermal sensors

The baby is alerted to cold stress when thermal receptors in the skin, particularly the face, are stimulated. The responses of the skin surface are determined by the skin temperature, the rate and direction of temperature change and the size of the area stimulated. In the human newborn, cooling of the skin has been shown to increase metabolic heat production without any change in the core temperature (Darnall, 1987). The posterior hypothalamus is thought to be the area which processes signals from the various thermal sensors located over the body.

Heat production and brown adipose tissue (BAT)

A cold-stressed baby depends primarily on mechanisms that cause chemical thermogenesis. In the neonate the main process of heat production is by non-shivering thermogenesis. When stimulated by cold, noradrenaline and thyroid hormones are released, inducing lipolysis in brown fat. This process can be affected by pathological events such as hypoxia, acidosis and glycaemia.

Brown adipose tissue (BAT) is believed to comprise 2–7% of the newborn's weight, depending on gestation and weight. Brown fat starts to be deposited in the fetus from 26 weeks' gestation (Bruck, 1978). The brown adipocyte is uniquely suited to the role in newborn thermogenesis. This tissue differs from white adipose tissue in that it is capable of rapid metabolism, heat production and heat transfer to the peripheral circulation.

The total amount of heat produced in the neonate is unknown, but it may be up to 100% of its requirements. It is controlled by the sympathetic nervous system and hormone mediators. The sympathetic nervous system stimulates the adrenal gland to release adrenaline which increases the metabolism of brown fat and catecholamines which result in an increase in available glucose that is required for these metabolic processes. The thyroid gland is also stimulated by the pituitary to release thyroid-stimulating hormone and then produces thyroxine (T4). Thyroxine is known to enhance heat production from brown adipose tissue.

Heat production within brown adipose tissue is not yet fully known or understood, but what is known is that brown adipose tissue contains:

▶ a high concentration of complex mitochondria;
▶ electron transport compounds which are said to be responsible for the colour of brown fat.

Brown adipose tissue is especially prominent in the mammalian fetus and its anatomical distribution is important to its function. By far the largest mass of tissue envelops the kidneys and adrenal glands. Many smaller masses are present around the blood vessels and muscles in the neck, and there are extensions of these deposits under the clavicles and into the axillae. Further extensions accompany the great vessels entering the thoracic inlet. The proximity of brown adipose tissue to large blood vessels and vital vascular organs provides the ability for rapid transfer of heat to the circulation (Polk, 1988).

It is important to note that if a baby is exposed to cold stress, the nape of the neck is felt to be warmer than the rest of the body. The midwife should be aware of this when giving parents education and advice on the care of their baby. The best area for the mother/partner to check the baby's temperature is the skin of abdomen. Midwives, students and parents need to also be aware that the extremities, i.e. the hands and the feet

of the neonate, are often colder than the rest of the body, and this is not normally significant to well-being.

The baby may generate heat by crying and becoming hyperactive when cold stress is severe enough to cause jitteriness, although shivering does not appear to occur. If cold stress is not eliminated at this point the baby may become extremely hypothermic, hypoglycaemic, hypoxic, acidotic, lethargic and eventually death will ensue, caused by cold injury. The full-term baby can flex his body to the 'fetal' position which can provide some protection against cold stress. However, the lack of muscle tone and flaccid posture of the immature or ill baby means that he is fully exposed to the environment and has a higher heat loss. Babies can also reduce shunting of internal heat to body surfaces by vasoconstricting peripheral vessels.

Feeding

From the time of birth, the baby requires water, glucose and certain electrolytes. Calories are required for the baby's growth and energy needs in order to maintain body temperature and metabolism. The method of feeding the neonate, whether orally, by nasogastric tube or intravenously, and the frequency and volume of feeds depends on the gestational age and physical condition. When gastric feeds have to be delayed for days and certainly if more than a week, such as in a case of a baby with severe respiratory distress, parenteral nutrition will be required in order that adequate calories are given. It is important to remember that milk contains far more calories than dextrose given intravenously or orally (Klaus and Fanaroff, 1979).

Drugs

Medication given to pregnant women can affect the ability of the neonate to thermoregulate. Analgesia in labour such as pethidine given intramuscularly or intravenously, and the use of bupivacaine for epidurals, will cause vasodilatation and heat loss in the mother which in turn is passed to the fetus, rendering it vulnerable to heat loss after birth. Other drugs which may adversely affect the neonate's temperature control are tranquillizers, and antidepressants and hypnotics in large doses. These drugs will tend to affect the neonate's muscle activity and thus lead to flaccidity and a resulting hypothermia. General anaesthetics and muscle relaxants during Caesarean sections also produce the same effect.

A problem which is sadly on the increase is substance abuse, such as heroin addiction. Mothers addicted to drugs may give birth to babies who are hyperactive and subsequently have a higher metabolic rate, and this can upset the thermoregulatory balance, which may cause the baby to become hyperthermic.

The Role of the Midwife in Thermoregulation

The midwife is in control of the neonate's environment and, therefore, the actions that she takes prior to labour and delivery may determine the neonate's well-being. It is important for the midwife not to merely focus upon the temperature of the delivery room and the warmth of the towels used for wrapping the baby, but also to take into account other aspects that will interact and influence the neonate's well-being.

DURING PREGNANCY

The midwife will have a role in counselling and advising the woman on maintaining a stable temperature, especially during the period of cell division and differentiation in the first trimester of pregnancy.

It has been found that there is a higher risk of delivering a baby with congenital abnormalities in women who use a sauna, especially if this is a new activity to which the mother's physiology has not adapted (Cohen, 1987; Smith *et al.*, 1988; Tikkenhan and Heinonen, 1991). Care should be taken with other activities, such as hectic exercise, which significantly increase the maternal temperature.

Many women complain of the heat during their pregnancy. The midwife needs to be able to offer realistic and practical advice to the woman which includes wearing natural fabrics, such as cotton, thin wool, silk and linen, and having cool baths/showers. However, in offering this advice, the midwife should assess whether the woman is well, as she may be suffering from an infection and/or pyrexia. If infection or a pyrexia is identified, it is vital that action is prompt and effective for the sake of both mother and fetus.

DURING LABOUR

Part of the midwife's role and function is 'to care for and assist the mother during labour' (UKCC, 1994). This involves effective monitoring of her temperature on a regular basis. The temperature may be measured four hourly and recorded on the mother's partogram. Any deviations from the normal should be acted upon. A raised temperature may be an indication of infection or maternal ketosis (see Chapter 29) and the midwife needs to appreciate the effect on the fetus and later on the neonate, as well as on the woman.

Delivery room – preparation

To a certain extent the midwife is in control of the environment which the neonate will enter. If the woman is going to deliver her baby in the home, the midwife needs to ensure that the woman and her family know the importance of preparing the room in terms of warmth and absence of draughts. In the hospital, the midwife needs to ensure that there is adequate warmth and lack of draughts, whilst explaining to the mother and her partner why the room needs to be so warm.

The midwife should prepare the towels and blankets by warming them. In some units this may be achieved by placing these articles under the radiant heater of the resuscitaire. In other units there may be a warming cupboard or radiator that fulfils the same purpose. The midwife should ensure that, though the blankets are warm, they are not hot enough to cause any trauma to the neonate.

Risk factors in labour

The midwife will monitor the fetus for any signs of hypoxia or distress in order to effectively prepare for delivery. She needs to understand the implications of the maternal–fetal unit, because the following aspects may lead to neonatal hypothermia or hyperthermia:

▶ Maternal distress – resulting in pyrexia.
▶ Maternal infection resulting in pyrexia or hypothermia.
▶ Epidural anaesthesia in labour.
▶ Substance abuse.

Part of the preparation for delivery and resuscitation should include checking and preparing the equipment for resuscitation of the newborn.

The midwife will also need to inform the paediatrician and the staff in the special care baby nursery before delivery should the neonate be considered to be at high risk.

DURING THE NEONATAL PERIOD

Initial care of the neonate

The midwife's role then extends into understanding the implications of the neonate being exposed to heat or cold stress. She needs then to relate her knowledge and understanding of physiology to the care of the baby at birth to prevent hypothermia. As the midwife uses her knowledge of the factors which contribute to heat loss she will work to minimize these factors. She will dry the neonate's head as it enters the cooler delivery environment, or this could be done by the mother or father while the midwife is checking the neck for the presence of the umbilical cord. The neonate's head is the largest surface and is liable to rapid heat loss.

As the neonate is then helped into the world he may, if the mother wishes, be placed on her abdomen because this is a source of heat and probably comfort to the newborn baby. The midwife can then supervise the drying of the baby's skin, and cover or wrap him in warm, dry towels or blankets.

Examination of the neonate

The midwife usually performs an examination of the neonate in the delivery environment. Whilst she performs this examination, she needs to continue to ensure a warm and draught-free environment, as whilst the neonate is being examined he may lose precious heat rapidly. The examination may be performed in a cot by the bedside, or while the baby is on the resuscitaire under the radiant heater. If these strategies are used, the midwife must ensure that the parents can clearly see their baby, and can hear a running commentary on the examination. The ideal place to perform the examination is whilst the neonate is in his mother's or father's arms. This serves two purposes. First it keeps the neonate warm through the warmth of his parent's skin, and secondly this is an ideal opportunity for the midwife to educate the parents about what she is looking for and why. It is a time for parents to wonder at the miracle that is their baby, and for the midwife to assist in this and not to rush or bustle, or make it seem an everyday episode in their lives. It is also a time for parents to express their fears and anxieties and gives an opportunity for them to be alleviated. If done well, and thoroughly, the parents can use the framework provided by the midwife to be able to examine their own baby and thus work in partnership with the midwife in the hospital or community.

Temperature   If the maternal temperature is 37°C immediately after delivery of the baby, the neonate could be expected to reflect that and a temperature of 38°C would therefore be acceptable. The temperature will begin to adjust to the environment outside the uterus within a fairly short timescale.

The taking of the temperature by means of the rectal route is no longer a justifiable procedure. Historically by doing this procedure, the patency of the anus was established. However, this can be more effectively proved by the passing of a lubricated catheter or awaiting the passage of meconium (see Chapter 75). To effectively measure the temperature by the rectal route involves inserting the thermometer up to 3–5 cm into the anal sphincter. This ensures that the mercury within the thermometer bulb is well within the rectum. A knowledge of the anatomy of the rectum will inform the midwife that the rectum bends sharply to the right, and thus the passing of a hard, 3–5 cm object may perforate the rectum. It could also be envisaged that psychologically, from the neonate's point of view this is not the most ideal welcome to the world! The measuring of temperature via the axilla is now considered to be preferable.

Nutritional needs

It is widely accepted that breast milk is the ideal food for babies. The advantage to thermoregulation is that this food is already warmed and calorie controlled perfectly to fulfil the neonate's nutritional requirements. It is also immediately metabolized and therefore available to the neonate as energy for cellular function.

It has been found that the ideal time to feed the neonate is in the wakeful period after birth. The neonate's previous pre- and intranatal history will influence his nutritional needs and will need to be assessed prior to feeding. For instance an intrauterine growth-retarded baby, with limited stores of glycogen who has been asphyxiated and required resuscitation may have become cold during the resuscitation process and will first require a BMStix to measure his blood glucose level. Then, based on this, the neonate will be fed either gastrically or intravenously. The BMStix will then need to be monitored to ensure that the neonate has not depleted his glucose stores in improving his temperature.

Warding/change of environment

When the neonate is moved from one environment to another, there is an increased risk of temperature loss in transit. The midwife in charge of such a transfer must review the neonate's temperature on arrival. She should also place the neonate's cot away from draughts, or large expanses of window.

Maintaining and Monitoring the Temperature

The routine use of incubators or radiant warmers for the well baby is to be discouraged. This equipment should be used only for those babies who are ill, or likely to become ill, or less than 1.800 g, or less than 2.000 g requiring phototherapy. At birth, the well baby should be quickly dried, wrapped in warm blankets and given to his parents. If it is often found that babies are cold following delivery due to the environment, factors such as room temperature, draughts and resuscitation procedures should be investigated and corrected.

Modern incubators now have double walls to stop radiant heat loss, although this has not been proven in practice. In these incubators the air temperature can be controlled manually or automatically. Incubators and radiant warmers also have an automatic servo-control skin probe attachment. The probe is placed on the baby's abdomen or exposed skin surface and the temperature is set at 36.5°C. With smaller babies the desired skin temperature may need to be increased to a maximum of 37°C. The incubator heater will heat up or cool down to keep the skin temperature at the preset level. Care must be taken that the probe does not become detached and that the baby does not lie on it, resulting in overheating or cooling of the body.

When employing the servo-control mode, the incubator temperatures and radiant heater output must be noted because this mode may mask temperature instability. If the incubator temperature is higher than appropriate for the baby's weight, this could indicate hypothermia; a cold incubator on the other hand would indicate a febrile baby.

The addition of sterile water to the incubator humidity reservoir is not generally necessary or recommended because it can cause the growth of hydrophilic organisms such as *Pseudomonas*. Sterile water may need to be added for temperature stabilization of the baby weighing less than 1 kg; this is best accomplished by a humidifer system that can be changed daily.

Phototherapy

A baby undergoing phototherapy for jaundice who is nursed naked in a cot must *not* be assumed to be warm enough. The temperature should be checked 3–4 hourly, via the axilla, and recorded. Current practice allows phototherapy to be delivered to the baby either in an incubator, in a cot or in an 'Ohio' (i.e. open incubator with overhead radiant heating). Whatever the environment chosen for phototherapy, the midwife should ensure that the neonate's temperature remains stable, as the baby can become hyper- or hypothermic during this treatment.

Heat pads/mattresses

Heat pads or mattresses may be used and, if so, they must be checked every 6–12 months by the medical physics department, or equivalent organization within the health service.

Heat shields

Perspex heat shields should be used with one end blocked to stop the wind tunnel effect. They should be checked to see that they are not cracked, are wide enough to allow the baby to move inside and must be positioned correctly, to avoid injury to the baby. The incubator or cot should be in a warm room (22–24°C) and away from draughts. Heat shields should be used when nursing a baby naked in an incubator, as well as in other situations to prevent, or help treat, hypothermia.

Oxygen therapy

When oxygen is given in greater percentages than 30% it should be humidified and warmed. If given via an endotracheal tube, it should be given at body temperature; if given via a head box, it should be the same as the incubator temperature to avoid instability caused by confusing information being received by the neonate's hypothalamus. Cases have been reported in which ventilated babies were given oxygen at a high temperature because of a faulty humidifier system, and their lung tissue was severely damaged, leading to their death.

The surgical patient

The surgeon sees more variations of body temperature because all known general anaesthetics inactivate the thermoregulatory system and the patient becomes poikilothermic. The neonate should be nursed during the operation on heat pads and parts of the body not being operated on should be securely covered. The environment temperature needs to be maintained at between 24 and 26°C.

The artificial cooling of the neonate during a surgical procedure such as open heart surgery will have little long-term sequelae on the neonate's well-being. This is because the neonate is cooled rapidly, the situation is controlled, and the baby monitored and nourished throughout. Therefore there is little risk of actual tissue damage. This is a similar mechanism to that found in cases where children or babies have been accidently immersed in freezing water, and have 'miraculously' survived.

Minimizing the Risks of Hypothermia

Wrapping and swaddling

Warm towels or blankets and clothing for the baby are a necessity; swaddling of babies so tightly that it restricts their movements should be discouraged. Also, when the baby is left in its cot it should not be swaddled as it may have a detrimental effect on thermoregulation and respiration when the baby is asleep. The *silver swaddler* is used when transporting a baby from one place to another and is used to retain heat. However, the midwife should ensure that the silver swaddler is used correctly. First, the baby should be dried, then wrapped in a warmed blanket or towel. The silver swaddler can then be used, ensuring that there are no sharp edges in contact with the baby's skin. The swaddler will only *maintain* the temperature of the neonate, *not* increase it, as it will not allow heat transfer either in or out. The midwife needs to be aware of this, as even placing the neonate in a warmed incubator will not affect the temperature if he is wrapped in a silver swaddler.

Hats and clothes

The use of hats for the newborn, especially those who are small for gestational age and preterm, has proven effective in reducing heat loss from the largest surface area of the baby.

If the baby is wearing clothes, the midwife should ensure that these are of natural fabrics and are not too close fitting. It is better to use several layers of thin clothing rather than one or two thick layers. The midwife needs to also ensure that there are no loose threads which may become wrapped around the neonate's fingers or toes, as these can cause considerable trauma if not discovered quickly.

Hot water bottles

Hot water bottles should only be used to warm a cot and must always be *removed* when the baby is placed in the cot. The midwife should explain the use of hot water bottles to the mother and partner, and establish the rationale for removing them prior to putting the baby in the cot. A more effective and convenient method of warming the neonate is the mother, as she is a great source of heat to her baby when he is in her arms. This is so whether she breast- or bottle-feeds her baby. The midwife should therefore encourage the mother to hold her baby close to her body to promote warmth and also engender a greater sense of intimacy. This method of maintaining temperature was investigated in a study performed at the Hammersmith Hospital in 1987 and it has earned the term 'Kangeroo care' when used for very small neonates (Whitelaw *et al.*, 1988). A similar approach to care was used in a study in Colombia, in which very preterm and small-for-gestational-age babies were nursed inside their mothers' clothing, between their breasts (Sleath, 1985). There was a 95% survival rate for babies of 500–2000 g. Other benefits of this care were an improved rate of breastfeeding and closer maternal-baby interaction. Similar good outcomes have been found by using the same approach in London.

EDUCATION OF PARENTS

Educating parents in the care of their babies at home to provide warmth includes giving advice on suitable clothing for the baby with regard to the material and the number of layers required to maintain both heat and ventilation. The midwife may find a checklist useful for educating parents of small babies going home, which includes practical advice on helping babies keep warm indoors and outdoors (see example included in Table 1). This should be translated into the appropriate language for those whose first language is

Table 1 Advice sheet to mothers on the prevention of hypothermia

It is well recognized that small, or preterm babies need careful protection against getting cold. What is less well known is that the normal term baby can become seriously cold in the first weeks of life and that this can be, in extreme cases, fatal.

Babies are most at risk during the winter and spring months, or when it is particularly cold. It is important to be aware of the temperature inside and outside the home.

All babies lose heat easily and have rather poor food and fat stores in the early days of life. They also cannot shiver and tend to lie immobile for a large part of the day. Activities such as feeding, crying and limb movements normally increase heat production. Therefore tight swaddling should be avoided, especially when the baby is sleeping.

SERIOUS CHILLING
Temperature may fall to below 32°C (90°F) or lower.

The baby may become
- difficult to rouse
- difficult to feed
- cold to touch
- oedematous (swelling)

Unfortunately, the baby's skin may appear quite pink or red, which may mask the seriousness of the situation. This can mislead parents who mistake the rosy appearance for a healthy glow.

Babies who have an infection or who are feeding poorly, are more prone to chilling.

PREVENTION
The house or at least the preterm baby's room should be kept evenly warm if possible at 21°C (70°C) (see Chapter 72). Draughty windows and doors should be attended to, and additional background heating provided. Insulation can be provided by stretching 'clingfilm' over the windows in the baby's room. Social services can give financial assistance for heating the home in cases of need.

The cot should not be placed by an outside wall or by large windows, as heat may be lost.
Warm, light cot coverings and clothing for the baby should be used and extra clothing put on the baby if it is taken outside or to a colder room.

As babies lose heat through the large surface area of the head, in cold weather it is advisable for the baby to wear a bonnet if taken outside.

The baby should be bathed in a thoroughly warm room and dried very thoroughly and dressed in warm clothes immediately afterwards. Baths should not be given if the baby is unwell in any way. The room temperature should not be allowed to fall too low during the night hours.

NEVER
- put a hot water bottle in the cot with the baby. Only use to heat the cot and remove *before* the baby is placed in the cot.
- use unguarded open fires or paraffin heaters
- use mittens where an unstitched seam can damage the baby's fingers

N.B.
If you are at all worried about your baby, contact your general practitioner, midwife or health visitor.

not English, particularly for those who have little knowledge of caring for neonates in the UK climate.

Teamwork involves liaison with the community health care professionals. Social workers can be mobilized in circumstances where financial help is needed to assist with heating bills and adequate home insulation or ventilation.

The Sick Neonate

Hypothermia

Hypothermia should be anticipated in low birthweight babies and low-grade thermometers (from 33.8°C) should be used, as identifying a temperature below 34.4°C can be missed using the routine clinical thermometer. It is also important to note that core temperature drops only when the baby's effort to produce heat has failed. A rectal temperature in the normal range does not therefore indicate that a baby is not cold stressed.

Thermometer and means of taking the neonate's temperature

The normal temperature of the newborn should be:

▶ Rectal 36.5 – 37.0°C.
▶ Skin   36.0 – 36.5°C.

The temperature can be measured in the axilla or rectum. Routine use of the rectal route is no longer recommended because of the risk of perforation. Axillary temperatures are therefore preferred. In cases of suspected hypothermia or a very ill baby the rectal route may be used. Studies have recently shown that rectal temperatures taken with a mercury thermometer took five minutes to stabilize, and eight minutes in the case of the axillary route (Dodman, 1987). The thermometer should not be inserted more than 3–5 cm into the rectum of the term baby and no more than 2 cm in the preterm. It should be well lubricated with Vaseline or soft paraffin prior to insertion.

Cold stress

Hypothermia is seen, in particular, following resuscitation of asphyxiated and/or preterm babies. This may be due to poor management of the thermal environment by the carers or it could be an early sign of sepsis, cerebral haemorrhage or severe central nervous system anomalies.

The consequences of hypothermia may be devastating to the neonate. The chronically cold stressed baby may lose, or fail to gain weight because of the increased metabolic rate. In the acutely stressed baby, oxygen consumption will be increased and the baby may become hypoxic, acidotic and show signs of respiratory distress. The increased metabolism will result in rapid depletion of glycogen stores, which may result in hypoglycaemia. Pulmonary vasoconstriction may develop, resulting in right–to–left shunting of blood, aggravating the baby's hypoxia. If allowed to become severely cold stressed, the neonate may develop shock, disseminated intravascular coagulation, sclerema and ultimately die.

Management of cold injury

There is no general agreement on the management of hypothermia. Clearly prevention is the best treatment. Rewarming the mildly hypothermic neonate is no great problem, but debate continues about the virtues of rapid versus slow rewarming and their respective advantages and disadvantages. Slow rewarming is the usual practice.

The main aim is to maintain a thermal environment in which the baby is not required to increase its basal metabolic rate. Therefore the baby is rewarmed slowly to avoid hypotension, due to vasodilatation of the peripheral circulation, and acidosis. Apnoea and cardiac failure may be induced by rapid rewarming. Because oxygen consumption is minimal with gradients of less than 1.5°C, the incubator temperature is set at 1.5°C higher than the baby's core temperature and adjusted every 30–60 minutes. The baby must be naked to allow the heat from the incubator or radiant warmer to warm him. The baby should preferably not be fed gastrically as hypothermia reduces gastric evacuation of contents and reduces peristalsis. Intravenous fluids ensure adequate fluids and glucose intake.

Hyperthermia

Hyperthermia can be defined as a temperature of more than 37.4°C. This is a less common complication in the care of the neonate but can still be problematic. The pyrexia may be due to excessive environmental temperatures, incubator overheating (or the greenhouse effect of an incubator in the sunlight), infection, dehydration or a change in central control by drugs or cerebral damage. As with cold stress, hyperthermia results in increased metabolism and oxygen consumption. It is important that the baby is cooled slowly. This means removing woollens or leaving the baby with only one blanket. Extreme measures, such as leaving the baby in thin clothes and only one sheet should be avoided.

The midwife/neonatal nurse should monitor the temperature and blood sugar closely.

Conclusion

Although a homeotherm in the true sense of the word, the neonate has higher heat and water losses compared to the adult which require the carer to provide a thermal environment which allows a minimal resting metabolic rate. Midwives caring for neonates must give special attention to the maintenance of a 'normal' temperature, particularly in the 'at risk' neonate. Therefore an understanding of the physiology of temperature control and its application to practice is vital for the midwife and includes the means of providing a safe transition to extrauterine life. A knowledge of calorific intake related to thermoregulation is vital.

The midwife will apply her physiological knowledge to monitor normal temperature variances, identify when these become abnormal and the possible causes of the deviations from normal. These include sepsis, cerebral malfunction or simply an inadequate stable thermal environment.

The midwife needs to pay the same attention to the care of the neonate as she does to the mother, if not more. If there is a problem, a worry, or individual needs, the woman is given the opportunity to express them. The neonate is not able to speak, and sometimes not able to cry. He is at the mercy of those who care for him to recognize his needs and meet them. It is therefore important to learn to understand the language of the neonate through physiology and his behaviour in order to fulfil his needs.

References

Adamsons, K. (1966) The role of thermal factors in fetal and neonatal life. *Paediat. Clin. North Am.* **13**: 599.

Baldino, F. & Geller, H.M. (1982) Electrophysiological analysis of neuronal thermosensitivity in rat preoptic and hypothalamic culture. *J. Physiol.* **327**: 173.

Bruk, K. (1978) Heat production and temperature regulation. In Stave, U. (ed.) *Perinatal Physiology*, pp. 455–498. New York: Plenum.

Cohen, F.L. (1987) Neural tube defects: epidemiology, detection and prevention. *J. Obstet. Gynaecol. Neonatal Nurs.* **16**(2): 105–115.

Darnal, R.A. (1987) The thermophysiology of the newborn infant. *Med-Instrum.* **22**: 33–38.

Dick, D. (1987) *Yesterday's Babies (a History of Baby Care)*. London: Bodley Head.

Dodman, N. (1987) Newborn temperature control. *Neonatal Network* **5**: 19–23.

Doumanis, M. (1983) *Mothers in Greece: From Collectivism to Individualism*. London: Academic Press.

Dunn, P.A., York, R., Cheek, T.G. & Yeboah, K. (1994) Maternal hypothermia: implications for obstetric nurses. *Gynaecol. Neonatal Nurs.* **23**: 238–242.

Guyton, A.C. (1979) *Textbook of Medical Physiology*, 8th edn. Philadelphia: W.B. Saunders.

Hammarlund, K. & Sedin, G. (1986) Heat loss from the skin of preterm and full term newborn infants during the first weeks after birth. *Biol-Neonate* **50**: 1–10.

Klaus, M.H. & Fanaroff, A.A. (1979) *Care of the High-Risk Neonate*. London: W.B. Saunders.

Mitchell, D. & Laburn, H.P. (1985) Pathophysiology of temperature regulation. *Physiologist* **28**: 507–517.

Morishima, H.O., Yeh, M.N., Niemann, W.H. & James, L.S. (1977) Temperature gradient between fetus and mother as an index for assessing intrauterine fetal condition. *Am. J. Obstet. Gynecol.* **129**: 443.

Polin, M.D. & Fox, W.W. (1992) *Fetal and Neonatal Physiology*, Vol. 1, pp. 447–483. Philadelphia: WB Saunders.

Polk, D-H. (1988) Thyroid hormone effects on neonatal thermogenesis. *Clinics in Perinatology.* **12**: 151–156.

Rutter, N. (1988) *A Guide to Radiant Warmer Care of Infants.* Air-Shields (S & W Vickers, Sidcup, Kent, UK).

Rutter, N. (1985) The Evaporimeter and emotional sweating in the neonate. *Clinics in Perinatology.* **12**: 63–77.

Sinclair, J.C. (1992) Management of the thermal environment. *Effective Care of the Newborn Infant.* Oxford: Oxford Medical Publications.

Sleath, K. (1985) Lessons from Colombia. *Nursing Mirror* **160**(14): 14–16.

Smith, M., Upfold, J. & Edwards, M. (1988) The dangers of heat to the newborn. *Patient Management* **3**: 157–165.

Tikkenhan, J. & Heinonen, O. (1991) Maternal hyperthermia during pregnancy and cardiovascular malformations in the offspring. *Eur. J. Epidemiol.* **7**(6): 628–635.

Tucker Blackburn, S. & Lee Loper, D. (1992) *Maternal, Fetal and Neonatal Physiology.* London: W.B. Saunders.

UKCC (UK Central Council for Nursing, Midwifery & Health Visiting) (1994) *The Midwife's Code of Practice.* London: UKCC.

Whitelaw, A., Heisterkamp, G., Sleath, K., Acolet, D. & Richards, M. (1988) Skin to skin contact for very low birthweight infants and their mothers. *Arch. Dis. Child.* **63**: 1377–1381.

Further Reading

Alistair, G.S. & Philip, M.B. (1980) *Neonatology*, 2nd edn. Medical Examination Publishing.

Babson, S.G. & Pernoll, M.L. (1980) *Diagnosis and Management of the Fetus and Neonate at Risk*, 4th edn. St Louis: CV Mosby.

Flant, Michael & Cloherty, John P. (1988) *Manual of Neonatal Care Joint Programme in Neonatology*, 2nd edn. Harvard Medical School, Beth Israel Hospital, Brig- ham and Women's Hospital, The Children's Hospital Boston.

Kelnar, C.J.H., Harvey, D. & Simpson, C. (1995) *The Sick Newborn Baby*. London: Baillière Tindall.

Korongs, Sheldon B. (1976) *High-risk Newborn Infants*, 2nd edn. St Louis: C.V. Mosby.

Robertson, N.R.C. (1981) *A Manual of Neonatal Intensive Care*. London: Edward Arnold.

Simbruner, G., Weninger, M. & Popow, C. (1985a) Regional heat loss in newborn at various environmental temperatures. *S. Afr. Med. J.* **68**: 940–944.

Simbruner, G., Weninger, M. & Popow, C. (1985b) Heat loss in newborns with various diseases. A method of assessing local metabolism and perfusion. *S. Afr. Med. J.* **68**: 645–648.

Stothers, J.K. (1981) Head insulation and heat loss in the newborn. *Arch. Dis. Childh.* **56**: 530–534.

67

The Preterm Baby

A baby weighing 2.5 kg or less is said to be of *low birthweight*. Low birthweight babies may be either:

1 *preterm*, if born before 37 completed weeks of pregnancy; or
2 *small-for-gestational-age* (SFGA) if the birthweight is below the tenth centile for gestational age (Figure 1).

Some babies are born preterm and small-for-gestational-age and therefore may have problems from both these aspects. SFGA babies are discussed in Chapter 68.

Although only about 7–8% of babies born in the UK fall into the low birthweight group, more than half of all neonatal deaths occur among these small infants.

With the development of special and neonatal intensive care in recent years, the survival of low birthweight infants above 1500 g has become commonplace. High mortality rates are now found predominantly in those under 1500 g (very low birthweight) and particularly in

those under 1000 g (extremely low birthweight) (Yu *et al.*, 1986a).

Assessment of Gestational Age

All low birthweight babies are examined by a paediatrician soon after birth and their gestational age is assessed. The obstetrician will have based the assessment of gestation on such factors as the date of the last normal menstrual period, the size of the growing uterus and tests such as ultrasonography and amniocentesis. After birth it is possible for gestational age to be determined within two weeks on the basis of physical characteristics and neurological development.

Several scoring systems have been devised to aid accurate assessment. Points are awarded for each characteristic and the total number of points scored used to assess gestational age. The *Dubowitz scale* (Dubowitz *et al.*, 1970) is the best established in the UK but has the

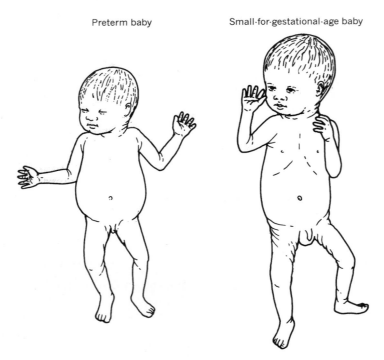

Preterm baby   Small-for-gestational-age baby

Figure 1   Low birthweight babies.

drawback that it involves measures of neurological state (e.g. muscle tone) as well as external criteria. It may therefore be inappropriate for use with sick, ventilated infants. Providing the baby is well and examined at a few hours of age, this assessment is accurate within two weeks. An abbreviated scale that relies solely on external criteria, the *Parkin score* (Parkin *et al.*, 1976), avoids these limitations (Table 1). The Parkin score is quicker to perform than the Dubowitz assessment but may not be quite as accurate.

Characteristics of the Preterm Baby

Preterm babies are immature and not ready to adapt to extrauterine life. Their characteristics are related to gestational age. The head is large in proportion to the body and the baby has a small triangular face with a pointed chin and worried expression. If very immature the eyelids may be fused or the eyes opened infrequently. Owing to poor ossification the sutures and fontanelles are widely spaced and skull bones soft. The skin is red due to the absence of subcutaneous fat, surface veins are prominent and the body is covered with varying amounts of soft downy hair called lanugo. The limbs are thin, the nails soft, the chest small and narrow with little or no breast tissue and the abdomen large; the umbilicus appears to be low set. The genitalia are small, the labia majora does not cover the labia minora and the testes may not have descended into the scrotum. Muscle tone is poor and the more immature the baby, the greater the degree of extension of the arms and legs. The baby may be feeble and drowsy with a poor or absent sucking reflex. At 28 weeks the baby weighs 1–1.25 kg and measures about 37 cm. At 36 weeks the baby weighs 2.25–3.75 kg and measures about 47 cm.

Causes

No cause can be found for 40% of preterm births, but the commonest known causes are pre-eclampsia and antepartum haemorrhage. Serious general disease of the mother such as pyelonephritis, chronic nephritis or essential hypertension and illness associated with a high temperature may also cause preterm birth. Cervical incompetence, though usually a cause of late abor-

Table 1 The Parkin score for assessment of gestational age (Parkin *et al.*, 1976)

Skin texture. Tested by picking up a fold of abdominal skin between finger and thumb, and by inspection.

0 very thin with a gelatinous feel
1 thin and smooth
2 smooth and of medium thickness, irritation rash and superficial peeling may be present
3 slight thickening and stiff feeling with superficial cracking and peeling especially evident on the hands and feet
4 thick and parchment-like with superficial or deep cracking

Skin colour. Estimated by inspection when the baby is quiet.

0 dark red
1 uniformly pink
2 pale pink, though the colour may vary over different parts of the body, some parts may be very pale
3 pale, nowhere really pink except on the ears, lips, palms and soles.

Breast size. Measured by picking up the breast tissue between finger and thumb.

0 no breast tissue palpable
1 breast tissue palpable on one or both sides, neither being more than 0.5 cm in diameter
2 breast tissue palpable on both sides, one or both being 0.5–1 cm in diameter
3 breast tissue palpable on both sides, one or both being more than 1 cm in diameter

Ear firmness. Tested by palpation and folding of the upper pinna.

0 pinna feels soft and is easily folded into bizarre positions without springing back into position spontaneously
1 pinna feels soft along the edge and is easily folded but returns slowly to the correct position spontaneously
2 cartilage can be felt to the edge of the pinna though it is thin in places and the pinna springs back readily after being folded
3 pinna firm with definite cartilage extending to the periphery and springs back immediately into position after being folded.

Score each external sign in turn. Add them up. Read off the baby's gestational age on the following chart:

| Score | Gestational age | |
	days	weeks
1	190	27
2	210	30
3	230	33
4	240	34½
5	250	36
6	260	37
7	270	38½
8	276	39½
9	281	40
10	285	41
11	290	41½
12	295	42

tions, may result in the birth of a live very preterm infant. Smoking, drug and alcohol abuse in pregnancy are associated with preterm labour and the birth of small babies. Other causes are multiple pregnancy, polyhydramnios, rhesus incompatibility and congenital abnormalities. Preterm births are more common amongst social classes IV and V and mothers of short stature and this illustrates the effect of nutrition and physique upon pregnancy. Other social factors which contribute to the birth of preterm babies are maternal age below 20 and multiparity.

Early Management

There are many physiological functions that a preterm baby is unable to perform adequately. These are related to the immaturity of the various systems or of the nerve centres controlling them. Neonatal care is an attempt to compensate for these deficiencies until such time as the infant is able to cope unaided. Accurate assessment of the baby's condition at birth and prompt resuscitation are therefore essential. Subsequently meticulous care and close observation are required to detect even small departures from normal physiological function which can lead to serious complications.

CARE IN LABOUR

Every effort should be made to deliver the mother in a consultant maternity hospital with a neonatal unit since it is generally safer to transfer the fetus *in utero* rather than after birth. Care must be taken during labour to avoid giving the mother drugs which will depress the fetal respiratory centre at birth. Adequate relief of pain is essential, however, and may be achieved by epidural anaesthesia. An episiotomy may be necessary to shorten the perineal phase of the second stage of labour and thus reduce the risk of intracranial injury which may occur due to poor ossification of the skull bones and fragility of the blood vessels. Some obstetricians also recommend elective forceps delivery to shorten the second stage and reduce the risk of intracranial injury, particularly for breech presentations. Elective Caesarean sections are now more widely used in preterm deliveries, to prevent the likelihood of trauma to the baby.

Once labour is established, the paediatrician, midwifery and nursing staff in the neonatal unit must be informed to allow preparations to be made for the admission of the baby. The paediatrician and midwifery staff who are to care for the baby also have the opportunity to meet the parents before the delivery.

Preparation for the baby in the delivery room

The midwife is responsible for ensuring that all equipment required to resuscitate a baby at birth is available, functioning and prepared. The delivery room must be warm for the reception of a preterm baby, thus draughts are minimized and fans are turned off. Equipment which must be prepared includes the following:

1 The resuscitaire is prepared and checked and the overhead heater is turned on.
2 A portable incubator is heated and prepared to receive the baby.
3 Warm blankets are prepared.
4 The oxygen supply is checked and turned on. A second source of oxygen which can be connected directly to an endotracheal tube via a pressure-limiting device (traditionally a column of water) should be available.
5 Suction apparatus is turned on and checked. A range of sizes of suction catheters is required. For example, 10 G catheters are used to remove tenacious meconium, 6 G catheters are required to pass through a small endotracheal tube and 8 G for suction of the baby's nose and throat.
6 Resuscitation bag and face masks must be available. A range of small masks should be at hand.
7 At least two laryngoscopes with blades of a suitable size for a small baby must be present and checked. Spare batteries and bulbs should be readily available.
8 A selection of oral endotracheal tubes should be at hand. A clean stethoscope should be available.
9 A box of neonatal drugs for resuscitation must be checked ready for use.
10 Equipment to establish an intravenous infusion of dextrose, saline or plasma is prepared.

CARE AT BIRTH

Establishment of respiration

An experienced paediatrician should always be present at birth to resuscitate the baby. If this is not possible a midwife or doctor skilled in resuscitation should attend. The more preterm the baby, the less developed are all the physiological functions. The baby born at term has strong respiratory muscles and the nerve centre in the medulla controlling respiration is fully developed. In the preterm baby the muscles may be weak and the respiratory centre incompletely developed. Thus it may, in the first place, be difficult to establish satisfactory breathing.

Some paediatricians advocate elective intubation immediately following delivery for resuscitation of all low birthweight babies. Studies have shown that this improves the mortality and morbidity rates for this group (Drew, 1982). In some circumstances the baby may initially appear well, breathing regularly and becoming pink, but later develop expiratory grunting, apnoeic attacks and poor colour, deteriorating in condition rapidly. Resuscitative measures are as for the mature baby.

The paediatrician will require trained assistance to resuscitate an asphyxiated baby and extra help may be required if cardiac massage and intravenous fluids are necessary.

Warmth

The temperature of the delivery room should be increased to at least 24°C immediately prior to delivery, to help prevent cold stress to the newborn baby. Following delivery the baby is dried with warm towels, paying particular attention to the head as up to 80% of heat loss occurs through this area. Once breathing is established and the baby is in good condition, the mother may wish to cuddle or have skin-to-skin contact with her baby. Covering them with warm blankets will help to reduce heat loss. If resuscitative measures are necessary, the baby is placed on a preheated resuscitaire under an overhead radiant heater after being quickly dried and wrapped in warm blankets. During resuscitative procedures some exposure of the baby will be necessary, but great care must be exercised to avoid chilling.

Parent–baby relationship

It is most important that the parents have an opportunity to see and hold their baby, even if only briefly, before transfer to the neonatal unit. The paediatrician will usually see the parents later to give them an account of their baby's condition, care and prognosis. Often the mother can be taken to the neonatal unit to see her baby again when she is transferred from the labour suite to the postnatal ward.

Other essential procedures include labelling the baby and attending to the umbilical cord before transfer to the neonatal unit. Weighing, measuring and a detailed examination can wait until after the baby's transfer.

The baby should be given an initial dose of phytomenadione (Konakion) 0.5–1 mg to reduce the risk of haemorrhage (see Chapter 72).

Admission to the neonatal unit

On arrival in the neonatal unit the baby is quickly weighed and then transferred into a preheated incubator. Weighing is important because drugs and fluid requirements are calculated according to this weight.

A baseline set of observations are made on admission, including temperature, respiratory and heart rates, blood glucose and oxygenation levels. The appropriate monitors are connected to the baby and any urgent procedures necessary are performed. These may include siting of an intravenous infusion to correct or prevent hypoglycaemia, or the administration of oxygen.

If the baby is in a headbox (Figure 2) to increase the oxygen concentration of inspired air, an oxygen analyser will also be required. An arterial line may be inserted for blood gas sampling and blood pressure monitoring. Some preterm babies with respiratory problems may require mechanical ventilation. In these cases an endotracheal tube is inserted, if a suitable one is not in position already, and ventilation is established.

An intravenous infusion of 10% dextrose is set up if the baby cannot be fed. Prophylactic antibiotics are usually prescribed for those with respiratory problems and are given intravenously. Before the first dose is administered, however, samples of blood, gastric aspirate and swabs from the nose, mouth and umbilicus are taken to screen the baby for infection.

Subsequent Observations and Care

The nursing care given to the preterm baby is of vital importance as survival depends on the quality of care received. The care is supervised by a paediatrician in the neonatal unit.

In the early stages continuous observation is necessary and frequent records are made of the baby's condition.

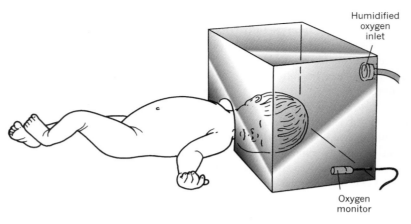

Humidified
oxygen
inlet

Oxygen
monitor

Figure 2   Baby being nursed in a headbox (incubator not shown).

Control of body temperature

The aim is to maintain body temperature in the thermoneutral range. At this temperature oxygen consumption is less and energy requirements to maintain body temperature are reduced to a minimum. In order to achieve this the temperature within the incubator must be controlled. The incubator temperature is set at between 33 and 37°C, the higher temperature usually being required for very small babies. Alternatively, the desired body temperature for the baby may be set, 36.8–37°C, and a servofeedback mechanism is used to maintain it. In the latter case a skin probe is attached to the baby and the incubator temperature automatically adjusts in response to changes in the skin temperature. Whichever method is used, both the incubator and baby's temperature must be checked and recorded regularly. The skin probe may become detached from the baby's skin, or if the baby lies on it or skin perfusion is poor, record inaccurately, and thus cannot be relied on as the sole means of recording the baby's temperature. The room temperature must be maintained at about 24°C, and occasionally needs to be even higher if there is difficulty in maintaining a very small baby's temperature.

Although brown fat in very low birthweight infants is active in cold stress, it is often quite inadequate to maintain such an infant's core temperature. The high surface area of preterm infants in relation to their size and their thin skin permit rapid heat loss.

Infants born before 30 weeks' gestation have an additional problem in that their skin is porous as well as thin. This allows water to pass through and evaporate, thereby increasing heat loss. To reduce this evaporative heat loss, these babies may be nursed in a humidified incubator for the first week of life. Radiant heaters may exacerbate this problem by increasing the evaporative heat loss, thus their use is inappropriate for these small babies.

To prevent heat loss by radiation the baby may be covered with a Perspex radiant heat shield, enveloped in a bubble-blanket or wrapped in polythene sheets (e.g. clingfilm). Attempts to make the skin less permeable by rubbing in sunflower seed oil has been tried and may also be of nutritional value. Hats, boots and other garments may be worn to prevent heat loss, provided they do not prevent adequate observation of the baby.

Respiration

The respiratory rate should be between 40 and 60 per minute and the baby's colour pink all over. Continuous monitoring of respiratory rate and pattern is performed with an electronic monitor which also records heart rate. The apnoea alarm is usually set at 20 seconds so that any resuscitative measures required can be carried out promptly should respiration cease. If this equipment is not available an apnoea alarm mattress or monitor may be used, but these are less reliable.

Transient tachypnoea occurs when the fluid is slow to clear from the lungs after birth and may be the result of asphyxia temporarily impairing cardiac function. Subsequently tachypnoea may be an early sign of many problems, particularly lung disease, but also of sepsis and acidosis.

Oxygen therapy   Oxygen therapy is frequently required by preterm babies to relieve cyanosis where there are respiratory problems, but it must be realized that oxygen is a dangerous drug when given in excess. It is one of the main factors in the aetiology of *retrolental fibroplasia*, also called retinopathy of prematurity (Prendiville and Schulenberg, 1988), which may lead to blindness and pulmonary damage. The aim is therefore to maintain normal arterial oxygen tensions:

7–10 kPa (60–80 mmHg) in a mature baby
6–9 kPa (50–70 mmHg) in a preterm baby

Inadequate oxygenation may result in hypoxic brain damage. Careful monitoring is therefore essential to maintain normal arterial oxygen tension. If the baby is in a headbox with extra oxygen, an oxygen analyser must be used to monitor the oxygen concentration of inspired air. In addition the arterial oxygen tension is monitored using a *transcutaneous oxygen monitor* or via an arterial catheter. A heated electrode applied to the skin is used for the continuous monitoring of transcutaneous oxygen which approximates to the arterial oxygen tension. The electrode should be re-sited every 3–4 hours to prevent first-degree burns.

A sudden drop in transcutaneous oxygen levels may indicate a sudden deterioration following handling of the baby, or complications such as pneumothorax or periventricular haemorrhage.

Transcutaneous oxygen monitoring becomes less reliable as the baby gets older and in term infants, as the skin is less permeable. *Oxygen saturation monitoring* is now more widely used. An infrared probe attached to the hand or foot gives a continuous reading. This method is preferred in small and very preterm babies as it causes no skin damage and is non-invasive. Transcutaneous oxygen monitoring and oxygen saturation monitoring give different information, and both may be useful in some situations (Southall *et al.*, 1987).

Arterial cannulation is also necessary in the ill baby so that blood specimens can be obtained to measure blood gases and pH. The commonest site for an indwelling arterial catheter is in the umbilicus, but if this is not possible a peripheral artery is used. Some arterial catheters allow the continuous monitoring of oxygen tension, thus transcutaneous oxygen monitoring can then be dispensed with.

Blood sugar

The blood sugar should be checked every 4–6 hours during the first 48–72 hours after birth using Dextrostix paper strips or BMStix, since hypoglycaemia is a common problem in preterm babies. Oxygen deprivation may have caused them to consume much of their available energy stores during the perinatal period. In addition, their stores of brown and white fat and glycogen are too small to maintain their blood sugar level at a time when their energy requirements are particularly high.

Preterm babies expend more energy for their weight than term infants because of the heat loss from their large surface area, the increased effort of breathing which accompanies respiratory difficulties and their greater rate of growth. The problem may be further exacerbated by an inadequate energy intake during the first few days of life.

Hypoglycaemia is not a diagnosis but a sign of an underlying disorder. The definition of hypoglycaemia is widely accepted as a plasma glucose level less than 1.7 mmol/l; although recent evidence has suggested that prolonged blood glucose levels of less than 2.6 mmol/l may cause problems (Lucas *et al.*, 1988). If severe (blood sugar usually under 1.1 mmol/l), it will cause problems such as apnoea and convulsions. Urgent treatment with intravenous dextrose is necessary followed by a 10% dextrose infusion to maintain the blood sugar at a safe level.

About 30% of babies who have suffered severe hypoglycaemia in the early neonatal period will have long-term damage such as cerebral palsy and/or mental retardation (Halliday *et al.*, 1989).

Hyperglycaemia will result in glycosuria and this increases fluid loss because a certain quantity of water is lost with sugar. This makes the control of the baby's fluid balance more difficult.

Heart rate

The heart rate is electronically monitored and should be within the normal range of 120–160 beats per minute. It is also checked by listening to the apex beat at regular intervals, the frequency being determined by the condition of the baby. Mild bradycardia may occur during the recovery from asphyxia when there is raised intracranial pressure. Later it may be associated with apnoea and indicate the need for stimulation and resuscitation.

If a baby on a ventilator develops bradycardia, it could be caused by a blocked or misplaced endotracheal tube, a pneumothorax, a periventricular haemorrhage or septicaemia. Tachycardia is an indication that the baby is responding to some stress. It may occur during the early stage of one of the complications mentioned above, or be due to a fever or an excess of a cardiac stimulant drug such as dopamine.

Blood pressure

The blood pressure is monitored in a preterm baby and/or ill baby and may be continually monitored via an arterial catheter. It is important to recognize that the normal range for blood pressure varies with birth-weight and gestational age. A mean diastolic blood pressure of 30 mmHg may be acceptable in a baby weighing 1 kg who is well, whereas in a baby of 4 kg the mean would be nearer 40 mmHg.

Hypotension results in insufficient blood flow to vital organs. This may cause irreversible damage to organs such as the brain and heart and other organs, such as the kidneys, may fail. Whilst peritoneal dialysis can tide the baby over a period of renal failure, the infant may not withstand this additional complication.

Hypotension is treated with blood products and/or drugs. Blood or plasma is usally given if the cause is thought to be an inadequate blood volume and drugs such as dopamine or isoprenaline may be prescribed to increase the power of the heart's contraction.

Hypertension may also occur, especially when the baby is subjected to stressful procedures like the discontinuation of ventilation during suction via an endotracheal tube, and when complications such as pneumothorax develop. Hypertension may lead to periventricular haemorrhage, especially in babies of less than 32 weeks' gestation, because the capillary network in the brain is very fragile in such immature infants. Hypertension also occurs in response to painful stimuli.

Urine

The baby is expected to pass urine within 24 hours of birth. As feeding is established the volume of urine excreted increases.

Any baby receiving intensive care should have each urinary output measured and samples tested for glucose and osmolality. Glycosuria may indicate a reduced renal threshold for glucose and the amount of glucose administered should be reduced, as it may lead to dehydration. Glycosuria may be an early sign of an underlying infection. Osmolality of the urine indicates whether the baby's kidneys are retaining fluid by concentrating the urine, or excreting excess water by passing a dilute urine, and thus gives a guide to the fluid intake required. A prismatic device is available that gives an accurate measurement of the specific gravity of the urine, this being equivalent to knowing the urine osmolality. The aim is to achieve a specific gravity of between 1010 and 1015.

Oliguria of less than 0.5 ml/kg per hour occurs in some ill neonates who fail to micturate. It may also be associated with hypotension, acute renal failure or urinary obstruction.

Meconium/faeces

The passage of meconium in small, preterm babies may be delayed, particularly if they are not fed and/or if they have respiratory distress syndrome. This delay may contribute to hyperbilirubinaemia as the bilirubin in the meconium may be reabsorbed. Once milk feeds are started it is important to observe the faeces for signs of blood and mucus which may indicate the onset of *necrotizing enterocolitis*. This condition is most likely to occur in babies recovering from asphyxia and respiratory distress syndrome.

Hygiene and prevention of infection

Very small preterm babies should be handled as little as possible and with great gentleness.

Daily toilet should be carried out including washing the face, hands and skin folds with warm water. The napkin area needs particular attention. Oral hygiene is necessary for babies with an endotracheal tube *in situ* and for others unable to suck. During this procedure the baby is carefully examined for signs of infection and the cord is treated like that of the mature baby.

Special precautions must be taken to reduce infection. The nurseries should be well ventilated and thoroughly cleaned each day using vacuum cleaners and scrubbing machines for the floor and damp dusting for other surfaces. Soiled linen and dressings should be collected in disposable bags and removed from the nursery as soon as possible.

All staff and visitors should be free from infection and well trained in the technique of hand-washing which must be carried out before and after handling each baby using an antiseptic soap such as providone-iodine or chlorhexidine. Each baby should have individual equipment which is stored in the incubator or cot cupboard. The incubator is cleaned regularly both inside and out using an antiseptic solution and is changed weekly. After use incubators are dismantled and thoroughly cleaned and aired before being used again.

FEEDING

The method of feeding depends on the size, maturity and condition of the baby. Well babies of any size or gestation may show signs of sucking and therefore can be tried with breast or bottle feeds, although careful supervision will be necessary to ensure that they are having adequate fluid intake and are not becoming too tired by prolonged attempts to feed. Immature babies may have poor suck and swallow co-ordination and thus tube feeding may be necessary. If the baby is bottle fed, breast milk is the milk of choice but if this is not available a low birthweight formula milk should be given. Small babies tire easily and may benefit from having a regime of mixed bottle and tube feeds initially, until they can cope with more and eventually all bottle feeds. Ill babies are given an intravenous infusion of 10% of dextrose initially and later total intravenous nutrition may be necessary.

Total intravenous feeding

Babies who are being ventilated are fed exclusively by the intravenous route initially. This is for four principal reasons:

1   There is a substantial risk of milk aspiration which intubation does not abolish since the endotracheal tubes used for neonates are uncuffed.
2   There is an ileus for the first few days of respiratory distress syndrome so that milk placed in the stomach or small bowel will accumulate as if the bowel were obstructed.
3   Milk in the stomach increases the work of breathing. In an infant suffering from respiratory distress, any factor that increases the work of breathing, or that increases oxygen demand, should be avoided.
4   During the course of respiratory distress syndrome many infants have periods of hypotension and/or hypoxia. This is hazardous in any circumstances, but if there are bacteria proliferating in the bowel because the infant has been fed, then the risk of septicaemia or bowel disease (necrotizing enterocolitis) is greatly increased. This risk is significantly reduced if the baby is fully or partly fed on breast milk (Lucas and Cole, 1990).

The nutritional requirements of sick infants are considerable but there are constraints as to what can be given. Thus the volume of fluid in which their nutrients are administered is restricted by what their kidneys can cope with. The various nutrients must also be compatible with each other and with any drugs being given simultaneously.

For the first day or two, ventilated infants are usually given intravenous water and dextrose, with the addition of some minerals, particularly sodium and calcium. If the ventilation has to be continued, amino acids are added to prevent the breakdown of the infant's proteins which could otherwise be used as an energy source. If feeding is still not possible for another day or two, lipids (fats) will also be given. Fat is the most dense source of energy available and allows the maximum input of calories in the smallest fluid volume. Fats are also needed as some fatty acids cannot be synthesized by the body (i.e. are essential) and because some vitamins are fat soluble.

A preterm infant on total intravenous nutrition receives a mixture of water, salts (including sodium, potassium, calcium, chloride and phosphate), amino acids, lipids and vitamins. Trace elements are also given. These foods are given as a mixture prepared in sterile conditions in a pharmacy as a 24-hour bag, or the various components may be blended in the intravenous infusion tubing. Strict aseptic precautions must be taken in all manipulations of the system, and a bacterial filter will be incorporated in the line, although the lipids cannot pass through these filters and must join the line nearer the baby. The whole circuit, except for the intravenous cannula, is changed daily.

Naso/orojejunal feeds

Enteral feeding (into the bowel) will commence once the baby's condition improves. The intravenous intake is gradually reduced as the enteral intake is increased until finally it is discontinued altogether. A radio-opaque jejunal tube 5 G is marked at the length of mouth to ankle of the baby. It is then passed into the stomach and its position confirmed by aspiration of acidic stomach contents. The baby is then turned on to the right side to encourage the tube to go through the pylorus. It is passed a further centimetre every 15–20 minutes until the mark previously measured is at the mouth or nostril. The correct location of the tube (Figure 3) is determined by the aspiration of bile-stained, alkaline fluid, and by failing to aspirate water from the stomach if a few millilitres are passed down the jejunal tube. The position of the tube may need to

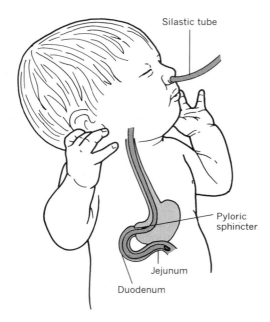

Silastic tube

Pyloric
sphincter

Jejunum

Duodenum

Figure 3   Baby with nasojejunal tube *in situ*.

be confirmed radiologically. Once the correct position is confirmed the tube is secured and jejunal feeds can be started.

An infusion pump is usually used to regulate the amount of milk given. It is important to rotate the syringe periodically to mix the fat, or to place the nozzle uppermost. A gastric tube is left in place and aspirated regularly so that pooling of milk in the stomach is detected, as is the presence of bile. These signs could indicate necrotizing enterocolitis or other sepsis, so the paediatrician must be informed. Once the baby's condition has improved (i.e. intermittent positive pressure ventilation is no longer required), the tube may be removed and naso/orogastric feeding commenced.

Intragastric feeding

A naso/orogastric tube is used. It is measured from the bridge of the nose to the tip of the sternum and marked before being gently introduced into the stomach until the mark made reaches the baby's nostril or mouth. The tube is then securely attached to the face with Micropore tape. To check that the tube is in the stomach a little gastric juice is aspirated and tested with litmus paper. An acid reaction indicates that the tube is in the correct position.

Feeds are given slowly via the tube using a syringe.

At the end of each feed the tube is carefully spiggotted and the head of the cot left raised for 20–30 minutes. The baby must be observed for vomiting and any changes in colour or apnoea. The cardiac sphincter is poorly developed in the preterm baby and thus, if the stomach is overdistended, regurgitation and inhalation may occur, especially as the cough reflex is poorly developed or may be absent. Small frequent feeds are therefore advisable and may be hourly initially and then extended to two- and eventually three-hourly.

Continuous intragastric feeding   Because of the risks of overdistending the stomach and subsequent regurgitation and inhalation, continuous milk feeds may be the most suitable method of feeding very small, immature babies. Milk in a large bottle is attached to a paediatric intravenous giving set which is attached to the nasogastric tube. An infusion pump may be used to regulate the number of millilitres of milk per hour. The baby usually progresses from continuous naso/orogastric feeding to intermittent feeds. The interval between feeds is gradually increased until the baby is having three-hourly feeds. Bottle and breast feeds are gradually introduced when the baby shows signs of sucking. Positioning the baby at the breast during tube feeds may encourage rooting and early sucking.

Choice of milk

The rate of growth in preterm babies is greater than that in their mature counterparts and thus they require a greater energy intake. To achieve a rate of growth similar to that *in utero*, the preterm baby needs 540–600 kJ per kilogram body weight per day. This equates to approximately 180–200 ml/kg/day of standard formula milk or breast milk. This energy intake may be achieved by giving smaller volumes of low birth-weight formula milk, or by adding calorific supplements to milk. Larger babies will gain weight on smaller volumes but may also need over 200 ml/kg body weight.

Minerals and nutritional supplements

The advantages of breast milk over formula milk for both term and preterm babies are widely documented, particularly in terms of immunological properties (Lucas and Cole, 1990; Howie *et al.*, 1990). Research has also suggested that breast milk may be advantageous in the development of the central nervous system and subsequent intelligence quotient in preterm infants (Lucas *et al.*, 1992). Wherever possible a mother's own fresh expressed breast milk is the milk of choice.

Although preterm breast milk has a higher sodium content than mature breast milk, it lacks adequate energy, protein and some minerals to be the sole diet of the very preterm and low birthweight infants. Human milk fortifiers containing carbohydrate, protein, vitamins and minerals (Warner *et al.*, 1993) are becoming more widely used for these babies to supplement expressed breast milk.

Low birthweight formula milks are also available, the constitution of which provides the baby with more energy, protein, vitamins and minerals per millilitre than term formulas or breast milk. These now have long-chain polyunsaturated (LCP) fatty acids added to them, as these have been identified in human milk, term and preterm, as being important for normal development of the eye and brain (Carlson *et al.*, 1992; Uauy *et al.*, 1990).

Current Department of Health recommendations are that all infants should receive daily vitamin supplements, such as children's vitamin drops – vitamins A, C and D, from the age of one month to two years. These are especially important for preterm babies as they have small stores of fat-soluble vitamins and are at risk of vitamin deficiency.

Vitamin K is given to all newborn babies to help prevent haemorrhagic disease of the newborn. There has been some controversy over the route of administration for sick and preterm babies. Further studies are necessary to ascertain whether there is any link between intramuscular injection of vitamin K and the incidence of childhood cancers. Current studies are conflicting in their findings (Golding *et al.*, 1992; Hull, 1992; Report of an Expert Committee, 1992).

Vitamin C is required for efficient iron absorption as well as for growth and healing. Preterm babies have inadequate stores of iron at birth and these become depleted further as the baby grows over the next few weeks. There is also a delay in the production of red blood cells by the immature bone marrow. All preterm babies are therefore supplemented with iron from the age of 4 weeks and this continues until they are weaned. Very preterm and ill babies may need frequent blood transfusions, but whilst these boost the haemoglobin level they may also temporarily further suppress the baby's own formation of new red blood cells. Excessive or early iron supplementation can be harmful, since free iron in the bowel reverses the anti-infective properties of lactoferrin, enabling *E. coli* to multiply.

Very preterm babies of low birthweight also require folic acid to prevent macrocytic anaemia developing later. Blood alkaline phosphatase, calcium and phosphate levels should be regularly checked in very preterm babies, as they are at risk of developing osteopenia or metabolic bone disease (rickets of prematurity). Extra vitamin D, calcium and phosphate supplements may be needed, particularly in babies fed on breast milk (Bishop, 1989). Calcium and phosphate supplements are continued until 42–43 weeks post-term as there is an increased rate of bone mineralization at this stage (Congdon *et al.*, 1990).

MOTHER–BABY RELATIONSHIP

A mother may feel quite bereft in a postnatal ward without her baby, especially when she is surrounded by other mothers who have their babies beside them and are busily involved in their care. In addition, she will be anxious about her baby's condition and concerned about what is happening in the neonatal unit when she is not there. There should be good communication between the neonatal unit and the postnatal ward staff so that the staff can answer the mother's questions and give her the support she needs. If the mother is unable to visit her baby a member of the neonatal staff should visit her and give first-hand information about her baby's condition. It is important for the parents to have as much contact with their baby as possible and thus they are encouraged to visit frequently and are kept fully informed of their baby's progress.

Intensive care of the baby is usually a very distressing experience for parents. Their anxiety may be relieved a little by explaining in simple terms the purpose of all the equipment and the treatment their baby is receiving. The parents must be involved as much as possible in the care, even when their baby is in an incubator or being ventilated.

Parents and siblings should be encouraged to wash their hands and touch or stroke their baby gently. Very few babies are too sick to be wrapped warmly, taken out of the incubator and given to the parents to cuddle for a while. The opportunity to hold their baby is both exciting and frightening for many parents. It is important in establishing a relationship with their baby. Siblings, grandparents and friends of the family are welcome to visit the baby with the parents' consent, providing they do not have a cold, sore throat or any other infection.

If the mother wishes to breastfeed she should be encouraged to express her milk within a few hours of delivery, if she is well enough. The sooner this is initiated, the greater the chance of establishing breastfeeding successfully. She should be taught how to express her milk by hand and using a pump, how to store the milk and should be encouraged to express at least six times in 24 hours.

Many preterm babies are in hospital for several weeks or months before they are ready to be discharged home. During this time the parents do an increasing amount of their baby's care and will gradually gain confidence. Before discharge, many parents find it helpful to stay in hospital to care for their baby day and night, either on the neonatal unit or in a transitional care ward.

Complications

Various complications are more likely to occur in the preterm baby than in the mature infant and these are related to the immaturity of the various systems or of the nerve centres controlling them, in proportion to the period of gestation. Prematurity is a major cause of perinatal death; thus it is important to prevent complications occurring, where possible, and to detect early and treat those which cannot be prevented.

Birth asphyxia (hypoxic ischaemic encephalopathy)

The respiratory centre, respiration system and muscles of respiration are all immature and thus the initial establishment of respiration may be difficult, especially if the respiratory centre is depressed by drugs given to the mother in labour.

The fetus only begins to lay down stores of brown fat from 22 weeks, of white fat from 28 weeks, and of glycogen from 36 weeks. Therefore at birth the preterm infant has little energy reserve if there is any interruption to the oxygen supply and in this event the heart will not continue pumping for long. It is cardiac glycogen stores which allow the heart to continue in cases of asphyxia and continued cardiac function is required to remove the accumulating lactic acid from the brain. Since glycogen stores are reduced, the

capacity of the preterm baby to withstand asphyxia is reduced (see Chapter 69).

Other respiratory problems

Many preterm babies develop respiratory difficulties at birth or within the next few hours (see Chapter 69). In the very preterm, 24 weeks' gestation, this may be due to the fact that the *lungs have not developed sufficiently* to support life without assistance. Gaseous exchange may be insufficient because the alveoli are lined by cuboidal epithelium and surrounded by an inadequate capillary network. *Respiratory distress syndrome* develops when there is insufficient surfactant and so more effort is required to re-inflate the alveoli after each breath. Other causes of respiratory problems include *meconium aspiration* and *damage to the respiratory centre* in the medulla at birth, or following long periods of apnoea and hypoxia. *Atelectasis* may occur when the alveoli have failed to expand or, having done so, have collapsed and air cannot enter due perhaps to inhalation of vomit or feeds.

Mechanical intermittent positive pressure ventilation is employed to overcome many of these problems. The survival of very preterm infants has greatly improved in recent years with the introduction of different methods of ventilating, such as patient-triggered ventilation or rapid oscillating ventilation using rates of up to 2000 per minute (Greenough *et al.*, 1987). There are many complications associated with ventilation, however, and these include pneumothorax and bronchopulmonary dysplasia (see Chapter 69). Treatment with pancuronium which induces muscle paralysis has been shown to prevent pneumothorax in babies actively expiring against ventilator inflation (Tarnow-Mordi and Wilkinson, 1986). Sedation should always be prescribed for babies who are paralysed, and adequate explanation given to the parents.

Patent ductus arteriosus

The ductus arteriosus fails to close in a number of very low birthweight babies, partly because of immaturity and partly because the chemical conditions are not suitable in babies who are hypoxic and acidotic. Hence the baby becomes more hypoxaemic and a vicious circle ensues. This situation may also develop in some term babies who have been severely asphyxiated and is called *persistent pulmonary hypertension* or persistent fetal circulation. One circumstance in which persistent ductus arteriosus is of use is in the presence of certain cardiac malformations. In transposition of the great arteries, for instance, the only routes for oxygenated blood to reach the systemic circulation are through the ductus and the foramen ovale. Thus in these cases a prostaglandin infusion may be used to keep the ductus open until intervention at cardiac catheterization is possible.

Care is taken to minimize the risk of patent ductus arteriosus in ventilated preterm infants. Prostaglandin synthetase inhibitors such as indomethacin may be used to close the ductus chemically. Frusemide may be given as well because indomethacin often causes oliguria (Kelnar *et al.*, 1995). If this treatment fails, surgical ligation or division and anastomosis of the ductus may be performed.

Periventricular haemorrhage

This may occur in preterm babies even after what has seemed an easy delivery. Its occurrence is facilitated by intrauterine hypoxia, poor skull ossification and fragile blood vessels. Preterm babies are specially liable to haemorrhage into one of the lateral ventricles of the brain (*intraventricular haemorrhage*), which may well be fatal (Figure 4).

Episodes of hypotension, hypertension or hypoxia may result in intraventricular haemorrhage. If the haemorrhage extends into the parenchyma of the brain, there is a high chance of brain damage resulting in cerebral palsy. Other factors which contribute to intraventricular haemorrhage include the obstruction of venous return from the skull causing distension of intracerebral veins and any abnormality in clotting.

The aim of *management* is to prevent the occurrence of a major periventricular haemorrhage. The majority of extremely low birthweight babies have some degree of haemorrhage which usually appears within a few hours of birth, but it may be possible to prevent further bleeding by providing excellent supportive care. This includes control of blood pressure, of blood gases and of coagulation. The prevention of asphyxia at delivery and of respiratory failure at any time is crucial. Active resuscitation of all very low birthweight babies at birth and elective ventilation of most of these babies has proved helpful in reducing this problem. The prevention of pneumothoraces is another factor of great importance. Episodes of deterioration associated with a pneumothorax often lead to the extension of a periventricular haemorrhage.

Complications of periventricular haemorrhage include shock, disseminated intravascular coagulation and pressure on parts of the brain concerned with the autonomic system, thereby influencing respiration, blood pressure and temperature control. This occurs when the blood in the ventricles clots and obstructs the flow of cerebrospinal fluid, or when the viscosity of the cerebrospinal fluid is altered because it contains debris from the haemorrhage. The result is the development of acute hydrocephalus. Drugs such as isosorbide and acetazolamide reduce the rate of cerebrospinal fluid production and may thereby reduce hydrocephalus. Regular lumbar puncture may be performed to relieve excess pressure. If the problem persists, the insertion of ventricular shunts may be necessary.

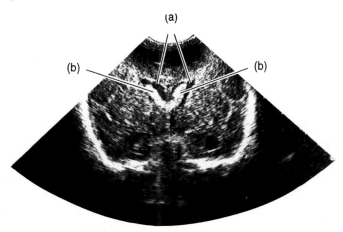

Figure 4   Coronal cranial ultrasound showing intraventricular haemorrhages (b) in dilated lateral ventricles (a). (Reproduced from Kelnar *et al.* (1995).)

Another cause of long-term problems which is often associated with periventricular haemorrhage is reduction in the white matter around the ventricles, that is periventricular leucomalacia which is caused by ischaemia and subsequent formation of cystic areas. Intrapartum events may predispose to the onset of periventricular haemorrhage and leucomalacia, which emphasizes the importance of preventing perinatal hypoxia (Doran, 1992). Periventricular haemorrhage and leucomalacia (cysts) can be diagnosed by ultrasound scanning. There is a very high incidence of spastic cerebral palsy associated with periventricular cysts (Fawer *et al.*, 1987), whereas a small confined periventricular haemorrhage may not cause any long-term neurological damage. The site of a haemorrhage or cyst formation appears to be relevant when considering the prognosis (Pidcock *et al.*, 1990).

Hypothermia

The preterm baby has difficulty in maintaining the body temperature because heat production is low and heat loss is high. This is because the heat-regulating centre is immature and the surface area is large in proportion to body weight. In addition there is a lack of subcutaneous fat and little brown fat which can be metabolized quickly to produce heat. Initially energy (calorie) intake may be poor and this exacerbates the problem.

Hypoglycaemia

This is a common problem in preterm babies in the first 48–72 hours because their stores of glycogen are low and, initially, energy intake may be inadequate. The problem is aggravated by asphyxia and hypothermia.

Hypocalcaemia

Early hypocalcaemia due to stress or illness may occur within the first 72 hours of life in preterm babies, and in those suffering from asphyxia, respiratory distress syndrome or sepsis, or in the babies of diabetic mothers. Asphyxia results in the excretion of high levels of calcitonin from the parathyroid glands and this reduces calcium mobilization from the bone. Vitamin D which is required for parathyroid hormone action on bone and gut is also deficient in the preterm baby.

Jaundice

Physiological jaundice is exacerbated in preterm babies as the liver is immature and therefore conjugation of bilirubin is further delayed. There is a greater danger of kernicterus.

Another factor which increases the incidence of hyperbilirubinaemia in preterm infants is any delay in the passage of meconium which allows bilirubin to be reabsorbed. This may occur if enteral feeds are not commenced for several days.

Anaemia

Anaemia is common in preterm babies. The shorter intrauterine period prevents the accumulation of an adequate iron store. An immature gastrointestinal system does not easily digest iron supplements. The rapid rate of growth and increase in circulation is too fast for the rather inactive bone marrow to manufacture the necessary red blood cells. Ill babies may have had much blood removed for sampling. A blood transfusion may be necessary, though some babies make good progress in spite of a low level of haemoglobin.

Haemorrhagic disease

Newborn babies are at risk of developing haemorrhagic disease due to a deficiency of the vitamin K-dependent clotting factors which include prothrombin and factors VII, IX and X. These factors fall markedly during the second and third day of life and rise when feeding has been established because vitamin K can then be produced in the intestines. Vitamin K_1 in the form of phytomenadione (Konakion) 0.5–1 mg is therefore given to all babies at birth to try to reduce the risk of haemorrhagic disease.

Secondary haemorrhagic disease of the newborn occurs mainly in preterm babies and is more likely to be intraventricular or pulmonary than gastrointestinal. The cause may be multifactorial and repeated small blood transfusions and the administration of vitamin K are given in an attempt to treat the condition successfully.

Infection

Infection occurring in a preterm baby is very serious for the baby has a poor resistance to infection. A preterm infant is more vulnerable because:

1   maternal IgG levels are low;
2   the skin is a less efficient barrier to invading bacteria;
3   the tears and saliva are less copious and contain fewer antibacterial factors;
4   the stomach produces less protective acid;

5 the immune cells are less numerous and efficient, and thus do not respond so effectively to stress;

6 the baby is subject to more invasive procedures and to multiple contacts with hospital staff.

Retrolental fibroplasia

Too much oxygen is a major factor in the aetiology of retrolental fibroplasia (retinopathy of prematurity), a condition in which an opacity forms behind the lens in the vitreous body (Prendiville and Schulenberg, 1988). The condition begins in the retina and later fibrous tissue forms in the vitreous body behind the lens, hence the name. Blindness will ensue, so great care must be taken in monitoring the concentration of oxygen given to babies and the arterial oxygen tensions which result. The aim is to maintain the latter between 6 and 9 kPa (50–70 mmHg) in a preterm baby. All preterm babies born before 32 weeks' gestation should have their eyes checked regularly by an ophthalmologist, until they are term.

Necrotizing enterocolitis

Necrotizing enterocolitis is an inflammatory disease of the bowel which is associated with septicaemia. It is thought to occur as a result of bacteria proliferating in the bowel and then penetrating the bowel wall at points where it has suffered ischaemic damage. Oedema, ulceration and haemorrhage of the bowel wall are found and may progress to perforation or peritonitis.

The condition typically develops in babies who have been ill with asphyxia, respiratory distress, hypoglycaemia, hypothermia or cardiovascular disease. Predisposing factors include variations in bowel perfusion associated with exchange transfusion, hypotension, patent ductus arteriosus, polycythaemia (when the blood is too thick to flow readily) and thrombosis or spasm of the mesenteric vessels from an umbilical catheter. Careful placement of the umbilical catheter may prevent this latter cause.

The problem usually declares itself within a few days of starting milk feeds because it is then that colonization of the intestine is more likely. It may present with non-specific malaise and indications of sepsis, with apnoea or septic shock, or with abdominal signs such as distension, bile-stained aspirate or the passage of blood and mucus per rectum. The diagnosis can be confirmed by the appearance of the bowel on radiography (Figure 5). This may show the bowel wall to be thickened due to oedema, a pattern of bowel obstruc-

tion, excessive or deficient quantities of gas within the bowel or the presence of gas bubbles. This last feature is virtually diagnostic of necrotizing enterocolitis.

The chance of developing the condition can be minimized by the cautious introduction of feeds using breast milk where possible because the intestines are then primarily colonized by lactobacilli (Lucas and Cole, 1990). If the baby develops early signs of sepsis or of necrotizing enterocolitis in particular, milk feeds are stopped and parenteral nutrition resumed. The baby is fully screened for infection, and antibiotics are administered parenterally. Strict isolation of the baby is essential to prevent cross-infection.

Further radiographs will be required to detect any early signs of bowel perforation. Surgery would be required in cases of bowel perforation but only minimal resection of damaged bowel is made since extensive resection leads to problems of short bowel malabsorption. Another later complication which may occur is stricture of the bowel as a result of scar formation. This may also require surgical treatment. Once the baby's condition improves milk feeds are very cautiously reintroduced, ideally starting with breast milk.

Necrotizing enterocolitis is now one of the commonest causes of neonatal surgery and is associated with a very high mortality (up to 40%). It is therefore essential to try to prevent the onset of the condition where possible or, failing that, to detect the earliest signs. Early treatment can then be instigated to prevent extensive damage and long-term problems.

Bronchopulmonary dysplasia

Bronchopulmonary dysplasia is a chronic respiratory disorder which occurs in about 20% of babies treated with intermittent positive pressure ventilation. It most commonly occurs after severe lung disease when high concentrations of oxygen and high ventilator pressures have been used for long periods. This results in serious disruption of lung growth. Examination of radiographs and lung specimens reveals patches of collapse and fibrosis (Figure 6). The lungs are stiff and difficult to ventilate.

Since the cause of the problem seems to be ventilation, it is essential to wean the baby off the ventilator even if the blood gases are outside the usual desired range, otherwise the condition will worsen. The peak pressure will be lowered and the rate of ventilation slowly reduced over hours or days. During this time regular endotracheal suction is performed, with lavage

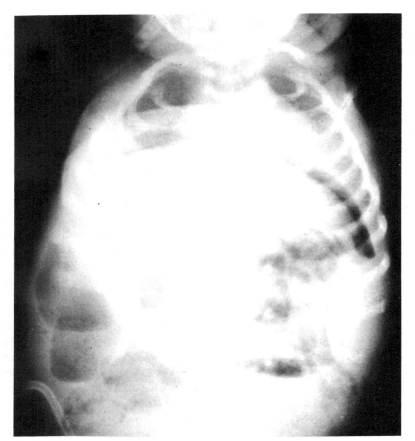

Figure 5   Necrotizing enterocolitis showing dilated loops of bowel. (Reproduced from Kelnar *et al.* (1995).)

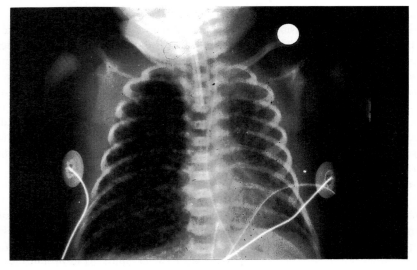

Figure 6   Chest radiograph showing early signs of bronchopulmonary dysplasia. (Reproduced from Kelnar *et al.* (1995).)

if necessary, to prevent secretions accumulating in the lungs and blocking the bronchi or endotracheal tube. Gentle physiotherapy is also employed. Steroid drugs may be given to assist in weaning the baby off the ventilator. Diuretics and fluid restriction may be required in the presence of cor pulmonale.

Once the baby is coping without ventilation continuous positive airways pressure (CPAP) may be needed for a few days. Supplementary oxygen will certainly be required for some weeks or even months to keep the arterial oxygen tension above 55 kPa. The baby may still be having oxygen therapy via a nasal catheter when discharged home.

Continuous negative extrathoracic pressure boxes are being used with some success to help wean babies from endotracheal ventilation.

The outlook for these babies is variable. Some die in infancy, whilst others recover gradually, but many continue to have problems with frequent chest infections and asthma which necessitate repeated hospital admissions (Powell et al., 1986; Berman et al., 1986).

Congenital malformations

Congenital defects are commoner in low birthweight babies than in mature babies. This is partly because malformed babies tend to be small for the period of gestation and partly because they are often preterm.

Follow-up Care

The midwife, health visitor or community neonatal sister will have been informed of the baby's impending discharge. Home visits will be made following discharge to give any advice and support required. Any problems requiring a medical consultation will be referred to the general practitioner who will also have been informed of the baby's perinatal course and discharge. The paediatrician usually follows up preterm babies after discharge from hospital to assess their progress, development, general condition and to detect a wide range of possible problems.

A *general examination* is carried out to note the colour, state of nutrition, any signs of infection, activity, behaviour, alertness and response.

A *neurological examination* is performed to detect any evidence of hypotonia, hypertonia or early signs of cerebral palsy.

The *chest* is examined for signs of chronic respiratory problems and evidence of patent ductus arteriosus or ventricular septal defect. The *eyes* are examined regularly by an ophthalmologist to detect evidence of retrolental fibroplasia or of congenital infection. It may be several months before retinal damage caused by a congenital infection becomes apparent.

Hearing must be carefully checked both on discharge from hospital and at follow-up visits. Preterm babies are at particular risk of hearing impairment due to hypoxia, sepsis, drugs (e.g. gentomicin, frusemide) and hyperbilirubinaemia.

The *haemoglobin* may be checked as anaemia is a common problem in preterm babies.

Outcome

Over the past decade there has been an increase in the survival rates for very preterm and low birthweight babies. Most follow-up studies consider the outcome of babies in relation to their birthweight rather than gestation. Recent research (Yu et al., 1986b; Wariyar et al., 1989a,b) has shown that for babies under 28 weeks' gestation, mortality rates depend on gestational age, whilst neurodevelopmental outcome relates more closely to birthweight.

Mortality rates are about 50% for babies under 29 weeks' gestation, as shown in the study by Johnson et al. (1993). Of the survivors 23% were found to have severe disabilities. The most common impairment in very low birthweight babies is cerebral palsy (Pharoah et al., 1990).

Stewart (1990) showed that 25% of survivors of extremely low birthweight babies, under 33 weeks' gestation, had minor impairments at the age of 4 years. These include varying degrees of cognitive, visuospatial, behavioural, language and motor difficulties. Another long-term study (Marlow et al., 1993) found that amongst children of birthweight 1250 g or below and with no major impairment, there is a high incidence of learning difficulties at the age of 8 years. These problems were more apparent with advancing age and further studies of these children at the age of 12 years are planned.

Although the number of very low birthweight babies surviving is increasing, the percentage with major disabilities appears to have changed little. Continuing studies into the mortality and morbidity rates for this group of babies may help to identify significant perinatal findings which will enable a more accurate prediction of the neurological outcome to be made. Findings from current methods of assessing babies, such as cerebral ultrasonography, do not correlate well with eventual outcome and severity of disabilities.

Ethical Issues

Many ethical issues arise in the intensive care of very preterm and very low birthweight babies, especially when complications occur which substantially increase the risk of long-term handicap, or if chromosomal abnormalities or major congenital malformations are present. Many of these babies die despite the efforts made to save them. Difficult decisions arise when the baby is surviving solely due to the supportive care being given, yet the risk of handicap is known to be extremely high. Then both professionals and parents need time to discuss the situation openly, and space to reflect on the possible consequences of continuing full intensive care as long as it is required, or of withdrawing such care to allow the baby to die in peace and dignity. This is one of the most agonizing and difficult decisions both parents and professionals have to face. Having decided on what appears to be the best course of action, it is important for parents to accept that they made the best decision possible given the information and advice available at the time. Situations change and retrospectively they may be beseiged by doubts and intense feelings of guilt if their baby dies, or perhaps survives despite discontinuing intensive care and is severely handicapped.

Cultural factors and the individual's personal values and beliefs are deeply challenged at times like this and will influence the decisions made. Sometimes parents appreciate the opportunity to discuss the situation with a minister of religion or with a counsellor who is not directly involved in the care of their baby. Such help can be invaluable during this extremely stressful period.

Individuals react differently to stress and staff in the neonatal unit need to learn to recognize the signs in parents and develop appropriate skills to enable families to cope during this difficult time. They must also recognize the signs of stress in themselves and in colleagues, and opportunities to share and discuss problems can be of immense benefit to all concerned. One of the factors which increases stress is lack of resources, which includes both manpower, cots and suitable equipment. This inevitably leads to further ethical problems as difficult choices have to be made. Effective personal coping strategies are therefore essential for those working under such pressures.

References

Berman, W., Katz, R., Yabek, S.M. *et al.* (1986) Long-term follow-up of bronchopulmonary dysplasia. *J. Pediat.* **109**: 45–50.

Bishop, N. (1989) Bone disease in preterm infants. *Arch. Dis. Childh.* **64**: 1403–1409.

Carlson, S.E., Werkman, S.H., Peeples, J.M. *et al.* (1992) Plasma phospholipid arachidonic acid and growth and development of preterm infants. In Koletzko, B., Okken, A., Rey, J. *et al.* (eds) *Recent Advances in Infant Feeding*, pp. 22–27. Symposium Leidschendam 1990. Stuttgart/New York: Georg Thième Verlag.

Congdon, P.J., Horsman, A., Ryan, S.W. *et al.* (1990) Bone mineral repletion in preterm infants after 40 weeks post-conception. *Arch. Dis. Childh.* **65**: 1038–1042.

Doran, L. (1992) Periventricular leucomalacia. *Neonatal Network* **11**(4): 7–13.

Drew, J.H. (1982) Immediate intubation at birth for very-low-birthweight infants. *Am. J. Dis. Child.* **136**: 207–210.

Dubowitz, L.M.S., Dubowitz, V. & Goldberg, C. (1970) Clinical assessment of gestational age in the newborn infant. *J. Pediat.* **77**: 1–10.

Fawer, C., Diebold, P. & Calone, A. (1987) Periventricular leukomalacia and neurodevelopmental outcome in preterm infants. *Arch. Dis. Childh.* **62**: 30–36.

Golding, J., Birmingham, K., Greenwood, R. *et al.* (1992) Childhood cancer, intramuscular vitamin K and pethidine given during labour. *Br. Med. J.* **305**: 341–346.

Greenough, A., Greenall, F., Pool, J. *et al.* (1987) Comparison of different rates of artificial ventilation in preterm infants with respiratory distress syndrome. *Acta. Paediat. Scand.* **76**: 706–712.

Halliday, H.L., McClure, G. & Reid, M. (1989) *Handbook of Neonatal Intensive Care*, 3rd edn. London: Baillière Tindall.

Howie, P.J., Forsyth, J., Ogston, S.A. *et al.* (1990) Protective effect of breast feeding against infection. *Br. Med. J.* **300**: 11–16.

Hull, D. (1992) Vitamin K and childhood cancer. The risk of haemorrhagic disease is certain; that of cancer is not. *Br. Med. J.* **305**: 326–327.

Johnson, A., Townshend, P., Yudkin, P. *et al.* (1993) Functional abilities at age 4 years of children born before 29 weeks of gestation. *Br. Med. J.* **306**: 1715–1718.

Kelnar, C.J.H., Harvey, D. & Simpson, C. (1995) *The Sick Newborn Baby*, 3rd edn. London: Baillière Tindall.

Lucas, A. & Cole, T.J. (1990) Breast milk and neonatal necrotizing enterocolitis. *Lancet* **336**: 1519–1523.

Lucas, A., Morley, R. & Cole, T.J. (1988) Adverse neurodevelopmental outcome of moderate hypoglycaemia. *Br. Med. J.* **97**: 1304.

Lucas, A., Morley, R., Cole, T.J. *et al.* (1992) Breast milk and subsequent intelligence quotient in children born preterm. *Lancet* **339**: 261–264.

Marlow, N., Roberts, L. & Cooke, R. (1993) Outcome at 8 years for children with birth weights of 1250 g or less. *Arch. Dis. Childh.* **68**: 286–290.

Parkin, J.M., Hey, E.N. & Clowes, J.S. (1976) Rapid assessment of gestational age at birth. *Arch. Dis. Childh.* **51**: 259.

Pharoah, P.O.D., Cooke, T., Cooke, R.W.I. *et al.* (1990) Birthweight specific trends in cerebral palsy. *Arch. Dis. Childh.* **605**: 602–606.

Pidcock, F. *et al.* (1990) Neurosonographic features of periventricular echodensities associated with cerebral palsy in preterm infants. *J. Pediat.* **116**: 417–422.

Powell, T.G., Pharoah, P.O.D. & Cooke, R.W.I. (1986) Survival and morbidity in a geographically defined population of low birthweight infants. *Lancet* **i**: 539–543.

Prendiville, A. & Schulenberg, W.E. (1988) Clinical factors associated with retinopathy of prematurity. *Arch. Dis. Childh.* **63**: 522–527.

Report of an Expert Committee (1992) *Vitamin K Prophylaxis in Infancy*. London: British Paediatric Association.

Southall, D.P., Bignall, S., Stebbens, V.A. *et al.* (1987) Pulse oximeter and transcutaneous arterial oxygen measurements in neonatal and paediatric intensive care. *Arch. Dis. Childh.* **62**: 882–888.

Stewart, A.L. (1990) Cerebral morbidity in the extremely low birthweight infant. In Duc, G., Huch, A. & Huch, R. (eds) *The Very Low Birthweight Infant*, pp. 3–9. Stuttgart: Georg Thième.

Tarnow-Mordi, W. & Wilkinson, A. (1986) Mechanical ventilation of the newborn. *Br. Med. J.* **292**: 575–576.

Uauy, R.D., Birch, D.G., Birch, E.E. *et al.* (1990) Effects of dietary ω3 fatty acids on retinal function of very low birthweight neonates. *Pediat. Res.* **28**: 485–492.

Wariyar, U., Richmond, S. & Hey, E. (1989a) Pregnancy outcome at 24–31 weeks gestation: mortality. *Arch. Dis. Childh.* **64**: 670–677.

Wariyar, U., Richmond, S. & Hey, E. (1989b) Pregnancy outcome at 24–31 weeks gestation: neonatal survivors. *Arch. Dis. Childh.* **64**: 678–686.

Warner, J.T., Lintou, H.R. & Cartlidge, P.H.T. (1993) Human milk fortification in preterm infants. Abstract. (Available from Milupa, Milupa House, Uxbridge Road, Hillingdon, Middx, UB10 0NE, UK).

Yu, V.Y.H., Wong, P.Y., Bajuk, B. *et al.* (1986a) Outcome of extremely low birthweight infants. *Br. J. Obstet. Gynaecol.* **93**: 162–170.

Yu, V.Y.H., Loke, H.L., Bajuk, B. *et al.* (1986b) Prognosis for infants born at 23–28 weeks gestation. *Br. Med. J.* **293**: 1200–1203.

Further Reading

Coster, D.D., Gorton, M.E., Grooters, R.K. *et al.* (1989) Surgical closure of the patent ductus in the neonatal intensive care unit. *Ann. Thorac. Surg.* **48**: 386–389.

ESPGAN Committee (1987) Nutrition and feeding of preterm infants. *Acta Paediat. Scand.* Suppl. 336.

Stewart, A.L. (1992) Follow-up studies. In Roberton, N.R.C. (ed.) *Textbook of Neonatology*, Chapter 4, pp. 49–74. Edinburgh: Churchill Livingstone.

Wharton, B.A. (1987) *Nutrition and Feeding of Preterm Infants*. Oxford: Blackwell Scientific.

68

Small-for-Gestational-Age Babies

A baby whose weight is below the tenth percentile for gestational age (Figure 1) is termed 'small-for-gestational-age'. One third of all babies of low birthweight fall into this category; the majority are born after the 37th week.

Characteristics

Babies who are small-for-gestational-age are categorized into two groups according to whether they are affected by:

1 asymmetrical growth retardation; or
2 symmetrical (global) growth retardation.

Asymmetrical growth retardation

In cases of asymmetrical growth retardation (*Clifford's syndrome*), intrauterine growth is normal until about the third trimester of pregnancy when complications such as pre-eclampsia develop, which adversely affect placental function and thereby lead to growth retardation from malnutrition. It is thus a relatively late phenomenon and the degree of growth retardation depends on the severity of the condition.

The head circumference is within normal limits for the gestational age of the baby, but birthweight is low in proportion to head circumference and length. Owing to lack of subcutaneous fat, the head appears large in relation to the wasted appearance of the body and limbs. The ribs are easily visible and the abdomen hollowed. The skin tends to be dry and loose and may be peeling and stained with meconium. Similarly, the umbilical cord is thin and may also be meconium-stained.

The baby may look wizened and old with an anxious, wide-awake expression. Muscle tone is usually good and the baby is active and tends to suck a fist as though ravenously hungry. Neurological responses usually correspond to gestational age.

The main problems with these small babies are related to their low energy stores. They are at special risk of intrauterine hypoxia, especially in labour, and early postnatal hypoglycaemia.

Symmetrical growth retardation

The underlying causes of symmetrical growth retardation are early intrauterine infections, such as cytomegalovirus, rubella or toxoplasmosis (Greenough *et al.*, 1992), chromosomal abnormality, malfor-

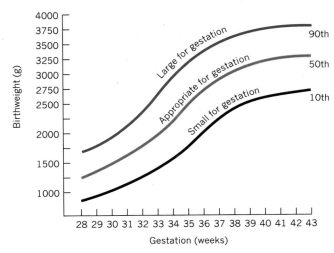

Figure 1   A centile chart, showing weight and gestation.

mation and maternal substance abuse (e.g. fetal alcohol syndrome). Intrauterine growth has therefore been affected since early in the pregnancy. This is recognized by the fact that the head circumference is in proportion to their overall size and weight. The prognosis for these babies is poorer than those asymmetrically grown.

Causes

The growing fetus is entirely dependent upon its placenta for nutrition, elimination and respiratory exchange. Any dysfunction of the placenta will cause retarded fetal growth and so lead to a small-for-gestational-age baby. Placental dysfunction is associated with conditions such as pre-eclampsia, essential hypertension and chronic nephritis. In all these conditions spasm of the spiral arterioles reduces the intervillous blood flow and so reduces the exchange across the placental barrier. Other conditions associated with placental dysfunction are smoking, severe anaemia, multiple pregnancy and prolonged pregnancy.

Following threatened abortion or antepartum haemorrhage, the fetus has to exist on less functioning placental tissue and therefore fetal growth is likely to be retarded. Maternal diseases such as asthma, chronic renal failure, sickle cell disease and phenylketonuria are all associated with intrauterine growth retardation. Some drugs which are prescribed to treat maternal

conditions may also adversely affect intrauterine growth. These include steroids, anticonvulsants, the antihypertensive drug methyldopa and cytotoxics. In addition a moderate or heavy intake of alcohol and other substance abuse may contribute to the problem. High altitude is another predisposing factor. Babies born with a congenital abnormality or who have had an intrauterine infection such as rubella or cytomegalovirus are commonly small-for-gestational-age. In many cases of placental insufficiency and consequent retarded fetal growth there is no known cause, although the condition occurs more commonly in mothers of low socio-economic status.

Management

The typical problems encountered by small-for-gestational-age babies are mainly due to the lack of energy stores laid down *in utero*. They have a relatively small liver with correspondingly small glycogen reserves, thus the transition through labour and the initial adaptation to extrauterine life is often traumatic.

Antenatal care
A detailed booking history is essential, as it may identify risk factors associated with intrauterine growth retardation. Careful assessment of the uterine size in relation to gestation is also important. Accurate measurement will enable early signs of a slow or reduc-

ing rate of growth of the fetus, possibly indicating the need for a more detailed assessment of fetal well-being.

Care during labour and delivery

The growth-retarded fetus has very small energy reserves in the form of both fat and glycogen. Chronic hypoxia (see Chapter 46) often results from long-term placental insufficiency and these babies rapidly become distressed during labour. The fetal heart rate should be closely monitored throughout labour and the liquor observed for meconium. In all cases of severe growth retardation or fetal distress, somebody skilled at resuscitation should be present at delivery – this may be a paediatrician or specially trained midwife or neonatal nurse. Expert and urgent resuscitation is vital, particularly if there is meconium-stained liquor, to prevent further hypoxia and respiratory complications, with possible neurological damage.

Small-for-gestational-age babies have only a thin layer of subcutaneous fat and subsequently lose heat very rapidly. The room temperature prior to delivery should therefore be about 24°C and the baby dried and wrapped in warm blankets quickly following delivery.

Complications

The majority of small-for-gestational-age babies are mature, having a gestational age of 37 weeks or more. It is not uncommon, however, for preterm babies to be small-for-gestational-age and many of the predisposing factors are the same in both situations. Growth-retarded infants should be carefully examined for congenital malformations, chromosomal abnormalities and intrauterine infections which may be the causative factors.

Perinatal asphyxia

The growth-retarded fetus is chronically hypoxic and subsequently tolerates the stresses of labour and delivery poorly, as the blood supply to the placenta is further interrupted during each contraction. The midwife should anticipate the possibility of fetal distress and careful fetal monitoring during labour is imperative. A paediatrician should be available to attend the delivery if the fetus is known to be preterm, growth-retarded or showing signs of fetal distress.

Hypoxic ischaemic encephalopathy (birth asphyxia)

This condition is mainly avoidable in countries with good antenatal care, careful monitoring in labour of high-risk pregnancies and early intervention to expedite delivery in the event of fetal distress. It must be remembered that even modern methods of assessing fetal well-being are relatively insensitive and the midwife must be vigilant.

It may, however, occur following prolonged or repeated episodes of prenatal or intrauterine hypoxia resulting in some degree of cerebral injury. Mild symptoms of hypoxic ischaemic encephalopathy may resolve after a few days with little or no residual cerebral damage. More severe injuries may result in neonatal fits and cerebral palsy (Finer et al., 1983).

Meconium aspiration syndrome

By 11 weeks' gestation the fetus shows signs of breathing movements, the rate of which increases over the subsequent trimester. These are seen as a sign of fetal well-being. Hypoxia results in a reduced rate of these movements, or in severe cases may cause them to cease completely. Hypoxia also increases the rate of gut peristalsis and relaxes the anal sphincter, allowing meconium to be passed into the liquor. The asphyxiated fetus gasps in utero which causes the thick, tenacious meconium to be inhaled into the bronchial tree.

With the first breath, more meconium is drawn into the trachea which may result in a chemical pneumonitis, respiratory distress syndrome, pneumothoraces or a secondary bacterial pneumonia. It is important to have a paediatrician, midwife or nurse skilled in resuscitation present at the delivery of all babies where there is meconium-stained liquor. As the head is born, the mouth and nose should be gently aspirated. Deep pharyngeal aspiration is not recommended. The practice of holding the chest tightly to prevent the first breath and allow aspiration of the pharynx is not only difficult, but may also be dangerous. If examination with a laryngoscope shows meconium in the larynx, the baby should be intubated and the trachea suctioned through the endotracheal tube (Linder et al., 1988).

Hypothermia

As with preterm babies, the growth-retarded baby has a deficit of both subcutaneous and brown fat. In addition, hypothermia is a risk due to the relatively high surface-area-to-bodyweight ratio. It is important that the baby is dried and wrapped quickly following delivery and the axillary temperature monitored carefully in the first 48 hours. If necessary the baby may be nursed in an incubator next to the mother in the postnatal ward.

Hypoglycaemia

This is a common problem for growth-retarded infants and in many cases can be prevented with early and regular feeding. These babies would particularly benefit from the advantages afforded by breastfeeding as they are also at a greater risk of neonatal necrotizing enterocolitis (Lucas and Cole, 1990). Low birthweight formula milks are now widely used with the advantage for these small babies that they are more energy-dense.

Small-for-gestational-age babies have small livers and correspondingly small glycogen stores. A large proportion of these energy reserves are used during labour, particularly if it is prolonged or difficult. Asphyxia and hypothermia will exacerbate the problem of hypoglycaemia.

Frequent recordings of the blood glucose level are important within the first 48 hours, at least four hourly until they are stable. As well as screening for hypoglycaemia these babies should also be monitored for signs of *transient neonatal diabetes mellitus*. This is a rare complication in which there is hyperglycaemia and glycosuria, but no ketones in the urine. The baby presents as being dehydrated and failing to thrive but is otherwise lively (Stirling and Kelnar, 1995).

Polycythaemia

This is defined as a venous packed cell volume of >65% and occurs in these small babies as a consequence of chronic intrauterine hypoxia. To improve the oxygen-carrying capacity of the blood the haemoglobin level may have risen to more than 20 g/dl. Haemoconcentration takes place leading to a high proportion of red blood cells and therefore increased viscosity of the blood. This situation results in high jaundice levels and cerebral irritation is possible in extreme cases. In this event an exchange plasma transfusion may be necessary, where 20–30 ml/kg of arterial blood is removed and replaced with fresh plasma into a peripheral vein. This reduces the viscosity of the blood and often helps to alleviate some of the symptoms of respiratory distress and cerebral irritation.

Polycythaemia is also a risk factor for necrotizing enterocolitis, especially when combined with perinatal asphyxia. The introduction of feeds is therefore often delayed and intravenous fluids prescribed to prevent dehydration and hypoglycaemia.

Poor feeding

This is not a problem for asymmetrically growth-retarded babies, who tend to feed eagerly and thrive from birth. Symmetrically growth-retarded babies, however, who have been starved for a prolonged period *in utero*, often continue the slow rate of growth once delivered and may always be small, although a degree of catch-up growth is often evident.

Pulmonary haemorrhage

This is another rare complication associated with small babies, the aetiology of which is uncertain. It may be due to left ventricular failure or a coagulation disorder, but appears to be largely preventable by eliminating other risk factors such as hypoglycaemia, perinatal asphyxia and hypothermia.

Neonatal abstinence syndrome

A high proportion of babies born to substance-abusing mothers are growth-retarded, particularly following the prolonged use of 'crack' cocaine (Kennard, 1990), heroin and alcohol (Spohr et al., 1993). It is often very difficult to obtain an honest and accurate history of drugs taken during pregnancy from the parents. These babies, as well as being at risk of withdrawal symptoms and future developmental problems, are often poor at withstanding labour and may suffer perinatal hypoxia (Chasnoff et al., 1986).

It is important that the baby of a substance-abusing mother is *not* given neonatal naloxone during resuscitation, as this will initiate rapid withdrawal symptoms as any narcotics in the baby's circulation are rapidly broken down.

Postnatal Care

A great deal of the care required in the first 48 hours by small-for-gestational-age babies centres around prevention and early recognition of any possible complications. In most cases therefore, these babies can be cared for in normal postnatal wards with their mothers and do not need admission to a neonatal intensive or special care unit. Transitional care wards are an ideal place to care for those babies with minor problems such as poor temperature control.

It is not uncommon for preterm babies to be small-for-gestational-age, as many of the predisposing factors are the same in both situations. Growth-retarded babies should be carefully examined for congenital malformations, chromosomal abnormalities and intrauterine infections which may be the cause.

Transitional care

Current practice in many maternity units is for small-for-gestational-age babies to be cared for in transitional wards together with their mothers, rather than in the cool nurseries of neonatal units. This reduces the length of time the mother and baby are separated and enables the mother to get to know her baby and gradually assume responsibility for care throughout the day and night. The mother has the company of other mothers with small babies and does not have to make many tiring visits to the neonatal unit to see and learn to care for her baby.

Ideally transitional wards are situated near the neonatal unit and are staffed by midwives with particular skills in caring for small-for-gestational-age babies. Once the baby is feeding and thriving well, arrangements are made for mother and baby to be transferred home. No longer is it the usual practice to keep babies in hospital until they weigh 2500 g. Indeed, in some areas, babies weighing well under 2000 g are discharged home provided the home conditions are suitable, the parents appear proficient in caring for their baby and adequate supervision is available at home by the community midwife or a neonatal nurse.

Follow-up care

It is important to monitor the progress of small-for-gestational-age babies both in the short term and long term. In particular, the symmetrically growth-retarded and cerebrally damaged babies will need close follow-up for several years in paediatric outpatient clinics, to assess their growth and development.

Outcome

In general, the outcome for the small-for-gestational-age babies is not as good as that of babies of the same weight or gestation, who are appropriately grown. The perinatal mortality rate increases with decreasing birth-weight of babies, regardless of gestation. The risk of sudden infant death syndrome is also greater for low birthweight babies, many of whom are mature but small-for-gestational-age.

The prognosis for these babies is dependent on many factors, including the cause of poor growth and the severity and duration of any complications experienced. The brain undergoes a growth spurt during the last trimester of pregnancy and is therefore particularly vulnerable to neurological damage at this time, as a result of prolonged or severe hypoxia and malnutrition. Epidemiological studies have shown growth-retarded babies to be at an increased risk in adult life of certain cardiovascular conditions, such as hypertension (Osmond et al., 1993) and diabetes mellitus (Barker, 1992). Thus poor intrauterine growth has major implications on mortality and morbidity throughout the individual's life.

Health education and informed encouragement to reduce risk factors during both the preconception and antenatal periods are therefore vital roles for the midwife.

References

Barker, D.J.P. (1992) *Fetal and Infant Origins of Adult Disease.* London: B.M.J. Publishing Group.

Chasnoff, I., Burns, K., Burns, W. *et al.* (1986) Prenatal drug exposure: Effects of neonatal and infant growth and development. *Neurobehav. Toxicol. Teratol.* **8**: 357–362.

Finer, N.N., Robertson, C.M., Peters, K.L. *et al.* (1983) Factors affecting outcome in hypoxic-ischemic encephalopathy in term infants. *Am. J. Dis. Child.* **138**: 21.

Greenough, A., Osborne, J. & Sutherland, S. (1992) *Congenital, Perinatal and Neonatal Infections.* London: Churchill Livingstone.

Kennard, M. (1990) Cocaine use during pregnancy: Fetal and neonatal effects. *J. Perinatal Neonatal Nursing* **3**(4): 53–63.

Linder, N., Aranda, J.V., Tsur, M. *et al.* (1988) Need for endotracheal intubation and suctioning in meconium-stained infants. *J. Pediat.* **112**: 613.

Lucas, A. & Cole, T.J. (1990) Breastmilk and neonatal necrotising enterocolitis. *Lancet* **336**: 1519–1523.

Osmond, C., Barker, D.J.P., Winter, P.D. *et al.* (1993) Early growth and death from cardiovascular disease in women. *Br. Med. J.* **307**: 1519–1524.

Spohr, H-L., Willms, J. & Steinhausen, H-C. (1993) Prenatal alcohol exposure and long-term developmental consequences. *Lancet* **341**: 907–910.

Stirling, H.F. & Kelnar, C.J.H. (1995) Neonatal diabetes (transient and permanent). In Kelnar, C.J.H. (ed.) *Childhood and Adolescent Diabetes*, pp. 419–426. London: Chapman & Hall.

Further Reading

Campbell, A. & McIntosh, C. (eds) (1992) *Forfar and Arneil's Textbook of Paediatrics*, 4th edn. Edinburgh: Churchill Livingstone.

David, T.J. (ed.) (1991) Infants of drug dependent mothers. *Recent Advances in Paediatrics*, Vol. 9. Edinburgh: Churchill Livingstone.

Kelnar, C.J., Harvey, D. & Simpson, C. (1995) *The Sick Newborn Baby*, 3rd edn. London: Baillière Tindall.

Scottish Low Birthweight Study (1992) 1. Survival, growth, neuromotor and sensory impairment. *Arch. Dis. Childh.* **67**: 675–681.

Sinclair, J.C. & Bracken, M.B. (eds) (1992) *Effective Care of the Newborn Infant*. Oxford: Oxford University Press.

69

Respiratory Disorders
of the Neonate

The Lungs *in Utero*

The lungs begin as epithelial tubes surrounded by mesoderm, which develop into primitive bronchioles and terminal air sacs. By 24–26 weeks the capillary network is developing and alveoli are forming from the terminal air sacs. The lungs are now capable of some gaseous exchange but this may not be adequate to support life (see Chapters 9 and 26).

A little before this, at about 22 weeks, a complex lipoprotein called *surfactant* begins to be produced and secreted in the lungs. The amount of surfactant continues to increase until birth, with a surge in production at around 33–35 weeks' gestation. The two main functions of surfactant are to reduce the surface tension in the alveoli, allowing them to expand more easily, and to help prevent atelectasis at the end of expiration.

Lung fluid is produced from about 13 weeks' gestation and is thought to play an important role in cell proliferation and differentiation. At birth, a surge in catecholamines causes the lungs to switch from secretion to absorption of lung fluid, which prevents the neonate drowning.

Fetal breathing movements occur from as early as 11 weeks' gestation. As the fetus develops, the strength and frequency of these movements increases until they are present between 40–80% of the time, at a rate of 30–70 breaths per minute (Davis and Bureau, 1987).

Establishing Respiration

As the fetal chest passes through the vagina it is squeezed, forcing lung fluid and liquor from the alveoli into the upper respiratory tract, where it may be gently aspirated by the midwife. As it is delivered, the chest re-expands, drawing in air. Peripheral stimulation from handling, the cooler atmosphere and the mucus catheter on the nasopharynx bombards the higher centres.

During the latter part of labour the fetus is hypoxic and when the placenta separates, with the birth of the fetal head, the oxygen content of the blood begins to decrease whilst the carbon dioxide tension rises. This causes chemoreceptors in the carotid arteries to set up a reflex stimulus in the respiratory centre. The respiratory centre is excited causing the baby to inspire; the lungs fill with air and intrathoracic pressure alters. The presence of surfactant aids the distension of the air sacs and facilitates the uptake of oxygen.

With the clamping of the cord, the right atrial pressure is reduced and left atrial pressure increased, resulting in closure of the foramen ovale. These circulatory changes ensure that blood is directed to the lungs for oxygenation, rather than the placenta, following birth. With increasing oxygenation, the pulmonary vascular resistance reduces and this in turn initiates closure of the ductus arteriosus.

Hypoxia then is the main stimulant to inspiration, but in a minority of babies the degree of hypoxia is so great that it depresses rather than stimulates the respiratory centre and asphyxia occurs.

In order to maintain effective oxygenation there are four essentials:

1 The air passages must be clear.
2 Adequate respiratory exchange must take place in the alveoli. The alveoli must be properly expanded and there must be no barrier between the air and the epithelium.
3 Circulation must be adequate to transport oxygen to the vital centres.
4 The respiratory centre must be active and not damaged or depressed by drugs.

The care given during labour and at delivery is all directed to this end.

Birth Asphyxia (Hypoxic Ischaemic Encephalopathy)

Birth asphyxia is the result of a failure of the baby to establish spontaneous respiration at birth, though a heart beat may be present. A depletion of oxygen and an accumulation of carbon dioxide will lead to acidosis unless respiratory function is quickly established.

Causes

The trachea and bronchi may be obstructed by mucus, meconium, blood or liquor. This is likely to be most marked when intrauterine hypoxia has occurred (see Chapter 46 for causes of intrauterine hypoxia). Chronic or severe hypoxia and the resulting rise of carbon dioxide will stimulate the respiratory centre. Fetal breathing patterns alter significantly in the hypoxic fetus, with gasping occurring initially. As a result, liquor, meconium, mucus and blood can be drawn into the trachea and bronchi. In more severe cases fetal breathing movements may cease completely (Kelnar et al., 1995).

Some of the drugs given to relieve pain in labour may depress the respiratory centre in the baby, e.g. pethidine, especially if given in large doses, morphine and papaveretum. General anaesthetics given for operative deliveries may do the same.

Periventricular haemorrhage, possibly resulting from a tentorial tear, may cause pressure on the cerebellum and medulla, which may reduce or even prevent medullary activity. As the respiratory centre lies in the floor of the fourth ventricle within the medulla, respiration is affected.

Congenital abnormalities may also result in asphyxia in the newborn baby. Choanal atresia may cause an obstruction of the airways. Hypoplastic lungs or a diaphragmatic hernia will prevent respiration being established, as may certain congenital cerebral abnormalities such as anencephaly.

In the preterm baby there are several factors which predispose to birth asphyxia. These babies are more likely to suffer intrauterine hypoxia. In addition they may have an inadequate amount of surfactant at birth, an immature respiratory centre and weak respiratory musculature.

Severe intrauterine infections, such as pneumonia or septicaemia, may inhibit respiration being established efficiently.

Overzealous resuscitation of a baby can cause a worsening of the condition. Overinflation with a bag and mask may result in a pneumothorax, or a reflex apnoea may be caused by deep pharyngeal suction. Expert resuscitation is essential and all midwives should receive regular updating in neonatal resuscitation techniques.

Recognition

In the past, birth asphyxia has been classified according to the colour of the baby (blue or white). A better and more meaningful classification is mild to moderate or severe. The Apgar score is recorded one minute after birth (see Chapter 63). A score of:

7 to 10	indicates no depression
4 to 6	indicates mild to moderate depression
3 or less	indicates severe depression.

Table 1 differentiates the two levels. The two states are merely differing degrees of the same condition. As mild hypoxia becomes more marked, the circulating oxygen is being used up and there is no replenishment. The medulla is affected by hypoxia, acidaemia occurs, there is cardiac arrest and death ensues.

If this sequence of events occurs before the baby is born, it would be clinically recognizable as fetal distress and the baby would be born with severe asphyxia or might be stillborn.

Table 1   Differentiation between mild/moderate and severe asphyxia

	Mild/moderate	Severe
Colour	Deeply cyanotic	Greyish white, lips and gums blue
Respiratory effort	Attempts to breathe	No attempt to breathe
Muscle tone	Fair to good	Fair to poor; pupils dilated
Reflex irritability	Fair to good	Poor or none
Heart rate	Strong, fairly slow	Slow, becoming weaker
Apgar score	4–6, indicating mild to moderate shock	1–3, indicating severe shock
Response to treatment	Usually good	Urgent resuscitation needed

TREATMENT

Before delivery the resuscitation equipment should always be checked and prepared ready for use. At birth the shocked baby is handled gently and skilfully, care being taken to avoid chilling. Start the stop-watch.

The initial treatment is the same whatever the degree of asphyxia:

1   Clear the air passages gently. Vigorous suction is dangerous because it can cause vagal stimulation with a reflex bradycardia and apnoea.
2   Quickly clamp and cut the cord.
3   Transfer the baby to a resuscitation table and place under a radiant heater in the supine position with the head extended.
4   Dry the baby, remove wet towel and wrap warmly.
5   Give oxygen. In cases of mild birth asphyxia this is gently directed around the baby's nose and mouth from a face mask. Oxygen does not stimulate respiration; but if the baby does gasp greater benefit is derived from this than from breathing air.

Mild/moderate birth asphyxia

Ensure the upper airways are clear by performing gentle suction. Start intermittent positive pressure ventilation using an Ambu or Laerdal resuscitation bag, which should be connected to an oxygen supply, and a round face mask of the appropriate size to form a good seal. The bag should have an inbuilt pressure-limiting valve to reduce the risk of pneumothoraces from overinflation. If there is no such valve fitted, the bag must be connected to a water manometer and a pressure of 30 cmH$_2$O should not be exceeded.

An initial rate of 15–20 per minute at a pressure of 30 cmH$_2$O, is chosen and the pressure sustained for 2 seconds with each breath. Once good air entry has been achieved, the duration of each breath can be reduced to 1 second and the rate increased to 30 per minute. The pressure may also be gradually reduced provided the baby's condition improves. As the baby begins to breathe spontaneously and the heart rate increases, the rate of intermittent positive pressure ventilation is reduced until it is no longer necessary.

Throughout this procedure the baby must be kept warm and the condition is constantly assessed by observing the heart rate, respiratory effort, colour, muscle tone and response to stimuli. Apgar scores must be assessed at one and five minutes of age and thereafter at five-minute intervals until the baby is breathing spontaneously.

If the mother has received pethidine or morphine derivatives within 2–3 hours of delivery, a narcotic antagonist may be given intramuscularly or into the umbilical vein. Naloxone hydrochloride (Narcan) (0.01 mg/kg) is the drug of choice now as it does not have the effect of depressing the respiratory centre.

In the majority of cases of mild to moderate birth asphyxia the baby begins to breathe and cyanosis disappears following this treatment.

Severe birth asphyxia

If the baby who is moderately asphyxiated does not respond to treatment in one minute, the midwife should send for a paediatrician. In cases of severe birth asphyxia, most of which should be anticipated from fetal monitoring, the paediatrician should be present at delivery or summoned immediately. In the meantime the midwife should initiate intermittent positive pressure ventilation using a bag and mask. When preparing the resuscitation equipment prior to a delivery, the midwife should ensure that equipment for *endotracheal intubation* is ready. In an emergency, when there is no doctor available, a midwife who has been taught and pronounced proficient may carry out this procedure.

A laryngoscope should be passed over the tongue to the posterior pharynx. The laryngoscope is then gently advanced over the epiglottis until the glottis comes into view. If the epiglottis cannot be seen gentle cricoid pressure may be applied or the blade may be gently inserted further and lifted forward with slightly more firmness whilst it is slowly withdrawn. The epiglottis will then usually slip into view (Figure 1). Further aspiration of mucus can then be carried out under direct vision. A size 2.5 or 3.0 endotracheal tube is passed 1–2 cm through the glottis into the trachea and the laryngoscope is gently removed. A fine suction catheter may be passed through the endotracheal tube to clear the trachea before the tube is connected to the oxygen supply. This is connected to a water manometer from which can be seen the pressure of the oxygen.

Intermittent positive pressure insufflation is commenced at a rate of 15 times per minute and at an initial pressure of 30 cmH$_2$O, later reduced to 25 cmH$_2$O. This directs oxygen into the baby's lungs and as it closely resembles ordinary respiration can be a life-saving measure. Insufflation should continue until spontaneous respiration is established and the heart rate exceeds 100 beats per minute.

Cardiac massage should be commenced if the baby's heart rate (monitored with a stethoscope) remains below 70–80 per minute despite efficient ventilation being established, or if the femoral and carotid pulses

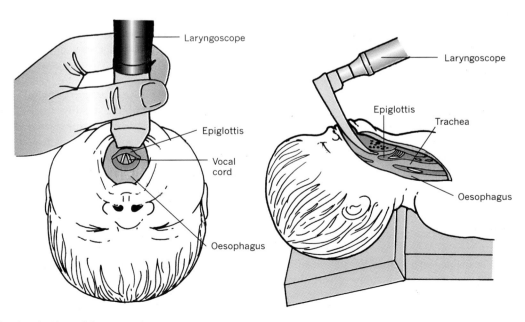

Figure 1   Intubation of the neonate.

are feeble or cannot be felt. With the baby supine on a firm surface (the resuscitation trolley), the midwife places two fingers just below the middle of an imaginary line drawn between the baby's nipples, on the sternum. Gentle pressure is applied to depress this area by 1.5–2 cm, at a rate of about 120 per minute. The pressure is released immediately and the efficacy of this procedure assessed by monitoring the femoral pulse.

DRUGS AND FLUIDS

Naloxone hydrochloride (Narcan) may be given if the mother has been given narcotics within 2–3 hours of delivery (see above). Subsequently the baby should be observed for periods of apnoea over the next 8–12 hours as pethidine lingers in the neonate for some days whereas the effect of naloxone lasts only for a few hours. *Adrenaline* may be administered via the endotracheal tube or intravenously if the heart rate is very slow or absent. The administration of *sodium bicarbonate* to counteract acidosis is controversial and generally not recommended. The administration of bicarbonate is associated with intraventricular haemorrhage in very preterm babies (Halliday *et al.*, 1985). *Calcium* may also be given intravenously for hypocalcaemia but it must be given very slowly. Intravenous *dextrose 10%* is given if hypoglycaemia has been confirmed. A peripheral vein is the route of choice, but if this is not possible a catheter is inserted into the umbilical vein. Finally the baby is given *vitamin K_1* in the form of phytomenadione (Konakion) intramuscularly or intravenously to reduce the risk of haemorrhagic disease of the newborn (Report of an Expert Committee, 1992).

Throughout these procedures the baby should be handled gently and kept as warm as possible. The baby's condition is repeatedly assessed by observing the heart rate, respiratory effort, colour, muscle tone and response to stimuli and accurate records are kept. The Apgar score at five minutes is considered of particular value in forecasting the long-term prognosis (Rehnke *et al.*, 1987). Cord blood pH is also of great value in assessing the degree of intrapartum asphyxia.

In community practice only simple resuscitation equipment is available and medical aid is often not immediately at hand. Fortunately severe birth asphyxia is not common in home births and for most purposes the Ambu or Laerdal resuscitation bag is adequate.

Mouth-to-mouth and nose breathing may be effective and should be attempted if better facilities are not available. The object is to direct air from the attendant's mouth into the baby's air passages and it is thus a very much cruder variant of endotracheal insufflation. The baby's nostrils may be pinched to prevent air escaping through the nose if mouth-to-mouth resuscitation is preferred.

After resuscitation, it is essential to discuss what has happened with the parents. If the baby has to be transferred to the neonatal unit this is explained. The parents should have the chance to touch and, if possible, hold their baby, before transfer. They should be reassured that they may visit their baby at any time.

AFTER-CARE

The baby who has been severely asphyxiated is transferred to the neonatal unit for careful observation. The ability of the baby to withstand asphyxia depends largely on the cardiac glycogen stores. These are likely to be deficient in the preterm and small-for-gestational-age, chronically asphyxiated babies. It is mainly the low birthweight babies and those who suffer severe, prolonged hypoxia who develop complications and are likely to need more supportive care. This includes maintenance of body temperature using an incubator, mechanical ventilation where indicated, control of convulsions, monitoring of fluid balance and parenteral nutrition. Regular monitoring of blood sugar, electrolytes and blood gases will be required and the following observations are carried out to monitor progress and ensure early detection of complications.

▶ *Signs of cerebral oedema or injury* include poor muscle tone initially which steadily resolves in babies who have been only mildly asphyxiated. Moderately asphyxiated babies may become tense and irritable, whereas a severely asphyxiated baby may develop an abnormal, high-pitched, irritable cry, abnormal eye movements, convulsions and periods of apnoea. In some cases death will ensue.

▶ The *blood sugar* is monitored at four- to six-hourly intervals to detect hypoglycaemia which is a common problem in asphyxiated babies, especially those who are preterm or small-for-gestational-age.

▶ The *temperature* is recorded regularly to detect hypothermia which again is a common problem following severe asphyxia.

▶ The *respiratory pattern and rate* are recorded to

detect any signs of respiratory distress. Severe asphyxia may cause the lung vasculature to spasm in response to the elevated carbon dioxide levels and this produces pulmonary hypertension (see Chapter 67).

▶ The *apex beat* is monitored since cardiac failure can occur (as in myocardial infarction in adults).

▶ *Oedema* is noted (see below).

▶ *Urinary output* is observed because fluid retention leading to oedema and fluid overload may occur. This may be due to the antidiuretic hormone which is produced in response to stress or the cause could be acute renal failure. In the former case the baby's fluid intake is restricted until urinary output returns to normal. Acute renal failure is treated by peritoneal dialysis until the problem resolves.

▶ *Meconium/faeces* are observed, especially once milk feeding is started since the passage of blood and mucus could indicate necrotizing enterocolitis, a possible complication of severe asphyxia.

FOLLOW-UP AND PROGNOSIS

Paediatric follow-up is essential to detect any long-term sequelae of perinatal asphyxia such as delay in development, mental retardation or cerebral palsy (Freeman and Nelson, 1988). It is extremely difficult to predict the outcome following birth asphyxia since many babies with prolonged low Apgar scores survive normally, although this scoring system alone is not a good indicator of outcome. The prognosis is worse for babies who have prolonged low Apgar scores, evidence of encephalopathy and who have had seizures (Nelson and Ellenberg, 1986). Factors such as birthweight, gestation and the degree of brain injury are all relevant in determining the outcome, but the level and duration of hypoxia which causes such injuries is still not known.

Acidosis

The normal blood pH in the adult is 7.35–7.45 and in the fetus 7.30–7.35, showing that blood is a slightly alkaline fluid. Minute alterations of pH are associated with serious disorders of metabolism. When the pH falls the blood is more acid and a state of 'acidosis' exists.

Acidosis is the presence of excess hydrogen ions in the body and this concentration of hydrogen ions is directly related to the ratio of carbon dioxide to bicarbonate. The more carbon dioxide, or the less bicarbonate, the more acid is the fluid.

Respiratory acidosis results from the accumulation of carbon dioxide as a waste product of aerobic metabolism; the circulation of the fetus, or the ventilation of the neonate, has allowed some oxygen to enter but is unable to remove the carbon dioxide. Metabolic acidosis is the loss of bicarbonate, caused either by the accumulation of acids (e.g. lactic acid) in the body during anaerobic metabolism, or by a renal problem that prevents the excretion of acids or allows a urinary leak of bicarbonate.

If the body suffers one sort of acidosis only, it can use the other system to compensate. Whereas the lungs are central in the control of the carbon dioxide level (in *respiratory acidosis*), the kidneys are central to the regulation of the bicarbonate level (*metabolic acidosis*). Thus, if excess carbon dioxide is retained, the kidneys will increase the bicarbonate level present in body fluids, and this will restore the hydrogen ions and thereby the pH, to normal.

These buffering systems (lung and kidney, respiratory and metabolic) may fail to cope in neonates, because acidosis at birth tends to be mixed (respiratory and metabolic) and because the whole metabolism is so fragile. When the supply of oxygen ceases, there is initially a pure respiratory acidosis, but as the metabolism changes to be anaerobic, lactic acid accumulates and a metabolic acidosis develops. Values in respiratory and metabolic acidosis are shown in Table 2.

The *base deficit* is a measure of circulating organic acids, the products of anaerobic metabolism, and is expressed as the deficiency of circulating bicarbonate.

Table 2 Values in respiratory and metabolic acidosis

	Normal range	Respiratory acidosis	Metabolic acidosis
pH	7.30–7.35	Falls	Falls
H$^+$	4.5–5	Raised	Raised
P_{CO_2} (mmHg) (kPa)	35–45 4.6–6	Raised over 45 Above 6	Little change
Standard bicarbonate (mmol/l) (mEq/l)	21–25	Little change	Low, 18
Base deficit (mmol/l) (mEq/l)	5–6	Unchanged	Raised, 15

There is much controversy over the administration of *sodium bicarbonate* to an infant at delivery. As an emergency measure, some paediatricians may give it to a severely asphyxiated baby without obvious lung disease who has failed to respond to ventilation and cardiac massage within a few minutes, but blood gas analysis should be undertaken first. It is not given where the primary problem is respiratory, unless blood gases can be measured to distinguish metabolic from respiratory acidosis. This is because the bicarbonate (HCO_3) combines with hydrogen ions to form carbonic acid (H_2CO_3) which dissociates to water (H_2O) and carbon dioxide (CO_2). If the carbon dioxide can leave the body via the lungs, there is no problem, but if there are respiratory difficulties it may accumulate. It then crosses cell membranes and the blood–brain barrier to cause a worsening of the acidosis within cells and within the brain, despite an improvement in the acidosis as measured in the blood. This happens because carbon dioxide crosses such membranes freely, lowering the pH, while the bicarbonate cannot follow to balance it.

The bicarbonate solutions also contain a high sodium concentration, and this can result in an overloading of the infant's vascular system, and in damaging fluxes of water and salts across cell membranes and the blood–brain barrier.

Respiratory Distress Syndrome

Respiratory distress syndrome is responsible for the largest number of neonatal deaths, from a single disease, in normal, liveborn babies. It most commonly affects preterm babies, especially those of less than 34 weeks' gestation, babies born by Caesarean section or after antepartum haemorrhage, and babies of diabetic mothers. Gestational age correlates to the incidence of respiratory distress syndrome, with those of low gestational age being at greatest risk. Approximately 25% of babies of 34 weeks' gestation are affected, whilst 90% of 26 weeks' gestation babies require treatment (Halliday *et al.*, 1985). There is also a significant morbidity rate from this syndrome.

Cause

The cause is a deficiency of surfactant in the lungs. Surfactant is a phospholipid which reduces surface tension in the alveoli where gas meets tissue, thereby facilitating lung expansion. It prevents their complete collapse during expiration, so that when there is a deficiency of surfactant a greater negative intrathoracic pressure is required to inflate the alveoli. As a result the baby has to work harder to breathe and soon becomes exhausted. *Atelectasis*, or imperfect expansion of the lungs, therefore occurs. In addition, blood flow to the lungs is reduced and right-to-left shunting of blood through the ductus arteriosus and foramen ovale occurs. The baby deteriorates further as less surfactant is produced during hypoxic and acidotic episodes. A vicious circle results and, unless appropriate intervention is instituted quickly, the metabolism spirals out of control.

At post-mortem, areas of atelectasis are found in the lungs and a hyaline membrane lines the alveoli and small bronchioles. This membrane is thought to be formed from a leakage of plasma from the pulmonary capillaries into the alveoli due to a lack of surfactant. These findings are known as *hyaline membrane disease*, the clinical syndrome of which is respiratory distress syndrome.

Prevention

The lecithin–sphingomyelin (L/S) ratio may be estimated before delivery (see Chapter 21). If low, the mother may be treated with betamethasone or other corticosteroids for at least 24 hours before delivery to increase the production of surfactant in the fetal lungs. The risk of respiratory distress syndrome and its associated complications occurring in the baby is thereby reduced (Doyle *et al.*, 1986).

Some maternal conditions such as hypertensive disorders (Szymonowicz *et al.*, 1987) and prolonged rupture of the membranes are associated with an increased production of surfactant and thus the incidence of respiratory distress syndrome is reduced.

Surfactant deficiency is not specific to respiratory distress syndrome, but also occurs in babies with congenital pneumonia and transient tachypnoea.

The production and use of bovine, porcine and artificial surfactant to prevent and reduce the severity of respiratory distress syndrome has been widely trialled, with excellent results, (Ten Centre Study Group, 1987; Collaborative European Multicentre Study Group, 1988).

Signs of onset

In some cases there has been hypoxia at birth, but in many breathing is established quickly. The onset of respiratory difficulty occurs within four hours of birth and the condition gradually worsens.

The baby tends to lie limply and makes little spontaneous movement. The respiratory rate is raised to 60–100 or more per minute, accompanied by paradoxical breathing, the abdomen rising while the chest sinks. There is flaring of the nostrils, intercostal and substernal recession and a noisy expiratory grunt. In severe cases there is cyanosis, initially relieved by oxygen. Oedema of the hands and feet becomes apparent and the heart rate increases.

Crepitations and reduced breathing sounds are heard on auscultation. The diagnosis is confirmed by a chest radiograph which shows a fine ground-glass mottling throughout both lung fields and, in contrast, a clear outline of the bronchial tree. The radiograph is also of value in excluding other conditions which could cause respiratory distress, such as meconium aspiration, emphysema, pneumonia, atelectasis, pneumothorax and diaphragmatic hernia.

Those babies most commonly affected are the preterm and may be electively intubated at delivery. Many of these signs and symptoms may not, therefore, be apparent.

Prognosis

In most cases there is a deterioration during the first 24–36 hours. Ventilation may need to be continued for a considerable time, but should be reduced as soon as possible to prevent further lung damage as a result of high pressures.

Complications are common and these, together with the birthweight and gestation of the baby, will influence the outcome.

MANAGEMENT AND NURSING CARE

All babies at risk of developing respiratory distress syndrome should be closely observed to detect early signs of the condition so that there is no delay in starting treatment. Those who develop the condition are nursed in the neonatal unit where they are in the constant care of skilled nurses, midwives and paediatricians.

Provision of warmth

It is essential to avoid hypothermia, not only because it leads to an increased consumption of oxygen and use of more energy to produce heat, but also as it may inhibit the production of surfactant. Thus the baby is nursed

in an incubator (see Figure 3) and may be covered with a 'bubble blanket' or Perspex heat shield to prevent radiant heat loss. The baby may also be partially dressed to conserve heat and later when the chest no longer has to be continuously observed, the baby is fully dressed. The baby's temperature is recorded at intervals of not less than four hours and should be maintained in the range of 36.5–37.0°C. The skin temperature may be continually recorded by attaching a skin probe to the abdomen. Incubator temperature must also be observed and, depending on the size and condition of the baby, is maintained at between 34 and 37°C.

Oxygen therapy

Relief of hypoxia is essential to prevent brain damage. It may be achieved by increasing the oxygen concentration of inspired air by placing a Perspex headbox over the baby's head and providing added humidified oxygen into the headbox. An oxygen analyser is used to measure the inspired air concentration in the headbox and the partial pressure of oxygen in arterial blood (P_aO_2) is monitored continuously with a transcutaneous oxygen monitor (see Chapter 67). The aim is to maintain arterial oxygen tension within the normal range of 7–10 kPa (50–75 mmHg) in a mature baby or 6–9 kPa (45–65 mmHg) in a preterm baby. Oxygen saturation levels may also be monitored. Accurate measurement of P_aO_2 is essential to avoid hyperoxaemia. Prolonged episodes of high P_aO_2 levels may lead to retinopathy of prematurity, resulting in retinal detachment and blindness. Hypoxaemia may cause irreversible brain damage.

Continuous positive airways pressure (CPAP)

Some babies with respiratory distress require more help than added oxygen in a headbox. They need to have the work of breathing done for them to some extent and this can be achieved with CPAP. It may also be used in preference to mechanical ventilation for babies with normal lungs who are having frequent apnoeic attacks.

CPAP prevents collapse of the alveoli on expiration by maintaining a positive pressure of about 5–10 cmH$_2$O in the airways whilst the baby breathes spontaneously. This effectively splints the airways open, thereby saving the baby much inspiratory effort and reducing the oxygen requirements. This continuous pressure can be maintained either by using an endotracheal tube, by nasal prongs, or through a short nasopharyngeal tube. If not applied via an endotracheal tube, a gastric tube must be left in place (oral or nasal) and on free drainage to prevent air accumulating in the stomach and causing gastric distension which could cause respiratory embarrassment. Humidified oxygen is given and blood gases are carefully monitored. As the baby's condition improves the oxygen concentration is reduced and is followed by a gradual reduction in the continuous positive airways pressure.

Possible dangers of CPAP are pneumothorax and ulceration of the nasal passages if prongs are used for a prolonged period. There is an increased incidence of periventricular haemorrhage, which leads to hydrocephalus in some cases.

Mechanical intermittent positive pressure ventilation (IPPV)

Very small babies, or those with severe respiratory distress syndrome, may require virtually all the work of breathing to be done for them. They require full ventilation. The indications for mechanical ventilation include severe apnoea, a Po_2 of less than 5 kPa (40 mmHg) despite a high concentration of oxygen in inspired air and a Pco_2 greater than 12 kPa associated with acidosis which fails to respond to treatment. Some paediatricians now ventilate all very low birthweight babies for 24 hours or so in the absence of frank respiratory distress because it is thought to prevent the development of the condition and to avoid such complications as periventricular haemorrhage.

Neonatal ventilators differ from those used for adults in that the controls preset the pressures generated, rather than the volume of each inflation. Since cuffed endotracheal tubes are not used, there is an unavoidable and variable leak around the endotracheal tube and a fixed volume machine would be unreliable. The flow through a neonatal ventilator circuit is constant, while the pressure in the circuit is controlled at a valve on the gas return port of the ventilator. The pressure required to open this valve varies with the ventilator settings, and determines the pressure generated in the endotracheal tube.

As discussed above, the small airways of an infant with respiratory distress syndrome collapse at the end of each breath and require excessive effort to reinflate them. Infants with respiratory distress adopt a strategy that reduces this collapse somewhat by grunting. This

is a partial *Valsalva manoeuvre* (breathing out against a closed larynx) that maintains a positive pressure in the chest even during exhalation, i.e. a positive end expiratory pressure (PEEP). Intubation prevents the baby from generating this PEEP, and causes a disadvantage unless positive pressure is applied externally; an endotracheal tube must never be left in place without a source of pressure applied.

The ventilation of such infants traditionally involves applying moderately high pressure for about 1 second at a rate of about 30 per minute, the pressure being adjusted to maintain the Pco_2 in a satisfactory range, and to ensure adequate oxygenation. In between these inflations, a background pressure (the PEEP) is applied to prevent alveolar collapse.

High pressures, particularly when sustained for relatively long periods of the respiratory cycle, cause damage to the lungs and may result in bronchopulmonary dysplasia, or pneumothoraces. These conditions, in turn, lead to a greater incidence of periventricular haemorrhages and the resulting sequelae.

There are many different techniques of ventilation now available. High-frequency ventilation allows short bursts of high pressure, with rates exceeding 60 per minute and an inspiratory-to-expiratory ratio (I:E ratio) of 1:1.5 or 1:2. An extension of this idea allows very high-frequency oscillation to be used, with rates over 1000 per minute, reducing damage to the lung tissue. *Synchronous intermittent mandatory ventilation* (SIMV) is a form of trigger ventilation, which allows the baby to trigger the ventilator in time with his own inspiration, but supplies a breath if there is a long apnoeic period.

Arterial oxygen tension is measured continuously with a transcutaneous oxygen analyser and is maintained at the optimal level of 7–10 kPa (50–75 mmHg) in the mature baby and 6–9 kPa (45–65 mmHg) in the preterm. Arterial cannulation is also necessary so that blood gases and pH can be regularly monitored. If adjustments are made to the ventilator controls further measurement of blood gases and pH is necessary. The aim is to keep the Pco_2 in the range of 5–6 kPa (40–45 mmHg) so that the pH remains about 7.25. The blood sugar is also monitored to detect hypoglycaemia. The removal of frequent blood samples from the baby can amount to a considerable blood loss and replacement transfusions may be required. Oxygen or air delivered via a ventilator should be humidified.

Complications of mechanical ventilation

Air leaks High pressures, and an infant struggling against the ventilator, predispose to air leaks within the lung. These leaks occupy space that is then unavailable for gas exchange, and they often physically obstruct the entry of gas into the functioning areas of lung. Leaks into the bronchial walls cause interstitial emphysema; this may then burst through into the pleural space around the lungs causing a pneumothorax. This can be catastrophic since air can accumulate rapidly in the pleural space and this compresses the lung and prevents it from functioning. Often, however, there is an initial gradual deterioration; if this is spotted, a chest drain may be inserted before too much harm is done. Air leaks may also burst into the pericardium causing tamponade, into the peritoneum, or into the bloodstream.

If a pneumothorax is suspected it may be confirmed on X-ray, by transillumination of the chest with a cold light source (using fibreoptics), or by needling the chest and finding gas that escapes readily into a syringe or through a butterfly tubing to emerge under water. If found, a pneumothorax is drained with a 10 G or larger chest drain and either an underwater seal or with a flutter valve. Adequate analgesia should be given and local anaesthesic used during the chest drain insertion.

Other complications

1 Oxygen is directly toxic to lung tissue, and concentrations of above 80% for more than a few hours should be avoided where possible.
2 Intubation with an endotracheal tube, and the lavage and suction required to keep the tube patent, may introduce infection and cause a secondary pneumonia.
3 The process of lavage and suction through the endotracheal tube is distressing for the baby and causes swings in blood pressure and oxygenation.
4 There are long-term problems associated with prolonged ventilation, especially bronchopulmonary dysplasia. In this condition lung growth has been disrupted not only by the disease process but also by the ventilation. Fibrosis and scarring occurs in the lungs and oxygen therapy may be required for many months. These children are susceptible to chest infections and to heart failure.
5 Retinopathy of prematurity is the formation of scar tissue in the posterior chamber of the eye in response to haemorrhages from excessive and unsupported new growths of retinal blood vessels. Their formation is related to the arterial partial pressures of oxygen and carbon dioxide as well as other factors (Prendiville and Schulenberg, 1988).
6 Excessive arterial oxygen can also cause specific patterns of damage to some areas in the brain.

Observations

The observations are listed here as they are similar to those described in detail in Chapter 67. Possible equipment is shown in Figures 2 and 3.

▶ *Temperature* is recorded rectally and via a skin probe. The incubator temperature is also recorded.
▶ A cardiac monitor is attached to the baby to record *heart rate* and *variability* continuously.
▶ *Respiratory rate* is continuously monitored.
▶ A transcutaneous oxygen monitor is attached to the infant to measure the *arterial oxygen tension. Oxygen saturation* may also be monitored.
▶ *Blood pressure* may be continuously monitored via an umbilical arterial line.

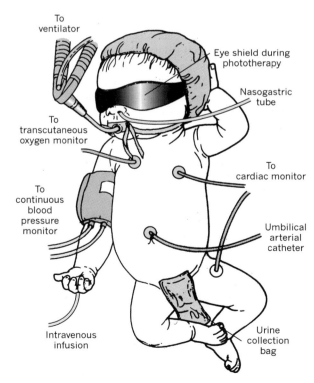

To ventilator

Eye shield during phototherapy

Nasogastric tube

To transcutaneous oxygen monitor

To cardiac monitor

To continuous blood pressure monitor

Umbilical arterial catheter

Intravenous infusion

Urine collection bag

Figure 2 Possible equipment for baby receiving intensive care (incubator not shown).

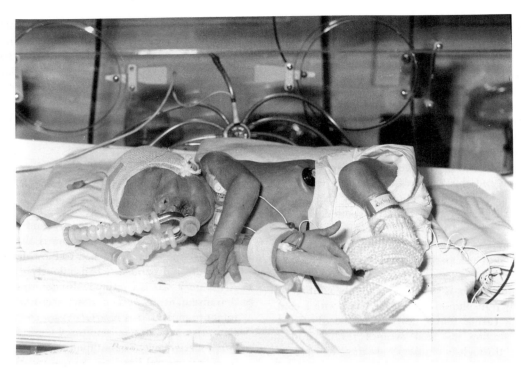

Figure 3   A baby having assisted ventilation.

▶ *Urinary output* is measured and samples are tested for glucose and osmolality.

▶ The presence and amount of *oedema* is noted.

▶ The passage and character of *stools* are observed.

▶ The baby's *general behaviour, muscle tone, colour, activity* and *response to stimuli* are important observations to make.

▶ *Attention* to the endotracheal tube, intravenous infusions, including parenteral feeding, and arterial catheter will also be required.

▶ *Blood tests* include:

Blood gases and pH.
Dextrostix strip tests for blood sugar estimation.
Bilirubin if the baby appears jaundiced.
Electrolytes.
Calcium levels.
Haemoglobin or packed cell volume.

Nursing care

Babies being nursed on a ventilator require constant, skilled nursing care. Suction to the endotracheal tube will be necessary using an aseptic technique, the frequency being indicated by the baby's condition. The baby's condition must be carefully observed during suction and, if there are any signs of deterioration, the procedure must be stopped at once. The risk of the endotracheal tube becoming blocked is minimized by maintaining a high humidity in the ventilator circuit. This also helps to reduce heat loss from the baby. The time when the tube is most likely to become blocked is during the recovery phase of the illness when thick secretions tend to accumulate in the bronchi. Physiotherapy and lavage before suction may help to relieve this problem.

Mouth care is also required. If temporary paralysis has been induced to prevent the baby 'fighting' the ventilator, the instillation of artificial tears into the eyes may be required to prevent corneal damage. All paralysed babies must also be sedated. Cleansing the skin is carried out gently, as required, and the baby's position is changed regularly. Careful positioning of preterm babies is important to prevent delays in their subsequent sensorimotor development.

The importance of preventing infection in these babies cannot be overemphasized. Frequent and effective handwashing is essential and high standards of care must be maintained at all times. No-one with an infection should attend these small infants.

Feeding

During the early stages of respiratory distress syndrome babies who are being ventilated cannot be fed via the gastrointestinal tract due to the risk of milk aspiration. There is a paralytic ileus during the first few days of respiratory distress syndrome, so milk in the stomach or bowel will just accumulate there. Consequently, the risk of milk aspiration is high and the full stomach may also cause further respiratory embarrassment. Another problem associated with milk feeding is that bacteria proliferate in the intestines once feeding is started and thus increase the risk of septicaemia and enterocolitis following periods of hypotension and/or hypoxia.

Parenteral (intravenous) feeding is therefore required for the first few days. Enteral feeding into the stomach or bowel will be started as soon as the baby shows signs of recovery, but great caution must be exercised in the introduction of such feeds. Gastric aspiration must be performed every few hours to detect any accumulation of milk which could indicate sepsis (including necrotizing enterocolitis), the continued presence of the ileus or bowel obstruction. Full or partial feeds of expressed breast milk reduce the risk of necrotizing enterocolitis. If milk feeds are absorbed the baby's intravenous intake is steadily reduced as the enteral intake is increased. The parenteral feeding can then be discontinued.

Weaning off the ventilator

The rates and pressures of ventilation are reduced at the earliest safe opportunity. Generally, the inspiratory time is left at a useful setting, and the expiratory time is steadily lengthened to allow the infant to take over the work of breathing. This process may take days, or even weeks. Gradually, the bulk of the work comes to be performed by the baby. Ventilation becomes CPAP. Extubation is possible once the infant has been stable with minimum CPAP. Each stage of this long process must be undertaken slowly, and the baby watched for clinical signs of inability to cope and for deteriorating blood gases.

COMPLICATIONS

Periventricular haemorrhage is a common complication of respiratory distress syndrome. Other complications include pneumothorax, patent ductus arteriosus, pulmonary infection, especially following CPAP or IPPV, pulmonary haemorrhage, bronchopulmonary dysplasia

and disseminated intravascular coagulation. Sepsis may also occur and lead to necrotizing enterocolitis. Oxygen therapy, unless carefully controlled, may cause retinopathy of prematurity and subsequent blindness. Close follow-up care is required to detect and monitor long-term problems, including neurological disorders. These complications are discussed more fully in Chapter 67.

Other Respiratory Disorders

BRONCHOPULMONARY DYSPLASIA

This condition occurs in babies who are ventilated and receiving oxygen therapy for prolonged periods. It is defined as the need for IPPV for at least three days in the first week, the baby still requiring oxygen therapy at the age of 28 days and characteristic changes on chest X-ray. With the increasing number of extremely low birthweight survivors, the incidence of this condition is increasing.

Both the toxic effects of oxygen and the pressure effects of ventilation are thought to play a part in the aetiology of bronchopulmonary dysplasia, with the latter being the more significant. New methods of ventilation may help to reduce the severity of these effects. Advances in antenatal steroid treatments and surfactant administration following delivery will reduce the severity of respiratory distress. This in turn may reduce the number of babies with chronic lung disease.

Some of these babies are given steroids to try to assist in weaning them from the ventilator (Ng, 1993). Low-flow oxygen may continue to be needed for several months after discharge home and the families need a great deal of support.

TRANSIENT TACHYPNOEA OF THE NEWBORN

This condition is commonly found in babies delivered by Caesarean section. During delivery there is no compression of the chest which assists in the expulsion of lung fluid in a vaginal delivery. The surge of catecholamines to initiate a switch in the lungs from secretion to absorption of lung fluid, is also impaired by an operative delivery. Consequently, excess lung fluid is present, which needs to be absorbed via the lymphatic system.

The baby has a respiratory rate of more than 60 per

minute, may have sternal or intercostal recession, with grunting and possibly cyanosis. A chest X-ray shows enlarged lymph vessels as characteristic streaks and signs of oedema between the lung lobes. The symptoms usually resolve within 24 hours, although tachypnoea alone may persist a little longer.

Nursing care involves providing adequate oxygen to eliminate cyanosis and maintaining a thermoneutral environment for the baby.

DIAPHRAGMATIC HERNIA

This is a congenital condition which presents as an emergency at birth. There is a defect in the diaphragm, usually on the left side, through which abdominal viscera herniate into the thoracic cavity. The lung on the affected side is often hypoplastic and immediate intubation for resuscitation is vital. Bag and mask ventilation will inflate the bowel in the thorax, causing increasing respiratory difficulty. This condition is discussed further in Chapter 75.

ATELECTASIS

This condition occurs in the newborn when there is imperfect expansion of the lungs following birth. The alveoli have failed to expand or, having done so, have collapsed and air cannot enter, due perhaps to inhalation of vomit or feeds.

MECONIUM ASPIRATION

This occurs when there has been intrauterine hypoxia causing the fetus to pass meconium *in utero*. The hypoxic fetus gasps *in utero* or at birth, thereby inhaling the thick tenacious meconium. This results in the obstruction of air passages, acts as a chemical irritant to the lungs and predisposes to infection. A pneumothorax may occur.

Meconium aspiration most commonly occurs in the baby who is small-for-gestational-age since intrauterine hypoxia is common in these infants. It may also occur

in postmature babies and following fetal distress in labour, whatever the cause.

If anticipated, a paediatrician should be present at birth to resuscitate the baby. The damage may be minimized by suction under direct vision and intubation. Admission to the neonatal unit is necessary in all but the very mildest cases and the level of care given depends on the condition of the baby. Those who are severely asphyxiated or develop respiratory distress will be managed as already described.

ASPIRATION PNEUMONIA

Aspiration of infected amniotic fluid may cause neonatal pneumonia.

Aspiration of meconium or infected amniotic fluid is likely to lead to severe irritation of the lungs, causing emphysema, atelectasis and secondary collapse. Treatment includes aspiration of the trachea and bronchi and maintenance of a clear airway, nursing the baby in an incubator to ensure adequate warmth and to facilitate easy observation, the provision of oxygen, as required, and the administration of a broad-spectrum antibiotic.

PNEUMOTHORAX

Rupture of the alveoli allows air to escape into the pleural cavities causing pneumothorax. It may follow meconium aspiration or be a complication of CPAP or mechanical ventilation. It is suspected when there is a sudden rapid deterioration in the baby's condition. A quick diagnosis can be made with a fibreoptic light which is used to transilluminate the chest and treatment can then be instigated immediately. A chest radiograph will also confirm the diagnosis. In mild cases the lung will re-expand spontaneously within a few days. Otherwise treatment includes inserting a needle into the pleural cavity and aspirating air or setting up underwater drainage of the pneumothorax.

References

Collaborative European Multicentre Study Group (1988) Surfactant replacement therapy in severe neonatal respiratory distress syndrome; an international randomized clinical trial. *Pediatrics* **82**: 683.

Davis, G.M. & Bureau, M.A. (1987) Pulmonary and chest wall mechanics in the control of respiration in the newborn. *Clin. Perinatol.* **14**: 551–579.

Doyle, L.W., Kitchen, W.H., Ford, G.W. *et al.* (1986) Effects of antenatal steroid therapy on mortality and morbidity in very low birth weight infants. *J. Pediat.* **108**: 287–292.

Freeman, J. & Nelson, K. (1988) Intrapartum asphyxia and cerebral palsy. *Pediatrics* **82**: 240–249.

Halliday, H.L., McClure, G. & Reid, M (1985) *Handbook of Neonatal Intensive Care*, 3rd edn. London: Baillière Tindall.

Kelnar, C.J.H., Harvey, D. & Simpson, C. (1995) *The Sick Newborn Baby*, 3rd edn, pp. 54–60. London: Baillière Tindall.

Nelson, K. & Ellenberg, J. (1986) Antecedents of cerebral palsy. Multivariate analysis of risk. *N. Engl. J. Med.* **315**: 81–86.

Ng, P.C. (1993) The effectiveness and side effects of dexamethasone in preterm infants with bronchopulmonary dysplasia. *Arch. Dis. Childh.* **68**: 330–336.

Prendiville, A. & Schulenberg, W.E. (1988) Clinical factors associated with retinopathy of prematurity. *Arch. Dis. Childh.* **63**: 522–527.

Rehnke, M., Carter, R.L., Hardt, N.S. *et al.* (1987) The relationship of Apgar scores, gestational age and birthweight to survival of low-birthweight infants. *Am. J. Perinatol.* **4**: 121–124.

Report of an Expert Committee (1992) *Vitamin K Prophylaxis in Infancy*. London: British Paediatric Association.

Szymonowicz, W., Yu, V.Y.H., Astbury, J. *et al.* (1987) Severe pre-eclampsia and the very low birthweight infant. *Arch. Dis. Childh.* **62**: 712–716.

Ten Centre Study Group (1987) Ten centre trial of artificial surfactant (artificial lung expanding compound) in very premature babies. *Br. Med. J.* **294**: 991–996.

Further Reading

Moore, K.L. (1988) *The Developing Human; Clinically Orientated Embryology*, 4th edn, Chapter 11. Philadelphia: W.B. Saunders.

Peliowski, A. & Finer, N. (1992) Birth asphyxia in the term infant. In Sinclair, J.C. & Bracken, M.B. (eds) *Effective Care of the Newborn Infant*. Oxford: Oxford University Press.

Yu, V.Y.H. (ed.) (1986) *Respiratory Disorders of the Newborn*. Edinburgh: Churchill Livingstone.

70

Neonatal Jaundice

Jaundice

Jaundice is a common physiological problem seen in both term and preterm infants (Blackburn, 1995). It is a symptom, not a disease, and is caused by deposits of *bilirubin* in the skin which becomes clinically apparent when the serum bilirubin rises above 85 µmol/l. The significance of jaundice in an infant may lie either in the harm that may be done by the bilirubin itself, or in the nature of the underlying cause of the jaundice. Thus, a high level of bilirubin may in itself be hazardous, or it may be harmless in itself but indicate the presence of a sinister underlying disorder.

When red cells are broken down, bilirubin is released into the bloodstream, where it is bound to the serum albumin and transported in this bound form. It is not sufficiently water-soluble to be transported in the free state. In the liver it is combined ('conjugated') with glucuronic acid to form *bilirubin glucuronide*. This compound is water-soluble, and is called *conjugated bilirubin*. It is also termed *direct bilirubin*, because the traditional chemical test for bilirubin detects it directly. In contrast, the unconjugated bilirubin is called *indirect* because an extra step in the test is required to measure it. The conjugated bilirubin can be excreted through the kidney and intestine and is eliminated.

Bilirubin bound to serum albumin (fat-soluble) + Glucuronic acid $\xrightarrow{\text{In the presence of glucuronyl transferase}}$ Bilirubin glucuronide (water-soluble)

Unconjugated bilirubin, on the other hand, because it is fat-soluble, cannot be eliminated and if for any reason conjugation does not take place the bilirubin is deposited in fatty tissues. Nervous tissue contains a high proportion of fat, particularly areas of the brain known as the basal ganglia. If bilirubin is deposited there it gives rise to irreversible changes resulting in spasticity. This condition is known as *kernicterus* and is characterized by muscular twitchings, hypertonicity of limbs and neck retraction and later some neuromuscular defects such as athetosis or possible mental retardation. Factors that may delay conjugation include:

- too much unconjugated bilirubin in the plasma to be bound by albumin;
- drugs such as salicylates, sulphonamides, heparin, diazepam and chloramphenicol because they are excreted by the same pathways as bilirubin;
- haematin formed during haemolysis;
- baby with metabolic acidosis or hypoalbuminaemia (Kelnar *et al.*, 1995).

Kernicterus

The signs of kernicterus in small, preterm infants may not be so obvious, and the diagnosis may only become apparent at follow-up or at post-mortem examination. Kernicterus can usually be prevented, except sometimes in sick, very low birthweight infants. In these babies, the highest 'safe' level for the bilirubin may not be known; intervention may therefore be called for at much lower levels than in term infants.

Most paediatricians are anxious if the serum bilirubin level rises above 250 µmol/l, but it is the quantity of unconjugated, fat-soluble bilirubin that is of most significance. A serum level of more than 350 µmol/l is liable to cause kernicterus in even a healthy, term baby. Lower levels may cause transient hearing impairment in such infants. Kernicterus can occur at lower levels than this in preterm, sick infants whose blood–brain barrier is defective.

Kernicterus may also occur at lower serum levels if the quantity of *free* bilirubin in the serum is increased for any reason. This makes it more likely for bilirubin to leave the serum and enter brain tissue. It occurs when the serum albumin level is low and when drugs displace bilirubin from its binding sites on albumin. Kernicterus also occurs more readily if the blood–brain barrier is injured by acidosis, osmolar shocks and other insults that occur in the sick neonate.

Causes of Jaundice

'Physiological' jaundice

In order to obtain sufficient oxygen from the placental circulation the fetus has a greater number of red cells than the adult, some 6–7 million/mm^3 instead of the 4–5 million/mm^3 of the adult. This large number of red cells is not required after birth and they are destroyed in the first few weeks of life. During the destruction of the red cells bilirubin is formed, conjugated by the liver and excreted. In the early days of life there is a high bilirubin load to excrete. Late clamping of the cord results in an increased blood volume and this exacerbates the problem (Kelnar *et al.*, 1995).

Liver function in the newborn may be immature, and this can also contribute to neonatal jaundice. In addition, there is much conjugated bilirubin in the bowel, both already present in meconium and also in fresh bile, and this may be broken down to release free bilirubin again which then re-enters the baby's circulation.

Physiological jaundice commonly appears about the third day, is slight and fades by the seventh or eighth day. The child is a typical orange-pink or bronzed colour and is clearly not anaemic. The general condition is good. If the jaundice conforms to this pattern, no anxiety need be felt. If, however, it arises earlier, becomes deep or the child's condition is adversely affected, a doctor must be consulted without delay. When jaundice is pronounced the serum bilirubin will be checked and if it reaches a level of 250 µmol/l the baby may be treated with phototherapy.

Jaundice of prematurity

This is an exaggeraton of the condition described above. In preterm babies it is not surprising that jaundice is deeper and more prolonged. Occasionally an exchange transfusion is necessary to prevent kernicterus.

Haemolytic jaundice

Haemolysis of the red cells due to iso-immunization to the rhesus factor or the ABO groups will result in jaundice which occurs in the first 24 hours of life.

ABO incompatibility   When ABO incompatibility occurs the mother is blood group O and the fetus A or B or AB. The anti A or B haemolysins present in the blood of a group O mother may cross the placenta to the fetus causing haemolysis of the fetal red blood cells. After birth jaundice appears within 24 hours (Schneider, 1993) but is rarely severe.

Infection

Prenatal viral infections such as rubella, syphilis, cytomegalovirus inclusion disease and toxoplasmosis may cause neonatal jaundice. After birth both viral and bacterial infections may lead to haemolysis of the red blood cells and subsequent jaundice. Umbilical infections, septicaemia and pyelonephritis are some of the infective conditions responsible for this.

Obstructive jaundice

This is an uncommon problem caused by an obstruction to bile flow. It may result from the obliteration of the bile ducts in biliary atresia, from compression on the ducts, or from various metabolic problems including cystic fibrosis, antitrypsin deficiency and some other enzyme disorders. A deep bronze jaundice develops in the second week of life or later (Schneider, 1993), stools are putty-coloured and the urine contains bilirubin. Operative treatment may be necessary and if so there is some urgency in establishing the diagnosis and the precise site of the obstruction since the outlook is better after early surgery.

There may also be difficulty in distinguishing various metabolic disorders, neonatal hepatitis and congenital infections from a surgical obstruction. These disorders may produce a similar conjugated hyperbilirubinaemia, or a mixed picture with both types of bilirubin elevated.

Metabolic disorders

There are many metabolic disorders that can cause jaundice. The important ones to detect are those which can be treated. *Hypothyroidism* causes mental retardation unless treated and then the effects are minimal. Nowadays most babies are screened for this condition at seven days with the phenylketonuria (Guthrie) test.

Persistent jaundice may also occur with *galactosaemia*, an inborn error of metabolism where there is a deficiency of the enzyme required for the conversion of galactose to glucose. It is diagnosed by an enzyme assay performed on red blood cells, but testing the urine may also detect it. The urine contains a non-glucose reducing sugar, galactose, so the urine is Clinitest positive but Clinistix negative.

Glucose-6-phosphate dehydrogenase is an enzyme necessary for the metabolism of glucose in the red blood cells. A deficiency of this enzyme may occur in Mediterranean, Asian and African people and results in haemolysis of red blood cells.

Breast milk jaundice

Breastfed infants are more likely to become jaundiced than are those fed on cows' milk (Brown, 1992; Brown

et al., 1993; Salariya and Robertson, 1993). This causes no ill-effects apart from the anxiety it produces. While it may be necessary to investigate an infant with breast milk jaundice, this is not because the jaundice causes any ill-effects, but to ensure that there is no other underlying cause of more sinister potential. The causes of breast milk jaundice are thought to be:

▶ inhibition of glucuronyl transferase and therefore diminished conjugation of bilirubin;
▶ delayed passage of meconium which allows more time for the conjugated bilirubin in the gut to be broken down and reabsorbed (Kelnar *et al*, 1995). According to a study conducted by Salariya and Robertson (1993), early and successful establishment of feeding helps to overcome this problem;
▶ the presence of β-glucuronidase which splits conjugated bilirubin and increases the absorption of unconjugated bilirubin.

Breast milk jaundice may persist but is not considered harmful. Brown *et al.* (1993) report jaundice still present on day 13 in a significant number of term breastfed babies. It is important, however, to exclude other serious causes of jaundice. The mother is informed about the condition and encouraged to continue breastfeeding.

Drugs

Drugs such as vitamin K (not vitamin K_1), sulphonamides, diazepam and salicylates contribute to jaundice and should therefore be avoided where possible in the first few weeks of life (see earlier in this chapter).

Haematoma

A haematoma or excessive bruising increases the amount of bilirubin to be conjugated, so that jaundice may be increased and more prolonged when these conditions exist.

Other factors

Some aspects of the management of labour are thought to have contributed to the increase in neonatal jaundice over recent years. Several studies have shown that neonatal jaundice is increased due to greater erythrocyte destruction following the administration of oxytocin for the induction of labour (Buchan, 1979; D'Souza *et al.*, 1979). Singhi *et al.* (1982) found a higher incidence of neonatal jaundice in babies born vaginally to mothers who received aqueous glucose solutions in labour. This treatment seems to lead to reduced cord serum sodium levels and low osmolality which probably results in a flow of water across the fetal cell membranes and consequent haemolysis of red cells.

Another factor which leads to increased haemolysis is trauma and this may be caused by operative deliveries which have increased markedly in recent years.

Investigations

The mother's notes are examined to check her blood group, Rhesus factor, antibody tests, medical history and the records of pregnancy and labour.

Bilirubin estimation

A test to estimate bilirubin using a jaundice meter may be carried out initially. The meter is pressed against the baby's forehead and a beam of light is seen which indicates the degrees of yellowness. It is presented as 'transcutaneous bilirubin index' (tcBl) and corresponds to the degree of skin jaundice only. The test is useful to determine whether a laboratory test for serum bilirubin is necessary (Kelnar *et al.*, 1995). A serum bilirubin will be required if the tcBl level rises significantly, or is high, or the condition of the baby gives rise to concern.

Other tests

In severe or persistent cases of jaundice further tests will be required:

▶ Serum bilirubin.
▶ Haemoglobin.
▶ Blood group and Coombs' antibody test.

Other tests which may also be carried out include:

▶ Screening for infection i.e. swabs are taken from areas, such as umbilical cord, eyes, nose, mouth, ears and skin lesions, where infection is likely. Urine is collected for culture, and blood culture and perhaps lumbar culture may be performed.
▶ IgM, cytomegalovirus, toxoplasma and rubella antibody titres should be estimated (Kelnar *et al.*, 1995). A raised IgM indicates intrauterine infection, especially if in cord blood.
▶ Thyroxine (T_4) and thyroid-stimulating hormone to diagnose or exclude hypothyroidism.
▶ Glucose-6-phosphate dehydrogenase (G-6-PD) assay.

Management of Jaundice

Physiological jaundice occurring on the third day is very common and, in most cases, mild, resolving spontaneously within about a week. As already discussed, the early establishment of successful feeding appears to be an important factor in reducing the incidence of this condition. Complementary feeds, however, should not be given to babies who are being breastfed, even if they are jaundiced, as they have an adverse effect on the establishment of lactation and cause nipple confusion for the baby which may delay the establishment of successful feeding.

If the jaundice persists and the bilirubin rises, phototherapy is usually the treatment of choice. In cases where there is a very rapid rise in bilirubin levels, or when it reaches dangerous levels, exchange transfusion is necessary. Sometimes the baby is given an intravenous infusion of albumin because this increases the bilirubin-binding capacity of the blood. This treatment is especially useful if there is a delay for any reason in giving an exchange transfusion (Kelnar *et al.*, 1995).

PHOTOTHERAPY (Figure 1)

Some 2–6% of babies in the UK receive phototherapy for the treatment of neonatal jaundice. If a baby shows increasing jaundice, the serum bilirubin is monitored so that treatment can be started well before it reaches a level of about 350 µmol/l when the risk of kernicterus arises. Many paediatricians now consider it safe to withhold treatment in term healthy babies until the serum bilirubin exceeds 320 µmol/l (Lewis *et al.*, 1982; Kelnar *et al.*, 1995; Torres-Torres *et al.*, 1994; Yau and Stevenson, 1995). The rate at which the serum bilirubin is rising is of significance. If the level is rising very slowly and the infant is well there may be no need for phototherapy.

In preterm babies lower serum bilirubin levels may cause kernicterus, so treatment is started earlier, possibly when the level reaches 150–180 µmol/l in babies of 28 weeks gestation, and 200–240 µmol/l at 34 weeks gestation (Kelnar *et al.*, 1995).

Phototherapy is not without its problems and should not be undertaken without good cause. Its main purpose is not to abolish jaundice but to prevent the need for exchange transfusion to prevent kernicterus. When the baby's skin is exposed to light of

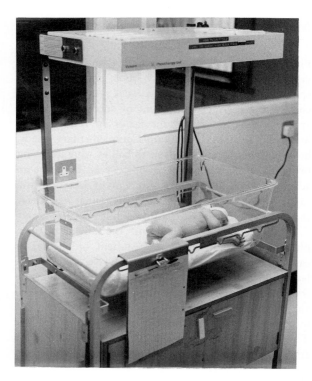

Figure 1   A baby receiving phototherapy.

wavelength 400–500 nm, the unconjugated bilirubin in the skin and superficial vessels is converted to a non-toxic, water-soluble substance which can be readily excreted.

Phototherapy may be given either continuously or intermittently. Lav and Fung (1984) gave a regimen of one hour of phototherapy and three hours off and found this was as effective as continuous treatment. The serum bilirubin is repeatedly monitored during treatment until it falls to a safe level and the jaundice fades.

During phototherapy treatment the baby lies exposed in an incubator or cot with eyes covered to prevent the white or blue light from damaging the retina (Messner *et al.*, 1975). It is important to record the baby's temperature three- or four-hourly, as the baby may become overheated or, if treated in a cot rather than an incubator, chilled. The baby is fed every 3–4 hours and adequate fluids are required to prevent dehydration. The stools are usually green and loose during treatment owing to the excretion of excess bilirubin.

The idea that breastfeeding should be temporarily stopped because of jaundice is false unless the infant is unwell and feeds are to be stopped anyway. Only if bilirubin levels were approaching 350 μmol/l may breastfeeding be temporarily suspended. The giving of water serves only to undermine the mother's confidence, reduce lactation and deprive the infant of calories. It has not been shown to help the jaundice (Carvalho *et al.*, 1981).

Summary of problems of phototherapy

1   Dehydration.
2   Interruption of feeds, and slower weight gain.
3   Trauma to the eyes from eye-pads (no retinal damage has been reported in humans).
4   Maternal distress and possibility of mother–infant separation.
5   Disturbed temperature control.
6   Polycythaemia.
7   Bronze discolouration. There is a theoretical risk of DNA damage in the skin.

Separation of mother and baby should be avoided where possible, phototherapy being given to the baby beside the mother's bed. The mother is encouraged to feed and care for her baby and is kept fully informed of progress. Most mothers are very anxious when their baby is jaundiced and requires phototherapy, thus the midwife will need to give them time to express their anxieties, ask questions and assimilate information. If the serum bilirubin continues to rise and reaches levels which are considered dangerous, an exchange transfusion will be required.

Drugs   Phenobarbitone 4 mg/kg per day may be prescribed for the baby as it promotes the production of the enzyme glucuronyl transferase. It takes four or five days to take effect and, therefore, is of limited value. It also makes the baby very sleepy and may intefere with effective feeding. In high-risk cases diagnosed antenatally (e.g. rhesus disease) phenobarbitone may be given to the mother from 32 weeks gestation and has been shown to result in babies who are less jaundiced (Kelnar *et al.*, 1995).

Rhesus Iso-immunization

The population can be divided into two groups by determining whether the red cells contain a protein antigen known as the *rhesus factor*. Of the European

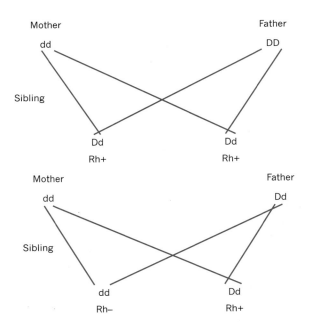

Figure 2   Inheritance of the rhesus factor.

population approximately 85% have this antigen and are rhesus–positive (Rh+) while 15% are without the antigen and are rhesus–negative (Rh–). In the Asiatic races the incidence of rhesus-negativity is less.

The rhesus factor is a complex antigen with three pairs of genes named *cde/CDE*. It is the pair named *D* which are likely to cause iso-immunization. They may be shown as follows:

Rhesus negative	*dd*	
Rhesus positive	*Dd*	Heterozygous
	DD	Homozygous

The rhesus grouping is genetically determined (Figure 2). A heterozygous father with one positive and one negative gene may transmit either to his children; his children may be rhesus-positive or rhesus-negative. A homozygous father with two positive genes will transmit only positive genes and all his children will be rhesus-positive and could be affected by haemolytic disease.

In 10% of all pregnancies the woman is rhesus-negative, but a problem arises in only about 0.5% of cases. This is accounted for first by some husbands being rhesus-negative and some being rhesus-positive heterozygous. Secondly, antibodies are rarely produced in a first pregnancy and it is the second or subsequent child who is affected.

How iso-immunization occurs

Very occasionally a rhesus-negative mother forms antibodies from a previous transfusion of rhesus-positive blood. This is unlikely nowadays as the consequences of such an action are known. Nevertheless one must always enquire in the antenatal period if the woman has ever had a blood transfusion. More usually sensitization occurs in some way from the rhesus-positive fetus (Figure 3).

It is known that fetal red cells do enter the maternal circulation in pregnancy, but in such small amounts that they are destroyed before iso-immunization can occur. There may be a larger transplacental haemorrhage if the mother has a hypertensive condition or if there is some placental separation in pregnancy, trauma to the placenta during amniocentesis or external cephalic version. In these circumstances the risk of iso-immunization is increased. In labour, particularly

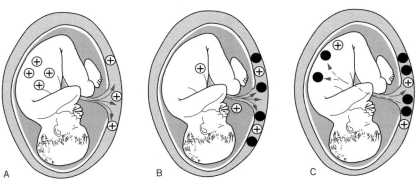

Figure 3   Antibody formation. **A**: Transfer of rhesus antigen (+) to the maternal circulation. **B**: Antibody formation (•) in the rhesus negative mother. **C**: Transfer of rhesus antibody to the fetus.

when the placenta separates, a much larger transfer may occur and this may provoke antibody production.

In a subsequent pregnancy antibodies circulating in the maternal bloodstream may pass through the placenta and destroy the fetal antigen, at the same time causing haemolysis of the fetal red cells (this will occur only if the fetus is rhesus-positive). This haemolysis leads to anaemia which may progress to a condition called *hydrops fetalis* where there is severe oedema, and enlargement of the liver and spleen which eventually results in intrauterine death. The placenta, too, is grossly oedematous, weighing about one third of the weight of the fetus.

Jaundice at birth is rare, but may appear during the first few hours. This is because until this time the mother has been dealing with the excess bilirubin from the broken down red cells. The bilirubin in the bloodstream at birth is unconjugated and must be dealt with by the baby. The quantities may be too great and the bilirubin rises to dangerous levels. There is a danger of kernicterus unless treatment is commenced.

Prevention of rhesus incompatibility

The *Kleihauer test* is carried out on a sample of maternal blood taken soon after delivery. The test estimates the number of fetal cells which have passed into the maternal circulation during the third stage of labour. All rhesus-negative mothers who are found to have rhesus-positive fetal cells in their blood are given an intramuscular injection of anti-D immunoglobulin 100 μg within 60 hours of delivery. This is the standard dose but may be increased if the Kleihauer test indicates an especially large leak of fetal cells into the maternal circulation. Anti-D immunoglobulin coats the fetal cells and thus prevents the formation of antibodies which could cross the placenta in a subsequent pregnancy and cause haemolysis of fetal red blood cells.

All rhesus-negative women who have an abortion should be given anti-D immunoglobulin within 60 hours of the abortion, otherwise iso-immunization may occur. The dose is usually 50 μg before the 20th week and 100 μg after. Similarly it is given in other circumstances when transplacental haemorrhage is likely, such as premature separation or trauma to the placenta following external cephalic version, chorionic villus biopsy and amniocentesis. Clarke *et al.* (1985) stress the importance of giving anti-D rhesus immuno-globin antenatally as well as postnatally. In studying deaths from rhesus haemolytic disease in England and Wales in 1982 and 1983, they conclude that about one third of the deaths could have been prevented only by giving anti-D rhesus immunoglobin antenatally as well as postnatally.

Investigations Certain routine investigations are made in the antenatal period. The maternal ABO and rhesus groups are determined and if the blood is rhesus-negative further specimens are examined during the third trimester for the presence of antibodies.

If no antibodies are detected there is nothing further to be done. If antibodies are present further investigation depends on the titre and whether or not they are increasing. The quantitation of maternal antibody levels has advanced, and these may now be used to defer an amniocentesis when the serum test can provide adequate reassurance that the fetus is not at risk. Maternal antibody titres of 1:16 in the indirect anti-globulin test (to detect free antibodies in maternal blood) is usually indicative of the need for further investigations (McDonald, 1992) because the risks to the fetus are increasing. After full discussion with the parents and having obtained their consent, amniocentesis is carried out to examine the liquor for bilirubin content. The amniotic fluid is scanned in a spectrophotometer to detect bile products, the optical density of which can be measured to provide an indication of the severity of the haemolysis of fetal red cells (Liley, 1961). The subsequent management depends on the severity of the disease and the period of gestation. When there is evidence of severe rhesus incompatibility before 33 weeks' gestation an intrauterine transfusion may be carried out. The aim is to prevent fetal death from severe anaemia and hydrops fetalis. At 33–34 weeks delivery can be expedited since the risks of prematurity are then less hazardous.

Intrauterine transfusion

The amount of blood given depends on the size of the fetus; this must be estimated as accurately as possible. Rhesus-negative blood of the same group as the mother is given via a cannula, using ultrasound for guidance, and the amount estimated at 60–70 ml/kg fetal weight. The donor blood is introduced into the fetal peritoneal cavity, where it is absorbed by the lymphatic system, transferred to the thoracic duct and so into the subclavian vein. The blood is absorbed quickly and by the third day is in the fetal circulation. Fetal blood transfusion by fetoscopy has been given in a few cases of severe rhesus iso-immunization (Rodeck *et al.*, 1981). The mother generally notices the increased fetal activity once the blood has been absorbed.

Method   The placenta is located with a scan and can then be avoided. On the previous day a contrast medium such as Urografin is introduced into the amniotic cavity. This will be swallowed by the fetus and become concentrated in the gut. The next day the woman is given a premedication such as pethidine and promethazine and taken to the X-ray department. After the skin has been prepared and anaesthetized, the skin is nicked and a Tuohy needle is inserted through the abdomen and uterine wall and into the amniotic cavity. The fetal gut can be seen on the viewing screen and the needle directed to the lower quadrant of the fetal abdomen. A fine nylon catheter is passed through the needle and when it is in place the needle is withdrawn. The blood is now given, taking about 30 minutes depending on the quantity. At the conclusion of the transfusion, the catheter is removed and the wound sealed with collodion. Careful record of the fetal heart is kept throughout.

The mother usually rests in bed for the next 24 hours and is closely observed for signs of preterm labour and infection. Transfusions may be repeated as necessary. Delivery will be induced at about 35 weeks, or before in severely affected cases, and later where the fetal health is satisfactory. Before preterm delivery, the lethicin–sphingomyelin ratio and phosphatidylcholine level are determined. Dexamethasone may be given, although rhesus haemolytic disease is technically a contraindication.

An alternative therapy is to give blood into the umbilical vessels and this can be performed from about 26–28 weeks gestation (McDonald, 1992). Fetal blood sampling by cordocentesis enables the fetal condition to be monitored accurately.

After delivery

Cord blood is taken and examined immediately for:

▶ Haemoglobin level and packed cell volume.
▶ ABO and rhesus group.
▶ Serum bilirubin level.
▶ Coombs' test.

Jaundice becomes apparent within 24 hours of birth in cases of rhesus and ABO incompatibility.

When there is ABO incompatibility between mother and fetus, fetal cells entering the maternal circulation are destroyed by the anti-A and anti-B haemolysis in the mother's blood before rhesus antibodies can be produced, with the result that the likelihood of haemolytic disease is reduced.

Coombs' direct antiglobulin test is carried out to detect the presence of maternal antibodies on the baby's red blood cells.

On the findings of the cord blood tests the future care is determined. The baby may be unaffected, but, if it is, careful observation will be required for the next few days. Most paediatricians agree that a positive Coombs' test, a serum bilirubin level of 88 µmol/l (5 mg/100 ml) or higher, or a haemoglobin level of less than 11 g/dl at birth warrants an immediate exchange transfusion.

The danger level of hyperbilirubinaemia leading to kernicterus depends on many factors and is the subject of much debate. This level is lower in preterm and ill babies who are acidaemic, especially if they have had drugs which compete with bilirubin for the albumin-binding sites (Kelnar *et al.*, 1995). Therefore, exchange transfusion would be carried out much earlier.

In cases of rhesus incompatibility the rate at which the serum bilirubin rises, the degree of anaemia and the condition of the baby are key factors in determining the need for exchange transfusion. The transfusion may be carried out well before the serum bilirubin reaches the danger zone because of the rapidity of the haemolysis and the increasing severity of the anaemia.

In cases of hyperbilirubinaemia in the term baby, perhaps associated with severe physiological jaundice, the trend now is to decrease intervention and carefully observe the baby (Torres-Torres *et al.*, 1994), allowing the serum bilirubin to reach 300–350 µmol/l, even up to 380 µmol/l in some cases, before performing an exchange transfusion. It is postulated that there may actually be beneficial effects of bilirubin at cellular level (Yau and Stevenson, 1995), and this has to be balanced against the dangers of severe hyperbilirubinaemia leading to kernicterus.

In a rhesus affected baby phototherapy should be started at birth; even if an exchange transfusion is planned phototherapy is given whilst preparations are being made for the transfusion. This action appears to reduce the number of transfusions required (Kelnar *et al.*, 1995).

Exchange Blood Transfusion

An exchange blood transfusion is carried out in haemolytic disease to avoid the dangers of kernicterus, by removing blood containing maternal antibodies and bilirubin from the baby's circulation, and to correct anaemia. The baby's blood is replaced with fresh rhesus-negative blood, the ABO group being compatible with the baby's. Usually a two-volume exchange is given, 170 ml/kg, so as to remove as much of the undesirable factors as possible. In other circumstances, as in an exchange transfusion carried out for severe sepsis or poisoning, a single-volume exchange may be used (85 ml/kg).

As much as 90% of the infant's blood may be removed and replaced with donor blood which will not be haemolysed by residual maternal antibody. This should be performed as soon as possible after the need for an exchange transfusion has become clear. Less haemolysis will then occur, the peak serum bilirubin level will be lower and risks of a dramatic rise in serum bilirubin level, with ill-effects occurring sooner than anticipated, will be minimized. In addition, there will be less risk of an acute anaemia and a deterioration in the general condition of a small or preterm infant.

Technique

The most efficient technique, and the safest, is to perform a two-site exchange transfusion. Blood is withdrawn from an artery, a peripheral artery by choice but an umbilical artery may be used if it is being cannulated for other reasons, and the donor blood is infused through a peripheral vein. The whole procedure should take about two hours, perhaps a little less in large, healthy infants or a little longer in sick babies. A precise record must be kept of the fluid balance at all times, and the baby's blood volume should be constant throughout because the two processes are done in parallel. An infusion syringe pump may be used for the donor blood, and that and the fluid balance chart may be the responsibility of one person and the withdrawal of blood from the arterial line the responsibility of another, either the doctor or midwife in each case.

Samples of blood should be checked for bilirubin, haemoglobin and serum sodium, potassium, calcium and glucose immediately before the exchange transfusion, after one hour, at the end of the procedure and again over the next hour. Blood gases may also need to be checked. These precautions are taken because the donor blood, if it is not fresh, may be acidotic and have a high potassium level. This is unsafe unless given slowly. The blood frequently contains dextrose in the anticoagulant, and a rebound hypoglycaemia may occur after the exchange transfusion. The anticoagulant may also bind calcium and cause hypocalcaemia which can result in convulsions during the procedure.

The traditional technique for exchange transfusion is to cannulate the umbilical vein. A three-way tap is used to withdraw 5–10–20 ml of blood into a syringe, to discard it, and then to replace it with the same volume of donor blood. The disadvantages of this approach include the cannulation of the umbilical vein itself which is associated with necrotizing enterocolitis. Other problems include the swings in central venous pressure that result from alternate removal and injection of blood into the inferior vena cava and the possible liver and bowel damage caused by the retrograde perfusion of these tissues with hypoxic, acidotic and hyperkalaemic blood. Since some babies tolerate the procedure so badly, it is wise to disturb the infant's bodily functions as little as possible.

Whatever technique is used, strict aseptic precautions must be taken.

Observations

Accurate records of the fluid exchange must be kept. Observations must include the continuous display of an electrocardiogram and regular recording of body colour, transcutaneous oxygen if in respiratory distress, temperature, blood pressure, respirations and movements. Any twitching will be noted. The procedure will usually be performed in an incubator to prevent excessive heat loss and full resuscitation equipment must be available.

Subsequent care

Sometimes two or three exchange transfusions are necessary in severe cases, although nowadays the baby is also treated with phototherapy and this helps to reduce the rise in serum bilirubin and the need for repeat transfusions. The baby is usually kept in the neonatal unit until it is certain that no further exchange transfusions are required. The mother should be encouraged to visit and handle her baby as much as possible.

Before discharge or possibly later a small top-up transfusion may be given if the haemoglobin falls below 8 g/dl. Anaemia occurs due to haemolysis of red blood cells and the reduced activity of the bone marrow. A top-up transfusion may further delay the activity of the bone marrow and consequently is given only in cases of severe anaemia. Oral iron should be given at an early date.

Prognosis

Provided the bilirubin levels have not risen too high, the danger of kernicterus and its sequelae of cerebral palsy, mental retardation and deafness should be avoided.

Follow-up is essential to assess developmental progress and to detect and treat anaemia.

References

Blackburn, S. (1995) Hyperbilirubinaemia and neonatal jaundice. *Neonatal Network* 14(7): 15–25.

Brown, L.P. (1992) Breastfeeding and jaundice: cause for concern? *NAACOGS Clinical Issues in Perinatal and Women's Health Nursing* 3(4): 613–619.

Brown, L.P., Arnold, L. & Allison, D. *et al.* (1993) Incidence and pattern of jaundice in healthy breastfed infants during the first month of life. *Nursing Research* 42(2): 106–110.

Buchan, P.C. (1979) Pathogenesis of neonatal hyperbilirubinaemia after induction of labour with oxytocin. *Br. Med. J.* 2: 1255–1257.

Carvalho, M. de, Hall, M. & Harvey, D. (1981) Effects of water supplementation on physiological jaundice in breastfed babies. *Arch. Dis. Childh.* 56(7): 568–569.

Clarke, C.A., Mollison, P.L. & Whitfield, A.G.W. (1985) Deaths from rhesus haemolytic disease in England and Wales in 1982 and 1983. *Br. Med. J.* 291: 17–19.

D'Souza, S.W., Black, P., Macfarlane, T. & Richards, B. (1979) The effect of oxytocin in induced labour on neonatal jaundice. *Br. J. Obstet. Gynaecol.* 86: 133–138.

Kelnar, C.J.H., Harvey, D. & Simpson, C. (1995) *The Sick Newborn Baby.* London: Baillière Tindall.

Lav, S.P. & Fung, K.R. (1984) Serum bilirubin kinetics in intermittent phototherapy of physiological jaundice. *Arch. Dis. Childh.* 59: 892–894.

Lewis, H.M., Campbell, R.H.A. & Hambleton, G. (1982) Use or abuse of phototherapy for physiological jaundice of newborn infants. *Lancet* ii: 408–410.

Liley, A.W. (1961) Liquor amnii analysis in management of pregnancy complicated by rhesus sensitization. *Am. J. Obstet. Gynecol.* 82: 1359.

McDonald, M. (1992) Rhesus incompatibility. *Nurs. Times* 88(19): 42–44.

Messner, K.H., Leure-Dupree, A.E. & Maisels, M.J. (1975) The effects of continuous prolonged illumination on the newborn primate retina (abstr). *Paediatr. Res.* 9: 368.

Rodeck, C.H., Holman, C.A., Karnicki, J. *et al.* (1981) Direct intravascular fetal blood transfusion by fetoscopy in severe Rhesus isoimmunisation. *Lancet* i: 625–627.

Salariya, E.M. & Robertson, C.M. (1993) Relationships between baby feeding types and patterns, gut transit time of meconium and the incidence of neonatal jaundice. *Midwifery* 9(4): 235–242.

Schneider, V. (1993) The differential diagnosos of neonatal jaundice. *J. Am. Acad. Physician Assistants* 6(8): 533–541.

Singhi, S., Choo Kang, E. & Hall, J. St. E. (1982) Hazards of maternal hydration with 5% dextrose. *Lancet* ii: 335–336.

Torres-Torres, M., Tayaba, R., Weintraub, A. & Holzman, I.R. (1994) New perspectives on neonatal hyperbilirubinaemia. *Mount Sinai J. Med.* 61(5): 424–428.

Yau, T.C. & Stevenson, D.K. (1995) Advances in the diagnosis and treatment of neonatal hyperbilirubinaemia. *Clinics in Perinatology* 22(3): 741–758.

Further Reading

Dennery, P.A., Rhine, W.D. & Stevenson, D.K. (1995) Neonatal jaundice – what now? *Clin. Pediatr.* 34(2): 103–107.

Dodd, K.L. (1993) Neonatal jaundice – a lighter touch? *Arch. Dis. Childh.* 68(5): 529–532.

Gartner, L.M., Catz, C.S. & Yaffe, S.J. (1994) Neonatal bilirubin workshop. *Pediatrics* 94 (4 Pt 1): 537–540.

Matthew, R. (1995) Nursing care of infants on phototherapy. *Nurs. J. India* 86(9): 197–198.

Murphy, B.N. & Welch, R. (1992) Home phototherapy for the jaundiced full-term newborn. *J. Home Health Care Pract.* 5(1): 26–33.

Rubaltelli, F.F. & Griffith, P.F. (1992) Management of hyperbilirubinaemia and prevention of kernicterus. *Drugs* 43(6): 864–872.

Tan, K.L. (1993) Neonatal jaundice: update on phototherapy management. *Ann. Acad. Med., Singapore* 22(2): 225–228.

71

Cardiac and Circulatory Conditions in the Newborn

Cardiac conditions account for about 30% of all congenital malformations; they are the commonest single group of congenital abnormalities. The incidence is approximately 8 per 1000 live births, with about a third of these being mild defects requiring no treatment.

Approximately 40% of babies with Down's syndrome have some form of congenital cardiac malformation. The commonest lesion is an atrioventricular defect. Tetralogy of Fallot, ventricular septal defects and patent ductus arteriosus are also common.

Mothers with diabetes mellitus have about a 5% greater risk of having a baby with a structural cardiac defect (Rowland et al., 1973), particularly ventricular septal defect, coarctation of the aorta or transposition of the great arteries.

Siblings of a baby with a heart defect have a 1–3% increased risk of a cardiac lesion, depending on the type of defect (Nora and Nora, 1978). The offspring of a parent with a cardiac abnormality are also at a greater risk of congenital cardiac conditions. The degree of risk depends on the lesion the parent has (Nora and Nora, 1978; Rose et al., 1985).

Aetiology

The cardiovascular system is the first system to be functional in utero, with blood beginning to circulate by the end of the third week. Development continues at a rapid rate to ensure that the growing embryo is adequately supplied with the necessary nutrients. The heart and circulatory system are therefore susceptible to teratogenic insults from very early in the pregnancy, before most women realize they are pregnant. The effects of any such insults will depend on which parts of the cardiac system are forming at that time (Nora and Nora, 1983).

The aetiology is thought to be multifactorial in 90% of cases, with both genetic and environmental factors implicated. Approximately 8% are caused by genetic factors alone, whilst the remaining 2% can be traced to an environmental factor, such as rubella infection in early pregnancy.

In order to recognize and understand the presentation and implications of cardiac conditions, it is important to have an understanding of fetal circulation and the changes which take place after birth. These are comprehensively explained in Chapters 9 and 63.

Investigations into Cardiac Conditions

General examination

In many conditions obvious clinical signs are not present in the early neonatal period. One of the first suggestions of a cardiac condition may be cardiac failure. Early signs and symptoms of cardiac failure are persistent, unexplained tachypnoea, tachycardia and hepatomegaly. A history of dyspnoea, feeding difficulties or vomiting are also common. Cardiomegaly, sweating, excessive weight gain from oedema and peripheral oedema are late signs.

Auscultation

Abnormal heart sounds may be identified, such as unusually loud sounds, a prolonged interval between them or extra noises such as clicks being heard. In addition to these, murmurs may be detected which are caused by blood flowing through an abnormal tract in the heart, such as a hole or malformed valve.

Chest radiography

The position, size and shape of the heart are noted on chest X-ray. An assessment of the relative positions and sizes of the heart chambers and great vessels is made.

Electrocardiography (ECG)

An ECG recording should be taken when the baby is quiet, preferably asleep. Accurate interpretation of the recording may give a great deal of information about the haemodynamic state of the baby, severity of the lesion and the need for further investigations.

Echocardiography

Ultrasound scanning may be used antenatally or post-natally to examine the anatomy of the heart chambers, valves, associated vessels and other structures. Doppler echocardiography allows measurement of the rate and direction of blood flow through the heart, detecting obstructions and shunting of blood through septal defects.

Detailed fetal ultrasound scanning, including Doppler assessment, is now routinely offered in most obstetric units in early pregnancy to screen for abnormalities. The vast majority of major cardiac defects can be identified by the 18th week of pregnancy. If the parents already have a child with a cardiac problem, have a congenital cardiac condition themselves or if the mother has diabetes mellitus, the midwife should ensure a detailed scan is offered usually between 18 and 20 weeks of pregnancy. The parents may wish to discuss the possible outcomes prior to the scan and will need much support if any abnormality is detected. They should have the opportunity to discuss what will happen once their baby is delivered. An antenatal visit to the neonatal intensive care unit may be helpful in their preparation.

Magnetic resonance imaging (MRI)

MRI scanning gives much clearer pictures of the anatomy of the heart and is becoming more widely used on the neonate. It is not as convenient as ultrasound scanning as it cannot be performed at the cotside. However, the quality of images produced makes this a worthwhile procedure, particularly in complex lesions.

Cardiac catheterization

As the quality of information available from non-invasive diagnostic techniques continues to improve, cardiac catheterization is more widely used as a method of treatment rather than diagnosis (Lock *et al.*, 1986). The procedure is performed under general anaesthetic and involves passing a catheter through the femoral vein into the right side of the heart, pulmonary arteries and its branches. In neonates it is often possible to pass the catheter into the left side of the heart through the foramen ovale or a ventricular septal defect if one is present.

Cardiac catheterization allows the identification of abnormal tracts and the measurement of blood pressure and oxygen saturation levels within the heart and great vessels. A radio-opaque dye can be injected into the heart using this procedure (angiography), which enables filming of the passage of blood to help identify abnormalities and obstructions more precisely. Treatment of some conditions, such as valve stenosis and small septal defects, may be carried out using special balloon catheters.

Types of Congenital Heart Disease

Congenital cardiac lesions may be separated into two groups – *acyanotic* and *cyanotic*. Cyanosis is not always present at birth, but may develop later as the ductus arteriosus closes. With an increase in the number of home and Domino deliveries, the midwife must be aware of early signs and symptoms of a cardiac defect. If the baby is breathless, dyspnoeic, failing to thrive, gaining weight excessively or showing signs of cyanosis, an urgent referral to a paediatrician is vital.

ACYANOTIC LESIONS

Patent ductus arteriosus (PDA)

The ductus arteriosus diverts blood *in utero* from the lungs into the descending aorta. Specialized contractile tissue forms in the ductus from about 25 weeks' gestation, which enables it to close. This is not fully mature and functional for about three months which partly explains the high incidence of patent ductus arteriosus in preterm babies (Clyman, 1986). In the term infant the ductus normally closes at 10–15 hours of age. Spontaneous closure in term babies after two weeks is rare, whilst closure in preterm infants may occur up to three months after birth as the contractile tissue of the ductus develops.

Symptoms of patent ductus arteriosus occur at about 3–7 days of age when the baby appears tachypnoeic, dyspnoeic and lethargic. The pulses are bounding and both systolic and diastolic murmurs can be heard. Readmission to hospital is necessary to treat this condition.

Treatment will include restricting fluids, giving adequate oxygen to eliminate hypoxia which maintains the patency of the ductus and possibly prescribing diuretics. Indomethacin may also be prescribed for preterm babies to close the ductus arteriosus (Rennie and Cooke, 1991). Surgical ligation of the duct is rarely necessary but may be indicated if medical management fails.

Ventricular septal defect (VSD)

This is one of the commonest defects to present in childhood, accounting for about one third of all lesions.

There is a hole in the membranous or muscular part of the septum between the ventricles which allows a left-to-right flow of blood through it (Sutherland and Godman, 1986). Although usually singular, multiple defects may be present and ventricular septal defects are often found in conjunction with other cardiac conditions.

The clinical presentation and prognosis depend on the size and position of the defect. Babies with small defects may be asymptomatic and the characteristic murmur is often not heard until the baby is a few weeks old; many are diagnosed at the six week examination. No treatment is needed for these as the vast majority of them close spontaneously over a period of several years. The parents will need the condition fully explained.

Larger defects may cause dyspnoea and difficulty with feeds in the early weeks of life. Surgical repair may be necessary if the symptoms are severe.

Atrial septal defect (ASD)

There are two types of atrial septal defects:

1   Simple defects in which there is a hole in the atrial septum.
2   Complex defects where there is also involvement of the mitral valve and in severe cases (atrioventricular defects) the ventricular septum, mitral and tricuspid valves.

A simple defect very rarely gives rise to symptoms until adult life and accounts for almost 9% of all cardiac lesions. Surgery to repair a small lesion is carried out at about 4–5 years of age, if required. If the mitral valve is involved, surgery is performed earlier, at about 2–3 years of age, as deterioration is more likely.

Babies with complete *atrioventricular defects* (AVD) have a poor prognosis and there is a high mortality associated with surgery. Babies usually present in the first few weeks with dyspnoea, poor feeding and failure to thrive. Mild cyanosis may occur and there are abnormal heart sounds including a systolic murmur. About 30% of babies with an atrioventricular defect also have Down's syndrome. This is the commonest cardiac defect found in babies with Down's syndrome, accounting for about 40% of associated cardiac lesions.

Coarctation of the aorta

In this condition, which accounts for 6% of all cardiac defects, there is a narrowing of the aorta where the ductus arteriosus joins the aorta (Allen *et al.*, 1988). Associated lesions are present in more than 50% of cases, most commonly ventricular septal defect, aortic stenosis and mitral valve abnormalities. A small narrowing may not produce symptoms for several years.

More severe strictures cause a neonatal emergency. There is a sudden onset of symptoms as the ductus arteriosus closes, usually between days 2–10. The baby becomes dyspnoeic and tachypnoeic with hepatomegaly and signs of renal and cardiac failure. Femoral pulses are weak or absent and the blood pressure in the arms is higher than in the legs. The baby needs urgent treatment with an intravenous infusion of prostaglandins to maintain the ductus arteriosus. Once the baby's condition is stable, surgery is performed to widen the constricted segment.

Pulmonary valve stenosis

This is a narrowing of the pulmonary valve and as an isolated condition accounts for about 8% of cardiac conditions. Even when severe narrowing occurs the only symptom in neonates is often a murmur.

Mild stenosis usually improves with growth, whilst severe stenosis worsens. Treatment, if needed, is by pulmonary valvuloplasty, where a balloon catheter is inflated inside the obstructed valve to widen the orifice (Ettedgui *et al.*, 1988).

Aortic valve stenosis

This is a narrowing of the aortic valve causing restricted bloodflow from the left ventricle into the aorta. Isolated cases account for 6% of cardiac conditions but this abnormality also occurs in association with about 6% of other conditions, especially coarctation of the aorta. It is four times more common in boys than girls.

Mild or moderate stenosis is usually asymptomatic in neonates although a murmur may be present. A severe obstruction may cause sudden collapse in the neonatal period. Initial treatment of severe stenosis is by surgical aortic valvotomy, but valve replacement is often subsequently required during the growing period of the child.

CYANOTIC LESIONS

Transposition of the great arteries

This defect accounts for 4% of all lesions. The pulmonary artery arises from the left ventricle and the aorta from the right ventricle, thus producing two independent circulations (Figure 1). A chest X-ray shows a typical 'egg-on-side' appearance of the heart due to the aorta overriding the pulmonary artery and enlargement of the right ventricle.

Whilst the foramen ovale and ductus arteriosus remain patent, blood mixes. Closure of the ductus arteriosus results in severe, worsening cyanosis, dyspnoea and cardiac failure. Urgent treatment with an intravenous infusion of prostaglandins is needed to maintain a patent ductus arteriosus, allowing mixing of the two blood supplies. This may be followed by definitive surgery in the next few days when the pulmonary artery, aorta and coronary arteries are 'switched' back to their normal anatomical positions

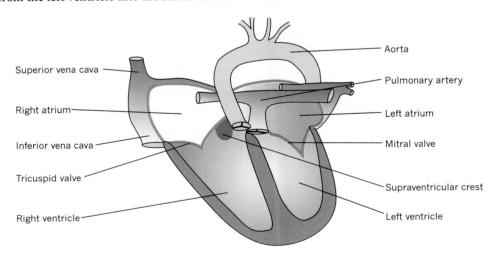

Figure 1   Transposition of the great arteries.

(Quaegebeur *et al.*, 1986). Some surgeons delay this operation for 6–9 months and perform an atrial balloon septostomy in the meantime. The inflated balloon of a cardiac catheter is pulled through the atrial septum forming a hole thus allowing blood to mix.

Approximately 20% of cases also have a ventricular septal defect. In these babies cyanosis is less severe and the 'switch' operation can be delayed for up to two years depending on the severity of symptoms.

Tetralogy of Fallot

Tetralogy of Fallot accounts for approximately 5% of cardiac lesions. There are four abnormalities:

1   Pulmonary stenosis.
2   Ventricular septal defect (VSD).
3   Right ventricular hypertrophy.
4   Overriding aorta, across the ventricular septal defect (Figure 2).

In the neonatal period this condition often presents with symptoms of a ventricular septal defect and mild pulmonary stenosis. The baby is pink at birth, gradually developing cyanosis on crying and dyspnoea as the pulmonary stenosis worsens which may take several months. Many babies present at the age of 4–6 months with cyanotic episodes, often in the morning, resulting in a loss of consciousness.

All patients require surgery to correct the abnormalities, the timing of which depends on the severity of the various defects and symptoms produced.

Total anomolous pulmonary venous drainage (TAPVD)

This is a rare condition, accounting for about 1% of cardiac abnormalities. Forty per cent of cases have associated cardiac defects. The pulmonary veins drain into the right atrium instead of the left. There is also a right-to-left shunt of blood with mixed oxygenated and deoxygenated blood being circulated.

In the obstructed form, pulmonary venous obstruction causes central cyanosis, dyspnoea and tachypnoea in the first few days. Urgent surgery is required to

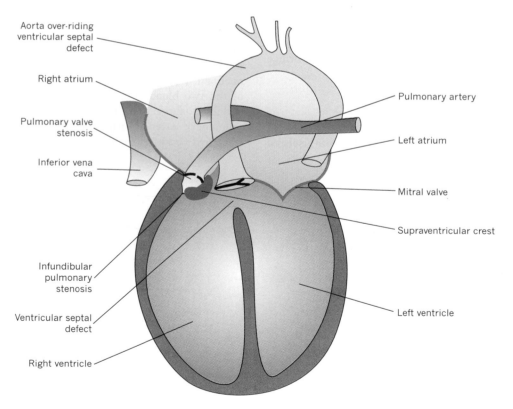

Figure 2   Tetralogy of Fallot.

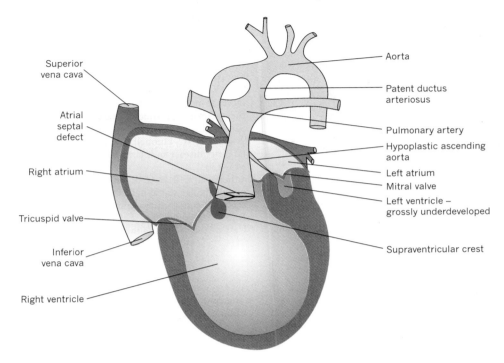

Figure 3 Hypoplastic left heart syndrome.

correct the anomaly. In the non-obstructed form, symptoms often do not develop for 2–3 months, sometimes longer, allowing surgery to be delayed.

Hypoplastic left heart syndrome

In this condition the whole of the left side of the heart is underdeveloped (Figure 3). It is the commonest cause of cardiac failure in the first 2–3 days of life and symptoms present much earlier than in other cardiac conditions. The ascending aorta and coronary arteries are hypoplastic with blood passing into the aorta through the patent ductus arteriosus. As the ductus closes the baby becomes increasingly cyanosed and dyspnoeic. The majority of babies die within the first week. Surgery is attempted in some cases (Barber *et al.*, 1988) but no long-term results are available to assess its effectiveness and most cardiologists do not recommend any treatment.

Follow-up and Support

Many babies are discharged home whilst awaiting non-urgent cardiac surgery; some will be cyanosed. Dyspnoea and tiredness may make feeding difficult and many babies require some nasogastric tube feeds. Weight gain is often slow but may be improved by offering small, frequent feeds or by adding calorific supplements to the milk. Early involvement of a dietician is important and the family will require much support from the midwife. Regular and accurate administration of medication will be vital to the baby's condition and the midwife must ensure the parents are confident and competent at giving these.

Information about local and national cardiac support groups may be helpful.

References

Allen, L.D., Chita, S.K., Anderson, R.H. *et al.* (1988) Coarctation of the aorta in prenatal life: an echocardiographic, anatomical and functional study. *Br. Heart J.* 59: 356–360.

Barber, G., Murphy, J.D., Piggott, J.D. *et al.* (1988) The evolving pattern of survival following palliative surgery for hypoplastic left heart syndrome. *J. Am. Coll. Cardiol.* 2: 139A.

Clyman, R.I. (1986) Pharmacology of the fetal and neonatal

ductus arteriosus. In Doyle, E.F., Engle, M.A., Gersomy, W.M. *et al.* (eds) *Pediatric Cardiology*, pp. 871–875. New York: Springer-Verlag.

Ettedgui, J.A., Martin, R.P., Jones, O.D.H. *et al.* (1988) Balloon dilatation of the pulmonary valve in neonates: technical considerations and results. *Br. Heart J.* 59: 118.

Lock, J.E., Keane, J.F. & Fellows, K.E. (1986) The use of catheter intervention procedures for congenital heart disease. *J. Am. Coll. Cardiol.* 7: 1420–1423.

Nora, J.J. & Nora, A.H. (1978) *Genetics and Counselling in Cardiovascular Diseases*. Springfield, IL: Charles C. Thomas.

Nora, J.J. & Nora, A.H. (1983) Genetic epidemiology of congenital heart disease. In Steinberg, A.G., Bearn, A.G., Motulsky, A.G. *et al.* (eds) *Progress in Medical Genetics*, Vol. 5., p. 102. Philadelphia: W.B. Saunders.

Quaegebeur, J.M., Rohmer, J., Ottenkamp, J. *et al.* (1986) The arterial switch operation: an eight year experience. *J. Thorac. Cardiovasc. Surg.* 92: 361–384.

Rennie, J.M. & Cooke, R.W.I. (1991) Prolonged low dose Indomethacin for the persistent ductus arteriosus of prematurity. *Arch. Dis. Childh.* 66: 55–58.

Rose, V., Gold, R.J.M., Lindsey, G. *et al.* (1985) A possible increase in the incidence of congenital cardiac defects among the offspring of affected parents. *J. Am. Coll. Cardiol.* 6: 376–382.

Rowland, T.W., Hubbell, J.P. & Nadas, A.S. (1973) Congenital heart disease in infants of diabetic mothers. *J. Pediat.* 83: 815–820.

Sutherland, G.R. & Godman, M.J. (1986) The natural history of ventricular septal defects. A long-term prospective cross-sectional echocardiographic study. In Hunter, A.S. & Hall, R.J.C. (eds) *Clinical Echocardiography*. Tunbridge Wells: Castle House Publications.

Further Reading

Moore, K.L. (1988) *The Developing Human. Clinically Orientated Embryology*. Philadelphia: W.B. Saunders.

Jordan, S. & Scott, O. (1989) *Heart Disease in Paediatrics*. London: Butterworths.

Roberton, N.R.C. (ed.) (1992) *Textbook of Neonatology*. Edinburgh: Churchill Livingstone.

72

Metabolic and Endocrine Disorders of the Newborn

Hypoglycaemia

There is much debate over what constitutes a normal plasma glucose value for both term and preterm infants, and therefore what constitutes a finite definition of hypoglycaemia (Koh *et al.*, 1988). It is now accepted that asymptomatic babies with a plasma glucose level of less than 2.6 mmol/l – particularly for a prolonged period – may suffer long-term neurological abnormalities (Lucas *et al.*, 1988; David, 1992). Plasma glucose levels should therefore be maintained above 2.6 mmol/l in both term and preterm babies.

Causes

Hypoglycaemia occurs most commonly in low birthweight babies and in babies of diabetic mothers. Low birthweight babies tend to have inadequate glycogen stores and those who are small-for-gestational-age also suffer from intrauterine malnutrition. The baby of the diabetic mother is subject to hypoglycaemia due to the continued overproduction of insulin for some hours after birth, even though the baby is no longer subject to the mother's high blood glucose levels.

Other babies at risk of hypoglycaemia are those who have been asphyxiated at birth or who have respiratory distress syndrome, hypothermia, cerebral damage, severe haemolytic disease or some rare inborn error of metabolism.

Signs

The signs are non-specific and could be attributed to a variety of conditions. They are:

- Lethargy.
- Hypotonia.
- Cyanosis.
- Periods of apnoea.
- Shallow respirations.

▶ Twitching leading to convulsions.
▶ Eventual coma.

In some cases, hypoglycaemia may be asymptomatic.

Management

Prevention Early feeding is essential to prevent hypoglycaemia in babies who are at risk. These babies are also regularly screened for hypoglycaemia by using Dextrostix or BM Stix strip tests during the first 2 or 3 days of life. A specimen of blood should be sent to the laboratory for estimation of true blood glucose if the Dextrostix reading is below 2.5 mmol/l or BM Stix below 2.2 mmol/l. Test strip readings are inaccurate at low levels and in polycythaemic babies it is important to maintain the baby's temperature within the normal range.

Treatment of mild hypoglycaemia In mild or asymptomatic cases where the true blood glucose level is more than 1.7 mmol/l, the baby should be given a feed of breast or bottle milk immediately. The baby's axillary temperature is checked and the environmental temperature adjusted as necessary. Repeat the Dextrostix or BM Stix one hour after the feed. If the level is still low an intravenous infusion may be required.

Treatment of severe hypoglycaemia If the true blood glucose level is below 1.7 mmol/l, an intravenous infusion of 10% glucose solution is commenced at a rate of 10 ml/kg per hour. Oral feeds are temporarily stopped. The Dextrostix or BM Stix levels are checked at half-hourly to hourly intervals until they are stable – Dextrostix above 2.5 mmol/l; BM Stix above 2.2 mmol/l. The blood glucose levels continue to be monitored closely and oral feeds are gradually reintroduced to replace the intravenous fluids.

If the baby is fitting with a blood glucose level less than 1.7 mmol/l, a bolus dose of 15% glucose solution, 2–3 ml/kg, is given intravenously. An infusion of 10% glucose is then commenced and close monitoring of the Dextrostix or BM Stix levels continues, as a rebound hypoglycaemia is likely.

Follow-up Careful follow-up is essential for babies who have had symptomatic hypoglycaemia because of the risk of neurological damage.

Hypocalcaemia and Hypomagnesaemia

Hypocalcaemia (neonatal tetany) is defined as a blood calcium level less than 1.7 mmol/l. The normal range in a newborn baby is 1.8–2.2 mmol/l. These levels fall over the first 48 hours then rise again and stabilize in response to an increase in parathyroid hormone levels after three days.

Early hypocalcaemia occurs in the first three days and is exacerbated in babies born preterm, asphyxiated, infected or with respiratory distress syndrome.

There is a close relationship between serum calcium and magnesium levels. Hypomagnesaemia is often associated with hypocalcaemia. The normal range is 0.6–1.0 mmol/l and hypomagnesaemia is defined as a serum level less than 0.6 mmol/l.

Late hypocalcaemia occurs between the 5th and 8th days. It is usually associated with feeding the baby unmodified cows' milk. In developed countries this is now rare due to the availability of modified baby milks.

The high phosphorus content of unmodified cows' milk causes a rise in the blood phosphate level and, in response, the serum calcium level falls. The excess phosphate cannot be excreted rapidly enough to prevent a drop in serum calcium because the kidneys of the newborn are immature.

Some immigrant mothers and those in low socio-economic groups may have been hypocalcaemic in pregnancy due to a deficient intake of vitamin D and calcium and their babies are particularly likely to develop tetany. In rare cases persistent neonatal tetany may be associated with maternal hyperparathyroidism.

Signs

The signs of neonatal tetany are irritability followed by twitching, periods of apnoea and sometimes repeated convulsions. Between convulsions the baby is alert when roused.

Management

Prevention Maternal hypocalcaemia in pregnancy should be prevented by encouraging mothers to have an adequate intake of vitamin D and calcium. Breast-feeding should be encouraged where possible. Modified baby milks should always be recommended if the baby is artificially fed because the amount of phosphorus in these milks is reduced.

Treatment If the baby is fitting, with a low calcium level, an infusion of 10% calcium gluconate, diluted 1:4 with sterile water or 10% dextrose, 0.2–0.5 ml/kg, is commenced. It must be given slowly and the baby's heart rate is constantly monitored throughout as bradycardias and arrhythmias may occur. It is important to monitor the infusion site closely as extravasation of calcium solutions may cause severe skin necrosis. Solutions containing calcium must not be given through umbilical vessels or mixed with bicarbonate, phosphate or parenteral solutions as precipitates may form.

Oral calcium supplements are given to asymptomatic, hypocalcaemic babies.

Persistent hypocalcaemia may be associated with hypomagnesaemia and a single intramuscular injection of 0.2 mmol/kg 50% magnesium sulphate solution will correct both conditions.

Prognosis Neurological development is usually normal in babies who have suffered from transient hypocalcaemia between the 5th and 8th day of life. The only sequela seems to be hypoplasia of the dental enamel in the first teeth which predisposes to dental caries.

Hypernatraemia

Hypernatraemia is defined as a plasma sodium level above 143 mmol/l. It may be caused by a failure to compensate adequately for large fluid losses in very preterm babies, for example during the use of phototherapy or radiant heaters and episodes of diarrhoea or vomiting. Excess sodium may be given unintentionally in the form of bicarbonate or in plasma infusions.

Prevention

All babies receiving intensive care should have plasma electrolytes checked at least daily, and adjustments made to their intake appropriately. All mothers should be encouraged to breastfeed if possible.

It is important to teach parents who choose to bottle-feed, to measure the milk powder accurately, as heaped or tightly packed scoops, or extra scoops, will increase the sodium content of the feed. Very often the baby is then thirsty and cries; if the parents respond by offering more milk, rather than boiled water, the situation is exacerbated. If the baby becomes dehydrated, perhaps in hot weather or due to an infection such as diarrhoea, the serum sodium levels will rise even further. The kidneys of the baby are immature and cannot cope with an excess sodium load, especially when there is insufficient water for excretion, so that hypernatraemia occurs. This condition may cause irreversible brain damage.

Signs

Initially the baby may be fretful and thirsty. Then oedema becomes apparent and the baby becomes dehydrated and pyrexial. In severe cases convulsions will occur, leading to death if untreated.

Treatment

The baby must be slowly rehydrated by an intravenous infusion of an isotonic solution such as 0.9% saline or plasma initially. This will reduce the risk of permanent damage caused by cerebral oedema. Sedation will be necessary to control fits and the baby will be screened for infection. Breast milk or a low-solute artificial milk will be given, great care being taken to reconstitute the milk correctly. No solids are introduced until the baby is 4–6 months old to reduce the solute load to the kidneys.

Prognosis

Neurological abnormalities may occur following hypernatraemia and thus the baby is followed up by a paediatrician.

Phenylketonuria

Phenylketonuria is an autosomal recessively inherited inborn error of metabolism which occurs in about 1 in 10 000 births. It is more common in the Irish population, where the incidence is about 1 in 4000. Owing to its recessive inheritance the parents have a 1 in 4 risk of producing a child with phenylketonuria. In this condition there is a deficiency of the enzyme phenylalanine hydroxylase which is necessary for converting the amino acid phenylalanine to tyrosine. This results in a raised level of phenylalanine in the blood and tissues which will lead to severe brain damage unless early treatment is instituted. Phenylpyruvic acid is excreted in the urine.

All newborn babies are routinely screened for this

condition, so it is rare to see older children or adults with long-term effects of seizures, developmental delay and severe eczema.

Diagnosis

In the past a urine test, the Phenistix colour test, was carried out at the age of 6 weeks to detect the presence of phenylpyruvic acid. Nowadays babies can be screened earlier by more accurate blood tests.

Guthrie test   This test is carried out between the 6th and 14th days of life when the baby has been taking milk feeds for more than 48 hours. Capillary blood from a heel prick is collected to cover four circles on a specially prepared absorbent card which is then sent to the laboratory. The Guthrie may be a bacterial inhibition test; thus if the baby (or the mother if breastfeeding) is receiving antibiotics the test should be deferred until 48 hours after the completion of treatment because antibiotics will destroy *Bacillus subtilis* and a false result is thus likely. However, *Bacillus subtilis* has largely been superseded by plasma amino acid chromatography.

Blood taken for the Guthrie test can also be used to screen for other conditions such as hypothyroidism, galactosaemia, maple syrup urine disease, histidinaemia and tyrosinaemia.

Other tests   Antenatal diagnosis using DNA analysis and gene probes is now possible.

Management

The baby is fed on a low phenylalanine milk such as Minafen (Cow & Gate). The requirement for phenylalanine (and tyrosine) which are needed for growth has to be balanced against the toxicity from high serum phenylalanine levels. Blood samples are checked regularly for phenylalanine levels and adjustments to the diet are made as necessary. With a low phenylalanine diet the child should develop normally. From the age of about 10 years strict adherence to the diet is no longer so important. However, there are advantages in maintaining the diet even if less rigorously, because mental function can still be mildly impaired by high phenylalanine levels.

It is important that mothers with phenylketonuria resume their low phenylalanine diet at least six months before pregnancy. High phenylalanine levels in the mother during pregnancy damage the developing fetus, so must be avoided. In some antenatal clinics all mothers are screened for phenylketonuria early in pregnancy by a urine test with Phenistix. Phenylpyruvic acid is excreted in the urine.

Hypothyroidism

Hypothyroidism affects 1 in 3500 infants. If untreated it results in cretinism with irreversible mental retardation. Early diagnosis and treatment with thyroxine prevents this tragedy occurring. Diagnosis is made by assaying the level of thyroid-stimulating hormone on the blood spots from the Guthrie test card, and is confirmed by triiodothyronine (T_3) and thyroxine (T_4) measurements.

Cystic Fibrosis

Cystic fibrosis is an autosomal recessively inherited inborn error of metabolism with a recurrence risk of 1 in 4. The incidence is currently quoted as 1 in 1600. It is a congenital abnormality of the mucus-secreting glands throughout the body, particularly the lungs and the pancreas. They become distended and dilated and this ultimately leads to obstruction and fibrosis.

Diagnosis

A family history of disease is always of significance. The thick tenacious secretions cause abnormally solid meconium which may result in meconium ileus, recurrent respiratory tract infections and failure to thrive. About 15% of babies with cystic fibrosis will present with meconium ileus.

The diagnosis is made by the serum immunoreactive trypsin (IRT) test. A sweat test, if carried out, shows a raised level of sodium chloride. Antenatal diagnosis is now possible using DNA analysis and gene probes.

Management

There is no cure for this condition but early diagnosis and treatment will greatly improve the prognosis. The control of infection, especially respiratory tract infection, is most important and thus long-term antibiotics may be prescribed together with regular physiotherapy to try and minimize lung damage. Pancreatic enzyme replacements to replace the absent pancreatic enzymes and also vitamin supplements are prescribed and have improved the prognosis for these children.

Galactosaemia

Galactosaemia is another autosomal recessively inherited inborn error of metabolism. It occurs in about 1 in 50 000 babies. There is a deficiency of the enzyme galactose-1-phosphate uridyltransferase which converts galactose to glucose. Lactose (milk sugar) is normally broken down to galactose and glucose in the intestine; in this condition further breakdown cannot occur causing galactose and galactose-1-phosphate to accumulate. These may damage the neonatal liver, brain, ovaries and lens of the eye.

Diagnosis
The condition is diagnosed by testing for galactose in the urine. The Clinitest on urine is positive but not the Clinistix. The diagnosis is confirmed by the estimation of galactose phosphate in the red cells. Signs of the condition will appear in the first week or so of life with persistent jaundice, overwhelming sepsis, reluctance to feed, vomiting, hepatosplenomegaly and failure to thrive. Cataracts may develop. Antenatal diagnosis is now possible.

Management
The baby is fed with lactose-free milk. The prognosis is improved with early diagnosis and treatment since sepsis may be prevented and damage to the brain, eyes and liver may be avoided.

In subsequent pregnancies heterozygous mothers should have a lactose-free diet. Siblings of affected babies must be given a lactose-free milk from birth whilst they are investigated for this condition.

Neonatal Convulsions

Convulsions in the neonatal period often consist of a collection of subtle signs such as fluttering of the eyelids, apnoea attacks, cycling movements of the limbs or lip-smacking. They may easily be overlooked. Jerky, repetitive movements of limbs, seen in clonic fits, may be focal or generalized. Tonic seizures can occur, where the body and limbs are hypertonic and extended, the eyes diverging and rolling downwards and the baby having apnoea attacks causing cyanosis.

Cause
During the neonatal period, convulsions may be caused by the following conditions:

- Hypoxia.
- Intracranial injury.
- Hypoglycaemia.
- Hypocalcaemia.
- Hypomagnesaemia.
- Hypernatraemia.
- Kernicterus.
- Hyperpyrexia.
- Drug withdrawal.
- Infections such as septicaemia and meningitis.
- Certain congenital anomalies.

Management
The paediatrician is called. The baby is turned on to its side and the airways gently suctioned. Intubation may be required or the administration of oxygen if the baby is breathing but cyanosed. Milk feeds are stopped and an intravenous infusion sited. The Dextrostix or BM Stix is checked and appropriate treatment given if the baby is hypoglycaemic. An anticonvulsant drug, such as phenobarbitone 10–20 mg/kg, is given. If fits recur, maintenance anticonvulsant treatment is started. Investigations into the cause of the convulsion include a full infection screen with a lumbar puncture, blood sugar, blood gases, electrolytes, packed cell volume, white cell and platelet count and a serum bilirubin estimation if the baby is significantly jaundiced. A cerebral ultrasound scan is performed and further, more detailed tests may be indicated.

Haemorrhagic Disease of the Newborn

This disease mainly affects breastfed babies between 24 and 72 hours of birth – although it may occur much later if vitamin K levels remain low for a prolonged period. During the first few days of life there is a deficiency of vitamin K which is necessary for the synthesis of clotting factors, including prothrombin. Vitamin K is synthesized by bacteria which colonize the gut once feeding starts. Plasma levels start to rise a few days later. This process takes longer in breastfed babies as breast milk contains very little vitamin K. It is also impaired by maternal phenobarbitone or phenytoin therapy and perinatal asphyxia.

Bleeding usually starts on the second, third or fourth day after birth. The baby may vomit dark blood (*haematemesis*), may pass altered blood in the stool (*melaena*) or sometimes bleeds from the mouth, nose or umbilical stump. Malaena is easily distinguished from meconium by putting the napkin in water. In malaena the water turns pink, while meconium causes a green stain. Prolonged bleeding will be noticed from puncture sites and a large cephalhaematoma may be noticed.

Management

Prevention Most paediatricians recommend that 0.5–1 mg vitamin K should be given to all babies soon after birth as a prophylactic measure. The route of administration has been of some debate in recent years. One study (Golding *et al.*, 1992) suggested a link between intramuscular injection in the first week of life, and an increased risk of childhood cancer. This has not been substantiated in a further study (Hull, 1992). It is therefore recommended that oral (0.5 mg) vitamin K is given to all low-risk, normal newborn babies and that the dose is repeated at about eight days for breastfed babies. Intravenous or intramuscular vitamin K (0.5–1 mg) is given to all preterm and high-risk babies at birth, including those needing surgery.

Treatment The baby with haemorrhagic disease is given vitamin K (Konakion) 1 mg by intravenous injection immediately.

If the bleeding has been severe a blood transfusion is given. In these ways the blood prothrombin is raised to a normal level and the baby's condition improves. Blood should be taken and checked for prothrombin time, partial thromboplastin time, thrombin time and fibrinogen level. The first two will be very prolonged, but the latter two are usually normal.

Cold Injury

All babies may become chilled if not kept in a reasonably warm atmosphere. Cold injury occurs when the body temperature falls below 35°C and may have serious consequences. It is not confined to the first month of life.

Causes

The cause may be chilling at birth or due to a prolonged period in a cold atmosphere. Preterm babies are especially at risk because of their immature heat-regulating centre and lack of subcutaneous and brown fat. Small-for-gestational-age babies are also at risk due to their large surface area and relatively low subcutaneous fat deposits.

Hypothermia may be secondary to other conditions, such as birth asphyxia, cerebral injury, infection and malnutrition.

Signs

The baby's temperature falls to below 35°C and there is slowing of the heart and respiratory rates. The baby tends to look red and rosy and unfortunately this is often mistaken for a sign of good health, but it is caused by reduced tissue metabolism, hence unused oxyhaemoglobin. The skin is cold to touch and may be solid with oedema (*sclerema*) which does not pit on pressure. Peripheral cyanosis is apparent and oliguria and proteinuria occur. The baby becomes increasingly lethargic and drowsy with a feeble cry. Death will ensue unless treatment is quickly instituted.

Management

Prevention To prevent excessive heat loss from the baby's relatively large surface area at birth, it is important to quickly dry and wrap the baby. Particular care must be taken to avoid chilling when an asphyxiated baby requires resuscitation or other procedures need to be carried out. Subsequently the baby must be nursed in an environmental temperature appropriate to the size, age and gestation. This is a room temperature of 18–20°C for babies under one month of age, and 16–18°C from one to six months. Preterm and small babies may need extra layers of clothing or blankets than term babies in these temperatures, and these should be adjusted to the needs of each baby. An adequate energy intake is necessary and care should be taken to protect the baby from infection. The baby's temperature should be measured using a low-reading thermometer whenever the skin feels cold. Baths and exposure for any other reason should be postponed if the baby is chilled or the atmosphere cold.

Treatment   The baby must be transferred to a neonatal unit and nursed in an incubator where gradual rewarming takes place over a period of several hours. In severe cases an intravenous infusion of 10% glucose is given. Dextrostix strip tests are carried out every 3–6 hours because hypoglycaemia may occur as the metabolic rate increases. Electrolyte imbalance is corrected and the baby is screened for infection before prophylactic antibiotic therapy is started.

Prognosis   Treatment is usually successful if not too long delayed. In some cases, however, death follows complications such as pulmonary haemorrhage.

References

David, T.J. (ed.) (1992) Hypoglycaemia. In *Recent Advances in Paediatrics*, Vol. 10. Edinburgh: Churchill Livingstone.

Golding, J., Birmingham, K., Greenwood, R. *et al.* (1992) Childhood cancer, intramuscular vitamin K and pethidine given during labour. *Br. Med. J.* **305**: 341–346.

Hull, D. (1992) Vitamin K and childhood cancer. The risk of haemorrhagic disease is certain; that of cancer is not. *Br. Med. J.* **305**: 326–327.

Koh, H.H.G., Eyre, J.A. & Aynsley-Green, A. (1988) Neonatal hypoglycaemia – the controversy regarding definition. *Arch. Dis. Childh.* **63**: 1386.

Lucas, A., Morley, R. & Cole, T.J. (1988) Adverse neurodevelopmental outcome of moderate neonatal hypoglycaemia. *Br. Med. J.* **97**: 1304.

Further Reading

Mann, I.M., Gibson, B.E.S. & Letsky, E.A. (eds) (1991) *Fetal and Neonatal Haematology*. London: Baillière Tindall.

73

Infections of the Newborn

Prenatal Infections

During intrauterine life the fetus is generally protected from extrauterine infection by the intact amniotic sac and the placenta which acts as a barrier to most bacterial conditons. Certain microorganisms, however, can cross the placenta from the mother's blood into the fetal circulation and infect the fetus. The commonest of these intrauterine infections are rubella, cytomegalovirus, toxoplasmosis and, more rarely, syphilis.

Prenatal infections are mostly viral and protozoal agents and the infections they produce share many features. This is probably because they exist as intracellular parasites. The acronym TORCH has been devised to list some of them (Nahmias *et al.*, 1971):

T *Toxoplasma gondii.*
O Other, e.g. syphilis.
R Rubella.
C Cytomegalovirus.
H Herpes simplex or hepatitis B.

These infections may present in one of several ways:

1 *Widespread and severe*: Stillbirth or malformation.
2 *Systemic*: Anaemia, jaundice, purpura, enlarged liver and spleen.
3 *Central nervous system*: Encephalitis, meningitis, ocular involvement. Infections in these areas are harder for the body to combat.
4 *Mild*: Isolated features, such as skin or bone involvement.

5   *Intrauterine growth retardation.*
6   *Subclinical*: Problems may arise later, especially with vision, mental retardation, deafness, seizures, microcephaly. This can be a progressive neurological syndrome, as with rubella.

Early diagnosis is important because treatment can sometimes be of value even after delivery. Immunization against hepatitis B or treatment for toxoplasmosis may be started at birth because in these cases transmission is often delayed until after delivery. Syphilis may be usefully treated after birth, too, and so may herpetic infection. Even where curative treatment is not possible, early diagnosis allows the best assistance to be provided for the child.

RUBELLA

The fetus develops a viraemia which inhibits cell division and causes defects of the organs which are developing at the time of the infection.

First trimester infections are the most serious, with up to 80% of babies being infected. Fetuses infected within the first eight weeks of pregnancy have a high risk of multiple defects affecting the eyes, cardiovascular system, ears and nervous system (Enders *et al.*, 1988). Spontaneous abortion may occur. Deafness may result from infection after 14 weeks' gestation and there is a risk of fetal damage up to 24 weeks' gestation.

Intrauterine growth retardation is usual and at birth hepatitis, thrombocytopenia and neurological disorders such as microcephaly or hydrocephaly may be present. In some cases the neurological disorders are not evident until later. It is important to realize that the baby may excrete rubella virus in the urine for months or even years after birth, so there is a potential danger to pregnant women.

Careful follow-up of these children is essential to detect hearing and visual impairment and neurological disorders. Relatively minor hearing defects may not be diagnosed until much later.

Prevention of rubella infection in pregnancy

Vaccination is offered to all schoolgirls between the ages of 11 and 13 in an effort to eliminate rubella occurring in pregnancy. Antenatal mothers are screened for rubella antibodies and, if non-immune, are offered rubella vaccination in the early postnatal period. Following the vaccination it is essential that a reliable method of contraception is used for three months. Despite the vaccination of schoolgirls, congenital rubella syndrome continues to occur at an unacceptable level. It is for this reason that a combined measles, mumps, rubella vaccine is now given to all babies at the age of one year. Selective vaccination of schoolgirls will continue until the circulation of rubella has ceased.

CYTOMEGALOVIRUS

Cytomegalovirus is the commonest prenatally-acquired fetal infection. It may produce a mild influenza-like illness in the mother, but is usually asymptomatic. Maternal viraemia may lead to fetal viraemia. Fortunately over 50% of pregnant women are already immune to cytomegalovirus and of those who are not immune only a small proportion of maternal infections leads to fetal disease. In some cases the baby is affected at the time of delivery from virus in the cervical secretions or later from breast milk (Johnson, 1985).

Unlike rubella the effects on the fetus are not limited mainly to the first 12–16 weeks of pregnancy but may occur at any time. They include intrauterine growth retardation, preterm delivery and, in very severe cases, stillbirth, or, if the baby is born alive, early neonatal death. Babies who are infected at birth but show no adverse effects are unlikely to suffer long-term developmental problems. Pearl *et al.* (1986) found that 90% of children with cytomegalovirus infection at 2 years old are neurologically and developmentally normal. Complications which may occur, however, include hepatitis, with or without jaundice, thrombocytopenia, meningoencephalitis and choidoretinitis. Severe mental subnormality and motor impairment may follow.

As with rubella, babies may excrete the virus in their urine for many months and thus are a potential danger to pregnant women (Advisory Committee on Dangerous Pathogens, 1990).

LISTERIOSIS

Listeriosis is caused by the Gram-positive bacillus *Listeria monocytogenes*. The mother is usually infected by eating soft cheeses or contaminated chicken (Jones, 1990). Infection in the first trimester often results in spontaneous abortion. Preterm labour is common and listeriosis infection in the baby causes pneumonia, general sepsis and meningitis.

TOXOPLASMOSIS

Toxoplasmosis is a protozoal infection which commonly occurs in children and young adults. It is caused by the organism *Toxoplasma gondii*, found in undercooked meat and the faeces of infected cats. The incidence of this infection is much higher in continental Europe than in the UK because of the cultural preference for rare meat.

If the mother develops the disease in pregnancy the protozoon can cross the placenta and infect the developing fetus. In early pregnancy fetal death and abortion may occur. In a later infection the effects on the fetus are similar to those of cytomegalovirus. The most severe effects are seen when the infection is acquired between 10 and 24 weeks' gestation. In some cases transmission is delayed until after delivery.

If toxoplasmosis during pregnancy is diagnosed, maternal treatment with the appropriate drugs may reduce the risk of fetal damage by 50%.

SYPHILIS

Congenital syphilis, caused by the organism *Treponema pallidum*, is rare in the UK due to serological tests on all pregnant women in early pregnancy and subsequent treatment where infection is present. Recently, however, concern has been expressed because the incidence of infectious syphilis in women is rising and several cases of congenital syphilis have been reported in children under the age of two (Nicoll and Moisley, 1994). Infection of the fetus does not occur before the 16th week and is more likely later in pregnancy, so that early treatment of the mother is important in the prevention of congenital syphilis (Centers for Disease Control, 1988).

Syphilis may result in abortion, stillbirth, premature delivery or congenital syphilis (see Chapter 43).

ACQUIRED IMMUNODEFICIENCY DISEASE (AIDS)

One of the routes of transmission for AIDS is from an infected mother to her fetus or newborn; this is known as vertical transmission (see Chapter 43). The risk of fetal infection is greater if the mother has AIDS, rather than being HIV positive alone. The infection can be acquired *in utero* or around the time of delivery. After birth, babies of HIV-infected mothers are tested regularly (with the mother's consent) preferably using a combination of tests. This usually enables

a diagnosis of HIV in the infant to be made by six months. A large number of infected babies will go on to develop AIDS or related disease, usually within 6–8 months of birth (Pinching and Jeffries, 1985). The incidence varies in different countries: the European Collaborative Study (1991) showed 13% infected, whilst this rate is much higher in parts of Africa. There also appears to be an increased incidence of congenital malformations, mainly of the central nervous system, among babies born to infected mothers.

Another possible route of infection for babies is from the breast milk of infected mothers (Thiry *et al.*, 1985). Breastfeeding should therefore be discouraged for these mothers (Lederman, 1992; Palasanthiran *et al.*, 1993). In developing countries, however, the risks of using breast milk substitutes may be greater than the risk of HIV or AIDS transmission, because of unclean water, inability to read the directions on how to prepare artificial feeds and inability to afford or obtain regular supplies of artificial milk. The World Health Organization therefore recommend breastfeeding in these circumstances, because the risk of HIV by breastfeeding may be low compared to the risks of artificial feeding (WHO, 1995).

In addition to the opportunistic infections which occur in children with AIDS, failure to thrive, hepatosplenomegaly, parotitis and interstitial lymphocytic pneumonitis may occur.

Pregnancy may also have an adverse effect on the woman infected with HIV in that it can increase the risk of her developing AIDS. Because of the risks to mother and fetus, women of childbearing age who have been infected with HIV are advised to avoid pregnancy. In cases where pregnancy does occur termination may be considered.

INFECTION DUE TO INVASIVE PROCEDURES CARRIED OUT IN PREGNANCY

Organisms may be introduced into the uterus in pregnancy during procedures such as amniocentesis, fetoscopy, cordocentesis and intrauterine blood transfusion. Intrauterine pneumonia is likely following the introduction of microorganisms into the uterus.

Perinatal Infections

Perinatal infections include ascending infections which mainly occur once the membranes have ruptured, and infection acquired during passage through the birth canal and during the first few days after birth.

Ascending infections in pregnancy

Ascending infections may follow premature rupture of the membranes and lead to intrauterine pneumonia. The microorganisms most commonly found are streptococci, Gram-negative bacteria such as *Escherichia coli* and *Listeria monocytogenes*. There also seems to be a link between chorioamnionitis and infection (e.g. group B streptococcus) and preterm rupture of the membranes (Möller *et al.*, 1984; Chaudhrey *et al.*, 1984; Newton and Clark, 1988). Group B streptococcus is now one of the commonest causes of neonatal infections.

Infections acquired in labour

Virulent microorganisms that are typically acquired during the birth process, and that produce infection in normal infants, include *Neisseria gonorrhoeae, Chlamydia trachomatis, Listeria monocytogenes* and the herpes simplex virus.

Gonococcal conjunctivitis is increasing in incidence again and used to be an important cause of blindness; it is preventable and treatable (see Chapter 43). *Chlamydial conjunctivitis* is the largest single cause of blindness in the world (trachoma), and is also readily treatable. Treatment with systemic antibiotics as well as with eyedrops is necessary because, unless eradicated, this organism can cause severe neonatal pneumonia and otitis media. It is also important to treat both the mother and her partner when gonorrhoea or chlamydia are diagnosed. *Listeriosis* can produce severe and widespread infection in the neonate, including pneumonia, septicaemia and meningitis. *Herpes infections* may cause a range of illnesses in the neonatal period from skin blisters to overwhelming viraemia and encephalitis. The baby may also develop a chronic and progressive disorder of the eyes and brain (Freij and Sever, 1988).

An otherwise normal baby may be compromised by such procedures as the application of a scalp electrode which, on rare occasions, may result in abscess formation. Similarly microorganisms may be introduced into the vagina during vaginal examinations and artificial rupture of the membranes unless strict aseptic precautions are taken when performing these procedures.

Infections acquired at birth

All babies become colonized or invaded by microorganisms during labour and after birth. The predominant organisms to which the baby is exposed at birth are those of the mother's vagina, perineum and rectum. Colonization includes staphylococci on the skin and umbilicus, streptococci in the upper respiratory tract and *Escherichia coli* in the lower gut.

The baby at birth has a limited defence mechanism to infection and must therefore be protected as much as possible. From the third month of pregnancy onwards there is a transfer of immunoglobulin IgG from the mother to the fetus. This gives the baby some immunity for the first few months of life to infectious diseases to which the mother has antibodies. Preterm babies have a lower serum concentration of IgG than term babies and are therefore more susceptible to these infections. These diseases may include such conditions as chickenpox, measles and mumps. Further immunity will be acquired if the baby is breastfed. Immunoglobulin IgA is produced by the fetus only in response to an intrauterine infection.

Problems arise for the newborn when exposed to a particularly heavy dose of normal bacteria, to particularly virulent organisms or to organisms against which the mother has no IgG antibodies. In the latter case this will occur if the mother has only recently contracted the infection. IgM molecules do not cross the placenta, but are synthesized in the fetus from about 20 weeks. This immunoglobin acts against Gram-negative bacteria such as *Escherichia coli*; but neonatal serum concentrations are relatively low, making newborn babies susceptible to these infections.

High standards of hygiene and cleanliness will limit the microorganisms to which the baby is exposed. Cross-infection can be avoided by enabling the mother to care for her own baby as much as possible, who will then be colonized mainly by her microorganisms.

Thrush is an infection caused by the fungus *Candida albicans*. It may be acquired at delivery if the mother has a vaginal infection, or from poor hygiene practices. Babies receiving antibiotics are more prone to oral thrush.

Postnatal Infections

Response to infection

The presentation of infection is highly variable in the newborn and is often subtle and difficult to recognize.

It is important that midwives learn to detect the early signs so that treatment can be started promptly.

Subtle presentations

The baby may initally manifest few signs. Reluctance to feed, lethargy and fretfulness are all associated with infection. Vomiting commonly occurs and this, together with poor feeding, causes loss of weight and failure to thrive. Poor temperature control (above 37.2 or below 36°C) is common and tachypnoea (respiratory rate above 60 per minute), apnoeas and bradycardias may be apparent. The baby looks pale or grey and the skin may appear mottled. Jaundice is frequently evident.

Dramatic presentations

These are mainly episodes of 'collapse'. The baby becomes pale or cyanosed, limp or rigid and apnoeic. In these cases the diagnosis is more difficult because the signs may be the result of sepsis or due to other conditions such as hypoglycaemia, aspiration of feed, congenital heart disease, an inborn error of metabolism or intracranial haemorrhage.

Management

As soon as infection in the newborn is suspected the midwife notifies the doctor so that a diagnosis is made and treatment instituted at the earliest opportunity. Treatment for specific conditions is included under the appropriate headings, but the principles of care for babies with severe infections are outlined here.

Resuscitation is promptly carried out, if required. Then the baby is screened for infection. This includes taking nose, throat, skin and umbilical swabs, collecting urine and stool samples and taking blood for culture. In some cases a lumbar puncture is also performed. A broad-spectrum antibiotic is prescribed until the causative organism is identified.

Help in maintaining a correct body temperature may be required and an adequate food and fluid intake must be assured. Vital signs will be monitored and additional assistance such as ventilation will be provided, if required.

OPHTHALMIA NEONATORUM

This term is used to describe a discharge from the eyes of an infant within 21 days of birth.

It became notifiable in England and Wales in 1914. The severe forms are preventable. It was the cause of 50% of blindness in children but now the incidence of severe ophthalmia has greatly diminished and it is an exceptionally rare cause of blindness.

Mild ophthalmia neonatorum is common and in many cases no bacteria are found. This is probably because they are small in number or have disappeared. The most commonly identified organisms include staphylococci, *Escherichia coli*, streptococci and *Chlamydia trachomatis*.

Causes

Predisposing causes are immaturity or illness lowering the baby's resistance to infection, and the fact that in the first few weeks of life the baby secretes no tears, so that dust and bacteria do not get washed away and may block the tear ducts.

Infection may arise from trauma during a face presentation or forceps delivery, which cause bruising or abrasion through which microorganisms enter. If the mother has a vaginal discharge, infective material in the birth canal may collect around the eyelids and lashes; when the baby's eyes open the bacteria gain entry. This is especially dangerous in gonorrhoea but may also occur in conditions such as chlamydial infections. Handling of the baby by an attendant with a cold or septic focus may infect the baby. Dust in the atmosphere containing bacteria, contaminated toilet requisites and poor standards of hygiene may also lead to infection.

Preventive treatment

Treatment is firstly preventive by the medical treatment of the mother during pregnancy in all cases of vaginal discharge. No one with a cold or with any other infective condition should be allowed in contact with the baby. Strict handwashing is important and the baby's eyes should not be routinely cleaned unless there is a discharge.

Signs

Slight discharge from one eye may occur at any time during the first 10 days of life, commonly about the 3rd or 4th day. The conjunctiva may be slightly inflamed. Rarely there is profuse purulent discharge, the conjunctiva and eyelids being grossly inflamed and oedematous.

Management

The midwife must report immediately any discharge from or inflammation of the eyes, however slight. This includes that commonest of all neonatal infections, the 'sticky eye'.

A conjunctival swab is sent to the laboratory to ascertain the infecting organism and the antibiotics to which it is sensitive. Meanwhile the eye is bathed with sterile water. Many authorities recommend the immediate use of chloramphenicol eyedrops 0.5% or chloramphenicol ointment 1% since it is effective against most conjunctival infections. Others prefer to await the laboratory's report before prescribing treatment. Often the culture is sterile and the baby's eye is clear within 48 hours. In more severe cases the appropriate systemic antibiotic is used as well as the frequent instillation of eyedrops. The baby should be nursed on the affected side to prevent the discharge running into the other eye. Clean head squares should be provided as necessary. The possibility of a blocked lacrimal duct must be considered if the problem recurs.

Neonatal chlamydial conjunctivitis is usually apparent between the 5th and 10th day of life, the average day of onset being 6.8 days (Clearkin, 1986). In cases where the mother has a genital chlamydial infection and/or the baby has discharging eyes, a smear should be taken to detect *Chlamydia trachomatis*. Specimens should be taken with a cotton-tipped swab which is stroked firmly over the upper and lower palpebral conjunctivae. The swab is then placed in a suitable transport medium and sent to the laboratory. The result is available within four days. Chlamydial ophthalmia is treated with tetracycline eyedrops or ointment 1% every 2–3 hours for 10–14 days. In addition systemic erythromycin is prescribed to prevent the infection spreading to the nasopharynx and respiratory tract. The mother and her partner should be referred to a specialist in genitourinary medicine for treatment of the condition.

The incidence of genital chlamydial infection has increased markedly in recent years. Many of the babies born to infected women will develop chlamydial conjunctivitis (Rettig, 1988).

INFECTION OF THE UMBILICAL CORD

Cord sepsis is uncommon since with good standards of hygiene it can be prevented. A study by Bain (1993) has shown that using alcohol wipes to clean the cord and using Sterzac powder reduces the time taken for the cord to separate and results in less cord infections. Other studies, however, have found no increase in infection when the cord is not treated (Lawrence, 1982; Barr, 1984; Rush *et al.*, 1989; Dignan, 1994),

but the method of treatment does affect the time of separation and healing of the umbilical stump. In a large, randomized trial conducted by Mugford *et al.* (1986) it was found that although the cord separated earlier when an antiseptic powder such as Sterzac was used, the time for the umbilical stump to heal was longer, and therefore the community midwives were required to make more postnatal visits. As in most other studies, there was no increase in infection. Further studies on cord care in the early postnatal period are required.

Signs of infection include slight periumbilical inflammation, the cord becomes moist and offensive and delay occurs in separation. A swab is taken and sent to the laboratory for culture and sensitivities. The organism most commonly responsible is *Staphylococcus*. Frequent cleaning of the infected cord with an antiseptic spirit and the application of an antiseptic powder may be sufficient to clear the infection. Exceptionally a case of severe cord infection occurs. The periumbilical inflammation worsens and there is a danger of abdominal cellulitis developing and the infection tracking along the umbilical vein to the liver. The baby becomes very ill with jaundice, vomiting, diarrhoea and rapid dehydration. Urgent treatment with systemic antibiotics and intravenous fluids is required.

INFECTIONS OF THE ALIMENTARY TRACT

Thrush

Thrush or candidiasis produces white plaques on the oral mucosa of the tongue, cheek and pharynx. These may be mistaken for milk curds which can be removed easily. True thrush spots are the result of the growth of a fungus *Candida albicans* (*Monilia albicans*), and if the infection is severe they may even bleed. The fungus tends to spread to the stomach and intestine and causes loose and offensive stools, giving rise to sore buttocks. There may be difficulty at feeding times, because the baby's mouth is sore. Treatment with nystatin 100 000 units (in 1 ml) four times a day for 4–7 days is effective. Nystatin cream may be applied to sore buttocks.

Thrush occurs fairly commonly in newborn infants, as often in breastfed as in artificially fed babies. It has been noted in the babies of mothers who have or have had monilial infections and for this reason special attention should be paid to handwashing and the techniques of sterilizing bottles and making up of feeds.

Preterm babies and those being given antibiotics are

at greater risk of candidiasis and the infection in these infants may be more severe. Prophylactic nystatin is often given to babies on antibiotics. Systemic candidiasis may develop and is indicated by positive urine cultures followed by blood culture. Both antifungal and antibacterial treatment are required as bacterial sepsis may coexist.

Gastroenteritis

This is uncommon but extremely dangerous. It is highly infectious and for this reason an outbreak in a nursery in which several babies are nursed is a catastrophe.

The causative organism may be one of the *Salmonella* group, especially if there is also an outbreak of diarrhoea and vomiting in adults. Certain strains of *Escherichia coli*, echovirus type II and rotavirus have been shown to cause gastroenteritis which spreads from one baby to another very rapidly and may have a high mortality. Severe infections by staphylococci are sometimes noted. Diarrhoea may arise in babies receiving antibiotic therapy for another infection. Often no pathogenic organism is discovered when the stools passed by the baby are examined in the laboratory. It is thought that a viral infection is responsible in these cases (Melnick, 1990).

Signs and symptoms   The baby's appetite is poor, and there is weight loss and pallor. Soon the stools become frequent and watery, yellow or green. Temperature instability is common and there may be an increase in the frequency of apnoea attacks and bradycardia. If vomiting occurs, the baby rapidly becomes dehydrated and extremely ill. The skin will be dry and inelastic, the eyes dull and fontanelles sunken.

Prevention   It is obvious that preventive measures are of the utmost importance in lowering the number of deaths due to this infection. Breastfeeding should be encouraged and, where it is abandoned, clean methods of preparing and giving feeds should be taught. Cross-infection must be prevented by staff and parents.

Treatment   A baby in hospital must be cared for as much as possible by the mother and should be strictly isolated. It cannot be emphasized too strongly that each affected baby, and everything used in its care, must be segregated from other babies and from equipment used for other babies. If more than one baby is affected the

closing of the department is essential. No newly born babies must be admitted until all the mothers and babies have been discharged and the department has been disinfected.

Specific treatment is ordered by the doctor. Dehydration occurs rapidly and it may be necessary to begin treatment with intravenous fluids. It is customary for a biochemist to examine the baby's blood and to recommend how the correct balance of blood electrolytes should be restored; antibiotics are needed to combat the infection. When the baby's condition improves, feeds may be restarted.

NECROTIZING ENTEROCOLITIS

See Chapter 67.

SYPHILIS

See Chapter 43.

INFECTION OF THE RESPIRATORY TRACT

The newborn child has little resistance to infection, even to organisms which have little serious effect on the adult. A 'cold' of no significance to an adult may lead to fatal pneumonia in a newborn baby. Organisms which do not usually cause pneumonia such as *Escherichia coli*, *Staphylococcus pyogenes* and *Streptococcus viridans* can become the responsible organism in the newborn.

If the mother has genital chlamydia the baby may develop a chlamydial respiratory tract infection. Pneumonia is common after amnionitis, and is difficult to distinguish from respiratory distress syndrome. Such infants are usually treated with prophylactic antibiotics as if they have pneumonia until the correct diagnosis is made. It may also arise as a complication of ventilator therapy that was initiated for another reason. Occasionally a virus is responsible for respiratory tract infections in the newborn. Respiratory syncytial virus causes bronchiolitis and may be fatal. The resistance of the lungs to infection may be lowered if meconium or vernix caseosa have been inhaled during birth. The aspiration of regurgitated milk has the same effect. The preterm baby has little resistance to infection and the cough reflex, which helps to clear the air passages and to keep the lungs expanded, may be deficient.

When infection of the respiratory tract has occurred the baby develops rapid respirations and may have cyanotic episodes. The temperature may be unstable.

The diagnosis may be confused by the occurrence of diarrhoea and vomiting, which may also cause further deterioration in the baby's condition. In severe cases, rapid deterioration and death occur.

Prevention of infection is of the first importance. Anyone with a cold or sore throat should be excluded from the care of the baby. Chlamydial infections in the mother or baby must be effectively treated.

If a baby should become infected, nursing in an incubator and humidified oxygen may be required. The doctor will probably order a broad-spectrum antibiotic which may be given intravenously initially. The baby should be handled as little as possible. Breast-feeding is continued if possible, although it may be necessary for the milk to be expressed and given by nasogastric tube. In cases of severe respiratory distress intravenous feeding will be required. Continuous monitoring of heart rate, temperature, oxygenation, blood pressure and respiratory rate is carried out where possible. Slight elevation of the head and shoulders may help breathing. In severe cases mechanical ventilation will be required (see Chapter 69).

URINARY TRACT INFECTION

Pyelonephritis can occur in the newborn baby. The infecting organism is usually *Escherichia coli*.

The signs are somewhat indefinite, but the child is clearly not well, refuses feeds and looks pallid or greyish in colour. Jaundice may also be apparent. Vomiting and frequent loose stools may occur. The temperature may be unstable but is often normal.

The diagnosis can be made only by the collection and examination of a specimen of urine. This is obtained in a sterile plastic bag fastened inside the baby's nappy. If the specimen is contaminated, a suprapubic aspiration sample will be required. Pus cells and bacteria will be found in the urine if urinary tract infection is present.

The nursing care is of great importance. The baby must be given sufficient fluid to overcome dehydration. Sulphonamides may be used to overcome the infection or an antibiotic to which the organism is sensitive. Recovery from the infection is usually rapid but sometimes it recurs and the possibility that there is a congenital abnormality of the urinary tract must then be considered. Ultrasound examination of the urinary tract is indicated whenever a urinary tract infection is diagnosed.

Follow-up by the family doctor or hospital and long-term trimethoprim may be prescribed until the doctor is satisfied the infection is not likely to recur and the urinary tract is normal.

INFECTION AND ABNORMALITIES OF THE SKIN

A rash is abnormal and should be regarded as potentially serious. A possible source of infection is a septic focus (ear, mouth, nose, skin) of the person caring for the baby. Infection may spread from another baby already affected and, occasionally, in the community, impetigo may spread from older children.

Pyoderma

Small spots or pustules appear on the skin, as a result, almost always, of staphylococcal infection. They must not be disregarded, as they may spread rapidly, especially in a preterm or ill baby. The baby should be isolated and a doctor notified.

Paronychia

This is a staphylococcal infection of the nail bed. The skin is broken, giving the bacteria a portal of entry. The baby should be prevented from sucking the fingers by wearing loose mittens, which are changed frequently. These mittens should be carefully made so that there are no loose cotton threads inside as these can wind around the fingers and cut off the blood supply. The doctor should be informed. Occasionally antibiotic drugs will be required to control the infection.

Pemphigus neonatorum

This is one of the most serious forms of infection in the newborn. Because of its seriousness and its highly contagious character, it is wise for the midwife to consider any skin lesion associated with the formation of a blister or pus as a possible case of pemphigus and to treat it accordingly. A doctor should be notified without delay if any such lesions appear.

The causative organism is a staphylococcus of a particular phage type, which probably comes from the skin of the attendant, but must gain entry through a broken skin surface.

Blisters, which soon become filled with pus and break, leaving a raw surface, appear on the head or trunk. This is often called the *staphylococcal scalded skin syndrome* since these thin blisters break easily and mimic scalded skin. The infection spreads in the superficial tissue, large areas soon become involved, and the blisters run into one another. The baby becomes very ill. Complete isolation of mother and baby is essential, and isolation techniques should be carried out conscientiously. In an epidemic it will be necessary to close down a maternity unit until no more cases are reported and the department has been thoroughly cleaned and disinfected.

After the exudate from the blisters has been cultured, systemic treatment with antibiotics will be necessary and efforts must be made to combat the dehydration which occurs. Fluid loss can be rapid and devastating and the infant may succumb to septicaemia and the ensuing shock. The baby must be kept warm in an incubator, and should be prevented from scratching the blisters or eyes.

Complications may arise since staphylococci can settle in the lungs, gut and liver producing osteitis and arthritis.

ARTHRITIS/OSTEITIS

These infections are usually caused by staphylococcus. The conditions are not clearly separable as they are in other age groups. Such infections often present non-specifically with general malaise, or crying when the affected limb is disturbed. Although early diagnosis is difficult, early treatment is necessary to prevent joint destruction. Changes will be seen on X-ray.

OTITIS MEDIA

This is another condition which is difficult to diagnose in the neonate. Babies who have a nasotracheal tube *in situ* are at particular risk because it blocks the Eustachian tube. It may be an important cause of meningitis or a focus of chronic sepsis. Chlamydia infection may also cause this condition.

SEPTICAEMIA

Septicaemia is the growth of bacteria in the bloodstream, as distinct from their presence in the blood (bacteraemia) which can be a transient phenomenon related to intubation or other invasive procedures. The cause of septicaemia is not always clear but it generally occurs when infection spreads from localized sites to the bloodstream. It indicates a failure of the baby's defences either at the specific site of infection or of the immune system as a whole and is most likely to occur in the sick, preterm baby. The organ-

isms most commonly found in blood culture are *Escherichia coli*, staphylococci, haemolytic streptococcus, *Proteus*, *Pseudomonas aeruginosa* and *Listeria monocytogenes*. Group B streptococcus is now the commonest infecting organism in neonates, and is probably of intrauterine origin.

The baby's response to infection is typically non-specific (see earlier in this chapter) and may be accompanied by an enlarged liver and spleen. If the subtle signs are not detected and treated the infant may have an episode of collapse. The diagnosis is confirmed by blood culture and the baby is then treated with the appropriate antibiotic. Shock is treated with intravenous fluids and perhaps drugs to improve the cardiac output. Apnoea may require ventilator therapy, and neutropenia (an inadequate number of neutrophils to fight infection) can be combated with transfusions of white blood cells.

Complications of septicaemia include disseminated intravascular coagulation and meningitis.

Disseminated intravascular coagulation

Disseminated intravascular coagulation is the result of simultaneous activation of the clotting (fibrin-generating) and clot-dissolving (fibrinolytic) pathways and can result in widespread capillary bleeding as well as major haemorrhages. It leads to impaired tissue function, shock and death. Platelets may be given if thrombocytopenia is causing haemorrhage and fresh frozen plasma for the clotting factors it contains and for the serum factors that help granulocytes fight bacteria. The underlying cause (e.g. sepsis) must be treated and full supportive care provided, as described in Chapters 67 and 69.

MENINGITIS

Group B streptococci and *E. coli* are the most common organisms in cases of meningitis. It may occur following septicaemia. Initially the signs are non-specific and it is only later that vomiting, a high-pitched cry, raised anterior fontanelle, convulsions and, possibly even later, neck rigidity occur.

Diagnosis is made by lumbar puncture and the condition is treated with antibiotics given intravenously or intrathecally.

Unless meningitis is diagnosed and treated early, there is a high risk of permanent brain damage or even death.

References

Advisory Committee on Dangerous Pathogens (1990) Appendix 1: Cytomegalovirus and the pregnant woman. In *Categorisation of Pathogens According to Hazard and Categories of Containment*, 2nd edn, pp. 54–55. HMSO: London.

Bain, J. (1993) Umbilical cord care. In *The Neonatal Nurses Year Book 1993*. Cambridge: CMA Medical Data.

Barr, J. (1984) The umbilical cord: to treat or not to treat? *Midwives' Chronicle and Nursing Notes* July: 224–226.

Centers for Disease Control (1988) Guidelines for the prevention and control of congenital syphilis. *Morbidity and Mortality Weekly Report* 37 (Suppl. 1): 1S–13S.

Chaudhrey, H., Nergesh, T., Uma, L.V. & Frank, A. (1984) Silent chorioamnionitis as a cause of preterm labour to tocolytic therapy. *Am. J. Obstet. Gynecol.* 149: 726–730.

Clearkin, L.J. (1986) Chlamydial ophthalmia neonatorum. *Midwives' Chronicle and Nursing Notes* August: 174–176.

Dignan, K. (1994) Is cord care really necessary? *Br. J. Midwifery* 2(2): 121–125.

Enders, G., Nickerl-Pacher, U., Miller, E. *et al.* (1988) Outcome of confirmed periconceptional maternal rubella. *Lancet* i: 1445–1447.

European Collaborative Study (1991) Children born to women with HIV-1 infection: natural history and risk of transmission. *Lancet* ii: 253–260.

Freij, B.J. & Sever, J.L. (1988) Herpes virus infections in pregnancy: risk to embryo, fetus and neonate. *Clin. Perinatol.* 15: 203–231.

Johnson, C. (1985) Cytomegalovirus infection. *Midwife, Health Visitor & Community Nurse* 21: 166–168.

Jones, D. (1990) Foodborne listeriosis. *Lancet* ii: 1171–1174.

Lawrence, C.R. (1982) Effect of two different methods of umbilical cord care on its separation time. *Midwives' Chronicle and Nursing Notes* June: 204–205.

Lederman, S.A. (1992) Estimating infant mortality from human immunodeficiency virus and other causes in breast-feeding and bottle-feeding populations. *Pediatrics* 89(2): 290–296.

Melnick, J.L. (1990). Enteroviruses: Polioviruses, Coxsackieviruses, Echoviruses and newer enteroviruses. In Field, B.N. & Knipe, D.M. (eds) *Virology*, 2nd edn, pp. 549–603. New York: Raven Press.

Möller, M., Thompson, A.C., Borsch, K., Dinsen, K. & Zdravkovicm, M. (1984) Rupture of fetal membranes and premature delivery associated with group B streptococcus in urine of pregnant women. *Lancet* ii: 69–70.

Mugford, M., Somchiwong, M. & Waterhouse, I. (1986) Treatment of umbilical cords: a randomized trial to assess the effect of treatment methods on the work of midwives. *Midwifery* 2(4): 177–186.

Nahmias, A.J., Walls, K.W., Stewart. J.A., Herrmann, K.L. & Flint, W.J. (1971) The TORCH complex–perinatal infections associated with toxoplasma and rubella, cytomegalo- and herpes simplex viruses. *Pediat. Res.* 5: 405–406.

Newton, E.R. & Clark, M. (1988) Group B streptococcus and preterm rupture of membranes. *Obstet. Gynecol.* 71: 198–202.

Nicoll, A. & Moisley, C. (1994) Antenatal screening for syphilis. *Br. Med. J.* 308: 1253–1254.

Palasanthiran, P. *et al.* (1993). Breast-feeding during primary maternal human immunodeficiency virus infection and risk of transmission from mother to infant. *J. Infect. Dis.* 167(2): 441–444.

Pearl, K.N., Preece, P.M., Ades, A. & Peckham, L.S. (1986) Neurodevelopmental assesssment after cytomegalovirus infection. *Arch. Dis. Childh.* 61: 323–326.

Pinching, A.J. & Jeffries, D.J. (1985) AIDS and HTLV-III/LAV infection: consequences for obstetrics and perinatal medicine. *Br. J. Obstet. Gynaecol.* 92: 1211–1217.

Rettig, P.J. (1988) Perinatal infections with *Chlamydia trachomatis*. *Clin. Perinatol.* 15: 321–350.

Rush, J., Chalmers, I. & Enkin, M. (1989) Care of the new mother and baby. In Chalmers, I., Enkin, M. & Keirse, M.J.N.C. (eds) *Effective Care in Pregnancy and Childbirth*, Vol. 2, pp. 1136–1139. Oxford: Oxford University Press.

Shepherd, C.M. (199) *HIV Infection in Pregnancy*, pp. 55–57. Hale: Books for Midwives Press.

Thiry, L. Sprecher–Goldberger, S. *et al.* (1985) Isolation of the AIDS virus from cell-free breast milk of three healthy virus carriers. *Lancet* ii: 891–892.

WHO (World Health Organization) (1995) Safe Motherhood. A newsletter of worldwide activity. Pregnancy, Childbirth and AIDS. WHO. Geneva, Issue 16: 4–8.

Further Reading

Remington, J.S. & Klein, J.O. (eds) (1990) *Infectious Diseases of the Fetus and Newborn Infant*, 3rd edn. Philadelphia: W.B. Saunders.

Greenhough, A., Oxborne, J. & Sutherland, S. (eds) (1991) *Congenital, Perinatal and Neonatal Infections*. Edinburgh: Churchill Livingstone.

74

Birth Injuries

While it is possible for the baby to sustain injury during normal labour, such injury is far more likely to occur in a labour complicated by some mechanical difficulty. Birth injuries range from small bruises and abrasions to tentorial tears causing intracranial haemorrhage. By good antenatal care and skilful labour management many birth injuries may be avoided (Liu *et al.*, 1984). At present they are still a major cause of perinatal death.

Head injuries are the most common. They include:

▶ Intracranial injury, i.e. tentorial tears causing intracranial haemorrhage.
▶ Cephalhaematoma.
▶ Nerve injury, causing facial paralysis.
▶ Fracture of the skull, either linear or depressed.

Other injuries include:

▶ Injury to brachial nerve roots, causing paralysis of the arm (Erb's palsy).
▶ Sternomastoid haematoma.
▶ Dislocation of joints.
▶ Fractured limbs and ribs.

▶ Injury to internal organs (occasionally the liver or kidneys, through faulty handling in a breech delivery).
▶ Injury to the skin.

Head Injury

INTRACRANIAL INJURY (Figure 1)

Intracranial haemorrhage may be caused by hypoxia or trauma. Intra- or extrauterine hypoxia is the commonest cause of the baby displaying signs of cerebral injury after birth. Hypoxia may result in cerebral oedema, petechial haemorrhages, intracerebral haemorrhage (into the brain substance), periventricular haemorrhage or subarachnoid haemorrhage. In some cases cerebral trauma may result in cerebral palsy, especially in cases of pregnancy complications such as pre-eclampsia and intrauterine growth retardation. This suggests that prenatal factors, perhaps associated with chronic hypoxia in the fetus, may result in damage to

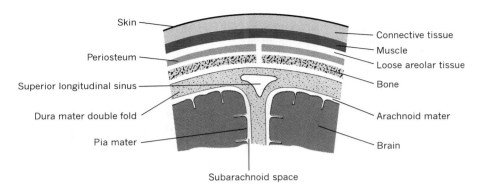

Figure 1　A cross-section through the skull.

the developing brain. The fetus may then be less able to cope with the stress of labour (Gaffney *et al.*, 1994). Preterm babies, especially those suffering from respiratory distress syndrome, are most likely to bleed into the ventricles of the brain or the subarachnoid space. Such haemorrhage is a common cause of cerebral problems in preterm babies with respiratory distress syndrome.

Intracranial haemorrhage due to trauma is usually due to a tear of the tentorium cerebelli or falx cerebri and the involvement of a venous sinus. Occasionally subdural haemorrhage may follow a tentorial tear.

Tentorial tears (Figure 2)

As the fetal head passes along the birth canal it is moulded by contact with the pelvis and the resistance of the pelvic floor, there being a certain amount of cranial stress during the process. The effect is to reduce some diameters and to elongate others. Normally the fetal skull can stand this moulding without

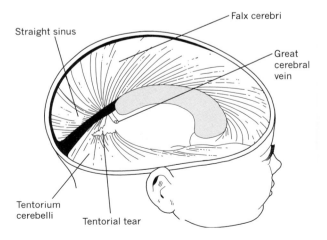

Figure 2　A tentorial tear.

any damage to the cranium, brain or supporting membranes, as during normal birth the compressing forces act gradually. If, however, the head is extended or larger in diameter than normal, or if the baby is preterm so that the bones are soft, or if the forces act suddenly (as in a precipitate labour or particularly in a breech presentation), then cranial injuries are more likely to occur. A limit of pressure is reached, so that further stress on the cranium results in something giving way, the most likely structure being the dura mater. The tentorium cerebelli lies at the back of the skull near the occipital region at right angles to the falx cerebri. The falx cerebri occupies a vertical and longitudinal position and divides the two hemispheres of the brain. The pressure on the front and back of the skull forces the bone of the cranium upwards, drawing the falx cerebri with them; this in turn pulls on the tentorium cerebelli, which tears. This tear is not usually the source of the bleeding; it is the tearing of a large vein, the great cerebral vein (the vein of Galen), which opens into the commencement of the straight sinus which lies at the junction of the falx cerebri and the tentorium cerebelli.

Predisposing causes

1　Preterm labour because the fetal skull bones are soft and afford little protection to the internal structures. There is also marked fragility of the blood vessels.
2　The prothrombin level is low during the first few days of life, thus increasing the risk of haemorrhage.
3　Prolonged labour is commonly associated with abnormal moulding and fetal distress.
4　Abnormal moulding. *Excessive* moulding may be

due to cephalopelvic disproportion or a larger pre-senting diameter as occurs with a big baby or an occipitoposterior position. *Rapid* moulding commonly occurs with precipitate labour. Rapid compression and decompression of the head occurs in a breech delivery. *Abnormal* moulding is associated with malpresentations.

5   Fetal distress/intrapartum asphyxia.
6   Operative deliveries.

Signs

The baby may be asphyxiated at birth, and recovers only slowly from the effects of birth, often remaining hypotonic for a while. Subsequently, the baby becomes hypertonic and irritable, does not suck well, sometimes vomits and may have apnoeic attacks. These babies are often unusually wakeful, though quiet, lying for long periods with eyes open and wrinkled brow. Even when asleep they may twitch and move restlessly; have a shrill cry and hold their hands clenched, with thumbs held inside the fist. The fontanelle may be tense.

Pallor is marked and the baby is lethargic and often hypothermic. Convulsions may occur and may be subtle or obvious (see Chapter 72).

Management

At birth, as always, the baby should be handled gently and skilfully resuscitated. The baby is nursed in an incubator, the head slightly raised, and kept absolutely quiet. The doctor may order phytomenadione (Kona-kion) 0.5–1 mg which is given intramuscularly or intravenously to make the blood clot more readily and thus help to prevent further haemorrhage.

Observations are made with minimal handling and include temperature, apex beat, respirations, blood pressure, oxygen saturation, colour, muscle tone, reflex irritability, movements, cry, feeding, vomiting and tension of the anterior fontanelle. Dextrostix strip tests are carried out six-hourly to detect hypo-glycaemia. Careful monitoring of the fluid input and output should be made. Oxygen is given if cyanosis occurs. The doctor may order sedation or anti-convulsant therapy as appropriate.

When the injury is slight, and is not accompanied by haemorrhage, the symptoms are probably due to cerebral oedema.

On discharge these babies require paediatric follow-up to detect neurological sequelae.

CEPHALHAEMATOMA

A swelling will be seen on the head, owing to the escape of blood between the skull and the periosteum from the rupture of small blood vessels during labour. This may occur during an apparently normal labour. It is usually situated over a parietal bone, but can never cross a suture because the periosteum under which the blood collects envelops each bone separately. Occasionally two swellings may be seen separated by the sagittal suture (Figure 3). Cephalhaematomae do occasionally overlie a fracture, thus a radiograph should be taken. The swelling does not as a rule appear until a few hours after birth and it may increase in size during the next day or so. No local treatment is required and aspiration is contraindicated, as the procedure may introduce infection. The swelling takes several weeks to disappear and because of this the parents will need reassurance.

It is important not to confuse cephalhaematoma (Figure 4) with caput succedaneum (Figure 5). The comparison in Table 1 may be helpful.

The midwife's duty in these cases is to reassure the parents by explaining that the condition is only a temporary one, that it does not affect the child's brain and is in fact outside its skull, and that it will eventually disappear.

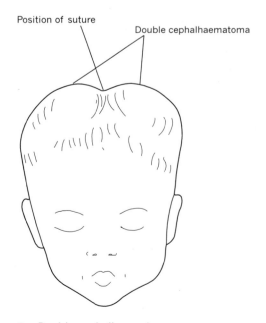

Figure 3   Double cephalhaematoma.

Table 1 Differentiation of cephalhaematoma and caput succedaneum

Cephalhaematoma	Caput succedaneum
Haematoma	Oedema
Caused by trauma	Caused by pressure
Appears after birth	Present at birth
Tends to increase in size	Tends to reduce in size
Does not pit on pressure	Pits on pressure
Cannot cross a suture line	May cross a suture line
Persists for 4–6 weeks	Disappears in 24 hours

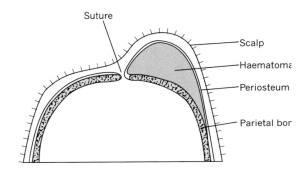

Figure 4 Cross-section of a cephalhaematoma.

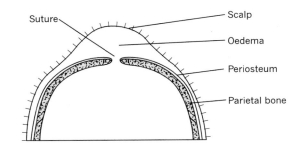

Figure 5 Caput succedaneum.

FACIAL PARALYSIS

This is a form of paralysis which arises owing to injury to a branch of the seventh cranial nerve. It is caused by a traumatic delivery when pressure is applied on the facial nerve as it emerges from the skull near the angle of the jaw. The affected side is not the one which is drawn up, but the opposite one, which shows no movement when the child cries; the eye remains open and the corner of the mouth droops (Figure 6). The baby may feed badly if the paralysis is extensive and usually unilateral. Full

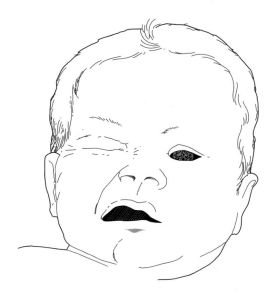

Figure 6 Left-sided facial palsy. The right side is active when the baby cries but the left side is relaxed.

movement of the face often returns within half an hour although it sometimes takes several hours, or even days. Artificial tears should be instilled into the open eye and care taken to prevent corneal damage. Almost always the baby recovers completely.

FRACTURED SKULL

This is uncommon. Occasionally the mother has an ankylosed sacrococcygeal joint and the immobile coccyx so compresses the head during delivery that when the head emerges a small depressed fracture is seen, usually of one frontal bone. The bone recovers its contour spontaneously.

Sometimes a head undergoes unusual moulding and a small linear fracture of a cranial bone is seen on the radiograph.

In neither case are symptoms likely to be present and these fractures need no treatment.

Other Injuries

ERB'S PALSY

This is caused by injury to the upper brachial plexus. The nerves derived from the brachial plexus control the arm and some of the neck and chest muscles. Dragging on the neck in cephalic or breech presenta-

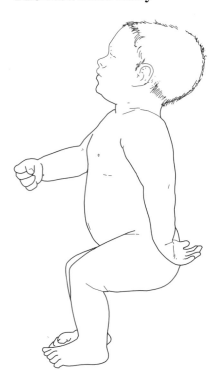

Figure 7 Erb's palsy.

tions may result in injury to the fifth and sixth cervical nerves, in which case the arm hangs loosely with the palm turned backwards ('waiter's tip' position) (Figure 7). Physiotherapy is of great value. Recovery is sometimes slow but usually complete.

KLUMPKE'S PALSY

Traction on the arm when delivering the shoulders may cause damage to the eighth cervical and first thoracic nerve roots – the lower brachial plexus. This results in paralysis of the hand and wrist drop. Physiotherapy is of great value. X-rays of the spine, shoulder and arm will diagnose or exclude a fracture. As with Erb's palsy, recovery is slow; surgical intervention may aid recovery (Hunt, 1988).

References

Gaffney, G., Sellers, S., Flavell, V., Squier, M. & Johnson, A. (1994) Case-control study of intrapartum care, cerebral palsy and perinatal death. *Br. Med. J.* **308**(6931): 743–750.

Hunt, D. (1988) Surgical management of brachial plexus birth injuries. *Devel. Med. Child Neurol.* **30**: 824–828.

DISLOCATIONS AND FRACTURES

The femur, humerus or clavicle may be fractured during a difficult delivery. In a mismanaged breech delivery the child's hip may be traumatically dislocated.

STERNOMASTOID HAEMATOMA

A swelling may occur in the sternomastoid muscle after traction has been used to deliver the head or shoulders. It may occur in a breech or cephalic delivery. A blood vessel is torn, very slow oozing of blood occurs and it may be a week before the swelling is noticed. It takes several weeks to subside, but it is very rarely that the child is left with permanent shortening of the muscle. Such shortening twists the head to one side causing *torticollis* (wry-neck).

INJURY TO ABDOMINAL ORGANS

Rupture of internal organs such as the liver and spleen is a rare complication of breech delivery when the baby is incorrectly grasped around the body.

MINOR SKIN INJURIES

There is commonly bruising on the presenting part whether the presentation is cephalic, breech or face. Occasionally small abrasions may be found on the face due to poor application of forceps blades. Abrasions on the scalp may be caused by a scalp electrode, fetal blood sampling or possibly vacuum extraction.

Small petechial haemorrhages in the skin of the head and neck give the appearance of cyanosis, though the body and mucous membranes are pink. It is called traumatic cyanosis and is caused by congestion of blood vessels in the head. The colour gradually improves and no treatment is required.

Fat necrosis may occur, especially on the face, and is detected by small, hard lumps in the subcutaneous tissue. These areas should be monitored closely to ensure secondary infection does not occur.

Liu, D.T.Y. & Fairweather, D.V.I. (1984) The management of preterm labour. In Elder, M.G. & Kendricks, C.H. (eds) *Preterm Labour*, pp. 231–259. London: Butterworths.

Further Reading

Roberton, N.R.C. (ed.) (1992) *Textbook of Neonatology.* Edinburgh: Churchill Livingstone.

Sinclair, J.C. & Bracken, M.B. (eds) (1992) *Effective Care of the Newborn Infant.* Oxford: Oxford Univerisity Press.

75

Congenital Malformations and Conditions

A congenital anomaly is a defect present at birth and occurs in approximately 5% of babies. Congenital anomalies are categorized into two groups: *malformations* and *deformations*:

▶ A malformation is a primary defect of organ or tissue development in the embryo or fetus.
▶ A deformation is damage caused by external factors influencing a previously normal structure.

Malformations and deformations occur in a ratio of 3:2. These conditions are an important cause in neonatal and perinatal mortality, accounting for about 40% of deaths.

Aetiology

In many cases the cause of a congenital anomaly is unknown, however, several factors are known to be associated.

Genetic factors These account for some abnormalities when a single defective gene causes conditions such as achondroplasia, cystic fibrosis and haemophilia. Neural tube defects and other fairly common abnormalities are caused by a combination of multiple defective genes and environmental factors. Chromosomal anomalies are also frequently associated with major congenital malformations.

Maternal infections Infections such as rubella, cytomegalovirus, toxoplasmosis and syphilis can cause severe congenital abnormalities (see Chapters 15, 43 and 73).

Drugs Drugs administered to the mother in pregnancy can affect fetal development. The most notorious example is, of course, thalidomide, but many other drugs are now suspect. Streptomycin can cause eighth nerve deafness, whereas tetracycline causes yellow staining of the teeth and enamel hypoplasia. There is an increase in the incidence of cleft lip and palate in babies of epileptic mothers treated with phenytoin. Heavy smoking, an excessive intake of alcohol or opiates may adversely affect mental and physical development of the fetus.

Irradiation Exposure to irradiation in early pregnancy may have a harmful effect on the developing fetus. Abnormalities may also occur in the next generation when the fetal gonads are exposed to radiation.

Maternal age and health These also affect fetal well-being. Older mothers are more likely to have a child with Down's syndrome and the incidence of congenital abnormalities is increased when the mother has diabetes mellitus.

Geographical factors These may also have some influence since the incidence of some abnormalities is higher in certain parts of the UK and the world (Knox and Lancashire, 1991).

Dietary factors There is now evidence to suggest that dietary deficiencies or excesses may cause certain congenital malformations. A deficiency of vitamins has been found to be associated with neural tube defects (MRC, 1991). Excess vitamin A in pregnancy is teratogenic (DHSS, 1990). There is also increasing concern that poor maternal nutrition adversely affects fetal growth and well-being *in utero*, and may lead to health problems in adult life (Luke, 1994; Godfrey *et al.*, 1994; Grey, 1994; Barker, 1993; Giotta, 1993; Wilkins, 1993) (see Chapter 16).

Abnormalities of the Central Nervous System

Spina bifida, anencephaly and hydrocephalus are the common abnormalities of the central nervous system and form a large percentage of all abnormalities. Improved antenatal detection, therapeutic termination and routine vitamin supplementation, specifically folic acid, preconception and for the first 12 weeks of pregnancy, has accounted for a dramatic drop in the incidence of neural tube defects.

Spina bifida

This is a congenital defect of the posterior laminae and spinous processes of one or more vertebrae. It may be a simple bony defect giving rise to no symptoms, and occasionally only found accidentally in later life when that part of the spine has been X-rayed for some reason. A sacral dimple or hairy patch may be evident. It may involve a protrusion of the meninges which is covered by skin – a *meningocele* – or the protrusion of the cord and meninges – a *meningomyelocele*. The latter is the most serious as often areas of spinal cord are found in isolated patches of the protruding meninges and restoration to normal function is unlikely.

The condition usually affects the lumbosacral region of the spine. Commonly the skin is stretched or completely absent over the bulging meninges. Cerebrospinal fluid may leak from the swelling. Talipes is often present and sometimes there is complete paralysis of the lower limbs. Hydrocephalus can also occur.

Surgical closure of these defects may be undertaken if there are few adverse features, such as paraplegia or associated anomalies. If a meningocele is present, it should be covered by a sterile saline-soaked dressing to minimize fluid loss, prevent garments sticking to the lesion and reduce the risk of infection. Adequate analgesia should be prescribed for the baby.

Cerebral meningocele

A meningocele may also occur in the skull. The meninges bulge through a defect in the skull bones, usually in the region of the posterior fontanelle.

Anencephaly

In this condition the vault of the skull is absent and there is almost no development of the brain, which is exposed and appears as a dark red mass of tissue. The incidence of anencephaly is approximately 1 in 1000. Spina bifida often accompanies anencephaly. The fetus has large protruding eyes and wide shoulders; the face presents during labour. There is polyhydramnios in about 50% of these pregnancies. Only 25% of the babies are born alive, they are usually female, and most die within a week.

Hydrocephalus

The head is unduly large as the result of an increase in the amount of cerebrospinal fluid, which distends the brain. The cranial bones are soft, the fontanelles large and the sutures wide. This condition may cause obstructed labour unless diagnosed early. On abdominal palpation the head feels large, and is above the brim or the breech may present. The diagnosis may be confirmed by ultrasound, radiographically or when making a vaginal examination. In severe cases the fetus cannot be delivered vaginally and a Caesarean section is necessary. In many cases this condition may be successfully treated surgically by the insertion of a valve and catheter from a lateral ventricle to the jugular vein and right side of the heart, thereby reducing the cerebral fluid pressure.

Microcephaly

This is a very small vault to the skull. There are two types, one in which the brain has failed to grow and the other in which the sutures have ossified prematurely and constricted the growth of the brain. The former type may be caused by intrauterine infections such as rubella, cytomegalovirus, toxoplasmosis or severe intrauterine hypoxia. Babies with microcephaly are usually mentally impaired.

Abnormalities of the Alimentary System

Cleft lip and cleft palate

These deformities often occur together, the incidence of just a cleft lip or the two together being 1 in 700 births. They may also be *unilateral* or *bilateral*. Cleft palate may involve the soft or hard palate or both and the incidence of this condition alone is 1 in 2000 births. Unless great care is taken it can easily be missed during routine examination if the deformity is slight. The baby's sucking powers vary according to the degree of the cleft. In mild cases the baby may feed normally but in those which are more severe a special teat (*Habermann teat*) may be used or the baby may be spoon-fed.

The surgeon may decide to repair the lip soon after birth and the palate at about three months of age. In the past the timing of surgery was considerably later, at three months for the lip and about 1 year for the palate. One of the advantages of earlier repair is that subsequent problems of hearing and speech are minimized. It also reduces the feeding problems which are associated with this condition. Before surgery a dental plate may be fitted to improve feeding and control the growth of the upper jaw. Early involvement of the orthodontist and speech therapist are important.

A midline cleft of the soft palate associated with

micrognathia (small mandible) is called *Pierre Robin syndrome*. Until this condition is repaired the baby has to be nursed in the prone position to prevent the tongue protruding through the cleft and obstructing the air passages. In severe cases a nasal airway may need to be kept *in situ* until surgical repair. Again a dental plate may be fitted and tube feeds may be necessary.

Congenital hypertrophic pyloric stenosis

During the 2nd or 3rd week of life a baby suffering from this condition – often a first-born male child – will begin to vomit. The incidence in boys is four times greater than in girls. Vomiting is projectile in character and not bile-stained, and on examination of the baby's abdomen the thickened pyloric sphincter may be felt. Weight loss and constipation are common. On feeding, peristalsis is visible.

Treatment is surgical (*Ramstedt's operation*) in which the sphincter but not the mucous lining is divided.

Duodenal atresia

In this condition the patency of the duodenum is interrupted and projectile, bile-stained vomiting occurs as soon as the baby begins to be fed. The incidence of duodenal atresia is 1 in 6000, making it the commonest site of atresia. In one third of cases it is associated with Down's syndrome. An abdominal X-ray shows a classic 'double bubble' appearance. Surgical correction is needed with a duodeno-duodenostomy being performed.

Oesophageal atresia

In this malformation (Figure 1) the upper end of the oesophagus ends blindly in a pouch. In about 87% of cases the lower end is connected with the trachea by a tracheoesophageal fistula. The condition should be suspected if there is a history of polyhydramnios in pregnancy or if the newborn baby regurgitates frothy mucus from the mouth. If this happens it is important not to give a feed as there is a risk of aspiration; the doctor should be notified. An orogastric tube is passed into the oesophagus and down towards the stomach. The tube should not be too soft or it may curl up at the back of the throat or in the blind pouch and give the appearance of having satisfactorily reached the stomach. If in doubt, and particularly if there has been

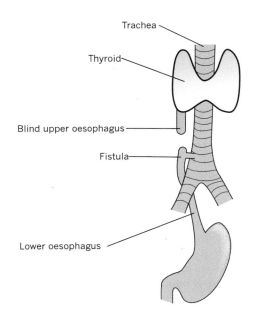

Trachea

Thyroid

Blind upper oesophagus

Fistula

Lower oesophagus

Figure 1 Tracheoesophageal atresia with fistula.

a history of polyhydramnios, a radio–opaque X-ray should be taken.

Early operation may be life-saving; thus it is important to recognize the abnormality early. While the infant is awaiting surgery, or is being transported to a neonatal surgical centre, a double lumen (Replogle) tube should be left in the upper pouch, and continuous suction applied. This prevents aspiration of the saliva. Care must be taken to ensure that the volume of fluid removed in this way is measured and recorded so that it can be replaced with intravenous fluids.

The baby is nursed with the head elevated. Surgery involves anastomosis of the ends of the oesophagus, and division of any fistula. If the gap between the oesophageal ends is too wide more than one operation may be necessary.

Oesophageal atresia commonly occurs in association with other anomalies (Chittmittrapap *et al.*, 1989).

Diaphragmatic hernia

In this condition the intestines and other abdominal organs pass through a defect in the diaphragm, usually the left side, into the chest. The incidence is about 1 in 2000 births. There is often a history of polyhydramnios in pregnancy and respiratory distress and cyanosis occur after birth. The maximal heart sounds are heard to the right and bowel sounds to the left of the chest. The abdomen is concave whereas the chest may appear

distended. Diagnosis is confirmed radiographically and immediate surgery may be a life-saving measure. Whilst awaiting surgery, respiratory support must be provided. An endotracheal tube must be used instead of bag and mask ventilation for resuscitation, as the latter distends the bowel and further compresses the lungs. A gastric tube should be passed to decompress the bowel as much as possible by removing air and fluid (Theorell, 1990).

Imperforate anus

The anal canal may end blindly or, more commonly, there is an abnormal opening or fistula. The fistula may open into the perineum or into the vagina in females and into the urethra in males. It may be associated with other malformations, thus careful examination and investigation are necessary.

Surgical treatment is necessary to correct this anomaly.

Meconium ileus

In this condition, obstruction occurs because the bowel is blocked with thick, dense (inspissated) meconium. Seventy five per cent of babies with this condition have cystic fibrosis (see Chapter 72).

Hirschsprung's disease

The colon is grossly distended because it lacks the ganglion cells of the nerve supply controlling peristalsis. Diagnosis is often made by the delayed passage of meconium, subsequent infrequent, offensive stools and abdominal distension.

Exomphalos (congenital umbilical hernia)

Exomphalos is a protrusion of the abdominal organs, chiefly intestine, through an opening in the abdominal wall at the umbilicus. The herniated organs are covered by a sac of peritoneum and amniotic membranes. It is present at birth and an operation to repair the hernia should be performed as soon as possible. As soon after birth as possible the protruding intestines should be placed in a sterile impermeable (plastic) bag to reduce fluid loss and infection risk. The whole lower body may be placed in the bag for ease. Cultures are taken and prophylactic antibiotics started.

Exomphalos is associated with other malformations in up to 75% of cases, so careful examination is required.

Acquired umbilical hernia

Following the separation of the cord a small protrusion may be seen at the umbilicus. This is due to a temporary weakness of the abdominal wall and no treatment is required.

The hernia gradually disappears as the child grows older.

Gastroschisis

Intestines and other abdominal organs protrude through a defect in the abdominal wall adjacent to the umbilicus. There is no covering membrane and owing to interference with the blood supply the organs are usually discoloured and may be gangrenous. Urgent surgical treatment is necessary. As soon after birth as possible (before transfer), the protruding intestines, or the whole lower body, should be placed in a sterile, impermeable (plastic) bag. Cultures should be taken and antibiotics commenced. Full supportive care, including intravenous fluids, will be required (Swift *et al.*, 1992).

Abnormalities of the Genitourinary System

Imperforate urethra

In rare cases the urethra, which leads from the bladder, is closed and retention of urine arises as a consequence. The bladder may become distended, but this condition must not be waited for. A doctor should be asked to examine the child if it does not pass urine within a few hours after birth.

Phimosis

This is a constriction of the prepuce of the penis, but it is very rare for the prepuce to be so tight that urinary retention occurs.

Hypospadias

A malformation in which the urethra opens on the undersurface of the penis. The nearer the urethral opening is to the tip of the penis, the less severe the problem, and less urgent the surgery providing there is no urinary obstruction. The stream of urine should be observed to ensure it is not impeded.

Epispadias

The urethra lies open anteriorly along the shaft of the penis.

Renal agenesis

Absence of the kidneys is a rare and fatal condition. If the baby fails to pass urine, has low set ears and furrows under the wide-set eyes (*Potter's facies*); renal agenesis should be suspected. It is commonly associated with only two vessels in the umbilical cord.

Polycystic disease of the kidneys

There are two main types of polycystic disease of the kidneys. One is inherited as an autosomal recessive characteristic. It is often accompanied by cystic disease of the liver and generally has a poor prognosis. The other type is transmitted as a dominant condition and renal function is usually satisfactory.

Problems of sex determination

True hermaphroditism, in which both male and female genital organs are present, is very rare. In *pseudo-hermaphrodites* a small penis can be confused with a large clitoris, while a bifid scrotum may resemble the labia majora. Chromosome analysis is necessary to establish the sex of the baby. The possibility of congenital adrenal hyperplasia must be considered. This may cause an Addisonian crisis, with vomiting and dehydration. It is corrected with intravenous saline and steroids.

Abnormalities of the Heart and Blood Vessels

These abnormalities are described fully in Chapter 71. The midwife should recognize the signs of cardiac problems and seek immediate medical help for the baby.

Signs of cardiac failure

The early signs are tachypnoea, tachycardia, feeding difficulties and failure to thrive. Later dyspnoea, cyanosis, enlargement of the liver and excessive weight gain due to oedema may occur.

Management

Medical management includes nursing the baby in a semi-upright position, in oxygen, and the administration of digoxin and a diuretic. Tube feeding may be necessary.

Initial investigations include a chest radiograph and an electrocardiogram. The baby should be transferred to a regional centre for further investigations such as cardiac catheterization and possible surgery.

Abnormalities of the Limbs

Talipes

This deformity is due to the contraction of certain muscles or tendons. In some cases, especially the milder ones, it is positional, related to the fetal position in the uterus, with restriction of movement. With early treatment by the physiotherapist, these minor deformities are quickly cured. If the deformity cannot be corrected by passive movement it may be of genetic origin and present as one of three types:

1 *Talipes equinovarus* is the commonest form of talipes with the foot pointing downwards and inwards (Figure 2).
2 In *talipes calcaneovalgus* the foot points upwards and outwards (Figure 3).
3 *Talipes metatarsus varus* affects only the forefoot, which turns inwards.

In all these cases one or both feet may be affected. Whereas talipes equinovarus is usually mild, easily

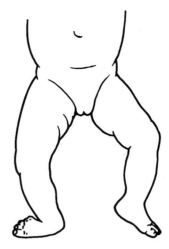

Figure 3   Talipes calcaneovalgus.

correctable and requires only physiotherapy and splinting, the situation for talipes calcaneovalgus is different. This is less common, but is more likely to require prolonged splinting or surgery. An underlying neurological lesion may also be present.

A few cases of apparent talipes will be vertical talus, also a serious condition often requiring surgery.

Syndactyly (webbed fingers and toes)

In this condition the fingers or toes are held together by folds of skin (Figure 4), or in serious cases there may be bony fusion.

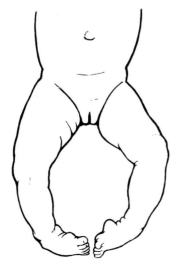

Figure 2   Talipes equinovarus.

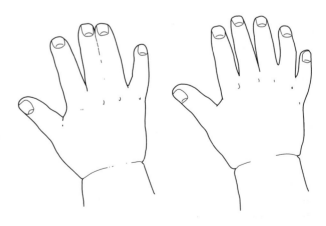

Figure 4   Syndactyly (*left*) and polydactyly (extra digit) (*right*).

Polydactyly (extra fingers and toes)
There is a tendency for these abnormalities to be hereditary.

Missing or deformed fingers, toes or limbs
In the minor degrees the deformity is confined to one or more fingers or toes, but in severe degrees the whole limb may be small or deformed. The most severe and tragic cases of limb deformity occurred in the babies of mothers who had been given the drug thalidomide in early pregnancy. Other drugs, including some tranquillizers, abused drugs such as cocaine (Hadeed and Siegel, 1989), and steroids, may cause abnormal limb development.

Some terms for missing limbs are as follows:

▶ *Amelia*:   Absence of one or more limbs.
▶ *Ectromelia*:   Absence of part of a limb.
▶ *Phocomelia*:   Absence of the long bones of a limb (there may be a rudimentary or well-developed hand or foot springing from the shoulder or hip respectively).

Congenital dislocation of the hip
The incidence is approximately 1 in 1500 births. In this condition one or both hips are abnormally developed and thus the head of the femur is partially or wholly displaced from the acetabulum. It is of genetic origin since it is commoner in girls and children of affected families, but may also be associated with environmental factors such as breech presentation and oligohydramnios.

Many babies have some instability of the hips at birth and should be examined a few days later. If the instability persists they should be referred to an orthopaedic surgeon, but most recover spontaneously within a month or two.

Diagnosis   Congenital dislocation of the hip is suspected when flexion and abduction of the hip to 90° is not possible.

Ortolani's and Barlow's tests are usually carried out on all babies at birth by the midwife and later by the paediatrician (see Chapter 63). If the hip is dislocated a click is felt as the head of the femur slips into the acetabulum.

Ultrasound scanning of the hip joint confirms diagnosis (Berman and Klenerman, 1986).

Management   Early treatment is essential. The baby is referred to an orthopaedic surgeon and a van Rosen, Aberdeen or Pavlik harness splint is applied to keep the hips flexed and abducted. It is worn continuously for about three months, being adjusted at intervals to keep pace with growth. This treatment is usually very effective.

In cases where the condition is not diagnosed early it may cause serious problems later when the child begins to walk. Without treatment the adduction contracture becomes more marked; there is apparent leg shortening, a protruding hip and asymmetrical skin folds. Treatment may include six months to a year in a hip spica or, in the older child, long periods of traction and an open reduction of the hip. All this can be avoided with early diagnosis in the neonatal period and the institution of prompt treatment.

Abnormalities of the Skin

Naevus or birth mark
This is a congenital blemish of the skin due either to dilatation of small blood vessels in the skin or to a pigmented area of the skin. 'Strawberry' naevi are small, red, raised and clearly outlined. They usually appear after birth and often grow over the next year, though they finally disappear spontaneously. The parents should be reassured on this point.

'Port wine stains' are flat purplish areas, often extensive and, if on the face, disfiguring. They do not disappear, but special make-up foundations make them less obvious. Laser surgery is being used with some success now.

'Mongolian blue spots'
These are slate-blue patches usually found over the sacral area, although they may be found elsewhere. They occur in children of African and Asian parents and sometimes those of Mediterranean parents. No treatment is required.

Bullae/blisters
If these appear after birth they may be staphylococcal in origin, but if they are present at birth they may be due to an inherited disorder of the epidermis. Some forms of this epidermolysis bullosa are fatal.

Chromosomal Abnormalities

Down's syndrome (Figure 5)

Down's syndrome is more common in the children of older women when the incidence can be as high as 1 in 40. There are two forms of Down's syndrome which can be distinguished after studies of the chromosomes. The more common one, *trisomy 21*, when 47 chromosomes are present, is associated with increasing maternal age. In the other form a translocation occurs, usually between chromosomes 14 and 21, as a de novo structural arrangement in the child, although the parents have normal chromosomes. In these cases there are 46 chromosomes, because the extra chromosome (number 21) is joined to another chromosome (i.e. translocation) (see Chapter 4). At other times the translocation occurs as a result of a similar translocated chromosome in the parents. This latter variety has about a 10% chance of recurring in a further pregnancy.

The characteristic features of a baby with Down's syndrome are:

▶ prominent epicanthic folds;
▶ white flecks in the iris called *Brushfield's spots*;

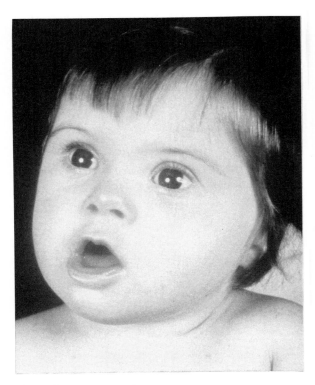

Figure 5   Down's syndrome.

▶ a small head with a flattened occipital region;
▶ small mouth;
▶ thick gum margins;
▶ protruding tongue;
▶ broad, flat nose;
▶ short hands, particularly the terminal phalanx of the little finger;
▶ a deep single crease across the palm; and
▶ broad, short feet with wide deviation of the great toe and a plantar crease between the first and second toes.

The skin tends to be dry and the muscles hypotonic. Congenital heart defects occur in about 50% of these babies and there is an increased incidence of duodenal atresia.

Children with Down's syndrome will have learning difficulties which may range from mild to severe, and may need care or supervision all their lives. With good care and stimulation in infancy and childhood they should attain their maximum potential.

Other trisomies

In these conditions there is an extra chromosome attached to a certain pair of chromosomes.

Edwards' syndrome (trisomy 18)   The incidence is about 1 in 8000 births. An extra chromosome is attached to number 18. Trisomy 18 is less common than trisomy 21 but results in well-recognized clinical features. The baby is small-for-gestational-age and has typical facies, hands and feet. The jaw is poorly developed, the ears malformed and low-set and the occiput prominent. The fingers are characteristically crossed and flexed and the infant also has prominent heels and rocker-bottom feet. Most of these children have severe congenital heart disease, a single umbilical artery and all are mentally retarded. Most die soon after birth.

Patau's syndrome (trisomy 13)   The incidence is about 1 in 14 000. An extra chromosome is attached to number 13. This is a relatively rare chromosomal abnormality characterized by certain clinical features. The baby is small-for-gestational-age and has typical facies, hands and feet. The face is abnormal with a sloping forehead, bilateral cleft lip and/or palate and malformed ears. Polydactyly is a common feature. Like trisomy 18 (Edwards' syndrome) the infant has prominent heels and rocker-bottom feet and a single umbilical artery. The brain is poorly developed and mental retardation occurs. The prognosis for these children is poor.

Cri du chat syndrome

Deletion of a portion of chromosome number 5 results in *cri du chat* syndrome. During infancy the infant has a typical mewing cry due to softening of the larynx and it is this which gives the syndrome its name. Again there are typical features, a moon-shaped face with wide-set eyes, small jaw and low-set ears. The child is mentally retarded.

X chromosomal abnormality

Turner's syndrome (XO)   The incidence is 1 in 2500 live girls. An X or Y chromosome is missing. Spontaneous abortion is a common outcome of pregnancy. The baby is a female and often has a webbed neck and oedema of the lower limbs. Growth is stunted and there is an increased incidence of congenital heart disease (particularly coarctation of the aorta).

Klinefelter's syndrome (XXY)   In Klinefelter's syndrome there are at least two X chromosomes as well as a Y. This condition may not be recognized. There is a risk of mental retardation and the man is always infertile.

References

Barker, D.J. (1993) Maternal nutrition and cardiovascular disease. *Nutr. Health* 9(2): 99–106.

Berman, L. & Klenerman, L. (1986) Ultrasound screening for hip abnormalities: preliminary findings in 1001 neonates. *Br. Med. J.* 293: 719–722.

Chittmittrapap, S., Spitz, L., Kiely, E.M. *et al.* (1989) Oesophageal atresia and associated anomalies. *Arch. Dis. Childh.* 64: 364.

DHSS (1990) *Vitamin A and Pregnancy.* PL/CMO (90)11/PL/CNO (90)10. London: DHSS.

Giotta, M.P. (1993) Nutrition during pregnancy: reducing obstetric risk. *J. Perinatal Neonatal Nursing* 6(4): 1–12.

Godfrey, K.M., Forrester, T., Barker, D.J. *et al.* (1994) Maternal nutrition status in pregnancy and blood pressure in childhood. *Br. J. Obstet. Gynaecol.* 101(5): 398–403.

Gray, J. (1994) Maternal nutrition, fetal environment and adult disease. *Modern Midwife* 4(8): 13–16.

Hadeed, A.J. & Siegel, S.R. (1989) Maternal cocaine use during pregnancy: effect on the newborn infant. *Pediatrics* 84: 205–210.

Knox, E. & Lancashire, R. (1991) *Epidemiology of Congenital Malformations.* London: HMSO.

Luke, B. (1994) Nutrition in pregnancy. *Curr. Opin. Obstet. Gynaecol.* 6(5): 402–407.

MRC (Medical Research Council) (1991) Prevention of neural tube defects. Results of the Medical Research Council Vitamin Study. *Lancet* 338: 131–137.

Swift, R.I., Singh, M.P., Ziderman, D.A. *et al.* (1992) A regime in the management of gastroschisis. *J. Pediat. Surg.* 27(1): 61–63.

Theorell, C. (1990) Congenital diaphragmatic hernia: a physiological approach to management. *J. Perinatal Neonatal Nurs.* 3(3): 66–79.

Wilkin, T.J. (1993) Early nutrition and diabetes mellitus. *Br. Med. J.* 306: 283–284.

Further Reading

Jones, K.L. (1988) *Smith's Recognizable Patterns of Human Malfunction*, 4th edn. Philadelphia: W.B. Saunders.

Long, W.A. (1990) *Fetal and Neonatal Cardiology.* Philadelphia: W.B. Saunders.

76

Neonatal Surgery and Pain

Many of the major conditions requiring surgical correction can be identified antenatally, many within the first or early second trimesters, with the use of ultrasound scanning. A family history of certain conditions, or specific problems in the pregnancy, may indicate the need for more detailed investigation and aid early diagnosis of some conditions.

Wherever possible, *in utero* transfer of the baby is advised to ensure that delivery takes place in a regional, specialist centre. In many instances this will mean the family travelling many miles to be with their baby and every neonatal unit should have facilities for families to be resident, including siblings. There is a tremendous difference in the outcomes in relation to the place of delivery (Stoodley *et al.*, 1993). Most ill babies do not withstand transportation between hospitals very well and often arrive in a poorer condition than they were born. In addition to this, valuable time is lost by the need to transfer the baby, particularly if the journey is prolonged.

Prenatal Surgery

In utero surgery is now possible for the treatment of certain conditions. The aim is either to correct the defect, or to alleviate symptoms and eliminate the need for elective preterm delivery, thus improving the baby's chance of survival. An example of such treatment is the repair of urethral valves which may cause renal damage from back pressure, as a result of the obstructed flow of urine (Kullendorff *et al.*, 1984). Another example of prenatal treatment is the provision of blood transfusions for babies severely affected by rhesus disease, where blood is injected into the fetal peritoneal cavity and is gradually absorbed from there.

Pre-operative Care

Neonatal conditions requiring surgery fall into two main categories:

1 those which are life-threatening and need immediate surgery; and
2 those which may be postponed until the baby is in the optimum condition for surgery.

With modern technological advances, most procedures can be delayed for a short while by the implementation of a temporary measure to alleviate some of the symptoms. This gives the neonatal team valuable time in which to stabilize the baby with regard to his temperature, respiratory state and blood electrolytes. The better the condition of the baby at the time of surgery, the better the chances of survival.

Much of the pre-operative care will be specific to the condition, but the general principles are as follows (not in order of priority, as each baby's needs will vary):

1 Stabilize the baby's temperature within normal limits. Hypothermia and hyperpyrexia have dramatic effects on metabolism. Cold stress in particular will greatly increase the oxygen requirements of a baby.
2 Ensure the respiratory state is as stable as possible. This includes the ventilation, oxygen requirements and blood gas values.
3 Correct acidosis or electrolyte imbalances.
4 Ensure the baby is well hydrated with the administration of intravenous fluids.
5 Ensure vitamin K is administered to the baby, as prescribed, to help prevent haemorrhagic disease of the newborn.
6 Screen the baby for signs of infection and begin treatment with antibiotics if appropriate.
7 Ensure adequate pre-operative and post-operative analgesia is prescribed for the baby and administered as appropriate.
8 Check that the consent forms are signed and contact telephone numbers obtained from the parents.
9 Explain all events and situations to the family using appropriate terminology. Wherever possible they should be prepared in advance for all changes to care and how their baby will look on return from theatre, with an explanation of the equipment which will be used.
10 Be aware of the religious and cultural beliefs of the family and treat them with respect and understanding. For example, Jehovah's Witnesses do not allow blood or blood products to be transfused and artificial substitutes should be available. Another situation which may be relevant with preterm babies in particular, is the use of bovine surfactant with babies of Muslim families. Porcine and artificial surfactants are also available and have been shown to be effective in clinical trials.
11 If the baby's condition permits, the parents should have the opportunity to cuddle their baby before surgery. In the event of the baby dying, this contact will play a very important part in the grieving process.

Post-operative Care

The principles of post-operative care are very similar to those of pre-operative care, particularly with regard to the involvement of the family. The mother should be encouraged to express her breast milk for the baby, as it is much better tolerated than formula milk, may enable feeds to be started sooner and significantly reduces the risk of necrotizing enterocolitis developing (Lucas and Cole, 1990). The main aims are to promote a good recovery, the early identification and treatment of complications, prevention of infection by aseptic techniques and strict hygiene, establishment of adequate nutrition and to ensure the baby is pain free.

Specific Conditions

DIAPHRAGMATIC HERNIA
(incidence approx. 1 in 2000)

This condition develops very early on embryologically, as the result of a defect in the formation of the diaphragm, usually on the left side. As a consequence the bowel and abdominal viscera herniate through the diaphragm and continue to develop in the thoracic cavity. The lung does not have room to grow properly and is therefore usually hypoplastic. This abnormality can be identified by early ultrasound scans, allowing time to prepare the parents and formulate a plan for delivery in conjunction with paediatric and obstetric staff. It should be suspected in the event of polyhydramnios. Most of these babies are born at term and the condition is more common in male infants.

At delivery the hypoplastic lung fails to inflate and the baby presents with increasing dyspnoea and cyanosis. Bowel sounds are heard in the chest, the heart beat can be auscultated on the right hand side of the chest as it is displaced by the inflated bowel and the abdomen looks hollow. Bag and mask resuscitation should not be used as it will overdistend the stomach and bowel with air, further restricting breathing. Endotracheal intubation and ventilation is imperative for these babies who present one of the most urgent neonatal surgical emergencies.

Surgery involves replacing the bowel, stomach and any other herniated viscera in the abdominal cavity and repairing the diaphragmatic defect. The baby will remain ventilated post-operatively and the prognosis will depend to a great extent on the amount of functional lung tissue and the baby's ability to sustain its own oxygenation.

OESOPHAGEAL ATRESIA AND TRACHEOESOPHAGEAL FISTULA
(incidence approx. 1 in 3000)

Oesophageal atresia is a condition where there is a blind ending to the upper end of the oesophagus, usually at the level of the third or fourth vertebrae. There is no connection between the upper and lower portions of the oesophagus. In about 90% of cases there is also an oesophageal fistula, where there is a connection between one or both portions of the oesophagus and the trachea. Associated anomalies are present in about 50% of cases (Chittimittrapap et al., 1989). As the oesophagus is obstructed the fetus is unable to swallow amniotic fluid, which leads to polyhydramnios.

At birth there are often copious, frothy oral secretions and, if a fistula is present, aspiration of these secretions into the lungs will cause cyanotic episodes. It is important to pass a nasogastric tube to assess the patency of the oesophagus in all cases of polyhydramnios. Oral feed *must not* be offered until a fistula has been excluded. The prognosis for a baby is much worse once milk has been aspirated.

Surgery involves rejoining the ends of the oesophagus if they are close enough, but if the gap is too large definitive surgery may be delayed or grafts used. The fistula is removed and a feeding tube inserted through the anastomosed segment to protect it whilst healing takes place. In the long term, these babies often need frequent dilatations of the oesophagus as they grow, due to scar tissue restricting the lumen.

EXOMPHALOS AND GASTROSCHISIS
(incidence approx. 1 in 5000–6000)

Both of these anomalies occur at the end of the first trimester and involve a herniation of abdominal contents either through the base of the umbilical cord (*exomphalos*), or through a defect in the anterior abdominal wall (*gastroschisis*). There are raised alpha-fetoprotein levels and diagnosis can be confirmed early by ultrasound scan.

In exomphalos, there is a covering of fused peritoneum and amnion which may rupture during delivery. In a large percentage of cases there are associated congenital abnormalities, particularly those of the alimentary tract, heart and genitourinary system. Exomphalos is one of the features of *Beckwith's syndrome*, another feature of which is a large, protruding tongue.

The herniated viscera in gastroschisis is not protected by a covering sac and may appear oedematous or inflamed at birth. The blood supply may be disrupted to parts of the gut due to rotation or malpositioning of the viscera. This may result in necrosis and necessitate resection of the affected parts. If large lengths of bowel are involved, malabsorption syndrome may result.

At delivery, the care of babies with both of these conditions is the same. The main aims are to avoid overhandling of the herniated contents, which may cause damage or introduce infection and to reduce heat and evaporative fluid loss from the large exposed bowel. The best way of achieving this is to cover the defect in sterile, warm, saline-soaked gauze swabs, then place the baby's legs and abdomen, up to its armpits, in a sterile plastic bag.

Surgery will attempt to replace as much of the abdominal contents as possible, but may need to be performed in stages over subsequent months or years, due to the comparative size of the hernia and abdomen.

CLEFT LIP AND/OR PALATE
(incidence approx. 1 in 1200 cleft lip; 1 in 2500 cleft palate)

A cleft lip is one of the most immediately noticeable and distressing of the congenital abnormalities, but with modern surgical techniques can be repaired extremely skilfully. There is often a family history of such abnormalities and genetic counselling should be offered to parents who themselves have a cleft lip or palate, or who have a child with these defects. The recurrence risk (Kelnar *et al.*, 1995) can be discussed with them and early detailed ultrasound scanning should be arranged in the next pregnancy.

Feeding problems may occur with these defects but breastfeeding is not impossible. Adequate support for the mother and referral to a feeding specialist can help tremendously. The mother may wish to express her milk for the baby until the first operation has been performed and feeding is easier. Special-shaped teats or the use of a Habermann bottle or cup feeding can also ease the problems, which are often related to the baby being unable to form a seal around a normal teat.

Surgical repair of a cleft lip is often undertaken at the age of about three months. Repair of the palate is frequently left until the baby is about 9–11 months old. Future operations are also likely to refine the original repair as the child grows. Referral to an orthodontist and speech therapist should also be made at the appropriate stages. The parents will require much support and may benefit from information about local and national self-help organizations.

PYLORIC STENOSIS
(incidence approx. 1 in 500)

In this condition the muscle of the pylorus, in the stomach, hypertrophies over a number of days or sometimes weeks, causing increasing obstruction. The baby begins to posset regularly and this gradually worsens until projectile vomiting occurs immediately after all feeds. This may begin within the first week but more commonly presents at the age of 3–6 weeks. The baby shows signs of failure to thrive. Peristalsis may be visible during feeds and a mass can be felt at the site of the obstruction.

Surgery is performed to divide the relevant muscle thus resolving the problem. There may be a family history of this condition, which is five times more common in boys than girls.

HIRSCHSPRUNG'S DISEASE
(incidence approx. 1 in 5000)

There may be a family history of this condition in which there is congenital absence of ganglionic cells in one or more parts of the distal colon. It is most common in term, male infants. Development of this part of the alimentary tract occurs at about the same time as fusion of the palate and lips takes place, therefore a common associated condition is a cleft lip or palate.

The earliest characteristic sign is a delayed passage of meconium. Any baby who has not passed meconium within 24–48 hours should have a rectal examination. Another way in which this condition presents is by bowel habits alternating between constipation and diarrhoea within the first week of life.

Initial surgery forms a colostomy and removes the aganglionic segments of bowel. Once the gut has grown and developed, anastomosis may be undertaken, which is usually at about one year of age.

IMPERFORATE ANUS
(incidence approx. 1 in 15 000)

As part of the general examination of the newborn baby the anus must be examined for patency. Meconium-stained liquor is not indicative of a patent anus as a fistula may be present allowing the passage of meconium, in which case the following signs and symptoms may not present. In the absence of a fistula the baby will fail to pass meconium, there will be abdominal distension and bile-stained vomiting.

The surgical procedure depends on the exact anatomical abnormalities found and whether a fistula is present or not.

Pain

There has been much controversy amongst clinicians, over the years, on the subject of neonatal pain. Topics of debate have included:

▶ whether or not the neurological systems of preterm and term babies are developed and mature enough to sense pain;
▶ the efficacy of various methods of assessing response to pain;
▶ the effects and safety of different forms of pain relief on the neonate.

NEUROLOGICAL DEVELOPMENT

In recent years, numerous studies have conclusively proven that neonates of all gestations *do* feel and react to painful stimuli (Anand and Hickey, 1987; Fitzgerald

1987; Fitzgerald and McIntosh, 1989). Although considerable maturation of the central nervous system takes place postnatally, basic pathways between the spinal cord and primary sensory neurones are present in the early stages of fetal development. Evidence has shown the whole of the nervous system to be functional in the prenatal period (Flower, 1985). Complete myelination of neurones is not necessary for perception of pain; the lack of myelination in immature neonates merely slows the rate of conductivity of nerve impulses (Anand and Hickey, 1987).

ASSESSING RESPONSES TO PAIN

Babies react in many ways in response to stimuli. Not all stimuli are painful, some may cause discomfort or a disturbance as opposed to an actual pain. Examples would include heel pricks as painful, physical examination as a discomfort and bright lights as a disturbance. However, all negative stimuli should be minimized or alleviated wherever possible.

There are numerous variable factors to be considered when assessing an individual baby's level of response to a stimulus. These include the gestational age and health of the baby and the intensity and duration of the stimuli. Frequent or prolonged episodes of pain may result in the baby becoming listless with reduced limb activity and an abnormal, stiff posture.

Responses may be in the form of *behavioural*, *physiological* or *metabolic* changes. Many methods of quantifying these are currently used in order to make an assessment of the degree of pain experienced by the baby (Craig *et al.*, 1993; Lawrence *et al.*, 1993).

1   *Behavioural* effects include crying, grimacing, increased agitation (Broome and Tanzello, 1990), withdrawal of limbs, Moro reflex and acute irritability.
2   *Physiological* changes include tachycardia or bradycardia, tachypnoea, hypertension, increased oxygen requirements and palmar sweating in babies over 37 weeks' gestation (Harpin and Rutter, 1982).

3   There is an increased rate of metabolism of fats and carbohydrates in response to a decreased insulin secretion and a release of corticosteroids, following prolonged painful procedures. This leads to hyperglycaemia. Other *metabolic* changes include glycosuria, proteinuria, ketonuria and a raised urine pH.

PAIN RELIEF

There are many methods of relieving pain and discomfort. Careful attention to the neonatal environment, expertise at performing techniques and careful choice of equipment used, can all help to reduce trauma to babies. For example, high levels of noise and bright lights are known to be detrimental to babies in neonatal intensive care units, and the use of automated machines to perform heel-prick tests has been shown to be less painful and reduce the risk of long-term damage (Harpin and Rutter, 1983).

Interventional techniques which may be used during or following procedures to comfort the baby, should be taught to parents. These may include comfortable positioning post-operatively, talking or providing music, gentle massage or stroking of the limbs, cuddling, breastfeeding or non-nutritive sucking.

Pharmacological methods of alleviating pain should also be considered. The dose, method and frequency of administration of each drug will need careful consideration. The half-life and absorption rates of a drug are affected by the gestation, age and condition of the baby.

Some form of anaesthesia should routinely be given prior to any invasive procedure, and adequate analgesia given postoperatively as a matter of course, as with adults (Spear, 1992). Narcotic drugs may depress respiratory effort and their use is often limited to those babies already receiving respiratory support. Morphine and fentanyl are the most commonly administered opioids, with morphine favoured for its greater sedation effects. Sedation on its own has no place in the relief of pain and it is important to distinguish between pain and irritability before prescribing (Broome and Tanzello, 1990).

References

Anand, K.J.S. & Hickey, P.R. (1987) Pain and its effects in the human neonate and fetus. *New Engl. J. Med.* 317: 1321–1329.

Broome, M.E. & Tanzello, H. (1990) Differentiating between pain and agitation in premature neonates. *J. Perinatal Neonatal Nurs.* 4(1): 53–62.

Chittimittrapap, S., Spitz, L., Kiely, E.M. *et al.* (1989)

Oesophageal atresia and associated anomalies. *Arch. Dis. Childh.* **64**: 364.

Craig, K.D., Whitfield, M.F., Grunau, R.V.E. *et al.* (1993) Pain in the preterm neonate: behavioral and physiological indices. *Pain* **52**: 287–299.

Fitzgerald, M. (1987) Pain and analgesia in neonates. *Trends Neurosci.* **10**: 344–346.

Fitzgerald, M. & McIntosh, N. (1989) Pain and analgesia in the newborn. *Arch. Dis. Childh.* **64**: 441–443.

Flower, M. (1985) Neuromaturation of the human fetus. *J. Med. Phil.* **10**: 237–251.

Harpin, V.A.H. & Rutter, N. (1982) Development of emotional sweating in the newborn infant. *Arch. Dis. Childh.* **57**: 691–695.

Harpin, V.A.H. & Rutter, N. (1983) Making heel pricks less painful. *Arch. Dis. Childh.* **58**(3): 226–228.

Kelnar, C.J.H., Harvey, D. & Simpson, C. (1995) *The Sick Newborn Baby.* London: Baillière Tindall.

Kullendorff, C.M., Larsson, L.T. & Jorgensen, C. (1984) Advantages of antenatal diagnosis of intestinal and urinary malformations. *Br. J. Obstet. Gynaecol.* **91**: 144–147.

Lawrence, J., Alcock, D., McGrath, P. *et al.* (1993) The development of a tool to assess neonatal pain. *Neonatal Network* **12**(6): 59–66.

Lucas, A. & Cole, T.J. (1990) Breast milk and neonatal necrotising enterocolitis. *Lancet* **336**: 1519–1523.

Spear, R.M. (1992) Anesthesia for premature and term infants: Perioperative implications. *J. Pediat.* **120**(2): 165–176.

Stoodley, N., Sharma, A., Noblett, H. *et al.* (1993) Influence of place of delivery on outcome in babies with gastroschisis. *Arch. Dis. Child.* **68**: 321–323.

Further Reading

Kenner, C., Harjo, J. & Brueggemeyer, A. (1988) *Neonatal Surgery: A Nursing Perspective.* Orlando: Grune & Stratton.

Sudden Infant Death Syndrome

The definition of 'sudden infant death syndrome' (SIDS) is a sudden infant death, unexpected by history and unexplained by post-mortem examination. 'Cot death' is the sudden and unexpected death of a baby for no obvious reason. Some deaths may be explained by post-mortem examination. Those which remain unexplained after post-mortem may be registered on the death certificate as SIDS, sudden infant death, sudden unexpected death in infancy or cot death.

Following much debate over the definition of SIDS in recent years (Limerick and Gardner, 1992; Gordon, 1992), the term sudden infant death syndrome is now recommended to be used only in those cases where it is the only cause of death stated on the death certificate. The data collected by the Office of Population Censuses and Surveys (OPCS) contains statistics for deaths where other causes are also mentioned on the death certificate (OPCS, 1994).

Different studies into this condition have used differing definitions, some including deaths within the first week, some only deaths occurring after the 7th day and some including deaths beyond the first year (of which there were 18 in the UK in 1993). About 90% of sudden infant deaths occur in the postneonatal period (between 1 month and 1 year), and all the studies include this period.

Incidence and Trends

During the 1970s and early 1980s in the United Kingdom, interest in the topic of sudden infant deaths increased considerably. Deaths previously attributed to other causes, particularly unspecified respiratory illnesses, were more frequently diagnosed as sudden infant death on death certificates. There was a corresponding steady rise in the SIDS rate for England and Wales to a rate of 2.1 per thousand live births in 1982. A peak rate of 2.3 per thousand live births was recorded in 1988.

At the end of 1991 campaigns to reduce the risks were launched by the Foundation for the Study of Infant Deaths and the Department of Health. These made the following four main recommendations to parents:

1   Do not place babies on their fronts to sleep.
2   Do not expose babies to cigarette smoke.
3   Do not overheat babies.
4   Seek medical advice early if babies are unwell.

Between 1991 and 1992 there was a 47% reduction in the SIDS rate. The UK SIDS rate for 1993 was 0.7 per thousand live births – a reduction of 72% from 1988 to 1993.

There is a wide variation in the incidence throughout the country and indeed worldwide. The rate for the Maori population of the South Island of New Zealand is one of the highest in the world (6.9 per thousand live births), compared to the very low rate of 0.3 per thousand live births in Hong Kong in the same year.

The peak incidence of cot death occurs at the age of 2–3 months. It occurs more commonly in the winter months, in boys (61% of cases between 1989 and 1993), in preterm and low birthweight babies.

Risk Factors and Advice

The aetiology of SIDS is multifactorial and research into many aspects of its nature continues. Certain factors have been identified as being associated with an increased risk of SIDS.

SLEEPING POSITION

This was first considered in 1965 (Carpenter and Shaddick, 1965), but the association of sleeping position and SIDS was not found to be statistically significant at this time. Different cultures and communities have different practices in childcare and comparison of cot death rates in different communities in the mid-1980s showed lower rates when babies were placed on their backs to sleep (Davies, 1985; Beal, 1986). Prone sleeping became popular in The Netherlands in the early 1970s, following which there was a three-fold increase in their SIDS rate.

Since 1988 various studies into the prone sleeping position and subsequent cot death rates have been undertaken throughout the world (Beal, 1988; Wigfield et al., 1991; Engelberts et al., 1991; Mitchell et al., 1991a; Taylor et al., 1991). They have consistently shown this position to be a significant risk factor, and

recorded dramatic falls in SIDS rates when babies are put to sleep on their backs or sides. A study in Avon (Fleming et al., 1990) found the risk of SIDS to be 8.8 times higher if a baby slept prone compared to supine or on its side.

Although safer than prone sleeping, babies lying on their sides appear to have almost twice the risk of SIDS as those lying supine. This may be partly due to the increased likelihood of these babies rolling on to their stomachs. For this reason, it is advised that the lower arm is extended forwards to prevent rolling if the baby is placed in this position.

SMOKING

Smoking during pregnancy has been widely identified as a significant risk factor for SIDS (Mitchell et al., 1991b, 1993; Schoendorf and Kiely, 1992). The baby of a mother who smokes is twice as likely to die from a cot death as the baby of a non-smoking mother, even after allowing for other influencing factors. The risk increases three times for every 10 cigarettes smoked (Haglund and Cnattingius, 1990).

The effects of passive smoking on the risk of cot death are more difficult to prove. A Tasmanian study (McGlashan, 1989) shows a significant risk increase if both parents smoke as opposed to just one, and an American study (Malloy et al., 1988) concludes that passive smoking may be related to SIDS and respiratory deaths.

TEMPERATURE AND WRAPPING

Overheating of a baby may occur if the room temperature is inappropriately high, if there is an excessive amount of clothing and bedding in use or if the baby's ability to lose heat is impaired – for example, if swaddled tightly, the head is covered, prone sleeping or the baby has a high temperature due to illness.

Fleming et al. (1990) demonstrated that SIDS babies in their Avon study were more likely to have been heavily wrapped, sleeping prone and to have had heating on all night. The risk from such overheating was found only to be significant in babies over 70 days of age. Each of these situations is recognized as a risk factor on its own, but when combined with one or more other factors it becomes much more significant.

Parents tend to increase the amount of bedding if their baby is ill. This is another factor which, when combined with those already mentioned, increases the risk of SIDS substantially (Gilbert *et al.*, 1992; Ponsonby *et al.*, 1992).

ILLNESS

Evidence of minor illnesses, insufficient to cause death, are found at post-mortem examination on many babies who die from SIDS. The severity of an illness may be underestimated – one retrospective study (Cole *et al.*, 1991), showed that 8% of SIDS babies had signs of serious illness before they died. As a result of such findings, a scoring system of signs and symptoms has been devised, called Babycheck, to aid parents and professionals in assessing the severity of illness in a baby under six months of age (Morley *et al.*, 1991).

OTHER FACTORS

Evidence to support the idea that bottle feeding is a risk factor for SIDS is inconclusive. The New Zealand study (Mitchell *et al.*, 1991b) showed a significant association between not breastfeeding and cot death. However, in Hong Kong, which has one of the lowest SIDS rates in the world (Lee *et al.*, 1989), the rate of breastfeeding is extremely low. It is generally accepted that breastfeeding should be encouraged for all babies, as its benefits to both mother and baby are numerous.

There is thought to be a greater risk to babies who sleep with their parents, but this again is not supported by conclusive evidence. An increased risk may be afforded by overheating of babies in this situation, as they will gain heat from both parents and their bedding, which may be a heavy duvet. Advice to parents who wish to sleep with their baby is to make up a separate 'bed' for the infant between their pillows. They must ensure the baby's head is not covered, not swaddle the baby, ensure there is no risk of suffocation from the parent's pillows and use thin sheets or blankets to cover the baby. If either parent has been drinking or using drugs the advice is that they should not sleep with the baby.

ADVICE

Advice regarding reducing the known risk factors of cot death needs to be given to potential parents before conception. This gives them the opportunity to stop smoking and improve their own health prior to conception. Unfortunately, in the UK at present, preconception advice and screening is mainly available to those who request or pay privately for it, and these parents are often those who are low risk anyway.

General advice to parents is as follows:

▶ Lie the baby on his back to sleep, never his stomach. When lying on his side, the baby's lower arm should be extended forward to prevent the possibility of rolling on to the stomach.
▶ Stop smoking before or during pregnancy. If this is not possible, reduce the number of cigarettes smoked to as few as possible.
▶ Always keep the baby in a smoke-free environment.
▶ Discuss the appropriate number of layers of clothing and bedding needed for the baby with the midwife, health visitor or doctor. In the recommended room temperature of 18–20°C, babies under one month of age require 6–8 layers. A vest, stretch-suit, cardigan and a single blanket each count as one layer. A room temperature of 16–18°C is recommended for babies between the ages of 1 and 6 months. Babies born preterm or small may need one or two extra layers until they are able to regulate their temperature. More detailed recommendations of tog values are given in Wigfield *et al.* (1993).
▶ Do not swaddle the baby tightly or cover the baby's head with bedding.
▶ Do not use pillows, cot bumpers or duvets for babies under one year old.
▶ Get used to feeling the baby's temperature on the back or chest. A wall thermometer may help to monitor the room temperature.
▶ If the baby appears ill or has a high temperature, take layers of bedding or clothing off and contact a doctor. Paracetomol elixir may be given to babies over four months of age.

A leaflet containing this information must be given to all parents.

Apnoea Alarms at Home

There is no evidence to show that the use of apnoea monitors at home reduces the incidence of cot death. Over 50 000 monitors are in use in America, but there has not been a significant drop in the cot death rate since their use became so widespread (National Institutes of Health, 1987).

It is widely accepted that monitoring normal,

healthy babies is impractical and undesirable. There is a high rate of false alarms with apnoea monitors, which heighten the parents' anxieties. Many parents become reliant on the monitors as a measure of the well-being of their baby and may miss early signs of illness. Resuscitation of an apnoeic baby is not always successful and some will have sustained irreversible brain damage by this time.

The breathing patterns of babies are erratic and short apnoeic spells are normal. Occasionally babies have longer periods of apnoea which result in hypoxia, leading to cyanosis, hypotonia and choking or gagging. These are known as *apparent life-threatening events* (ALTEs) and may require stimulation or resuscitation to correct them. Not all apparent life-threatening events are associated with prolonged apnoeic periods, some are caused by infection or aspiration of feed or vomit. The relevance of apparent life-threatening events with regard to SIDS is uncertain, with an American study showing that less than 7% of SIDS babies had a history of such episodes (National Institutes of Health, 1987). Like SIDS however, apparent life-threatening events are more common in male infants, preterm babies and occur more frequently in the same age ranges.

Trials are being conducted on the use of monitors for home use which detect a drop in oxygen saturation (Kelnar *et al.*, 1995). At present evidence of their effectiveness is insufficient to recommend for home use.

The current recommendations from the British Paediatric Association Respiratory Group (Davies *et al.*, 1990) are that home monitoring may be appropriate for two groups of babies:

1   Babies who have had one or more apparent life-threatening events, depending on whether a cause is known.
2   Subsequent siblings of a SIDS baby.

Care of the Family

SIDS is a tragedy which brings devastation to a family. The unexpected nature of the death, usually in a previously healthy baby, and the lack of explanation as to the cause, deepens the distress. Great care and sensitivity are required by those professionals in contact with the family at this time. The parents, siblings and other family members may wish to see and hold the baby before he is taken away. They should be supported in doing this and given as much time as they wish to say goodbye to their baby. For fuller details on bereavement care see Chapter 78.

All sudden infant deaths are investigated by a coroner which can also be very distressing for the parents. It is important to warn them of the possibility of an inquest. A post-mortem examination will be necessary to try to establish the cause of death. This should be carefully explained to the family in terms of the benefits of having a definite diagnosis. If the death occurred at home the parents should be told that the police will visit and that they will be required to make a statement about the death at some stage. The police may remove bedding and clothes for further examination and this needs to be explained gently to the parents. Advice on funeral arrangements, registering the death and financial issues may also be required.

Parents may find it helpful to talk to a social worker or minister of religion at this time. The cultural and religious beliefs and rituals of the family must be considered at all times. It is important to notify the members of the primary health care team of the baby's death, so that continued support can be given and insensitive errors, such as sending immunization reminders, prevented.

Siblings and grandparents will also need support and explanations. Their grief is different to that of the parents and they are all too often forgotten. Support groups, locally or nationally, may be helpful to the family.

FOLLOW-UP

Parents will have many questions about their baby's death and it is important that they have the opportunity to discuss these with the paediatrician involved. Once all the results of the tests and post-mortem examination are available, the parents should be offered an appointment with the paediatrician. It is very common for parents of SIDS babies to feel that their care was in some way inadequate and that they caused the death of their baby, and where possible reassurances must be given that this was not the case. It is likely that several appointments will be helpful to the family and this may be particularly relevant if they are planning another pregnancy, to discuss risks and care of the next baby.

SUBSEQUENT PREGNANCIES

Families who have suffered the death of a baby often have mixed feelings about subsequent pregnancies.

The pregnancy and first few months after the birth can be very anxious times, particularly around the age when the last baby died. The Foundation for the Study of Infant Deaths has set up a programme of support for these families called 'Care of Next Infant' (CONI). This uses the skills and support of the paediatrician, family doctor, midwife, health visitor and a local Care of Next Infant co-ordinator. It involves the parents themselves in deciding the level of care they require throughout the pregnancy and following months. The support offered may include weekly visits to the health visitor, a set of weighing scales to monitor the baby's weight regularly, a wall thermometer to monitor the room temperature, a symptom diary for the parents to note any changes in their baby and an apnoea monitor. Discussion and advice about reducing known risk factors is of great importance.

References

Beal, S.M. (1986) Sudden infant death syndrome: epidemiological comparisons between South Australia and communities with a different incidence. *Aust. Paediat. J.* **22** (Suppl.): 13–16.

Beal, S. (1988) Sleeping position and sudden infant death syndrome. *Med. J. Aust.* **149**: 562.

Carpenter, R.G. & Shaddick, C.W. (1965) Role of infection, suffocation and bottlefeeding in cot death. An analysis of some factors in the histories of 110 cases and their controls. *Br. J. Prevent. Soc. Med.* **19**: 1–7.

Cole, T.J., Gilbert, R.E., Fleming, P.J. *et al.* (1991) Babycheck and the Avon infant mortality study. *Arch. Dis. Childh.* **66**: 1077–1078.

Davies, D.P. (1985) Cot death in Hong Kong: a rare problem? *Lancet* ii: 1346–1349.

Davies, P.A., Milner, A.D., Silverman, M. *et al.* (1990) Monitoring and Sudden Infant Death Syndrome: an update. Report from the Foundation for the Study of Infant Deaths and the British Paediatric Respiratory Group. *Arch. Dis. Childh.* **65**: 238–240.

Engelberts, A.C., de Jonge, G.A. & Kostense, P.J. (1991) An analysis of trends in the incidence of sudden infant death in The Netherlands 1969–89. *J. Paediat. Child Health* **27**: 329–333.

Fleming, P.J., Gilbert, R., Azaz, Y. *et al.* (1990) Interaction between bedding and sleeping position in sudden infant death syndrome: a population based case-control study. *Br. Med. J.* **301**: 85–89.

Gilbert, R., Rudd, P., Berry, P.J. *et al.* (1992) Combined effect of infection and heavy wrapping on the risk of sudden unexpected infant death. *Arch. Dis. Childh.* **67**: 171–177.

Gordon, R.R. (1992) What counts as cot death? *Br. Med. J.* **304**: 1508.

Haglund, B. & Cnattingius, S. (1990) Cigarette smoking as a risk factor for Sudden Infant Death Syndrome: a population-based study. *Am. J. Public Health* **80**(1): 29–32.

Kelnar, C.J.H., Harvey, D. & Simpson, C. (1995) *The Sick Newborn Baby*, p. 393. London: Baillière Tindall.

Lee, N.N.Y., Chan, Y.F., Davies, D.P. *et al.* (1989) Sudden infant death syndrome in Hong Kong: confirmation of low incidence. *Br. Med. J.* **298**: 721.

Limerick, S.R. & Gardner, A. (1992) What counts as cot death? *Br. Med. J.* **304**: 1176.

Malloy, M.H., Kleinman, J.C., Land, G.H. *et al.* (1988) The association of maternal smoking with age and cause of infant death. *Am. J. Epidemiol.* **128**(1): 46–55.

McGlashan, N.D. (1989) Sudden infant deaths in Tasmania, 1980–1986: a seven year prospective study. *Soc. Sci. Med.* **29**: 1015–1026.

Mitchell, E.A., Taylor, B.J., Ford, R.P.K. *et al.* (1991a) Further evidence supporting a casual relationship between prone sleeping position and SIDS. In *Founding Congress, Rouen. Workshop Abstracts. The European Society for the Study and Prevention of Infant Death 1991*.

Mitchell, E.A., Scragg, R., Stewart, A.W. *et al.* (1991b) Cot Death Supplement. Results from the first year of the New Zealand cot death study. *N.Z. Med. J.* **104**(906): 71–76.

Mitchell, E.A., Ford, R.P.K, Stewart, A.W. *et al.* (1993) Smoking and the sudden infant death syndrome. *Pediatrics* **91**: 893–896.

Morley, C.J., Thornton, A.J., Cole, T.J. *et al.* (1991) Babycheck: a scoring system to grade the severity of acute systemic illness in babies under six months old. *Arch. Dis. Childh.* **66**: 100–105.

National Institutes of Health Consensus Development Conference on Infantile Apnea and Home Monitoring, 1986 (1987) Consensus Statement. *Paediatrics* **79**(2): 292–299.

OPCS (Office of Population Censuses and Surveys) (1994) *Sudden Infant Deaths, 1989–93.* DH3 94/1. London: HMSO.

Ponsonby, A.-L., Dwyer, T., Gibbons, L.E. *et al.* (1992) Thermal environment and sudden infant death syndrome: case-control study. *Br. Med. J.* **304**: 277–282.

Schoendorf, K.C., Kiely, J.L. (1992) Relationship of sudden infant death syndrome to maternal smoking during and after pregnancy. *Pediatrics* **90**(6): 905–908.

Taylor, B.J., Nelson, E.A.S. & Mackay, S. (1991) Changing child care practice in an area with high post neonatal mortality. In *Founding Congress, Rouen. Workshop Abstracts. The European Society for the Study and Prevention of Infant Death 1991*.

Wigfield, R.E., Gilbert, R.E., Fleming, P. *et al.* (1991) Prone sleeping position and sudden infant death syndrome (SIDS): The effect of changing practice. In *Founding Congress, Rouen. Workshop Abstracts. The European Society for the Study and Prevention of Infant Death.*

Wigfield, R.E., Fleming, P.J. *et al.* (1993) How much wrapping do babies need at night? *Arch. Dis. Childh.* **69**: 181–186.

Further Reading

Foundation for the Study of Infant Deaths (1994) *Factfile 1: Cot Death – Facts, Figures and Definitions.* FSID, 35 Belgrave Square, London SW1X 8QB.

Stewart, A. & Dent, A. (1994) *At a Loss: Bereavement Care When a Baby Dies.* London: Baillière Tindall.

Grief and Bereavement

Stages of Grief

Grieving is a normal emotional, mental, physical and societal reaction to bereavement. One of the first people to record grief reactions was Darwin (1872), although he was mainly interested in the emotional reactions of the bereaved person and the muscles used to express those reactions. He concluded that the facial expressions displayed were analogous to those of an infant screaming.

Bowlby (1980) presents four processes involved in healthy, as opposed to pathological, mourning:

1 Numbness.
2 Yearning.
3 Disorganization and despair.
4 Reorganization.

He states that these processes attempt to effect a withdrawal of emotional investment in the lost person, which may prepare the bereaved person for making a relationship with another person. The phase of *numbness* can last from a few hours to a week, and is followed by a persistent and insatiable *yearning* for the lost person, which causes pain. Along with the feeling of pain can be those of fear, guilt, anger, hatred, anxiety and despair. There is a searching for the one lost, a strong desire for other people to help with this, and yet at the same time there may be a rejection of help. The third phase is one of *disorganization and despair* and the final phase, *reorganization*.

Kubler-Ross (1970) describes five stages of grieving in her work with terminally ill patients:

1 Denial.
2 Anger.
3 Bargaining (with the doctor, with God).
4 Depression.
5 Acceptance.

In the first stage the shock of the deeply distressing news seems to cause a *denial* of the truth of the news. This stage may last for seconds, minutes or days and appears to act as a buffer to protect the person from the resulting pain. At this time the person cannot seem to hear, or register what is being said; there may be no sign of emotion and a frozen immobility.

The stage of *anger* brings with it the question 'Why me?' and is a stage during which emotions are usually freely expressed. In the case of a stillbirth or neonatal death the father of the baby is usually the first to respond with anger, which he may direct at the doctor, midwife, God or even his wife. She will usually respond with tears – in fact, if she does not do so, she may still be denying the baby's death and refusing to grieve. Her tears may initially be a 'calling weeping' (Bowlby, 1980) indicative of her desperately wanting her live baby back. Subsequently the weeping may be related to frustration, anger, bitterness, resentment, fear, panic or guilt. This loss of emotional control may be strongly resented. It brings with it a feeling of helplessness and regression to childhood, but crying, weeping, even screaming is an essential part of grieving, and without this early show of emotion many authors maintain that the grieving, or grief work, is likely to be incompletely resolved (Parkes, 1972; Kubler-Ross, 1989).

Leick and Nielsen (1991) maintain that human beings have an innate ability to reduce stress by weeping, although this ability is often obstructed and may be all but removed as people grow up. In Western society men are actively encouraged not to cry, but instead to 'be strong', as if crying is an expression of weakness.

The stage of *bargaining* in the case of a perinatal death is probably a short phase and may not be expressed verbally. The bereaved mother may, however, bargain with God, promising perhaps that she will dedicate her baby to Him if only He will let her have the baby back. Some mothers develop the idea that their baby has been mixed up with another, particularly if the baby has been taken away from them to a neonatal unit perhaps in another hospital; these mothers may well resort to bargaining in an attempt to retrieve their baby.

The fourth stage of *depression* may follow on from the failure of the bargaining stage, but may also occur concurrently with bargaining, episodes of anger and even a reversion back to periods of denial – 'They got my baby mixed up, it wasn't my baby who died'.

Although distinct stages of grieving are described, no one stage may be paramount at any one time, certainly until acceptance of the loss has been reached and recovery is in sight. During the stage of depression, which Bowlby (1980) refers to as disorganization, often a variety of unhappy emotions are felt by the one

bereaved. The woman who has had a miscarriage, stillbirth or neonatal death may experience a feeling of loss of status, low self-esteem, inadequacy and guilt at her failure to become a mother and her consequent failure to be a 'good wife'. An enormous sense of loneliness and isolation may take her over – no one, not even her husband, can fully share in her pain of unfulfilled motherhood. Leick and Nielsen (1991) suggest that losing a child is like losing a part of one's own body, particularly so soon after birth. The just-born baby has had so little time, or none at all, to become a separate entity and the mother has to grieve not only at her never-to-be-fulfilled dreams of motherhood (with this pregnancy), but also at the loss of a living, possibly moving and perhaps communicating, hitherto healthy and differentiated structure inside her own body. This experience has been compared with amputative grief (Brenkley, 1991).

During a period of depression, for whatever cause, many people experience a replay of other unhappy or unsuccessful times in their lives, and the woman bereaved of her child is no exception. The grief and mourning of the present reality is compounded by that of the memory of past losses. Often the social withdrawal, loss of purpose in life and feeling of helplessness is accentuated to a point at which neither the company nor comfort of her husband or other children bring any sense of pleasure or indeed of relief.

The fifth and final stage of the grieving process as described by Kubler-Ross (1970) is that of *acceptance*, called reorganization by Bowlby (1980). During this stage, the loss begins to be accepted as a reality, attachment to the lost individual begins to be broken and emotional energy is gradually withdrawn from the one lost. The capacity to enjoy life again and receive pleasure from other individuals is restored. The loss needs to be worked through to achieve a positive psychological outcome (Miller, 1985; Schneider, 1984). Recovery from the grief of a miscarriage, stillbirth or neonatal death may take many months, years or even a lifetime. Most people recover sufficiently to resume a normal lifestyle, some, however, suffer from the consequences of unresolved, or pathological, grief and a few slide into a psychiatric condition for which they require treatment, perhaps for the rest of their lives.

Help for the Recently Bereaved

How can midwives help to initiate, facilitate, ease, accentuate and complete the grieving process?

Many people reach middle age without ever having been in the presence of death and dying has become isolated from everyday life, as death rarely occurs at home. Kubler-Ross (1989) states that ours is a death-denying society; any society which rates materialistic values highly creates individuals who find the idea of death difficult. Mother Frances Dominica (1987) considers that the more sophisticated our society becomes and the more it pays homage to the powers of intellect and reasoning, the more ill at ease it is with death and that which lies beyond. Death is not commonplace, and when it does occur it is usually hidden from view. Death, therefore, to the average young couple is unexpected, unexperienced and unthought of. Little wonder that the first reaction is usually denial.

The midwife often has the task in the case of a stillbirth of reversing that denial. A continuation of this stage of the grieving process ultimately leads to avoided grief which in turn can lead to psychosomatic or psychological symptoms such as anxiety, dependence or isolation (Leick and Nielsen, 1991). Many authors (Klaus and Kennell, 1982; Pepper and Knapp, 1980; Leon, 1990; SANDS, 1991) advocate encouraging the parents to see, touch and hold their stillborn baby, although they would respect the parents' wishes if they refused to do so. In the latter case a photograph of the baby should be taken and left in the medical records so that at a future date the parents can have it, if they so request.

Leon (1990) makes the point that although most mourning is retrospective, perinatal mourning is prospective: the parents have to relinquish all hopes, wishes and dreams that they may have had about the future of this infant. In view of this, it is helpful to the parents, especially to the mother, to give them as much to remember as possible. If they will see and hold the baby, it is kindest to leave them together with the baby for as long as they wish, with frequent but brief visits to the room to give comfort and support. As many mothers have remarked, 'It's my baby'. Mothers often like to create a book of remembrance for their babies which helps the grieving process. To facilitate this, a lock of the baby's hair may be given to the parents, as may the baby's name bracelet, the cot card or a foot or hand print. A photograph may be taken of the whole family with the stillborn baby, and other siblings may wish to touch or hold their baby brother or sister (SANDS, 1991). The whole family, and especially the mother, need to have memories to last a lifetime.

However short the baby's lifespan, it is invariably of importance to the mother for a professional person to acknowledge that this baby was alive and that the baby's life had some meaning to it. One mother who had a normal delivery after a previous Caesarean section told her obstetrician that she was so grateful to the tiny stillborn baby for giving her the experience of a normal birth.

If the professional becomes the object at which the father's or mother's anger is directed, she/he should try not to take it personally, even if involved in the delivery. It is important not to get angry in return but see the anger as a symptom of acute need.

Parkes (1986) describes the physical effects of grief and states that the initial effect relates to the 'fight or flight' syndrome, in which the fight may be expressed as anger and the flight as withdrawal or denial. With this emotional reaction usually comes the familiar autonomic disturbances of a dry mouth, rapid beating of the heart, sighing respirations and restlessness. C.S. Lewis (1961) wrote after his wife died 'no one ever told me that grief felt so like fear . . . the same fluttering in the stomach, the same restlessness, the yawning. I keep on swallowing'. Parkes (1986) also states that the loss of a child causes a high state of alarm, and as a result of this, physical symptoms include increase in muscle tension, loss of appetite, weight loss, digestive disturbances, palpitations, headaches, exhaustion and difficulty in sleeping. In relation to the last symptom, however, automatic sedation may not be the correct management as it might delay the grief process and ultimately create more distress.

At any stage of the grieving process, the parents, especially the mother, might suddenly burst into tears. In Western society, men are taught not to cry and with the loss of a baby, the father may be encouraged by other relatives not to express emotion so that he shows himself strong and supportive of his wife. Mother Frances Dominica (1987) is highly critical of a society in which everyone, as she states, is afraid of emotional behaviour. She states that face to face with grief we feel inadequate or embarrassed, make ourselves scarce and fervently hope that there is an 'expert' around to handle the situation. Kubler-Ross (1989) advises that when seeking to help a grieving parent the professional should just be herself; even to say 'I don't know what to say' or 'I'm so sorry' shows a caring attitude, and just to hold a hand in silence during an emotional outburst gives a feeling of security in knowing that someone is there. Some mothers feel that they should not show emotion, and need 'permission' to cry. Just to say 'It's all right to cry' may start the healing process.

In a time of such acute sadness, midwives have a vital role of fulfilling the meaning of their named profession, 'with mother'. To stay with the grieving mother, to comfort her, to encourage her to accept the reality of the death of her baby and to help her cry is to assist in the creation of the grieving and healing process. The midwife who was present at the delivery and who has shared the pain of the loss is usually the best person to do this.

Stillbirth

The Stillbirth (Definition) Act (1992) states that it would be, from October that year, a legal requirement to recognize any stillbirth where the gestation period has been 24 weeks or more. The definition of stillbirth, therefore, in the Births and Deaths Registration Act (1953) will now be as follows: 'Stillborn child' means a child which has issued forth from its mother after the 24th week of pregnancy and which did not at any time after being completely expelled from its mother breathe or show any other signs of life.

Following a stillbirth a certificate must be signed by the doctor or midwife who was present at the delivery, or who examined the body, certifying that the baby was not born alive. This is usually taken by the parents to the Registrar of Births and Deaths. The stillbirth must be registered by 42 days; if it is still not registered by three months, the Registrar has the power to compel any qualified informant in writing to do so. The doctor or midwife who was with the woman during her delivery must notify the prescribed medical officer of the stillbirth within 36 hours of birth.

The Registrar of Births and Deaths issues a Certificate of Registration and a Certificate for Burial or Cremation of the stillborn child. The latter certificate is required before a burial or cremation can take place and is taken either to the funeral director or, if the hospital authorities are arranging the funeral, to the appropriate hospital administrator. If the parents employ a funeral director, then he or she will normally make all the arrangements, which include the service,

contact with the cemetery or crematorium, flowers, organist and arrangements for collection of the baby. If the burial is arranged by the hospital the baby may be buried with other babies in unconsecrated ground. The parents should be encouraged to attend the funeral service or burial and be told that, if they wish, they may bring their other children with them.

The hospital chaplain will often visit bereaved parents and, if they do not have a minister of their own, he may offer to take the funeral service. If the parents are not of the Christian religion, the chaplain may offer to undertake a naming and/or blessing ceremony.

If a post-mortem is required, one of the parents is asked to sign the consent form. If they refuse to do so, their wishes must be respected, unless the death has been referred to the coroner, as occurs in the case of any suspicious or unusual circumstances. The coroner has the right to order a post-mortem.

The midwife must inform her/his supervisor of midwives of the stillbirth (UKCC, 1994).

Neonatal Death

A neonatal death is a baby who dies within four weeks of birth. A baby who lives for even a few minutes after birth must be counted as a live birth and therefore registered as a birth and a death.

If a baby who is born *under* 24 weeks of gestation breathes, or shows other signs of life, then that baby must be registered as a live birth. If an abortion is performed for medical reasons after 24 weeks' gestation, which under the amendments to the Abortion Act 1967 by the Human Fertilisation and Embryology Act 1990 it may be in specified circumstances, and that baby is born alive, then that birth, too, must be registered.

Registration of a neonatal death must take place, as with any death, within five days, and is normally undertaken by one of the parents. A medical certificate will have been issued by the doctor and this must be taken to the Registrar of Births and Deaths. The parents should be encouraged to name the baby if they have not already done so, as forenames cannot be entered at a later date.

The midwife must inform her/his supervisor of midwives of the neonatal death if she/he is responsible for the care of that mother and baby (UKCC, 1994).

When a baby lives for a short time, the parents often want to have a service either in the hospital chapel or in a church. If it has been known that the baby is near death, then the parents may have had the opportunity to stay in a hospital room especially designated for the purpose with their dying baby (SANDS, 1991). They will then have formed a closer bond with their baby, and may have asked their minister or other religious leader to visit them and the baby. Baptism may be arranged before the baby dies, if it is the parents' wish.

Miscarriage

A miscarriage may be spontaneous or induced. It is said that 10% of pregnancies fail as a result of natural causes. A woman who has experienced a miscarriage will almost always see herself as having lost a baby, however early the miscarriage occurred. A period of grief is experienced, the stages of which are similar to grief from any other cause, although there are certain unique features about grieving following an early pregnancy loss (Bansen and Stevens, 1992). There is often a distinct lack of professional and community support (Hill, 1989); a miscarriage is frequently seen as an insignificant event from which a couple can quickly recover with no lasting psychological effects (Conway, 1991). Parents may be encouraged not to grieve, cry or talk about their loss, and there is often an absence of ceremony in relation to what happens to the baby's body or products of conception. A survey of disposal arrangements for fetuses lost in the second trimester found that in over half of the 28 hospitals they surveyed no single method of disposal was employed, but most of the fetuses were incinerated (Batcup et al., 1988). Facilities offered by some of the hospitals to the bereaved parents were a burial or cremation, a special religious service, a photograph of the baby, a blessing card and a record in a book of remembrance. In some cemeteries or crematoria a special plot of land was reserved for stillbirths and younger fetuses and a few hospitals offered the services of a bereavement counsellor.

Oakley (1984) emphasizes the need for parents to grieve following a miscarriage and states that a key social identity, that of parenthood, has been challenged.

David et al. (1988) describes a plan of support for grieving families following a medical abortion carried out because of a diagnosed serious fetal malformation, which cannot be treated either in utero or following delivery. This is a unique type of pregnancy loss in which the couple have made a deliberate decision to end the pregnancy. As part of the plan, he suggests that the mother should hold or touch the fetus and that a photograph should be taken which should be available for the parents if they request it. The opportunity and advisability of parents seeing, holding and photographing their baby is also presented in a booklet specifically written for parents by the organization Support After Termination for Abnormality (SAFTA, 1990). David et al. (1988) also advocate a funeral service and the issuing of a certificate of birth, thereby symbolically registering the child within the family history. The importance of a doctor being available to talk to the parents and the need for genetic counselling is also emphasized. These parents are likely to experience both grief and a feeling of relief, which can be emotionally exhausting.

When in vitro fertilization (IVF) fails most women and their partners will experience a grief reaction, which appears to be most intense following the first attempt. The intensity of the grief reaction appears to correlate with the intensity of attachment to the expected pregnancy, which may be increased according to the extent of the involvement with, and exposure to, IVF technology. The grief response following a failed IVF is said by Greenfeld et al. (1988) to be analogous to the reaction experienced following a miscarriage. IVF often constitutes an enormous investment of time, money and emotional energy, and failure is very likely to cause acute disappointment, a feeling of inadequacy, fragility and grief, deprivation and loss (Friedman and Gradstein, 1992). Leon (1990) states that infertility may lead to profound grief, depression, anger, guilt, despair and yearning, and has been called a 'hidden' bereavement. A sympathetic approach can do much to help and support couples with this problem (Winston, 1994).

Faiths Other Than Christian

Rituals in relation to death and dying vary according to people's faiths and whether or not there is a belief in life after death, reincarnation or re-birth of some type.

Judaism
The Jewish faith does not normally allow for full mourning until a baby has lived for at least 30 days (Neuberger and White, 1991). The stillborn baby or neonate is traditionally buried in an unmarked grave after a simple ceremony. Parents may, however, request

full funeral rites, which they will arrange (Jolly, 1987). Jewish mourning encourages the passionate expression of grief extending to tearing of the clothes, which can be an approved way of expressing anger and anguish, and may also symbolize a tearing away from the relationship with the deceased (Kubler-Ross, 1989).

There is a seven-day pattern of mourning, known as Shiva, during which family members stay with the bereaved parents, cook for them, care for them and listen to them talking about their lost baby. Following this there are 30 days of gradual readjustment to normality and one year of remembrance and healing.

Sikhism

Families of the Sikh faith will usually take responsibility for arranging the last offices, and the whole family goes into mourning. Stillborn babies are usually buried. There is no restriction about who touches the baby, but if any jewellery has been put on, then it should be left unless discussion with the parents indicates otherwise. About 10 days following the death a special ceremony is held to mark the end of the official mourning (Neuberger, 1987).

Hinduism

Hindu parents may object to anyone who is not a Hindu touching their baby after death. A Hindu priest, known as a pandit, may visit the parents and a ceremony is held. Babies and young children are normally buried. The parents may refuse to have a post-mortem. Grief is usually expressed openly (Neuberger, 1987).

Islam

Muslim parents may lie their baby with the head pointing towards Mecca following death, and may object to anyone who is not a Muslim touching the body. They may want to take the baby home or to a mosque. Burial usually takes place within 24 hours. A post-mortem is usually refused unless it is a legal requirement.

The mourning period is usually about one month, the first three days of which the parents would stay at home. The mother may try to accept the death of her baby without crying and therefore may not want to hold her baby (Jolly, 1987).

Buddhism

Families who are Buddhists may face death with a calmness and acceptance; grieving is allowed as a natural occurrence, but is not dwelt on (Neuberger, 1987). There appear to be no restrictions on who touches the baby and no firm feelings about the performance of a post-mortem. The baby is usually cremated.

A Handicapped Child

Giving birth to a child with a malformation results in a grieving for the loss of the perfect baby which the parents visualized during pregnancy. The mother may feel a personal failure, experience a sense of inadequacy and loss of self-esteem (Leon, 1990). Both parents have to cope with the emotions of guilt, anger and shame towards the child (Leick and Nielsen, 1991). The grief may not resolve, but may continue as the child grows and the disability becomes more obvious.

Adoption

Adopted children are often termed 'relinquished children'. Howe (1992) states that women who lose a baby through adoption have many experiences in common with those who lose a baby through death. Raphael (1983) believes that the grief of these mothers is often poorly resolved, as they suppress their longing for their babies so that they have the strength to continue with the decision. Also, because the child is living, the mother may continue to experience 'calling weeping' particularly at each birthday. She may attempt to visualize the child growing up.

Mander (1991) undertook a study of midwives' care of mothers who relinquished their babies by adoption. She found that the midwives showed a reluctance to burden the women with what they saw as mundane decisions about their care. The midwives were adamant, however, that the woman should make her own decision about whether or not she should see and care for her baby. Mander (1991) states that in this study a discrepancy between the midwives' theoretical knowledge of grieving and their reported practice existed.

Death of a Twin

The death of a twin puts the parents in a position of having to cope with mutually incompatible feelings: of the celebration of new life and yet at the same time sadness, resentment, guilt, shame and despair (Lewis and Bryan, 1988). The second twin can be a constant and growing reminder of the loss of the other (Raphael-Leff, 1991).

SANDS (1991) advocates that the parents see and hold both babies together. A photograph may be taken of the dead baby with the live baby. It is important that the parents have as many memories as possible of the lost baby.

Grief of the Other Children

Young children tend to see death as a temporary occurrence. Explaining death to very young children, especially those under 5 years of age, is difficult because they cannot understand the concept (Lansdown and Benjamin, 1985). When children reach the age of 8–9 years, however, they begin to see that death is permanent (Kubler-Ross, 1981; Stewart and Dent, 1994). Grief for small children may be a mixture of loneliness and terror (Randall, 1993). They may be confused because of their parents' grief and somehow feel responsible for the loss and disappearance of 'their' baby. The child may not show his or her grief by crying and needing to be comforted, but parents may notice a change in behaviour. The child may become quiet and withdrawn, panic at any change in routine, easily get angry or return to an earlier stage of behaviour such as bed-wetting (Black, 1993; Randall, 1993; Stewart and Dent, 1994). Older children may also show a change in attitude to attending school and a drop in their school work.

In order to facilitate the grief work, the parents should be encouraged to include their children so that the family grieve together. The children may then somehow share their parents' mourning instead of mourning alone (Stewart and Dent, 1994; Black and Urbanowicz, 1985). It is important to listen to the children and provide reassurance that the baby's death was not their fault. Questions should be answered as fully as possible and the parents' tears and grief should not be hidden. Unanswered questions and unexplained silences are much more difficult for children to accept than tears. Many writers advocate taking the other children to the funeral service (Stewart and Dent, 1994), so allowing them to become involved in this important family ceremony and, as a consequence, encouraging them to develop positive memories of their lost brother or sister.

References

Bansen, S. & Stevens, H.A. (1992) Women's experiences of miscarriage in early pregnancy. *J. Nurs. Midwifery*, 37(2): 84.

Batcup, G., Clarke, J.P. & Purdie, D.W. (1988) Disposal arrangements for fetuses lost in the second trimester. *Br. J. Obstet. Gynaecol.* 95: 547–550.

Black, D. & Urbanowicz, A. (1985) Bereaved children – family intervention. In: Stevenson, J.E. (ed) *Recent Research in Developmental Psychopathology*. Oxford: Pergamon Press.

Black, P.A. (1993) Neonatal death and the effect on the family. *Prof. Care Mother and Child* 3: 19–21.

Bowlby, J. (1980) *Attachment and Loss*. Vol. 3: *Loss, Sadness and Depression*. London: The Hogarth Press.

Brenkley, W. (1991) Understanding bereavement. *Paed. Nurs.* 3(1): 18–21.

Conway, K. (1991) Miscarriage (psychological aspects of bereavement in the aftermath of miscarriage). *J. Psychosomatic Obstet. Gynaecol.* 12(2): 121–131.

Darwin, C. (1872) *Expressions of the Emotions in Man and Animals with Illustrations*. London: John Murray.

David, D.L., Stewart, M. & Harmon, R.J. (1988) Perinatal loss: providing emotional support for bereaved parents. *Birth* 15(4): 242–246.

Dominica, Mother Francis (1987) Reflection on death in childhood *Br. Med. J.* **294** (6564): 108–110.

Friedman, R. & Gradstein, B. (1992) *Surviving Pregnancy Loss. A Complete Source Book for Women and their Families*. Boston: Little Brown and Co.

Greenfeld, D.A., Diamond, M.P. & De Cherney, A.H. (1988) Grief reactions following in vitro fertilisation treatment. *J. Psychosomatic Obstet. Gynaecol.* 8(3): 169–174.

Hill, S. (1989) *Family*. London: Penguin Books.

Howe, D., Sawbridge, P. & Hinings, D. (1992) *Half a Million Women*. Harmondsworth: Penguin.

Jolly, J. (1987) *Missed Beginnings. Death Before Life has been Established*. London: Austin Cornish Publishers in Association with the Lisa Sainsbury Foundation.

Klaus, M.H. & Kennell, J.H. (1982) *Parent–Infant Bonding* St. Louis: C.V. Mosby.

Kubler-Ross, E. (1970) *On Death and Dying*. London: Tavistock.

Kubler-Ross, E. (1981) *Living with Death and Dying* London: Macmillan.

Kubler-Ross, E. (1989) *On Death and Dying*. London: Tavistock.

Lansdown, R. & Benjamin, B. (1985) The development of the concept of death in children aged 5–9 years. *Child Care Health Dev.* **11**: 13–20.

Leon, I.G. (1990) *When a Baby Dies. Psychotherapy for Pregnancy and Newborn Loss.* New Haven: Yale University Press.

Leick, N. & Davidson–Nielsen, M. (1991) *Healing Pain: Attachment, Loss and Grief.* London: Routledge.

Lewis, C.S. (1961) *A Grief Observed.* London: Faber & Faber.

Lewis, E. & Bryan, E. (1988) Management of perinatal loss of twins. *Br. Med. J.* **297**: 1321.

Mander, R. (1991) Midwifery care of the grieving mother: How the decisions are made. *Midwifery* **7**(3): 133–142.

Miller, B. (1985) Maternal–fetal attachment, loss and grief. *Br. J. Midwifery* **3**(1): 16–18.

Neuberger, J. (1987) *Caring for Dying People of Different Faiths.* London: The Lisa Sainsbury Foundation, Austin Cornish.

Neuberger, J. & White, J. (1991) *A Necessary End. Attitudes to Death.* London: Macmillan.

Oakley, A., McPherson, A. & Roberts, H. (1990) *Miscarriage* London: Fontana.

Parkes, C.M. (1972) *Bereavement: Studies of Grief in Adult Life.* London: Tavistock.

Parkes, C.M. (1986) *Bereavement: Studies in Grief in Adult Life.* Tavistock: London.

Pepper, L.G. & Knapp, R.J. (1980) *Motherhood and Mourning* New York: Praeger.

Randall, P. (1993) Aspects of bereavement: young children grieve differently from adults. *Prof. Care Mother and Child* **2**: 36–37.

Raphael, B. (1983) *The Anatomy of Bereavement.* New York: Basic Books.

Raphael–Leff, J. (1991) *Psychological Processes of Childbearing.* London: Chapman & Hall.

SANDS (1991) *Guidelines for Professionals. Miscarriage, Stillbirth and Neonatal Death.* London: Stillbirth and Neonatal Death Society.

SATFA (1990) *A Parents' Handbook.* London: Support After Termination for Abnormality.

Schneider, J. (1984) *Stress, Loss and Grief: Understanding Their Origins and Growth Potential.* Baltimore: University Park Press.

Stewart, A. & Dent, A. (1994) *At a Loss – Bereavement Care When a Baby Dies*, pp. 175–182. London: Baillière Tindall.

UKCC (UK Central Council for Nursing, Midwifery and Health Visiting) (1994) *A Midwife's Code of Practice.* London: UKCC.

Winston, R. (1994) *Infertility, a Sympathetic Approach.* London: Optima.

Further Reading

Bourne, S. & Lewis, E. (1984) Pregnancy after stillbirth or neonatal death: psychological risks and management. *Lancet* **ii**: 31–33.

Davis, D.L., Stewart, M. & Harmon, R.J. (1988) Perinatal loss: providing emotional support for bereaved parents. *Birth* **15**(4): 742–746.

Hutti, M.E. (1988) A quick reference table of interventions to assist families to cope with pregnancy loss or neonatal death. *Birth* **15**(1): 33–35.

Lloyd, J. & Laurence, K.M. (1985) Sequelae and support after termination of pregnancy for fetal malformation. *Br. Med. J.* **290**: 907–909.

Moscarello, R. (1989) Perinatal bereavement support services: three year review. *J. Palliat. Care* **5**(4): 12–18.

SANDS (1995) *Pregnancy Loss and the Death of a Baby: Guidelines for Professionals.* London: Stillbirth and Neonatal Death Society.

Theut, S., Henderson, F., Zaslow, M., *et al.* (1989) Perinatal loss and perinatal bereavement. *J. Psychiatry* **146**(5): 635–639.

Tschudin, V. (1995) *Counselling Skills for Nurses*, 4th edn. London: Baillière Tindall.

Warnock, M. (1985) *A Question of Life.* Oxford: Blackwell.

Worden, W. (1982) *Grief Counselling and Grief Therapy.* London: Tavistock Publications.

Useful Addresses

Miscarriage Association
P.O. Box 24,
Osset,
West Yorks.,
WF5 9XG
Tel: 01924 830515

National Childbirth Trust
Alexandra House,
Oldham Terrace,
Acton,
London, W3 6NH
Tel: 0181 992 8637

SAFTA (Support after termination for fetal abnormality)
29–30 Soho Sq.,
London, WIV 6JB
Tel: 0171 439 6124

SANDS (Stillbirth and Neonatal Death Society)
28 Portland Place,
London, W1 4DE
Tel: 0171 436 5881

Compassionate Friends, (An international organization for bereaved parents)
6 Denmark St.,
Clifton,
Bristol, BS1 5DQ
Tel: 0117 9292778

Health and Social Services

The National Health Service

This chapter seeks to identify how the health services in the United Kingdom have developed and briefly considers the events leading up to the implementation of the National Health Service Act in 1948. It then outlines the many changes which have taken place since that time and how they have affected midwives and the maternity services. It is a brief overview only and readers are strongly recommended to look at more detailed accounts, some of which are referenced at the end of this chapter, and to explore the many sources available on the development of the maternity services in the UK.

Health Provision Before the National Health Service

The National Health Service (NHS) emerged from a health care system that was fragmented and favoured those who could afford to pay. In 1946 the National Health Service Act was passed and it became operative in 1948. This Act, together with the National Insurance Act of 1946 provided a complete health and welfare package, unique at the time, that was free and open to all, although those in employment pay National Insurance contributions to help pay for the service and benefits.

Until 1930 there were three main providers of hospital services:

1 The Poor Law Medical Service provided infirmaries which were noted for the practice of subsistence medicine and responsible for the chronic sick from the poorer sections of society. Later the Poor Law scheme was administered by local authorities.

2 Voluntary hospitals supported by charitable trusts were the main providers of hospitals. They had a good reputation for their high standards of care and for advancing the knowledge of medicine. Exam-

ples of voluntary hospitals are Guy's, St Thomas' and St Bartholomews. In addition to large teaching hospitals, there were also smaller cottage hospitals in the voluntary sector.

3   Local authority hospitals were mainly provided for special needs, for example, isolation and children.

Inadequate funds to run the hospitals and widely varying standards of care led to mounting pressure to unify the system. The public health services were the responsibility of the Ministry of Health.

General practitioners were in private practice and they therefore received payment for their services from all patients until 1911. Then the National Health and Unemployment Insurance Act was passed which created a health insurance scheme for the working man whose earnings were below a certain level. The contributions, which were shared by employee, employer and the state, entitled the individual to receive free treatment from a general practitioner, but excluded hospital treatment and treatment for dependants who were expected to obtain help from the Poor Law Medical Service.

The Introduction of the National Health Service

In the years prior to the introduction of the National Health Service Act (1946) a number of reports, including the Beveridge Report (1942), highlighted the shortcomings of the existing health services and recommended unification and access for all, irrespective of circumstances. There was general support for a freely accessible health service, but not for the structure of such a service. Government policy on this issue was influenced by three pressure groups who had vested interests in the structure of the service. These groups were:

1   the local authorities who owned hospitals and had administrative expertise to offer;
2   the charitable trusts who owned hospitals but needed substantial public money to survive; and
3   the doctors, a powerful body whose co-operation was essential as they provided the skills needed at that time to operate the system.

The consequences of trying to meet the demands of

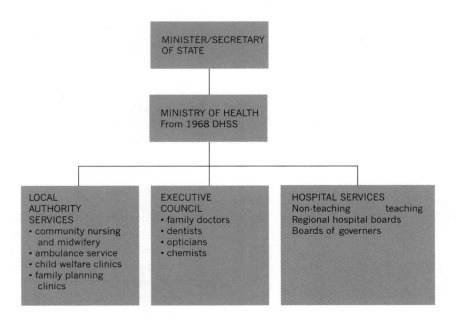

Figure 1   The tripartite system introduced under the National Health Service Act 1946.

these three groups meant that the government was forced to abandon trying to develop a unified system of health care and created a tripartite system (Figure 1).

In 1946 the National Health Service Act was passed and it became operative in 1948. This Act was supplemented by other Acts that together form the social security measures which provide security and care for all classes of the community. In effect three health care systems were created, making co-ordination difficult and resulting in a fragmented service and inefficient use of resources. The National Health Service Act 1946 split health care services into three parts. The three parts of the midwifery and maternity services were as follows:

1   A hospital maternity service.
2   A community midwifery service under the control of local authorities. The local authorities were also the Local Supervising Authorities responsible for the supervision of midwives.
3   General practitioners who remained separate, but increasingly took on more midwifery care now that the service was free to all patients. The general practitioners, together with the pharmaceutical, dental and ophthalmic services were administered by local executive councils.

Midwives practising in hospitals and the community began to lose their autonomy as more doctors became involved in the provision of midwifery care. Another effect of this tripartite service was that the care of mothers became fragmented and continuity of care became increasingly difficult to achieve. There was also duplication of care by the different professional groups involved in the maternity services.

A review of the maternity service bed needs in 1970 (DHSS, 1970) found that the tripartite system was ineffective and emphasized the need for those providing care to work together in teams, comprising the midwife, obstetrician and general practitioner. It also recommended 100% hospital confinement on the grounds of safety, although valid evidence to support this recommendation was not available. The government accepted this recommendation and increased the number of maternity beds to enable all women to have their babies in hospital. This policy further fragmented the service and eroded the autonomy of midwives and, indeed, the women in their care. By this time there were many critics of the tripartite system for the delivery of health care because it was found to be cumbersome, inefficient and costly. Plans were there-

fore being made to reorganize the structure of the National Health Service after it had been in existence for 25 years. The build up to the new structure of the National Health Service is shown in Figure 2 which illustrates some of the complexities involved in policy formation and the continuing influence of a powerful medical profession.

National Health Service Reorganisation Act 1973

A reorganized structure for the National Health Service was finally agreed and the National Health Service Reorganisation Act was passed in 1973 and implemented in 1974 (Figure 3). This Act enabled the existing services of hospitals and local authorities to be integrated under a single management. General practitioner, dental, pharmaceutical and ophthalmic services continued to be administered separately by the Family Practitioner Committees.

Under the new Act the NHS had a three-tiered structure which consisted of Regional and Area Health Authorities and Health Districts. The structure theoretically enabled the integration of community and hospital services. Midwives were therefore responsible to one employer and administration. This reduced some of the divisions in the provision of care and made co-ordination of the service easier. The Regional Health Authorities became the Local Supervising Authorities and appointed local supervisors of midwives.

In the 1970s and 1980s childbirth became increasingly medicalized and hospital delivery became the norm. Early transfer home after delivery to the care of the community midwife became common practice and an integrated maternity service certainly made this easier to administer effectively. Many obstetric interventions became routine and there was increasing use of technology, some of which had not been fully evaluated. These interventions, which were under the control of the medical staff, further eroded the autonomy and role of the midwife. Choice of place of birth became severely restricted as an increasing number of health districts reduced the community midwifery service. There was also little choice for women in the care provided and continuity of care became almost non-existent.

There was widespread criticism about the three-tiered structure of the reorganized NHS, mainly because there were too many layers of management

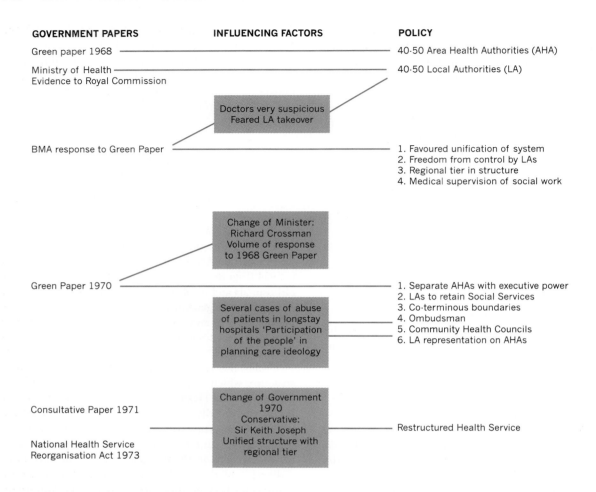

Figure 2   The build up to the 1974 reorganization of the NHS.

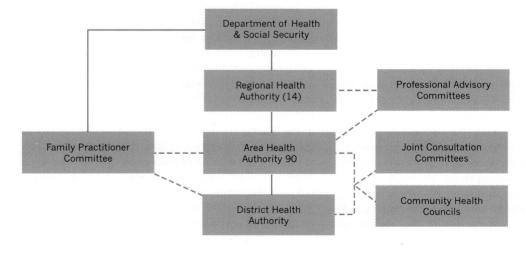

Figure 3   The structure of the NHS following the National Health Service Act 1973.

and it was costly to administer. In 1979 a Royal Commission was therefore set up and concluded that there was one tier too many. A new NHS structure was therefore planned.

Health Services Act 1980

A consultative document on the structure and management of the National Health Service, named *Patients First*, was published by the Department of Health and Social Security in December 1979. This document suggested that the organization of the NHS should be streamlined and that a tier of administration should be removed. Following a period of consultation, the plans for the new structure and management of the NHS were announced and incorporated in the Health Services Act 1980.

All Area Health Authorities and Health Districts were removed and replaced by 200 *District Health Authorities* (DHAs). The 14 *Regional Health Authorities* (RHAs) remained.

Family Practitioner Committees remained and continued to be responsible for the administration of the family practitioner services, dentists, pharmacists and ophthalmic services.

Community Health Councils, which were set up in each district in 1974, were retained, one for each DHA.

Shortly after the 1980 Act was implemented in 1982 the Government established an NHS Management Inquiry which reported in 1983.

NHS Management Inquiry 1983

The NHS Management Inquiry team (leader of Inquiry: Roy Griffiths) was set up to give advice on the effective use and management of manpower and related resources in the NHS. Their recommendations on management action were reported in October 1983. The recommendations of this report (DHSS, 1983) were implemented in 1984 and fundamentally affected the management style of the NHS, changing it from consensus 'team' management to it being the overall responsibility of one person, the general manager. The general manager would be the final decision-maker for decisions previously delegated to the consensus team.

The Government publication *The Next Steps* (DHSS, 1984) states:

> By establishing a general management function in health authorities, the concern shared by all working in the health service for the quality and efficiency of patient services will be more easily translated into effective action; the available resources will be better used and those working in the service will obtain greater satisfaction from their work. The patient, the community, the tax payer will all benefit.

The Next Steps (DHSS, 1984) included the government's national development programme from 1982 to 1984 and the changing structure within the Department of Health and Social Security, namely the establishment of a Health Services Supervisory Board and a full-time NHS Management Board. The role of the Health Services Supervisory Board was mainly to determine the overall objectives and direction for the NHS; to approve the overall budget and resource allocations; to make strategic decisions; and to monitor performance. The NHS Management Board was under the direction of the Supervisory Board. Its main responsibilities were to plan implementation of the policies approved by the Supervisory Board; to give leadership to the management of the NHS; to control performance; and to achieve consistency and drive.

Greater freedom was given to organize the management structure of a health authority in the most effective way to suit local circumstances, thus different structures emerged at district level up and down the UK. Each health district was divided into units of management and each unit is headed by a unit manager and has a budget.

Midwives endeavoured to maintain an integrated midwifery service by supporting units of midwifery comprising hospital and community midwifery headed by a senior midwife at unit level, but in some cases the midwifery service was again fragmented. The senior midwife or nurse at unit level reports to the general manager, now called the chief executive. There is little opportunity therefore for midwives to influence policy at a higher level. Doctors were seen as the controllers of resources and this was reflected in many of the new management structures.

A recommendation of the NHS Management Inquiry states that general managers should be appointed regardless of discipline, the main criteria for their appointment being their general management skills and experience. They are appointed for a fixed term of three years and their re-appointment is not automatic, but depends on their performance.

Underfinancing of the health service between 1982 and 1989 led to long delays in patients receiving hospital care and many other inadequacies of the service were highlighted. Further reforms of the NHS were therefore planned during the latter part of the 1980s. One of these was the division of the Department of Health and Social Security into two separate departments: the Department of Health and the Department of Social Security. Further changes in the health service were influenced by two key factors, namely value for money and containment of costs (Abel-Smith, 1992).

National Health Service and Community Care Act 1990

A White Paper entitled *Working for Patients* (DOH, 1989) outlined the proposed changes in the NHS and stated that it would continue to be funded through central taxation, although there would be major changes in resource allocation. This White Paper was followed by the National Health Service and Community Care Act in 1990 which included many far-reaching reforms. They introduced a competitive market for health services and separated the two functions of purchasers and providers of health services which were previously both the role of the District Health Authorities. The Districts and the general practitioners who became fundholders were the purchasers and the hospitals and various community services were the providers. Hospitals, community and other health services (e.g. ambulances) were encouraged to become self-governing trusts and now virtually all have acquired trust status. Until trust status was achieved the term Directly Managed Units was used to describe services which were still the responsibility of the District Health Authorities. Figure 4 shows the structure of the NHS following the implementation of the NHS and Community Care Act.

One of the essential roles of the District Health Authorities (now Health Authorities) is to assess the health care needs of their population. This information is required to enable them to make appropriate decisions about the services they purchase for their population. The health targets specified in *The Health of the Nation* White Paper which was published by

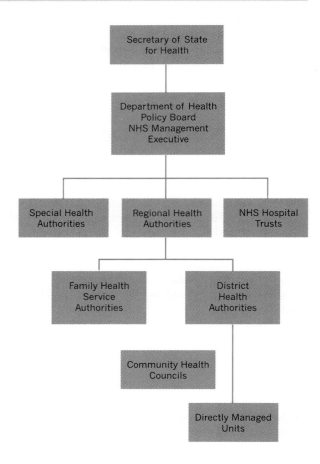

Figure 4   The structure of the NHS following the National Health Service and Community Care Act 1990.

the Department of Health in 1992 has helped to provide a focus for the needs assessment (Levitt *et al.*, 1995).

Another major role of the Health Authorities is to draw up and negotiate contracts which include details of the services to be provided, prices, quality and any other requirements. The Health Authorities obviously wish to purchase the most efficient and cost-effective services for their local population and so there is usually competition for contracts between providers. Fundholding general practitioners also purchase services for their patients and can specify the type of service which they require. Competing for contracts has had a marked effect on the provision of services. Trusts generate income by selling their services and therefore in many cases competition has resulted in

Table 1   Freedoms and Benefits of Trust Status for a Women's Services Unit

Freedoms for management	Benefits to women and babies
Ability to create local management structure	Services will be managed by people who understand and are committed to women's services
Ability to develop own plans in conjunction with Health Authorities and GPs	Development of services designed to meet the needs of women and babies
	Services accessible to the women of local area and beyond
Ability to determine own employment policies	Staff will be motivated to continually improve services
Increased financial flexibility and control	All resources will be used for the benefit of women and babies
	Efficiency savings will be re-invested in further developing services

higher standards and a more cost-effective service as they compete for contracts. In some instances, however, it may also lead to a reduction in the provision of a service if a trust fails to obtain a contract and therefore cannot afford to maintain the service. The Government has specified core services, however, which trusts are required to provide (these do not include the maternity services). Most contracts are for one year and then have to be re-negotiated. Some contracts have been awarded to private hospitals, especially when there are long waiting lists in a particular specialty and a concerted effort is being made to reduce it by using other services which are available.

Extra-contractual referrals occur when a patient is referred by a general practitioner or admitted as an emergency to a provider which does not have a contract with the district in which the patient normally resides (Levitt *et al.*, 1995). In non-emergency cases approval for extra-contractual referrals has to be obtained by the provider from the district in which the patient lives. In some cases this may be refused.

Although it was emphasized that choice for patients was a central part of the health service changes, the system of block contracts and restrictions on extra-contractual referrals mitigates against a major element of choice. In the maternity service, for instance, women are expected to have their baby in the hospital to which the Health Authority has given the contract, or have a home birth in the district in which the woman normally resides. Extra-contractual referrals are not always possible, mainly because of lack of funds at Health Authority level.

Trust status for the maternity services, however, can provide opportunities for midwives to provide the service which women are now demanding. Table 1 summarizes the freedoms and benefits of a self-governing trust for a Women's Services Unit which includes midwifery, obstetrics, gynaecology and neonatal services. The roles of executive members of the trust are indicated in Table 2. With the implementation of the recommendations of *Changing Childbirth* (DOH, 1993a) and the opportunities afforded by self-governing trusts, the future maternity services should more fully meet the needs and aspirations of childbearing women.

In the document *A Vision for the Future* (DOH, 1993b), the NHS Management Executive summarizes the main changes following the implementation of the NHS and Community Care Act as follows:

▶ make explicit responsibilities for identifying the health needs of local people and securing health care to meet them;

▶ implement a contract system between purchasers and providers;

▶ give general practitioners greater ability to act on behalf of their patients;

▶ give hospitals and other units more control over their own affairs;

▶ better integration of primary and secondary care, leading to a better balance between prevention, health improvement and treatment.

(DOH, 1993b)

Table 2   Roles of the Executive Members of a Women's Services Unit

---

Chief Executive

Overall management of the Trust
Development, implementation and review of the business plan
Overall performance in financial and service terms
Advice and support to the chairman
Principal advisor to the trust
Direction of the other executives and senior managers
The Trust's public affairs policies

Director of Patient Services

Provide the board with professional advice on midwifery and nursing
Development of nursing and midwifery practice through the clinical programmes
Develop the Trust's Quality Strategy, including the Patient's Charter
Monitor service delivery

Director of Finances and Information

Ensure an effective financial strategy for meeting the Trust's financial targets and duties
Provide accurate and timely financial and patient activity information to the Trust and its managers
Support the Director of Service Development in setting and managing contracts
Ensure effective financial systems, including cash and treasury management
Provide financial advice to the Trust

Medical Director

Acquire and provide medical advice to the Trust Board
Ensure effective communications with hospital doctors and GPs
Assist the Chief Executive and the Personnel Director with medical staffing and contracts issues
Support Medical Audit

Director of Personnel

Develop a Human Resources Strategy to underpin the Unit Business Plan
Lead on organizational development issues, particularly relating to service integration
Develop the Training Strategy
Develop the Trust as an employer

Changes in the NHS in Scotland, Wales and Northern Ireland

The Scottish Home and Health Department is responsible for the administration of the NHS at central level in Scotland and is accountable to the Secretary of State for Scotland.

Scotland had 15 Health Boards which were directly responsible to the Secretary of State for Scotland for the planning and provision of an integrated health service in their area (Levitt *et al.*, 1995). Ten of the 15 Boards were divided into Districts. In 1983 the Districts were abolished, leaving only the Health Boards and the new Unitary structure headed by Unit General Managers. There has never been a separate authority for the family practitioner services in Scotland.

The NHS and Community Care Act 1990 applies to the whole of the United Kingdom and Part 11 refers particularly to Scotland. The implementation of the Act in Scotland is in the process of taking place.

In Wales the system of health care is more like England. There were nine District Health Authorities and no Regions. In 1996 these were replaced by five new Health Authorities. The NHS Community Care Act 1990 is being implemented with an increasing number of units becoming self-governing trusts, Health Authorities changing their role, as described above, and general practitioners becoming fundholders.

Northern Ireland has four Health and Social Services Boards which are accountable to the Secretary of State for Northern Ireland. Unitary management is now in place and the 1990 NHS Community Care Act is in the process of being implemented.

Managing the New NHS – Further Changes

Following a Department of Health review of the functions and manpower of the NHS, a paper *Managing the New NHS* was published in 1993 which specified further changes in its organization and management (DOH, 1993c). These changes are:

1   The abolition of the 14 Regional Health Authorities in England.
2   Changes in the NHS Management Executive.
3   Mergers of the District Health Authorities and Family Health Services Authorities (FHSAs).

The legislation for formally abolishing Regional Health Authorities and for merging Family Health Services Authorities was set to come into effect in 1996. In April 1994, however, the 14 Regional Health Authorities were abolished and replaced by eight Regional Offices

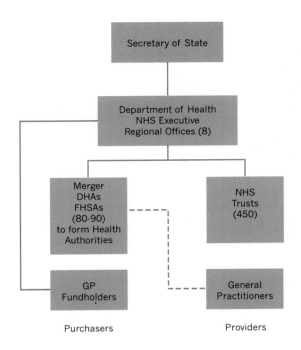

Purchasers   Providers

Figure 5 Changes to the NHS in England announced in October 1993 and implemented by 1996.

The District Health Authorities and the Family Health Service Authorities merged in April 1996. The structure of the NHS from 1995/96 is represented in Figure 5. The District Health Authorities and Family Health Service Authorities are replaced by Health Authorities and some changes in boundaries were necessary. Some of the functions of the former Regional Health Authorities are transferred to Health Authorities, including the supervision of midwives. The new Health Authorities are the Local Supervising Authorities for midwives in the Health Authorities Act, 1995.

According to the Department of Health, the NHS now only has two tiers: central and local. The changes appear to have strengthened the Department's control over the local level because the Regional Directors are directly accountable to the Chief Executive of the NHS, and all staff at regional level are now civil servants.

A major aim of the NHS is to improve the quality of the service which it offers and to reduce unnecessary costs, including those associated with litigation. Risk management has therefore been introduced to try and achieve these aims.

(Figure 5). These incorporate the former NHS Management Executive outposts. Each Regional Office is headed by a Regional Director who is directly accountable to the Chief Executive at the Department of Health. The eight Regional Directors are on the Board of the NHS Executive (NHSE), formerly called the NHS Management Executive. Eight non-executive directors have also been added to the Board to aid communications between the Secretary of State and the Chairmen of the Health Authorities and Trusts. The role of the NHS Executive is both central at national level, and it now also has a new local role at regional level. The central role is concerned with implementing Government policy and the provision of support and advice to Ministers. Responsibilities at regional level include the following:

▶ Managing the performance of purchasers and providers. This includes monitoring that they function within the regulations, arbitrating in contractual disputes and further developing the role of purchasers.
▶ Approving applications from general practitioners for fundholding and budgets.
▶ Contributing to the work on policy and resources.

Risk Management

In 1993 a manual giving guidance on risk management was produced by the National Health Service Executive for the attention of chief executives in NHS Trust hospitals (DOH, 1993d) and as a result many trusts are forming risk management groups. Risk management can be described as a process to reduce or eliminate loss due to accident or misadventure and a Risk Management Group should have two main aims:

▶ To improve the quality of the service.
▶ To reduce the costs associated with litigation.

These two elements are closely linked as improving quality of care will reduce cost and vice versa.

Risk management covers all aspects of activity within a hospital but can be divided into two large areas:

1 Clinical aspects.
2 Health and safety aspects.

Although health and safety risks are very important, it is the clinical risks that will more frequently affect the midwife in her daily activity.

Setting up a Risk Management Group to review cases where a clinical risk exists should be seen as a method of avoiding, not evading, litigation (Clements, 1992). The overall knowledge gained from such reviews should be used to improve the quality of care given to mothers and babies. An obstetric Risk Management Group will be composed of:

▶ Senior obstetricians, one or two.
▶ Senior midwives, one or two.
▶ A person with legal knowledge.
▶ A co-ordinator with a midwifery or medical background.
▶ A paediatrician or anaesthetist co-opted as necessary.

Each area within the maternity unit should have a list of 20 or more conditions where a risk factor may be present and examples of such conditions are:

▶ An Apgar score of four or less.
▶ A baby unexpectedly admitted to the neonatal unit.
▶ A mother who receives injury to other organs during an operation.

If such a condition occurs, the patient's name and brief clinical details should be referred to the Risk Management Group co-ordinator by the midwife or doctor. An initial review of the casenotes can then be undertaken by the co-ordinator who will discuss the case with the relevant staff and make a written summary. The Risk Management Group will discuss the case and make a decision as to whether formal statements should be taken from all staff involved, even though there may not be any question of litigation at this stage.

Statements made at this early stage will be more accurate than if they were made months or years after the event and, if it becomes necessary to defend the case in court, this accuracy will assist the staff involved in recalling the details.

Examples of implementing a risk management system in a maternity unit and how a risk management cycle was introduced following debriefing after childbirth are given by Dineen (1996) and Smith and Mitchell (1996).

Part of the risk management process is to recognize where quality of care can be improved. A booklet produced by the Royal College of Obstetricians and Gynaecologists (Chamberlain, 1992) lists ten key points for good practice. These can be described under three main headings: *communication, record-keeping* and *staffing issues.*

Communication

In order that the best possible care is received by mothers and babies it is important that communication systems are effective at all levels of the service. This includes good interaction between the community and hospital services, between all relevant departments within the hospital and between all relevant professional groups.

An example of where all systems of communication failed is described in *Risk and Injury to Patients Arising from Failure of Communication in Risk Management in the NHS* (DOH, 1993e).

Communication with parents must include clear information on all aspects of care and, if consent for treatment is required, risk factors must be clearly explained (Dimond, 1994).

Record-keeping

Writing a contemporaneous record of the care and treatment given to a mother is an essential part of a midwife's duty (UKCC, 1993). The midwife's records should be of such a quality that a reader will be able to gain a clear understanding of all events, even when reading the notes some 25 years later.

All entries should be written in black ink, be dated and have a clear signature. The time of the event should be recorded, not the time the entry is being written, and midwives should encourage their medical colleagues to adopt this system. Each sheet should be identified with the patients name and hospital number.

Staffing issues

Induction programmes for new staff and clear policies to assist staff should exist in every maternity unit. Adequate numbers of appropriately skilled midwives and doctors should be available at all times and staff must recognize their level of skill and not work beyond it. Adequate, well-maintained equipment must be available for staff to use, when required.

In order that the quality of the service is constantly improved the Risk Management Group should audit identified failures in communication, record-keeping and staffing issues, and inform the staff of the action taken to prevent recurrence. The Risk Management Team can then be seen as an effective mechanism for reducing risk and acting as an aid to protecting the staff.

Risk management is one of the ways in which the NHS is striving to achieve high-quality and cost-effective standards of care. The fundamental changes which are taking place in the NHS with the implementation of the NHS and Community Care Act 1990 and the Health Authorities Act 1995 will require careful and objective evaluation. These changes affect the provision of all services in the NHS, including those for mothers and babies. Midwives, together with their medical colleagues, are also in the process of implementing major changes in the provision of

midwifery and obstetric care to fulfil the recommendations of the report *Changing Childbirth* (DOH, 1993a) which has been accepted as government policy. With both the NHS reforms and the blueprint for the maternity services specified in *Changing Childbirth*, midwives have the opportunity to provide women with a truly woman-centred, accessible service that meets their needs and fulfils their expectations.

References

Abel-Smith, B. (1992) The reforms of the health service. *Quality Assurance Health Care* **4**(4): 263–272.

Beveridge Report (1942) *Report on Social Insurance and Allied Services*. London: HMSO.

Chamberlain, G.V.P. (ed.) (1992) *How to Avoid Medicolegal Problems in Obstetrics and Gynaecology*. London: Royal College of Obstetrics and Gynaecology.

Clements, R.V. (1992) Defensive medicine – is this where risk management leads? *Health Service J.* April.

DHSS (Department of Health and Social Security) (1970) *Domiciliary Midwifery and Maternity Bed Needs* (Peel Report). London: HMSO.

DHSS (1979) *Patients First*. London: HMSO.

DHSS (1983) *National Health Service Management Inquiry*, Chairman: Sir Roy Griffiths. HMSO: London.

DHSS (1984) *The Next Steps*. London: HMSO.

Dimond, B. (1994) *The Legal Aspects of Midwifery*. Hale: Books for Midwives Press.

Dineen, M. (1996) Clinical risk management – a pragmatic approach *Br. J. Midwifery* **4**(8): Supplement.

DOH (Department of Health) (1989) *Working for Patients: The Health Service Caring in the 1990s*. London: HMSO.

DOH (1992) *The Health of the Nation. A Strategy for Health in England*. London: HMSO.

DOH (1993a) *Changing Childbirth*. Report of the Expert Maternity Group, Part 1. London: HMSO.

DOH (1993b) *Vision for the Future*. London: HMSO.

DOH (1993c) *Managing the New NHS*. London: HMSO.

DOH (1993d) *Risk Management in the NHS*. London: HMSO.

DOH (1993e) *Risk and Injury to Patients Arising from Failure of Communication in Risk Management in the NHS*. London: HMSO.

Levitt, R., Wall, A. & Appleby, J. (1995) *The Reorganised National Health Service*. London: Chapman & Hall.

Smith, J. & Mitchell, S. (1996) Debriefing after childbirth – a tool for effective risk management. *Br. J. Midwifery* **4**(8): Supplement.

UKCC (United Kingdom Central Council for Nursing, Midwifery and Health Visiting) (1993) *Midwives' Rules*. London: UKCC.

Further Reading

Ball, J., Leighton, J. & Mayes, G. (1992) *The National Health Service – Midwifery Update Series*. London: Distance Learning Centre, South Bank University.

Clark, J. (1991) *A Case Study of a Unit/Area of Practice*. Block 4 Year 2 Professional Perspectives (2). London: Distance Learning Centre, South Bank Polytechnic (now University).

Connah, B. & Pearson, R. (1991) *NHS Handbook*. London: NAHAT Macmillan.

DOH (Department of Health) *NHS Management Executive News*. Room 8E64, Quarry House, Quarry Hill, Leeds LS2 7UE.

Leathard, A. (1990) *Health Care Provision, Past Present and Future*. London: Chapman & Hall.

Levitt, R., Wall, A. & Appleby, J. (1995) *The National Health Service*, 5th edn. London: Chapman & Hall.

St Leger, A.S., Schnieden, H. & Walsworth-Bell, J.P. (1992) *Evaluating Health Services' Effectiveness*. Milton Keynes: Open University Press.

80

Community Health and the Social Services

Historical Perspectives

The World Health Organization states categorically that health services should be made available as close to people's homes as possible (WHO, 1991). The United Kingdom can rightly be proud of its long-standing history of community-based services which provide a high level of expertise in health care in the home and in the community health centre or surgery of the general practitioner.

The local authorities were recognized as pioneers in the provision of public health services during the nineteenth century. This included the basic but crucial provision of a clean water supply and drainage. After 1900, the local authorities took the initiative in health education and curative medicine and, from 1906, the school medical service. The provision of sanatoria for the care of patients with tuberculosis in 1911 was an important step in the prevention of the spread of disease. Welfare clinics for mothers and children which proliferated after the First World War formed the basis of the community-based maternal and child health care system with which we are familiar today.

From this time there was a gradual concentration of responsibility focusing on the local authority which appeared to provide a democratic way forward when the National Health Service was introduced. It has been stated that prior to 1939 'progressive councils' held the ideal that:

Each neighbourhood should have a health centre to co-ordinate the 'primary care' provided by individual practitioners, clinics and the public health service, and that from these centres patients requiring more specialist treatment should be referred to the 'secondary' level of district hospitals.

(Lowe, 1993)

Adequate provision of public or community health and social services are undeniably important factors in promoting the health and well-being of a population. McKeown (1976) concluded that the reduction in mortality rates could be attributed largely to the impact of factors associated with public health and the environment, economic and social issues rather than to medical and surgical interventions. McKeown, in a historical analysis of the reasons for population growth in England and Wales, reflected the ideas of Sigerist (1941), Ryle (1948) and Morris (1975, 1980) when he purported that high mortality rates in the past were largely due to infectious diseases and nutritional problems combined with other environmental factors. In presenting his hypothesis, McKeown estimated that 80–90% of the reduction in total deaths between the eighteenth and twentieth centuries was effected by reducing the incidence of infection, especially tuberculosis and chest infections along with a reduction in disease transmitted in food and water (McKeown, 1976).

This historical aspect serves to emphasize the need for community-based health care and attention to social issues in the promotion of health. It could be argued that it is the balance between the provision of and access to community-based services and a secondary level of specialist care to which clients may be referred which is important. Excellence at either the primary level or the secondary level without the effective functioning of the other will result in a deficit in health care. This chapter concentrates on health care in the community, but recognizes the crucial importance of a specialist obstetric and paediatric service and an efficient referral system which links the two.

Today, community health services are offered in partnership with social services with the overall aim of providing a comprehensive care and support network for every member of the community and particularly for the most vulnerable. Maternal and child health issues are a priority in the health and social system which can begin in the home and provide a referral system to specialist care in hospital for mother and baby. Community health care is provided free of charge under the National Health Service which is described in Chapter 79. This chapter focuses on specific community-based maternal and child health care provisions and the social services which are of particular concern to the midwife. The next chapter (Chapter 81) details the system of social security, including financial benefits which are available to the pregnant woman, mother and family.

The quality and effectiveness of community health care and social services provided in the community are dependent upon many factors. These include the skills and approach of the professionals who form the primary health care team and those who provide the social services, the resources which assist them to function effectively, the organization of the health and social services and the uptake of care by the population who stand to benefit from those services which are available to them at community level.

In spite of the increasing range of skills and services which are available in the community, it has been claimed that in certain areas of the UK, particularly in inner city and peripheral public housing estates:

The gap between the health experience of different social classes has continued to increase. In particular, there is a general lack of what might be called the epidemiological or population view of primary health care as espoused by Hart and Kark (in 1981) and there is a great need for the injection of epidemiological skills into the normal functioning of primary health care teams.

(Ashton and Seymour, 1988: 35–36)

There is reason to believe that this gap still exists almost a decade later.

The Primary Health Care Team

The Primary Health Care Team provides the first line of approach to health care and medical services in the community. The team currently consists of a wide range of health care professionals usually based at the surgery of a general practitioner or in a health centre. The midwife will form part of this team, sometimes working totally in the community, sometimes working as part of a midwifery team in hospital as well as in the community. Chapter 33 details the role and function of the midwife in the community. The role and function of the other members of the primary health care team who may contribute to maternal and child health are described below and summarized in Figure 1.

The general practitioner (GP) obstetrician

The general practitioner obstetrician is a doctor who, having had recognized post-registration obstetric experience, is on the obstetric list and is thus qualified to provide an obstetric service to women in the community. The general practitioner may provide this service in the home or based at their own practice surgery, health centre, in general practitioner units or in consultant obstetric units where agreement has been reached for general practitioners and community midwives to deliver women whom they have agreed to attend during labour and delivery. Nowadays, the general practitioner and the community midwife provide the majority of the antenatal care and postnatal

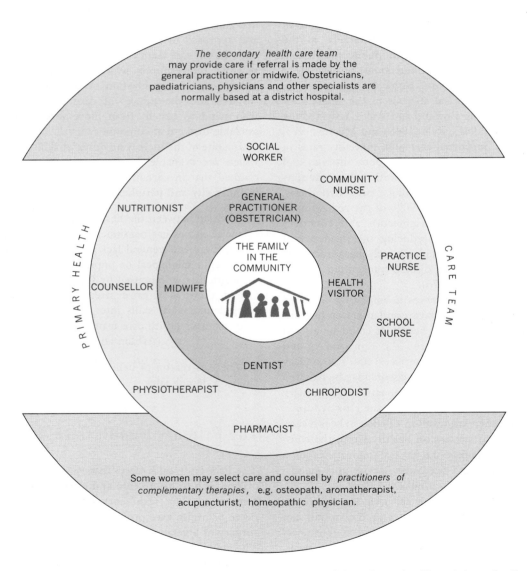

Figure 1 The primary health care team. Blue shading: Key members of the primary health care team for the pregnant woman and her child. Red shading: Other members of the primary health care team accessible for those with special needs.

follow-up care, including the six-week check-up, referring those identified as being at risk or with complications to a consultant obstetrician.

Differing professional attitudes combined with varying public demands echoed in the document *Changing Childbirth* (DOH, 1993) may well make greater demands upon both the general practitioner obstetrician and the community midwife as home births may again become more usual.

Currently there is an increasing tendency for general practitioners to work in group practices. Large group practices can have the advantage of promoting medical cover by a doctor from the same practice instead of using a doctor's deputising service, but can have the disadvantage of making continuity of care with the same doctor much more difficult. Consequent to the implementation of the NHS and Community Care Act of 1990, some general practitioners' practices have become fundholding practices whilst others continue to receive funds from the Family Health Services Authority. The advantages and disadvantages of these administrative changes to the utilizers of the community health services are likely to be debated for a long time to come.

The health visitor/public health nurse

The health visitor is a registered nurse who will have completed a short programme of approximately one month in maternity and neonatal care as part of her nurse training. Some will have also completed midwifery training and all are now required to have two years experience in community nursing. The health visitor will have undertaken a post-registration course, usually of one year's duration, in an institute of higher education in order to qualify as a health visitor. This programme consists of core modules which are shared with community and school nurses, as well as modules which are specific to her role as a health visitor. These programmes are now at degree level.

The work of the health visitor has five main aspects:

1   The prevention of mental, physical and emotional ill-health and its consequences.
2   Early detection of ill-health and the surveillance of high-risk groups.
3   Recognition and identification of need and mobilization of appropriate resources where necessary.
4   Health promotion.

5   Promotion of care, which will include support during periods of stress and advice and guidance in cases of illness as well as in the care and management of children.

Health visitors are usually based at a health centre or general practitioners' surgery; they run Child Health Clinics, make home visits and may also visit schools. Health visitors currently may specialize in certain areas of practice, some may participate in sessions which provide opportunity for parent preparation during pregnancy. Health visitors take over the care of the mother and baby when discharged by the midwife between the 10th and 28th day after delivery. They will provide health screening, education and advice throughout infancy, run immunization programmes for the pre-school child and will liaise with the school nurse in the monitoring and health care of children once they enter school between the ages of 3 and 5 years.

Community nursing staff

Nurses working in the community may be those who provide care in the home, practice nurses based at the health centre or general practitioner surgery or school nurses based in educational institutions. Nurses will have undergone specialist courses in their particular area of nursing, sharing core modules of their programme with health care workers from other disciplines. They may continue the care of a mother or baby in certain cases, for example, when there is infection, long-term illness or accident if it is considered inadvisable for the midwife to continue care from the point of view of cross-infection or where the condition requires specialist nursing care. A midwife will, however, always fulfil the statutory requirement of attending the newly delivered mother and baby (UKCC, 1993) and monitor their progress at least for the first 10 days after delivery.

The school nurse has an important role to fulfil in respect of the health care of children. In the context of maternal and child health, this will vary from assisting in promoting the uptake of immunizations in both primary and secondary schools to the support and referral of teenagers who are pregnant. School nurses may assist in health promotion, sex education and AIDS awareness programmes.

Practice nurses should not undertake maternity care unless they are also practising midwives. They may assist the doctor or health visitor, for example in the provision of immunizations or in health promotion.

The social worker

Social workers may be attached to a community health centre or general practitioners' practice. They work in close co-operation with general practitioners and midwives to promote the social well-being of mothers and young families. They will assist through providing emotional support and counselling, advising regarding available benefits, accessing appropriate resources and referring as appropriate to other professionals. Social workers have a particular role in assisting disadvantaged families who may be struggling against poverty or lack of family support. Preparation of the social worker is through study for the Certificate of Qualification in Social Work (CQSW). This is normally a two-year course but will be reduced to one year for a student who has graduated with a degree in sociology or related subject. Undergraduate studies in sociology may include study for the CQSW, thus qualifying the graduate to practise as a social worker.

The counsellor

A counsellor may also be based at the community health centre or general practitioners' surgery. A counsellor will have undergone specialist training in counselling skills and will hold a diploma or degree which is approved by one of the professional bodies, for example, the British Association of Counselling. Counsellors specialize in providing a counselling service and clients may be referred to the counsellor in preference to or as a follow-up after receiving psychiatric care. They can provide skilled emotional support and guidance to families and the midwife may work in partnership with the counsellor.

A counsellor may assist in providing care for those who, for example, are contemplating or have undergone termination of pregnancy, experienced a miscarriage, have been bereaved, are HIV positive or fear that they may be so, are distressed by actual or anticipated abnormalities or handicap of their baby. The counsellor may be asked to assist couples who may be seeking advice about infertility, repeated miscarriage or the problem of inherited disease. In the latter instance, the couple are normally referred to a genetic counsellor who will usually be a doctor with a special interest and expertise in inherited disorders and usually has a postgraduate qualification in genetics. The midwife

acts as a counsellor in many aspects of her work, but an important part of counselling is to recognize the limits of one's own skills and therefore to refer to the appropriate colleague when necessary.

The nutritionist

Dietary advice in pregnancy and the postnatal period is inevitably offered by the midwife. However, some women may require specialist help and the nutritionist may form part of the primary health care team and is able to assist in such cases. Women who are known diabetics or incur gestational diabetes will require skilled dietary advice, women who are very obese or undernourished and those with anaemia can also benefit from the specialist assistance of the nutritionist. The nutritionist is a specially trained professional who holds a diploma or degree in nutritional studies or dietetics and will be a State Registered Dietician. The nutritionist will also help in cases of metabolic disorder in babies and children and will provide skilled assistance in conditions such as phenylketonuria or coeliac disease.

The physiotherapist

A physiotherapist is a professional who has studied for a minimum of three years to qualify as a State Registered Physiotherapist. Some practitioners have specialized as obstetric physiotherapists having undergone a specialist postgraduate course to prepare them for their particular role in assisting pregnant and newly delivered women. A physiotherapist may work in partnership with the midwife to assist women preparing for labour. She may provide sessions in parent preparation and postnatal groups or classes.

The dentist

The dentist may be based at the health centre or may work from a separate surgery. Dentists are qualified dental surgeons and provide free care under the National Health Service for children and pregnant women and those who have given birth within the past year. The midwife should encourage women to take advantage of this care at the earliest opportunity during pregnancy. The dentist will encourage all members of the population to attend for regular check-ups, usually at six-monthly intervals. The dentist is usually assisted by a dental nurse or dental hygienist who will have undergone a recognized training.

The chiropodist

The chiropodist is a practitioner who, having undergone specialist training and holding a qualification as a State Registered Chiropodist, is able to provide skilled assistance in the care of the feet. The pregnant woman may benefit from care by a chiropodist if she is unable to attend to her feet in the later stages of pregnancy or if she encounters particular problems. Increase in body weight and an alteration of weight distribution and posture may cause foot problems which the woman has not previously experienced. The midwife may suggest that the woman attends for chiropody. The chiropodist may be based at a health centre or may work in private practice.

The pharmacist

The pharmacist has received education and training, normally to graduate level, in pharmacology and related subjects and will be skilled in the dispensing of medicines and other pharmaceutical substances. Some of these may be sold directly to the public, others will be available only on the prescription of a registered medical practitioner. The pharmacist provides a valuable service to the community not only in dispensing medicines but also in providing free advice concerning ailments, recommending medical consultations as appropriate. Women receive medicines on prescription free of charge during pregnancy and for one year after giving birth. Children under 16 years are also entitled to free prescriptions; this entitlement will extend to 18 years if the young person is in full-time education.

Practitioners of complementary therapies

In modern society there is an increasing trend towards holistic care. Practitioners of complementary medicine and other therapies form the backbone of this system of care and may work in partnership with other members of the primary health care team. The midwife should familiarize herself with the advantages and disadvantages of the various complementary therapies and advise women to seek appropriately qualified practitioners when they require such care (UKCC, 1994; Dimond, 1995a, b). Complementary practitioners may include osteopaths, acupuncturists, medical herbalists, homeopathic physicians, aromatherapists and hypnotists. Chapter 22 discusses complementary therapies and their implications in midwifery practice. Public libraries carry lists of qualified practitioners in the area.

Child Health Care and Surveillance

Boucaud (1989), in making the case for a European convention on children's rights, points out in the context of the child and the community that the emphasis in considering the rights of the sick or handicapped child lies as much on prevention as on treatment. It could be argued that a child in Europe should be born with the expectation that preventable conditions will be prevented and this is congruent with the Alma Ata Declaration which shares the vision of Health for All by the Year 2000 with the whole world (WHO, 1978). Midwives will be aware that appropriate child health care starts long before birth in the preconception and antenatal periods. Healthy children are more likely to become healthy parents of the next generation and some health deficits of childhood can never be compensated for in later life.

The Select Committee of Experts on Child Health Surveillance set up within the Council of Europe urged social service departments to pay attention to two basic principles:

▶ First, that child health surveillance must not only be regarded as a service available to the community, but one which is used by the community. Since people cannot be compelled to use services provided by the State, appropriate ways of encouraging uptake of care must be discovered.
▶ Secondly, that the community itself and the families which comprise that community must be regarded as involved in and responsible for health surveillance (Strasbourg, 1985).

These principles could be applied not only to child health surveillance but also to all aspects of maternal and community health. The first principle of community utilization is fundamental if a country's health services are to be effective in health promotion and disease prevention. It is in harmony with the first three questions which Currell (1990) states may be asked of any system of maternity care, namely whether it is available, accessible and acceptable to those who need it. These issues are discussed further below in the context of health promotion.

The midwife has a key role in encouraging the uptake of health services. The notion that people are responsible for their own health may arguably have become less fashionable with the introduction of the National Health Service in 1948 and the growth of the social security system with its numerous financial benefits and concessions. Health care and social systems in the UK are the envy of much of the world, but the negative aspect centres around a confusion between the rights of the citizen to utilize it and creating a dependency which may make claiming those rights a priority over the individual taking responsibility for his or her own health. However, the move away from the paternalistic approach to medical care towards increased client involvement should, in theory, make communities more aware of their responsibilities as they become partners in their health care. The reality of the situation may be very different and broad generalizations are inappropriate.

The Health Visitors' Association, in harmony with the World Health Organization objectives for child health (WHO, 1985) identified four essential components in child health surveillance. These were (HVA, 1985):

1 *Screening tests*: These are procedures carried out to detect specific abnormalities or disorders (see Chapter 63).
2 *Health promotion support*: This includes advice on all aspects of child health, including immunization.
3 *Developmental screening*: This involves examination of the child at determined intervals in order to detect any deviation from the normal range of development.
4 *Developmental assessment*: This involves the assessment of abnormal findings identified during developmental screening.

CHILD HEALTH CLINICS

The Maternal and Child Welfare Act of 1918 empowered local authorities to provide maternal and child health clinics for expectant and nursing mothers and for children under 5 years of age. In 1936 the Public Health Act made notification of all births compulsory and therefore made it possible for all babies to be followed-up. In the National Health Service Act 1946, local authorities were responsible for providing child health clinics, but in April 1974 when the National Health Service Reorganisation Act came into force, this responsibility was transferred to the Area Health Authorities. With the implementation of the National Health Service and Community Care Act of 1990, care providers including those providing a

service in the community could apply for NHS Trust status (see Chapter 79).

Child health clinics are mainly held in health centres and doctors' surgeries and are staffed by health visitors, a doctor for some sessions, clinic nurses and sometimes voluntary helpers. They offer free medical advice but not treatment. Regular developmental screening is carried out with assessment divided into five parts:

1 Posture and large movements.
2 Vision and fine movements.
3 Hearing and speech.
4 Social behaviour and play.
5 Physical examination including weight and height measurements.

Development assessment is usually carried out at 6 weeks, 6–7 months, 12 months, 18 months and 2 years.

Other functions of the child health centres are health promotion, vaccination and immunization and the sale of welfare foods. They also give mothers the opportunity to meet others with young children and share experiences.

VACCINATION AND IMMUNIZATION

In order to realize the aim of the World Health Organization to eliminate neonatal tetanus, polio, measles, diphtheria and congenital rubella by the year 2000, a target of 90% uptake of immunization for these diseases was set for all children under 2 years in Europe by 1990. It has been contended that whilst the immunization targets may be achievable, the total eradication of these diseases may not actually be possible (Begg and Noah, 1985). Smith and Jacobson (1988) in considering a strategy for health for the 1990s suggest that the USA has set more realistic goals simply by specifying that there should be a major reduction in the incidence of these diseases but not an elimination of them by 1990 (USDHHS, 1980). They concluded that:

> The European targets – with the exception of past rubella policy – are all translatable into UK policy. But the DHSS has only so far set a firm target for 95% of measles vaccine by 1990, with the aim of total elimination by 1995.
>
> (Smith and Jacobson, 1988)

Uptake of immunization and therefore prevalence of infectious diseases will be affected by numerous factors which are not always predicted. For example, recent controversy about the mode of production of the measles vaccine affected uptake of this on ethical or religious grounds by a proportion of the population.

A summary of the recommended immunization schedule is provided in Table 1.

Health Promotion in the Context of Community Health

The midwife has an important role in health promotion, especially as it relates to reproductive health. The term 'health education' has given way to the term 'health promotion' as midwives and other health professionals are seen more as catalysts within a process rather than teachers in the school of life. Whatever the term used, the issue is one of raising awareness and encouraging a healthy lifestyle for the benefit of the community and the individuals comprising that population (see Chapter 23).

Health promotion has been described as:

An activity whose basis resides in gaining change, change to promote health. The methods of change are its subject. It draws on the skills and practice of change that are found well established in politics, economics, the media, therapy, education, advocacy, legislation etc.

(Ashton and Seymour, 1988)

Change is rarely easy and not always acceptable, neither is it always necessary. In health promotion there is a need to assess the health status and lifestyle of the individual, family or community, provide encouragement where there are positive findings and approach the negative with sensitivity and skill. Preferably, the midwife encourages those with whom she works to want to undertake their own assessment of their health status and lifestyle and motivates them to introduce the changes which they perceive as necessary. The midwife encounters the woman and her family at a time when they are experiencing a major life event. The woman will be making many changes to adapt to her pregnancy and her new or altered role as a mother. The midwife can be influential in promoting health and works in this context alongside the health visitor and other health care workers. Her 'public' role in health promotion may be seen in parent preparation groups and in providing information and counselling during the antenatal and postnatal periods.

Table 1   Recommended immunization schedule

	Vaccination	To protect against	Given at	Route
1	Triple vaccine	Diphtheria Tetanus Whooping cough	2, 3 & 4 months	Injection
2	Poliomyelitis vaccine	Poliomyelitis	2, 3 & 4 months	Oral
3	MMR (combined vaccine)	Measles Mumps Rubella	12–18 months	Injection
4	Booster	Diphtheria Tetanus Poliomyelitis	4–5 years	Injection Oral
5	Rubella vaccine	Rubella	girls 10–14 years – who have not had MMR	Injection
6	BCG vaccine	Tuberculosis	10–14 years if tuberculin negative	Injection
7	Booster	Tetanus	15–19 years	Injection

Note: Hepatitis B vaccine will be given to babies whose mothers are carriers of the hepatitis B surface antigen. This will be given by injection at birth, 4 weeks and at 6 months.

Rubella vaccine will be offered to women before pregnancy or postnatally if they are not immune to this disease as it can cause congenital abnormalities if contracted during pregnancy.
Source: DOH, 1990.

However, the midwife's effectiveness and that of any of the primary health care team in promoting health will be influenced by other more subtle issues, emphasizing the need for:

▶ a sound *knowledge* which is up to date and whenever possible based on relevant and critically evaluated research;
▶ a high level of *interpersonal skills*, an ability to listen being more important initially than an ability to provide guidance and information;
▶ an *awareness and sensitivity* that enables the midwife to provide stimuli that will engender change relevant and appropriate to the client and the situation;
▶ an ability and determination to function as a *role model* for healthy living. This can be a challenge to professionals in a variety of ways, but a midwife who promotes a particular aspect of health by her words but is a poor example of the application of the truth may have difficulty in convincing a reluctant client to adopt the change which could affect the length or quality of her life as well as that of her unborn or newborn child.

How midwives work to promote health may be determined to a large extent by their personal philosophy of care and that of the organization for which they work. Arnstein suggested a 'ladder of community participation' (Figure 2) and maintained that most professionals as well as welfare bureaucracies functioned largely on the bottom half of the ladder (Arnstein, 1969). It could be challenging for the midwife to identify a particular professional function which she fulfils, whether in health promotion, care provision or in providing social support, and critically evaluate how far up Arnstein's ladder her practice usually ascends.

There is much spoken about partnership at present, but the character of the partnership between the woman and the midwife, health visitor or doctor may be very variable and rightly so in differing situations. Doubtless the increased tendency towards litigation will affect ascent of this ladder. The frequency with which the top rung of 'citizen control' is encountered may be the cause or effect of changing public and professional attitudes, along with a redefining of rights and expectations. In focusing on Arnstein's ladder, Ashton points out that: 'in wishing for people to take increased responsibility for their own health it is necessary to recognize the close relationship between risk taking behaviour and lack of empowerment' (Ashton, 1983). The midwife may profitably reflect on issues of

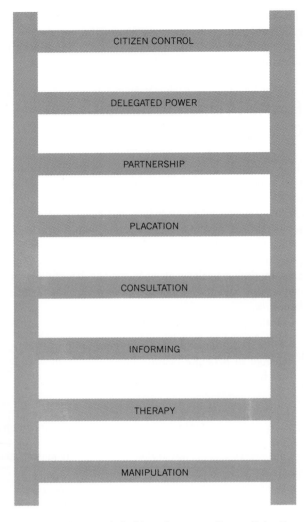

Figure 2 Arnstein's ladder of community participation. On which rung of the ladder does your midwifery practice usually rest? (After Arnstein, 1969).

risk taking in the context of midwifery care as well health promotion. It could be appropriate to ask such questions as:

▶ Does lack of empowerment promote or mitigate against risk-taking behaviour?
▶ How should my attitude and philosophy of care and/or that of my team or organization be modified in order to further:
  – minimize risk-taking behaviour?
  – assist families to take increased responsibility for their own health?

– increase or introduce empowerment at individual, family or community level?

Poverty and Pregnancy

Poverty has been recognized as one of the major factors influencing mortality and morbidity rates worldwide (Townsend and Davidson, 1982; Royston and Armstrong, 1989) and is a curse in any society. It is therefore important to explore the issue in the context of community health and social services. In the UK, the debate about poverty is frequently controversial and the status may be termed relative rather than real, though even relativity and reality are in a constant state of flux and one must be careful to avoid value judgements on the issue.

Poverty may be described in many ways and one cannot relate it totally to monetary income. In conducting a systematic synthesis of available literature and research on social, financial and psychological support in the context of childbearing, Enkin et al. (1990) concluded that: 'When resources of money, time and energy are limited, the possibilities of making choices that promote health are also limited'.

The existence of a welfare state theoretically eliminates poverty, but in practice, although the condition is minimized by comparison with many other countries, it is obvious that poverty has not been eliminated in the UK. Falling into 'the poverty trap' is an acknowledged situation affecting members of the community who have an income which disqualifies them from claiming benefits, but may be inadequate to meet all their needs. Chapter 81 addresses issues of social security and benefits and the reader can consider a variety of situations in which women may not be entitled to benefits which they appear to need.

At the bottom of the social spiral of need lie the homeless who may be victims of injustice, inequality, abuse or for want of a better word, misfortune. Unfortunately, homelessness may be consequential to the implementation of the National Health Service and Community Care Act 1990 since some who live on the streets suffer mental handicap, instability or illness and they may fall between the diminishing provisions made in institutions and those provided within the community. Concern has also been expressed recently about teenage girls who become victims of prostitution. These, technically, may be girls in the care of the local authority or from various home backgrounds having experienced emotional poverty or sexual abuse. Research and investigations by government and charitable organizations like the Children's Society (1995) tend to reveal further causes for concern from time to time. The whole topic of homelessness presents a vast area of social concern to the midwife, health visitor, social worker and others, the details of which are beyond the scope of this book. This chapter attempts only to raise awareness of an increasing problem in Britain today.

Greve and Currie (1990) recognize that 'there is no universally accepted definition of homelessness' and acknowledge that the condition may range between 'rooflessness' to a statement on the quality of accommodation. An examination of population statistics reveals that, of the total number of homeless people in a national census in 1991, the vast majority were male. Of the 2827 homeless people, little more than 15% (430) were women (OPCS, 1993). It must be acknowledged that homelessness is inherently difficult to quantify, but it can be concluded that: 'It remains true that rough sleeping is not a common route for women to take' (Greve and Currie, 1990).

However common or uncommon homelessness may be amongst women, it relates to a group of people amongst the most vulnerable of those whom the midwife will encounter. Add to these, women who may have appalling accommodation or live with a 'bed and breakfast' type of arrangement, some women and young families find themselves, for all practical purposes, homeless or on the streets for a significant proportion of any 24 hours. In a study examining young women and homelessness in south-east Northumberland, Gilroy and Douglas (1994) challenge the concept that homelessness is 'only a big city problem'. Whenever homelessness exists and regardless of the degree of poverty or inferior accommodation which may officially classify the woman as homeless, it is obvious that a pregnant or newly delivered woman in such circumstances is at considerable risk. Researchers focusing on two pilot schemes in the London area, studied the particular problems of health care for the single homeless and point out that:

Homeless people do not belong to a homogenous group for policy makers to focus on and there is no all-embracing solution to ensure that all homeless people get primary health care when they need it.

(Williams and Allen, 1989)

Maybe some quotes from the data collected by these workers serve to illustrate the different perspectives from which homelessness is viewed and provide food for thought for the health professional:

'Many single homeless people don't have access to primary health care' (Voluntary sector worker)

'It's almost as if they don't count because they're homeless and rootless' (Social worker)

'The problem is their mobility which creates extra work for us' (General practitioner)

'If you're homeless they don't want to know' (Homeless person)

(Williams and Allen, 1989)

It could be a salutary exercise for the midwife to express her own view of the homeless, remembering to reflect on all those situations in which a woman may be deemed 'homeless' even though she may not be 'roofless'. The result should be not an idealistic but a realistic statement which could be the basis of a primary health care policy.

Legislation relating to homelessness was provided in the Homeless Persons Act of 1977 which is now enacted in Part III of the Housing Act 1985. Without question a pregnant woman and a person with whom dependent children reside are considered 'priorities' under the Act in respect of homelessness. The midwife may be the first person in the professional chain to act as an advocate for such a family. Those who exist in accommodation which less clearly identifies them as 'homeless' may be more difficult to help, but the midwife will work in co-operation with the social worker and health visitor in order to facilitate the optimum outcome for the disadvantaged family.

Child Care: Legislation and Relevant Issues

The Children Act of 1989 which came into force on 14 October 1991 was predicted to bring about: 'The most fundamental change of child law this century' (Preface to the Children Act 1989). In commending the Bill to parliament, Sir Geoffrey Howe described it as: 'The most comprehensive and far reaching reform of this branch of law ever introduced. It meets a long felt need for a comprehensive and integrated statutory framework to ensure the welfare of children' (Howe, 1989).

Table 2   Summary of content of the Children Act 1989

Part	Content
I	Introductory
II	Orders with respect to children in family proceedings: – general – financial relief – family assistance orders
III	Local Authority support for children & families
IV	Care & supervision
V	Protection of children
VI	Community homes
VII	Voluntary homes & voluntary organizations
VIII	Registered children's homes
IX	Private arrangements for fostering children
X	Child-minding & day care for young children
XI	Secretary of State's supervisory functions & responsibilities
XII	Miscellaneous & general: – notification of children accommodated in certain establishments e.g. health authorities, residential care – adoption (section 88) – paternity tests (section 89) – criminal care & supervision orders (section 90) – effect & duration of orders etc. – jurisdiction & procedure etc. – search warrants – general

The content of the Children Act is summarized in Table 2 and it can be noted that the legislation covers practically all issues relating to the care and upbringing of children along with relevant social rules and services. The Children Act 1989 amends other Acts such as the Adoption Act, and repeals some earlier legislation, for example: the Guardianship of Minors Act 1971, the Children Act 1975 and the Child Care Act 1980. It has been claimed that the Act will: 'revolutionise the law to be applied by courts hearing all kinds of children cases, whether in divorce or other family proceedings, care proceedings or wardship' (White et al., 1990).

The following provisions for child care which were transferred to the Department of Health and Social Security from the Home Office in 1971 will be of particular interest to the midwife. The local authority social services departments assume responsibility for children's services. Their responsibilities include:

1   The provision of day nurseries in many instances.
2   Supervision of children in private playgroups, day nurseries, with child-minders, in foster homes and children placed for adoption.
3   The reception of children into care when necessary and ensuring that they are well looked after.
4   Arranging for children to be adopted.
5   Initiating court proceedings, where appropriate in respect of children and young persons, and ensuring that the interests of children and young people are looked after following court orders.

DAY CARE

Day nurseries

Day nurseries may be provided by the local authority social services departments or privately by voluntary organizations or private bodies. Private day nurseries must be registered with and supervised by the local authority social services department. The purpose of day nurseries is to care for preschool children whose parents are working or ill or need particular help with the care of young children. Since the number of places is invariably insufficient to meet the demand, priority is given to the children of one-parent families, the handicapped and those at risk of child abuse or whose home circumstances are unsatisfactory.

Day nurseries are staffed by nursery nurses and visited regularly by a health visitor. They open early and close late from Monday to Friday to allow parents to leave children before they go to work and collect them at the end of their working day. Charges are made according to the parents' means, or there may be a minimal flat-rate charge. In cases of very low income or a handicapped child the charge is waived altogether.

Child-minding

A child-minder is a person who minds a child under the age of 8 years in her own home for two hours or more a day for a fee or reward. Registration of child-minders was made compulsory by the Nurseries and Child-Minders Regulation Act 1948 and amended by the Health Services and Public Health Act 1968 and Children Act 1989. Under the Local Authority Social Services Act 1970 responsibility for the registration and supervision of child-minders was transferred to the social services departments.

The local authority inspect the premises to be used for child-minding and may impose conditions regard-ing facilities and safety and limit the number of children to be cared for. They have a duty to inspect the premises at least once a year. The local authority ensure that the child-minder is in good health and will check with police records whether an applicant has been convicted of any offences listed in the schedule to the Disqualification Regulations. The authority may also refuse or cancel registration if they consider that the child-minder is seriously inadequate to meet the child's needs, especially regarding religion, race, culture or language. Many local authorities provide training schemes for child-minders. Arrangements are made for medical supervision of children being minded.

The child-minder must keep a register of attendances. Payment is a private arrangement between the child-minder and the parent. There is a National Association of Child-Minders.

Playgroups

Preschool playgroups are provided by groups of parents or voluntary organizations for normal children between the ages of $2\frac{1}{2}$ and 5 years. They were started in 1961 by parents in an attempt to compensate for the lack of nursery schools. Local authorities may provide financial aid to playgroups and in many areas have established their own schemes.

Children usually attend for between two and five sessions weekly, each of about $2\frac{1}{2}$ hours duration.

All playgroups have to be registered and supervised by the social services department. Parents pay a fee and may be encouraged to assist in running the playgroup. There is a Preschool Playgroups Association.

Education for the preschool child

Nursery schools for children between the ages of 2 and 5 years are provided by the Local Education Authority under the Education Act of 1944. They provide nursery education and there is no payment. There are limited places available in nursery school and thus priority is given to children with special needs. There is an increasing demand for nursery school places and currently mounting public pressure for the right of parents who wish their children to attend from 3 years of age. This has resulted in the government now providing vouchers to enable parents to 'purchase' nursery school education for children between the ages of 3 and 5 years.

RESIDENTIAL CARE

Under the Children Act 1989, local authorities are required to provide accommodation for children who require it because:

▶ no one has parental responsibility for them;
▶ they are lost or abandoned;
▶ their carers are prevented from providing care or suitable accommodation.

The authority is also required to provide accommodation for 16- and 17-year-olds whose welfare may be seriously prejudiced if they do not provide this. Care proceedings enable the courts to authorize local authorities to take action if a child is considered otherwise to be significantly at risk. Such proceedings may be brought by the local authority or the National Society for the Prevention of Cruelty to Children (NSPCC) in respect of a child under 17 years of age or under 16 years if they are married.

A child may initially be admitted to a reception centre where his or her physical, psychological and educational condition is assessed before a placement is made. The views of social workers, teachers and psychiatrists and the wishes of the child and the child's family are considered before a placement is made. Acceptance of the accommodation offered is voluntary and unless the child has a residence order, the local authority may not provide or continue to provide accommodation for a child under 16 years of age against the wishes of the person with parental responsibility if they are willing and able to provide accommodation or arrange for this. Once 16 years of age, the child must be consulted and agree to the accommodation.

Fostering

To 'foster' a child means to look after a child with whom there is no blood or legal relationship for 28 days or more whether or not there is any payment. A foster child is under 16 years of age, or under 18 years in the case of a disabled child. The Children Act 1989 and the Children (Private Arrangements for Fostering) Regulations 1991 (SI 1991/2050) apply. A foster parent is required to notify the local authority social services department at least six weeks but not longer than 13 weeks before placement unless it is an emergency when there must be notification within 48 hours of reception of the child. The number of children who may be fostered by a foster parent as well as their ages and sex may be restricted.

Individuals wishing to become foster parents must be approved by the local authority and may be disqualified if, for example, they have been convicted of certain criminal offences. The premises also will be inspected and the local authority has a duty to ensure the welfare of foster children. Foster parents do not have parental rights over the children but natural parents may designate certain responsibilities to the foster parents, for example, the right to authorize medical treatment.

There are training programmes for foster parents in many areas and efforts are being made to place disturbed and handicapped children with skilled foster parents. Foster parents have formed the National Foster Care Association.

ADOPTION

Legal adoption means that the legal relationship between parents and child is severed and all parental rights and duties are transferred to the adoptive parents. An adopted child has the same legal status in relation to the adoptive parents as any other child born in marriage, except that he or she cannot inherit titles.

The Adoption Act 1976 consolidates former Adoption Acts and the provisions for adoption in the Children Act of 1975. The Children Act 1989 amends the Adoption Act of 1976 but the latter remains the only statute governing adoption. The Adoption Agencies Regulations 1983 (SI 1983/1964) should now be read in conjunction with Arrangements for Placement of Children (General) Regulations 1991 (SI 1991/890). A recent government announcement indicates that changes are to be made to the process of adoption which will remove some of the present restrictions.

All local authorities are adoption agencies, sometimes in partnership with another local authority or with an approved voluntary society. Voluntary adoption societies have to be approved by the Secretary of State every three years. A child under 18 years of any nationality who has not married may be placed for adoption by an adoption agency, that is an approved adoption society or local authority. Private placements made in Great Britain are illegal except if the proposed adopter is a relative or the placement is as a result of an order of the High Court.

Application to adopt

A married couple or single person can apply to adopt. A man may not normally adopt a female but a woman may adopt a male or a female. A married person cannot apply singly unless the couple are permanently separated, the spouse cannot be found, or he or she is incapable because of mental or physical illness. A sole parent cannot adopt unless the other parent is dead or missing or there is some other good reason. The minimum age for applicants for adoption is 21 years unless the applicant is a parent adopting his or her own child, together with his or her spouse. In the latter case the applicant must be at least 18 years of age. A couple applying to adopt must be married and a sole adopter single with the exception of special circumstances. One of the adopters must normally reside in the UK, Channel Isles or Isle of Man. If they are not domiciled as specified they must have a home in Great Britain. The local authority in the area in which the applicant is living must be notified when the application is made.

Placing a child for adoption

A child placed for adoption must be cared for continuously for a period of three months after the age of six weeks before an adoption order can be made. During this time the local authority is responsible for supervising care. Agreement for adoption must be obtained in writing from the mother or parents after the child is six weeks old. The mother or parents may withdraw their agreement until the adoption order is made, but cannot remove the child from the prospective adoptive parents without the court's permission once application has been made for adoption and the agreement signed. The court may dispense with parental agreement under certain circumstances such as serious ill-treatment of the child.

The agreement of the father of an illegitimate child is not required but when he is paying maintenance he must be given notice of proceedings to adopt the child and may oppose them. With the introduction of the Child Support Agency, an increasing number of putative fathers are paying maintenance. Putative fathers who have legal custody of the child have the same status as parents and guardians as regards agreeing to adoption.

The mother or parents may consent to free their child for adoption which means that they transfer all legal rights to the child to the adoption agency before arrangements for adoption are made.

If an older child is to be adopted the child's wishes must be taken into consideration.

Responsibility for applying to the court for an adoption order lies with the prospective adopters. Those who wish to adopt a child in their care who was not placed with them by an adoption agency are required to notify the local authority of their intention to adopt. The child then becomes a protected child and the local authority is required to report on the application to the court.

After an application for an adoption is made the court must appoint a guardian ad litem who may be an officer of the local authority or a probation officer. The function of the guardian is to safeguard the interests of the child and to investigate all circumstances relating to the proposed adoption, interview all the parties concerned and make a detailed report to the court with recommendations.

No payments, other than those sanctioned by the court, are given or received in respect of the child.

Adoption order

When the court makes an adoption order the rights and duties of natural parents are transferred to the adoptive parents. The adopted child's new name is entered in the Adopted Child's Register which is kept by the Registrar General. A certificate is issued which takes the place of a birth certificate.

The Children Act 1975 gave adopted persons over the age of 18 years the right to access their original birth records. A counselling scheme is available for those who seek information about their natural parents.

CUSTODY

Custody provides a means by which relatives and others looking after children on a long-term basis can apply for and obtain legal custody of the children. It may be an alternative to adoption. Certain parental rights and duties are invested in the custodian. A person having legal custody cannot effect or arrange for the child's adoption unless they are a parent or guardian of the child.

The Handicapped or Disabled Child

A handicap is a temporary or permanent disability or disadvantage which adversely affects normal growth and development and/or the ability to adjust to a normal life. The handicapping condition may be present at birth or may become evident or occur later. It may be a physical or mental condition or both.

With the advance of science and technology and as neonatal intensive care facilities improve, the babies who survive with conditions that in earlier years would have proved fatal are increasing. The degree of morbidity which may accompany survival is always a matter of concern and follow-up of babies cared for in neonatal special and intensive care units is the responsibility of paediatricians and specialist paediatric nurses and health visitors. Risk factors which have been identified as associated with infant mortality include accidents, infections and non-accidental injury (Goodwin, 1991; Chadwick, 1994). These factors are inevitably linked with child handicap too. The increasing incidence of child abuse in modern society leaves individuals with a health deficit which may be emotional and/or physical and which is inevitably long term.

Identifying the baby at risk to handicap from the family, medical and obstetric history and from complications which may occur during the prenatal and perinatal period remains an important responsibility of the midwife. Every effort can then be made to ensure that these women and their babies receive the best possible antenatal, intranatal and postnatal care in an attempt to reduce perinatal death and to improve the quality of life of those who survive.

Most parents experience some anxiety in pregnancy about having a malformed child, but the shock when this fear is realized is distressing to all involved in the birth. One of the first questions the mother asks after delivery is whether the baby is alright. If there is an obvious malformation the midwife will tell the parents as gently as possible that something is wrong and initiate the process of referral which will result in the best possible specialist opinion and treatment. Sometimes an abnormality is not as clearly obvious yet the midwife suspects a problem and does not want to alarm the parents unnecessarily. She must then initiate a paediatric consultation earlier than would otherwise be arranged as part of the neonatal screening process, taking care not to give any information to the family which she might later have to contradict.

When the doctor has examined the baby he or she will usually see the parents together and talk to them about the baby's condition. The couple are often too stunned and distressed to absorb much of the information given at this first interview, thus further interviews are essential. The parents should be given time and opportunity to ask questions and to express their feelings. The midwife initially provides much of the help and support which the parents require. Ultimately, however, they need constant access to someone such as their family doctor, counsellor or social worker to whom they can turn for guidance and support as they learn to cope with their handicapped child. Depending on the condition and on its severity, the baby may need to be cared for in a special or intensive care nursery, or it may be possible for the child to remain at the mother's bedside in a postnatal ward. Where possible there is much to commend the latter to help the mother form a relationship with her handicapped child, but the condition and individual situation will inevitably influence these decisions.

Handicapped children have the same basic needs as other children, but require more help and support from sources outside the family if their needs are to be met and they are to achieve the best physical, mental and social performance possible. The current approach endeavours to promote the concept that a person may be disabled but is not necessarily handicapped as a result.

SERVICES FOR HANDICAPPED OR DISABLED CHILDREN

Medical assessments will include frequent assessments of the degree of handicap throughout infancy and childhood and the provision of treatment as appropriate. At the age of 2 years a detailed medical examination and comprehensive assessment is made to decide which children have special educational needs. Education authorities are empowered to require parents to submit their children over the age of 2 years for medical examination under the 1944 Education Act.

Education

Wherever possible, handicapped children attend ordinary schools. Efforts to encourage this trend have increased in recent years with only the more severely handicapped attending special schools where there are teachers who are specially trained to meet their needs. Sometimes a special helper who may be a qualified nursery nurse will be appointed to augment the care provided for a handicapped child who is receiving education at a normal school. In a special school teaching staff will be supported by nursing staff who can take care of the more complex problems of a child's handicap. Education is aimed at enabling the child to lead as normal a life as possible in the community.

Wherever education of the handicapped child takes place, there is close liaison between the school, medical staff and a disablement resettlement officer to find suitable employment for disabled young people on leaving school. Some undergo training and work in sheltered workshops, whilst others find suitable employment in the community or go on to further education. An increasing awareness of the need for access to buildings and transport for the disabled, as well as supportive legislation, means that an increasing number of handicapped children may expect in the future to be educated, live and work in the community alongside their able-bodied peers, though much yet needs to be done to achieve an equality which is desirable. Some handicapped individuals are too seriously disabled for any kind of employment and may require help from the social services department.

Social services

The social services department provides social workers to help and support the handicapped and their families. To enable the handicapped to remain in the community as far as possible the social services department provides supporting services such as home helps. A community care grant may be awarded at the discretion of a Social Fund Officer to assist the parents of a disabled child where laundering costs are higher than normal because of the child's disability. This may facilitate the purchase or repair of a washing machine, tumble or spin drier. The community care grant may also be awarded if the child suffers from behavioural problems arising from mental illness or handicap. This will help in offsetting the cost incurred due to excessive wear and tear on clothing or house redecoration. The handicapped may also qualify for housing grants for home alterations solely on the grounds of their disability. A disability living allowance is tailored to meet a person's care and mobility needs. Details of financial help available are provided in Chapter 81. Other services provided by the social services department include day care, training centres, workshops, recreational facilities, holiday schemes and respite care. More permanent residential care is also provided where needed.

VOLUNTARY AND SUPPORT GROUPS

There are an ever-increasing number of support groups which are specifically designed to help and support those with particular disabilities and their families. Examples of these include the Down's Syndrome Association, the National Society for Phenylketonuria (NSPKU), the Association for Spina Bifida and Hydrocephalus (ASBAH) and Scope (formerly, the Spastics Society).

The Abused Child

Child abuse may take the form of physical, emotional, sexual or mental cruelty. Children may suffer a form of abuse as a result of neglect as well as wilful ill-treatment. All professional health personnel have a responsibility in the course of their work to be alert to the possibility of child abuse and to take appropriate action where indicated (DOH, 1991, 1992). The midwife in her close contact with the family, especially in the home, may have reason to suspect that a child is at risk and therefore in need of protection.

Predisposing factors

These are numerous and may be associated with the parents' age and physical and emotional health, their own background and experience, their current social or economic status. The increased risk may relate to issues associated with the birth, health or immediate care of a newborn baby. Maybe a positive statement issued by the Department of Health in a recent report provides a focus on this topic: 'Child abuse is less likely if there is an affectionate and positive relationship between parents and baby' (DOH, 1992). Beyond acknowledging a statement of the obvious here, it could be useful for the midwife to reflect upon what it is that contributes to 'an affectionate and positive relationship' and conversely what is likely to interfere with this. It is the breaking down or failure to nurture a positive relationship within a protective environment which predisposes to the risk of child abuse. It is therefore of paramount importance that the midwife does all within her ability to foster this positive relationship from the earliest possible opportunity. In this context Clarke (1993) emphasizes that:

Postnatal care should promote positive parenting, especially when babies are more vulnerable e.g:

those who require neonatal or special care, or are congenitally abnormal or in need, as these babies are at increased risk to abuse.

(Clarke, 1993: 29)

A poor experience of mothering or actual experience of abuse for the parent concerned may well contribute to factors which predispose to child abuse. Other factors include poor housing, unemployment, marital problems, drug or alcohol abuse. Whatever the predisposing factors, the National Society for the Prevention of Cruelty to Children estimate that, on average, 3–4 children die in the UK every week following abuse or neglect (NSPCC, 1995).

Warning signs

There are well-documented warning signs which should alert the midwife. The mother may reject her pregnancy and subsequently her baby. She may handle and talk to her baby roughly, make unrealistic demands on the baby or make no effort to communicate with the child at all. As a result the baby is insecure, often fretful and fails to thrive. Poor mother–child attachment is particularly likely when mother and baby have been separated in the early postnatal period.

Diagnosis

The diagnosis is made on the history, the injuries reported and evidence of other injuries found on clinical examination. Minor injuries such as facial bruising, damage in the mouth area or small burns may be the first signs. More extensive bruising may indicate that the child has been gripped tightly and possibly shaken. The child may show signs of failure to thrive or actual neglect and slow social development. There may also be evidence of fractures or sexual abuse.

Suspicion is aroused by the injuries, especially if the parents delay in seeking advice about them and there is inadequate explanation or a discrepancy between the parents' explanation and the actual injuries found on examination of the child. The parents may exhibit disturbed behaviour or an unusual reaction to the child's injuries. Sometimes they make frequent visits with the child to the doctor or an accident and emergency department of a hospital without convincing reasons.

Management

If child abuse is suspected a full examination is essential and a consultant paediatrician should be called immediately. If it is confirmed that abuse is likely, the paediatrician will inform the social services department.

Section V of the Children Act 1989 provides for the 'Protection of Children' (Table 2). This enables a Child Assessment Order and subsequently an Emergency Protection Order to be made. In emergency, the police are authorized to remove a child to suitable accommodation for protection for a maximum of 72 hours.

The Children Act 1989 also requires the establishment of an Area Child Protection Committee (ACPC) to organize 'inter-agency cooperation' to protect children at risk. Local authorities must also maintain a Child Protection Register. This register contains data related to all children who are subject to a Child Protection Plan and is to ensure that such a plan is reviewed formally at six monthly intervals.

Occasionally the midwife or other health worker may suspect child abuse but their suspicions are not firm enough to warrant arranging for the child's admission to hospital or to initiate Assessment and Emergency Protection Orders, as Dimond points out: 'to make a diagnosis of suspected child abuse is a weighty matter' (Dimond, 1994: 292). In these circumstances the midwife should consult the family doctor and her supervisor or senior colleague without delay. All midwives and other health workers should have knowledge of the implications of the Children Act 1989 and the local practice and procedures for the protection of children who may be victims of any form of abuse.

Voluntary Organizations and Pressure Groups

Although the State provides a comprehensive range of social services and social security, the voluntary organizations augment the services and make a valuable contribution to the needs of special groups. They are non-profit-making organizations and most are registerd charities under the Charities Act legislation. Many voluntary organizations receive financial aid from government grants and local authorities and work in close liaison with the statutory services. In some cases they provide a statutory service for the local authority, for instance day nurseries.

Sometimes support groups will provide assistance of a particular kind by those who have experience in dealing with specific issues themselves. Associations for the handicapped cited above are examples of this kind of support. Others exist to provide support for parents who have multiple births, for example, the Multiple Births Foundation and the Twins and Multiple Births Association (TAMBA). Some groups provide support and practical assistance, for example in instances such as domestic violence or rape. Women's Aid and Victim Support Schemes are examples of these. Some telephone networks exist to help people who require such advice, the Samaritans being perhaps one of the best-known examples of telephone counselling services organized on a national and even international basis by volunteers.

A similar network for children has been developed in the form of Childline which provides a telephone counselling service for those who are being physically, emotionally or sexually abused. Support groups for those who are victims of drugs, alcohol or gambling are also available across the country.

Numerous pressure groups have arisen in recent years which represent the interests of women or their families. These groups have many and varied functions and often succeed in raising government and/or public awareness on certain issues and rights. The National Childbirth Trust and the Maternity Alliance are examples of such pressure groups which increasingly work in partnership or co-operation with the midwife for the benefit of the woman and her family. Some support groups also function as pressure groups and numerous such organizations promote research into the causes, prophylaxis and treatment of serious or fatal diseases. The Cystic Fibrosis Trust and the British Heart Foundation serve as examples here.

It is important for the midwife to know of the voluntary organizations which provide services for families in her area so that she can inform parents of these groups when appropriate. The Yellow Pages of the local telephone directory is a useful source of addresses and contact numbers for such organizations. The Citizens' Advice Bureau is another source of useful information and advisers are able to provide information of both local and national organizations.

References

Arnstein, S. (1969) A ladder of public participation. *J. Am. Inst. Planners.* Cited in Wates, N. & Nevitt, C. (1987) *Community Architecture.* London: Penguin Books.

Ashton, J. (1983) Risk assessment. *Br. Med. J.* **286**: 1843.

Ashton, J. & Seymour, H. (1988) *The New Public Health.* Milton Keynes: Open University Press.

Begg, N.T. & Noah, N.D. (1985) Immunisation targets in Europe and Britain. *Br. Med. J.* **291**: 1370.

Boucaud, P. (1989) *The Council of Europe and Child Welfare: The Need for a European Convention on Children's Rights.* Human Rights Files No. 10. Counseil de l'Europe. Statutory Council of Europe Publications & Documents Division, Strasbourg.

Chadwick, J. (1994) Perinatal mortality and antenatal care. *Modern Midwife* **9(4)**: 18–20.

Clarke, E.J. (1993) The Children Act 1989: implications for midwifery. *Br. J. Midwifery* **1(1)**: 26–30.

Currell, R. (1990) The organization of midwifery care. In Alexander, J., Levy, V. & Roch, S. (eds) *Antenatal Care: A Research Based Approach.* London: Macmillan Education.

Dimond, B, (1994) *The Legal Aspects of Midwifery.* Hale: Books for Midwives Press.

Dimond, B. (1995a) Complementary therapy and the midwife. *Modern Midwife* **5(2)**: 32–34.

Dimond, B. (1995b) Complementary therapy and the mother's wishes. *Modern Midwife* **5(3)**: 34–35.

DOH (Department of Health) (1990) *The new immunization schedule and the 1990 edition of the memorandum, 'Immunization against infectious disease'* EL (90) P/78. FPCL 91/90. London: DOH.

DOH (1991) *Working Together under The Children Act – A Guide to Arrangements for Inter-Agency Co-operation for the Protection of Children from Abuse.* London: HMSO.

DOH (1992) *Child Protection: Guidance for Senior Nurses, Health Visitors & Midwives.* The Children Act 1989. London: HMSO.

DOH (1993) *Changing Childbirth.* Report of the Expert Maternity Group (Cumberlege Report). London: HMSO.

Enkin, M., Keirse, J.N.C. & Chalmers, I. (1990) *A Guide to Effective Care in Pregnancy and Childbirth.* Oxford: Oxford University Press.

Gilroy, R. & Douglas, A. (1994) Young women and homelessness. In: Gilroy, R. & Woods, R. (eds) *Housing Women*, pp. 127–151. London & New York: Routledge.

Goodwin, S. (1991) Breaking the links between social deprivation and poor child health. *Health Visitor* **64**: 375–380.

Greve, J. & Currie, E. (1990) *Homelessness in Britain.* York: Joseph Rowntree Foundation.

Hart, T.J. (1981) A new kind of doctor. *J. R. S. Med.* **74**: 871–873.

Howe, G. (1989) House of Commons Debate, 26 October 1989, Vol. 158. Col. 1071.

HVA (Health Visitors' Association) (1985) *The Health Visitor's Role in Child Health Surveillance: A Policy Statement.* London: HVA.

Kark, S.L. (1981) *The Practice of Community Orientated Primary Health Care.* New York: Appleton, Century, Crofts.

Lowe, R. (1993) *The Welfare State in Britain since 1945.* Basingstoke & London: Macmillan.

McKeown, T. (1976) *The Role of Medicine – Dream, Mirage or Nemesis*. London: Nuffield Provincial Hospitals Trust.

Morris, J.N. (1975) *Uses of Epidemiology*. Edinburgh: Churchill Livingstone.

Morris, J.N. (1980) Are health services important to the people's health? *Br. Med. J.* **280**: 167–168.

NSPCC (1995) Promotional literature. National Society for the Prevention of Cruelty to Children, London.

OPCS (1993) *Census for 1991*. London: Office of Population & Census Statistics. Crown copyright.

Royston, E. & Armstrong, S. (1989) *Preventing Maternal Deaths*. Geneva: World Health Organization.

Ryle, J.A. (1948) *Changing Disciplines*. Oxford: Oxford University Press.

Sigerist, H. (1941) *Medicine and Human Welfare*. Oxford: Oxford University Press.

Smith, A. & Jacobson, B. (eds) (1988) *The Nation's Health: A Strategy for the 1990s*. A report from an independent multidisciplinary committee chaired by Professor Alwyn Smith. King Edward's Hospital Fund for London. King's Fund Publication Office.

Strasbourg (1985) *Child Health Surveillance Council of Europe*, Strasbourg.

Townsend, P. & Davidson, N. (1982) *Inequalities in Health* (Black report). Harmondsworth: Penguin.

UKCC (UK Central Council for Nursing, Midwifery & Health Visiting) (1993) *Midwives' Rules*. London: UKCC.

UKCC (1994) *Register. Complementary therapies: The UKCC's Principles on the Use of Complementary Therapies*. No. 15. London: UKCC.

USDHHS (US Department of Health & Human Services) (1980) *Promoting Health, Preventing Disease, Objectives for the Nation*. Washington DC: Public Health Service.

White, R., Carr, P. & Lowe, N. (1990) *A Guide to the Children Act 1989*. London: Butterworths.

WHO (World Health Organization) (1978) *Alma-Ata 1978: Primary Health Care*. Report on the international conference, Alma Ata, USSR, 6–12 September 1978. Geneva: WHO.

WHO (1985) *Targets for Health for All*. European Health for All Series, No. 1. Copenhagen: WHO Regional Office for Europe.

WHO (1991) *Essential Elements of Obstetric Care at First Referral Level*. Geneva: WHO.

Williams, S. & Allen, I. (1989) *Health Care for Single Homeless People*. London: Policy Studies Institute, Pinter Publishers.

Further Reading

Allen, N. (1990) *Making Sense of the Children Act 1989*. London: Longman Group.

Ashton, J. & Seymour, H. (1988) *The New Public Health*. Milton Keynes: Open University Press.

Boucaud, P. (1989) *The Council of Europe and Child Welfare: The Need for a European Convention on Children's Rights*. Human Rights Files No. 10. Conseil de l'Europe. Statutory Council of Europe Publications & Documents Division, Strasbourg.

Cullen, D. (1992) *Child Care Law: A Summary of the Law of England and Wales*, 3rd edn. London: British Agencies for Adoption & Fostering.

Smith, A. & Jacobson, B. (eds) (1988) *The Nation's Health: A Strategy for the 1990s*. A report from an independent multidisciplinary committee chaired by Professor Alwyn Smith. King Edward's Hospital Fund for London. King's Fund Publication Office.

The Children's Society (1995) *The Game's Up: Redesigning Child Prostitution*. London: The Children's Society.

WHO (World Health Organization) (1978) *Alma-Ata 1978: Primary Health Care*. Report on the international conference, Alma Ata, USSR, 6–12 September 1978. Geneva: WHO.

WHO (1991) *Health for All Targets. The Health Policy for Europe*. Target 7: Health of children and young people, pp. 36–40. Copenhagen: WHO Regional Office for Europe.

Useful Addresses

Child Support Agency (CSA)
DSS, PO Box 55, Brierley Hill, West Midlands DY5 1YL
Enquiry line. 0345 133433

Citizens Advice Bureau
(See local telephone directory/Yellow Pages)

CRY-SIS
B.M. Cry-sis, London WC1N 3XX
Tel. 0171 404 5011

Family Welfare Association
501–505, Kingsland Road, Dalston, London E8 4AU
Tel. 0171 254 6251

Gingerbread
35 Wellington Street, London WC2E 7BN
Tel. 0171 240 0953

National Childbirth Trust (NCT)
Alexandra House, Oldham Terrace, Acton, London W3 6NH
Tel. 0181 922 6762

National Children's Home
85 Highbury Park, London N5 1UD
Tel. 0171 226 2033

National Council for One Parent Families
255 Kentish Town Road, London NW5 2LX
Tel. 0171 267 1361

National Society for the Prevention of Cruelty to Children (NSPCC)
42 Curtain Road, London EC2A 3NH
Tel. 0171 825 2670

Parentline
Rayfa House, 57 Hart Road, Thundersley, Essex SS7 3PD
Tel. 01268 757077

Scottish Council for Single Parents
13 Gayfield Square, Edinburgh EH1 3NX
Tel. 0131 556 3899

81

Social Security and Benefits

Social System and Statutory Framework

The Department of Social Security (DSS) is directly responsible for the system of social security throughout the United Kingdom. The Benefits Agency was established in April 1991 as a wing of the DSS and is responsible for administering the national benefits system. In 1995 the Benefits Agency employed 63 000 people who process about 12 million claims and a billion benefit payments each year. These benefits amount to £70 billion annually and account for about 35% of public expenditure (BA/MG 1, 1995).

The Social Security Act 1986 constituted a major revision of social security in the United Kingdom. Subsequent modifications to legislation have given rise to further changes in rights and benefits. A recent Act of Parliament affecting maternity and other benefits is the Social Security Contributions and Benefits Act 1992. The other relevant legislation is as follows:

▶ Social Security Contributions & Benefits Act 1992 (Chapter 4)
▶ The Statutory Maternity Pay (General) Regulations 1986
▶ The Social Security (Maternity Allowance) Regulations 1987
▶ The Social Security (Claims & Payments) Regulations 1987
▶ Affiliation Proceedings Act 1957
▶ Congenital Disabilities (Civil Liability) Act 1976
▶ Employers Liability (Compulsory Insurance) Act 1969
▶ Employment Protection (Consolidation) Act 1978
▶ Employment Act 1990
▶ Health & Safety at Work Act 1984
▶ Health & Safety at Work Regulations 1992
▶ Trade Union & Labour Relations (Consolidation) Act 1992
▶ European Pregnant Workers Directive 1992
▶ Trade Union Reform & Employment Rights Act 1993
▶ Vaccine Damage Payments Act 1979.

Table 1   Leaflets and other benefit information of interest to the midwife

Leaflet		Information and benefit
I *Child and maternity*		
CH	1	Child Benefit
NI	17 A	A Guide to Maternity Benefits*
FC	47	Advisor Briefing (Family Credit)
NI	261	A Guide to Family Credit*
FC	1	Family Credit (claim pack)
NI	14	Guardian's Allowance
FB	8	Babies and Benefits
PL	958	Maternity Rights
CH	11	One Parent Benefit
CSA	2001	For parents who live apart
SF	100	Social Fund Maternity Payments
II *No income and low income*		
FB	9	Unemployed?
NI	12	Unemployment Benefit
IS	1	Income Support
IS	26	Income Support if you are 16–17
IS	20	A Guide to Income Support*
SB	16	A Guide to the Social Fund*
F2	022	Assisted Prison Visits
CTB	1	Help with Council Tax
RR	1	Housing Benefit – help with your rent from the local council
RR	2	A Guide to Housing Benefit & Council Tax Benefit*
AB	11	Help with NHS costs
SF	300	Budgeting Loans
CWP	1	Cold Weather Payments
III *Sickness and disability*		
NI	224	Statutory Sick Pay – check your rights
HB	3	Payment for people severely disabled by a vaccine
IB	202	Incapacity Benefit
DS	704	Disability Living Allowance
HB	5	A Guide to non-contributory benefits for disabled people*
DS	703	Disability Working Allowance
HB	4	A Guide to Disability Working Allowance*
NI	252	Severe Disablement Allowance
SDA	1	Severe Disablement Allowance (claim pack)
IV *Death and widowhood*		
D	49	What to do after a death
NP	45	A Guide to Widows' Benefits*
S	200	Funeral payments

* Indicates detailed guide.

Information is available from local social security offices, post offices or Benefits Agency.

The midwife is advised to frequently update her knowledge on this topic by seeking advice from a local Benefits Agency. Leaflets and booklets provide helpful information and the midwife may receive regular mailings of literature by requesting that her name be entered on the Benefits Agency Publicity Register (Tel. 01645 540 000).

Benefits may be classified into three main categories namely, those which are:

1   available as of right;
2   income related and are means tested;
3   employment related and dependent on payment of National Insurance contributions.

Information about leaflets and claim forms relating to the various social security benefits which may be of interest to the midwife are summarized in Table 1.

Benefits Available as of Right

Non-monetary benefits

Maternity care   This is one of the major benefits available free of charge to every woman in the United Kingdom entitled to treatment under the National Health Service. It includes antenatal, intrapartum and postnatal care for the mother and care for the baby. The provision of the services of a midwife are mandatory (see Chapter 84). Access to other members of the primary health care team aims to meet the varied health and social needs of women and their families. Referral to specialist care is also available without payment where the need exists. Details of the care available under the National Health Service are explained in Chapter 79.

Free prescriptions   National Health Service prescriptions are free for pregnant women and mothers who have a child less than 12 months old. The doctor or midwife gives the woman Form FW8 which is sent to the Health Authority (or Health Board in Scotland) and the woman then receives an exemption certificate.

Free dental treatment   Dental treatment is free of charge for pregnant women and those who have had a baby within the last 12 months. The woman notifies her dentist of the pregnancy.

Monetary benefits (see Table 1, section I)

Child Benefit   This is a weekly tax-free cash benefit which is paid for all children under the age of 16 years and under the age of 19 years if still receiving full-time education. A claim form can be obtained from a local social security office and, once completed, is returned there together with the child's original birth or adoption certificate; a copy is not acceptable. The payment is usually made by credit transfer directly into a bank or building society account. This is recommended because of the security it offers to clients and because it costs less to administer. The benefit is normally paid every four weeks in arrears, however, special arrangements can be made to receive the payment weekly with a post office order book. Child benefit is currently paid at a rate of £10.20 for the eldest child and £8.25 for other children.

Income-related Benefits

Income-related benefits are listed as follows under the Social Security Contributions and Benefits Act of 1992:

(a)   income support;
(b)   family credit;
(c)   disability working allowance;
(d)   housing benefit; and
(e)   community charge benefits.

(DSS, 1992)

A means test is used to establish whether persons are eligible for these benefits. Those who receive income support may also be entitled to certain other benefits.

Income support   Income support provides a weekly income for claimants who are normally over 18 years of age or, in prescribed circumstances for a prescribed period, it may be available to those over 16 years of age. The benefit provides financial assistance for those who are not in full-time employment and whose income falls below a certain level. The claimant must be available for work and taking reasonable steps to find a job, but pregnant women and lone parents are amongst those exempt from this requirement. The amount received will depend on several factors including age, whether the person has a partner, the number and age of dependent children, whether anyone in the family has a disability, and whether anyone in the family has a weekly income and savings. Payment is made up of personal allowance, premiums and housing

costs. Help with mortgage interest payments may be included in certain circumstances. A claim for income support should be made on the prescribed leaflet, a separate leaflet being used by 16–17 year olds. Further information is available in a detailed guide on income support available from a social security office or post office (see Table 1).

Family credit   This is paid to people who are working at least 16 hours a week for a low or moderate wage and who have at least one child under 16 years or under 19 years of age if in full-time education. The amount paid depends on the family's income and the number and age of the children. The personal message on the second page of the child benefit book will help parents decide whether they are entitled to family credit. A detailed guide and special claim packs are available from a social security office or post office. Further information supplied in a separate leaflet on 'Advisor Briefing' may also be of assistance to the midwife in advising families concerning these issues (see Tables 1 and 2).

Table 2   Specialized help and information

For those who have sensory disabilities
Social Security information is available in:
– large print
– Braille
– audiotape
– videotape
– teletext (dial freephone: 0800 24 33 55)

(Details available in DSS leaflet CAT 1)

* *For those whose mother tongue is not English*

Leaflets on Social Security and Council Tax Benefits are available in the following languages:

Arabic	Gujarati	Turkish
Bengali	Hindi	Urdu†
Chinese†	Punjabi†	Vietnamese
Greek	Somali	Welsh†

† Free telephone helplines are also available in these languages

For professional advisers

Persons may request that their name be added to:

The Benefits Agency Publicity Register (Tel. 01645 540 000)

Members receive the full catalogue of Social Security information materials, leaflets, posters & other mailings relevant to their area of interest.

Disability working allowance   This benefit is for people who are able to work at least 16 hours a week but have an illness or disability which puts them at a disadvantage in getting a job. A claimant must be aged at least 16 years and have a qualifying benefit. The amount payable depends on the personal situation including whether the person has a partner, the age and number of children living with them, their weekly income and savings; their capital must not exceed £16 000.

Housing benefit   The local authority may provide financial assistance in paying rent to those receiving income support or who are assessed by a means test as being on a sufficiently low income to warrant this.

Community charge benefit   A person may be entitled to benefit in respect of community charges in certain circumstances. Regulations prescribe the manner in which the appropriate maximum benefit is determined in any case.

Other benefits for those on low income (see Table 1, section II)

The midwife will need to enquire periodically about changes in the benefit system, but the following serve to illustrate other benefits to which the woman may be entitled if she has a low income or is in receipt of income support.

Free milk and vitamins   Tokens are issued to enable the woman to obtain seven pints of milk a week during pregnancy and after the baby is born until the child reaches the age of 5 years. In the first year of the baby's life, if not being breastfed these tokens may be exchanged for 500 g of powdered baby milk each week at a clinic or health centre.

Vitamins are issued free of charge to the mother during pregnancy, whilst the baby is being breastfed and for the child until the age of 5 years is reached.

Optical services   Vouchers are issued to those receiving income support or family credit to enable them to have free eye tests and to help towards the cost of spectacles or contact lenses if indicated.

Repayment of travel costs   Travel costs to and from hospital for the purpose of receiving NHS treatment can be claimed.

One-parent benefit   Parents bringing up children on their own may be entitled to this benefit on top of child benefit. It is payable for the eldest child only and is currently paid at a rate of £6.30 a week. It is tax free.

The Social Fund   This fund provides a more flexible means of responding to needs which cannot immediately be met from regular weekly benefit. There is a fixed allocation of funding to each Benefits office and applicants are means tested to assess whether they are eligible for the following benefits:

Maternity payment   This is a lump sum of up to £100 available to people getting income support, family credit or disability working allowance and with savings under £500. It is intended to assist with essential purchases for the expected baby.

Cold weather payment   This is a payment made to families with special needs, for example if a person and their partner are receiving income support, including some disability premiums, or if the family includes a child under 5 years, a cold weather payment of £8.50 may be made automatically to these families during a declared period of cold weather where the temperature is 0°C or below. This is intended to help to reduce the risk of hypothermia which is a particular risk to the newborn. The payment is also available to the elderly.

Funeral payment   In the case of a stillbirth or neonatal death, the parents may be entitled to a funeral payment if they are receiving income support, family credit, disability working allowance, housing benefit or council tax benefit. This is intended to provide some help with the costs of burial or cremation.

Community care grant   This is a grant to help particular groups, for example, the disabled, to lead independent lives in the community. They must be eligible for income support in order to be eligible for a community care grant.

Loans

There are two types of payment which may be made, but must be repaid as an interest-free loan. Requests and applications should be made at a social security office.

Budgeting loan   These are intended to help people spread the cost of items which are difficult to budget for, e.g. cooker, bed, over a longer period. Those wishing to apply for a budgeting loan must have been on income support for at least 26 weeks.

Crisis loan   These are intended to help people who cannot meet their immediate short-term expenses in an emergency or following a disaster when there is serious risk to the family. The loan may be needed to meet essential expenses in the home or incurred in travelling.

Employment-related Benefits

Non-monetary benefits

Maternity leave   Under European Commission regulations all women whose babies were due after 16 October 1994 became eligible for 14 weeks maternity leave which can be taken before or after the birth of the baby. During this period of leave, the woman does not lose entitlement to pension and other rights including holiday entitlement. All continuous service rights and benefits are maintained. The woman is entitled to return to work after taking maternity leave, but must give her employer written notice of this if so requested. She should do this not sooner than 21 days before the maternity leave is due to end.

Maternity absence   This is an additional right which may be claimed by a woman who has been employed for two years full time or for five years part time by the 11th week before the expected date of confinement. The woman is allowed to take a longer period of maternity leave extending up to 28 weeks after the birth of the baby.

Leave to attend clinics   Regardless of her employment status and length of service, every woman is entitled to time off without loss of earnings in order to attend clinics for the purpose of receiving antenatal care. The employer may require written evidence of the clinic appointment having been made as well as the maternity certificate (MAT B1) verifying the pregnancy.

Relevant legislation   Relevant legislation on employment rights during pregnancy includes:

▶ The Employment Protection (Consolidation) Act 1978
▶ The Trade Union Reform and Employee Rights Act 1993 (this resulted from the European Pregnant Workers Directive 1992).

Under current legislation a woman has the right not to be dismissed or suspended from employment due to her pregnancy. Where health and safety regulations indicate, she also has the right to be offered alternative suitable employment where necessary during pregnancy, if she has recently given birth or if she is breastfeeding.

Monetary benefits

Statutory maternity pay   Women who work may be entitled to statutory maternity pay (SMP); the amount and type of benefit will depend on how long the woman has been working with her present employer. In order to qualify for statutory maternity pay the woman must fulfil the following requirements:

▶ She must have been employed continuously for 26 weeks up to the qualifying week (i.e. the 15th week before the baby is born).
▶ Earnings in the eight weeks before the qualifying week must, on average, be at least £57 per week. This is the lower earnings limit for the payment of National Insurance contributions.
▶ She must have given her employer advance notice of her intention to take maternity leave at least 21 days before her absence. This should be in writing if the employer so requests. The woman should supply a maternity certificate (MAT B1) signed by a doctor or midwife.
▶ She must have become pregnant and reached (or delivered the baby before reaching) the commencement of the 11th week before the estimated date of confinement (i.e. 29th week of pregnancy).

Statutory maternity pay is paid by the employer for a maximum of 18 weeks and is paid weekly. The amount may be paid at the higher or lower rate. The higher rate constitutes 90% of the woman's average earnings for six weeks (subject to a minimum of £52.50), then £52.50 for 12 weeks.

Statutory maternity pay will be paid regardless of whether the woman intends returning to work. The time when the woman is receiving this payment is known as the *maternity pay period* which can start any time after the 11th week before the expected date of confinement, i.e. the 29th week of pregnancy. It is not now necessary for the woman to stop work prior to the sixth week before the expected confinement in order to qualify for statutory maternity pay. If the baby is stillborn after the start of the 16th week before the expected date of confinement (the 25th week of pregnancy) the woman will be entitled to statutory maternity pay, but not if the stillbirth occurs earlier than this. The baby being born later than the expected date does not affect the payment.

Maternity allowance Women who are not able to claim statutory maternity pay may be able to claim maternity allowance (MA) if, for example, they are self-employed or have recently changed or left their job. The following criteria will help a woman to decide if she may be entitled to maternity allowance:

▶ She is not entitled to statutory maternity pay because she has not been working for long enough or has been earning less than £57 per week.
▶ She has paid National Insurance (NI) contributions for at least 26 out of the 66 weeks preceding the week in which her baby is due. This could either be as an employee or as a self-employed person.
▶ She will not be working during the time she is claiming maternity allowance.

Maternity allowance will be paid weekly for up to 18 weeks at the lower rate of £44.55 to non-employed or self-employed women or at the higher rate of £52.50 to employed women.

In order to claim maternity allowance, the maternity certificate (MAT B1) signed by a doctor or midwife should be submitted along with the claim form MA 1 which is available from a social security office.

Disability and sickness benefits

(See Table 1, section III)
There are a number of payments which may be available if a woman is sick or disabled. These include:

Statutory sick pay (SSP) This may be claimed by employed persons. The woman may not, however, claim both statutory maternity pay and statutory sick pay. She may be entitled to the latter if she is ill during the pregnancy but will not be entitled to statutory sick pay if she becomes sick whilst receiving statutory maternity pay.

Incapacity benefit This may be paid to people who are incapable of work and are employed and cannot get statutory sick pay from their employer. The benefit may be claimed by people who are self-employed or unemployed providing they have paid enough National Insurance contributions.

The effect of statutory maternity pay on other benefits

Other benefits may be affected on the receipt of statutory maternity pay. Details are provided on request from social security offices.

Special Needs

Benefits which may be claimed for a child with special needs

A child may have special needs because of physical or mental disability or because of circumstances which threaten the financial security of the parent or guardian.

Child maintenance The Department of Social Security Child Support Agency was set up in 1993 to assess, collect, review and enforce the maintenance of children in various circumstances. Taking into account the income and basic expenditure of both parents, a formula is used to calculate how much maintenance should be paid to support a child.

Spousal maintenance A person may be entitled to spousal maintenance from an absent husband or wife.

Disability living allowance This is intended for people who need help with personal care or getting around. A disabled mother or child may be eligible and there are special rules which may be applied to enable the terminally ill to obtain the benefit quickly. The rates paid will depend on the person's care and mobility requirements and are paid separately in these two categories. Both care and mobility needs are classified in order to qualify the claimant at a higher, middle or lower rate. Weekly rates vary between £46.70 and £12.40.

Vaccine damage People who have become severely disabled as a result of specified vaccinations may be eligible for a tax-free lump sum payment of £30 000. Further information may be obtained from: Vaccine Damage Payments Unit, Fylde Benefits Directorate, DSS Benefits Agency, Norcross, Blackpool FY5 3TA. Claims should be made to the Directorate.

Widows' benefits

(See Table 1, section IV)

Widowhood for the pregnant or newly delivered woman is inevitably a tragedy and one which, fortunately, the midwife does not deal with frequently. Nevertheless, as well as the counselling and emotional support which a woman in such circumstances will need, there are practical issues which have to be addressed. Various social security benefits may be available. These include: widow's payment, widow's pension and widowed mother's allowance. Certain conditions as well as National Insurance contributions must be satisfied when claiming widow's benefits. The widow's payment is tax free and is a lump sum of £1000, whereas a widowed mother's allowance is paid to the mother of at least one child qualifying for child benefit at a basic rate of up to £58.85 a week with additions for each child who is eligible for child benefit. This allowance is also paid if the widow is expecting a child by her late husband or as a result of artificial insemination or *in vitro* fertilization.

Other Services

Other services provided by the Department of Social Security Benefits Agency include the following:

Special communication services Interpreters and signers as well as special telecommunication facilities and literature are available. These exist to assist families with special needs, whether they require translation because they are not English speaking or signing because of hearing impairment. Telephone helplines providing specialized assistance for people who have sensory disabilities and for those whose mother tongue is not English are summarized in Table 2.

Customer service managers These people have the responsibility in each locality of liaising with community organizations. In order to assist people to understand the benefits to which they may be entitled they may arrange for displays in areas easily accessible to the community, for example, in shopping or community centres. They will also speak to professional groups such as midwives to assist them in their advisory role in this area. Complaints about the services which are provided can also be made to customer service managers of the Benefits Agency.

Home visits Social security officers will arrange to visit clients in their own homes when this is the only satisfactory way of dealing with their needs.

Helplines Expansion of telecommunications across the country has enabled the public to access information by telephone with ease. There are some freephone numbers and some local rate telephone numbers. A list of telephone helplines which may be of assistance to the midwife and her clients is provided at the end of this chapter.

Accessing Benefits and Meeting Individual and Family Needs

This chapter has attempted to introduce the midwife to the benefits to which families in her care may be entitled. It must be appreciated that broad generalizations sometimes have to be made in this context and that the situations which the midwife meets in practice are likely to be very variable. For this reason the reader is invited to consider the situations presented below and decide on the social security benefits and other sources of help which may be available to such individuals or families. Ten social situations are presented below (Examples 1–10). Suggested assistance is then outlined for each of the examples given. In order to consider the total social situation before completing these exercises, it may be helpful for the reader to refer also to other chapters in this book, for example Chapter 80 on Community health care and social services, Chapter 82 on Sociology, Chapter 78 on Grief and bereavement, Chapter 85 on The law and the midwife and Chapter 84 on The statutory framework and control of the practice of midwives in the UK.

Social Situations

Example 1

Anna is 17 years old and 32 weeks pregnant. Six months ago she moved out of local council care and into bed and breakfast accommodation. Now she is moving into a flat where she wants to set up home independently. This is her first baby. Anna is unemployed and single. What benefits and other assistance may be available to Anna?

Example 2

Beverly is 25 years old and has just given birth to her second child. Her husband was a soldier and was killed during active service with the British army three weeks ago. Her army accommodation will now no longer be available to her and she has no other close relatives. What benefits and other assistance may be available to Beverly?

Example 3

Ching Chee moved to the UK from Hong Kong a year ago to join her husband who has worked here in a restaurant for the past two years. They have two children aged 5 and 3 years. Ching Chee is now 20 weeks pregnant and speaks no English. What benefits and other assistance may be available to Ching Chee?

Example 4

Debbie is a 28-year-old teacher. She has one child aged 3 years who attends nursery school and she is now 33 weeks pregnant. Her husband, Dave, is unemployed and so Debbie is the family 'breadwinner'. You diagnose that Debbie has pregnancy-induced hypertension and you advise her to rest. She is anxious about the mortgage repayments. A recent robbery deprived the family of some valuables including their Visa cards resulting in thefts from their bank accounts. What benefits and other assistance may be available to Debbie and Dave?

Example 5

Elizabeth is a 24-year-old mother of three and is 34 weeks pregnant. She works in a canteen and there is currently an industrial dispute. She is worried that strike action will affect the statutory maternity pay to which she is entitled. What benefits and other assistance may be available to Elizabeth?

Example 6

Fiona is 14 years old and lives with her parents. She concealed her pregnancy until she delivered a stillborn baby. The family want to arrange a funeral for the baby, but the parents are unemployed and live in temporary accommodation. What benefits and other assistance may be available to Fiona and her parents?

Example 7

Gwyneth has just given birth to twins. She has a child, Gareth, aged 4 years suffering with spina bifida. She tells you that she cannot afford a washing machine and she is worried about how she will cope. Her husband is in prison more than 100 miles away and she wants to be able to take the babies for him to see them. Her first language is Welsh and she tells you that she has difficulty filling in forms in English. What benefits and other assistance may be available to Gwyneth?

Example 8

Hope lives in a caravan on the outskirts of the town. She belongs to an itinerant community. She has delivered a baby weighing 2.5 kg at home. It is January, the roads are icy and the ambient temperature has been below zero for the past week. What benefits and other assistance may be available to Hope?

Example 9

Jacky is 16 years old and lives on the streets. She arrived at the maternity unit in labour and delivered a healthy baby boy. She says that she wants the baby fostered until she can find a place to live and a way to support herself and the baby. She confides in you that she ran away from home because she had been sexually abused and that this pregnancy was the result of rape. What benefits and other assistance may be available to Jacky?

Example 10

Kate is 18 years old and has given birth to a baby suffering with Down's syndrome. It is her first baby and her husband has recently filed for a divorce because he has returned to live with a previous partner. Kate's 14-year-old sister Karen lives with her and recently told her that she is pregnant. What benefits and other assistance may be available to Kate and Karen?

SUGGESTED ASSISTANCE

Example 1

Benefits

Anna would be entitled to income support and housing and council tax benefits. She would receive child benefit when her baby is born and this would be supplemented with the one parent benefit. Provision from the Social Fund would allow Anna to claim a lump sum maternity payment. She may also be assisted to settle into her flat by claiming the community care grant or she may wish to take advantage of a budgeting loan.

Other assistance available

Anna may wish to seek help from such organizations as Gingerbread or the National Council for One Parent Families. The welfare rights officer based at the local social security office would be able to advise Anna about the help available to her or Anna may have a personal social worker who will continue to monitor her well-being since she moved out of council care.
(Source: BA/FB 8, 1994; BA/MG 1, 1995)

Example 2

Benefits

Beverly would be entitled to a war widow's pension with an increase for her dependent children, but a state widow's pension will not be paid at the same time. Child benefit will be paid for both the children. Providing that she does not have more than £16 000 in savings, Beverly would be entitled to housing benefit if she finds

---

rented accommodation or to a council tax benefit if she finds accommodation which requires her to pay this herself.

Other assistance available

Beverly may wish to receive bereavement counselling from a voluntary organization such as Cruse. As a lone parent, Beverly may find it helpful to seek assistance from such organizations as Gingerbread or the National Council for One Parent Families. The army may be able to offer their own welfare assistance to help the family resettle.
(Source: BA/FB 27, 1994; BA/MG 1, 1995)

Example 3

Benefits

Ching Chee would be entitled to child benefit for the two children and for the baby after the birth. She may be entitled to family credit. The latter will depend on an assessment of their situation, including whether she or her husband are regarded as being normally resident in Great Britain (England, Scotland or Wales) and whether her husband is engaged in remunerative work which averages at least 16 hours a week.

Other assistance available

A free telephone helpline in Chinese would be helpful to Ching Chee and her husband in obtaining information. They may utilize this by dialling 0800 25 24 51. The social security office will also arrange for the help of an interpreter.
(Source: BA/FB 27, 1994; BA/NI 261, 1995; BA/MG 1, 1995)

Example 4

Benefits

Debbie would be entitled to statutory sick pay when she submits a medical certificate followed by statutory maternity pay. These benefits are available providing she has paid the necessary National Insurance contributions. Dave may be entitled to unemployment benefit providing that he is capable of and actively seeking work and has paid enough standard rate Class 1 National

Insurance contributions at the right time to make him eligible now. Depending on their precise circumstances they may be able to claim income support. Recent amendments to the rules mean that no help will be available to assist with mortgage interest for at least eight weeks and possibly 39 weeks. A crisis loan may help them through the period of difficulty inflicted on them as a result of the robbery.

Other assistance available

Because Debbie is advised to rest she will need some help in the home. If her family cannot provide the necessary support she may need to call on the Home Help Service though availability of a home help or a home aide will vary according to the district in which Debbie lives. A social worker could advise and help initiate this assistance if required. If the 3-year-old child does not attend nursery school full time, it may be possible to increase this or to consider child-minding services for some of the time to ease the responsibility on the family.
(Source: BA/FB 27, 1994; BA/NI 17A, 1994; BA/MG 1, 1995)

Example 5

Benefits

Elizabeth's statutory maternity pay will be affected by the weeks she is away from work on industrial dispute unless she can show that she had no direct interest in the dispute. She should consult leaflet NI 17A and discuss the matter with the welfare rights officer at her local social security office. Elizabeth will receive child benefit for her three children and for the fourth on application after birth.
(Source: BA/FB 8, 1994; BA/FB 27, 1994)

Example 6

Benefits

Fiona would not be entitled to any benefits in her own right, but her parents will be receiving child benefit for her. If they get income support the parents will be able to claim housing benefit or council tax benefit, depending on their type of accommodation. They can also apply to the

Social Fund for a funeral payment on form SF 200 and the leaflet D 49 'What to do after a death' may be helpful to them. These are available from a local social security office.

Other assistance available

The hospital chaplain or other clergyman known to the family will provide help in conducting a funeral and may also provide or advise on bereavement counselling. The undertaker will otherwise contact a Christian clergyman or person in a leadership position from another religious group, depending on the wishes of the family. Fiona, and possibly her parents too, will need someone who can help them come to terms with the loss of the baby; the organization Cruse may be helpful here. The general practitioner will be able to refer Fiona for professional counselling if she wishes as she may have issues which she needs to discuss in confidence following the traumatic experience of a concealed pregnancy which ended with a bereavement.
(Source: BA/SB 16, 1994; BA/FB 27, 1994; BA/MG 1, 1995)

Example 7

Benefits

Gwyneth will be entitled to child benefit for each of her children, additionally, she can claim the 'care component' of the disability living allowance for Gareth. Gwyneth will be able to obtain income support and because of Gareth's needs she could claim for the purchase of a washing machine from the Social Fund. The Assisted Prison Visits Unit of the Department of Social Security will consider help towards the cost of prison visits. Leaflet F2 022 available from social security offices explains the help available to the relatives of prisoners.

Other assistance available

Gwyneth can use the free telephone helpline in Welsh by ringing 0800 289011. Many social security information leaflets and claim forms are bilingual and available from social security offices, benefits agencies or post offices in Wales. there is also help available to her in completing the necessary forms.

The specialist paediatric services and those of a health visitor would be made available to monitor Gareth's progress and advise on his care. Voluntary organizations which may be able to offer support include local branches of the Association of Spina Bifida & Hydrocephalus (ASBAH). Also contact with Twins Clubs or the Twins and Multiple Births Association (TAMBA) may be helpful. Special day-care centres or nurseries could help with Gareth's day-to-day care and education and she may need respite care for him at times.

Voluntary organizations which provide support for prisoners' families may also be able to provide some assistance. Advice could best be obtained through a social worker who would consider the total needs of this family.
(Source: BA/SB 16, 1994; BA/FB 27, 1994; BA/MG 1, 1995)

Example 8

Benefits

Hope should be entitled to income support and a maternity payment from the Social Fund. She will receive child benefit for the baby which may be supplemented by the one parent benefit for her first child if she is a lone parent. Due to the severe weather conditions Hope will be entitled to a cold weather payment of £8.50 which may be paid automatically during this declared period of cold weather. More information on this payment is available on leaflet CWP:1: 'Extra help with heating costs when its very cold'.

Further reading in this context which may be of interest to the midwife: Maternity Alliance (1991) Information pack: *Safe Childbirth for Travellers*.
(Source: BA/SB 16, 1994; BA/FB 27, 1994; Maternity Alliance, 1991)

Example 9

Benefits

Jacky could claim income support utilizing the special rules for 16–17 year olds who are unable to live at home for safety reasons. Details are provided on leaflet IS 26: 'Income support if you are 16–17' available from social security offices or post offices. The foster parents will receive a special payment and child benefit whilst they are caring for Jacky's baby.

Other assistance available

Jacky will have numerous needs both physical and emotional. Foster parents will be found by a social worker to care for the baby until Jacky is able to make provision for herself and her baby. As a single homeless mother, Jacky would rate as a priority in acquiring some form of accommodation and the social worker will help her in this. Jacky is likely to benefit from skilled counselling following her experiences of sexual abuse and rape. A general practitioner with whom Jacky should register may refer her to a counsellor in the practice or she may prefer to seek help from a specialist organization or support group for example: Victim Support schemes, Women's Aid, the Samaritans, the National Society for the Prevention of Cruelty to Children (NSPCC).
(Source: BA/MG 1, 1995; BA/FB 27, 1994; HMSO, 1985)

Example 10

Benefits

Kate would be entitled to income support, child benefit and one parent benefit. She would also be able to claim the 'care component' of the disability living allowance for her baby. Depending on the circumstances, she may be able to claim guardian's allowance for Karen who may also be eligible for a maternity payment from the Social Fund.

Other assistance available

Kate may be able to obtain some assistance through the Child Support Agency whereby her estranged husband would be required to pay a contribution for the upkeep of his child. She could ring the CSA Enquiry Line: 0345 133 133 about this. Kate and Karen may find it helpful to contact organizations such as Gingerbread or the National Council for One Parent Families. The welfare rights officer based at the local social

security office would be able to advise them in detail about the help available in their situation. The health visitor and social worker would provide health and social support and advice. There would be access to specialist paediatric help as required. A local support group of the Down's Syndrome Association would be able to offer Kate emotional and practical support in bringing up her baby.
(Source: BA/MG 1, 1995; BA/FB 27, 1994; BA/SB 16, 1994)

References

BA/MG 1 (1995) *A Guide to Benefits: A Concise Guide to Benefits & Pensions. MG 1 from April 1995*. Heywood, Lancs: The Benefits Agency, Department of Social Security.

BA/NI 261 (1995) *A Guide to Family Credit from April 1995*. Heywood, Lancs: The Benefits Agency, Department of Social Security.

BA/FB 8 (1994) *Babies & Benefits from August 1994*. Heywood, Lancs: The Benefits Agency, Department of Social Security.

BA/SB 16 (1994) *A Guide to the Social Fund from August 1994*. Heywood, Lancs: The Benefits Agency, Department of Social Security.

BA/NI 17A (1994) *A Guide to Maternity Benefits: Statutory Maternity Pay & Maternity Allowance from June 1994*. Heywood, Lancs: The Benefits Agency, Department of Social Security.

BA/FB 27 (1994) *Bringing Up Children? A Guide to Benefits for Families with Children from April 1994*. Heywood, Lancs: The Benefits Agency, Department of Social Security.

DSS (Department of Social Security) (1992) *Social Security Contributions & Benefits Act*, Chapter 4. London: HMSO.

HMSO (1985) *The Housing Act. Part III*. London: HMSO.

Maternity Alliance (1991) *Safe Childbirth for Travellers: An Information Pack*. London: Maternity Alliance.

Further Reading

Dimond, B. (1994) Maternity benefits. In *The Legal Aspects of Midwifery*, Chapter 11. Hale: Books for Midwives Press.

European Commission (1995) Sickness & maternity (Articles 18–25, 35, 36) and Family benefits (Articles 72–76). In *Compendium of Community Provisions on Social Security*, 4th edn, European Commission Directorate-General for Employment, Industrial Relations & Social Affairs. Social Europe DGV. Luxembourg: Office for Official Publications of the European Communities.

Lowe, R. (1993) *The Welfare State in Britain since 1945*. Basingstone & London: Macmillan.

Maternity Alliance (1991) *Safe Childbirth for Travellers: An Information Pack*. London: Maternity Alliance.

Thompson, R. & Thompson, B. (1993a) *Women at Work*. London: R. Thompson & Partners, B. Thompson B. & Partners.

Thompson, R. & Thompson, B. (1993b) *Dismissal: A Basic Introduction to your Legal Rights*. London: R. Thompson & Partners, B. Thompson B. & Partners.

Telephone Helplines

Benefit Enquiry Claim Form Completion Service 0800 44 11 44

Benefits for the disabled & their carers 0800 88 22 00
  Disability Living Allowance 0345 123 456

Child Support Agency: Child maintenance & support 0345 133 133

Child Support Agency: Leaflet request line 0345 830 830

Family Credit advice and claims 01253 500 050

Family Credit leaflet & claim form request line 0800 500 222

Health-related information 0800 66 55 44

Health literature request line 0800 555 777

Social Security (general advice) 0800 666 555

Winter warmth line 0800 28 94 04

Winter warmth line (Scotland) 0800 83 85 87
  Note: Telephone calls are charged as follows:
  Those beginning: 0800 are free
                   0345 at local rate
Others are at normal rates.

Part Sixteen

The Sociological Context of Childbirth

82

Sociology and the Social Context of Childbearing

Sociology is the study of social interaction among people in a society over a particular time span. A sociological perspective is one that looks beyond the commonsense assumptions that are made about a society and questions events as they appear at face value. Sociology provides interpretive frameworks through which various forms of social organization may be understood. This perspective involves a critical and systematic appraisal of the accepted norms, power structures, social inequalities and the differences between groups.

Historical Developments

Western sociology had its origins in the Industrial Revolution during the late eighteenth and nineteenth centuries, a time that witnessed enormous social change. Significant changes in the organization of economic production were brought about through capitalism and new social relationships were developed in relation to private ownership of the means of production. This refers not only to the means of production of material goods but also to the social relations that developed between producers (Giddens, 1993). One of these significant social changes was the move away from a population that was predominantly agrarian to one that became largely urban. New populations emerged as large conglomerations of people gathered around cities and a new male workforce developed to work in the large-scale industries.

The social commentators during this time included philosophers such as Auguste Comte and political economists such as Adam Smith and Karl Marx. The sociologists Max Weber and Emile Durkheim also considered the changing world around them and tried to make sense of it by constructing theoretical explanations of different aspects of industrial life. Durkheim was concerned about moral values and social cohesion and Weber's interests lay in the bureaucratic organization of large institutions (Giddens, 1993). Their influential ideas and theories about social action, social change and social order led to new ways of thinking about society and laid the foundations for sociology as a social science.

Subsequently, many other sociologists have commented upon, and accounted for, social action and social organization. The different ways of seeing things gave rise to a variety of theories, which provided explanations for the structures that developed and for the events that occurred. However, many sociologists shared two main concerns: *social control* and *social change*. Sociology has been informed by philosophy, social history, economics, politics, natural sciences and more recently by feminism (Mitchell and Oakley, 1986; Pascal, 1986; Ramazanoglu, 1989; Abbot and Wallace, 1990). Yet these disciplines are not discrete schools of thought. There is an overlap, as each one draws on aspects of another's theory.

As recognition of the complexity of Western societies developed, their study has been divided up into smaller parts, into categories for analysis. Such categories may include *social class* and the institutions of *marriage*, the *family* and *childbearing*. However, these categories are often presented as if they are naturally emerging rather than categories that are generated out of the perceptions of the authors. The philosopher Michel Foucault considers that these categories have no intrinsic meaning. He argues that reality does not exist independently of perception. For example, the categorization of people into groups such as social class is only significant because meaning has been ascribed to the relationship that individuals have to the labour market (Cousins and Hussain, 1984).

Since sociology has gained most of its material from Western industrial societies, it has developed in a narrow European social context and therefore cannot claim to provide any universal description of human action. Joseph *et al.* (1990) criticize the dominance of European ideas and concepts in all social science disciplines. They argue that Eurocentrism in the social sciences neglects alternative sources of knowledge and it legitimizes international systems of inequality. For example, the theory of child development, developed by Jean Piaget, is based on Western rational and scientific reasoning. It has been a universally applied theoretical yardstick for cross-cultural comparisons of 'natural' cognitive development. Joseph *et al.* (1990) argue that such a notion is Eurocentric not only because it overlooks the values and histories of non-Western societies, but also because it fails to acknowledge its own social origins.

Sociology and Midwives

For midwives, sociology is not just about observing social action and being social commentators; it is also about being part of the action itself and having an influence upon it. As the daily work of a midwife is essentially social, midwives cannot be immune to the social lives of their clients, nor can they be immune to their own social relationships that influence their practice.

Many sociological themes impinge on midwives. The themes that will be dealt with here are those that consider the social changes and the social constructs that are pertinent to midwives themselves coupled with those that are relevant to childbearing women.

In *Thinking Sociologically* Bauman (1990) is enthusiastic about sociology. As he guides readers through his book he wants 'to show how the apparently familiar aspects of life can be interpreted in a novel way and seen in a different light' (Bauman, 1990: 18).

For midwives, the relevance of sociology may be examined in the light of thinking,

> not to 'correct' your knowledge, but to expand it; not to replace an error with an unquestionable truth, but to encourage critical scrutiny of beliefs hitherto held; to promote a habit of self-analysis and of questioning the views that pretend to be certainties.
> (Bauman, 1990: 18)

Women, Midwives and Medicine

Midwives or analogous figures have existed in all societies. In the sixteenth and seventeenth centuries women as healers were seen as a threat, particularly to men (Ehrenreich and English, 1974b; Versluysen, 1980; Donnison, 1988). Men organized themselves into the profession of *medicine*, which originally formally excluded women. Medicine gained ascendancy through the legitimization of 'science'. It gradually encroached into aspects of people's lives and this was characterized in the nineteenth century by the medicalization of madness (Szasz, 1971; Showalter, 1987) and the medicalization of 'women's conditions', especially of pregnancy and childbirth (Ehrenreich and English, 1974a, b, 1979; Oakley, 1984; Towler and Brammall, 1986; Donnison, 1988). According to Gabe and Calnan (1989: 223) medicalization may be defined as 'the way in which the jurisdiction of modern medicine has expanded in recent years and now encompasses many problems that formerly were not defined as medical entities'.

By the early twentieth century the regulation and control of women, and in particular women's sexuality, had passed from Church to State to medicine (Ehrenreich and English, 1979; Bland, 1982; Turner, 1987). The control of pregnancy, childbirth and motherhood had passed from a primarily social domain to a primarily medical domain (Oakley, 1980, 1984). The locus of control in childbirth had also changed from the sphere of women to that of men (Oakley, 1976a; Stacey, 1988).

It has been argued that medical authority and control continues to encroach into many aspects of life (Zola, 1972; Illich, 1975; De Swaan, 1990). However, this is not necessarily a conscious design to accrue power, but a growth of technologies has been increasingly applied over different aspects of life and moreover, over formally social areas of life (Illich, 1975; Turner, 1987).

The expansion of medical control in pregnancy and childbirth was characterized by a view of women that separated their physical and reproductive lives from their social and emotional lives. The metaphor of the body, and specifically the uterus, as machine and the doctor as mechanic helps to explain the early development of obstetrics. Hereby, a woman's body is fragmented and reduced into component parts. It becomes an 'object'. It is seen as a machine that is not working and is in need of repair (Donnison, 1988; Arney, 1982; Rothman, 1982; Martin, 1987; Oakley, 1989).

Martin (1987) argues that although this metaphor alone does not continue to dominate medical practice, it is the underlying ideology of the discourses on technology around birth. Arguably, such themes are especially significant in the arena of 'reproductive technologies' (Arditti et al., 1984; Corea et al., 1985; Overall, 1989; Scutt, 1990). Moreover, Martin challenges the popular idea that technology develops autonomously through the process of evolution and she comments that 'Our focus on technology, its everchanging needs and demands, diverts our attention from the social relationships of power and domination

that are involved whenever humans use machines to produce goods in our society' (Martin, 1987: 57).

Ways of Looking at the World

A sociological perspective demonstrates that the world around us is not a 'given fact' but that it is socially created and given meanings. Views of biological processes are also related to specific social settings. As Stacey (1988: 1) comments,

> The ways in which a society copes with the major events of birth, illness and death are central to the beliefs and practices of that society and also bear a close relationship to its other major social, economic and cultural institutions.

Sociology examines the ways in which certain assumptions about social thought and social organization are made. For example the nature of *knowledge* itself is a social construct. Scientific knowledge cannot be regarded as a collection of objective facts. Generally created in a masculine form, it is transmitted through culture and it legitimates the status, control and authority of those in power (MacCormack and Strathern, 1981; Rueschemeyer, 1986; Turner, 1987). For example, Ehrenreich and English (1979) described how, during the early medical developments in the late nineteenth to the early twentieth century, ideas about women's health were based on the understanding that the female body and female functions, particularly menstruation, were inherently pathological.

However, it has been argued that there are different ways of seeing the world that make sense in women's lives (Rose, 1986; Hagell, 1989; Stanley, 1990). Women's own writing of their experiences of health, children, motherhood and sexuality are examples from bodies of knowledge through which women understand and explain their lives (Dowrick and Grundberg, 1980; Rossiter, 1988; Breen, 1989; Gieve, 1989; Phillips and Rakusen, 1989; McNeill et al., 1992)

In contrast, Marshall (1991) analyses the authoritative, medical and 'expert' tone of some childcare and parenting manuals. She argues that,

> there is an essentially consistent medical/psychological discourse which presents one version of the meaning of motherhood. Alternative ways of viewing motherhood or contradictory meanings of motherhood are either omitted or discounted. The

discourse ensures that women turn to the 'experts' – both medical and psychological professionals – for the definition and understanding of motherhood.
(Marshall, 1991: 83–84)

The notion of discourse introduced here is not just about the formalities of knowledge, such as statements; it also incorporates a variety of alternative and competing practices and disciplines.

Similarly, Spender (1985) explores the social construction of language, particularly in the context of women's subordination. The language of obstetrics and midwifery is equally socially constructed and value laden (Schwarz, 1990; Bastian, 1992; Leap, 1992; Hewison, 1993). Language changes as it imparts meanings, expresses attitudes and illuminates the balance of power. Leap (1992) suggests a reconsideration of such words as 'confinement', 'management', and 'allow' in the context of caring for pregnant women. Value is also imputed by phrases such as 'the advances in perinatal medicine' and 'the fashion of waterbirth'. By becoming conscious of the language, midwives can become conscious of the practice that generated it. Therefore, attempts to change words are attempts to change practice.

The assumption of the objectivity and neutrality of science has also been challenged (Rose and Rose, 1971). Many authors have argued that science can be seen as socially constructed knowledge (Burke *et al.*, 1980; Rose, 1982; Harding, 1986). The dilemmas of the scientific method have been explored by Oakley (1990) and McNabb (1989) with regard to research concerning childbearing women. McNabb (1989) questions the use of the randomized controlled trial (the epitome of the objective scientific method) to investigate activity during labour, by attempting to isolate 'parts' of labour such as ambulation and positions in labour. She argues that, 'it is a completely inappropriate research method when applied to a dynamic process such as labour'. The subtle interplay between the physical, psychological and cultural dimensions of labour does not lend itself to reductionist methods that attempt to isolate discrete 'parts' for observation, manipulation and control.

Biological events are also socially constructed and culturally controlled. Menstruation (Weideger, 1975) and childbirth are biological processes that find cultural expression in their 'rites of passage'. The experience of miscarriage is also a social phenomenon (Oakley *et al.*, 1990). Weideger (1975) and Greer (1991) describe the biological process of menopause and they critically assess the ways in which it has been socially constructed in such a way that creates negative stereotypes of older women. Furthermore, in citing a cross-cultural study of the menopause between Japanese and Canadian women, Lock (1991) emphasizes that physiological events cannot be divorced from their social meanings.

Events are described and conceptualized in different ways by a variety of people and this is often contingent on the balance of power in any one situation. This is particularly evident in situations around pregnancy and childbearing.

Graham and Oakley (1981) describe how women and doctors have a 'qualitatively different way of looking at the nature, context and management of reproduction'. They argue that this is more than a difference of opinion. This difference is indicated by the use of the concept 'frame of reference'. It is about a system of values and attitudes and the influences that other individuals have on these. In describing the ways in which women view their pregnancies, Graham and Oakley (1981) identify four dimensions of conflict that arise between them and doctors. These are: issues of the status of reproduction as health or illness; who is the expert; decision-making and communication. Roberts (1985) further raises these issues in her work describing the relationships between women and doctors. These differences arise from the different positions in a society that women and doctors occupy, whereby any knowledge women have is deemed to be of lesser value than that of men (Rowbotham, 1973; Ehrenreich and English, 1979; Rose, 1986). Similarly, in their study describing the roles and responsibilities of the midwife, Robinson *et al.* (1983) demonstrated that the doctors and midwives had different frames of reference when they made decisions about the care of pregnant women.

In the area of antenatal screening tests, particularly for Down's syndrome, Farrant (1985) highlights the differences in perspective between doctors and pregnant women. She suggests that the impetus for screening comes from the medical profession which is guided by its preoccupation with ideology and social control. Arguably, due to the influence of dominant (medical) ideas, women themselves have favoured some of these developments. But Farrant (1985) considers that their attitude towards disability is shaped by their understanding of their role as primary care-givers and their perceptions of women's responsibility towards children and adults with disability, combined with a recognition of personal hardship.

The Meanings of Birth

Childbirth is a socially significant and universal event and the different meanings that are ascribed to it vary over periods of time and between cultures. Herein, culture does not solely refer to the practices, values and attitudes of racial groups but also to cultures within and between the occupational groups of midwives and obstetricians (Arney, 1982; Kitzinger *et al.*, 1990).

Macintyre (1977: 18) argues that childbirth has always been socially controlled. She comments that 'In no society is the process of pregnancy and parturition treated as simply a physiological process, untouched by the cultural context, prescriptions, proscriptions, and customary practices.' Moreover, in reference to birth itself, Macintyre (1977: 18) continues,

> childbirth itself is surrounded by rules, customs and prescriptions. Where the birth is to take place, who is to be present, the position in which the woman labours and delivers, how she is to behave during childbirth – these matters are rarely left to the discretion of the parturient woman but are the subject of social controls and sanctions.

The culture of control around birth in Western societies in present times may be exemplified firstly through the *institutionalization* of birth. Such changes were premised on the 'increasing tendency to see pregnancy and childbirth as hazardous events in which medical assistance and intervention are often required' (Campbell and Macfarlane, 1987: 12).

In Britain, the move from birth at home to birth in an institutional setting started in the 1920s and the rates of births in institutions increased throughout the years until the present day. At present over 90% of women give birth in a hospital (Campbell and Macfarlane, 1987; Tew, 1990). However, this trend may be reversed since the publication of a government report *Changing Childbirth* (DOH, 1993). This document recommended that pregnant women should be able to exercise more choice with regard to the place of birth and that birth at home may be an appropriate choice for some women.

Secondly, birth has become industrialized through *technology*. This may be illustrated not only by the use of machinery itself but also, in some instances, by the engineering of childbirth. For example, in 'active management of labour' the activity and progress of labour is measured according to set criteria over a given time span (O'Driscoll and Meagher, 1980). It is the obstetrician or midwife who is active, in so far as they may or may not intervene in labour in order for progress to be 'normal'. The cultural milieux of such labours are in sharp contrast to the culture of 'active birth' whereby the woman herself and not her objectified uterus is the focus of labour (Balaskas, 1981).

Notwithstanding the disputed efficacy of the dominant culture of obstetrics in childbirth (Campbell and Macfarlane, 1987; Chalmers *et al.*, 1989; Tew, 1990), Macintyre (1977) cautions against romanticized notions of childbirth in pre-modern times and in non-Western cultures. She acknowledges that many women are dissatisfied with their experiences of modern practice but she considers that, 'The point is not what childbirth was once like . . . but what it *could* be like in our society now or in the future' (Macintyre, 1977: 22).

The Social Construction of Motherhood

The way in which women become mothers is culturally determined and socially controlled (Oakley, 1976b, 1981, 1985, Kitzinger, 1981; Holdsworth, 1988; Rossiter, 1988). Girls are strongly socialized to become mothers (Sharpe, 1976; Walkerdine and Lucey, 1989) and motherhood remains the proof and hallmark of adulthood, womanhood, and femininity (Oakley, 1980).

Central to the issues that surround motherhood is that of 'maternal instinct'. Macintyre (1976) challenges the assumptions that are made about the desire of women to have children as 'natural, normal and instinctive'. She considers that normal reproduction has been taken for granted and it has not been the subject of theoretical attention. Areas that have aroused interest have been those that have deviated from the 'norm' and these may currently include 'teenage pregnancy' (Murcott, 1980; Phoenix, 1991), 'older mothers' (Berryman, 1991) and reproductive technologies (Saffron, 1986; Stanworth, 1987; Overall, 1989; Stacey, 1993).

Despite the interest generated in these areas, Macintyre (1976) argues that this interest obscures the view that normal reproduction is socially constructed, particularly with regard to marital status. There has been little interest in why white, married, and middle-class women have or want to have children. This may be attributed to the notion that certain values are presented as 'normal' and they become the yardstick by which everything else is measured. These 'normative values' are rarely examined.

Social Differentiation

The use of broad categories such as race, social class and gender tends to infer homogeneity within groups. Such an oversimplification ignores the complexities of individual lives. These categories do not account for differences in life events and an individual's quality of life. For example, the experiences of pregnancy and childbirth may be very different between working-class women who live in a rural village and those who live in an inner city area.

RACE

'Race' is social construct that has more to do with social structures and power relationships than with biology (Phillips and Rathwell, 1986). The imbalance of power in society enables dominant ethnocentric ideologies to prevail and for racism to develop. It is within this context that the issues relating to racial groups are often seen in terms of individual pathology rather than as a result of inequalities in the social structure. Often the differences are seen as problematic and are conceptualized as deviant (Pearson, 1986; Phoenix, 1988; Douglas, 1992). Phoenix (1990) asserts that Asian women are socially constructed as socially inferior to white people; features perceived to be representations of their culture are negatively stereotyped as strange and exotic, and hence devalued.

Much of the work on race has concentrated on areas concerning health and on family life in general (Westwood and Bachau, 1988) and particular interest has been shown in diet, maternity care and diseases affecting certain racial groups (Rocheron, 1988; Phoenix, 1990; Torkington, 1991; Douglas, 1992). Moreover, Phoenix (1990) argues that the experiences of black and Asian women in the health service as both clients and as health workers reflects the racial discrimination that is institutionalized in British society.

Phoenix (1990) maintains that Asian women are perceived by the health services to have extraordinary needs and are thus regarded as causing a problem. She considers that some of these needs are shared by all women regardless of their cultural background. She illustrates this by considering that many women do not like hospital food and that many women find it difficult to understand what the medical staff say to them. Moreover, a lot of women dislike internal examinations, particularly by male doctors.

Similarly, in a study which investigated the provision of maternity care to women of South Asian descent, Bowler (1993) describes how midwives used stereotypes of women to make judgements about them and in order to provide care. She identified four main themes in the stereotype: communication; failure to comply with care and service abuse; making a fuss about nothing; a lack of normal maternal instinct. She also reported that the midwives tended to see Asian women as a homogeneous group with the same needs. Bowler (1993) suggested that service delivery can be affected, particularly in the areas of family planning, pain control and breastfeeding.

These issues of race do not stand alone. For women, they are closely related to the concerns of gender and of class. And, as a corollary, of sexism and inequality. Moreover, there is an increasing body of knowledge, borne out of black and Asian women's experiences of everyday life (Wilson, 1978; Amos and Parmar, 1982; Carby, 1982; Parmar, 1982; Bryan et al., 1985; Werbner, 1988). The maternity services have also been the focus of discussion (Rocheron, 1988; Phoenix, 1990). Such recognition has thus rendered the lives of black and Asian women more individual and visible.

SOCIAL CLASS

Social class remains an enduring theme within sociology. Class differentials have been constructed within a capitalist society according to an individual's relationship to the labour market. Hence, in this respect the notion of class is derived from economic events and as such it is an economic category.

The use of class as a social category has often been accepted uncritically and taken for granted as a 'natural' category. For example, in a comparative study of kinship between working-class and middle-class families in East London in the 1950s (Young and Willmott, 1957) the use of social class categorization is largely descriptive and the authors do not perceive class as problematic.

Oakley (1992) describes how social class can be regarded as a designation introduced by statisticians to describe occupational and social differences between people. Clearly, there are differences, but as Oakley emphasizes, 'What social class differences do not do is *explain* anything' (Oakley, 1992: 5).

This new science of 'vital statistics' developed in the mid-nineteenth century. At that time there was concern amongst politicians and economists over civil unrest in both rural and urban areas. Civil servants collected information about individuals' home ownership, occupation, marital status and other social distinctions. From this time onwards successive government regulations on all areas of public provision have been informed by demographic data.

The categorization of individuals into social class according to occupation by the British Registrar General is a commonly used classification (see Table 1). Using official government categorizations sociologists have conducted studies that have provided an array of descriptive data including lifestyle differences between occupational groups (Blaxter, 1990). The rates of births and deaths are also delineated according to social class, as well as more specific information such as the rate of perinatal mortality.

The empirical use of data using social class differentials has been useful in producing evidence of social inequalities between groups of individuals (Oppenheim, 1993). Inequalities in health were clearly revealed in the Black Report in 1980 and reiterated in *The Health Divide* in 1987 (Townsend *et al.*, 1988). Subsequent evidence demonstrates how such inequalities continue to prevail (Davey Smith *et al.*, 1990; Delamothe, 1991; Shiell, 1991; Whitehead and Dahlgren, 1991; Townsend, 1991). Moreover, Arber (1987) argues that the class differences in ill-health are further accentuated by unemployment. Yet, the awareness of these differences has not been translated into policy to redistribute wealth through, for example, improvements in social security and in reforming taxation (Parker, 1989; Quick and Wilkinson, 1991).

The inequalities in women's health have been primarily obscured by the conventional view of determining women's social class. A married woman is ascribed the same social class as her husband and for other women class is based on their own current or last occupation. This is a poor measure of a woman's material circumstances and thus renders many women's poverty invisible. Furthermore, the conventional approach to the construction of social class ignores the complex relationship between gender, health and inequalities (Doyal, 1984; Graham, 1984; Glendinning and Millar, 1987; Millar and Glendinning, 1989; Payne, 1991).

The narrowness of social class divisions has been the subject of debate and Arber (1990a, b) criticizes the conceptualization of social class based upon men's occupations. She considers that major changes in the patterns of employment of both men and women have made invalid the assumption that the material circumstances in a household are determined by a man's position in the labour market (Arber, 1990b).

For midwives, one significance of social class categorization is that it has led to the development of class stereotypes of women using the maternity services (Cartwright, 1979; Macintyre, 1982; Kirkham, 1989; Green *et al.*, 1990). Essentially, these stereotypes undermine good communication between pregnant women and their care-givers. The stereotype portrays women in a negative light and assumptions are made by midwives and doctors about women's understanding and their wants. Through changes in the organization of care, the assumptions upon which the stereotypes are founded may be challenged. As Green *et al.* (1990) argue, 'Systems of care which allow midwives and mothers to get to know each other (preferably before the birth) could do much to reduce the reliance on stereotypes, with beneficial results for all concerned.'

Table 1 The Registrar General's social class categories

Class	Occupation
I	Professional and managerial, e.g. lawyers, doctors, accountants, surveyors
II	Managerial and semi-professional, e.g. teachers, midwives, nurses, sales managers
IIIN	Skilled non-manual, e.g. clerical workers, secretaries, shop assistants
IIIM	Skilled manual, e.g. builders, taxi drivers, electricians
IV	Semi-skilled, e.g. agricultural workers, postal workers, telephone operators
V	Unskilled, e.g. cleaners, labourers

GENDER

As social roles, social activity and health status are linked to race and class, they are also inextricably bound to issues of gender. While anatomical and physiological differences between the sexes are biologically determined, gender may be described as the socially or culturally prescribed status of women and men in a society. The associated concepts of femininity and masculinity are similarly socially constructed and as such, they are not fixed.

Ideas about a person's gender roles and behaviour may be ascribed before birth. Rothman (1986) uses the phrase 'fetal sons and daughters' as she describes how women who know the sex of their child after amniocentesis describe fetal activity in a way that is gender stereotyped. The movements of the males were more often described as 'strong' and 'vigorous' and females were described as 'lively'. Gender stereotyping continues soon after birth as appearance and behaviour are gender related. For example, Rothman (1986: 129) contrasts the 'firm grip' of the boy's 'adorable little fists' to the 'tight cling' of the girl's 'delicate . . . tiny fingers'.

As part of the ideology of motherhood and the gendering of childcare, women and mothers are seen as the unique carers of young children. The ideas of maternal/infant attachment were primarily espoused by Bowlby (1953) who argued that the quality of the early relationship between a mother and her child was significant for the child's development. Despite challenges to this theory (Rutter, 1981), it remains pervasive and underpins the gendered division of labour in the home and in the workforce.

In practice this amounted to difficulties for women seeking paid employment outside the home. Furthermore, when women did, and still do seek paid employment, the opportunities are constrained by the gender-prescribed role of women as carers and nurturers (Finch and Groves, 1983). This is illustrated by the over-representation of women in part-time, low-skilled and low-paid jobs, the paucity of nursery provision and the uneven career development between women and men (Davies, 1990).

Rossiter (1988) argues that pregnancy, lactation and early infant attachment have acted as a justification of childrearing arrangements. She considers that they have been created in response to the changing needs of the economy, not those of dependent children. Such a situation was particularly evident in Britain during the Second World War when the needs of the economy resulted in an increase in the numbers of women in the paid workforce. This significant change was a concession to women's 'proper' and 'natural' role. It was conditional upon a return to the status quo after the war. A key element of the post-war propaganda was to encourage women to return to the hearth and for men to go back to their jobs (Holdsworth, 1988).

The pattern of work in the United Kingdom has changed since the 1970s (Davies, 1990) and this is having an impact on the gendered division of labour. These changes have been characterized by a general decline in employment and especially in male employment. Also, since the 1970s larger numbers of women are in paid employment than in previous years, but this employment is coupled with the work of childrearing (Joshi, 1989). Davies (1990) argues that the organization of work is likely to change. Individuals will no longer be in conventional lifetime full-time careers but will work for a number of employers in small organizations that will contract with each other. With reference to health service occupations, she discusses how, with flexible and contractual patterns of work, part-time work could lose its low status and become a more accepted feature of occupational organization.

As motherhood is socially prescribed, so too is fatherhood. The traditional gendered role for a father is to provide financially for his children. Generally, his involvement with babies and children is mediated through the mother; he rarely assesses a child's needs and he ends up being a helper. Lewis (1986) comments that men are initially excluded from the magic circle and they later take on the role as playmate. Mothers are the decision-makers. Yet, Brannen and Moss (1988) believe that this is a pseudo power. Women have control in the home by virtue of it not being very important.

Although its development is unclear, the most widespread and significant change in fathers' involvement has been their attendance at the birth of their children, but this has not been matched by their involvement in the antenatal and postnatal period (Barbour, 1990). There is a statement of good intent rather than a practical plan of action. Kitzinger (1989) suggests that men are poorly prepared for fatherhood and that they are presented with an image which they cannot match.

In spite of the rhetoric surrounding the 'New Man', there is little evidence to challenge situations that render childraising inequitable (Lewis and O'Brien, 1987). This may in part be attributed to the poor level of paternity leave and benefits, particularly in comparison to other European countries. Men in paid employment are given few opportunities to engage in sharing childcare on a basis comparable to women. Once again, inequalities arise from social structures and expectations are rooted in the processes of socialization.

As Lewis (1986: 190) concludes,

> truly participant fatherhood will not become the norm until great changes are made outside the family – in child-care arrangements and in the sexual division of labour in the workplace. . . . Certainly true symmetry between spouses cannot occur without major societal organisation.

In summary, for midwives to think sociologically is for them to think critically and systematically about the social context of their own lives and the lives of the women and families around them. It is about how different groups of people understand their world and the meanings it has for them. Pregnancy, childbirth and childrearing are all social events and as such they are not fixed, but changing. Traditionally, midwifery has tended to ignore sociology and it has not made a significant contribution to it. However, with greater insights into the social organizations and social structures of their world, midwives as a unique group have an important contribution to make to sociology that is not contingent on a reliance on the dominant medical model of childbearing.

References

Abbot, P. & Wallace, C. (1990) *An Introduction to Sociology: Feminist Perspectives.* London: Routledge.

Amos, V. & Parmar, P. (1982) Resistance and responses: The experiences of black girls in Britain. In McRobbie, A. & McCabe, T. (eds) *Feminism for Girls: An Adventure Story.* London: Routledge & Kegan Paul.

Arber, S. (1987) Social class, non-employment, and chronic illness: continuing the inequalities in health debate. *Br. Med. J.* **294**: 1069–1073.

Arber, S. (1990a) Opening the 'Black Box': Inequalities in women's health. In Abbot, P. & Payne, G. (eds) *New Directions in the Sociology of Health*, pp. 37–56. Hampshire: Falmer Press.

Arber, S. (1990b) Revealing women's health: reanalysing the general household survey. In Roberts, H. (ed.) *Women's Health Counts*, pp. 63–92. London: Routledge.

Arditti, R., Klein, R.D. & Minden, S. (eds) (1984) *Test Tube Woman: What Future for Motherhood?* London: Pandora.

Arney, W.R. (1982) *Power and the Profession of Obstetrics.* Chicago: University of Chicago Press.

Balaskas, J. (1981) *Active Birth: A Concise Guide to Natural Childbirth.* London: Unwin.

Barbour, R.S. (1990) Fathers: The Emergence of a New Consumer Group. In Garcia, J., Kilpatrick, R. & Richards, M. (eds) *The Politics of Maternity Care: Services for Childbearing Women in Twentieth Century Britain*, pp. 202–216. Oxford: Clarendon Press.

Bastian, H. (1992) Confined, managed and delivered. *Br. J. Obstet. Gynaecol.* **99**: 92–93.

Bauman, Z. (1990) *Thinking Sociologically.* London: Blackwell.

Berryman, J.C. (1991) Perspectives on later motherhood. In Phoenix, A., Woolett, A. & Lloyd, E. (eds) *Motherhood: Meanings, Practices and Ideologies*, pp. 103–122. London: Sage Publications.

Bland, L. (1982) 'Guardians of the race' or 'Vampires upon the nation's health'? Female sexuality and its regulation in early twentieth century Britain. In Whitelegg, M., Arnot, E., Bartels, E. *et al.* (eds) *The Changing Experience of Women*, pp. 373–378. Milton Keynes: Open University Press.

Blaxter, M. (1990) *Health and Lifestyles.* London: Routledge.

Bowlby, J. (1953) *Child Care and the Growth of Love.* Harmondsworth: Penguin.

Bowler, I.M.W. (1993) Stereotypes of women of Asian descent in midwifery: some evidence. *Midwifery* **9**(1): 7–16.

Brannen, J. & Moss, P. (1988) *New Mothers At Work.* London: Unwin Paperback.

Breen, D. (1989) *Talking With Mothers*, 2nd edn. London: Free Association Books.

Bryan, B., Dadzie, S. & Scafe, S. (1985) *The Heart of the Race: Black Women's Lives in Britain.* London: Virago.

Burke, L., Faulkner, W., Best, S., Janson-Smith, D. & Overfield, K. (1980) *Alice Through the Microscope.* London: Virago.

Campbell, R. & Macfarlane, A. (1987) *Where to be Born: The Debate and the Evidence.* Oxford: National Perinatal Epidemiology Unit.

Carby, H.V. (1982) White women listen! Black feminism and the boundaries of sisterhood. In *The Empire Strikes Back*, pp. 212–235. Centre for Contemporary Cultural Studies. London: Hutchinson.

Cartwright, A. (1979) *The Dignity of Labour.* London: Tavistock.

Chalmers, I., Enkin, M. & Kierse, M.J.N.C. (eds) (1989) *Effective Care in Pregnancy and Childbirth.* Oxford: Oxford University Press.

Corea, G., Klein, R.D., Hanmer, J. *et al.* (1985) *Man Made Woman: How New Reproductive Technologies Affect Women.* London: Hutchinson.

Cousins, M. & Hussain, A. (1984) *Michel Foucault.* London: Macmillan.

Davies, C. (1990) *The Collapse of the Conventional Career: the future of work and its relevance for post-registration education in nursing, midwifery and health visiting.* London: English National Board for Nursing, Midwifery and Health Visiting.

Davey Smith, G., Bartley, M. & Blane, D. (1990) The Black Report on socioeconomic inequalities in health 10 years on. *Br. Med. J.* **301**(18–25 August): 373–377.

De Swaan, A. (1990) *The Management of Normality. Critical Essays in Health and Welfare.* London: Routledge.

Delamothe, T. (1991) Social inequalities in health. *Br. Med. J.* **303**: 1046–1050.

DOH (Department of Health) (1993) *Changing Childbirth.* Report of the Expert Maternity Group. London: HMSO.

Donnison, J. (1988) *Midwives and Medical Men: A History of Interprofessional Rivalries and Women's Rights*, 2nd edn. London: Heinemann.

Douglas, J. (1992) Black women's health matters: putting black women on the research agenda. In Roberts, H. (ed.) *Women's Health Matters*, pp. 33–46. London: Routledge.

Dowrick, S. & Grundberg, S. (1980) *Why Children?* London: The Womens Press.

Doyal, L. (1984) Women, health and the sexual division of labour: a case study of the women's health movement in Britain. *Critical Social Policy* **3**(1): 21–33.

Ehrenreich, B. & English, D. (1974a) *Complaints and Disorders: The Sexual Politics of Sickness.* London: Compendium.

Ehrenreich, B. & English, D. (1974b) *Witches Midwives and Nurses: A History of Women Healers.* London: Compendium.

Ehrenreich, B. & English, D. (1979) *For Her Own Good: 150 years of the expert's advice to women.* London: Pluto Press.

Farrant, W. (1985) Who's for amniocentesis? The politics of prenatal screening. In Homans, H. (ed.) *The Sexual Politics of Reproduction*, pp. 96–122. Aldershot: Gower.

Finch, J. & Groves, D. (eds) (1983) *A Labour of Love.* London: Routledge & Kegan Paul.

Gabe, J. & Calnan, M. (1989) The limits of medicine: women's perception of medical technology. *Social Sci. Med.* **28**: 223–231.

Giddens, A. (1993) *Sociology.* Oxford: Polity Press.

Gieve, K. (ed.) (1989) *Balancing Acts: On Being a Mother.* London: Virago.

Glendinning, C. & Millar, J. (eds) (1987) *Women and Poverty in Britain.* London: Wheatsheaf Books.

Graham, H. (1984) *Women, Health and the Family.* London: Harvester Wheatsheaf.

Graham, H. & Oakley, A. (1981) Competing ideologies of reproduction: medical and maternal perspectives on pregnancy. In Roberts, H. (ed.) *Women, Health and Reproduction*, pp. 50–74. London: Routledge & Kegan Paul.

Green, J.M., Kitzinger, J.V. & Coupland, V.A. (1990) Stereotypes of childbearing women: a look at some of the evidence. *Midwifery* **6**: 125–132.

Greer, G. (1991) *The Change: Women, Ageing and the Menopause.* London: Penguin.

Hagell, E.I. (1989) Nursing knowledge: women's knowledge. A sociological perspective. *J. Adv. Nurs.* **14**: 226–233.

Harding, S. (1986) *The Science Question in Feminism.* Milton Keynes: Open University Press.

Hewison, A. (1993) The language of labour: an examination of the discourses on childbirth. *Midwifery* **9**: 225–234.

Holdsworth, A. (1988) *Out of the Dolls House: The Story of Women in the Twentieth Century.* London: BBC Publications.

Illich, I. (1975) *Medical Nemesis: The Expropriation of Health.* Harmondsworth: Penguin.

Joseph, G.G., Reddy, V. & Searle-Chatterjee, M. (1990) Eurocentrism in the social sciences. *Race & Class* **31**(4): 1–26.

Joshi, H. (1989) The changing form of women's economic dependency. In Joshi, H. (ed.) *The Changing Population of Britain*, pp. 157–176. Oxford: Blackwell.

Kirkham, M. (1989) Midwives and information giving in labour. In Robinson, S. & Thompson, A. (eds) *Research, Midwives and Childbirth*, Vol. 1, pp. 117–138. London: Chapman & Hall.

Kitzinger, S. (1981) *Women as Mothers.* Glasgow: Fontana.

Kitzinger, S. (1989) *The Crying Baby.* London: Penguin.

Kitzinger, J., Green, J. & Coupland, V. (1990) Labour relations: midwives and doctors on the labour ward. In Garcia, J., Kilpatrick, R., & Richards, M. (eds) *The Politics of Maternity Care: Services for Childbearing Women in Twentieth-Century Britain*, pp. 149–160. Oxford: Oxford University Press.

Leap, N. (1992) The power of words. *Nursing Times* **88**(21): 60–61.

Lewis, C. (1986) *Becoming a Father.* Milton Keynes: Open University Press.

Lewis, C. & O'Brien, M. (eds) (1987) *Reassessing Fatherhood: New Observations on Fathers and the Modern Family.* London: Sage Publications.

Lock, M. (1991) Contested meanings of the menopause. *Lancet* **337**: 1270–1272.

MacCormack, C.P. & Strathern, M. (eds) (1981) *Nature, Culture & Gender.* Cambridge: Cambridge University Press.

Macintyre, S. (1976) 'Who wants babies?' The social construction of 'instincts'. In Barker, D.L. & Allen, S. (eds) *Sexual Divisions and Society: Process and Change*, pp. 150–173. London: Tavistock.

Macintyre, S. (1977) Childbirth: the myth of the Golden Age. *World Medicine* **12**(18): 17–22.

Macintyre, S. (1982) Communications between pregnant women and their medical and midwifery attendants. *Midwives' Chronicle* November: 387–394.

Marshall, H. (1991) The social construction of motherhood: An analysis of childcare and parenting manuals. In Phoenix, A., Woollett, A., & Lloyd, E. (eds) *Motherhood: Meanings, Practices and Ideologies*, pp. 66–85. London: Sage.

Martin, E. (1987) *The Woman in the Body: A Cultural Analysis of Reproduction.* Milton Keynes: Open University Press.

McNabb, M. (1989) The science of labour? *Nursing Times* **85**(9): 58–59.

McNeill, P., Freeman, B. & Newman, J. (eds) (1992) *Women Talk Sex.* London: Scarlet Press.

Millar, J. & Glendinning, C. (1989) Survey article 'gender and poverty'. *J. Social Policy* **18**(3): 363–381.

Mitchell, J. & Oakley, A. (1986) *What is Feminism?* Oxford: Basil Blackwell.

Murcott, A. (1980) The social construction of teenage pregnancy: a problem in the ideologies of childhood and reproduction. *Sociol. Health Illness* **2**(1): 1–23.

O'Driscoll, K. & Meagher, D. (1980) *Active Management of Labour.* London: W.B. Saunders.

Oakley, A. (1976a) Wisewoman and medicine man: changes in the management of childbirth. In Mitchell, J. & Oakley, A.

(eds) *The Rights and Wrongs of Women*, pp. 304–378. Harmondsworth: Penguin.

Oakley, A. (1976b) *Housewife*. Harmondsworth: Penguin.

Oakley, A. (1980) *Woman Confined: Towards a Sociology of Childbirth*. Oxford: Martin Robertson.

Oakley, A. (1981) *Subject Woman*. London: Fontana.

Oakley, A. (1984) *The Captured Womb: A History of the Medical Care of Pregnant Women*. Oxford: Blackwell.

Oakley, A. (1985) *Sex, Gender and Society*. Aldershot: Gower.

Oakley, A. (1989) Who cares for women? Science versus love in midwifery today. *Midwives' Chronicle* July: 214–221.

Oakley, A. (1990) Who's afraid of the randomised controlled trial? Some dilemmas of the scientific method and 'good' research practice. In Roberts, H. (ed.) *Women's Health Counts*, pp. 167–194. London: Routledge.

Oakley, A. (1992) *Social Support and Motherhood*. Oxford: Blackwell.

Oakley, A., McPherson, A. & Roberts, H. (1990) *Miscarriage*. London: Penguin.

Oppenheim, C. (1993) *Poverty: The Facts*. London: Child Poverty Action Group.

Overall, C. (1989) *The Future of Human Reproduction*. Toronto, Canada: The Women's Press.

Parker, H. (1989) *Instead of the Dole: An Enquiry into the Integration of the Tax and Benefit System*. London: Routledge.

Parmar, P. (1982) Gender, race and class: Asian women in resistance. In *The Empire Strikes Back*, pp. 236–275. Centre for Contemporary Cultural Studies. London: Hutchinson.

Pascal, G. (1986) *Social Policy: A Feminist Analysis*. London: Routledge.

Payne, S. (1991) *Women, Health and Poverty*. London: Harvester Wheatsheaf.

Pearson, M. (1986) Racist notions of ethnicity and culture in health education. In Rodwell, S. & Watt, A. (eds) *The Politics of Health Education*, pp. 38–56. London: Routledge.

Phillips, D. & Rathwell, S. (1986) *Health Race & Ethnicity*. London: Croom Helm.

Phillips, A. & Rakusen, J. (eds) (1989) *The New Our Bodies Ourselves: A Health Book By and For Women*, 2nd edn. Harmondsworth: Penguin.

Phoenix, A. (1988) Narrow definitions of culture: The case of early motherhood. In Westwood, S. & Bachau, P. (eds) *Enterprising Women*, pp. 153–176. London: Routledge & Kegan Paul.

Phoenix, A. (1990) Black women and the maternity services. In Garcia, J., Kilpatrick, R. & Richards, M. (eds) *The Politics of Maternity Care: Services for Childbearing Women in Twentieth-Century Britain*, pp. 274–299. Oxford: Clarendon Books.

Phoenix, A. (1991) *Young Mothers?* Cambridge: Polity Press.

Quick, A. & Wilkinson, R. (1991) *Income & Health*. London: Socialist Health Association.

Ramazanoglu, C. (1989) *Feminism and the Contradictions of Oppression*. London: Routledge.

Roberts, H. (1985) *The Patient Patients*. London: Pandora.

Robinson, S., Golden, J., & Bradley, S. (1983) *A Study of the Role and Responsibilities of the Midwife*. Nurse Education Research Unit, University of London, Kings College.

Rocheron, Y. (1988) The Asian mother and baby campaign: The construction of ethnic minorities' health needs. *Critical Social Policy* 22: 4–23.

Rose, H. (1982) Making science feminist. In Whitelegg, E. *et al.* (eds) *The Changing Experience of Women*, pp. 352–372. Milton Keynes: Open University Press.

Rose, H. (1986) Womens' work: womens knowledge. In Mitchell, J. & Oakley, A. (eds) *What is Feminism?*, pp. 161–183. Oxford: Basil Blackwell.

Rose, H. & Rose, S. (1971) The myth of the neutrality of science. In Fuller, W. (ed.) *The Social Impact of Modern Biology*, pp. 283–294. London: Routledge & Kegan Paul.

Rossiter, A. (1988) *From Private to Public: A Feminist Exploration of Early Mothering*. Ontario: The Women's Press.

Rothman, B.K. (1982) *In Labour: Women and Power in the Birthplace*. New York: W.W. Norton.

Rothman, B.K. (1986) *The Tentative Pregnancy: Prenatal Diagnosis and the Future of Motherhood*. London: Pandora.

Rowbotham, S. (1973) *Woman's Consciousness, Man's World*. Harmondsworth: Penguin.

Rueschemeyer, D. (1986) *Power and the Division of Labour*. Oxford: Polity Press.

Rutter, M. (1981) *Maternal Deprivation Reassessed*, 2nd edn. London: Penguin.

Saffron, L. (1986) *Getting Pregnant Our Own Way: A Guide to Alternative Insemination*. London: Women's Health Information Centre.

Schwarz, E.W. (1990) The engineering of childbirth: A new obstetric programme as reflected in British obstetric textbooks, 1960–1980. In Garcia, J., Kilpatrick, R. & Richards, M. (eds) *The Politics of Maternity Care: Services for Childbearing Women in Twentieth-Century Britain*, pp. 47–60. Oxford: Clarendon Paperbacks.

Scutt, J.A. (ed.) (1990) *The Baby Machine: Reproductive Technology and the Commercialisation of Motherhood*. London: Green Print.

Sharpe, S, (1976) *Just Like a Girl: How Girls Learn to be Women*. Harmondsworth: Penguin.

Shiell, A. (1991) *Poverty and Inequalities in Health*. Discussion Paper 86. Centre For Health Economics, Health Economics Consortium, University of York, York YO1 5DD.

Showalter, E. (1987) *The Female Malady: Women, Madness and English Culture, 1830–1980*. London: Virago.

Spender, D. (1985) *Man Made Language*, 2nd edn. London: Pandora Press.

Stacey, M. (1988) *The Sociology of Health and Healing*. London: Unwin Hyman.

Stacey, M. (ed.) (1993) *Changing Human Reproduction*. London: Sage Publications.

Stanley, L. (ed.) (1990) *Feminist Praxis: Research, Theory and Epistemology in Feminist Sociology*. London: Routledge.

Stanworth, M. (ed.) (1987) *Reproductive Technologies: Gender, Motherhood and Medicine*. Cambridge: Polity Press.

Szasz, T. (1971) *The Manufacture of Madness*. London: Routledge & Kegan Paul.

Tew, M. (1990) *Safer Childbirth? A Critical History of Maternity Care*. London: Chapman & Hall.

Torkington, N.P.K. (1991) *Black Health: A Political Issue*. Catholic Association for Racial Health and Liverpool Institute for Higher Education.

Towler, J. & Brammall, J. (1986) *The Midwife in History and Society.* London: Croom Helm.

Townsend, P. (1991) Deprivation and ill health. *Nursing* 4(43): 11–15.

Townsend, P., Davidson, P. & Whitehead, M. (eds) (1988) *Inequalities in Health: The Black Report & The Health Divide.* Harmondsworth: Penguin.

Turner, B.S. (1987) *Medical Power and Social Knowledge.* London: Sage Publications.

Versluysen, M.C. (1980) Old wives' tales: women healers in English history. In Davies, C. (ed.) *Rewriting Nursing History,* pp. 175–199. London: Croom Helm.

Walkerdine, V. & Lucey, H. (1989) *Democracy in the Kitchen: Regulating Mothers and Socialising Girls.* London: Virago.

Weideger, P. (1975) *Female Cycles.* London: The Womens Press.

Werbner, P. (1988) Taking and giving: working women and female bonds in a Pakistani immigrant neighbourhood. In Westwood, S. & Bachau, P. (eds) *Enterprising women: Ethnicity, Economy and Gender Relations,* pp. 177–202. London: Routledge.

Westwood, S. & Bachau, P. (eds) (1988) *Enterprising Women.* London: Routledge & Kegan Paul.

Whitehead, M. & Dahlgren, G. (1991) What can be done about the inequalities in health? *The Lancet* 338: 1059–1063.

Wilson, A. (1978) *Finding a Voice: Asian Women in Britain.* London: Virago.

Young, M. & Willmott, P. (1957) *Family and Kinship in East London.* Harmondsworth: Penguin.

Zola, I.K. (1972) Medicine as an institution of social control. *Sociol. Rev.* 20: 487–504.

83

History and Development of the Midwifery Profession

Early History

The history of midwifery is a long and interesting one. Women of all ages and countries have done noble work as midwives throughout the centuries. In records from ancient Greece several references are made to midwives. Socrates' mother was a midwife and he considered it 'a most respected profession'. Plato referred to midwives as 'excellent matchmakers'. Aristotle gives a comprehensive description of a midwife:

> of middle age, neither too young nor too old and of good habit of body. Not subject to disease, fears or sudden fright. A lady's hand, a hawk's eye and a lion's heart. Sober and affable, not subject to passion, bountiful and compassionate and her temper cheerful and pleasant. A midwife is a most necessary and honourable office, being a helper of nature.

Biblical references to midwives have always been to their honour. We read in Genesis and Exodus of a maternal death, of a case of obstructed labour and of babies born before the arrival of the midwife. In Genesis 35:17–18, the death of Rachel, Jacob's wife, is recorded. She went into labour while journeying from Bethel to Ephrath and had a hard labour. The midwife said to her 'Do not be afraid, this is another son for you'. Her son Benjamin was born alive, but Rachel died.

Later, in Genesis 38:27–29, we read of a midwife attending Tamar, the daughter-in-law of Judah, in labour. Tamar was expecting twins and we read that during labour one child put out its hand (transverse lie with prolapsed arm). The midwife 'took a scarlet thread and fastened it around the wrist' to identify the first twin. The child withdrew his hand, however, and his brother was born first. Afterwards, the second child was born with the scarlet thread round his wrist.

In Exodus 1:16–21, it is recorded that Pharaoh, the King of Egypt, said to the Hebrew midwives Shiphrah and Puah 'When you are attending the Hebrew women in childbirth, watch as the child is delivered and if it is a boy, kill him, if it is a girl, let her live'. The midwives were God-fearing women, however, and did not do as the King of Egypt commanded but let the boys live. When summoned to the King to explain why they had not carried out his command they replied, 'that Hebrew women were not like Egyptian women. When they were in labour they gave birth before the midwife could get to them.' Therefore, 'God made the midwives prosper'. He gave them 'homes and families of their own, because they feared Him'.

In the second century Soranus of Ephesus wrote a book for midwives and for 14 centuries it was the only book to which they could refer. Midwifery knowledge and the birthing stool were passed from one generation to the next. In the sixteenth century *The Birth of Mankind* was published, based on the earlier writings of Soranus of Ephesus, but it had limited use because few midwives could read.

Until the end of the sixteenth century midwifery was practised entirely by women; and men could be severely punished – indeed there are records of them being burned at the stake – for attending women in childbirth. A Doctor Willoughby records that in 1658 his daughter, a midwife, consulted him about a case in which the breech was presenting. Unknown to the woman, he crept into the chamber on his hands and knees and examined her without attracting her notice. He advised his daughter to bring down a foot, which she did, but as she was aware of the possible complications, she asked her father to carry out the rest of the delivery.

In the seventeenth century men began to take up midwifery, though there was great opposition from the midwives and from some of the general public. Before the time of Henry VIII the medical profession was controlled by the Church. Doctors were licensed by the Bishops, as also were the apothecaries and the midwives. Later the medical faculty began to manage their own affairs and gradually the midwives were excluded. The Chamberlens, a renowned family of male midwives, campaigned unsuccessfully for the recognition of midwives. They also introduced the obstetric forceps but kept the design secret for 150 years to prevent other midwives and doctors from using it. Eventually, however, in 1733, after the death of the last of the Chamberlens, a description of the forceps was published and ultimately, in 1819, a number of forceps were discovered hidden beneath the floorboards of an attic in a house that had been owned by the family.

By the middle of the eighteenth century the number of male midwives had increased, and amongst them was William Smellie, from Lanark. Smellie came to London and, while attending many hundreds of poor women in labour, made detailed studies of normal labour. He gave practical and theoretical teaching to many doctors and midwives, using models for his demonstrations, and was the first person to describe accurately the relation of the fetal head to the mother's pelvis and the mechanism of labour. The numerous case histories he wrote are, even today, remarkably accurate. The midwives, already resentful of the intrusion of male midwives into their domain, were at first particularly opposed to Smellie, on account of his interest in normal cases. Queen Victoria is thought to have been the first Queen of England to be delivered by a medical man. It was because Princess Charlotte, daughter of George IV, died in childbirth, and her son was stillborn, that Victoria eventually ascended the throne of England.

In the nineteenth century further unsuccessful attempts were made to obtain the recognition of midwives and the popularity of midwives was at an all-time low, with the image of the gin-swilling Sairey Gamp created by Charles Dickens in Martin Chuzzlewit influencing public opinion. On the other hand, a fine description of a village midwife is given by Laurence Sterne in *Tristram Shandy*.

From time to time educated women, daughters of medical men and clergymen, became midwives and the Ladies Obstetrical College was founded in London in 1864. Florence Nightingale was a pioneer in the efficient training of midwives. In 1862 she organized a small training school in connection with King's College Hospital but the wards were inconvenient and the scheme was not a success due to outbreaks of puerperal fever. At about this time Semmelweiss introduced handwashing with chlorine and lime before attending women at childbirth. As a result of this simple measure there was a dramatic fall in maternal mortality due to puerperal sepsis in his maternity unit where handwashing was practised. Sadly he was ridiculed by his colleagues in the medical profession for his work and it was many years before it was accepted (Thompson, 1969).

In 1869 the London Obstetrical Society undertook to investigate and report on the causes of infant mortality. One recommendation of the report was that an Examining Board should be established, so that midwives might be tested and be granted a diploma. The government failed to act so the Society decided to issue a diploma to successful candidates after training and examination in midwifery. A Board for the examination of midwives was constituted and the first examination was held in 1872, for which six candidates sat. This training and examination was voluntary and the diploma was not recognized by the government. The requirements for the London Obstetrical Society examination were as follows:

- A certificate of moral character.
- Age not under 21 or over 30.
- Proof of having attended no fewer that 25 cases under supervision satisfactory to the Board of Examiners.
- Proof of having attended a course of approved lectures.
- A written and an oral examination.

The General Medical Council from 1872 onwards made great efforts to secure State recognition of midwives. The Midwives Institute was set up in 1881 with the object of gaining for midwives some form of state recognition. It promoted and obtained the introduction of the first Bill to Parliament in 1890 (Cowell and Wainwright, 1981). The Bill reached its second reading but was blocked at its third reading. A further seven Bills were introduced, unsuccessfully, the last of these in 1900 by Mr Heywood Johnstone. He introduced it again in 1902 and, this time, it passed all stages and received the Royal assent on 31 July 1902.

Midwifery in the Twentieth Century

The 1902 Midwives Act established the Central Midwives' Board which was authorized to frame rules regulating the training and practice of midwives, to conduct examinations, to issue certificates and to maintain a roll of certified midwives. Thus the title of midwife was, for the first time, protected. Midwives certified with the London Obstetrical Society were allowed to register with the Central Midwives' Board during its first three years, as were other, non-certified midwives of good character who were called 'bona fide' midwives (Donnison, 1988).

Despite the introduction of statutory control of midwives at the beginning of the twentieth century, the maternal mortality rate remained high. The Government therefore commissioned reports in 1924 and 1929. The first report by Janet Campbell (1924) recommended an increase in the number of midwives and higher standards of competence. The second report was from a Departmental Committee on the Training and Employment of Midwives (1929) which was established to review the working of the 1902 Midwives Act. It reported that one of the causes of the high maternal

mortality rate was the shortage of midwives in some rural areas because doctors allowed unsupervised handy women (who were untrained) to attend women in childbirth. The Committee recommended a State maternity scheme with free care from midwives and doctors to overcome the problem.

As a result of these reports, the 1936 Midwives Act addressed some of the issues. Amendments were made to the main Act of 1902 in 1918, 1926, 1927, and 1936. The 1936 amendments allowed midwives to add SCM (State Certified Midwife) after their names; training was increased to one year for State Registered Nurses and to two years for Enrolled Nurses. Local authorities were required to provide all expectant mothers with the domiciliary services of a qualified midwife – and it became illegal for anyone other than a midwife or doctor to attend a woman in childbearing, except in an emergency. The status of midwives was greatly enhanced by these changes and by the inception of midwife-teacher training.

A shortage of midwives and nurses caused by the demands of the Second World War led to an enquiry into their conditions, status and salary, and the publication, in 1943, of the Rushcliffe Report with its proposals for improved salaries and conditions of service (HMSO, 1943). A further report in 1949 of the Stocks Working Party on the Recruitment and Training of Midwives made recommendations for enhancing the status and training of midwives and midwife teachers (HMSO, 1949).

The implementation of the 1946 National Health Service Act in 1948 meant that, for the first time, mothers having a home or hospital delivery could receive free medical and midwifery services.

The 1951 Midwives Act consolidated all previous acts into one and remained the only legal framework for the midwifery profession in Britain until 1979 when the Nurses, Midwives and Health Visitors Act replaced the Central Midwives' Board and other statutory bodies with the United Kingdom Central Council and four National Boards. Further amendments to the Act were made in 1992 (see Chapter 84).

Factors Influencing the Contemporary Midwifery Profession

As can be seen from the above account of the history of midwifery, changes have occurred in both the delivery of the maternity services and in the status of midwives, particularly in the last hundred years.

Sociopolitical factors in the twentieth century have, however, greatly influenced the current maternity services. The Second World War largely contributed to the move towards hospital delivery, as women were encouraged to move away from their homes, which were at risk of being bombed, to a more central hospital site, where 24-hour attention could be given. By the late 1940s, the home birth rate had decreased to about 50% (Campbell and Macfarlane, 1987). This trend was completed in the 1970s following the publication of the Peel Report in which 100% hospital 'confinements' were advocated in an attempt to reduce perinatal mortality (Robinson, 1990: 71). Added to this, fragmentation of the maternity services occurred with the division between hospital and community midwifery, thus reducing continuity of care by midwives.

Schwarz's fascinating discussion of the 'engineering of childbirth' (Schwarz, 1990) explores the changes in midwifery and obstetric practices in the light of related textbooks of the middle and late twentieth century. He traces the evolution of the art of midwifery, as practised by doctors, into the science of obstetrics, in line with the technological advances that have been made. Schwarz postulates that obstetricians in the seventeenth, eighteenth and nineteenth centuries were merely 'mechanics', called on to extricate fetuses from difficult delivery situations, with an emphasis on recognizing and dealing with complications of the second stage of labour. However, scientific discoveries and developments in the late nineteenth and twentieth centuries, such as the use of chloroform for analgesia, gave obstetricians the beginnings of power over childbirth. As their ability to understand better the intrauterine environment increased, for example, with the advent of ultrasound scanning in the 1950s, so this facilitated the development of the obstetrician's role into one of anticipating potential problems during pregnancy. This inevitably led to increased intervention – and eventually the ultimate control of childbirth with the active management of labour, pioneered by men such as O'Driscoll and Friedman – so that obstetric practice became based on the philosophy that birth was only normal in retrospect. As maternal mortality rates reduced during the latter part of the twentieth century, the focus was placed firmly on improving perinatal outcomes, and the acknowlegement of needing to care for two 'patients'. This was often at the expense of maternal satisfaction, although conversely, parents' expectations of achieving a live healthy baby had increased considerably.

In addition, a power struggle was developing between obstetricians and midwives, which was not only based upon the division of labour, but also on gender. In the 1970s and 1980s, the midwife was often little more than a maternity nurse, adhering to obstetricians' and unit policy. This may have been exacerbated by the fact that most obstetricians were men, whilst almost all midwives were women, and the traditional cultural view of the dominant man prevailed (Morrin, 1992). The midwife's responsiblity in caring completely for a woman from booking to the end of the puerperium seemed lost forever, reducing both the mother's and the midwife's satisfaction in the process, and for a time midwifery appeared to be without direction, aimlessly attempting to rediscover its place.

Gradually, in response to the need to provide more holistic care to meet the needs and expectations of woman, training programmes for midwives included subjects such as psychology and sociology. In the 1980s women themselves began to rebel against the mechanization of childbirth, and midwives once again learnt how to be the mother's advocate, and developed new skills in counselling, advising, educating and facilitating successful parenthood.

The Sex Discrimination Act of 1975 eventually opened the doors of midwifery to men in 1983. This change was necessary, not only to meet the demand of men in the UK who wished to train as midwives, but also to avoid the contravention of EEC legislation which is non-discriminatory, although the EEC Midwives Directives were not agreed until 1981. McKenna (1991) believes that the increasing numbers of men in the profession works in favour of midwives in general as they are often better than women in negotiating terms and conditions of service, including salary structures, although Downe (1987) urges that men should not use midwifery simply as a strategy to develop their (nursing) careers.

The proposals in the 1980s to implement new nurse education programmes in the form of Project 2000 caused great concern for midwives. Initially there were plans to include midwifery as a fifth branch of nursing, but due to the overwhelming protest from Britain's midwives, the profession retained its own training programmes. Other health professionals were forced to acknowledge that midwifery was not a branch of nursing but a separate profession in its own right, with its own body of knowledge which is increasingly based on research. The Project 2000 Report (UKCC, 1986) did recommend that experimentation should be undertaken with a three-year midwifery programme and this was accepted but not with a Common Foundation Programme with nurses, and midwifery is not a branch programme. Shared learning with nurses may take place however for some subjects during the first year or so of training, but application to midwifery is required. These courses were initially called 'direct entry', then 'pre-registration' courses, but further confirmation of the discrete identity of midwifery has come in 1995, with a change in terminology for all midwifery preparation programmes. Anyone training to become a midwife is now considered to be undertaking a pre-registration course, with those who are qualified nurses undertaking a shortened course. Midwifery preparation programmes are either at diploma or degree level, and many midwives are choosing to follow their initial education with studies at Masters and PhD level. Consequently, the amount of research which is directly related to midwifery is growing as a result of these advanced programmes of study.

European Community legislation recognizes that midwifery is a profession separate from nursing. The European Community Midwives Directives were agreed in 1981 and implemented in January 1983. The 'Activities of a Midwife' are defined in the EC Midwives Directive 80/155/EEC Article 4 and are published in the *Midwife's Code of Practice* (UKCC, 1994). Member states of the European Community are required to ensure that midwives are trained to undertake these activities. It is the responsibility of the UKCC, as the Competent Authority for the Midwives (and indeed Nurses) Directives, to ensure that the requirements of the Directives are fully met.

For most countries of the European Community midwifery is a three-year programme (direct entry) and initially there was some reluctance by the other member states to recognize midwives who had completed a shortened programme following general nurse training. This problem was overcome by the extension of the shortened programme from one year to 18 months and the requirement for one year's practice as a midwife in the UK before being allowed to practice within the community. Freedom of movement within the community is then permitted, provided the language requirements are met. Similarly, midwives who are naturals of, and have trained in other member states have freedom of movement under the Midwives Directives.

The ability of midwives to examine critically new developments, to reflect on experiences and to evaluate their practice has resulted in improved services for mothers and babies. Midwifery had developed from being merely a group of handy women who help other mothers to give birth, into a well-educated and respected profession in which there are many opportunities. Midwives may deliver care in a variety of ways, for instance they may be attached to a midwifery team, or a 'one-to-one' service (Page *et al.*, 1994), or some prefer to work in independent practice (Demilew, 1994). Whatever the pattern of care, the aims are the same, to give women choice, continuity of high-quality care and control.

Changing Childbirth (DOH, 1993) proposes that all women should, as far as possible, know the person who delivers them, and that midwives should be the lead professional in at least one third of cases, with obstetricians and general practitioners taking responsibility for the other two thirds of women. Davis (1994) feels that this is an exciting time for midwives, who will be able to utilize the full range of their skills and expertise, in a variety of ways. She does, however, suggest that in order to fulfil the new role, midwives will need to redefine the relationship they have with the women in their care. It will also, surely, require a change in relationship with medical colleagues, both obstetricians and general practitioners. The locus of power may need to be renegotiated, with each professional involved in maternity care confident enough in their own role to work in equal partnership with other members of the team.

The future of the midwifery profession will be influenced by Government policies, and to some extent by the political influence of organizations such as the National Childbirth Trust, and various financial constraints, but one thing is guaranteed: there will always be pregnant women delivering babies and becoming parents. They will require professional assistance – and increasingly it is the consumers of the services who dictate what those services should be and how they should be delivered. Midwives will need strength and insight to act as the mothers' advocates, whilst recognizing the need to relinquish a degree of power to the parents. This new relationship should, however, facilitate a return to the literal meaning of the word 'midwife' – of being 'with woman'.

References

Campbell, J.M. (1924) *Maternal Mortality.* Reports on Public Health and Medical Subjects No. 25. London: HMSO.

Campbell, R.T. & Macfarlane, A. (1987) *Where to be Born – The Debate and the Evidence.* Oxford: National Perinatal Epidemiology Unit.

Cowell, B.T. & Wainwright, D. (1981) *Behind the Blue Door.* London: Baillière Tindall.

Davis, K. (1994) Responsibilities of choice. *Nursing Standard* 8(44): 20–21.

Demilew, J. (1994) South East London Midwifery Group Practice. *MIDIRS Midwifery Digest* 4(3): 270–272.

Departmental Committee on the Training and Employment of Midwives (1929) Report. London: HMSO.

DOH (Department of Health) (1993) *Changing Childbirth.* Report of the Expert Maternity Group. London: HMSO.

Donnison, J. (1988) *Midwives and Medical Men – A History of the Struggle for the Control of Childbirth.* London: Historical Publications.

Downe, S. (1987) Male midwives – a historical perspective (correspondence). *Assoc. of Radical Midwives Magazine* 31 (Winter): 5.

Ministry of Health (1943) *Report of Midwives' Salaries Committee* (Rushcliffe Committee). London: HMSO.

Ministry of Health (1949) *Report of Working Party on Midwives* (Stocks Report). London: HMSO.

McKenna, H.P. (1991) The developments and trends in relation to men practising midwifery: a review of the literature. *J. Adv. Nurs.* 16(4): 480–489.

Morrin, N. (1992) Unequal partners. *Nursing Times* 88(22): 58–60.

Page, L., Jones, B., Bentley, R. *et al.* (1994) One-to-one midwifery practice. *Br. J. Midwifery* 2(9): 444–447.

Robinson, S. (1990) Maintaining the independence of the midwifery profession: a continuing struggle. In: Garcia, J., Kilpatrick, R. & Richards, M. (eds) *The Politics of Maternity Care.* Oxford: Oxford University Press.

Schwarz, E.W. (1990) The engineering of childbirth: a new obstetric programme as reflected in British obstetric textbooks 1960–1980. In Garcia, J., Kilpatrick, R. & Richards, M. (eds) *The Politics of Maternity Care.* Oxford: Oxford University Press.

Thompson, M. (1969) *The Cry and the Covenant.* London: Pan Books.

UKCC (UK Central Council for Nursing, Midwifery and Health Visiting) (1986) *Project 2000 A New Preparation for Practice,* p. 50. London: UKCC.

UKCC (1994) *The Midwive's Code of Practice.* London: UKCC.

Further Reading

Leap, N. & Hunter, B. (1993) *The Midwife's Tale: An Oral History from Handywoman to Professional Midwife.* London: Scarlett Press.

Marland, H. (1993) *The Art of Midwifery: Early Modern Midwifery in Europe.* London: Routledge.

Tew, M. (1990) *Safer Childbirth? A Critical History of Maternity Care.* London: Chapman & Hall.

Towler, J. & Brammall, J. (1986) *Midwives in History and Society.* London: Croom Helm.

84

The Statutory Framework and Control of the Practice of Midwives in the UK

The first Midwives Act of 1902 sanctioned the establishment of a statutory body, the Central Midwives' Board for England and Wales, and prescribed its constitution and laid down its duties and powers. This Act was amended in 1918, 1926, 1934, 1936 and 1950. The Midwives Act of 1951 consolidated all previous acts. The Nurses, Midwives and Health Visitors Act of 1979 established a new statutory structure for nursing, midwifery and health visiting in the United Kingdom, and the UK Central Council and four National Boards were set up (Figure 1). Following a review, commissioned by the Health Departments in 1989, of the functioning of the 1979 Act (Peat Marwick McLintock, 1989), most of the recommendations made were embodied in the Nurses, Midwives and Health Visitors Act of 1992.

The United Kingdom Central Council for Nursing, Midwifery and Health Visiting (UKCC)

In 1980, the United Kingdom Central Council for Nursing, Midwifery and Health Visiting, and the four National Boards were established and worked alongside the existing statutory bodies until 1 July 1983. The Central Midwives' Boards, Northern Ireland Council for Nurses and Midwives, General Nursing Councils and Council for the Education and Training of Health Visitors were then dissolved and the United Kingdom Central Council and four National Boards for Nursing, Midwifery and Health Visiting took over their functions. The 1992 Nurses, Midwives and Health Visitors Act was implemented on 1 April 1993. Under this Act, the United Kingdom Central Council consists of a maximum of 60 members, with two thirds being elected by the three professions to serve on the Coun-

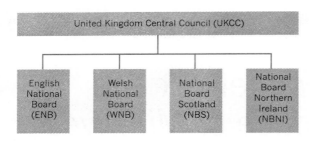

Figure 1   Statutory bodies for nursing, midwifery and health visiting.

cil: these are called the 'elected members' and they are also appointed by the Secretary of State. The one third of members who are unelected are appointed directly by the Secretary of State. Members must live or work within one of the four countries of the United Kingdom, and must either be registered nurses, midwives, health visitors or medical practitioners, or have qualifications and experience in education or other suitable fields to make their contributions pertinent to the work of the Council. A proportion of the Council members are required to be actively involved in the teaching of nursing, midwifery or health visiting. Council members elect a president and vice-president for themselves from those appointed.

Under the 1992 Act, only registered nurses, midwives and health visitors may vote for council members, or, indeed, be voted for by their peers to serve on the UK Central Council. Elections to the UK Central Council are held every five years, with separate electoral categories for nurses, midwives and health visitors. This means that both candidates and voters have to declare which of the three professions they wish to represent or vote for in the elections. Direct election of two thirds of Council members is one of the major changes introduced in the 1992 Nurses, Midwives and Health Visitors Act.

FUNCTIONS OF THE UK CENTRAL COUNCIL

The United Kingdom Central Council is responsible for establishing and improving standards of education and of professional conduct for all nurses, midwives and health visitors; these standards must comply with any European Community obligations of the United Kingdom. The Council makes Rules which set out the prerequisites for entry to pre-registration education, and the kind, content and standard of education

programme to be undertaken, both prior to registration, and as ongoing education.

The Council also provides a framework for expected standards of professional conduct across the three professions and throughout the United Kingdom by the provision of statutory *Rules* which govern practice, and *Codes* to guide practitioners.

The functions of the UK Central Council are to:

1   determine regulations regarding education of midwives, nurses and health visitors;
2   maintain a professional register of all practising midwives, nurses and health visitors;
3   maintain records of ongoing education of practitioners;
4   establish Preliminary Proceedings, Professional Conduct and Health Committees to investigate cases of alleged misconduct;
5   formulate Rules relating to midwifery practice, and publish Codes of Practice and advisory documents for its practitioners;
6   establish a Standing Midwifery Committee to deal with all matters relating to midwifery.

Education – preparation and continuing development of midwives

The UK Central Council is responsible for ensuring the highest possible standards of education for all midwives, nurses and health visitors. It specifies the kind, standard and content of initial education across the three professions and the four countries of the United Kingdom, and is a means of assuring the public of the safety and quality of practitioners at the point of registration.

Maintenance of a professional register of all practising midwives, nurses and health visitors

The Central Council maintains a 'live' register of all midwives, nurses and health visitors currently in practice in the United Kingdom; Part 10 of the register relates to midwives. Midwives are eligible to have their names recorded on the Register if, in addition to payment of the appropriate fee, they can produce documentary evidence of the relevant professional qualification and can satisfy Council that they are of good character. It is an offence in law to claim falsely to have a registration with the Council, either verbally, in writing, by the use of an assumed name, or by wearing a badge or uniform with the intent to deceive.

Midwives who have successfully completed their midwifery education in Britain at an approved institution are eligible for entry to Part 10 of the UK Central Council register. Midwives from European Community countries which have training programmes deemed to be equivalent to that available in the United Kingdom may also register with the UK Central Council. Midwives who have trained in countries other than Britain and the European Community may, in certain instances, be able to register immediately with the Central Council. However, if that training does not equip the midwife to practise British midwifery, she may be required to undertake an adaptation course before registering, or even to retrain completely in the United Kingdom. In addition, non-British nationals may be required to demonstrate a level of knowledge of the English language suitable for caring for people in the United Kingdom, or to undertake language training within a specified period of time.

All practising midwives are required to complete an annual Intention to Practise form which they send via their supervisor of midwives to the Local Supervising Authority (LSA) in which they intend to practise. The Local Supervising Authority forwards the forms to the UK Central Council in April each year for the information to be recorded on the professional register of practising midwives. Other changes are notified to the UKCC monthly.

Records of continuing professional education

Midwives have a long history of being required to undertake periodic refreshment to keep their knowledge and practice up to date. The 1936 Midwives Act included the introduction of statutory refresher courses, but implementation of this clause of the Act was delayed until after the Second World War. Since the 1950s midwives have been required to attend a minimum of five consecutive days, or, more recently, have the choice of seven accumulated study days every five years. From 1995, with the implementation of the Post Registration Education and Practice (PREP) regulations, this is in the process of changing to a minimum of five days every three years, and includes all practitioners on the professional register, not only midwives. Although PREP legislation came into effect on 1 April 1995, it is to be phased in over five years. By

the year 2001 all practitioners must meet all the requirements (see Chapters 1 and 86).

Establish and improve standards of professional conduct

It is the duty of the Central Council to establish and improve standards of professional conduct of all practitioners on its register. The Central Council makes rules which determine the circumstances which constitute misconduct, and the means by which a practitioner may have their name removed or suspended from, or restored to the register.

If a midwife, nurse or health visitor is accused of committing some act in the course of her or his duties which may have endangered patient or client wellbeing, or which is viewed as professional misconduct in any way, the practitioner may be summoned before the Professional Conduct Committee, which acts similarly to a court of law (Figure 2). Dimond (1995) defines misconduct as 'conduct unworthy of a registered nurse, midwife or health visitor . . . and includes obtaining registration by fraud'. Cases in which midwives, nurses and health visitors have been found guilty of misconduct include not only those situations in which clients or patients have been put at risk, but also instances outside work which reflect adversely upon the individual and the profession, for example, drugs offences or shoplifting. Minor offences such as traffic or parking offences are not normally placed in the same category.

The Preliminary Proceedings Committee (PPC) was transferred from the National Boards to the UK Central Council in the 1992 Nurses, Midwives and Health Visitors Act. It is convened from members of Council to investigate alleged misconduct. The Preliminary Proceedings Committee must decide if it is appropriate to:

1 refer a case to the Professional Conduct Committee, with a view to removal of the practitioner's name from the register;
2 refer the case to the professional screeners of the Health Committee to assess the practitioner's fitness to practise; or
3 if the case is not to be referred to the Conduct Committee or professional screeners, and the practitioner has admitted the alleged misconduct, consider issuing a caution to the practitioner.

The midwife, nurse or health visitor is called to account before a public hearing, with the Preliminary

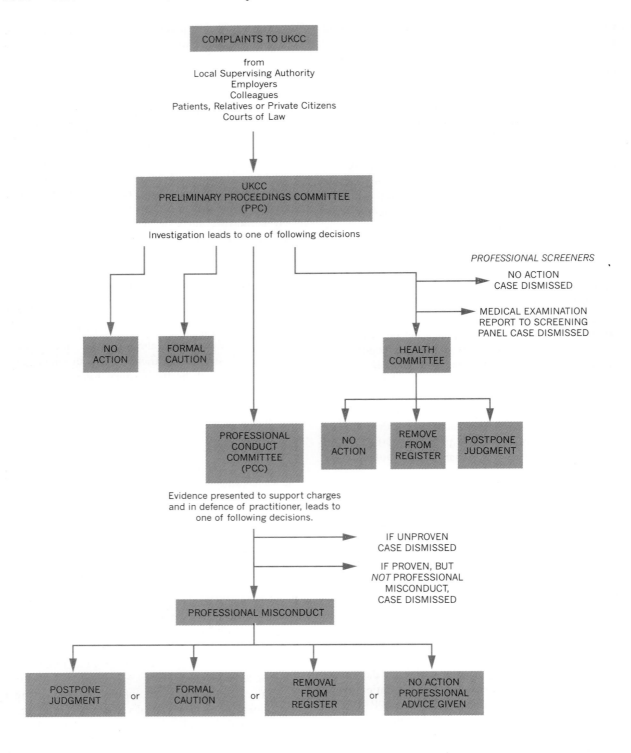

Figure 2   Procedures and possible outcomes of Preliminary Proceedings Committee, Professional Conduct Committee and Health Committee.

Proceedings Committee constituted from members of Council and the Vice President of Council acting as Chairman. Some of the Preliminary Proceedings Committee members must be from the same profession as the practitioner. Therefore, if a midwife is summoned before the Preliminary Proceedings Committee, some of the members will need to be midwives. The Preliminary Proceedings Committee can, at any time, decline to proceed, adjourn the hearing, or undertake further investigations into the matter, through the solicitor. The Preliminary Proceedings Committee is not required to justify its decision in the event of a case not being referred to the Professional Conduct Committee.

The Professional Conduct Committee is constituted by the Central Council and includes Council members, with a proportion being from the same profession as the complainant, and the President of Council acting as Chairman. Council members who have considered a case as a member of the Preliminary Proceedings Committee, or who have acted as professional screeners, are not allowed to be members of the Conduct Committee considering the same case.

The Professional Conduct Committee must decide whether or not the midwife, nurse or health visitor is guilty of misconduct. A public announcement of the Committee's decision is made.

If the practitioner is found guilty of misconduct, the Committee may decide to:

1 postpone judgment (except where the practitioner has been found guilty of misconduct, when the hearing will be resumed at a later date);
2 remove the name of the person from the Central Council register;
3 issue a caution to the practitioner about expected future conduct; this is retained on their records for five years (the power to caution is contained in the 1992 Act);
4 take no further action, professional advice given.

Midwives, nurses or health visitors who have their names removed from the register are prohibited from practising, either for a specified period of time, or indefinitely. Where the period of time is identified, the practitioner may apply to have her/his name restored to the register in accordance with Rule 22.

The Health Committee is responsible for ascertaining whether or not a practitioner's health status may have contributed to an incident which has resulted in the individual's case being reported to the UK Central Council. This may include cases of alleged misconduct when the midwife, nurse or health visitor may have been under the influence of alcohol or drugs.

The power of interim suspension of registration is available to the Preliminary Proceedings Committee, the Health Committee and the Professional Conduct Committee. Strict procedures are laid down related to the exercise of this power, including three monthly reviews of suspension.

Formulation of rules relating to midwifery practice

The UK Central Council is responsible for the protection of the public who may come into contact with its practitioners, and for upholding the good name of the midwifery, nursing and health visiting professions in Britain. The Council therefore frames *Rules* to facilitate midwives (as well as fever nurses; Dimond, 1995: 42) to practise within specified boundaries. It is when an individual acts outside these parameters that they may be called before the Preliminary Proceedings Committee. Unlike the Codes of Practice, the Rules relating to midwifery practice are legally binding (although the Codes may be used in evidence in cases of alleged professional misconduct).

The Midwives' Rules (UKCC, 1993) identify the responsibilities of midwives and their sphere of practice, and specify requirements for the education of midwives, throughout the four countries of the United Kingdom.

Section A relates to the education of midwives, and specifies prerequisites for entry to midwifery education programmes including a minimum age of 17 years and six months, and the minimum educational requirements. Strict rules are laid down regulating the length and the broad content of initial midwifery education programmes, as well as the arrangements for students who interrupt their studies, or who wish to transfer to another educational institution. The National Boards must maintain an index of all student midwives, and are responsible for overseeing the conduct of assessments and examinations for midwives.

Section B sets out rules for midwives in practice, including the notification of intention to practise, statutory periodical refresher courses, and criteria for suspension from practice. Rule 40 sets out the responsibility and sphere of practice of midwives, and other rules relate to administration of medicines, record-keeping, the duty to be medically examined to prevent the spread of infection, and for inspection of the midwife's professional premises and equipment.

Rules 44 and 45 refer to criteria for appointments of supervisors of midwives and requirements of local supervising authorities in discharging their statutory functions (see below).

Midwifery Committee of the UK Central Council

Section 4(3) of the 1979 Nurses, Midwives and Health Visitors Act required the Central Council to establish two standing committees to provide specific advice to the Council: these are the *Finance Committee* and the *Midwifery Committee*. The UK Central Council Midwifery Committee was retained and enlarged under the 1992 Act, but the National Boards are no longer required to set up Midwifery Committees. Also, the UK Central Council is not required to consult the National Boards before acting on any reports of its Midwifery Committee, as the National Boards are now executive bodies. Other standing committees can only be constituted by the Secretary of State on the request of Council members.

The Midwifery Committee has increased in size since the implementation of the 1992 Act, and the majority of members must be practising midwives. There must now be at least eight practising midwives who are also Council members, plus two registered medical practitioners. Other members may be appointed who are not Central Council members, but the Chairman of the Committee must be a member of Council.

The Midwifery Committee must be consulted by Council on all matters related to midwifery, and 'the Committee shall, on behalf of the Council, discharge such of the Council's functions as are assigned to them either by the Council or the Secretary of State' (Nurses, Midwives and Health Visitors Act 1979, section 4(2)). The Acts also require Council to assign to the Midwifery Committee any proposals to make, alter or revoke rules relating to midwifery practice; similarly, the Secretary of State cannot approve rules relating to midwifery practice unless they are framed in accordance with recommendations of the Council's Midwifery Committee.

Non-statutory documents published by the UK Central Council

In addition to the publication of Rules governing practice, which are statutory instruments, other documents are published by the UK Central Council which are intended as advisory documents. However, midwives, nurses and health visitors should always work within the parameters set by these Codes, and in the event of a practitioner being called before the Preliminary Proceedings Committee, Health Committee or Professional Conduct Committee, failure to comply with the standards expounded in the documents could be used in evidence against the individual.

The UK Central Council publications are available to all midwives and act as a source of reference for their practice. These include:

▶ *The Midwife's Code of Practice* (UKCC, 1994) – defines the duties and activities of a midwife and sets out standards for practice, including clarification of the *Midwives' Rules* (UKCC, 1993) and issues related to relevant Acts of Parliament.

▶ *The Code of Professional Conduct* (UKCC, 1992a) relates to all midwives, nurses and health visitors and offers a code of conduct which is primarily aimed at protecting the public; the safety and interests of the patient and society are paramount and practitioners must act always in a manner which 'justifies public trust and confidence' and which 'upholds and enhances the good standing and reputation of the professions'.

▶ *The Scope of Professional Practice* (UKCC, 1992b) recognizes the diversity of practices which contribute to client care and facilitates midwives in expanding their roles to encompass new aspects of care, where they are in the interests of clients, whilst remaining cognisant of personal professional accountability. Dimond (1995: 44) discusses the implications for midwives of this document, suggesting that there is an indistinct division between the roles of midwives and obstetricians/paediatricians, and that midwifery practice is only constrained where Acts of Parliament require specific professionals to perform a duty, for example, abortion.

▶ *The Standards for the Administration of Medicines* (UKCC, 1992c) builds on basic principles considered during education for registration and advises practitioners on certain aspects pertaining to medicines which may arise during their practice.

▶ *Guidelines for Professional Practice* (UKCC, 1996) provides a guide for reflection on statments within the Code of Professional Conduct. It replaces and updates the information provided in the following documents: *Exercising Accountability* (1987); *Confidentiality* (1987); and *Advertising by Registered Nurses, Midwives and Health Visitors (1985)*.

▶ *With a View to Removal from the Register* (1990), and
▶ *Complaints about Professional Conduct* (UKCC, 1993) explain issues related to professional conduct.

National Boards

The National Boards of the four countries of the United Kingdom are responsible for the approval and monitoring of educational institutions and the provision of programmes of education for both the initial preparation of midwives, nurses and health visitors, and their continuing education and development. The Boards must ensure that any courses which they approve comply with the requirements of the UK Central Council as regards content and standard. This responsibility includes holding, or arranging for others to hold, examinations, where appropriate, now normally organized by approved educational institutions, since the devolution of the final examinations. The Boards are also responsible for providing support and guidance to Local Supervising Authorities on the supervision of midwives in accordance with UK Central Council Rules, and for any other functions relating to midwives, nurses and health visitors which are prescribed by the Secretary of State.

The functions of the National Boards in relation to midwifery are to:

1 approve institutions in relation to the provision of initial and continuing education of midwives.
2 ensure that education programmes meet the requirements of the UK Central Council as to their content and standard.
3 hold or arrange for institutions to hold examinations.
4 support and provide guidance on supervision of midwives to Local Supervising Authorities.
5 carry out other functions prescribed by the Secretary of State.

Local Supervising Authorities

The Regional Health Authorities in England, Area Health Authorities in Wales, Health Boards in Scotland, and Health and Social Services Boards in Northern Ireland have been the Local Supervising Authorities since 1974. On 1 April 1996, Health Authorities took over the responsibilities of Local Supervising Authorities due to reorganization of Regional Health Authorities. According to the English National Board (1995), a 'strong midwifery input' will be essential at Health Authority level to enable the Local Supervising Authority functions to be carried out effectively. The National Boards give advice and guidance to the Local Supervising Authorities related to the supervision of midwives but, according to the 1992 Act, must comply with the standards prescribed by the UK Central Council.

The functions of the Local Supervising Authorities are laid down in the *Nurses, Midwives and Health Visitors Acts* of 1979 and 1992 and the *Midwives Rules* of 1993.

The Local Supervising Authorities (LSAs) are responsible for (STRHA, 1994):

1 Supervision of all midwives working within the area of the LSA.
2 Reporting cases of alleged misconduct by midwives working within its area to the UK Central Council.
3 Suspending from practice any midwife who may be a source of infection, or, if appropriate, any midwife who has been reported by the LSA to the UK Central Council, or referred to either the Professional Conduct or Health Committee.
4 Receiving annual notifications of intention to practise from all midwives working within the LSA (which are forwarded to the UK Central Council), and ensuring that all midwives provide evidence of appropriate professional education within the last five years.
5 Provision of professional support for all midwives, with the appointment of local supervisors of midwives.
6 Ensuring that midwives comply with their statutory duties under the following acts:

– Births and Deaths Registration Acts 1926
– Notification of Births Act 1936
– Public Health Acts 1936 – Part VII Notification of Births
– Population Statistics Act (Causes of Stillbirths) 1960
– Misuse of Drugs Act 1971 and Amendments
– Congenital Disabilities (Care Liability) Act 1976
– Nursing Homes and Mental Homes Regulations 1981: (SI 1981/832 HC (81)B)

- The Children Act 1989
- Misuse of Drugs Regulations 1985: (SI 1985 No. 2066)
- Human Fertilisation and Embryology Act 1990.

SUPERVISION OF MIDWIVES

The LSA appoints appropriately qualified midwives as supervisors of midwives in a local area. Supervisors must be registered midwives, eligible to practise, and with a minimum of three years experience, of which at least one year must have been in the immediate past two years. Most supervisors are midwifery managers although there is a move towards senior clinical midwives and midwifery lecturers taking on supervisory duties. Managers who are supervisors of midwives can sometimes find themelves in conflict when they are trying to balance the economic demands of service provision with the legal requirements for safe midwifery practice.

Local supervisors work with a co-ordinating supervisor who is usually the head of the midwifery service. It is the intention of the UK Central Council that each supervisor is responsible for no more than 40 midwives.

All supervisors are required to undertake a course of preparation by distance learning produced by the English National Board (1992), which must be completed within the three years preceding appointment as a supervisor; these preparation courses are now accredited by an institution of higher education. Further instruction at intervals of not more than five years is also required (UKCC, 1993).

Duties of the supervisor of midwives include:

1   To receive from midwives over whom she exercises supervision their annual intention to practise forms and forward these to the LSA. The supervisor must at all times be able to identify every midwife working within the geographical district, including those employed in private institutions, educational establishments, agencies and those in independent practice.
2   To identify midwives from amongst those who have notified their intentions to practise who are in need of statutory refresher courses, including Return to Practice courses.
3   To ensure that all midwives maintain contemporaneous records, and to store the records of any midwife unable to do so for herself, for the man-

datory 25-year period. The supervisor also obtains records of any cases where medical aid has been summoned.
4   To provide midwives with a signed supply order form to enable them to obtain pethidine (or other permitted controlled drugs) which are necessary for their professional practice. The supervisor is responsible for checking the midwife's drug register, record of cases and her remaining stock of controlled drugs. The level of stock held by a midwife is determined by the supervisor, who should also ensure that the midwife is able to store drugs correctly. Any request from a midwife to surrender drugs to the pharmacist is made after authorization by the supervisor of midwives, who may also act as an authorized person for the destruction of a controlled drug (see Chapter 88).
5   To act as a 'friend' and support for midwives, offering professional advice and guidance, to enable them to achieve high standards of practice and ensure the safety of the mother and baby. The UK Central Council wishes to develop this aspect of the supervisor's role further, and to reduce the perceived emphasis on 'policing' of practice.

Conclusion

Midwifery is a profession where art and science blend together to make a fascinating, stimulating and interesting career. Midwives undergo a rigorous training, they are carefully selected and they are required to prove that they are maintaining and developing their knowledge and expertise.

(Greenwood, 1992)

Midwifery is unique amongst health professions in having a system of supervision which is determined in statute. Each midwife is personally accountable for her or his own practice, within the boundaries of the statutory framework. Supervisors of midwives not only act to ensure safe local standards of practice, but also to provide support and guidance for midwives. Supervisors report to the Local Supervising Authority which communicates directly with the UK Central Council. The National Boards are executive bodies who provide guidance to Local Supervisory Authorities on the supervision of midwives.

Midwives occupy a responsible and respected position in society and are privileged to attend childbearing women and their families. The statutory framework supports midwives in providing a safe and satisfying experience for childbearing women, and should be viewed as a constructive framework for good practice.

References

ENB (English National Board) (1992) *Preparation of Supervision of Midwives.* Distance learning pack. London: ENB.

ENB (1995) *Communication re: Transfer of Local Supervising Authority function from Regional Health Authorities DCL/11/MT/May.* London: ENB.

Dimond, B. (1995) *The Legal Aspects of Midwifery.* Hale: Books for Midwives Press.

Greenwood, J. (1992) *Supervision – the Whys and Wherefores. London: Association of Supervisors of Midwives.*

Peat Marwick McLintock (1989) *Review of the UKCC and Four National Boards for Nursing, Midwifery and Health Visiting.* London: Management Consultants Peat Marwick McLintock.

STRHA (South Thames Regional Health Authority) (1994) *Midwives' Arrangements for Supervision.* NHS Executive.

UKCC (UK Central Council for Nursing, Midwifery & Health Visiting) (1985) *Advertising by Nurses, Midwives and Health Visitors.* London: UKCC.

UKCC (1987) *Confidentiality.* London: UKCC.

UKCC (1989) *Exercising Accountability.* London: UKCC.

UKCC (1990) *. . . with a View to Removal From the Register?* London: UKCC.

UKCC (1992a) *Code of Professional Conduct for Nurses, Midwives and Health Visitors.* London: UKCC.

UKCC (1992b) *Standards for the Administration of Medicines.* London: UKCC.

UKCC (1992c) *The Scope of Professional Practice.* London: UKCC.

UKCC (1993) *Complaints about Professional Conduct.* London: UKCC.

UKCC (1993) *Midwives' Rules.* London: UKCC.

UKCC (1994) *The Midwife's Code of Practice.* London: UKCC.

UKCC (1995) *PREP and You.* London: UKCC.

UKCC (1996) *Guidelines for Professional Practice.* London: UKCC.

Further Reading

Butterworth, A. (1993) *Delphi Survey of Optimum Practice in Nursing, Midwifery and Health Visiting* (Executive Report). Manchester: University of Manchester.

Friedman, S. & Marr, J. (1995) A supervisory model of professional competence: a joint service/education initiative. *Nurse Education Today* **15**: 239–244.

Hawkins, C. & Shohet, P. (1989) *Supervision in the Helping Professions.* Milton Keynes: Open University Press.

NHS Management Executive (1993) *A Vision for the Future: The Nursing, Midwifery and Health Visiting Contribution to Health and Health Care.* London: Tavistock.

The Law and the Midwife

It is important that midwives should understand some of the basic principles of law, because so much of their practice is defined in terms of the law. Midwifery is governed by statute – the Nurses, Midwives and Health Visitors Act 1979, details of which are described in Chapter 84. Other chapters describe in detail other legislation that the midwife should be aware of: drugs legislation, legislation regarding the welfare of children, the abortion legislation and the law on assisted reproduction.

As well as statutory law, law is also created by judges when making decisions on cases. Case law provides the legal principles for negligence, consent to treatment and confidentiality that are important protections for users of the health services. As a practitioner, the midwife can be held personally accountable if these principles are disregarded.

This chapter describes the main sources and structures of the law. It briefly outlines the main legal principles relating to negligence, consent to treatment and health records. Differences between the English and Scottish legal systems are described.

How The Law is Created

PARLIAMENTARY LAW

Green and White Papers

Before starting the formal procedure for passing an Act of Parliament, the Government may consult on the content and effect of a future law or may publish its proposals for future legislation.

A consultation document on future legislation is called a *Green Paper*. This is designed to encourage public debate so that the Government can be guided on the way to frame proposed legislation. Green Papers are usually widely circulated in full or summary form to individuals and groups who have an interest in the proposed law. The *Health of the Nation* (DOH, 1992) was a recent example of a Green Paper.

A *White Paper* is a statement of intent about an impending Act. It does not invite consultation but gives Parliament and the public the opportunity to scrutinize its proposals. *Working for Patients* (DOH, 1989) was the White Paper that preceded the National Health Service and Community Care Act 1990.

Both these stages offer an opportunity for the public to influence the legislative process either by direct response to a Green Paper or by lobbying Members of Parliament (MPs) to consider submitting amendments to the legislation.

How an Act is passed

A Bill, which is a draft of proposed legislation, passes through three stages in the House of Commons and the House of Lords before it becomes law. The First Reading in the House of Commons briefly introduces the Bill; the Second Reading takes the form of a debate on its contents. After this it passes to an all-party committee which examines the content in detail amending it where necessary. As it has a majority on this committee, amendments are usually acceptable to the Government. From here the Bill passes to the House of Lords where it again has a First and Second Reading and a Committee Stage. It finally goes back to the House of Commons for a Third Reading and a vote is taken. If passed, it receives the Royal Assent and becomes an Act.

Primary and secondary legislation

An Act that passes through Parliament in this way is known as *primary legislation*. It can only be changed by the passing of another Act or amendment.

Much legislation however is very detailed and technical and may need frequent amendment. The use of *secondary legislation* simplifies this process. The Primary Act will be worded to allow for future changes to be made without detailed reference back to Parliament and will designate responsibility for the formulation of these changes. This subsequent secondary legislation is called a *Statutory Instrument*. When it has been prepared, it is presented to Parliament by the appropriate Secretary of State and is automatically passed. The *Midwives' Rules* are an example of this process. The primary legislation is the Nurses, Midwives and Health Visitors Act 1979. This Act gives responsibility to the United Kingdom Central Council (UKCC) to formulate Rules from time to time. The

Rules are then passed through Parliament as a Statutory Instrument.

A private member's bill

Most legislation is presented by the Government. However it is possible for an MP to introduce a Bill. The limited opportunity to do this is decided by ballot. Unless there is general agreement in Parliament to its principles, these Bills often fail to reach the Statute Book but it can be a useful way to introduce legislation which is difficult for a Government to support because of its sensitive or ethical nature. The 1967 Abortion Act is an example of this.

CASE LAW

Case law is developed by judges as they make their decisions on the cases they hear. There are certain rules which have developed to enable the operation of legal precedent.

A judge is bound by decisions of previous courts. This brings some certainty to the outcome of a case, although it is possible for a judge to decide that the facts of a case he or she is hearing are different from a previous, similar case, which can then be disregarded.

A judge is bound by decisions made in a higher court to the one in which he or she is sitting (Figure 1).

Case Law can be used to:

▶ create new law;
▶ amend existing law; or
▶ clarify the terms of a statute.

The person or organization bringing a case is called the *plaintiff* and the other party to the case, the *defendant*. Cases are reported with the name of the plaintiff first and the defendant second. Thus in a case against a health authority, the authority's name will appear second.

Many areas of the law now depend upon a mixture of case law and statute as the later section on negligence shows.

EUROPEAN LAW

European law is an increasingly important source of law, the basis of which is laid down in the Treaty of Rome. The United Kingdom became a signatory of the Treaty when it entered the Common Market. The Council of Ministers and the European Commission formulate European law. The European Parliament has

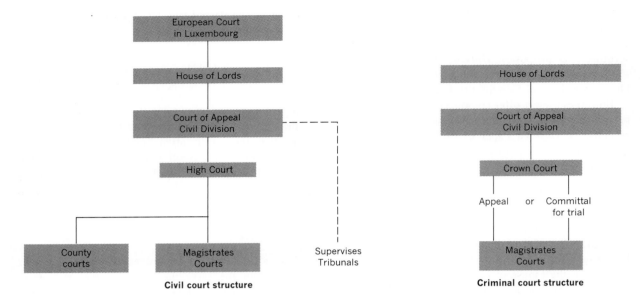

Figure 1   The English Court System.

a minor role in the process although this was strengthened in the 1993 Maastricht Treaty.

Community laws consist of Regulations and Directives. A *Regulation* applies immediately it is passed whereas member countries are required to change their laws to meet the requirements of *Directives*. European law can now override UK law with final reference to the European Court of Justice in Luxembourg. As an example, the Midwives Directive applies to all member states. In the UK it is incorporated into legislation in the Midwives' Rules.

The Structure of the Law

There are two main divisions within the legal system: civil law and criminal law. It is not always easy to define the difference between them, but generally the *civil law* deals with disputes between individuals and the *criminal law* with disputes between an individual and society. In some instances a problem can be referred to both systems. For example, assault can be either a civil or criminal offence.

Each system requires a different burden of proof. A criminal case requires proof beyond reasonable doubt. A civil case requires proof on balance given the circumstances of the case. Each system imposes different sanctions. The civil law usually awards damages whereas the criminal system imposes 'punishment' in the form of a custodial sentence, community service or a fine.

Civil law has many divisions including the law of contract which encompasses some principles of employment law; torts (civil wrongs) of negligence, nuisance and defamation; family law, administrative law, commercial law and property law. Each system relies upon its own hierarchical court structure (Figure 1).

Fortunately it is rare for health service cases to go to the criminal courts. Litigation cases are civil matters. Whether they are heard in the County Court or the High Court depends upon the possible level of damages that might be paid out.

Before a case is heard the lawyers for the defendants and the plaintiff meet, exchange all relevant information and attempt to reach a settlement. Most cases are settled before a formal trial. Cases go to court if there is a continuing dispute over the facts or the liability of the defendant. They may also go to court if the facts are not disputed but there is no agreement about the level of damages to be paid.

The coroner's court

This court examines the circumstances of suspicious deaths to determine the cause of death. 'Suspicious' can be interpreted widely and includes unexplained deaths in hospital. A coroner is medically or legally qualified and in some cases will sit with a jury.

Occasionally midwives are called to give evidence at a coroners court. They will be there as a witness and may not be represented in court, although they are often supported by their professional organization.

Tribunals

Court cases can be complex, lengthy and costly. For many matters of a technical nature it is now more usual to go to a tribunal. Tribunals hear disputes specific to their sphere of responsibility. Hearings are more informal than in court and it takes less time for problems to be resolved. Typically a tribunal consists of a Chairman who may be legally qualified and two other members who are experts in the relevant field. Some examples are industrial tribunals, medical appeals tribunals and rent tribunals.

Legal personnel

The Lord Chancellor This is the highest legal appointment in the UK. As President of the House of Lords and a member of the Cabinet, he advises Government on legal matters and appoints judges and magistrates.

Barristers These legally trained personnel have the right to argue cases in all levels of court. Judges in the higher courts are always barristers by training, as are most lower court judges.

Solicitors These legally trained personnel offer a range of legal services although many of them specialize, some in health service related work. They give legal advice and offer services such as conveyancing and will executorship. They do the preparation work before a case comes to court. Solicitors can be appointed as lower court judges and can present cases in these courts. Health Authorities and Trusts usually receive their legal advice from solicitors employed by the Regional Offices or from officially appointed firms of solicitors.

Magistrates Justices of the Peace are appointed by the Lord Chancellor. They hear first level criminal cases. They also have powers to issue emergency child protection orders.

The Legal System in Scotland

The courts and court officers differ in Scotland. The highest criminal court is the High Court of Justiciary and the highest civil court, the Court of Session. Scotland is divided into six sheriffdoms each with a sheriff's court and 49 districts each with a district court.

The principal law officer in Scotland is the Lord Advocate. The Procurator Fiscal is responsible for all prosecutions in the sheriff and district courts and for the investigation of all suspicious deaths. There is no separate coroner's court in Scotland.

Negligence

There is a legal principle that people have a duty not to harm others. If their negligence causes harm, the person who is hurt may apply to the courts to obtain damages as recompense. Rules governing the operation of negligence claims have been developed mainly through case law. In a famous case (*Donoghue* v. *Stevenson* 1932) Lord Atkin set out these rules:

> You must take reasonable care to avoid acts or omissions which you can reasonably foresee would be likely to injure your neighbour. Who then in law is my neighbour? the answer seems to be – persons who are so closely and directly affected by my act that I ought reasonably to have them in contemplation as being so affected when I am directing my mind to the acts or omissions which are called in question.

For a case to be successful, three conditions must be met:

1 there must be an existing duty of care;
2 a breach in that duty of care must be proved; and
3 the breach must have caused damage.

In almost all circumstances professionals have a duty of care towards the people they are looking after. This is rarely disputed in a court action. Proving they have failed in that duty usually depends on identifying a reasonable standard of care and assessing whether they have fallen below that standard. The judgment in the case of *Bolam* v. *Friern Hospital Management Committee* (1957) described how that standard of care should be defined:

where you get a situation which involves the use of some special skill or competence, then the test as to whether there has been negligence . . . is the standard of the ordinary skilled man exercising and professing to have that special skill.

To decide whether a professional has met the standard of the ordinary practitioner, the court uses the evidence of expert witnesses from the relevant profession.

Showing the link between a negligent act and subsequent damage is not always easy but must be proved if damages are to be awarded. It is not always possible for example, to link a child's cerebral palsy with poor management in labour. It may have been caused by antenatal events outside the control of the professionals.

Congenital Disability (Civil Liability) Act 1976

This is an example where statutory law and case law contribute to an overall legal principle. Until this Act was passed only living people could sue for negligence. That the fetus had no rights was highlighted when children affected by thalidomide were unable to sue the pharmaceutical company.

This Act gives the child limited rights to sue for negligence occurring before its birth. The main provisions of the Act are that:

▶ A fetus enjoys a duty of care if there is a pre-existing duty of care towards its mother and may therefore sue for damages.
▶ It may not sue if either or both its parents knew of a pre-conception risk, although it may sue its father if he knew of such a risk but its mother did not.
▶ It may not sue its mother except if she was negligent when driving a car.

The baby and Legal Aid

Legal Aid is available to children in their own right. Their finances are assessed independently of their parents when deciding whether to grant aid. As most children have no money of their own, most obtain aid which greatly facilitates their access to the law.

THE LIABILITY OF THE MIDWIFE

As independently accountable practitioners, midwives are liable for their actions when caring for clients. This liability exists whether they are employed or self-employed and they can be personally sued if they have been negligent.

The liability of the student midwife

If properly trained and competent in a procedure, students are liable for their actions. In the case of *Wilsher* v. *Essex Area Health Authority* (1988), however, it was established that students have the right to be supervised properly and have their work checked. The professional responsible for a student would be negligent if this supervision were not provided and a client suffered damage as a result. Equally if a health service failed to provide a system of supervision for students it could be held liable.

Vicarious liability

This legal principle allows a third party to indemnify the actions of others under certain circumstances. The law allows that an employer may be vicariously liable for the actions of his or her employees and that a partner may be liable for the actions of other partners.

Midwives and other professionals in the National Health Service are indemnified by the NHS. A person bringing a case is more certain to obtain financial recompense from an employer, so the employer is commonly sued, hence the cases quoted in this chapter name Health Authorities rather than individuals. This does not, however, protect the professional from being described as negligent in court.

OBSTETRIC LITIGATION

There has been an increase in obstetric litigation in recent years which has affected both obstetricians and midwives, but it should be emphasized that these cases are still rare and that most practitioners will never find themselves involved in litigation. For those who are, it can be a difficult experience and some knowledge about what happens can help to allay anxiety.

If a woman claims that negligence has occurred, her solicitors will first make contact with the Authority or Trust managers. Midwives first hear from them that there is a case pending. They are then asked by the employer's legal advisers to make a statement. Statements should always be prepared with reference to the case notes and with a copy of the first complaint available. The manager should be asked to obtain both of these. Often cases are brought some years after the event and midwives would be very unwise to rely on their memory of the events. They should also seek the immediate advice of their professional organization. When the statement is complete, this along with the case notes and any other relevant information becomes part of the evidence.

At this stage the lawyers for the two parties meet and try to reach a settlement out of court. This is the usual outcome and the midwife will hear no more about it. This does not, however, mean that midwives will not be disciplined by their employers if practice has fallen below standard, nor does it protect them from having their names forwarded to the United Kingdom Central Council. Each course of action can be taken independently of the other.

If the case comes to court, invariably it will be the Authority who is the defendant and will be represented. The professionals involved will be there as witnesses. Although witnesses do not have the right to representation, it is usual for the midwives to have support from their professional organization. The Authority's lawyers will also be there to give advice. When giving evidence, witnesses are able to seek advice and clarification from the trial judge.

AVOIDING LITIGATION

Litigation can occur when a woman or her family believe they have sustained damage because of the actions of a health care professional. The first way to avoid litigation and one clearly in the public interest, is to practise according to the recognized standard of the 'ordinary skilled practitioner'. To do this, midwives should be able to relate any of the care given to relevant research or good empirical evidence. They should be confident that, if asked, a significant number of their colleagues would agree with the clinical care they have given.

A number of defences fail, not because the midwives' actions are unacceptable, but because they cannot prove what they did as their record-keeping is poor. Notes should not just contain facts such as monitoring outcomes but should reflect any clinical decisions made and the reasons for them. This would include decisions not to act as well as decisions to do something. For example, a midwife may see an irregularity in a cardiotocograph recording but decide to watch it for a while before calling for a doctor. The decision not to call a doctor, and why it was taken, should be noted.

Practising according to acceptable standards and making good records do not necessarily protect the woman or her baby from an adverse pregnancy outcome. They should ensure that any health problems are not caused by the actions of the practitioner and that the practitioner can prove this to be the case.

Professional indemnity insurance

To give themselves additional protection, professionals frequently take out insurance to meet claims made against them. Although there is no legal requirement to be insured, there is a moral obligation to offer such cover. This is particularly the case when a midwife is self-employed. Indemnity insurance can often be obtained through membership of a professional organization, but this is not always the case (RCM, 1996).

Consent to Treatment

Consent must always be obtained before any treatment is given. If not obtained the professional may be prosecuted for criminal assault, or the patient may sue for assault under civil law. This applies not just to invasive treatments but to anything a professional does for a patient which involves physical contact.

Consent can be given in three ways:

1 Written consent.
2 Verbal consent.
3 Implied consent.

The law accepts all three as equal although verbal and implied consent are more difficult to prove. When obtained for difficult or invasive treatment, it is wise for the midwife to record such consent in her notes. She should make her own judgement about when to record consent. For example, she would not be expected to record implied consent for blood pressure estimation, but should record verbal or implied consent to an episiotomy.

A prerequisite of obtaining valid consent is that the person has had sufficient information about the implications of the treatment to be able to make a free choice about treatment.

Who may give consent

Any adult of sound mind may give consent to treatment. In the case of children, if they are able to understand the implications of the treatment, they may also give consent even if their parents do not agree.

If a woman's judgement is impaired because she has had drugs or is unconscious, it will be for the professional to decide whether she is capable of giving consent. In such circumstances it would be wise to discuss the treatment with the woman's partner, but consent given by someone else is not legally accepted. If consent cannot be obtained and immediate treatment is required for the woman's future well-being, the law recognizes the defence of 'necessity' and under this protection the professional should continue with the treatment.

Just as people of sound mind may give consent, they may also withhold consent. If a woman withholds consent to treatment, even if it may be harmful to her unborn child, the law upholds the woman's rights over that of her baby.

Giving information

Although consent should be obtained as near to the time when the treatment is to be carried out, it is possible to give information and advice about possible treatments when the woman is pregnant. In its booklet on consent to treatment (DOH, 1990) the Department states:

> It is important that the proposed care is discussed with the woman, preferably in the early antenatal period, when any special wishes she expresses should be recorded in the notes, but of course the patient may change her mind about these issues at any stage, even in labour.

Problems relating to consent

There may be problems in obtaining consent: a woman's judgement impaired by pethidine; a child who does not understand the proposed treatment; a woman making an inappropriate decision even though the implications have been explained. In these and similar circumstances, the midwives should carefully record the facts in their notes and at the earliest opportunity discuss the problem with the supervisor of midwives. The action taken when trying to obtain consent, the information given to help the woman make her decision and the reasons why consent was not obtained should all be recorded. Any subsequent course of action, including when and with whom the problem was discussed, should also be noted in the midwifery record.

The Law Relating to Health Records

Confidentiality

Health professionals have a duty to keep information that they have obtained from their clients confidential. If they break confidentiality they may be sued for negligently communicating information.

There are exceptions to this. Information may be passed on:

- ▶ if the person consents to it;
- ▶ on a 'need to know' basis. This applies to giving clinical information to other health service staff so that they can properly look after patients;
- ▶ because there is a statutory obligation – the notification of communicable diseases comes under this category;
- ▶ if required by a court: the Supreme Court Act 1981 requires that medical notes should be available to the court and lawyers when there is a case pending;
- ▶ in the public interest. This is seldom used, but would apply if a professional became aware of a serious criminal offence. It may apply to reporting suspected child abuse.

If a midwife is required to give clinical information in court, she should seek guidance from her employer's legal advisers about how much she may safely divulge.

Ownership of medical records

The medical and midwifery record belongs to the person or institution that produces the document on which the record is made. Records used in the NHS belong to the NHS, while the record made by a self-employed midwife or a record made by a midwife and kept privately by her, belongs to the midwife. Records do not belong to the patient even though they may be carried by women using the maternity services.

The format of medical records

The law does not require any specific format for medical records which may be manually or electronically created and stored. The midwife is required by the Rules to keep records, but again the format is not defined. In its document on record-keeping (UKCC, 1993) the UKCC states that records can be held as paper or computer records, but the usual rules of confidentiality must be preserved.

Medical record: patient's rights

The Access to Health Records Act 1993 gives people the right to see their medical records. Information which is likely to cause serious harm or which identifies a third party may be withheld. If this is the case, the professional who generated the information (who may be a midwife) should be consulted when deciding what can be disclosed and what should be withheld.

References

Bolam v. *Friern Hospital Management Committee* (1957) 2 All ER 118, (1957) 1 WLR 582.

DOH (Department of Health) (1989) *Working for Patients.* London: HMSO.

DOH (1990) *A Guide to Consent for Examination or Treatment.* Health Circular HC (90) 22. London: DOH.

DOH (1992) *The Health of the Nation: a Strategy for Health in England.* London: HMSO.

Donoghue v. *Stevenson* (1932) AC 562.

Royal College of Midwives (RCM) (1996) Response of the RCM to criticisms regarding independent midwives' insurance. *Midwives* **109**: 63–64.

UKCC (United Kingdom Central Council) (1993) *Standards for Records and Record Keeping.* London: UKCC.

Wilsher v. *Essex Area Health Authority* (1988) 1 All ER 871, (1988) 2 WLR 557.

Further Reading

Dimond, B. (1994) *The Legal Aspects of Midwifery.* Hale: Books for Midwives Press.

Jenkins, E.R. (1994) *The Law and The Midwife.* Oxford: Blackwell Scientific.

Mason, D., Edwards, P. & Capstick, B. (1993) *Litigation. A Risk Management Guide for Midwives.* London: Royal College of Midwives.

The Midwife and her Education

It has been said that midwifery is the oldest profession in the world. Certainly from the beginning of time, women have been producing offspring. Initially, personal experience was the only means they had of knowing what childbirth was all about. Today this would be called 'experiential learning' and it was this which equipped some mothers to help other women deliver their babies. Unfortunately such knowledge is always subjective, and these 'handy women' as they were known, did not always act wisely or well. History abounds with examples of unhelpful, if not dangerous, practices which developed through women, such as these, assuming power and passing on their 'wisdom' in the form of folklore; traditional remedies and potions; cutural ritual and superstitious customs. Some of these traditions still hold sway in parts of the world today.

Charles Dickens, in an attempt to alert British society to the plight of the poor, immortalized the midwives of his day, by caricaturing them as 'Sairey Gamp', in his classic novel *Martin Chuzzlewit*. During the nineteenth century, doctors became increasingly concerned about the high maternal and perinatal mortality rates. These were attributed to the standard of

care being given to mothers, especially those who delivered their babies at home and were too poor to afford the services of a doctor. The London Obstetrical Society therefore considered it worth their while to initiate a three-month training for women wishing to assist mothers in childbirth. Although a certificate of proficiency was awarded, it was recognized that the numbers involved were very small, so the effect of these midwives on the standard of maternity care overall was negligible.

It was against this backdrop that the Midwives' Institute started to campaign for the legalization of midwifery practice. Their objective was eventually achieved for England and Wales in 1902, with the passing of the first Midwives Act. Other parts of the United Kingdom were to attain registration of midwifery practice at a later date: Scotland in 1915 and Ireland in 1918. Given the situation at that time, it is not surprising that the purpose of this legislation was 'to safeguard the public' from the practices of uneducated and untrained women, who continued to assist those who were too poor to pay for medical care during childbirth.

The Central Midwives' Board, established by the

1902 Act, was charged by Government with responsibility for training midwives and conducting their examinations. This was no mean task when it is realized that many 'bona fide' midwives at that time were not able to read or sign their name. Many had to supply a thumb print or signature by proxy. The initial training established by the Board lasted just three months. Antenatal care was not known at this time and midwives were called only when the mother went into labour. They continued to visit her and supervise feeding and care of the baby during the postnatal period. Training concluded with a three-hour written midwifery exam and a 15-minute viva conducted by an obstetrician.

Length of training was increased to six months in 1916, but anyone already qualified as a nurse was granted a two-month exemption. Ten years later, non-nurses or 'direct entrants' had to undergo 12 months of training. It would appear that by this time, length and content of training was at last keeping pace with the standard of knowledge and degree of practical proficiency required. However, in 1938, midwifery training was separated into two parts:

► *Part 1*, 12 months for non-nurses and six months for registered nurses, consisted of midwifery and obstetric theory and hospital-based practice.
► *Part 2*, a further six months for all, was essential if midwifery was to be practised professionally.

However, this latter six months was frequently not undertaken by many who wished to have a midwifery qualification for career purposes only, such as entry into health visiting. It consisted mostly of clinical experience based in the community with some lectures from the Local Medical Officer of Health. Examinations at this time included practical assessment and submission of a set number of case histories.

Single-period midwifery training was established in 1968, by which time the so-called medicalization of midwifery was well underway. This training lasted 12 months for registered nurses, and 24 months for non-nurses. The change in format was intended to enable the curriculum to mirror practice and allow 'normal' midwifery to be mastered before student midwives (formerly pupil midwives) moved on to study more complicated obstetrics.

However by 1980, in line with other European countries, it was necessary to increase midwifery training to 18 months for registered nurses. Three years was required for the diminishing number of pre-registration student midwives to assimilate the vast amount of

new knowledge and gain sufficient experience in practical skills related to new technologies. Practical midwifery examinations were discontinued in favour of a 20-minute 'discussion' with a midwife teacher. Written examinations were set nationally and consisted of two three-hour papers in midwifery/obstetric practice and neonatal paediatrics respectively. A set number of 'doctors' lectures' were still required by the Board, although obstetricians and paediatricians eventually stopped marking examination papers.

The increase in the length and content of midwifery training was mirrored by a reduction in the time student nurses spent learning about maternal and child care. A 12-week obstetric course had been introduced into general nurse training in the early 1960s. Eventually this was made compulsory, but it decreased first to eight weeks and later to just four weeks, largely because it was not possible to accommodate the large number of nursing students in maternity wards and the community, when this was made compulsory for all nursing students.

Winds of Change – Setting the Scene for the Future

In 1970 the Peel Report (DHSS, 1970) was published with its recommendation for 100% hospital confinement. Its implementation reinforced medical domination of the maternity services, continued existing patterns of care practices and confirmed obstetric policies already in operation. Twenty years later, a medical statistician was to demonstrate the false assumptions on which this report had been based (Tew, 1990). By this time, however, midwifery care and organization of the maternity services had been moulded by the far-ranging effect of this influential report.

In 1974, Sir Keith Joseph, Minister of Health, introduced a major reorganization of the Health Service, the National Health Service Reorganisation Act 1974, which resulted in the creation of a unified and integrated midwifery service. This helped to accelerate the development of midwifery as a profession, by uniting the three previously distinct parts of the tripartite maternity services:

1 the domiciliary midwifery service under the control of local health authorities;

2   the hospital midwifery services administered by central government; and

3   the general practitioners' services.

Nursing education at this time was undertaken in schools organized separately from their clinical areas. Midwifery education, however, continued to be the responsibility of the midwifery manager. Although this may have caused some conflicts of interest for midwife teachers working under managers with little or no education background, generally it was a very satisfactory arrangement which worked well for the education of midwives and the organization of care given to mothers and their babies.

It was about this time that national and international legislation challenged the female-only concept of midwifery being 'woman with woman' in childbirth. A pilot scheme for potential male midwives proved successful and as male midwives were found to be equally acceptable as women to most mothers, the female stranglehold on midwifery was broken. In 1983, in response to the Sex Discrimination Act (1975) and the EEC Midwives Directives (EEC, 1980) based on the non-discriminatory Treaty of Rome, all restrictions on men practising midwifery were lifted. However, the majority of midwives and student midwives in training continued to be women.

Another report which was to have a significant effect on the direction which nursing and midwifery education were to take was published in 1972 by the Committee on Nursing (Briggs Report). They recommended that 'nursing [including midwifery] must become a research based profession'. At that time research by midwives was almost unheard of and the curriculum made little or no reference to whatever obstetric and paediatric research was available.

The Nurses, Midwives and Health Visitors Act (1979) arose out of recommendations made by the Committee on Nursing (1972). It made possible the incorporation of the Central Midwives' Board and eight other statutory bodies into a new United Kingdom Central Council. Separate but related National Boards for each of the four countries in the UK were also established and came into being in 1983. Keen to establish the academic credibility of health care and raise the professional status of practitioners, the UKCC launched 'Project 2000'. This was their blueprint for educating nurses and equipping them to meet the changing demands of the next millennium.

The original UKCC vision entailed a 'Common Foundation Programme' where student nurses, whatever their specialty, and student midwives, would learn core subjects, such as health sciences, approaches to care and interpersonal skills, together. After 18 months, specialization into separate 'branches' would occur. It was initially suggested that one of these branches should be 'Midwifery'. However, this would have relegated midwifery to being a 'branch' of nursing and not a profession in its own right, with a distinct history, different philosophy and defined legal parameters for practice. After a well-fought battle, midwifery was eventually recognized as a separate, though allied, profession to nursing. Pre-registration training for nurses and midwives remains distinct, although shared learning, as opposed to common core education, does take place.

The impact of Project 2000 on education for nurses was enormous. It was a catalyst for midwifery, helping to crystallize the decision to make pre-registration midwifery the model of education for the future. This had a number of advantages. It fitted in well with European requirements, where very few practitioners in European countries hold both qualifications. It avoided a great deal of repetition, allowing considerable savings in the time and cost of midwifery education. The most important outcome, however, was that it strengthened the uniqueness of the midwife and confirmed the distinctness of midwifery as a profession.

The new pre-registration midwifery curriculum enabled student midwives to learn the philosophy and absorb the ethos of midwifery from the outset. It was no longer necessary for would-be midwives to train as nurses and become socialized into nursing culture before having to commence midwifery education, with its emphasis on health, normality and midwife autonomy.

Another change to be introduced by the UKCC was the decentralization of education for nursing and midwifery. This meant that each nursing and/or midwifery training institution approved by a National Board became responsible for designing its own curriculum and setting, marking and moderating its own clinical and theoretical assessments.

At the same time, an attempt was made to standardize all health care education courses and bring them in line with higher education. Certificate level, the equivalent of former nursing and midwifery courses, corresponded with the first year of a university degree course. The new education courses were set at a minimum of diploma level, that is similar to the second year of a degree course. Degree courses in nursing and midwifery had been in existence for some time, and were already the equivalent of a university honours degree. However, from 1990 onwards, nurses and midwives qualifying with a Diploma in Higher Education (Nursing or Midwifery) or a specialist degree as well as a professional qualification, became the rule rather than the exception.

In order to cope with this enormous development, it was necessary for tutors and clinical midwives to be developed further in order to meet the training demands of the new practitioner. Experienced midwives needed to apply themselves to research appreciation and study of the behavioural sciences while midwifery tutors began to study for degrees in midwifery or related subjects or higher degrees and doctorates in midwifery studies. The statutory bodies are working towards a graduate status for all practitioners for the next millennium (ENB, personal communication).

Given this scenario, it was probably inevitable that midwifery and nurse education were required to move out of the health service into institutions of higher education. Although this has undoubted advantages in education terms, the close link between midwifery practice and education has been severed. This can only be detrimental to the quality of education provided. An old maxim states 'every midwife is a teacher' and in many ways this is correct. Midwifery, unlike nursing, never had clinical teachers. All midwives were expected to transfer their skills to students by teaching in the clinical environment all the time. However, as new knowledge became available, new research was undertaken with implications for practice and a more flexible practitioner was required. It became increasingly difficult for clinical midwives to keep up to date with the theoretical demands of teaching. Similarly, teachers separated from the clinical areas, quickly lost their practical skills so that the theory–practice interface in education is in danger of becoming even weaker.

Although the move of midwifery education into higher education establishments can be justified in education terms, and will help to raise the credibility of midwifery education for both midwifery teachers and practitioners, the resulting dichotomy between education and clinical midwifery will need to be evaluated before the profession enters its second century. The advent of trust status and new management structures in the National Health Service has further reduced the voice of midwifery within the health care

debate, because due to smaller numbers, midwives are sometimes not adequately represented at management meetings. However, the approved midwife teacher, usually the senior midwife educator in an ENB Approved Midwifery Training Institution, has been granted special powers so that she may report direct to the Chief Executive or Head of the College or University. This provision is helping to safeguard the rights of midwives and the provision and quality of midwifery education for the future.

Finally, although the NHS and Community Care Act 1990 did not have a major impact on midwifery practice as such, this legislation did help to create an entirely new climate which set the scene for further changes in midwifery education. The Act authorized and accelerated an existing trend whereby normal care of low-risk mothers can be undertaken in the community, leaving hospital settings available for high-risk or complicated obstetrics.

This in turn created the necessary conditions for the implementation of *Changing Childbirth* (DOH, 1993) where the three concepts of 'choice' and 'control' for mothers and 'continuity' of care by a named midwife (*Patients' Charter*, House of Commons, 1993), will have major implications for the management of the maternity services and thereby for the organization of student midwife education.

The Current Situation

INITIAL MIDWIFERY EDUCATION

There are two possible routes by which a midwife may be admitted to Part 10 of the UKCC Professional Register:

1 A non-nurse may complete a pre-registration midwifery course lasting a minimum of three years in order to receive a Registered Midwife qualification.
2 A Registered Nurse (adult branch) may undertake a further 18-month period of practical and theoretical education before being able to practise as a midwife (pre-registration, shortened programme).

Either of these routes may result in the award of a diploma or a degree depending on the nature of the course undertaken. The midwifery practice competencies to be achieved are identical. In addition to essential midwifery, obstetric and neonatal paediatric theory, the curriculum also includes the application of the behavioural and biological sciences to midwifery, research appreciation and the study of medical ethics.

The philosophy of midwifery education differs fundamentally from that underpinning nursing. It is now generally accepted that childbirth is a normal human function, which is often planned and usually undertaken by parents who are themselves healthy. For this reason any model of care or education that is sickness-orientated is totally inappropriate.

Similarly, because each midwife is an autonomous practitioner who is fully accountable for a legally defined sphere of professional practice, any medically orientated framework of care or education is also unsuitable.

The clientele of midwifery are mostly responsible adults who have a right to be able to make further decisions about the management of the pregnancy, labour and care of the child they have conceived. For this reason the role of the midwife is usually that of educator/assistant, working in partnership with parents, and able to provide total care for each one in any available setting (UKCC, 1993).

The organization of midwifery differs markedly from that of nursing. Although education is no longer under the umbrella of midwifery management, midwifery hospital and community services are fully integrated, and likely to become more so as the recommendations of *Changing Childbirth* (DOH, 1993) are implemented. This will have significant effects on the pattern of midwifery education, the relation of theory to practice and the organization of clinical experience for student midwives.

The UKCC (1994b) *Report of the Future of Professional Practice and Education* also distinguishes between nursing and midwifery. 'Specialist practice' is not recognized in midwifery as it is in nursing. A midwife is competent to practise from the date of registration. The only additional skill she is required to acquire is the topping up of epidural analgesia, although all midwives must gain competence in new skills and technologies as they become available (UKCC, 1994a). The midwife therefore progresses from a safe competent practitioner to one whom, with further practice and continuing education, gains increased knowledge and expert skill (Benner, 1986).

Consequently, post-basic and continuing education in midwifery contains some features that are different from nursing and other health care professions. For nurses after registration there are two levels of qualification recordable on the UKCC register, those of specialist and advanced practice. Midwives giving continuity of care to a caseload of clients need to increase their knowledge and skills in all areas of practice, rather than developing specialist skills. Therefore for midwives after registration, there is only one level of recordable qualification on the register and that is Advanced Practice. Continuing education programmes below advanced level will be essential.

CONTINUING PROFESSIONAL EDUCATION IN MIDWIFERY

PREP

The UKCC introduced its Post-Registration Education and Practice (PREP) project in 1990. After consultation with the professions and some modification, the implementation started in April 1995. PREP includes three major sets of requirements:

1 a period of support under the guidance of a preceptor for newly qualified midwives;
2 maintenance of effective registration;
3 specialist qualifications (UKCC, 1995).

Preceptors In the UKCC Model for Nursing and Midwifery Practice, primary practice 'begins at the point of registration and is the period in which the midwife can assume responsibility for meeting patient, client and health care needs competently' (UKCC, 1993). However in order to enable practitioners to achieve confidence in the early months of registered practice a preceptor will be appointed to act as a role model in day-to-day practice. The period of support is expected to be between 3 and 6 months depending on the practitioner's experience and ability. This will be concluded when the practitioner can satisfy herself and the preceptor that she can meet the criteria for primary practice, that is

> accept responsibility with confidence, in cooperation with other practitioners and disciplines required, for the individual's or groups' health care needs. This involves care which is comprehensive, appropriate and where possible, research based. (UKCC, 1991)

Midwives selected to act as preceptors will have 'substantial' clinical experience and associated experiential knowledge. They will need to demonstrate appropriate teaching, supervision and assessment skills. To achieve this expertise, specialist preparation and practice opportunities will be developed and provided by midwife educators, who will need to be satisfied that potential preceptors have been effectively equipped to fulfil competently the role that is required of them.

Maintenance of registration Initially, midwives working in isolated situations could keep up to date with increasing skills and knowledge by attending postcertificate courses. Recognizing this need, the third Midwives Act of 1936 was ahead of its time by providing for a mandatory, five-day, residential refresher course for all practising midwives. Midwives who failed to complete such a course within each five-year period had their names removed from the roll. The distinct nature of midwifery practice has meant that former post-basic midwifery education was designed to meet statutory requirements for continuing education (in the form of refresher courses). It did not need to utilize the acquisition of specific skills achieved through specialist courses.

The UKCC (1993) has recently introduced a similar updating requirement for nurses and health visitors, although provision of funding to enable its implementation has not been made available. From April 1995, each practitioner must attend five study days in each three-year period in order to be allowed to re-register with the UKCC. These study days are required to cover five identified areas:

1 Reducing risk.
2 Care enhancement.
3 Education development.
4 Practice development.
5 Patient/client and colleague support.

This overall model of statutory continuing education is also to be adopted for midwives. However, an important new development is that study days can be utilized for individual study. Thus a midwife could visit 'a centre of clinical excellence or spend a day in a professional library' (UKCC, 1993).

Midwifery refresher courses Until the new arrangements are fully introduced, every midwife is still required to maintain her practice by undertaking a week-long, National Board approved, midwifery refresher course within each five-year period. Alternatively, with the approval of her supervisor of midwives, a midwife may accumulate seven National Board

approved midwifery-related study days within a five-year period.

Other National Board approved refresher courses available to midwives in England are:

1 *A practice-based refresher course*: This is a two-week period, designed for midwives who have been specializing in a particular aspect of midwifery, such as antenatal clinic or neonatal special/intensive care. It enables them to update their clinical skills in delivery suite or the community, for example. Similarly it is an ideal opportunity for midwifery tutors to practise what they teach! A learning contract is developed between the supervisor of midwives, the midwifery tutor and the individual midwife, which will identify specific theory and related practice relevant to each midwife's needs and interests.

2 *Return to Midwifery Practice course*: Midwives who have allowed their registration to lapse, for whatever reason, can only have their names re-entered on the professional register by undertaking a Return to Midwifery Practice Course. The length of this is determined by the National Board and depends on the period of time during which the midwife has been 'out of practice'. The theory and practice components of the course can be tailor-made to suit individual requirements. The approved midwife teacher and supervisor of midwives will notify the Board and UKCC only when they and the midwife are satisfied with his/her competence, confidence and knowledge of current midwifery practice and related research-based theory. At the present time such courses are few and far between. Therefore it is important that midwifery registration is maintained if at all possible, otherwise it may be very difficult for a name to be restored to Part 10 of the register.

National Board approved courses, such as the 'Teaching and Assessing in Clinical Practice', 'Advanced Diploma in Midwifery' and 'Special and Intensive Care of the Newborn', have given midwives remission from attending a refresher course for a further five years.

Advanced midwifery practice The integrated nature of the midwifery service requires midwives to provide safe, effective, total care for mothers in all settings. As changes and developments in practice occur, they are incorporated into initial preparation of the midwife. Qualified midwives, however, are required to maintain their own education and practice (UKCC, 1993) through recognized midwifery programmes for professional development and other relevant further education opportunities.

Advanced midwifery practice, therefore, is not concerned with acquiring specialist competencies, but with the development of future practice by pioneering and developing new roles responsive to changing needs and, with advancing clinical practice, research and education, aiming to enrich professional midwifery practice as a whole (UKCC, 1994b).

It is anticipated that midwives who have attained the UKCC recordable qualification of advanced practitioner will make a contribution to health policy and management and assist with the process of determining the health needs of mothers and babies. To do this, advanced midwives will need to have developed management skills and be effective in co-ordinating midwifery and multidisciplinary teams as well as deploying resources cost effectively. They will be required to implement and evaluate standards of care and quality assurance programmes. Advanced midwives will also need to be thoroughly grounded in the principles of research in order to assist with the identification, initiation, collation, utilization and dissemination of published research relevant to midwifery practice.

From a more clinical perspective, advanced midwives will undertake counselling, teaching and supervisory skills, and be responsible for ensuring an effective learning experience and environment for students of midwifery. It will be the responsibility of advanced midwives to identify development needs for themselves and others as well as providing appropriate support and encouragement for practice initiatives to be fostered and implemented.

To achieve the combined level of knowledge and skill necessary to meet the requirements of an advanced practitioner, additional education will be essential. This is unlikely to take the form of a specific course but may incorporate clinical projects, as with the English National Board Framework and Higher Award or consist of a variety of individually selected academic modules. The resulting credit is expected to be equivalent to a Masters Level qualification.

Credit for Prior Academic Learning (APL) and Experiential Learning (APEL)

It is not difficult to appreciate that the changes being introduced into midwifery education as a result of the

UKCC initiatives are having a profound effect on existing midwifery practitioners. As the academic climate and requirements increase it has become evident that being updated in midwifery practice alone is insufficient. All qualified midwives need to be research minded and able to appreciate the application of biological health and the social sciences to midwifery if they are to be able to keep pace with, and effectively teach, diploma and degree level student midwives in the clinical learning environment. Midwives with years of clinical experience are realizing that they also need to obtain academic credit if they are to progress professionally.

Clinical experience can now be credited through a process of Accreditation of Prior Experiential Learning (APEL). Any courses previously undertaken which were not credit-rated can also be assessed and utilized through Accredited Prior Learning (APL) using the Credit Accumulation and Transfer Scheme (CATS). The CATS Officer in each institution will assess the credit-worthiness of previous learning and experience of an individual midwife and state what further general and/or specific credit has to be obtained in order to attain diploma, ordinary or honours degree status. Therefore, it is essential that a personal professional profile or portfolio is maintained, in which all theoretical and experiential learning undertaken is recorded. In addition, it is necessary to demonstrate, through reflection, exactly what knowledge and skills have been obtained through these means.

In this way midwives with a certificate-level qualification, may be able to obtain prior standing on some diploma-level courses. Most universities, however, are currently requiring all level-three credit, and possibly some level-two credit, to be undertaken through their own institution if an honours degree is to be awarded.

However, in order to obtain a midwifery-specific, as opposed to a generic degree, the programme of study selected must include a significant proportion of midwifery-specific modules facilitated by a midwife teacher. Care needs to be taken when selecting continuing education programmes, because although credit rating may be identical, only those courses carrying National Board approval, with sufficient specific, as opposed to general credits, will enable midwives to have their qualification recorded on the UKCC Professional Register. It is these qualifications which are expected to carry greatest weight in relation to skill mix and career development in the future.

Consequently, purchasers (Trusts, Health Authorities and individual practitioners) are requiring providers (colleges and universities delivering education programmes) to meet the needs of their staff. A plethora of modularized health-related and other education courses are rapidly becoming available. Modularization of courses has increased flexibility, is responsive to purchasers' and providers' requirements, promotes shared learning between varied health professionals and encourages effective use of resources by preventing repetition.

Thus qualified practitioners should be able to select a particular course of study which will meet their personal needs and preferences and match their credit requirements.

Specialist midwifery courses

Continuing professional education in midwifery may be achieved by undertaking a National Board-approved course which is recorded on the UKCC Professional Register when successfully completed. Those currently available to midwives include the following.

ENB 997: Teaching and Assessing in Clinical Practice Course   Sometimes run concurrently with the equivalent course for nurses (ENB 998), this provides the theory of teaching and learning in a clinical environment and develops a practitioner's skills in supervision and assessment of learners in their work setting. It is not intended to develop mini-lecturers for the classroom! Because midwives are competent to educate parents when they register, midwives may only use student midwives, nurses, medical students or health care assistants for their teaching experience.

ENB 405: Special and Intensive Care Nursing of the Newborn Course   In some places this course is no longer under the auspices of midwifery education, although it has a significant amount of midwifery theory content. It is intended for midwives or nurses who wish to specialize in this aspect of neonatal care.

The Advanced Diploma in Midwifery Course   Also called the Diploma in Professional Studies in Midwifery Course. Until recently, this has been the only course available for broadening and deepening a midwife's knowledge of her own professional practice, but it is now being subsumed among a number of modularized education programmes at honours degree and

Masters level. Although it is no longer the essential prerequisite to become a midwife teacher, advanced knowledge is still required and the ENB has decided to continue with this recordable qualification for the foreseeable future. All midwife teacher students are now required to be graduates, or to enter an undergraduate programme to ensure that they will be graduates on completion of their teacher preparation. It is likely that some or all of these courses will be incorporated into larger educational frameworks in order to comply with the UKCC (1993) PREP intentions.

The ENB Framework and Higher Award   The ENB has to translate the UKCC legislation into practical reality and has introduced its Higher Award and Framework. This makes it possible for non-graduate midwives to accumulate credit with successfully completed midwifery practice-related modules. The equivalent of 120 credits are required at certificate, diploma and degree level, making a total of 360 credits, before an honours degree can be awarded (Rogers, 1991).

The intention of this qualification is to provide a mechanism to link academic credit with summatively assessed innovation in clinical practice. A tripartite agreement involving a midwifery manager, midwifery educationalist and a practising midwife is required to design an individual learning contract. Each midwife has to complete a personal portfolio detailing her professional and academic qualifications, clinical experience and continuing professional education. She also has to demonstrate how each of the 10 key characteristics, delineated by the ENB, have been achieved. This may involve specific clinical or managerial projects which will be supervised by a named preceptor as well as attaining an honours-level degree.

Conclusion: The Future of Midwifery Education

It is not easy to look into a crystal ball but certain trends are becoming clear. Education is already a life-long occupation. Not only is it obligatory for continued professional practice, it is essential if practitioners are to keep abreast of rapidly developing knowledge and new technological skills within an ever-changing social climate.

The *Changing Childbirth* report (DOH, 1993) has

set targets to be achieved within five years'. It will be interesting to see whether they will be able to be met within the stated deadline. If, or when they are, a very different midwifery climate and type of midwifery practitioner will exist. An evaluation of the relationship between parents and practitioners at that time will make a fascinating sociological study. Without doubt, midwifery practice and education will become increasingly research based and focused.

The UKCC has largely adopted the American model of education for the United Kingdom. It is to be hoped that British midwives will be able to avoid the theory–practice gap that appears to have been created on the other side of the Atlantic. It is expected that, as in America, more doctors and professors of midwifery will be created. Methods of open and distance learning are expected to assume even greater importance, while the need to be computer literate will become essential as technology will be increasingly utilized in the development of independent learning. In America, at least one college of nursing and midwifery education is already advertising a 'classroom without walls', where students communicate with each other and their tutors only by electronic mail and their computers. The need for undertaking a course in order to 'update' theory and practice will become a thing of the past, continuous, independent self-development will be the norm.

To date, most midwifery refresher courses and much other post-registration professional education has been funded by a midwife's employing authority, but increasingly midwives will be expected to contribute all or part of the costs and time as they become increasingly accountable for their own continuing education, including refresher courses.

Houle (1980) wrote 'Everyone must expect constant change, and with it new goals to be achieved and new understanding and skills to be mastered.' However, all the learning in the world, all the qualifications that there are, will count for nothing unless these changes result in midwives providing sensitive, personalized care so that mothers feel that their childbirth experience has been safe, satisfying and personally fulfilling. It is for each individual midwife to ensure that her personal practice achieves this worthy outcome.

References

Benner, P. (1986) *From Novice to Expert*. Menlow Park, CA: Addison Wesley.

Committee on Nursing (1972) *Report of the Committee on Nursing*. London: HMSO.

DHSS (Department of Health and Social Security) (1970) *Domiciliary Midwifery and Maternity Bed Needs* (Peel Report).

DOH (Department of Health) (1993) *Changing Childbirth*. Part 1 Report of the Expert Maternity Group. London: HMSO.

EEC (1976) EEC Nursing Directives. *Official J. Eur. Communities* No. 20: 176.

EEC (1980) EEC Midwives Directives. *Official J. Eur. Communities* No. L33.

ENB (English National Board for Nursing Midwifery and Health Visiting, Council for National Academic Awards Credit Acumulation and Transfer Scheme) (1989) *Allocation of Credit Ratings to Nursing Courses*. London: ENB.

Houle, C (1980) *Continuing Learning in the Professions*. London: Jossey Bass.

House of Commons (1993) *Patients' Charter*. London: HMSO

Rogers, J. (Ed.) (1991) *Framework for Continuing Professional Education for Nurses, Midwives and Health Visitors*. London: ENB.

Tew, M. (1990) *Safer Childbirth – a Critical History of Maternity Care*. London: Chapman & Hall.

UKCC (UK Central Council for Nursing, Midwifery & Health Visiting) (1990) *Discussion paper on PREPP*. London: UKCC

UKCC (1991) *The Report of the Post-Registration Education and Practice Project*. London: UKCC.

UKCC (1993) *The Council's Proposed Standards for Post Registration Education*. London: UKCC.

UKCC (1994a) *A Midwife's Code of Practice*. London: UKCC.

UKCC (1994b) *The Future of Professional Practice – The Council's Standards for Education and Practice following Registration*. London: UKCC.

UKCC (1995) *PREP and You*. London: UKCC.

87

Ethics in Midwifery Practice

Ethics is now recognized as a major part of both midwifery education and practice; it permeates all professional relationships. Many childbearing women are no longer willing to be passive recipients of care; they expect to be fully informed of all aspects of their care so that they, rather than the professionals, make informed decisions, thereby retaining their autonomy and control. A knowledge of ethics will enable midwives to have a clear understanding of issues related to their practice and, in particular, of their role in empowering women to achieve a pleasurable, fulfilling experience of childbirth.

What is Ethics?

Ethics is basically moral philosophy, or at least the vehicle by which we transport moral philosophy into practical, everyday situations. There is a tendency to consider 'moral' to be related to matters of sexuality, however, here it relates to the 'rights and wrongs' or the 'oughts and ought nots' of any situation. There are three levels of ethics:

1 *Meta-ethics* involves the deeper philosophy of examining everything in abstract, for instance, what do we mean by 'right' and 'wrong'? In everyday situations we do not have time for this level of consideration.
2 *Ethical theory* aims to create mechanisms for problem-solving, much as mathematicians created formulae for solving problems related to their field. Whether such theories are of use to midwives will be discussed later.
3 *Practical ethics*, as the term suggests, is the active part where the work of the moral philosophers is put into practice. It is also the area on which this chapter will generally concentrate.

For readers who wish to know more about some of the philosophers, a list of further reading is given at the end of this chapter.

In everyday life, ethics underpins our actions, particularly those which involve other people and their possessions. It is translated into our thoughts and actions by principles and concepts which we have learned since early childhood, such as truth-telling. This obviously should start within the family but there are outside influences, for example, educational and religious institutions, the media and peer groups. This is not to say that all adults will behave within a given ethical code. As is all too obvious, there are those who never receive the principles and concepts in the first place and others who choose to take a different path. However, these individuals will still be judged according to the code which is generally accepted by society at the time of the incident. Everyone has the right to expect that moral principles will be upheld; these, therefore, become 'moral rights'.

There are numerous moral principles and concepts, some of which are listed here. Further reading in relation to these principles and concepts is suggested at the end of the chapter, as they cannot all be discussed in depth here. Autonomy is discussed later in the chapter.

▶ Accountability.
▶ Autonomy.
▶ Quality of life.
▶ Status of the fetus.
▶ Extraordinary/ordinary means.
▶ Confidentiality.
▶ Paternalism.
▶ Sanctity of life.
▶ Acts and omissions.
▶ Truth telling.
▶ Justice.
▶ Consent.
▶ Value of life.
▶ Killing/letting die.
▶ Doctrine of double effect.

Why is Ethics Important in Midwifery?

Clients do not surrender their moral rights once they seek care; these rights have to be observed within their new experience, in any setting. In midwifery, care is very intimate – from the handling of personal information through the spectrum of physical, psychological, social and educational care. Added to this there is

another dimension: there is no other field of human care where there is one person at the first point of contact and more than one at the end (obstetrics is considered with midwifery here). This transition itself is the source of great complexity when decisions have to be made. An understanding of ethics will not only assist the carer to make decisions, it will also help with the empowerment of the clients to make informed decisions and assist the carer in understanding the basis of those decisions.

There are ethical issues (i.e. debate/concern regarding the right and wrong actions) in all areas of midwifery. It is fairly easy to construct a list of the various areas from preconception care, through fertility and screening issues, to the end of the puerperium. Most people's lists would consist mainly of the highly emotive areas which gain media coverage, but there are many issues involved in the care of 'normal' pregnancy, labour and puerperium. Where there are ethical issues there are *conflicts* and *dilemmas*; it is important to understand the difference.

MORAL CONFLICT

According to Johnson (1990), moral conflict could be considered to be a show of strength within a moral principle, for instance the autonomy of the client versus that of the midwife or, more commonly, the autonomy of two or more professionals (Castledine, 1994). Both of these situations can be seen with regard to *Changing Childbirth* (DOH, 1993). The recommendations are intended to create choice and flexibility (among other things) for those clients who want such a service. At the same time, many midwives are anxious because the flexibility required by clients may not fit in with their own family commitments. In some areas there is also tension between midwives, general practitioners and obstetricians. It could be argued that there has been this tension for many years, but it is more acute now that the balance of power has to be seen to change. Eventually, when the consequences of implementing or not implementing the changes are fully thought through, a reasonable solution will be found, one which will benefit those for whom the service is provided (UKCC, 1989: H 1,2,3,7).

A conflict could also arise between two or more different principles. On closer examination of the conflict, one side becomes a clear winner. An example of this could be where, on immediate visual examination, a neonate is thought to have Down's syndrome and the mother's first question is: 'Is he alright?'. Do you protect her (non-maleficence) and answer 'yes', on the grounds that the Apgar scores were good and chromosome studies need to be performed for confirmation; or do you tell the truth and explain that tests are required to confirm it? Ethically, telling the truth wins. The mother has the right to know, especially as a positive test will indicate to her that she was initially deceived and this could affect her ability to trust midwives in future encounters. Added to which, the mother's permission should be sought regarding tests performed on her baby; she cannot consent unless she has the information. It is hoped that readers can see, from this example, that a conflict is logical in resolution once thought through properly. It is also acknowledged that in some units, in circumstances similar to the example, not all practitioners take this particular action; they obviously find that their clear solution is to protect the mother. Beauchamp and Childress (1989) feel that it is often this initial conflict which goes on to create the dilemma.

MORAL DILEMMA

This starts as a conflict between principles but, on further examination, there is no obvious solution as the choices are equally weighted but neither is satisfactory (Campbell, 1984; Johnson, 1990). The following is one such dilemma:

> A primiparous woman is admitted in established labour. She has a birth plan which states that under no circumstances will she give consent to an episiotomy. During the second stage of labour progress is slow but positive, however, the perineum remains thick and rigid. This is explained to the woman but she maintains her position regarding episiotomy. As time progresses the fetal heart shows signs of slight distress, to the point where most midwives would consider episiotomy to be the action of choice, but still the woman withholds consent. The midwife could either continue and hope that the fetus will survive (obviously notifying appropriate personnel), or she could perform the procedure without consent, in order to protect the fetus. If she carries out the episiotomy without consent she could face a claim of battery against her. Neither is the ideal solution. This is further complicated, however, by a British court decision, in 1992, to overrule a

> mother's wishes in favour of her fetus.
> (Dimond, 1993: 15–16; Jones, 1994)

This case is under further discussion within the legal network (Thomson, 1994: 132).

It is amazing that this type of situation does not happen more frequently than it appears to, as the *Code of Professional Conduct* (UKCC, 1992), in trying to protect the public, actually creates the possibility of dilemma. Sometimes it would be difficult to observe both of the following at one time:

> As a registered nurse, midwife or health visitor, you are personally accountable for your practice and, in the exercise of your professional accountability, must:
>
> 1 act always in such a manner as to promote and safeguard the interests and well-being of patients and clients;
>
> 2 ensure that no action or **omission** on your part, or within your sphere of responsibility, is detrimental to the interests, condition or safety of patients and clients. (UKCC, 1992)

What the client feels is in her best interests may not correspond with the midwife's view, and it could be detrimental to the woman's condition, or that of her fetus.

How are Dilemmas Solved?

This is where level two of ethics is required – ethical theory. There are probably as many theories as there are philosophers but, generally speaking, their views fit broadly into major theories. Two such theories, at either end of the spectrum, are *utilitarianism* and *deontology*.

Utilitarianism

This is a consequentialist theory, where possible actions are considered in terms of their probable consequences. The aim for the actions is to create the greatest 'good' or 'happiness' for the greatest number of people; this would obviously describe the essential outlook of those managing the National Health Service. It would also describe the intentions of Hitler in the Second World War, with his views of improving the human race as, unfortunately, the catchphrase for this theory is 'the end justifies the means'.

There are two forms of the theory: *act-utilitarianism*

and *rule-utilitarianism*. The first is the purer form, developed in the eighteenth and nineteenth centuries by Bentham, Mill (Norman, 1988: ch. 7) and others, where every action was assessed according to its outcome in terms of benefit. The second form does not look directly at the actual benefit of each act, rather it has developed rules which are intended to ensure the greatest benefit, and each act is assessed as to whether it fits into one of the rules (Smart and Williams, 1988).

Deontology

This is a duty-based theory. Consequences are not considered, as deontologists believe that what is good in the world is brought about by people doing their duty. This theory divides into three 'camps', each competing with the others, as well as with utilitarianism. A well-known name in philosophy is Immanuel Kant (Norman, 1988: ch. 6). He developed *rational monism* which he believed was how people already thought – that one's actions should be rational and stem from 'good will'; he believed in duty for its own sake – the 'categorical imperative'. He used two tests for the moral value of an action. The first was whether it would be suitable if universalized, i.e. if everyone was to do it. The second test involved whether the act would use anybody as a means to an end, which would not be acceptable, or as an end in himself, which would be acceptable as this is the basis of autonomy.

The second 'camp' is that of *traditional deontology* (Jones, 1994a); this is firmly seated in a belief in God and the sanctity of life. Each religion has its own model for behaviour, for instance Christians have the Ten Commandments. With this system there is little room for conflict as it is possible to carry out all the commands at one time.

The third form is *intuitionistic pluralism*, where it is believed that there are a number of moral rules which are of equal importance; unfortunately the possibility of rule conflict exists. To minimize this, W.D. Ross considered seven prima-facie duties which he felt were reasonable for people to abide by (Gillon, 1986):

1 *Duty of fidelity* – this involves keeping promises, being loyal and not deceiving.
2 *Duty of beneficence* – the obligation to help others.
3 *Duty of non-maleficence* – not harming others; this, says Gillon (1986: 18), is more stringent than the previous duty.
4 *Duty of justice* – to ensure fair play.
5 *Duty of reparation* – an obligation to make amends.
6 *Duty of gratitude* – to repay in some way those who have helped us (owed to special people such as parents), this also includes loyalty.
7 *Duty of self-improvement*.

(Jones, 1994)

As these duties are equal in importance, it is possible for conflict to arise between them. There is a system which can assist in such conflict – *casuistry*; this allows for the duties to be weighted or ordered according to the circumstances.

Readers have probably already identified that, although the NHS is generally essentially utilitarian, midwifery, medicine and other similar disciplines, tend towards a deontological approach. In fact the duty with which we are most familiar – the duty of care – would appear to encompass at least the first four of the above duties. This is certainly apparent in the *Code of Professional Conduct* (UKCC, 1992) which lists 16 of its own duties; here too there can be conflict. Most commonly for midwives, the conflict occurs between the following:

1. act always in such a manner as to promote and safeguard the interest and well being of patients and clients;

6. work in a collaborative and co-operative manner with health care professionals and others involved in providing care, and recognise and respect their particular contributions within the care team.

(UKCC, 1992: 2)

To assist understanding of the different focus of utilitarianism and deontology when faced with a dilemma, the following non-midwifery story from Smart and Williams (1988) is offered; readers are invited to determine the end:

Jim is a botanist on expedition in South America. He finds himself in a small town where twenty Indians are tied up ready for execution, following acts of protest against the government. The captain, Pedro, having explained the situation, offers Jim a guest's privilege of killing one of the Indians himself. If he accepts, as a special mark of the occasion, the other Indians will be freed. If he refuses, then there is no special occasion and Pedro will have them all killed as previously planned.

(Smart and Williams, 1988: 98–99)

You are Jim – what will you do? If you are utilitarian then your decision would be to shoot one (which one is another problem), thus saving the other 19 as a consequence. As a deontologist, however, you would feel a duty 'not to harm' each man; you would not think through the consequences, nor would you don a mantle of responsibility and guilt for Pedro's actions.

Do We Need the Theories?

Many theorists would suggest that we do, that we would not be able to make decisions effectively without them. It must be remembered, however, that most people have to deal with conflicts and dilemmas in their lives without any knowledge of these theories. When considering the fundamentals of the opposing theories, it is difficult to understand how someone could make a deontological decision on one day, but a utilitarian one on another; yet this happens all the time in hospital. A midwife on duty in a ward, but not responsible for ward management on that day, would have a number of clients to care for. She would hopefully treat these clients as individuals, carrying out her 'duty of care' for each one in line with the 'activities of a midwife' (UKCC, 1994: 5): this approach would be basically deontological. The next day, that same midwife could be responsible for the general ward management. On this occasion, the decisions which she makes must be for the good of the ward as a whole: the utilitarian principle of 'the greatest good for the greatest number'. While clinicians at the bedside, or in people's homes, can be deontological in their approach, the further up the management tree that is considered, the more it becomes obvious that a utilitarian approach is essential. It would not be acceptable to society, for instance, if the NHS purse were to be emptied by caring for the few; the limited resources are expected to do as much as possible for as many as possible.

There are some philosophers, known as *particularists*, who do not accept the formal theories. They believe in a more flexible approach (McNaughton, 1988) where people should learn about morality (rights and principles) through the usual routes of socialization, from childhood, and then apply it as is appropriate at the time. For instance, when faced with a situation where telling the truth could offend someone, a deontologist would be duty bound to tell the truth and so offend the listener. A particularist, however, might tell 'a white lie' in order to prevent causing

offence, so long as no other harm was created (Jones, 1994a). This could allow more than flexibility, it could enable a swifter response, as conducting a utilitarian exercise can be time-consuming. This viewpoint could be very attractive; it appears to be based on the balance between common sense and morality. It also suggests that it would be sufficient to teach rights and principles while omitting the formal theories. This idea is not supported by Hanford (1993: 979–982) who feels that teaching principles in place of theories (principlism) is 'reinforcing a sense of professional superiority among health care professionals', rather than creating 'a learning environment that promotes and enhances caring'. Whether we wish to embrace the formal or the informal approaches, it is important for health care professionals to know something about each of them, if only to understand how and why some decisions are made. It is also useful to have some idea of the approach which managers or clinicians might take when proposals for implementing schemes or changes are being made.

It is interesting to note that it is not only the philosophers who cannot agree on the content and method of ethics teaching. A survey, conducted between November 1993 and January 1994, of 66 institutions in England which offer midwifery courses, from Pre-registration (3 years) to Masters Degrees, appeared to show great disparity in the ethics input. The 50% response indicated great differences, in the number of hours and the actual content, between similar courses in different institutions (Jones, unpublished).

The Duty of Care

As health professionals, midwives have a duty of care to those persons who could be affected by their actions or omissions (Dimond, 1994). In midwifery it is important to note that 'persons' relates directly to the mother and the neonate. (Legally the fetus is not yet a 'person'; readers may wish to pursue the subjects of 'personhood' and 'potential' in other texts.) This duty of care would include at least the first four deontological duties listed earlier; failure in the duty of care could result in a civil law case for negligence (Clark and Stephenson, 1991).

The duty of fidelity

The duty of fidelity requires us to avoid deceiving our clients and their families; this suggests, therefore, that promises should not be made if they cannot be kept and that truth-telling is paramount. An example used earlier, to illustrate a moral conflict, involved a baby with suspected Down's syndrome. If the practicitioners involved were to withhold the truth from the mother, then they would be failing in their duty of fidelity, however good their motives might be. Verbal reports by students and qualified midwives suggest that this deception does occur sometimes, in the belief that the mother is being protected.

The duty of beneficence

The duty of beneficence creates the obligation to help our clients. This is a positive duty which covers numerous activities, ranging from the various ways of helping to make them comfortable, to the educational aspects of caring for their babies. What this duty does not include is the paternalistic attitude so often experienced within the health service, where practitioners feel that they 'know what is best'. This attitude, although generally well-meant, deprives the client of her right to self-determination (autonomy).

The duty of non-maleficence

The duty of non-maleficence is a negative duty – to do no harm. On the surface this would suggest that conducting unpleasant or painful procedures breaches this duty; this would be the case if the intention was to hurt the client. If the intention is to eventually benefit her and, knowing that she might experience pain or discomfort, she is in agreement, then there is no breach in duty. Administration of analgesic injections, the siting of an epidural analgesic or urinary catheterization would come into this category. This duty, although negative in its statement, can have a positive aspect: that of safety and protection from harm. This includes, among other things, consideration of the environment, observance of drug policies and adequate education and training of practitioners.

The duty of justice

The duty of justice requires us to treat our clients equally, without discrimination. For many people, the word 'discrimination' is immediately associated with terms such as race, skin colour or ethnic origin. While it is essential that we consider these areas, it is also important that we are aware of the other forms of discrimination which can occur, such as between articulate and less articulate clients. It is often easier to spend more time with the articulate clients, giving as much information and as much choice as possible, than it is with those who require greater explanations or who ask less questions. It could be argued that, to consider equality, we should aim to get all clients to the same endpoint; this would then necessitate that more time be spent with the less articulate clients. This is an area of great concern for many midwives who offer a limited Domino scheme. While they are pleased to offer the service, they are aware that inequality occurs, in that many women are denied the opportunities that the few are fortunate to be offered. This is mainly due to the financial and manpower constraints of service provision. Domino schemes offer clients continuity of care by their community midwife who provides hospital care for delivery and ante- and postnatal care in the community. Other schemes offering continuity of care are now more widespread.

Principles

Contrary to Hanford's opinion (1993), the view being taken here is that knowledge of the underlying moral principles is important, if only to ensure that practitioners are 'talking the same language'. It is not possible, in one short chapter, to consider each of the major principles, but in the author's opinion, one of the most basic moral principles is that of autonomy, since an understanding and observance of this principle should automatically lead professionals into the understanding and observance of many other principles.

AUTONOMY

> To be an autonomous person is to have the ability to be able to formulate and carry out one's own plans and policies . . . the ability to govern one's conduct by rules and values.
>
> (Downie and Calman, 1987: 51)

This suggests that autonomy involves self-control of one's actions and destiny. It could be argued that it is impossible to be totally autonomous, as society imposes certain rules, often sitting in judgement on the actions of individuals. However, there is a broad band of acceptability in most areas of life, at least in democratic societies, which gives individuals varying degrees of freedom of choice. What is expected of individuals is that their actions and decisions should be rational, i.e. based on sound reasoning. These decisions should then be accepted, whether or not they match the views of others, such as midwives and doctors.

For midwifery clients to make rational decisions about their care, the carers must ensure that sufficient information is given at the level and pace required by the individual. Many factors need to be considered: the *environment* should be conducive to the giving and receiving of information; the *language* that is being used should be in the 'mother tongue' of the client, with the avoidance of jargon and abbreviations; the *circumstances* in which a decision is required, for example, whether there is time for contemplation or whether a fairly urgent situation is faced. Having given the information, it is also important for professionals to assess the client's understanding of it.

Having determined that a client has made an informed decision based on what she thinks is sound reasoning, i.e. an autonomous decision, health professionals have no right to overrule that decision. This principle is inextricably bound to informed consent: if the client is autonomous then nothing should be done to her without her prior consent; to do so would be to commit a trespass against the person, i.e. battery (Kennedy, 1992: 320). If her consent is being sought then she is being considered to be autonomous, therefore a situation should not arise where, on her refusal to consent to a procedure, professionals attempt to overrule her. There are two groups of people who might be deemed to be not autonomous, therefore unable to give consent. One group includes children, but there is no longer a set age, it depends on the circumstances and degree of rationality of the child (DOH, 1989). The other group includes those who are mentally incapacitated, either by disability or by severe mental illness. With both groups consent by proxy would be sought. There is also the possibility of temporary mental incompetence in cases of unconsciousness or possibly the effects of drugs (including alcohol); in such cases the professionals would be expected to act out of necessity in the best interest of the client, unless there was sound evidence that the client would refuse consent if aware of the situation (such as a Jehovah's Witness carrying a card refusing blood products).

It is the author's firm belief that, if client autonomy was truly considered, then it would be unlikely that the

varying aspects of the duty of care would be breached. This would not remove situations of conflict and dilemma, but it would make decision-making more straightforward, with all practitioners working to the same ground rules. The use of reflective practice would assist in this area, by midwives analysing and reflecting upon their actions, particularly with regard to their observance of autonomy, then using this experience to formulate their plans for future decision-making.

Practitioner Activity

At the end of a shift, consider the clients for whom you cared. In each case consider:

▶ Which aspects of her care did you discuss with her?
▶ Which aspects of her care did you *not* discuss with her?
▶ What information did you give her?
▶ What decisions did she make?
▶ What decisions did you make?
▶ Did you accept *her* decisions or did you try to change them?
▶ What did you write in the records?
▶ Did you enable her to be autonomous?
▶ In light of this exercise, what will you do in similar circumstances in future?

If you are working in a delivery suite, conduct the same exercise with regard to one client for whom you cared.

Conclusion

This chapter is intended to help readers to accept the need for awareness of moral rights along with the will of individual practitioners to uphold them. An understanding of ethics will help midwives to make decisions in difficult circumstances, even if they do not choose to directly follow the theories outlined. The author firmly believes that observance of ethical principles, in particular autonomy, is the most direct route to assisting childbearing women to have the degree of choice and control which each individual feels is right for her. It is possible that the woman who achieves control in childbearing is better placed to do so in the parenting years ahead of her. By practising in this way, the midwife will also be fulfilling personal, professional accountability.

References

Beauchamp, T.L. & Childress, J.F. (1989) *Principles of Biomedical Ethics*, 3rd edn, p. 35. Oxford: Oxford University Press.

Campbell, A.V. (1984) *Moral Dilemmas In Medicine*, 3rd edn, p. 2. London: Churchill Livingstone.

Castledine, G. (1994) Is respect for patient autonomy declining? *Br. J. Nurs.* 3(16): 847.

Clark, P. & Stephenson, G. (1991) *Law of Torts*, 3rd edn., Chapters 3 & 4. London: Blackstone Press.

Dimond, B. (1993) Client autonomy and choices. *Modern Midwife* 3(1): 15–16.

Dimond, B. (1994) The duty of care. *Modern Midwife* 4(8): 17–18.

DOH (Department of Health) (1989) *The Children Act*, Report of the Expert Committee. London: HMSO.

DOH (1993) *Changing Childbirth*, Report of the Expert Maternity Group. London: HMSO.

Downie, R.S. and Calman, K.C. (1987) *Healthy Respect – Ethics in Health Care*. London: Faber & Faber.

Gillon, R. (1986) *Philosophical Medical Ethics*. Chichester: Wiley & Sons.

Hanford, L. (1993) Ethics and disability. *Br. J. Nurs.* 2(19): 979–982.

Johnson, A.G. (1990) *Pathways in Medical Ethics*. London: Edward Arnold.

Jones, S.R. (1994) *Ethics of Midwifery*. London: C.V. Mosby.

Jones, S.R. (unpublished) *Report of a Survey of Ethics Input to Midwifery Courses in England 1993/4*.

Kennedy, I. (1992) *Treat Me Right*. Oxford: Oxford University Press.

McNaughton, D. (1988) *Moral Vision*. Oxford: Blackwell.

Norman, R. (1988) *The Moral Philosophers*. Oxford: Clarendon Press.

Smart, J.J.C. & Williams, B. (1988) *Utilitarianism For and Against*. Cambridge: Cambridge University Press.

Thomson, M. (1994) After *Re S. Med. Law Rev.* 2(2): 132.

UKCC (UK Central Council for Nursing, Midwifery & Health Visiting) (1989) *Exercising Accountability* (H 1,2,3,7). London: UKCC.

UKCC (1992) *Code of Professional Conduct*. London: UKCC.

UKCC (1994) *The Midwife's Code of Practice*. London: UKCC.

Further Reading

Faulder, C. (1985) *Whose Body Is It?* London: Virago Press.

Norman, R. (1988) *The Moral Philosophers*. Oxford: Clarendon Press.

UKCC (1987) *Confidentiality*. London: UKCC.

UKCC (1989) *Exercising Accountability*. London: UKCC.

UKCC (1990) *. . . With a View to Removal from the Register . . . ?* London: UKCC.

UKCC (1993) *Midwives' Rules*. London: UKCC.

UKCC (1996) *Guidelines for Professional Practice*. London: UKCC.

88

Drugs and the Midwife

Drugs used in pregnancy are selected with extreme care as they may affect not only the mother but also her unborn child. The medical practitioner when prescribing must remember that in the early weeks of pregnancy drugs may give rise to serious congenital defects or even death of the embryo. The Committee on Safety of Drugs (Scowen Committee) was set up in the UK following the thalidomide disaster to ensure that such a tragedy should never occur again.

Drug use in pregnancy has fallen since the mid-1960s from nearly 80% to 35%, but in the first trimester of pregnancy only about 6% of women now take drugs (Rubin, 1987). Most drugs are transferred across the placenta to the fetus in due course, except for heparin.

A major problem is the effect of the *physiological changes* of pregnancy on blood concentrations of certain drugs. Because the total blood volume increases so markedly in pregnancy, drugs are diluted in a larger volume of fluid and so may be less effective than in non-pregnant women (Hytten and Leitch, 1971; Pirani *et al.*, 1973). Serum proteins are also affected by the increased fluid volume in pregnancy, for example, serum albumin is decreased and this affects the binding of acidic drugs such as phenytoin (Studd, 1975). The effect of this change leads to a reduction in the measured concentrations of drugs which are highly bound (e.g. phenytoin), but there will be higher levels of unbound drugs. Thus laboratory results on plasma concentrations of some drugs require careful interpretation by medical staff who prescribe drugs in pregnancy (Rubin, 1987), and the midwife needs to understand the reasons for these tests and why drug dosages may need to be increased as pregnancy advances.

Another factor which affects some drugs in pregnancy is the increased *rate of liver metabolism*. As a result, drugs which rely on the activity of liver enzymes are eliminated more quickly, for example, phenytoin (O'Hare *et al.*, 1984). There is no change in the rate of elimination of drugs which rely on blood flow in the liver. There is a change, however, in the rate of drug elimination in pregnancy due to increased blood flow in the kidney. This results in some drugs being excreted more quickly, mainly those which are eliminated unchanged by the kidney (Rubin, 1987).

Because of the changes in serum concentrations and the rate of elimination of some drugs in pregnancy, careful monitoring of plasma concentrations is necessary for drugs such as phenytoin, both during pregnancy and the postnatal period. Increases in doses are usually required as pregnancy advances and the dose is decreased in the postnatal period.

Drugs may also affect the *neonate*, as certain substances are passed in varying concentrations in breast milk. Sometimes, as with aperients and phenobarbitone, this is relatively harmless; but drugs which suppress thyroid activity, such as carbimazole or thiouracil, may have much more serious effects upon the baby.

The midwife must be familiar with statutory obligations, the rules of the UKCC (1993) and the local policies of her employing authority regulating the control and administration of drugs.

Legislation

CONTROLLED DRUGS

The possession and administration of controlled drugs by midwives is covered by the Misuse of Drugs Regulations 1985 (SI 1985 No. 2066), the Misuse of Drugs (Northern Ireland) Regulations (SR 1986 No. 52) and the Medicines Act 1968. These Acts are concerned with the control of narcotic drugs and other substances which can cause drug dependence.

Under these regulations a registered midwife who has notified her intention to practise is provided with a supply of pethidine (and any other controlled drug listed in Schedule 3 Parts I and III of the Medicines (Products other than Veterinary Drugs) (Prescription Only) Order 1983 S.I. 1983 No. 1212 and subsequent orders using the supply order form procedure. Supply

order forms are supplied by the midwife's supervisor of midwives). There are five Controlled Drug schedules:

▶ *Schedule 1:* Drugs which are often used illegally such as cannabis and hallucinogens.
▶ *Schedule 2:* Addictive drugs including diamorphine, pethidine and morphine.
▶ *Schedule 3:* Some of the barbiturates, including pentazocine which may be used by midwives.
▶ *Schedule 4:* This includes 33 benzodiazepine tranquillizers, some of which are commonly used in obstetric practice, e.g. diazepam (Valium), nitrazepam (Mogadon) and temazepam (Euhypnos).
▶ *Schedule 5:* This contains medicines which include only a limited amount of a controlled drug, e.g. some analgesics and cough mixtures.

Drugs in Schedules 3, 4 and 5 do not have to be kept in a controlled drug cupboard, nor do they have to be entered in a Controlled Drug Register.

Supply of controlled drugs to midwives

The midwife uses the supply order procedure to obtain these controlled drugs. Drugs obtained by this procedure can only be used by a midwife for women having a home birth. The midwife caring for women in hospital must use drugs supplied in the hospital and follow the agreed policies relating to the administration of drugs. These may allow midwives to follow the same practice as those working in the community.

To obtain pethidine (or other permitted controlled drugs) using the supply order procedure the following requirements must be met:

1   The midwife must obtain a midwife's supply order signed by the supervisor of midwives. Before providing the midwife with a supply order the supervisor will wish to see the midwife's:

▶ register of drugs;
▶ record of cases;
▶ remaining stock of controlled drugs.

2   The midwife will take the supply order to a pharmacy where prior arrangements have been made for her to obtain pethidine.
3   She shall not obtain any amount greater than that specified in the midwife's supply order.
4   The order must specify:

▶ the name of the midwife;
▶ the name of the drug;

▶ the purpose for which it is required;
▶ total quantity to be procured.

5   The midwife must enter in her drug book:

▶ the name of the drug and the quantity supplied;
▶ the name and address of the supplier;
▶ the date, name of mother, quantity administered.

6   She must keep every drug in a locked receptacle which can be opened only by her.
7   Midwives may not lend or borrow controlled drugs.

Destruction of controlled drugs obtained by a midwife through a supply order procedure

The Misuse of Drugs Regulations lay down a procedure by which midwives may surrender stocks of unwanted controlled drugs and a procedure for the destruction of pethidine (or other controlled drug approved in accordance with the Medicines Act 1968) which is no longer required. Stocks of unwanted controlled drugs may be surrendered to an authorized person, but not to a supervisor of midwives.

Controlled drugs may be destroyed by the midwife herself but only in the presence of an authorized person who may be either:

1   a supervisor of midwives in England, Wales and Northern Ireland;
2   a regional pharmaceutical officer in England;
3   a pharmaceutical adviser, Welsh Office;
4   a chief administrative pharmaceutical officer of health boards in Scotland;
5   in Northern Ireland an Inspector appointed by the Department of Health and Social Services under the Misuse of Drugs Act 1971;
6   medical officers of the regional medical services in England, Scotland and Wales;
7   an inspector of the Pharmaceutical Society of Great Britain;
8   a police officer; or
9   an inspector of the Home Office Drugs Branch (UKCC, 1994).

In some cases controlled drugs are supplied to a woman on prescription from her family practitioner for use in a home birth. The responsibility for the destruction of any unused drugs in this case lies with the woman to whom in law the drugs belong. The midwife should advise the woman to destroy the drugs and may suggest that she does so in her presence. The midwife should record in the mother's notes any advice she has given and action taken (UKCC, 1994).

Controlled drugs and medicines in hospital

The Aitken Report (DHSS, 1958), Section VI, paragraphs 84 and 85 states that midwives working in an institution are subject to the same rules related to the administration of controlled drugs and medicines as nurses. This means that drugs and medicines must not be administered unless prescribed by a doctor and obtained from the institution's pharmacy.

The former Central Midwives' Board for England and Wales made representation to the then Ministry of Health on behalf of midwives practising in maternity units, particularly in respect of the administration of pethidine. This resulted in a letter from the DHSS to health authorities permitting block authorization (standing orders) to be made by the appropriate registered medical practitioners particularly in respect of pethidine. This letter was operative in England and Wales and the same policies were adopted by Northern Ireland. The Roxburghe Report in Scotland was similar to the Aitken Report but subsequent provision for standing orders has not been made.

Since the publication of the Duthie Report (DOH, 1988), however, local policy can be more flexible. The Duthie Report on the 'Safe handling of medicines' carried out a total review of the security of medicines in the custody of health authorities. As a result the Department of Health recommended that the findings should be used either as a framework for setting up a system for the safe and secure handling of medicines or for evaluating the existing system. It also indicated that local policy could allow midwives practising in hospitals to follow the same practice as midwives in the community as regards the administration of medicines.

Supply of prescription-only medicines to midwives

In accordance with Part III of the Medicines Act 1968 the midwife may be supplied with certain medicines which are normally available only on prescription issued by a doctor. These medicines may be obtained from a retail or hospital pharmacist by a midwife who has notified her intention to practise. They may only be used in her professional practice.

Preparations for use by midwives are listed below.

These are included in Schedule 3 (Parts I and III) of the Medicines (Products other than Veterinary Drugs) (Prescription only) Order (1983) (Statutory Instrument No. 1212) and any subsequent orders:

Part 1

▶ Ergometrine maleate (tablets).
▶ Chloral hydrate derivatives – but Welldorm (formerly dichloralphenazone) is no longer recommended for use in pregnancy because the chemical composition has been changed (UKCC, 1991).

Part 3 (for parenteral use)

▶ Pentazocine lactate ⎫ These drugs have to
▶ Pethidine hydrochloride ⎭ be kept locked in a
                          controlled drug cup-
                          board and be entered
                          in a Controlled Drug
                          register.
▶ Promazine hydrochloride (Sparine).
▶ Lignocaine hydrochloride.
▶ Phytomenadione (vitamin K).
▶ Naloxone hydrochloride (Narcan).
▶ Oxytocin.
▶ Ergometrine maleate.

The law is different in Scotland because a midwife can only administer oxytocic drugs such as ergometrine and Syntometrine, and naloxone and lignocaine without a doctor's prescription.

Midwives' Rules (UKCC, 1993)

1   A practising midwife shall not on her own responsibility administer any medicine, including analgesics, unless in the course of her training whether before or after registration as a midwife, she has been thoroughly instructed in its use and is familiar with its dosage and methods of administration or application.

2   A practising midwife shall not on her own responsibility administer any inhalational analgesic by the use of any type of apparatus unless:

▶ that apparatus is for the time being approved by the Council as suitable for use by a midwife; and
▶ the midwife has ensured that the apparatus has been properly maintained.

3   Unless special exemption is given by the Council to enable a particular hospital or other institution to investigate new methods, a practising midwife must not administer any form of pain relief by the use of any type of apparatus or by any other means other than that approved by Council unless on the instructions of a registered medical practicioner (see Rule 41(3)).

4   The midwife must keep detailed records of medicines or other forms of pain relief administered by her to all mothers and babies.

A mixture of 50% nitrous oxide and 50% oxygen may be administered to mothers by midwives on their own responsibility using one of the following apparatus which are currently approved by the UKCC (1995):

▶ Entonox apparatus.
▶ PneuPac Apparatus.
▶ SOS Nitronox – midwifery model.
▶ Peacemaker apparatus.

The mother may obtain the analgesia by the use of a mouthpiece or facemask.

The Midwife's Code of Practice for Midwives Practising in the United Kingdom (UKCC, 1994)

The section headed 'Medicines, including analgesics (Rule 41)' contains information and guidance on:

▶ the supply, possession and use of controlled drugs;
▶ the destruction of controlled drugs obtained by a midwife through a supply order procedure;
▶ the surrender of controlled drugs (These can only be surrendered to the pharmacist who supplied them, or to an appropriate medical officer.);
▶ controlled drugs obtained by a woman on prescription from a family practitioner;
▶ prescription-only and other medicines used by midwives;
▶ the administration of homeopathic or herbal substances;
▶ administration of controlled drugs and medicines and audit of records.

The Duthie Report (1988) indicated that local policy could allow midwives practising in hospitals to follow the same practice as midwives in the community as regards the administration of medicines, or they may be governed by local standing orders, except for Scotland where there is no provision for standing orders.

Standards for the Administration of Medicines (UKCC, 1992)

This document outlines the standards for the administration of medicines which are expected of nurses, midwives and health visitors. Every practising midwife should have a copy of this paper and is responsible for maintaining the standards specified in it.

Local policies

The particular controlled drugs and medicines which a midwife may use will be determined locally and a midwife should obtain details from her supervisor of midwives.

A midwife working in the NHS should comply with locally agreed health authority or trust policies and procedures. These may include standing orders for the administration of controlled drugs and medicines for use by the midwife in a hospital. These drugs and medicines would be similar to those carried by a midwife in her practice in the community.

Aperients

Aperients must be given with care at any time, the idea being to augment the normal rhythm not disturb it. In pregnancy because progesterone reduces the activity of plain muscle, constipation occurs. Aperients are sometimes necessary but they must be gentle because of the predisposition of haemorrhoids. More roughage in the diet should be encouraged.

Isogel

Indications	Constipation
Action	Bulking agent
Dose	Two 5 ml teaspoonfuls in water once or twice daily with meals.
Route	Oral
Contraindications	None in normal pregnancy
Side-effects	None.
	Bulking agents for the treatment of constipation are preferable to irritants because the latter may cause high levels of abdominal discomfort (Hay-Smith, 1994).

Liquid paraffin

Indications	Constipation (short term)
Action	Aperient/faecal softener
Dose	10–30 ml
Route	Oral
Contraindications	(Children less than 3 years of age)
Side-effects	Continuous use in pregnancy can cause seepage and soiling of clothing. Long-term use may interfere with absorption of fat-soluble vitamins A, D and K.

Bisacodyl BP (Dulcolax)

Bisacodyl is a 'contact' aperient, which softens faecal mass. It is effective and safe in pregnancy and the puerperium as it is not absorbed. Bisacodyl may also be given in the form of suppositories.

> *Dose* 5–10 mg orally
> 10 mg per rectum

Haematinic Substances

IRON

Iron is an essential component of haemoglobin and is necessary not only for the mother but also for the growing fetus. In pregnancy there is an increase in the absorption of iron from food (Barrett *et al.*, 1994). Women who have a good diet therefore should not develop anaemia in pregnancy. If anaemia is diagnosed, however, the woman will require iron supplements. Iron often causes nausea and it is therefore wiser to begin its administration in the second trimester with meals when the symptoms of morning sickness have passed. Where the haemoglobin is very low or the date of delivery imminent, intramuscular or intravenous preparations may be used.

Ferrous sulphate compound tablets BPC (Fersolate)

Indications	Iron deficiency anaemia
Action	Increases haemoglobin regeneration
Dose	200 mg up to three times a day

Route	Oral
Contraindications	Antacids and tetracycline reduce absorption
Side-effects	Nausea, gastrointestinal irritation, diarrhoea, and, with continued administration, constipation, black-coloured stools.

Folic acid BP

Folic acid is a member of the vitamin B group and is necessary for maturation of the red blood cells.

Indications	Folate deficiency, prevention of neural tube defects
Action	Necessary for maturation of red cells
Dose	5 mg daily for prevention of recurrence of neural tube defect
	400 µg daily to prevent first occurrence of neural tube defect
	Both doses till 12th week of pregnancy (MRC, 1991)
Route	Oral
Contraindications	Caution in epilepsy – folic acid occasionally reduces plasma phenytoin concentration
Side-effects	None in short-term use.

Antihypertensive Drugs

These drugs may be used in the last trimester of pregnancy to treat severe pre-eclampsia or throughout pregnancy where essential hypertension exists.

Hydralazine hydrochloride (Apresoline)

Hydralazine is a vasodilator antihypertensive drug. One of the side-effects is tachycardia, thus it may be used together with a beta-blocker which reduces tachycardia.

Indications	Moderate–severe hypertension, hypertensive crisis
Action	Vasodilator antihypertensive
Dose	5–50 mg oral twice daily
	Slow IV – 5–10 mg over 20 min repeated after 20–30 min
	IV infusion – 200–300 mg/min initially → maintenance 50–150 mg/min
Contraindications	Idiopathic systemic lupus erythematosus, severe tachycardia, high output heart failure, myocardial insufficiency due to mechanical obstruction, cor pulmonale, dissecting aortic aneurysm, porphyria
Side-effects	Tachycardia, fluid retention, nausea and vomiting, systemic lupus erythematosus-like syndrome after long-term high-dose therapy.

Labetalol hydrochloride

Labetalol combines alpha- and beta-adrenoreceptor blocking activity. Alpha-blocking activity in peripheral arteries lowers peripheral resistance and helps to reduce the blood pressure.

Indications	Hypertension, hypertensive crisis
Action	Alpha- and beta-receptor blocking activity
Dose	50–800 mg depending on route
	Usual 100 mg twice daily to maximum 2.4 g daily. 50 mg over 1 minute IV – maximum 200 mg
	Pregnancy dose – IV infusion 20 mg/hour → 160 mg/hour
	Abrupt withdrawal to be avoided
Route	Oral, IV
Contraindications	Asthma or history of obstructive airways disease, heart failure, second- or third-degree heart block, cardiogenic shock, after prolonged fasting, metabolic acidosis
Side-effects	Postural hypotension, tiredness, weakness, headache, rashes, scalp-tingling, difficulty in micturition, epigastric pain, nausea, vomiting.

Methyldopa BP (Aldomet)

Methyldopa is a centrally acting antihypertensive drug. Vasodilators and beta-adrenoreceptor drugs are now preferred for the treatment of hypertension.

Indications	Hypertension, hypertensive crisis
Action	Centrally acting, antihypertensive drug
Dose	500–3000 mg depending on route Oral 250 mg 2–3 × daily → maximum daily dose of 3 g IV 250 mg–500 mg infusion repeated after 6 hours if required
Route	Oral, IV
Contraindications	History of depression, active liver disease, phaeochromocytoma, porphyria.

Magnesium sulphate

Magnesium sulphate is now considered the drug of choice to treat eclampsia (Neilson, 1995). The findings from the Eclampsia Trial Collaborative Group (1995) indicate that women who develop eclampsia and are treated with magnesium sulphate are less likely to suffer recurrent fits and to die.

Indications	Eclampsia
Action	Prevention of convulsions
Dose	There are different regimes and the following is one example: 5 g magnesium sulphate over a period of 20 min via an IVAC by adding 8 ml of 50% magnesium sulphate solution to 200 ml normal saline Continue to infuse 2 g magnesium sulphate in normal saline per hour for 24 hours Monitor magnesium levels after 1 hour and then 4 hourly. Maintain the therapeutic range at 2–3 mmol/l
Route	Intravenous
Contraindications	Renal failure
Side-effects	Magnesium is mainly excreted by the kidneys therefore is

retained in renal failure. Risk of toxicity.

Myometrial Relaxants

Beta-adrenoreceptor stimulants relax uterine muscle and may be used in selected cases in an attempt to inhibit preterm labour. The effect is brought about mainly by their influence on the receptors stimulated by the sympathetic nervous system. Large doses cause a rise in heart rate and a fall in blood pressure and therefore the pulse and blood pressure should be checked frequently, especially during intravenous administration. In the event of a marked fall in blood pressure it is recommended that the woman be turned into a lateral position. Other side-effects include nausea, vomiting, flushing, sweating and tremor.

Treatment is usually commenced by slow intravenous infusion followed, as contractions cease, by intermittent intramuscular doses and finally oral administration. The drug most commonly used now is ritodrine hydrochloride.

Ritodrine hydrochloride (Yutopar)

Indications	Uncomplicated preterm labour, fetal asphyxia due to hypertonic uterine action
Action	Beta-2-adrenoceptor stimulant
Dose	10–120 mg depending on route IV: Initial 50 µg/min increased to usual dose 150–350 µg/min IM: 10 mg 3–8 hourly Oral: 30 minutes prior to the termination of IV therapy Oral maintenance: First 24 hours 10 mg every 2 hours; thereafter 10–20 mg every 4–6 hours maximum 120 mg daily
Route	Oral, IM, IV
Contraindications	Haemorrhage, hypertension, pre-eclampsia, cord compression, infection, eclampsia, antepartum haemorrhage which demands immediate

	delivery, maternal cardiac disease
Side-effects	Nausea, vomiting, flushing, sweating, tremor, and, with high doses, hypokalaemia, tachycardia and hypotension.

Drugs Used in Labour

ANALGESICS

Pethidine hydrochloride

Pethidine is a powerful analgesic and antispasmodic; it is the most widely used analgesic in the obstetric field, relieving the pain of labour without diminishing the force of uterine contraction. It is used during the first stage of labour to produce analgesia and relaxation and, when given intramuscularly, takes effect in 10–15 minutes.

Pethidine crosses the placenta and may depress the fetal respiratory centre, thus if given within 2–3 hours of delivery it may cause birth asphyxia. In most normal deliveries a total of 200 mg (usually in doses of 100 mg) should prove adequate and therefore many health authorities and trusts insist that a medical practitioner is called if more than this amount is required.

In some cases pethidine may be given intravenously for rapid action and effective pain relief in labour.

Pethidine should not be given to mothers being treated with amino oxidase inhibitors as these drugs potentiate the action of pethidine about ten times, thus the combination is highly dangerous.

Indications	Moderate to severe pain, obstetric analgesia
Action	Opioid analgesic (used in labour due to being associated with less respiratory depression than other opioids)
Dose	SC or IM injection 50–100 mg repeated 1–3 hours later if necessary Oral 50–150 mg every 4 hours
Route	SC, IM, oral
Contraindications	Severe renal impairment, raised intracranial pressure, head injury; treatment with amino oxidase inhibitors

Side-effects	Nausea and vomiting, constipation, drowsiness, respiratory depression, hypotension.

Pentazocine (S.4B) (Fortral)

Pentazocine is a powerful analgesic, similar in its action to morphine but apparently free from its addictive properties. It is effective in labour and has been approved by the UKCC for the use of midwives although it is rarely used nowadays. The effect on the maternal blood pressure, pulse and uterine activity and on the fetal condition is similar to that seen with pethidine.

Indications	Moderate to severe pain
Action	Opioid analgesic
Dose	Oral 50 mg every 3–4 hours after food (dose range 25–100 mg) SC, IM, IV 30 mg for moderate pain, 45–60 mg for severe pain, every 3–4 hours
Route	Oral, SC, IM, IV
Contraindications	Avoid in patients dependent on opioids, or with hypertension or porphyria
Side-effects	Occasional hallucinations, nausea and vomiting, constipation, drowsiness. Can cause abstinence syndrome in fetus.

TRANQUILLIZERS

Tranquillizers are sometimes given in pregnancy, labour or postpartum. They are antiemetic, potentiate the analgesic (if given), relieve anxiety and apprehension and help the overanxious mother to rest. Tranquillizers which may be used in midwifery practice include the following.

Promazine BP (S.4B) (Sparine)

Indications	Short-term adjunctive management of psychomotor agitation
Action	Anti-psychotic
Dose	Oral 100–200 mg four times daily IM 50 mg for short-term adjunctive management

Route	Oral or IM
Contraindications	Coma caused by CNS depressants, bone marrow depression, phaeochromo-cytoma. Cardiovascular and cerebrovascular disease
Side-effects	Drowsiness, apathy, pallor, hypothermia, nightmares, insomnia, depression.

Diazepam (Valium)

Diazepam is a tranquillizer and an anticonvulsant and may be administered by intravenous infusion in cases of severe pre-eclampsia and eclampsia.

Indications	Anxiety, insomnia, anti-convulsant, may be used for treatment of severe pre-eclampsia and eclampsia
Action	Anxiolytic (sedative), anti-convulsant
Dose	2 mg → depending on need and route for pre-eclampsia and eclampsia 5–10 mg IM or by IV infusion (40 mg/500 ml) to a maxi-mum of 3 mg/kg over 24 hours
Route	Oral, IM, IV, rectal
Contraindications	Respiratory depression, acute pulmonary insufficiency, phobic or obsessional states, chronic psychosis, porphyria
Side-effects	Drowsiness and lightheaded-ness the next day, confusion and ataxia, amnesia, depen-dence.

HYPNOTICS

Chloral hydrate

Indications	Insomnia (short-term use)
Action	Hypnotic
Dose	0.5–1 g (maximum 2 g) at bedtime with plenty of water
Route	Oral
Contraindications	Severe cardiac disease, gastri-tis, marked renal or hepatic impairment, respiratory disease

Side-effects	Gastric irritation, flatulence, occasionally rashes, headache, dependence.

LOCAL ANAESTHESIA

Local anaesthetic drugs act by causing a temporary block to conduction along nerve fibres. Toxic effects associated with local anaesthetics may occur as a result of very high blood levels or too rapid an injection. Signs of toxicity include excitability of the central nervous system which is characterized by nausea and convulsions, followed by depression. The cardiovascu-lar system may also be depressed. Urgent resuscitative measures are necessary. The anaesthetics most com-monly used in obstetrics are as follows.

Lignocaine hydrochloride

Indications	Anaesthesia, nerve blocks, epidural and caudal block
Action	Local anaesthetic. Reversible block to conduction along nerve fibres
Dose	Adjusted according to site and response. For infiltration of the perineum prior to episiotomy up to 10 ml of 0.5% solution. Epidural and caudal block – with adrenaline 1 in 200 000, 1% to a maximum of 50 ml
Route	Topical or SC or epidural
Contraindications	Inflamed or infected tissues (may cause a systemic rather than a local reaction). Hypo-volaemia, complete heart block
Side-effects	Hypotension, bradycardia, cardiac arrest, agitation, euphoria, respiratory depres-sion, convulsions.

Bupivacaine (Marcain)

Bupivacaine is widely used for continuous epidural analgesia in labour. It takes up to 30 minutes to take full effect but then lasts for 2–3 hours.

Indications	Epidural and spinal anaes-thesia
Action	Local anaesthetic

Dose	According to the site of operation and response of the patient
Route	Into epidural space, e.g. in labour: Lumbar 0.25–0.5% maximum 12 ml Caudal 0.25% maximum 30 ml 0.5% maximum 20 ml (0.75% solution contraindicated for epidural use in pregnancy)
Contraindications	Hypovolaemia, complete heartblock, avoid in porphyria, intravenous regional anaesthesia, caution in epilepsy
Side-effects	Hypotension, bradycardia, cardiac arrest. CNS effects include agitation, euphoria, respiratory depression, convulsions.

Oxytocic Drugs

Oxytocin BP (Syntocinon)

Oxytocin was synthesized in 1954 by Du Vigneaud. In 1961 Embrey succeeded in combining ergometrine with oxytocin to form Syntometrine (Dumoulin, 1981). Syntometrine is now widely used for the active management of the third stage of labour. Administered intramuscularly it takes effect in 2–3 minutes.

Oxytocin may also be given diluted in an intravenous infusion to induce or augment labour. The uterine contractions and fetal heart are continuously monitored, as hyperstimulation can cause fetal distress leading to intrauterine fetal death. In the presence of malpresentation or cephalopelvic disproportion such contractions can cause rupture of the uterus. Intravenous oxytocin can cause a transient but marked fall in blood pressure (Hendricks and Brenner, 1970) with tachycardia and an increased stroke volume which increases the cardiac output. It also has an antidiuretic action.

Indications	For prevention or treatment of haemorrhage during third stage of labour. Induction and augmentation of labour
Action	Stimulates uterine contractions
Dose	For induction and augmentation of labour: 1–3 mU/min, adjusted according to response by slow IV infusion For missed abortion: As a solution containing 10–20 units/500 ml given at a rate of 10–30 drops/minute, increased in strength by 10–20 units/500 ml every hour to a maximum strength of 100 units/500 ml For postpartum haemorrhage: 20–40 units per 500 ml Hartmann's solution.
Route	IM, slow IV infusion
Contraindications	Hypertonic uterine action, mechanical obstruction to delivery, failed trial labour, severe hypertension, fetal distress, placenta praevia
Side-effects	High doses cause violent uterine contractions which may lead to rupture and fetal asphyxiation, arrhythmias, maternal hypertension and subarachnoid haemorrhage, and pulmonary oedema.

Ergometrine maleate BP (S.4B)

Ergometrine was introduced to obstetric practice in the 1930s by Chassar Moir. Since then it has proved to be of immense value in the prevention and treatment of postpartum haemorrhage. It has a powerful action on the uterus especially immediately after labour, when it produces rhythmic contractions. Its action is less rapid but more prolonged than that of oxytocin. Ergometrine is given to prevent and control haemorrhage during childbirth, especially if an anaesthetic has been used and hence uterine action is poor. It is most usually injected intramuscularly with the crowning of the head or the birth of the anterior shoulder, or intravenously when there is increased risk such as antepartum haemorrhage, postpartum haemorrhage or poor muscle tone which occurs with such conditions as grande multiparity and multiple pregnancy. It may be injected into the uterine wall by the surgeon during Caesarean section. Ergometrine may be given orally postpartum to ensure good contraction of the uterus.

There are complications associated with the use of ergometrine, particularly if given intravenously (Dumoulin, 1981). Hypertension has been reported by many researchers, including Hendricks and Brenner (1970), Johnstone (1972) and Moir and Amoa (1979). Cases of pulmonary oedema in cardiac patients, cardiac arrest and cerebral haemorrhage have also been reported (DHSS, 1986). It has been shown to cause a reduction in serum prolactin levels and thus could reduce the production of breast milk. Finally there is a high incidence of vomiting especially following the administration of intravenous ergometrine (Moodie and Moir, 1976). Midwives should therefore avoid giving ergometrine to women with hypertensive disorders (DOH, 1994) and those suffering from cardiac and respiratory conditions, unless the drug is prescribed by a doctor.

Indications	Prevention and treatment of haemorrhage
Action	Oxytocic, i.e. stimulates uterine contractions
Dose	Third stage labour: 500 µg IM, usually with oxytocin 5 units
	Prevention in high risk cases: 125–250 µg IV
	Secondary postpartum haemorrhage: 500 µg orally three times daily for three days
Route	IM, IV, oral
Contraindications	First and second stages of labour (only with crowning of head or birth of anterior shoulder in second stage), vascular disease, hepatic and renal impairment, severe hypertension, sepsis. Caution with multiple pregnancy, pre-eclampsia, eclampsia
Side-effects	Nausea, vomiting, transient hypertension, vasoconstriction, stroke.

Oxytocin and ergometrine (Syntometrine (S.4B))

This is a proprietary preparation containing oxytocin 5 units and ergometrine 500 µg in 1 ml. Intramuscular Syntometrine takes effect in 2–3 minutes. Syntometrine is said to combine the best of two constituents: it acts quickly because of the oxytocin and the action is prolonged by the ergometrine. Its use is confined to the prevention and treatment of postpartum haemorrhage. Syntometrine 1 ml is usually injected intramuscularly with the crowning of the head or the birth of the anterior shoulder. It causes a powerful contraction of the uterus which aids placental separation and the control of bleeding.

Indications	As for ergometrine maleate. Used for active management of third stage of labour or routine prevention or treatment of postpartum haemorrhage
Action	As for ergometrine maleate
Dose	1 ml IM
	0.5–1 ml IV
Route	IM, IV
Contraindications	As for ergometrine maleate.
Side effects	As for ergometrine maleate.

Prostaglandins

Prostaglandins are substances found in extracts and secretions of human prostate and seminal vesicles and in many other parts of the body. There are several preparations similar in action but slightly different in their chemical structure. Certain prostaglandins cause contraction of uterine muscle and are used in therapeutic abortion and to induce labour.

Prostaglandins are contraindicated in the same situations as oxytocin and should be used with caution in patients with raised intraocular pressure or a history of asthma.

They may cause nausea, vomiting and diarrhoea.

Prostaglandin E_2 (PGE_2) may be administered vaginally, extra-amniotically or orally to ripen the cervix, when necessary, or to induce labour. Vaginal PGE_2 may be given in a gel, tablets or lipid-based pessaries. A PGE_2 polymer vaginal pessary (3 mg) is now available. Extra-amniotic instillation can be either intermittent or by continuous infusion through a transcervical catheter. Prostaglandin $F_{2\alpha}$ may also be administered vaginally to ripen the cervix, although some studies have shown it to be less effective for ripening the unfavourable cervix than PGE$_2$

Oral preparations of prostaglandins for routine induction of labour are satisfactory provided the cervix is favourable and particularly in multiparous women. Prolonged treatment, however, such as may be required to ripen the cervix may cause side-effects.

Prostaglandins are not administered intravenously because of their unpleasant side-effects which include nausea, vomiting, diarrhoea, local tissue reaction and erythema.

Respiratory Drugs

Respiratory stimulants which are antidotes to pethidine and other narcotics may be used if the baby shows signs of respiratory depression at birth.

Naloxone hydrochloride (Narcan Neonatal)

Naloxone hydrochloride is a narcotic antagonist which is given intramuscularly or intravenously to a baby suffering from respiratory depression at birth. It has replaced earlier antidotes such as nalorphine and levallorphan because they are also partial agonists and can thus cause respiratory depression themselves.

Indications	Reversal of opioid-induced respiratory depression
Action	Competitively binds to opioid receptors
Dose	IV 100–200 µg. If response inadequate, increments of 100 µg every 2 min. Further doses by IM injection after 1–2 hours if required *Neonate*: 10 µg/kg by SC, IM, IV route repeated every 2–3 min or 200 µg (60 µg/kg) by IM as a single dose at birth
Route	SC, IM or IV
Contraindications	Acute opioid withdrawal may be precipitated in opioid-dependent patients
Side-effects	Not a problem at therapeutic doses.

Coagulants

Phytomenadione (Vitamin K)

Indications and action	Production of blood clotting factors and proteins necessary for normal calcification of bone
Dose	See policy agreed locally for neonatal use, e.g. prophylactic dose 0.5 mg orally or by injection If mother is breastfeeding, the dose is repeated on 7th and 28th day of life
Route	Oral, IM or IV
Contraindications	None reported
Side-effects	Associated with development of haemolytic anaemia; hyperbilirubinaemia and kernicterus have been reported.

Anticoagulants

Anticoagulants are widely used in the prevention and treatment of deep vein thrombosis.

Heparin

Heparin is given to start anticoagulation and is rapidly effective although its effects are of short duration. It is therefore best given by continuous infusion. If given intermittently, the interval should not exceed six hours. Oral anticoagulants are started at the same time as heparin and heparin is discontinued after three days.

Dose	5000 units initially, followed by continuous infusion of 40 000 units over 24 hours or 10 000 units by intravenous injection every 6 hours.

Warfarin sodium

Oral anticoagulants take 36–48 hours to take effect. The dose of oral anticoagulants is adjusted to prolong the prothrombin time.

Oral anticoagulants are teratogenic and therefore should not be given in early pregnancy. They cross the placenta and thus are not given in the last few weeks of pregnancy.

Protamine sulphate

Protamine sulphate is used to counteract an overdose of heparin. It is given by slow intravenous injection, the maximum dose being 50 mg. An overdose of protamine sulphate has an anticoagulant effect.

Other Drugs Used in Obstetrics

OPIUM DERIVATIVES

Narcotics may be prescribed by a medical practitioner. Morphine is rarely administered in labour now because labours are shorter and regional analgesia is preferred. Narcotics cross the placental barrier and will depress the fetal respiratory centre, thus should not be given if delivery is expected within the next two hours. They are more likely to be prescribed post-operatively or in conditions causing severe shock.

Morphine BP (CD)

Dose 10–15 mg subcutaneously or intramuscularly.

Drugs and Breastfeeding

Most drugs pass into the breast milk but reach the baby in much smaller quantities than the dose given to the mother. Many factors affect the amount of drug received by the baby in breast milk. These include dosage, duration of drug therapy, age of the infant, quantity of milk consumed and degree of oral absorption by the baby (Anderson, 1991). In addition to the effect of drugs on babies, the possible effect on lactation should be considered. Some drugs decrease the secretion of prolactin and therefore the milk yield which may lead to an early cessation of breastfeeding (Ostrom, 1990). Others may reduce oxytocin which affects the milk flow.

Drugs which should be avoided are listed below (Rubin, 1987):

▶ Laxatives, apart from bulking agents such as preparations containing bran, ispaghula, or methylcellulose.
▶ Barbiturates.
▶ Benzodiazepines.
▶ Bromide salts.
▶ Ephedrine.
▶ Amiodarone.
▶ Lithium.
▶ Opiates.
▶ Carbimazole.
▶ Iodine, apart from propylthiouracil.
▶ Cytotoxics and immunosuppressant drugs.

Expert advice should be obtained about the selection of suitable drugs for the mother who is breastfeeding. Very often there are safe alternatives which may allow the mother to continue breastfeeding. A detailed source of information on this topic is the book *Drugs and Human Lactation* which was compiled by the World Health Organization (Bennett *et al.*, 1988).

References

Anderson, P.O. (1991) Drug use during breastfeeding. *Clin. Pharm.* 10: 594–624.

Bennett, P.N., Matheson, I. & Dukes, N.M.G. *et al.* (1988) *Drugs and Human Lactation.* Amsterdam: Elsevier.

Barrett, J.F.R., Whittaker, P.G., Williams, J.G. & Lind, T. (1994) Absorption of non-haem iron from food during normal pregnancy. *Br. Med. J.* 309: 79–82.

DHSS (1958) *Controlled Drugs and Medicines in Hospital* (Aitken Report). HM (58) 17. London: DHSS.

DHSS (1986) *Report on Confidential Enquiries into Maternal Deaths in England and Wales 1979–1981.* London: HMSO.

DOH (Department of Health) (1988) *Guidelines for the Safe and Secure Handling of Medicines* (Duthie Report). London: DOH.

DOH (1994) *Report on Confidential Enquiries into Maternal Deaths in the United Kingdom 1988–1990.* London: HMSO.

Dumoulin, J.G. (1981) A reappraisal of the use of ergometrine. *J. Obstet. Gynaecol.* 1: 178–181.

Eclampsia Trial Collaborative Group (1995) Which anticonvulsant for women with eclampsia? Evidence from the collaborative eclampsia trial. *Lancet* 345: 1455–1463.

Embrey, M.P. (1961) Simultaneous intramuscular injection of oxytocin and ergometrine. *Br. Med. J.* i: 1387–1389.

Hay-Smith, J. (1994) Postpartum laxatives. In Enkin, M.W., Keirse, M.J.N.C., Renfrew, M.J. & Neilson, J.P. (eds) *Pregnancy and Childbirth Module.* Cochrane Database of Systematic Reviews: Review no. 03663. Cochrane Updates on Disk, Disk Issue 1. Oxford: Update Software.

Hendricks, C.H. & Brenner, W.E. (1970) Cardiovascular effects of oxytocic drugs used postpartum. *Am. J. Obstet. Gynecol.* **108**: 751–760.

Hytten, F.E. & Leitch, I. (1971) *The Physiology of Pregnancy.* Oxford: Blackwell Scientific.

Johnstone, M. (1972) The cardiovascular effects of oxytocic drugs. *Br. J. Anaesth.* **51**: 113–116.

Medical Research Council Vitamin Study Group (1991) Prevention of neural tube defects: Results of the Medical Research Council Vitamin Study. *Lancet* **238**: 131–137.

Moir, D.D. & Amoa, A.B. (1979) Ergometrine or oxytocin? *J. Anaesth.* **51**: 113–116.

Moodie, J.E. & Moir, D.D. (1976) Ergometrine, oxytocin or extradural analgesia. *Br. J. Anaesth.* **48**: 57.

Neilson, J.P. (1995) Magnesium sulphate: the drug of choice in eclampsia. *Br. Med. J.* **311**: 702–703.

O'Hare, M.F., Kinney, C.D., Murnaghan, J.A. & McDevitt, D.G. (1984) Pharmacokinetics of phenytoin during pregnancy. *Eur. J. Clin. Pharmacol.* **27**: 105–110.

Ostrom, K.M. (1990) A review of the hormone prolactin during lactation. *Prog. Food Nutr. Sci.* **14**: 1–44.

Pirani, B.B.K., Campbell, D.M. & McGillivray, I. (1973) Plasma volume in normal first pregnancy. *J. Obstet. Gynaecol. Br. Commonwealth.* **80**: 884–887.

Rubin, P.C. (ed.) (1987) *Prescribing in pregnancy.* London: British Medical Journal.

Studd, J. (1975) The plasma proteins in pregnancy. *Clin. Obstet. Gynaecol.* **2**: 285–300.

UKCC (UK Central Council for Nursing, Midwifery & Health Visiting) (1991) *Registrar's Letter 6/1991 Dichloralphenazone (Welldorm).* London: UKCC.

UKCC (1992) *Standards for Administration of Medicines.* London: UKCC.

UKCC (1993) *Midwives' Rules.* London: UKCC.

UKCC (1994) *The Midwife's Code of Practice.* London: UKCC.

UKCC (1995) Registrar's letter 31/1995. Approval of apparatus for the administration of inhalation analgesia by midwives. London: UKCC.

Further Reading

Lockie, A. (1989) *The Family Guide to Homeopathy*, p. 282–299. London: Hamish Hamilton.

Siney, C. (ed.) (1995) *The Pregnant Drug Addict.* Hale: Books for Midwives Press.

Tisserand, M. (1993) *Pregnancy and Childbirth, After the Birth*, pp. 102–116. London: Thorsons.

89

Vital Statistics

Notification and Registration of Births

The Public Health Act 1936 requires that the father, or any person in attendance at the birth or within six hours after, notify the birth to the Medical Officer within 36 hours. In practice this duty is commonly undertaken by the midwife, who is supplied by the health authority with printed cards and stamped envelopes, or completes a computerized notification.

All livebirths (even before the 24th week) and stillbirths must be notified.

The purpose of notification is to communicate information about the birth to the health visitor, including in particular any babies who may appear to be at risk. The information goes into a computer which is programmed to ensure recall at appropriate times for screening, vaccination and immunization. It is also used for statistical and epidemiological purposes.

Registration of births

The Registration of Births and Deaths Act 1953 requires all livebirths and stillbirths to be registered with the Registrar of Births and Deaths within 42 days of the birth of the baby. The baby has to be registered with the registrar of the district in which the child was born.

Registration is the responsibility of the child's parents. If the parents fail to register the birth, the duty falls on the occupier of the premises in which the birth took place, the midwife or some other person of authority. A short certificate giving the full name and sex of the child and the date and place of birth is issued free. A fee is charged for a more detailed certificate which includes information about the parents of the child.

An illegitimate child is registered by the mother. The father's name can be entered on the birth certificate only if he accompanies the mother and requests that his name be entered; or it may be entered without his consent on production of an order made under the Affiliation Proceedings Act 1957.

A stillbirth must be registered before burial and for this a certificate signed by a medical practitioner, or a midwife who was present at birth or examined the body afterwards must be produced.

Fertility Rate

The general fertility rate is described as the number of births per 1000 women aged 15–44 years. There was increasing fertility in the UK between 1952 and 1964 when it peaked at 94 births per 1000 women (DOH, 1994). The rate then gradually decreased until 1977 when it reached a minimum of 59. After a fluctuating rate for the next few years, there has been a slight annual increase since 1982. In 1990 the rate in the UK reached 64 (Craig, 1992).

Birth Rate

The birth rate is the number of registered livebirths per 1000 population. After a downward trend, there has been a slight increase in birth rate since the early 1980s. The live birth rate for England and Wales in 1994 was 12.9 per 1000 population.

Stillbirth

A baby who has issued forth from its mother after the 24th week of pregnancy and has not at any time after being completely expelled from its mother breathed or shown any sign of life is a stillborn baby.

The stillbirth rate is the number of stillbirths registered during the year per 1000 registered total (live and still) births. In 1994 the stillbirth rate for England and Wales was 5.7.

Causes

The main causes of stillbirth are:

▶ Fetal anoxia.
▶ Congenital abnormalities.

Conditions which may lead to intrauterine anoxia are cord prolapse, placental dysfunction or premature separation, abnormal uterine action, cephalopelvic disproportion, medical conditions such as diabetes, haemolytic disease, intrauterine infection and traumatic delivery.

Duties imposed on midwives by statute regarding stillbirths

Certain duties are imposed on midwives by statute regarding stillbirths. These include the following:

1   *Notification of stillbirth* (see previous page).
2   *Certification of stillbirth*: It is usual for the medical practitioner who was present at a stillbirth or examined the body to give the father or mother a certificate of stillbirth. Otherwise the midwife should give the certificate if she was present at the stillbirth or examined the body. Whenever possible the midwife should state on this certificate the cause of death and the estimated duration of pregnancy to the best of her knowledge and belief.
3   *Registration*: On receipt of the stillbirth certificate the Registrar of Births and Deaths issues a certificate for burial or cremation. The parents should be advised that the stillbirth certificate issued to them by the Registrar of Births and Deaths can, on request, include the chosen name of their stillborn baby. It is usual for the hospital or health authority to make arrangements for the baby's burial or cremation, although occasionally the parents prefer to do this personally.

Sometimes the coroner issues an Order for Burial and then a certificate is not required. The hospital or health authority meets the cost of the burial or cremation. There is no death grant for a stillborn baby.

Following a stillbirth the midwife must be prepared to provide much help and support to the mother and her family during the postnatal period. Her understanding of the family's grief and her skill as a counsellor can do much to comfort and support them (see Chapter 78).

Stillbirths are included in perinatal deaths.

Perinatal Mortality

The perinatal mortality rate comprises all stillbirths and all deaths in the first week of life per 1000 registered total births (Figure 1). The group includes all those children who have died 'around' the time of birth.

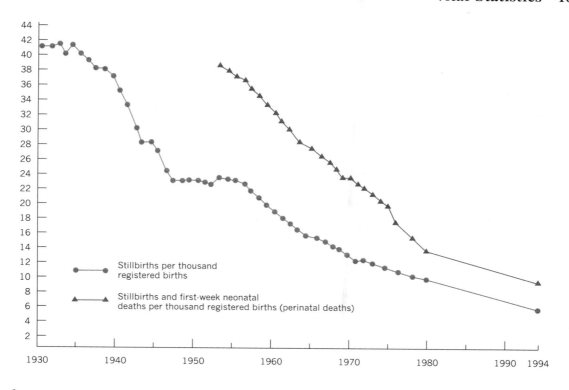

Figure 1   The stillbirth and perinatal death rates for England and Wales.

In 1958 and again in 1970 nationwide perinatal surveys were carried out to gain more knowledge of perinatal deaths and thus to reduce the number. Much valuable information was brought to light which analysed many factors which might in some way influence the survival of the child. The Report of the Committee on Child Health Services 1976 made unfavourable comparisons between perinatal and infant mortality in Great Britain and in other developed countries (DHSS, 1976). These were reiterated by the Department of Health and Social Security in *The Way Forward*, published in 1977 (DHSS, 1977).

Since then the perinatal mortality rate in the UK has fallen considerably and the Short Committee in 1984 welcomed the improvements in perinatal and neonatal mortality which had occurred since the publication of its earlier report in 1980 (Social Services Committee, 1980, 1984). The Committee expressed concern, however, that the highest fetal and infant mortalities are still mainly associated with the lower socio-economic groups. The Working Group on Inequalities in Health chaired by Sir Douglas Black made similar observations (DHSS, 1980).

Seven years later another report, *The Health Divide*,

found the problem of inequality still existed, although several local initiatives had been introduced in the intervening years to try and improve the care offered (Whitehead, 1987). Additional support and the provision of health care which is easily accessible and acceptable to the local community has been shown to improve mortality and morbidity rates (Davies, 1988; Armstrong and Royston, 1989; Currell, 1990; Chadwick, 1994; Keirse, 1994). Inequalities in health still exist, however, and are a cause of great concern. Despite this ongoing problem, the perinatal mortality rate in England and Wales fell from 19.3 per 1000 in 1975 to 8.9 per 1000 in 1994, but there are wide variations in rate between the different socio-economic groups, with markedly higher rates in the low socio-economic groups. Further initiatives are therefore required to address this problem.

Causes

The main causes of perinatal death are:

▶ Anoxia.
▶ Congenital abnormalities.
▶ Immaturity.
▶ Cerebral birth injury.

Predisposing causes

Social factors   The perinatal mortality rate is very much higher in the socio-economic groups IV and V and the gap among the social classes is widening rather than decreasing (DHSS, 1980; Social Services Committee, 1980, 1984; Whitehead, 1987). The social class differences in access to social and medical care also continue with the lower socio-economic groups still not fully utilizing the services available.

Several researchers have found that the decline in perinatal mortality may be attributed to an increase in birthweight, and this is regarded as an indicator of improved environmental and social factors rather than medical care (Editorial, 1986). Low birthweight is still more prevalent in lower socio-economic groups. Even if a low birthweight baby survives the perinatal period, recent studies have shown that those who are small or disproportionate at birth, or who have altered placental growth, are at an increased risk of developing coronary heart disease, hypertension and diabetes during adult life (Godrey and Barker, 1995).

The perinatal mortality rate for babies of unsupported mothers is nearly double that of their married (or supported) counterparts. Biological factors such as short stature, maternal age under 20 or over 35 years and first pregnancies or high parity all increase the risk. Similarly the risk is higher in most immigrant groups.

Obstetric factors   Conditions such as bleeding in pregnancy, hypertensive disorders, malpresentations, malposition, multiple pregnancy, cephalopelvic disproportion, prolonged labour, preterm and postmature labours, prolapsed cord and rhesus haemolytic disease all increase the perinatal risk.

Medical conditions   The risk of perinatal death is increased when the mother suffers from conditions such as diabetes mellitus, renal conditions, anaemia, respiratory conditions, epilepsy, infections such as rubella, cytomegalovirus, toxoplasmosis and syphilis and hyperpyrexia, whatever the cause.

Teratogenic factors   Some drugs taken by the mother, alcohol and smoking all increase the risk to the fetus. Dietary deficiencies such as folic acid deficiency during the preconception period and in early pregnancy have been shown to be a cause of neural tube defects (Smithels *et al.*, 1980; MRC, 1991; Wald and Bower, 1995). Periconception vitamin supplementation is therefore advised, especially when there is a history of these malformations. Poor intrauterine nutrition may also affect the long-term health of the individual into adult life (Godrey and Barker, 1995).

Measures to reduce the perinatal mortality rate

1   Better *social conditions*, such as improved nutrition and housing.
2   Improved *education*; including health education in schools and subsequently.
3   Better *antenatal care*, to include:

▶ individualized care to meet the particular needs of each woman, including the provision of additional support (Oakley *et al.*, 1990; DOH, 1993);
▶ early booking and proper selection of the appropriate place of confinement;
▶ identification and close supervision of all 'at risk' mothers;
▶ effective health education;
▶ screening tests to detect abnormalities;
▶ genetic counselling;
▶ early detection and treatment of complications.

4   Better *care in labour*, to include:

▶ induction, where appropriate, to avoid an unfavourable intrauterine environment;
▶ active management of labour, where necessary, to avoid prolonged labour;
▶ continuous fetal heart monitoring, if indicated;
▶ prompt and skilful management of intra- and extrauterine hypoxia;
▶ adequate neonatal special and intensive care facilities throughout the country;
▶ further improvements in the staffing levels and training of midwives and doctors involved in obstetrics and neonatal paediatrics.

The perinatal mortality rate is considered a good indication of the standards of obstetric and neonatal care, although, as discussed above, there are factors in addition to the health service which have an important influence. Nowadays there is concern not only about mortality, but also about the quality of the survivors. Some babies who survive perinatal complications may be left with a permanent handicap.

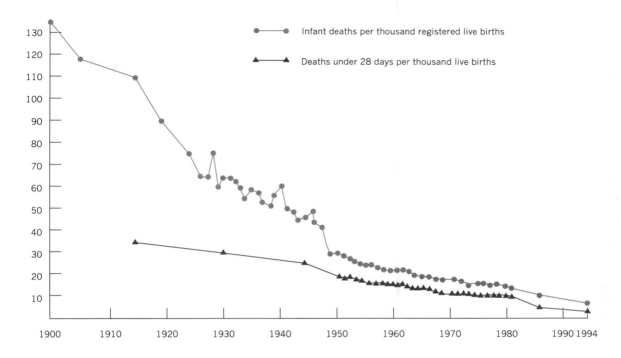

Figure 2 The infant and neonatal death rates for England and Wales.

Neonatal Mortality

The neonatal mortality rate (Figure 2) is the number of deaths of babies within four weeks of birth per 1000 registered livebirths. In 1994 the neonatal mortality rate was 4.1 per 1000.

The majority of neonatal deaths occur in the first day or two after birth, which closely relates the death of the baby to labour and delivery. The cause of perinatal and neonatal deaths occurring in the first week of life are obviously related and may also be responsible for later neonatal deaths, although other factors such as infection may then also be included.

The neonatal mortality rate, like the other mortality rates, is declining and fell from 11.0 in 1975 to 4.1 in 1994. The reasons for reduction in the neonatal mortality rate are similar to those responsible for the decline in perinatal mortality.

Infant Mortality

The infant mortality rate is the number of deaths of infants during the first year of life (including those occurring during the first four weeks) per 1000 registered livebirths in the year.

Although the infant mortality rate has declined greatly in the last 50 years, of the total number of deaths in the first year most still occur in the first four weeks of life. The majority of these neonatal deaths occur within a day or two of delivery.

The infant mortality rate for 1994 was 6.2, of which neonatal deaths accounted for 4.1. During this century there has been a remarkable decline in infant deaths from 140 per thousand livebirths in 1900 to 6.2 per thousand in 1994.

Causes

The main causes of death are:

▶ Infection, mainly acute respiratory and gastrointestinal infections.
▶ Accidents.
▶ Child abuse.
▶ Sudden infant death.
▶ All the causes of neonatal death already described.

The social factors discussed under perinatal mortality are predisposing causes of infant death. Children born

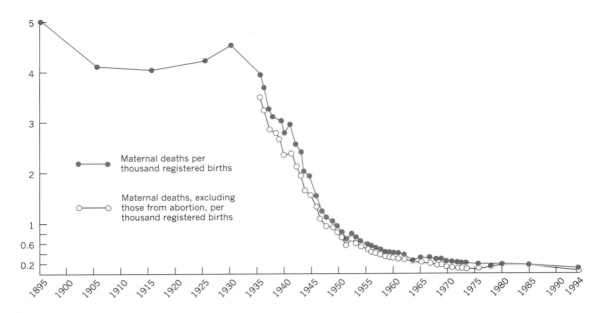

Figure 3 The maternal mortality rate for England and Wales.

into families in socio-economic groups IV and V are twice as likely to die between the end of the first month and the end of the first year of life since it is during this time that environment and other related factors have the most impact. However, the infant mortality rate is not related to class alone. It is also increased in children born to young mothers and to those who have inadequate antenatal care, smoke heavily, have low birthweight babies and live in inner city areas.

Measures to reduce the infant mortality rate

Measures to reduce the infant mortality rate include environmental improvements such as housing, improved preventive health services, education, including health education and social services. In parts of the country where the health services have changed their approach and go out and seek those in need, because it is these people who often do not use the services available, the results are encouraging (McKee, 1980; Reid *et al.*, 1983; Thomas *et al.*, 1987; Zander *et al.*, 1987; Davies, 1988).

Maternal Mortality

The maternal mortality rate (Figure 3) for any year is the number of deaths attributed to pregnancy and

childbearing per 1000 registered total births. In 1994 the maternal mortality rate in England and Wales was 0.07 (including abortions) per 1000 registered total births. Excluding abortions, the maternal mortality rate was 0.06.

Maternal deaths occurring more than 42 days after pregnancy or childbirth are no longer included in the figures, in line with the international definition of maternal deaths.

The International Classification of Diseases, Injuries and Causes of Death (ICD9) defines a maternal death as

the death of a woman while pregnant or within 42 days of termination of pregnancy, irrespective of the duration and the site of the pregnancy, from any cause related to or aggravated by the pregnancy or its management but not from accidental or incidental causes.

This definition is in accord with the definition adopted by the International Federation of Gynaecology and Obstetrics (FIGO).

The World Health Organization (WHO) Safe Motherhood Initiative was launched in 1987 and aims to reduce mortality and morbidity significantly among mothers and infants by the end of this century. Most of the annual total of 500 000 maternal deaths occur in developing countries, but women still die, albeit a small number, in the more affluent nations of the world. The maternal mortality rate is 7 per 100 000 births in the UK. In some parts of Europe it is lower, for example in Belgium 3.42 and in Sweden 4.78, whereas in some developing countries it is over 600 per 100 000 births (DOH, 1994).

In the UK a detailed report is published at three-yearly intervals on all maternal deaths reported.

Confidential enquiries into maternal deaths

A confidential enquiry into every maternal death is the responsibility of the Director of Public Health (DPH) in England and, in Wales, the Director of Public Health Medicine/Chief Administrative Medical Officer (DPHM/CAMO) of the District in which the woman usually resided.

When as much information as possible has been obtained from all the staff concerned with the care of the patient, the DPH or DPHM/CAMO sends the information to an assessor, who is a senior obstetrician in the same Region. In the case of anaesthetic deaths, or where there has been involvement of an anaesthetist, the case is also reviewed by an anaesthetic assessor. The assessor may require further information before commenting on the case and sending the completed form to the Chief Medical Officer at the Department of Health. In Scotland and Northern Ireland, the system of enquiry is similar, but one panel of assessors deals with all cases.

At the Department of Health, only advisors in obstetrics, gynaecology and anaesthetics see the forms. A *Report on Confidential Enquiries into Maternal Deaths in England and Wales* was published for each successive three-year period from the 1952–54 report until the 1982–84 report. The reports published on the years since 1985 have included all four countries of the UK.

In the latest report for the three-year period 1991–93 (DOH, 1996) there were 320 maternal deaths reported to the enquiry. Of these deaths, 46 occurred after 42 days postpartum and are therefore not included in the definition of maternal mortality. Maternal deaths are divided into *direct* deaths which result from obstetric complications of pregnancy, labour and the puerperium, and *indirect* deaths which are caused by either a previous existing disease, or from a disease which developed during pregnancy, or was worsened by pregnancy. *Fortuitous* deaths may also occur and are

the result of causes which are not at all related to pregnancy, for example, road traffic accidents.

In the 1991–93 enquiry there were 128 direct deaths, 100 indirect deaths and 46 fortuitous deaths.

Approximately one third (33%) of all maternal deaths in the 1991–93 report occurred before the 28th week of pregnancy. The main causes of direct deaths before 28 weeks were ectopic pregnancy and abortion.

Main causes of maternal death in the UK 1991–93

The main causes of maternal death are shown in Table 1.

Thrombosis and thromboembolism This is now the commonest cause of maternal deaths in the UK, with 35 deaths reported in the *Report on Confidential Enquiries into Maternal Deaths in the UK 1991–93* (DOH, 1996). There were 12 antepartum deaths, one intrapartum death and 17 postpartum deaths. Some of the deaths occurred in the second and third weeks after delivery, or even later. The significance of the symptoms of breathlessness and chest pain was not always recognized, especially when they occured late in the puerperium in low-risk women.

All 5 deaths due to cerebral thrombosis occured in the puerperium, and in 4 of the cases the women had been delivered by Caesarean section. Caesarean section is clearly an important risk factor in the development of venous thrombosis which may lead to thromboembolism. The Royal College of Obstetricians and Gynaecologists recommend that an assessment of risk should be made on all women undergoing Caesarean section and prophylaxis instituted, as appropriate (DOH, 1996: 58–59).

Table 1 Main causes of maternal death, UK 1991–93

Cause	No. of deaths
Thrombosis and thromboembolism	35
Hypertensive disorders	20
Early pregnancy deaths (including abortions)	18
Haemorrhage	15
Amniotic fluid embolism	10
Genital tract sepsis (excluding abortions)	9
Anaesthesia	8
Genital tract trauma	4

Hypertensive disorders of pregnancy These remain a major cause with 20 deaths due to this condition during 1991–93, a reduction from the previous report. Substandard care was evident in 80% of cases, compared with 81% in the previous report. This was mainly due to delay in taking appropriate action, failure to recognize the seriousness of the condition and inadequate consultant involvement.

Eclampsia occurred in 11 cases and severe pre-eclampsia in 9 of the maternal deaths. Cerebral complications, mainly intracerebral haemorrhage, is the commonest cause of death and this is followed by adult respiratory distress syndrome. Five women developed very severe pre-eclampsia between regular antenatal visits. One woman died undelivered and six died following a delivery that took place before 33 weeks. Twelve of the 19 patients who died in the puerperium were delivered by Caesarean section. In three of these cases the outcome was adversely affected by delay in expediting the delivery, the reason for this being the decision to wait for the availability of a cot in the neonatal unit in one of the cases. Delay in transferring the patients to an intensive care unit adversely affected the outcome in a further three cases. In six of the deaths poor control of fluid balance with circulatory overload was evident. The importance of maintaining an accurate fluid balance with one doctor coordinating clinical management is emphasized. In some cases serious symptoms such as headache, vomiting and epigastric pain are not recognized as being associated with severe pre-eclampsia, and therefore appropriate action is not taken early enough. All midwives must recognize the serious nature of these symptoms and take action when any one or more of them occur.

The *Report on Confidential Enquiries into Maternal Deaths in the UK 1991–93* stresses the importance of a system of referral to a regional consultant for advice and/or assistance for cases of severe hypertension in pregnancy. The occurrence of eclampsia or severe pre-eclampsia in the community is a serious emergency and the midwife should call ambulance paramedics immediately because they have been trained in cardiopulmonary resuscitation and the immediate management of obstetric complications. They can therefore give emergency treatment before the woman is transferred to hospital.

Haemorrhage Haemorrhage, both ante- and post-partum, is the third most common cause of maternal death in the UK. It is the major cause of maternal death in the world, the WHO estimating that nearly a quarter of all direct obstetric deaths are due to haemorrhage (WHO, 1994). The 15 deaths attributed to haemorrhage in the 1991–93 UK Report are nearly equally divided between ante- and postpartum haemorrhage. Coagulation failure (disseminated intravascular coagulation) occurred in about a quarter of the deaths due to haemorrhage.

Obstetric haemorrhage is still a significant cause of death in the UK, although the number of deaths from this cause has fallen since the previous *Report on Confidential Enquiries into Maternal Deaths in the UK, 1988–90*. Substandard care is still a cause of concern and the revised guidelines for the management of massive obstetric haemorrhage which are included in the 1988–90 Report are still relevant.

Early pregnancy deaths These include deaths due to ectopic pregnancy and abortion. In the 1991–93 Report there were 16 early pregnancy deaths, 8 due to ectopic pregnancy and 8 caused by abortion. Five of the deaths due to abortion were legal abortions and the other 3 were caused by spontaneous abortions. There were no deaths caused by illegal abortions.

The midwife should always refer a woman who complains of abdominal pain in early pregnancy to a doctor. Ectopic pregnancy is often a difficult condition to diagnose, especially as it may present with or without bleeding before the woman realizes that she is pregnant. Early investigations and appropriate treatment may be life-saving (see Chapter 40).

Other causes of maternal deaths

Amniotic embolism is a condition with a high mortality and was responsible for 10 maternal deaths in the 1991–93 report. Risk factors associated with this condition include higher maternal age and the use of oxytocic drugs to induce or augment labour (DOH, 1994). Sudden collapse during or after labour is a common feature of this condition.

There were eight deaths directly attributed to anaesthesia, an increase since the 1988–90 Report. It is a matter of concern that there are still deaths associated with sepsis during the three-year period 1991–93, a total of 15. This highlights the need to maintain high standards of hygiene and care and for vigilance to detect early signs and symptoms.

Throughout the Report cases of substandard care

are identified. This means that care fell short of generally accepted standards. Substandard care is still a major concern since it is identified in most sections of the Report.

Reasons for the reduction in maternal mortality

From 1900 until 1935 the maternal mortality rate was very high, varying between 4 and 5 per 1000 births, the commonest cause of death being puerperal sepsis. Other causes were haemorrhage, obstructed labour and eclampsia. Following the introduction in 1935 of the first of the sulphonamide drugs and in 1942 of penicillin, deaths from puerperal sepsis declined, at first with dramatic suddenness and then more gradually.

Blood transfusion, though a life-saving procedure, was at one time a hazardous and complicated operation. Gradually it became safer and simpler and blood banks were established, making blood more readily available, while more and more obstetric emergency services for the community were set up. Deaths from haemorrhage were thus fewer, oxytocic drugs such as ergometrine and Syntometrine having contributed further to the safety of the third stage of labour. Other drugs, such as anticoagulants, have also helped to reduce the maternal mortality rate.

The National Health Service provides complete maternity care for all childbearing women. Mothers are healthier and better nourished, and education, housing and other social conditions steadily improve. Doctors and midwives are better trained and they are supported by a substantial team of health workers of all kinds; most mothers receive good antenatal care. Deaths from eclampsia have declined, though hypertension remains a serious problem. With more skilled delivery and safer Caesarean section, many of the disasters resulting from obstructed labour and ruptured uterus are now avoided.

Women with medical complications come under the joint care of the specialist physician and obstetrician; anaesthetics are better and safer in the hands of skilled anaesthetists; and hospital delivery, with an experienced obstetrician at hand, good radiographic, ultrasound and laboratory facilities, and blood transfusion readily available, is strongly recommended for all mothers whose confinements may be anticipated to present special risk.

Since the implementation of the 1967 Abortion Act the number of deaths attributed to abortion has fallen considerably, whilst the provision of a free and widely available family planning service has reduced the number of unwanted pregnancies and the number of grande multiparous women.

Further efforts are required to improve the safety of childbirth and reduce the maternal mortality rate still more in the UK. A problem highlighted in the *Report on Confidential Enquiries into Maternal Deaths* is that some of the direct causes of death are so rare now that doctors and midwives have little experience of them and therefore may be slow to recognize the seriousness of the condition and instigate appropriate treatment. Vigilance must therefore continue in Britain and indeed worldwide to promote safe motherhood for all women.

References

Armstrong, S. & Royston, E. (1989) *Preventing Maternal Deaths.* Geneva: World Health Organization.

Chadwick, J. (1994) Perinatal mortality and antenatal care. *Modern Midwife* 4(9): 18–20.

Currell, R. (1990) The organisation of antenatal care. In Alexander, J., Levy, V. & Roch, S. (eds) *Antenatal Care. A Research-based Approach.* London: Macmillan.

Craig, J. (1992) Fertility trends in the United Kingdom. *Population Trends* No. 67. London: HMSO.

Davies, J. (1988) Cowgate Neighbourhood Centre – a preventative health care venture shared by midwives and social workers. *Midwives Chronicle* 101(1200): 4–7.

DOH (Department of Health) (1993) *Changing Childbirth,* Report of the Expert Maternity Group, Part 1. London: HMSO.

DOH (1994) *Report on Confidential Enquiries into Maternal Deaths in the United Kingdom 1988–1990.* London: HMSO.

DOH (1996) *Report on Confidential Enquiries into Maternal Deaths in the United Kingdom 1991–93.* London: HMSO.

DHSS (Department of Health and Social Security) (1976) *Fit for the Future. Report of the Committee on Child Health Services* (Chairman Professor S.D.M. Court). London: HMSO.

DHSS (1977) *The Way Forward.* London: HMSO.

DHSS (1980) *Inequalities in Health* (Chairman Sir Douglas Black). London: HMSO.

DHSS (1986) *Report on Confidential Enquiries into Maternal Deaths in England and Wales 1979–1981.* London: HMSO.

Editorial (1986) Perinatal care: organisation and outcome. *Lancet* April 5: 777–778.

Godrey, K.M. & Barker, D.J.P. (1995) Maternal nutrition in relation to fetal and placental growth. *Eur. J. Obstet. Gynecol. Reprod. Biol.* 61: 15–22.

Keirse, M.J.N.C. (1994) Maternal mortality: stalemate or stagnant? *Br. Med. J.* **308**: 344–345.

McKee, I. (1980) Community antenatal care: The Sighthill community antenatal care scheme. In Zander, L.I. & Chamberlain, G. (eds) *Pregnancy Care for the 80s*. London: Royal Society of Medicine/Macmillan Press.

MRC (Medical Research Council) (1991) Vitamin Study Research Group. Prevention of neural tube defects: results of the MRC vitamin study. *Lancet* **338**: 132–137.

OPCS (Office of Population Censuses and Surveys) (1995) Personal communication.

Oakley, A., Rajan, L. & Grant, A. (1990) Social support and pregnancy outcome. *Br. J. Obstet. Gynaecol.* **97**(2): 152–162.

Reid, M.E., Gutteridge, S. & McIlwaine, G.M. (1983) A comparison of the delivery of antenatal care between a hospital and a peripheral clinic. Social Paediatrics and Obstetric Research Unit, University of Glasgow.

Smithels, R.W., Sheppard, S., Schorah, L.J. *et al.* (1980) Possible prevention of neural tube defects by periconceptual vitamin supplementation. *Lancet* **i**: 339–340.

Thomas, H., Draper, J., Field, S. & Hare, M. (1987) Evaluation of an integrated antenatal clinic. *J. R. Coll. Gen. Pract.* **37**: 544–547.

Social Services Committee (1980) *Perinatal and Neonatal Mortality* (Chairman Mrs Renée Short). London: HMSO.

Social Services Committee (1984) *Perinatal and Neonatal Mortality: Follow-up* (Chairman Mrs Renée Short). London: HMSO.

Wald, N.J. & Bower, C. (1995) Folic acid and the prevention of neural tube defects. *Br. Med. J.* **310**: 1019–1020.

Whitehead, M. (1987) *The Health Divide: Inequalities in Health in the 1980s*. London: Health Education Council.

WHO (World Health Organization) (1994) *Mother–Baby Package: Implementing Safe Motherhood in Countries*. Geneva: WHO.

Zander, L., Lee-Jones, M. & Fisher, C. (1987) The role of the primary health care team in the management of pregnancy. In Kitzinger, S. & Davis, J. (eds) *The Place of Birth*. Oxford: Oxford Medical Publications.

90

Determining Effective Care: The Contribution of Midwifery Research

Many of the judgements about the value and safety of existing forms of obstetric care continue to be based on evidence that is likely to be invalid . . . . Similarly, the introduction of new forms of care is not accompanied by the kind of careful evaluation that history suggests would be a responsible and ethical way to proceed. . . . This is regrettable, not only because, in dealing with large numbers of basically healthy people, there is considerable potential for doing more harm than good on a very large scale; but also because the available evidence suggests that only a minority of innovations in health care turn out to be superior to existing practices.

(Chalmers, 1989: 3–4)

This extract highlights the crucial importance of evaluating alternative forms of care before practices become routinely accepted and adopted. For, as Chalmers reminds us, any treatment or therapy which has the potential to do good, also has the potential to do harm. This is especially significant when considering appropriate care for women, their babies and their families, since decisions and subsequent actions may have implications not just for the individual concerned, but also for future generations.

In this chapter, we will begin by exploring the sources of knowledge which influence the clinical decisions made by midwives whatever their sphere of practice or environment of care. We will then consider the role and specific contribution of research to the decision-making process and reflect upon why this link is important for professional accountability. Information sources unique to midwifery will be identified and we will consider ways in which current local and national initiatives within the UK offer unprecedented opportunities for the professional development of midwives and the development of midwifery practice.

Sources of Midwifery Knowledge

All decisions about midwifery care derive from specific sources of knowledge which are acquired through life experiences as well as through professional practice. They include ideas based on common sense, trial and error, tradition and ritual, in addition to lessons learned from personal and professional experience. In reaching a decision about which is the most appropriate care for a mother or her baby, it is unlikely that clinicians will draw upon only one source of knowledge. A decision is usually based upon a balance of influences which blend and fit together rather like pieces in a jigsaw to provide an overall picture of the whole situation (see Figure 1). We will now explore each of these sources of knowledge and consider their unique contribution to the development of midwifery practice.

Personal and professional experience

Personal or professional experience provides one piece of the jigsaw. These can be influential sources of knowledge which underlie personally held convictions about what constitutes 'best' care. Clearly, clinical impressions which stem from frequent contact with mothers and babies offer a vital source of professional knowledge; they can, however, also lead to false assumptions about the effects of care. Salmon (1985) cautions that 'the passing of the years does not necessarily bring gifts of understanding within one's own life. Twenty year's experience, it has been said, may be no more than one year's experience repeated 20 times'. What conclusions are we to draw when things are done one way by one midwife and a different way by a colleague? For example, there are those who frequently carry out episiotomies in the belief that, in so doing, they will

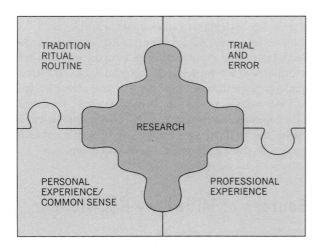

Figure 1   Sources of midwifery knowledge.

reduce the risk of severe maternal trauma, whilst other practitioners rarely reach for the scissors (Wilkerson, 1984).

Tradition, ritual and routine

Tradition, rituals and routines also play an important part in shaping midwifery practice. They exert a powerful influence largely because they are often handed down from one generation to another and in so doing achieve general acceptance. One such example is the way in which the pattern of antenatal visits has evolved over the years in such a way that it has become accepted practice in the UK for a women to attend for as many as 15 checks during pregnancy. Steer (1993) questions the effectiveness of such visits in detecting potential problems and suggests that the routine is perpetuated because 'midwives and doctors are haunted by the fear that they might miss something (or at least be accused of missing something) if they don't conform to the expected ritual'. Such rituals which clearly lack a sound rationale for their continuation need to be questioned. It is important, however, to differentiate between routines which are perpetuated because 'they have always been done that way', and those which may offer clearer benefits, such as listening to the fetal heart at regular intervals throughout labour.

Another way in which rituals and routines have been perpetuated is by using authority as a means of enforcing them. An example of this is the drafting of procedures and policies. Schön (1987) describes this as 'proceduralisation, that is, attempts to reduce professional practice to a set of absolutely clear, precise, implementable procedures'. You may be aware, in some units, of the imposition of a rigid time limit on the duration of the second stage of labour or restricting the time the baby is allowed to suck at the breast. Schön (1987) cautions that such authoritarianism 'invariably leads to the imposition of a rigid framework confining and limiting the actions of the professional, leaving little scope for individual judgement, skill, wisdom or artistry'. A further dimension is added when one compares policies across different maternity units, exposing considerable national variation (e.g. the policies relating to food and drink in labour). A survey of English maternity hospitals highlighted that units in the north of the country were more likely to allow women to eat at any time during labour than those in southern England (Garcia and Garforth, 1989). Differing practices such as these serve to highlight the lack of sound evidence to inform clinical decision-making.

Common sense and intuition

In many practice contexts, a midwife relies upon her intuition or 'gut feeling' in reaching a decision about what action would be in the mother's best interest. This is based on life experiences and on the kind of 'good sense' that does not depend upon being highly educated. Looked at in this way, Clark (1988) describes common sense as 'accumulated wisdom; it relies upon knowledge and judgement, and can, therefore, be considered as a way of thinking'. The problem is that it may reflect only the experience and feelings of one individual. Thus, in a given group of practitioners there may be a number of differing common-sense views of what constitutes appropriate care. For instance, one only has to reflect for a moment on the diversity of remedies used to soothe a crying baby to realize that there is no such thing as a common understanding. It is also important to remember how perceived wisdom can change for, as Luker (1986) reminds us, 'it used to be common sense to think that the world was flat and this could be confirmed by "just looking" or asking our neighbours. But, unfortunately, just looking or asking people who share our point of view, does not always provide valid conclusions'.

Trial and error

Historically, many developments in both obstetric and midwifery practice have been introduced on a trial-and-error basis. This applies equally to the use of new technologies (e.g. chorionic villus sampling and continuous electronic fetal monitoring in labour) to new therapies such as ultrasound and perineal massage, and to innovative patterns of care such as team midwifery. Very often, these innovations are adopted into practice without adequate evaluation, or on the basis of no evaluation at all. The problem lies not so much in the trial as in the possibility of error, for every time a new technique is used in a particular but uncontrolled situation with a given individual, this is tantamount to carrying out a poorly conducted experiment. Even if a treatment is found to be beneficial for a particular individual, the midwife could still not be confident that it would work for a different individual on a different occasion.

In addition, there is also a risk that an intervention may turn out to be positively harmful. Chalmers (1986) cautions against such an approach:

> When health professionals embark on uncharted therapeutic courses in their attempts to help individual patients, they tend to be judged by the worthiness of their intentions, not the lessons which should by now have been learned about the ways in which such uncontrolled experimentation has frequently led to clients receiving ineffective or positively harmful professional care.

A tragic example drawn from the past was the uncontrolled and widespread introduction of unrestricted oxygen into the care of respiratory distressed babies in the 1940s. Subsequently, thousands of newborn babies were irrevocably and permanently blinded due to retinopathy of the newborn, before the practice was challenged and systematically evaluated (Silverman, 1980).

Trial and error can also be exemplified in the way in which new products may be introduced into care; this is often on the basis of persuasive marketing or because clinicians believe that the products will be therapeutic. The introduction of glycerol-impregnated catgut (Softgut Braun) for perineal repair and the use of pramoxine/hydrocortisone foam (Epifoam, Stafford Miller Ltd) for the relief of perineal pain are examples of products which have gained widespread use on the basis of clinical impressions only. Clinicians firmly believed (or assumed) that they would prove beneficial to mothers. Only following formal evaluation through well-conducted, randomized controlled trials were both products found to be ineffective or, indeed, positively harmful to women (Spencer et al., 1986; Greer and Cameron, 1984).

To sum up, whilst each of the sources of knowledge described above is of undoubted value, it is important to recognize the dangers of drawing conclusions from untested individual experience that may well reflect personal bias. Knowledge gained from experience, common sense, intuition and trial and error is often haphazard and fallible, lacking the basis of sound evidence to support any claim of therapeutic potential. Little wonder that it can lead to the giving of diverse and often conflicting advice by health care professionals. Such sources of knowledge, useful as they are, need the underpinning of empirical evidence that can only be provided by scientific knowledge. How, then, does the latter differ from what has been described above?

Research-based knowledge

Science offers a means of generating new knowledge that is planned and systematic. This knowledge is generated through research which follows certain 'rules' and procedures. Research that is well conducted can provide midwives with sound evidence upon which opinions can be securely based, often challenging cherished beliefs and accepted practices. In short, it provides a means whereby midwifery practices and beliefs may be rigorously examined using scientific methods. Research could, therefore, be regarded as being 'subversive' in that it makes clinicians less sure that they possess all the right answers – it encourages midwives to challenge accepted wisdom. Furthermore, it empowers practitioners by providing a sound knowledge base upon which opportunities for change can be built, thereby providing well-founded confidence when making clinical decisions.

Where available, the results of sound research can provide the best guide in helping to identify the safest and most effective care. It is, therefore, vital to base the delivery of midwifery care on the best current knowledge available. At the same time, it is important to be mindful of the individualized needs of mothers and babies and of the fact that 'practice takes place in a context of continuing change and development' (UKCC, 1992a).

The Research Process

Before considering the main approaches used in midwifery research, we need to consider (a) what we mean by the term 'research', and (b) the steps that researchers usually go through when undertaking a study.

First, what is meant by the term 'research'? There are numerous definitions to be found in both the nursing and midwifery literature. However, rather than focusing on any single definition here, we suggest that it is more helpful to focus on the key ideas that are incorporated in the different definitions, thus enabling readers to create their own understanding of the term 'research'.

All definitions suggest that research *increases our knowledge and understanding of a subject*, and that this generation of new knowledge is achieved by undertaking some form of *scientific/systematic enquiry*. A further important point is that researchers *usually strive to be as objective as possible when undertaking research*. That is to say, they try to minimize the possibility of introducing their own prejudices and biases which could affect the data that are collected and the interpretation of those data. But, as you might imagine, it can sometimes be quite difficult to be entirely objective when studying aspects of clinical care. When reading published research, it is necessary, therefore, to decide how successfully you feel this has been achieved.

One of the key concepts mentioned above is that researchers study particular topics *systematically*. What precisely does this mean in terms of what researchers actually do? First, all research consists of three main phases:

1 a *planning phase*, during which the focus of the study is identified, an appropriate design selected and a method of data collection developed;
2 an *empirical phase*, during which data are collected;
3 an *analysis phase*, during which the data are analysed and interpreted.

Secondly, within each of the three main phases, researchers usually undertake a logical sequence of steps. These steps that investigators go through when carrying out a study are known as the *research process*. In order to make sense of published research, it is helpful to have some understanding of this process.

You will find that there is no general agreement in textbooks on the number of steps that make up the research process. Whilst this may initially appear confusing, it merely reflects differing amounts of detail and varying ways of categorizing specific research activities. The 11 main steps that we feel adequately describe the research process are listed below.

1 Identifying the research problem or research question.
2 Carrying out a literature search and review of the literature relating to the problem or question.
3 Defining/refining the research question or formulating a research hypothesis.
4 Choosing the research method and deciding on the overall design of the study.
5 Designing a data collection tool.
6 Identifying the group of subjects/participants to be studied.
7 Conducting a pilot study (that is, a 'dummy run' of the proposed study).
8 Collecting the data.
9 Analysing the data.

10 Interpreting the findings.
11 Disseminating the results.

The above series of steps should be regarded as being somewhat idealized. If you talk to anyone who has carried out research, you are likely to discover (or you may know from your own experience) that although it may seem that the research process follows a largely standardized and routine pattern, it is rather less 'tidy' and often far more creative than suggested by such neatly defined stages.

Different Approaches to Research

Although the research process highlights commonalities in what researchers actually do, it is important to realize that research may be designed and carried out in many different ways. The field and topic under investigation, its specific focus, and the precise nature of the research question will determine the most appropriate method to be used. Different approaches include:

▶ tightly controlled *experiments* in which the researcher evaluates or compares different clinical practices or patterns of organization of care;
▶ large- and small-scale *surveys* where the researcher designs a questionnaire or interview schedule in order to put a range of carefully worded questions to a sample of individuals to find out their views, beliefs, opinions or attitudes concerning a particular aspect of practice or approach to care;
▶ *qualitative* studies using in-depth, open-ended interviews or observation with small numbers of individuals which enable the researcher to understand the perspective of those being studied.

An example of each of these research approaches is given below to highlight some of the main characteristics of each approach.

EXPERIMENTAL RESEARCH

All experimental studies begin with a hypothesis. This is a testable statement which tentatively predicts the relationship between two or more variables. For example, one might predict that use of the Amnicot (a finger stalk with a plastic hook on the end) for amniotomy in labour would significantly reduce fetal scalp trauma compared with use of the Amnihook (a long rigid instrument with a hook at the end). An experiment is then designed to test rigorously whether the hypothesis can be supported or rejected (that is to say to test whether there is a relationship between the treatment variable and the outcome variable).

The experimenter does not merely observe what happens, but rather manipulates and controls the experimental situation and gathers objective, quantitative data which can be statistically analysed to see whether or not the evidence supports the hypothesis. Broadly speaking, the researcher manipulates the experimental situation by systematically varying one or more variables in the various 'treatment' conditions, whilst at the same time introducing some control over the experimental situation. This is achieved by eliminating the influence of variables other than those manipulated by the researcher. Ideally, the researcher will try to assign subjects randomly to the various 'treatment' conditions of the experiment to minimize from the outset the effect of possible differences between groups of subjects (e.g. age, parity, birthweight, etc.). Experiments, therefore, allow the relationship between variables to be investigated under conditions that are more tightly controlled than in any other research approach.

An interesting example of an experimental study is the randomized controlled trial carried out by Everett and her colleagues to assess the effectiveness of the use of ultrasound therapy as a means of treating persistent postnatal perineal pain and dyspareunia (Everett *et al.*, 1992). This multidisciplinary study investigated a common problem following childbirth – dyspareunia – which frequently goes untreated because the formal period of postnatal care is usually completed before it is recognized to be an ongoing problem. It highlights the need for midwives to be more aware of the longer term effects of care. Since the report of the research was published in the journal *Physiotherapy*, it also serves as a reminder of the importance of scanning journals other than the key midwifery publications, otherwise important studies can be missed. This is particularly pertinent with the increasing emphasis on multidisciplinary collaboration in research.

Sixty-nine women were approached to participate in this trial. Following a full explanation of the study and having given their consent, participants were randomly allocated to one of two groups – half the women received active ultrasound treatment, whilst the others received a placebo therapy. At the time of the trial, the researchers were not able to distinguish between the active and placebo treatments, thereby eliminating the possibility of researcher bias which could affect the results. In this instance, the women themselves were also unable to detect whether they were receiving active or placebo treatment. It was therefore a double blind trial. Participants completed a total of eight treatment sessions over a three-week period. Outcomes were assessed six weeks after starting the trial, using a self-determined questionnaire.

There was a reported improvement in symptoms for both groups of women over the course of the study, highlighting the importance of proper controls in order to evaluate the effectiveness of a treatment reliably. Although the small sample size must limit the generalizability of the results, these preliminary findings suggested there were no clear differences between the two groups in respect of reported perineal pain and dyspareunia. These results confirmed those of a previous, unpublished small trial of ultrasound undertaken by Sleep and colleagues which also failed to identify any benefit of ultrasound therapy for this distressing problem. Further larger scale placebo-controlled trials are, therefore, required in order either to confirm or refute the possible benefits of this electrical therapy.

This is just one example of the several thousand controlled trials that have been undertaken over the years to evaluate the effectiveness of different forms of midwifery and obstetric care. Systematic reviews of the results of such trials can be found in *Effective Care in Pregnancy and Childbirth* (Chalmers *et al.*, 1989a) and also the *Cochrane Collaboration Pregnancy and Childbirth Database*; both of these information sources will be discussed in the next section.

When reading experimental research, it is important to remember that the results from the study of groups of subjects can only show how the majority responded, based on the group data. That is to say, it can help to identify the form of care that is best for most women or for most babies. Such evidence can help to determine broad policies for midwifery care. For a particular individual, however, careful decision-making is needed whenever a midwife has to select which form of care is most appropriate. For, as Chalmers and colleagues (1989b) remind us: 'forms of care that appear to be desirable for the majority of women and babies may be wrong for some of them; conversely, forms of care that do not appear to be effective overall may be effective for some women or babies'. They go on to argue for advances in diagnostic accuracy which, they believe, would help care-givers to identify those

individuals most likely to respond in an atypical manner to specific forms of care. They concede, however, that 'tailoring care to meet the specific needs of individuals will continue to be more of an art than a science. This art can be improved by listening more carefully to what women have to say, and by involving them to a greater extent in decisions about their care'. This means that mothers should be given accurate and consistent information and treated as responsible adults, so that they can be helped to make their own decisions and can be supported in those decisions. What steps have you and your colleagues taken to establish a partnership between midwife and mother in decision-making and in care?

SURVEY RESEARCH

Nieswiadomy (1993) describes a survey as a form of investigation in which 'self-report data are collected from samples to describe populations on some variable or variables of interest'. Data are usually collected from a relatively large number of respondents using systematic and structured questions, either by interview or by questionnaire. Most surveys involve collecting data systematically from a sample of people, institutions or any other clearly identifiable group. As such, it is one of the most widely used methods of gathering data, particularly in the health care field. If the sample that is studied is representative of the wider group from which it was drawn – the target population – and the response rate (i.e. the proportion of those approached who agree to participate) is reasonably high, the research findings may be generalized to the wider population. Survey data can, therefore, provide useful overviews of midwifery practices and can play an important part in decision-making at both local and national levels.

An interesting example of a survey is the study by Jacoby (1988) looking at mothers' views of the information and advice they had received during pregnancy and childbirth. A random sample of 1508 women in England (79% response rate) completed a questionnaire they were sent four months after the birth of their baby. Whilst 59% of the women stated that they were generally satisfied with the information they had been given at the various stages, 20% said that they felt they had been given too little information and a further 20% stated that they had been given too much information about some things and not enough about others. Moreover, women who were in some sense socially disadvantaged appeared to experience the greatest difficulty in finding out what they wanted to know.

A further example is the study of midwives' management of postpartum pain by Sleep and Grant (1988). A random sample of 50 English maternity units (36 consultant and 14 general practitioner units) participated in a structured telephone interview (100% response rate). Oral analgesia was found to be the preferred first-line management for perineal pain in 78% of the units, whilst a few started by offering localized therapy using ice (10%), hydrocortisone and pramoxine foam (Epifoam) (10%) or witch hazel (2%). The first choice of oral analgesia for mild to moderate perineal pain was found to be paracetamol (in 96% of the units), whilst greater variation was found for more severe pain. The most commonly used included paracetamol + dextropoxyphene (18%), paracetamol + dihydrocodeine (12%), and aspirin and codeine phosphate (12%). The most frequently mentioned local treatments were ice packs (84% of the units), Epifoam (60%), and therapeutic ultrasound (36%). From this study it was evident that the effectiveness of many of the therapies that were being used had been poorly evaluated, highlighting the need for further randomized controlled trials to assess their usefulness in postnatal care. The results of this survey also drew attention to the fact that practice in this representative sample of units was not based on sound evidence. A similar conclusion was reached by Harris (1992) who also found that many of the treatments offered for the relief of perineal pain within a single district general hospital were not research-based.

QUALITATIVE RESEARCH

A range of more 'naturalistic' qualitative research approaches – including ethnography, phenomenology and grounded theory – with their emphasis on meaning have been used to study aspects of women's health and the impact of parenting.

Qualitative research aims to understand and explain social situations by incorporating participants' meaning and, therefore, can be used when little is known about a particular phenomenon. Data are usually gathered using participant observation and in-depth interviews. Field notes and interview transcripts are subsequently analysed for themes and concepts; the findings usually take the form of narratives and descriptive accounts. Data collection, coding and ana-

lysis are often undertaken alongside each other, so that the future direction of the research may be influenced by the data as they are collected. Since it is very time consuming to transcribe interviews and record and analyse detailed observations, only small numbers of individuals tend to be studied, thus making it inappropriate to generalize the findings.

Ethnography   This approach was first developed within anthropology as a means of trying to enter into the world of the individual or group being studied with an open mind and to try and understand the experience from the perspective of those involved. The researcher will usually start by recording everything he or she sees or hears and will then look for any patterns which emerge from the data. Thus, any categories that develop in the course of the research emerge from the observed behaviours, rather than from the presuppositions of the person undertaking the research. In some instances, the researcher may also feed back findings to participants and ask them to confirm that the interpretations made are correct.

An example of an ethnographic study is the work undertaken by Davies and Atkinson (1991) looking at the early experiences and coping strategies of a group of nine student midwives from one school of midwifery, who were undergoing the transition from experienced nurse to novice midwife. Data were collected during the first 18 weeks of their 18-month course, by means of unstructured individual interviews, observation, group discussions/interviews, a course diary kept by each student, and course documentation. The analysis of the informants' own concerns and interests, based on the data collected, showed that these student midwives tended to revert to carrying out routinized nursing activities such as 'doing the obs' in response to the uncertainties of their new role and status, and the strange midwifery environment in which they found themselves. The researchers commented that 'Based on their established recipes of knowledge and action they sought refuge in a restricted set of tasks and definitions of clinical work. The complexity of midwifery observation and monitoring may thus be translated into an unduly narrow set of physical concerns'. The students learned to be taciturn and expressed few definite opinions whilst they worked out the 'rules' of the various clinical settings in which they worked. They also 'sussed out' and 'sized up' clinical staff and the ward atmosphere quite competently and this, in turn, influenced the ways in which the students interacted with other members of the team.

Phenomenology   This approach is derived from the work of the German philosophers Husserl and Heidegger (Koch, 1995). Researchers working within this tradition are concerned with capturing essences and the lived experience. The main focus of enquiry is the 'essence' of being; the researcher seeks to understand the essence of an individual's being (their inner consciousness), acknowledging the uniqueness of individual experiences whilst searching for commonalities of meaning. It is a popular methodology for studying abstract concepts such as care, pain, suffering, empathy, parenting and infertility.

Patricia Benner, a North American Professor of Nursing, has helped to highlight the potential contribution of phenomenology to health care, through her well-known study of the development of expert nursing practice (Benner, 1984) and more recently her work on caring and ethics in health and illness (Benner, 1994). When you read an account of phenomenological data, you may find yourself reacting to the account with 'But it's like that for me, too'.

Grounded theory   This method derives its name from its approach of grounding theory in data in order to close the gap between theory and research. This approach was first promoted by two sociologists (Glaser and Strauss, 1967). Grounded theorists aim to develop theories that 'fit' the everyday realities of the research setting and the experiences of both the participants and the researcher. This makes it particularly well suited to the study of complex phenomena associated with health care.

In her address to the 1976 annual conference of the Association of Integrated and Degree Nursing Courses, Professor (later Baroness) McFarlane (1977) argued that grounded theory allowed theory to be developed from practice and was, therefore, an important research approach for a practice-based discipline such as nursing. This paper, which was published the following year in the *Journal of Advanced Nursing*, almost certainly helped to put grounded theory on the map as a suitable qualitative research approach for those working in healthcare settings. Beck (1993) used this approach to develop a theory of postpartum depression by talking to women about their experiences in the 18 months following childbirth.

The knowledge base of midwifery is continually being expanded as more and more research is undertaken and disseminated: keeping abreast of midwifery research is an ongoing process. In the next section, a range of information sources that enable midwives to keep up to date with new ideas is described.

Keeping Abreast of New Developments

So far in this chapter, we have considered the sources of knowledge which underpin decision-making in practice, and have explored ways in which sound research can strengthen that knowledge base, enabling clinicians to make informed decisions about what constitutes 'best care'. It is, however, important to recognize that scientific knowledge (i.e. research-based knowledge) is dynamic. As the findings from new studies are reported, so the knowledge base has to be re-evaluated and possibly modified. Keeping up to date with research is, therefore, a professional imperative. Midwifery is extremely fortunate in the range of unique resources and information services it currently has available. The most important of these are outlined below.

Effective Care in Pregnancy and Childbirth (ECPC)

In 1989 Chalmers and colleagues published a review of all randomized controlled trials in perinatal care. This was the first time that such a resource had been available providing a very important addition to the obstetric and midwifery literature. The two volumes contain 89 chapters and, when first published in 1989, provided an up-to-date, systematic overview of the evidence collected from more than 3000 clinical research studies which evaluated alternative forms of care. Each chapter includes recommendations for practice based on sound research findings, and highlights areas where further research is needed. The final chapter ends with four appendices:

1 Forms of care that reduce the negative outcomes of pregnancy and childbirth.
2 Forms of care that appear promising but require further evaluation.
3 Forms of care with unknown effects which require further evaluation.

4 Forms of care which should be abandoned in the light of available evidence.

These appendices provide a useful starting point for busy practitioners who are seeking ways of improving the efficiency and effectiveness of care. These volumes are now available electronically as they form the basis of the Cochrane Collaboration Pregnancy and Childbirth (CCPC) database.

A companion volume to ECPC, entitled *A Guide to Effective Care in Pregnancy and Childbirth* (Enkin *et al.*, 1989, 1995), provides an accessible summary of the contents of the above two volumes, but does not include any references to the research studies. It is important, therefore, for midwives to have ready access in their workplace to the two-volume publication and to the Cochrane Database (referred to below), so that they may follow up references to studies that are of particular interest. It is the authors' intention to produce regular revised editions of this Guide; a second edition was published in 1995.

Cochrane database

A Department of Health initiative led to the setting up, at the end of 1992, of the Cochrane Centre in Oxford, with Iain Chalmers as its Director. The remit of the centre is to undertake large-scale systematic reviews of the international evidence concerning the value of particular forms of health care derived from published and unpublished randomized controlled trials. Many traditional reviews that have been published tend to be based on data that are haphazardly selected. By contrast, these reviews are prepared methodically and describe clearly how the trials were identified, selected and evaluated. The *Cochrane Collaboration Pregnancy and Childbirth Database* was the first of the specialized resources to be developed by the Cochrane Centre to enable clinicians to gain easier access to reliable information about the effects of care. (Incidentally, the centre is named after Archie Cochrane who first stressed that reliable information from randomized controlled trials is vital for making sound decisions in health care.)

The database currently holds around 600 systematic reviews which are regularly updated. To avoid unnecessary duplication of effort, it also lists reviews that are being prepared or are planned. The database, therefore, provides an important extension to *Effective Care in Pregnancy and Childbirth* and an up-to-date overview of current experimental studies evaluating the care of mothers and their babies. Areas that have been reviewed include: the provision of antenatal care by midwives; the effect of social support in pregnancy; care during the first, second and third stages of labour; the immediate care of mother and baby; non-pharmacological methods of pain relief; and supporting the breastfeeding mother.

Each review consists of:

1 the title of the review, the name of the reviewer and contact details;
2 a structured report, comprising an introduction/ statement of objectives, information about the materials and methods used, the results of the review, and a discussion section that includes the implications for practice and for research;
3 tabulation of the results of the review, with a presentation of the syntheses of the statistical analyses (where these have been possible) in a standard format that allows the reader to identify very readily which outcomes are affected by the interventions;
4 a full listing of all the studies incorporated in the review.

The reviews can be used in various ways to provide more effective care for women and babies. For instance, they can be used by those responsible for developing guidelines for practice, for quality assurance and for audit so that these are based on sound evidence. They can also be used by women and their families (and organizations representing their interests) to make well-informed choices about maternity care. They enable standards to be set and specifications for service delivery. They also enable priorities for future research to be identified. We shall be considering one of the reviews in more detail in the next section.

The *Cochrane Collaboration Pregnancy and Childbirth Database* is available as a software package that can be loaded on to any IBM-compatible computer. Institutional and individual subscribers receive two annual updates on disk, providing more immediate access to updated information than is possible through published literature, thereby enabling clinicians to keep abreast of new developments on a regular basis and with the minimum inconvenience. It is important for every midwife to have access to the *Cochrane Collaboration Pregnancy and Childbirth Database*. Moreover, readers of the second edition of the *Guide to Effective Care in Pregnancy and Childbirth* will also find they need access to the Cochrane Database to follow up references to studies that are of particular interest.

The work of the Cochrane Centre is very much in line with several of the key initiatives proposed in the *Report of the Taskforce on the Strategy for Research in Nursing, Midwifery and Health Visiting* (DOH, 1993a). For example, this strategy acknowledges the need for expert review of the research literature in order to identify gaps in our current understanding. Recommendation 31 argues for the need to commission regular critical overviews of research in specific fields, whilst Recommendation 33 suggests that a feasibility study be initiated on 'how best to undertake systematic overviews across the entire field of research in nursing and to generate professionally credible protocols which encapsulate worthwhile research findings'.

MIDIRS

A further specialist database for midwives has been developed by the Midwives' Information and Resource Service (MIDIRS). Around 550 academic and professional journals are scanned regularly for material on midwifery, maternity services, pregnancy and childbirth. Most of the material entered on the databases dates from 1985 onwards, although some classic older material is also included. At the end of 1995, the database contained over 42 000 references, with between 600 and 700 new references added every month.

Of the material added to the database each year, some 20% of the articles are either reprinted in full or are presented in a shortened precis (abstract) followed by a reviewer's comments in a quarterly publication entitled *Midwifery Digest*. Information is organized under the following headings:

▶ Midwifery.
▶ Pregnancy.
▶ Labour and delivery.
▶ Maternity services.
▶ Childbirth trends.

In addition, MIDIRS provides an enquiry service on all aspects of midwifery care using the database. Midwives wishing to find information in order to provide evidence to support an argument, reassure a client, challenge policy, develop a standard of care, or write an essay can request relevant material from the MIDIRS database. During 1995, MIDIRS recorded nearly 16 000 enquiries. A list of all relevant references

is printed out and despatched within five working days (more quickly, if needed). All material listed on the database is also available at the MIDIRS office, should anyone experience difficulty in obtaining certain items locally.

In 1996 MIDIRS launched a new initiative in developing a series of leaflets, each of which provides information, based on current research evidence, on specific topics. For example, ultrasound scans, alcohol in pregnancy and support in labour. Each leaflet is aimed to provide informed choice for both women and the professionals responsible for their care. It is planned that the number of topics covered in this series will be increased each year.

MIRIAD

In 1989, *MIRIAD – a Database of Midwifery Research in the UK –* was established at the National Perinatal Epidemiology Unit in Oxford. This initiative, funded by the Department of Health, recognized that the care of mothers and babies should be informed by the results of sound research, and that midwives needed easier access to relevant research. MIRIAD was, therefore, set up with two key objectives:

1 to create a comprehensive, computerized record of both completed and ongoing studies in the field of midwifery so that information about research in midwifery was more easily available to all those involved in clinical care; and
2 to facilitate a network of researchers conducting studies of relevance to mothers, their babies and their families.

The 1996 Annual Report included details of 345 studies – 83% (285) of these had been completed, and 17% (60) were ongoing. At the time of publication of this report, 38% (70) of the studies had not been published and their details were not, therefore, available through any other source (McCormick and Renfrew, 1996). The studies fall into four main categories:

▶ Clinical.
▶ Educational.
▶ Management.
▶ Historical.

Every practising midwife in the 1990s should be fully aware of the excellent information services available, and should make good use of them whenever a question arises about an aspect of midwifery care. Clearly, the availability of these information resources offers midwives tremendous advantages not only in providing easy access to information, but also in helping to guide the reader towards an understanding of published research reports. Midwives are becoming more 'research aware' and are developing the skills and the confidence needed to read and evaluate research. It is important that objective criteria are used to judge the value of a particular study, rather than subjective assessments based on whether or not the reader agrees with the findings, or on perceptions of relative worth determined by the author's professional background.

In a small-scale experimental study, Hicks (1992) asked 18 registered midwives to evaluate two comparable research studies, using the following five criteria:

- clarity of expression.
- level of expertise on the topic.
- grasp of research methodology.
- understanding of statistical analysis.
- the articles contribution to current understanding.

Half the group were informed that the first paper was written by a midwife and the second by an obstetrician, whilst the authorship of the two papers was reversed for the remainder of the group. Hicks found, using the overall rating scores, that the midwives rated more highly the general quality of the paper they thought had been written by the obstetrician than the paper they believed to have been written by the midwife. She also found that whilst there were no significant differences on the first two criteria listed above, the paper believed to have been written by the obstetrician was rated more highly on each of the last three criteria. Following the integration of research into the midwifery curriculum at both pre- and post-registration levels, it is to be hoped that the outcome of a similar study undertaken in the future would be rather different. Midwives must value the research efforts of their midwife colleagues as highly as those of their medical colleagues, where this is warranted by the quality of the research.

The Midwife's Role in Research

What then, is the role of the midwife in research? Four main areas of responsibility can be identified:

1 To use research to inform practice and to improve standards of care.
2 To act as a collaborator and member of a multi-disciplinary team in supporting the conduct of research in a range of different settings.
3 To be the primary investigator in designing and conducting research of relevance to the care of mothers, their babies and their families.
4 To be an educator and facilitator in providing women and their partners with evidence to support decisions related to care.

Each of these will now be considered briefly in turn.

To use research to inform practice and to improve standards of care

The *Report of the Taskforce on the Strategy for Research in Nursing, Midwifery and Health Visiting* (DOH, 1993a) highlights the need for every health care practitioner to become 'research literate' as an essential step towards the development of knowledge-led practice. However, before clinicians can begin to use research to inform the knowledge base of practice and to improve standards of care, they must first develop a questioning approach to care by challenging accepted practices and traditional beliefs. They need to understand not only how to perform a task, but also, more importantly, *why* it is appropriate and *why* it may be in the mother and baby's best interests.

Professional accountability (UKCC, 1992b, 1994) requires midwives to examine the care they provide and to be answerable for their clinical decisions and actions. Clearly, a working knowledge and understanding of research can help midwives to exercise their accountability with some degree of confidence. Asking questions and being curious are important first steps. Midwives need then to be able to find answers to their questions. To do this, they need to be able to access appropriate library resources which offer a wide range of both UK and international refereed journals and also the range of information sources outlined above.

Accessing, critically reading and understanding published research are important prerequisites to planning any strategy for change. Kramer (1974) suggests that 'improvements in the quality of . . . care . . . will be brought about by [midwives] who truly care enough to work within the system to do something. On the other hand the status quo will be maintained and fostered, not by indolent, uncaring [midwives], but rather by good [midwives] who do nothing.'

Improvements in care are, therefore, more likely to succeed when those directly involved in providing the service are able to select the care they wish to improve, seek out the evidence and then take responsibility for developing a plan of action. This is the 'bottom up' approach. It enables clinicians to feel that they 'own' the change process and to develop a means of measuring the effectiveness of their actions.

The integration of research into practice needs, however, to be addressed at *all* levels within an organization in order to develop a culture of 'research awareness' or 'research mindedness'. Teamwork is an important part of this process and is also highlighted in the *Report of the Taskforce on the Strategy for Research in Nursing, Midwifery and Health Visiting* (DOH, 1993a):

> There is a need to create a climate where research is respected and used in practice. Managers, practitioners and educators should all be a part of this process. There is also a clear role for both purchasers and providers. Purchasers have a general concern with research and need to be concerned with investing, identifying and disseminating results of research. Providers need to agree treatment standards, and to have access to evidence of the use of research in practice so they can confidently choose particular care regimes. Practitioners involved in community and hospital practice are those who are ultimately responsible for the application of research in practice. Information should therefore be accessible, available and understandable.
>
> (Annex 3, para. 2.3 and 2.4)

The *Changing Childbirth* report (DOH, 1993b) also identifies a clear role for both purchasers and providers, but recommends that this collaboration is extended to include user groups. One of the identified action points advocates that 'purchasers and providers should provide clear information for users about the services available to them, and the standards they should expect. They should take a much more critical approach to the effectiveness of different practices and techniques' (para. 5.2.3). The report also endorses the view that purchasers have a key role to play in ensuring that providers implement practices of proven benefit and abandon those which have been demonstrated to be ineffective. Clearly, collaborative teamwork involving all professional groups with a responsibility for maternity care and well-informed users of the

service can greatly enhance the opportunity for the successful integration of research into practice.

An example of one such initiative is the strategy launched by the Research and Information Group of the National Childbirth Trust (NCT) entitled *Putting Research into Practice in Maternity Care* (NCT, 1993). This policy paper advocates the abandonment of practices which are still in common usage, despite research evidence of their ineffectiveness or even possible harm. For example, restricting maternal position during labour and delivery and the routine continuous monitoring of the fetal heart rate without fetal scalp blood sampling. The NCT launched their campaign by focusing on perineal care and enlisted the support of the professional organizations and the media in raising awareness of the existence of sound research to support good practice.

A further example of how research has been widely disseminated to help midwives (and, in this instance, mothers also) to use the results of research is in the area of breastfeeding. In 1989, Garforth and Garcia found that many of the current breastfeeding practices were inconsistent with the research evidence that was available at the time the study was undertaken. Indeed, the researchers indicated that there was a considerable confusion surrounding the whole area, and that some of the practices they observed would have been likely to hinder the establishment of successful breastfeeding. Two books have subsequently been published, combining the results of research with the clinical experience of midwives, and making a number of recommendations for practice that are helpful to both mothers and their babies (see Renfrew *et al.*, 1990; RCM, 1991).

For teamwork to succeed, it is important for standards of midwifery practice to be set, monitored and evaluated in each clinical setting, using the audit process. Formal audit of clinical practice is now being introduced throughout the National Health Service, following the 1990 NHS Act. Audit offers a method of systematically reviewing and evaluating the effectiveness of the service, using clearly defined, measureable criteria. It is expressly designed to:

▶ improve the quality of the service;
▶ make the most effective use of resources; and
▶ foster in midwives a critical questioning approach to their activities and the needs of mothers and their babies.

In order to achieve these aims, the audit results must be fed back and made available to clinicians so that they feel ownership of the data and view the process as a powerful and positive tool in recognizing areas for improvement. Audit may also help to identify instances where the outcome matches or exceeds the minimally acceptable standards of care. For example, drawing on current research evidence, a standard may be set to minimize the use of episiotomies conducted for maternal reasons during normal deliveries. The audit process can then be used to monitor the actual number of episiotomies performed and the indications for use. Another example of the way in which audit can provide a useful measure of the quality of care is in soliciting the views of users of the service. Auditing consumer satisfaction is another of the action points identified in *Changing Childbirth* (DOH, 1993b).

When considering the extent to which research evidence is currently being used in one's own practice area, it is important to be mindful of targets that have been set by the Department of Health. Two of the 12 targets outlined in *A Vision for the Future: The Nursing, Midwifery and Health Visiting Contribution to Health and Health Care* (National Health Service Management Executive, 1993) focus specifically on matters relating to research:

▶ *Target Eight*: 'At the end of the first year professional leaders should be able to demonstrate the existence of local networks to disseminate good practice based on research.'
▶ *Target Nine*: 'By the end of the year providers should be able to demonstrate at least three areas where clinical practice has changed as a result of research findings.'

Research is clearly on the health care agenda for the 1990s, and individuals working at all levels within the health care system are expected to make a contribution. What progress has there been in your practice area?

To act as a collaborator and member of a multidisciplinary team supporting the conduct of research in a range of settings

The midwife has an important role to play in supporting the conduct of research instigated by other health professionals. An example of such collaboration is the study referred to earlier in this chapter by Everett *et al.* (1992), where the principal investigator was a physiotherapist, supported by obstetric and midwifery colleagues.

In a multidisciplinary study, the midwife may be the professional who has the closest contact with mothers, their babies and their families. She may, therefore, be asked to select appropriate women and babies for recruitment into a study. She may also be the most appropriate carer to provide information to potential participants in a research study and to ensure that each woman is provided with an opportunity to raise questions and to clarify any issues of concern. The midwife may also be required to invite participation in the study and to solicit informed consent. It is important that the process of providing information and that of inviting women to consent to participate in a study should take place on separate occasions. This affords each mother adequate time to consider the implications of involvement, free from any coercion, and to be able to discuss the study with her partner and family. For this reason, it is not advisable or desirable that women are invited to participate in a study at the time they are admitted in labour.

Clearly, clinicians need to be fully informed about the nature and type of any research in which they are being asked to participate in any way, and to be provided with an opportunity to discuss any matters of concern with the research team. A copy of the research protocol should be available in the clinical area, as well as confirmation that the study has gained the necessary approval from the local research ethics committee.

Useful guidance regarding the ethical issues to be considered in such a situation are explored in a document prepared by the Royal College of Nursing entitled *Ethics Related to Research in Nursing* (RCN, 1993). Although the guidance relates specifically to nurses and to nursing, the issues are equally pertinent to midwifery and to midwives. For example, in considering the responsibilities of practitioners as data collectors, the following guidance is given:

Nurses asked to participate in research as data collectors in addition to their usual duties have an obligation to make it known if this extra responsibility might be, or has become, detrimental to their normal work. Nurses agreeing to assist with data collection must adhere to the ethical principles incumbent on all researchers. Integrity and accuracy in data collection are mandatory.

This document provides sound advice for any clinicians required to fulfil such a role.

To be the primary investigator in designing and conducting research

Close contact with women throughout the childbearing cycle places midwives in an uniquely advantageous position to identify research issues of importance to mothers and their families. Midwives are also rapidly gaining the skills necessary to undertake research as the primary investigators. Earlier in this chapter, we highlighted the increasing number of studies registered on MIRIAD – an increase from 267 to 345 within the two-year period between 1994 and 1996. Despite their clinical focus, the majority of these studies have addressed issues of personal interest to individual researchers, what Peckham (1993) describes as 'investigator-led rather than problem-led research'. However, midwife researchers have responded by mounting a national delphi survey to establish priorities for research in midwifery within the UK (Sleep et al., 1995). This survey solicited the views of midwives and maternity organizations as well as purchasers of the service to ensure that the resultant priorities reflected a range of differing perspectives. The 'top twenty' topics provide an agenda for future research which will address current needs identified from within the maternity services.

One of the prime responsibilities of the novice researcher is to seek out appropriate and adequate supervision from someone who has considerable experience in the application of the proposed research method. The guidance document *Ethics Related to Research in Nursing* (RCN, 1993) endorses the importance of this issue and the need for researchers to be adequately schooled in research methods: 'Each . . . researcher must possess knowledge and skills which are compatible with the demands of the proposed investigation. Researchers must recognise the nature and limits of their research competence and should not propose or accept work which they are not equipped to carry out'. The section of the guidelines headed 'Nurses undertaking research', also includes consideration of the integrity of the researcher, responsibility to subjects, and relations with sponsors, employers and colleagues, thus encompassing a wide range of important issues. It would be advisable to obtain a copy of this document and keep it somewhere that is readily accessible to all midwives working in your area.

To be an educator and facilitator in providing women and their partners with the evidence to support decisions related to care

Increasingly, women users of the maternity services are becoming more vocal in questioning the rationale for their care supported whenever possible by sound research evidence. The *Changing Childbirth* report (DOH, 1993b) identifies that 'tradition plays a large part in the way maternity care is provided. The Group saw a good deal of evidence that practice was not always based on measures known to be effective'. The report also calls upon providers to monitor and adjust services to reflect the needs of women.

The pro-active approach adopted by various maternity organizations has been instrumental in challenging midwives, general practitioners and obstetricians to reappraise the justification for their clinical decisions. Amongst the foremost of these organizations is the Association for Improvements in the Maternity Services (AIMS) and the National Childbirth Trust (NCT). The NCT has recently published a report entitled *The Perineum in Childbirth: A Survey of Women's Experiences and Midwives' Practices* (Greenshields and Hulme, 1993). This report highlights that wide variations in practice still exist, despite research evidence which provides a sound basis for care. Among the recommendations which conclude this report are that individual midwives should monitor their perineal injury rate, that there should be a strengthening of the informed partnership between midwives and women during delivery, and that suture materials and techniques for perineal repair should be based on current research evidence. A comparison is also made between current practice and published research and a number of topics are identified which need to be the focus of future studies. For example: Do women's views during pregnancy influence the perineal trauma they experience during childbirth? Does labouring and possibly giving birth under water affect perineal outcome? It is anticipated that this useful report will be widely available to women, thereby raising *their* awareness of these important issues.

Earlier in this chapter, we highlighted the major information resources, such as MIDIRS and MIRIAD, which are unique to midwifery. These resources offer enormous advantages to midwives in being able to access published research and systematic literature reviews which provide evidence on which practice can be based. This, in turn, enables clinicians to provide women with the opportunity for informed choice about their care. This role is best illustrated by drawing on a specific example from midwifery practice, namely, the support provided by care-givers during childbirth.

In recent years, there has been a steady movement within the UK towards giving women the freedom to decide who they wish to be present during the birth of their baby by choosing the people who they feel will provide them with the necessary emotional and physical support during labour. This may be her mother, a friend, the baby's father, or she may choose to depend entirely upon the midwife to fulfil this role. It is, however, important to recognize that this practice is by no means the accepted norm in all countries. For instance, in North America, it is comparatively rare for women to be offered a choice or opportunity for constant companionship at such a time. Indeed, it may be argued that we do not need research to tell us that offering women support at a time of stress is a basic act of human caring and kindness which can help to alleviate fear and anxiety, thereby enhancing the quality of the childbirth experience. It could also be argued that offering such companionship is an implicit and integral part of professional practice. As we shall see, recent evidence generated from sound research suggests that midwives may have grossly underestimated the value and profound influence that such support may provide.

The Cochrane Database includes a synthesis of the evidence taken from 11 randomized controlled trials designed to compare the effects of labour support provided by either a familiar or unfamiliar professional nurse, midwife or lay person, whether a paid or volunteer helper (Hodnett, 1993). These trials were conducted in a number of different countries including Guatemala, South Africa, Canada, the United States of America, as well as in European countries. Despite the differences in the environment of care and in the socio-economic status of the women, there was remarkable similarity in the nature of the experimental intervention, i.e. the support the women received. In all instances this included a continuous presence, if not for all of labour, then, at least, during the active phase. In the majority of these trials, the very least support offered to the women comprised comforting touch, words of praise and encouragement. Figure 2 details all the outcome measures used in the studies that were reviewed. It is important, therefore, to be able to

understand the significance of this method of presenting the results of research.

Almost all trials, however big they are, are carried out on only a comparatively small number (a small sample) of the total group (the population) to whom the results may be applicable. The results obtained must, therefore, be treated with some caution, because if the study were to be carried out again (replicated) with a different sample, it is unlikely that precisely the same result would be obtained. However, results from a single study may be used to calculate the range within which one can be 95% certain that the result would lie, if the entire population were to be included in the study. This is known as the 95% confidence interval and indicates the range within which the 'true' result for the population will lie. Thus, in Figure 2, the boxes indicate the actual result obtained in the study in question and each end of the horizontal line running through the boxes represents the 95% confidence interval (95% CI). The larger the sample size of a trial, the smaller the range of the 95% CIs will be, and if it were ever possible to study the entire population, there would just be one figure (the 'true' result) remaining.

An odds ratio compares the likelihood (the odds) of something happening in the one group with the likelihood (odds) of it occurring in the other. If there is no difference between the two groups in this respect, the odds ratio is 1; this 'point of no difference' is shown by the vertical line in Figure 2. Looking at Figure 2, it can be seen that all the trial results and most of the 95% CIs lie to the left of this vertical line, indicating that the outcome described in the left-hand column was less likely to occur in the groups who had received support from care-givers during childbirth than to occur in groups who had not; that is to say, the odds ratio was less than 1. Any result to the right of the vertical line would indicate that the event was less likely to occur in the unsupported group (the odds ratio being greater than 1). From the bottom two lines of Figure 2, it can be seen, therefore, that one can be 95% certain that support from care-givers will have a beneficial effect in reducing the likelihood of Apgar scores of less than 7 at five minutes. However, no such certainty exists in relation to their effect in reducing the likelihood of Apgar scores of less than 8 at one minute; since the upper end of the 95% CI range is greater than 1, the possibility exists that the unsupported group does better in relation to this.

The reviewer reports that there was remarkable consistency in the results of the trials and summarizes

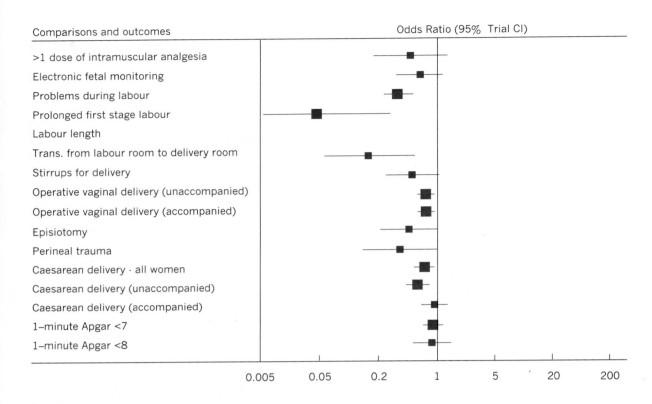

Figure 2 Basic care during childbirth: support from care-givers during childbirth. (Adapted from Hodnett, 1995.)

the overview thus: 'Regardless of whether or not a support person of the woman's own choosing could be present, the continuous presence of a trained support person who had no social bond with the labouring women reduced the likelihood of medication for pain relief, operative vaginal delivery, and a 5-minute Apgar score <7.'

In this chapter, we began by exploring the sources of knowledge which influence the decisions made by midwives in their everyday practice. We then considered the role and unique contribution of sound research evidence in informing and enhancing this decision-making process, whilst acknowledging that research is not a 'panacea for all ills'. Sound evidence needs to be combined with professional judgement, clinical experience and maternal preference in reaching an informed choice about the most effective care for each individual woman and her baby. To change practice and sustain innovation, however, requires collaborative support at all levels within the organization.

This should involve clinicians, educators and managers as well as users of the service. Midwives are in an uniquely privileged position to be able to influence both the standard of care and service provision for women, their babies and their families. Virginia Henderson (1987) powerfully summarizes the potential for practitioners to influence practice; although she is primarily referring to nurses and to nursing, her message is equally as appropriate for midwives and midwifery:

> When [midwives'] sensitivity to human needs (their intuition) is joined with the ability to find and use expert opinion, with the ability to find reported research and apply it to their practice, and when they themselves use the scientific method of investigation, there is no limit to the influence they might have on health care worldwide.

The future of the maternity services rests in their hands.

References

Beck, C.T. (1993) Teetering on the edge: a substantive theory of postpartum depression. *Nursing Res.* 42(1): 42–48.

Benner, P. (1984) *From Novice to Expert*. California: Addison-Wesley.

Benner P. (ed.) (1994) *Interpretive Phenomenology: Embodiment, Caring and Ethics in Health and Illness*. London: Sage.

Chalmers, I. (1986) Minimising harm and maximising benefit during innovation in health care: controlled or uncontrolled experimentation? *Birth* 13(3): 155–164.

Chalmers, I. (1989) Evaluating the effects of care during pregnancy and childbirth. In Chalmers, I., Enkin, M. & Keirse, M.J.N.C. (eds) *Effective Care in Pregnancy and Childbirth*, Vol. 1. Oxford: Oxford University Press.

Chalmers, I. (ed.) (1991) *Oxford Database of Perinatal Trials*. Oxford: Oxford University Press.

Chalmers, I., Enkin, M. & Keirse, M.J.N.C. (eds) (1989a) *Effective Care in Pregnancy and Childbirth*, Vols 1 & 2. Oxford: Oxford University Press.

Chalmers, I., Enkin, M. & Keirse, M.J.N.C. (1989b) Effective care in pregnancy and childbirth: a synopsis for guiding practice and research. In Chalmers, I., Enkin, M. & Keirse, M.J.N.C. (eds) *Effective Care in Pregnancy and Childbirth*, Vol. 2. Oxford: Oxford University Press.

Clark, E. (1988) Research and common sense. *Professional Nurse* 3(9): 344–347.

Davies, R.M. & Atkinson, P. (1991) Students of midwifery: 'doing the obs' and other coping strategies. *Midwifery* 7: 113–121.

DOH (Department of Health) (1993a) *Report of the Taskforce on the Strategy for Research in Nursing, Midwifery and Health Visiting*. London: DOH.

DOH (1993b) *Changing Childbirth* Part 1: Report of the Expert Maternity Group. London: HMSO.

Enkin, M., Keirse, M.J.N.C. & Chalmers, I. (eds) (1989) *A Guide to Effective Care in Pregnancy and Childbirth*. Oxford: Oxford University Press.

Enkin, M., Keirse, M.J.N.C. & Chalmers, I. (eds) (1995) *A Guide to Effective Care in Pregnancy and Childbirth*, 2nd edn. Oxford: Oxford University Press.

Everett, T., McIntosh, J. & Grant, A. (1992) Ultrasound therapy for persistent post-natal perineal pain and dyspareunia: a randomised placebo-controlled trial. *Physiotherapy* 78(4): 263–267.

Garcia, J. & Garforth, S. (1989) Labour and delivery routines in English consultant maternity units. *Midwifery* 5: 155–162.

Garforth, S. & Garcia, J. (1989) Breastfeeding policies in practice – 'no wonder they get confused'. *Midwifery* 5: 75–83.

Glaser, B.G. & Strauss, A.S. (1967) *The Discovery of Grounded Theory*. New York: Aldine Publishing.

Greenshields, W. & Hulme, H. (1993) *The Perineum in Childbirth: A Survey of Women's Experiences and Midwives' Practices*. London: National Childbirth Trust.

Greer, I.A. & Cameron, A.D. (1984) Topical pramoxine and hydrocortisone foam versus placebo in relief of postpartum episiotomy symptoms and wound healing. *Scottish Med. J.* 29: 104–106.

Harris, M. (1992) The impact of research findings on current practice in relieving postpartum perineal pain in a large district general hospital. *Midwifery* 8: 125–131.

Henderson, V. (1987) On the role of research in nursing, Paper circulated at the Third International Nursing Research Conference. Clinical Excellence in Nursing: International Networking, Edinburgh.

Hicks, C. (1992) Research in midwifery: are midwives their own worst enemies? *Midwifery* 8(1): 12–18.

Hodnett, E.D. (1995) Support from caregivers during pregnancy. In Keirse, M.J.N.C., Renfrew, M.J., Neilson, J.P. & Crowther, C. (eds) *Pregnancy and Childbirth Module*. Cochrane Database of Systematic Reviews. Cochrane Updates on Disk. Oxford: Update Software.

Jacoby, A. (1988) Mothers' views about information and advice in pregnancy and childbirth: findings from a national study. *Midwifery* 4: 103–110.

Koch, T. (1995) Interpretive approaches in nursing research: the influence of Husserl and Heidegger. *J. Adv. Nursing* 21: 827–836.

Kramer, M. (1974) *Reality Shock: Why nurses leave nursing*. St Louis: C.V. Mosby.

Luker, K.A. (1986) Who's for research? *Nursing Times* 82(52): 55–56.

McCormick, F. & Renfrew, M. (eds) (1996) *The Midwifery Research Database MIRIAD: A Source of Information about Research in Midwifery*, 2nd edn. Hale: Books for Midwives Press.

McFarlane, J.K. (1977) Developing a theory of nursing: the relation of theory to practice, education and research. *J Advanced Nursing* 2(3): 261–270.

National Childbirth Trust (1993) *Putting Research into Practice in Maternity Care*. London: Research and Information Group, NCT.

National Health Service Management Executive (1993) *A Vision for the Future: The nursing, midwifery and health visiting contribution to health and health care*. London: DOH.

Nieswiadomy, R.M. (1993) *Foundations of Nursing Research*, 2nd edn. Norwalk, Connecticut: Appleton & Lange.

Peckham, M. (1993) *Research for Health*. London: DOH.

RCM (Royal College of Midwives) (1991) *Successful Breastfeeding*. Edinburgh: Churchill Livingstone.

Royal College of Nursing (1993) *Ethics Related to Research in Nursing*. London: Research Advisory Group, Scutari Press.

Renfrew, M.J., Fisher, C. & Arms, S. (1990) *Bestfeeding: Getting breastfeeding right for you*. Berkeley, California: Celestial Arts.

Salmon, P. (1985) *Living in Time*. London: J.M. Dent.

Schön, D. (1987) Changing patterns of inquiry at work and living. *J. R. Soc. Arts* 135: 225–237.

Silverman, W.A. (1980) *Retrolental Fibroplasia: A Modern Parable*. London: Academic Press.

Sleep, J. & Grant, A. (1988) Relief of perineal pain following childbirth: a survey of midwifery practice. *Midwifery* 4: 118–122.

Sleep, J., Renfrew, M.J., Dunn, A. *et al.* (1995) Establishing priorities for research: report of a Delphi survey. *Br. J. Midwifery* 3(6): 323–330.

Spencer, J.A.D., Grant, A., Elbourne, D., Garcia, J. & Sleep, J. (1986) A randomised comparison of glycerol-impregnated chromic catgut with untreated chromic catgut for the repair of perineal trauma. *Br. J. Obstet. Gynaecol.* 93: 426–430.

Steer, P. (1993) Rituals in antenatal care – do we need them? *Br. Med. J.* 307: 697–698.

UKCC (United Kingdom Central Council for Nursing, Midwifery and Health Visiting) (1994) *The Midwife's Code of Practice*. London: UKCC.

UKCC (1992a) *The Scope of Professional Practice*. London: UKCC.

UKCC (1992b) *Code of Professional Conduct for the Nurse, Midwife and Health Visitor*, 3rd edn. London: UKCC.

Wilkerson, V.A. (1984) The use of episiotomy in normal delivery. *Midwives' Chronicle and Nursing Notes*, April: 106–110.

Further Reading

Abbott, P. & Sapsford, R. (eds) (1992) *Research into Practice: A reader for nurses and the caring professions*. Oxford: Oxford University Press.

Baker, M. & Kirk, S. (eds) (1996) *Research and Development for the NHS: Evidence, Evaluation and Effectiveness*. Oxford: Radcliffe Medical Press.

Chalmers, I., Enkin, M. & Keirse, M.J. (eds) (1989) *Effective Care in Pregnancy and Childbirth*, Vols 1 & 2. Oxford: Oxford University Press.

Clark, E. & Renfrew, M. (1992) *Research Awareness and the Midwife*. London: Distance Learning Centre, South Bank University.

Cormack, D.F.S. (ed.) (1996) *The Research Process in Nursing*, 3rd edn. Oxford: Blackwell Scientific.

Enkin, M., Keirse, M.J. & Chalmers, I. (eds) (1995) *A Guide to Effective Care in Pregnancy and Childbirth*, 2nd edn. Oxford: Oxford University Press.

Reed, J. & Proctor, S. (eds) (1995) *Practitioner Research in Health Care: The Inside Story*. London: Chapman & Hall.

Richardson, A., Jackson, C. & Sykes, W. (1990) *Taking Research Seriously: Means of improving and assessing the use and dissemination of research*. London: HMSO.

Robinson, S. & Thomson, A. (eds) (1988) *Midwives, Research and Childbirth*, Vol. 1. London: Chapman & Hall.

Robinson, S. & Thomson, A. (eds) (1991) *Midwives, Research and Childbirth*, Vol. 2. London: Chapman & Hall.

Robinson, S. & Thomson, A. (eds) (1993) *Midwives, Research and Childbirth*, Vol. 3. London: Chapman & Hall.

Robinson, S. & Thomson, A. (eds) (1995) *Midwives, Research and Childbirth*, vol. 4. London: Chapman & Hall.

Sapsford, R. & Abbott, P. (1992) *Research Methods for Nurses and the Caring Professions*. Milton Keynes: Open University Press.

91

Introduction to Statistics

Graphical Presentation of Data

The main purpose of graphical presentation of numerical data is to provide an immediate impression of the main features of the data. Detail may well be lost but bias should never be deliberately introduced. The eye will automatically assign importance to the amount of page used, that is the area, but can be unduly influenced by colouring or heavy shading. Data may be considered as being of two basic types: discrete, or categoric, and continuous, or measurable.

Categoric data

Categoric data are best displayed by either a bar chart or a pie chart. A *bar chart* consists of equal width bars clearly separated from each other, the length of the bars being proportional to the numbers in each category (Figure 1). It is usual to arrange the bars from most to least frequent, thus allowing immediate comparison between categories. We see therefore that amniotic fluid embolism accounted for about half as many deaths as haemorrhage. Bars may be arranged vertically or horizontally.

The same data are displayed as a *pie chart* in Figure 2. This presentation relates each category to the whole;

thus we see immediately that over half the recorded deaths are attributed to the first three categories and less than a quarter to the last three. Note that this presentation shows comparisons only and there is no indication of the actual totals involved.

Diagrams using pictures are really more for popular appeal than serious scientific usage and frequently can be of very doubtful validity.

Measured data

Measured data by their very nature take a great many values and so for other than a very small number of data will have to be grouped into class intervals. Such groups must be adjoining but not overlapping; for example birthweights are normally grouped as 2000 g to 2499 g, then 2500 g to 2999 g, and so on. Notice that the apparent gap between 2499 and 2500 does not exist since measurements would be made to the nearest gram. These data are presented in Figure 3 as a *histogram*, which is similar to a bar chart, but the 'category' scale is now a continuous one and the bars touch each other. Again conclusions can immediately be drawn from the graph.

To show how a total builds up, a *cumulative frequency graph* can be drawn, as in Figure 4. This is obtained by plotting the total from the start of the

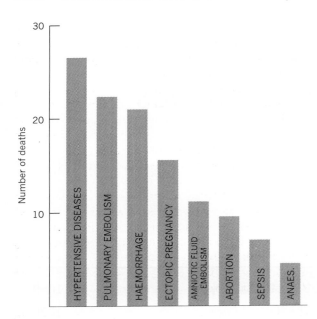

Figure 1   Bar chart showing major causes of maternal death in the UK 1988–90.

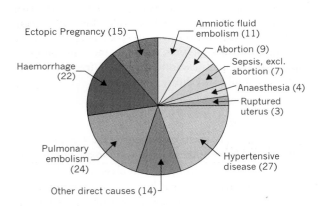

Figure 2   Pie chart showing major causes of maternal death in the UK 1988–90.

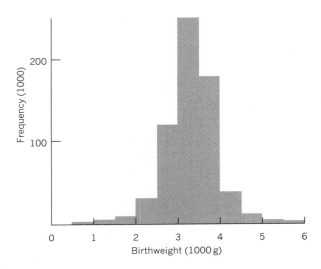

Figure 3   Histogram showing weight distribution of babies born in 1985.

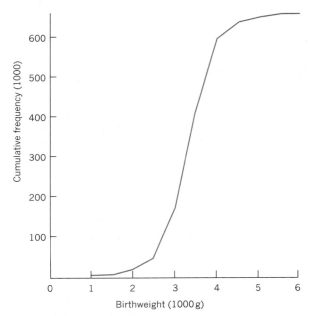

Figure 4   Cumulative frequency graph showing birthweights in 1985.

data up to the end of each class interval. We see that about 600 000 of the 656 000 births registered were of 4000 g or less.

Some data are not easy to determine as clearly categoric or measurable. For example, allocating births to the month in which they occur would at first sight appear to be categoric and can be treated as such.

However a bar chart might easily suggest that births were 10% more frequent in, say, May than in February, thus ignoring the difference in length of month. A true histogram of annual birth distribution would have widths of columns corresponding to the lengths of the months and then heights would have to be modified so that equal areas represent equal numbers of births. This is not really recommended as areas of unequal height and unequal width are hard to compare by eye.

Basic Statistics

In many situations it is convenient to be able to use a single item to represent a whole collection of data. Such representatives are referred to as *averages*, sometimes known as 'measures of central tendency'. The most commonly used averages are the mode, median and mean.

The *mode* is the item occurring most frequently; in the case of grouped data it will be its modal class. It is clearly seen as the highest column on either a bar chart or a histogram. The modal cause of maternal death is hypertensive disease and the modal class of birthweights is 3000–3499 g. For categoric data this is the only average which can be found.

The *median* is the middle item when all of the data are arranged in order. It can be read off from an accurately drawn cumulative frequency graph. From Figure 4 the median birthweight is that corresponding to a frequency of half the total of 656 000, that is at 328 000. Drawing a line to the graph and then down gives a median weight of about 3300 g. Exactly half of all values are above the median and half below the median.

The *mean* is that which most people think of as the only average, found by adding up all the data and dividing by the number of items. The mean age of a family whose ages are 30, 28, 8, 5 and 4 would be calculated by adding the ages together to give 75, then dividing by the number of people, 5, to give the mean age as 15 years. The mean birthweight from the values used to draw Figure 3 is 3321 g.

As well as an average of a set of data it is also of value to have some measure of how the data are spread about the average. For categoric data the only way to indicate this spread is to list all the categories.

For measurable data a similar method would be to quote the *range* from the smallest value to the greatest. Unfortunately, this is totally dependent on the most extreme values and so may be quite unrepresentative. Part ranges are quite widely used to show amounts of spread and are found in the same manner as the median. The *upper* and *lower quartiles* are the 25% and 75% values respectively and enclose the central

half of all values. Using the graph in Figure 4 we obtain the lower quartile by calculating a quarter of 656 000, that is 164 000, and reading the corresponding weight as 3000 g. The upper quartile is about 3700 g. Another much used measure is the percentile, usually the 10th and 90th percentiles, the values below and above each of which 10% of all values lie. From Figure 4 the 10th percentile is measured from 65 600 as about 2580 g and the 90th percentile at 590 400 is 3980 g. This range is used as a measure of the expected spread of normal children's weights.

For more detailed scientific work a measure of spread using all values is needed and this is the *standard deviation*. It is found by calculating how far each value is from the mean, squaring these figures, adding them together, dividing by the number of values and finally taking the square root. So for the family used to illustrate the mean we first calculate:

$$30 - 15 = 15, \quad 28 - 15 = 13, \quad 8 - 15 = -7, \quad 5 - 15 = -10$$
and $4 - 15 = -11$

Now square these and add together: $225 + 169 + 49 + 100 + 121 = 664$
then divide by 5 to give 132.8. The square root of this is about 11.5 and this is the standard deviation.

This is simply an illustration of how a standard deviation is calculated and in this illustrative case neither the mean nor the standard deviation are really very useful. For the full birthweight figures the standard deviation is 618 g.

The *variance* of a set of data is the square of the standard deviation.

Basic Probability

Many situations in life involve an element of randomness or chance. If a single die is thrown then there is no certainty as to what score will be shown. All we do know is that, if it is fair, then each of the scores 1 to 6 is equally likely to be obtained. The probability of each of these scores is said to be $\frac{1}{6}$ or 1 in 6. This certainly does not mean that in six rolls of the die each of the numbers will appear exactly once, but in the long run each score will turn up about the same number of times. In the short term, randomness is shown much more by lumpiness than evenness. Try throwing a single die and recording the score until each number has turned up at least once: only about once in every 60 tries will you get each score just once, and it is just as likely that one score has turned up more than 10 times. In the same way, if a midwife delivers on average one baby every other day these will not be evenly spaced, but it is very likely that on 5 days in a year there will be 3 or more arriving and about 20 occasions when 4 or more days in succession have no births. The probability of a Down's syndrome birth is 1 in 1350, but in random sets of 1350 births there will be no cases on about 1 in 3 occasions and more than one on about 1 in 4 occasions. Although the idea of long-term probability is not a difficult concept these patterns of clustering do require some mathematical theory to decide when the clustering is only to be expected and when it becomes something more and requires further investigation.

The Normal Curve

If a histogram like Figure 3 is drawn for a large number of data and with small class intervals then it will frequently look very like a smooth bell-shaped curve (Figure 5). This is known as the *normal* curve and is mathematically defined. It is symmetrical about the mean of the distribution and is scaled in standard deviations. For the normal curve 68% of all values lie within one standard deviation of the mean and 95% are within two standard deviations. In most experimental work one is consciously working with just a *sample* of

data and theory shows that random samples of data have mean values which do fit very well to the normal curve. This indicates the importance of standard deviation and shows why it is frequently desirable to express results in terms of how far they are from the mean in terms of standard deviations. This is known as *standardization* of values.

While many data do fit fairly closely to this curve it does not follow that all data will. In Figure 6 the data from Figure 3 are put on a normal curve: these data show a higher peak and rather less on the 'shoulders' of the curve than would be the case for truly normally distributed data.

As the above indicates, random samples can have quite widely spread values. Statistical testing for *significance* of results comes down to setting a probability level and if the chances of a result are smaller than this value then we will assume that it is not a random variation but the consequence of some other factor. The usual level fixed is 5% or only a 1 in 20 chance of being this different by random fluctuation. There is the implication that we shall be right 19 times to every once that we claim a random variation to be of significance.

This has been an attempt to give a fairly non-technical review of some aspects of statistics. For further reading the following titles have the same sort of approach. Three are general and one is specifically medical.

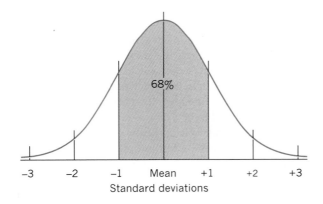

Figure 5   The normal curve.

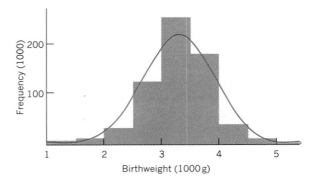

Figure 6   Data from Figure 3 put on a normal curve (see above).

Further reading

Clegg, F. (1990) *Simple Statistics*. Cambridge: Cambridge University Press.

Ingelfinger, J.A. (1983) *Biostatistics in Clinical Medicine*. London: Macmillan.

Moroney, M.J. (1969) *Facts from Figures*. Harmondsworth: Penguin.

Phillips, J.L. (1982) *Statistical Thinking – A Structured Approach*. Oxford: Freeman.

Management Issues in Midwifery Practice

The manager is the dynamic, life giving force in every business.

(Drucker, 1955).

Organization is used in the context of this chapter as the generic term for any unit such as a company, a freestanding division of a company or a unit in the public sector which provides products or services, for example a hospital. The term *structure* is used, as in management structure, to indicate the internal organization of such a unit.

Organizations bringing together the skills and effort of large numbers of people to achieve specific objectives are a distinguishing feature of modern society. The work of managers is essential in enabling organizations to function and achieve the objectives for which they have been established. This work differs from that of directly productive people, such as craftsmen, in that it is always done in an organization, that is in a network of human relationships (Drucker, 1977).

Management requires specific skills and techniques, as does the work of a craftsman, but with an additional dimension due to the interactive nature of the manager's work. Qualities of character, attitude and personality are required which facilitate interaction with and motivation of others and enable them to receive direction willingly from the manager.

Organizations

Organizations vary widely depending on the scale and nature of the activities in which they are engaged, but they are such a familiar feature of life in the industrialized world that daily interaction with them usually presents no problems. A letter is posted, a garment purchased or a light switched on without any need for the user to be concerned with the internal operation of the organizations concerned. However, appropriateness of their structure to the field of operation is very important to their effectiveness. Something is being achieved and the organization dictates, with greater or lesser degrees of prescription and control, what is done. Membership of organizations is important to individuals in contributing to a sense of identity and personal worth. Loss or impairment of these elements of self-perception is part of the scourge of unemployment (Lane, 1991).

Theory

In order to design and operate such a management structure it is necessary to understand the principles involved. A basis for the development of management theory was laid by Fayol (1916) who formulated his 14 principles of organization in the early years of this century. His ideas are still influential, so much so that a student coming fresh to the subject is likely to find most of these principles familiar. They may be summarized very briefly as follows:

1 Division of work – specialization.
2 Authority.
3 Discipline.
4 Unity of Command.
5 Unity of Direction – A single objective not to be split between managers.
6 Organizational interests take precedence over individual interests.
7 Remuneration – fair wages.
8 Appropriate devolution or centralization of decision-making.
9 Line of authority.
10 Orderly activity.
11 Equitable treatment of subordinates.
12 Stability of staffing.
13 Effort encouraged by freedom to innovate where possible.
14 Team spirit.

(Adapted from Pugh and Hickson, 1989)

Hierarchy

Fayol's principles are consistent with the hierarchic or pyramid structure of management. Authority branches from the *chief executive*, the senior person who is the source of authority in the organization, to a layer of *senior managers* each having a number of less senior managers or supervisors responsible to him or her and so on until all the employees are accommodated in the structure. The number of individuals reporting directly to a manager is known as the *span of control*. This is usually smaller at senior than at junior levels. The authority of the chief executive is devolved in such a way that each person in the organization has a single identified manager or supervisor to whom he or she is responsible.

The division of responsibility may be arranged on functional lines, that is by allocating the tasks to be performed to functional units and subunits. Many administrative and service tasks are common to a wide spectrum of organizations and the *finance function* is likely to include a staff payroll task, paying the organization's bills and receiving its income, and providing information on budgets and the financial status of the organization. There is usually a *services function* which may include maintenance of buildings, servicing of equipment, security, cleaning and catering, which may be done in house or contracted out.

The large majority of the staff are likely to be employed in '*operations*', that is in making the products and providing the services which are the reason for the existence of the organization. In a hospital all the medical, nursing, midwifery and other staff who interact to provide the service fall into this category. The structure of the organization may be illustrated by an organization chart as in Figure 1.

Organization charts

The purpose of a chart is to give a graphical representation of the formal system of relationships and of the flow of authority in the organization. Figure 1 is greatly simplified with the omission of detail to illustrate the principles. In a large organization there will usually be a family of such charts; a master giving the overall organization and subcharts for departments. It is usual also to include the names of managers with the position they hold. A box is provided, as illustrated, for the chief executive to show his or her name and title. This makes it more useful as a reference document, particularly for new staff joining the organization. The question of titles depends on the organization. While 'director' has a particular meaning in a limited company, it is often used without this special meaning to distinguish senior managers from managers in general.

Information technology has reduced the number of clerical and intermediate management staff required and made it possible for an individual to control more activities. This tends to flatten the hierarchy by enabling levels of intermediate management to be dispensed with. Thus there may not be an administrative director, in which case the finance manager and the personnel manager would report directly to the chief executive in Figure 1. Taken to its extreme this would lead to the Drucker (1993) analogy with an orchestra

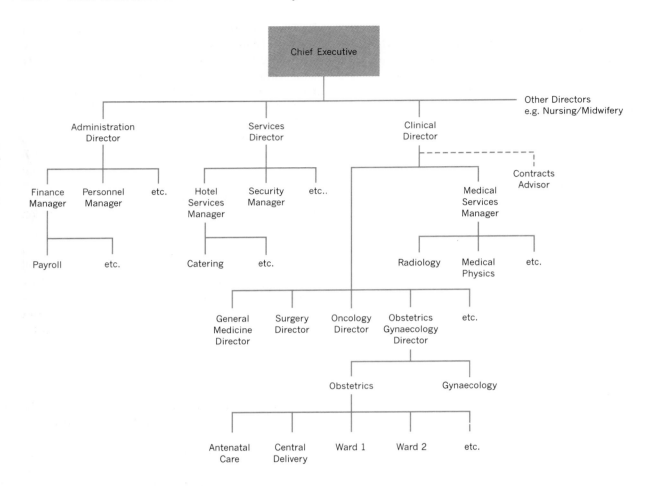

Figure 1   A hierarchy based on function.

and its conductor, where management is reduced to the chief executive who is in direct control of all the staff.

The mode of functioning of organizations is documented to varying degrees to provide a framework for disciplined operation. The documents may include policy statements, job descriptions, operating manuals including quality assurance manuals and procedures.

Alternative structures

Figure 1 is drawn almost entirely with solid lines, which means, in the convention of these diagrams, that all the relationships shown in this way are relationships of authority. This is not always satisfactory. As an example, the clinical director may wish to have specialist advice and to make it available to the directors of the clinical specialist areas on the best methods of negotiating contracts with the purchasers for the provision of health care. In these circumstances a contracts adviser might be appointed reporting to the clinical director and acting through him or her on commercial matters, but having no authority to instruct specialist clinical directors directly. Such an appointment would make this expertise available without infringing the autonomy of the specialist clinical directors. This is known as a 'staff' post as opposed to a 'line' post where the postholder is on the direct line of authority, giving and receiving executive instructions. In the convention, this would be shown on the organization chart by connecting the contracts adviser to the clinical director by a dotted line as shown in Figure 1. There may be a number of such staff posts in the organization which is then referred to as having a 'line and staff' structure.

Matrix organizations

A hierarchical structure has the merit of clarity of responsibilities but tends to suit static rather than dynamic organizations. A measure of flexibility may be added by introducing cross-connections within the management structure to form a matrix.

An organization which is developing new products, services or methods of operation is likely to need project teams drawn from various disciplines. Where there is a very large single customer for a service it may be appropriate to have a dedicated mixed-discipline team servicing the needs of this customer. Each team requires a leader with clearly established objectives: Fayol's fourth and fifth principles. Such teams may be built into a hierarchical structure in such a way as to confer increased flexibility and responsiveness without losing the stability of the hierarchy. Staff may be offered new challenges and widened experience more readily in a matrix than in a hierarchical structure.

Leadership Styles

Leadership

This is the combination of knowledge, skills, attitudes and personal qualities which enables the leader to co-ordinate the activities of a group and to motivate its members so that the objectives are achieved in a timely and efficient way. The knowledge and skills, as opposed to personal attributes, necessary for day-to-day success as a manager lie in two distinct areas: *specialism* and *administration*. The balance between them depends on the particular field of specialism and the seniority of the manager. The neophyte junior manager is likely to be directly involved as a practitioner, judged by the staff mainly on the facility with which problems are solved, guidance given and techniques demonstrated. Managers have to prepare by study and well-considered experiential learning for the gradual transition from predominant specialism to predominant administration in the course of their career.

Style

The traditional classification of style in this matter refers to *autocratic, bureaucratic, democratic* and *laissez-faire* leaders (Lewin *et al.*, 1939). These may be characterized briefly as follows:

▶ An *autocratic* leader monopolizes decision-taking and imposes the results on the group with little regard to the contribution individuals might make to the quality and acceptability of the decisions.
▶ A *bureaucratic* leader seeks to prescribe as much as possible of the work by means of written policies and procedures and to regulate the work by observance of approved methods.
▶ The *democratic* leader seeks to involve the members of the group in decision-making and thus to obtain their commitment to successful outcomes by giving them a degree of 'ownership' of the decisions.
▶ A *laissez-faire* leader is scarcely a leader at all, leaving the staff largely to their own devices.

The best style of leadership is a matter of opinion and depends on the circumstances in which leadership is being exercised. In a life-threatening emergency where time is of the essence the autocratic leader may be preferred. Where the activity is hedged about with legal requirements, hazard of litigation and a need for meticulous records the bureaucrat may be best. Where individual staff members require a certain amount of autonomy to do their job effectively a democratic style of leadership may be preferred. The democratic leader retains control and should not be confused with the laissez-faire leader who has effectively abdicated.

Situational leadership

The above considerations point to the need for leadership styles to be appropriate to the circumstances. The outline of autocratic, bureaucratic and democratic leadership given above concerns itself with the personal style of the leader and pays little regard to the reactions of the group. However, this reaction as indicated by productivity and morale is the test of the effectiveness of the leadership.

Robbins (1992) describes two recent studies seeking to establish whether management committed to straightforward pursuit of productivity or that pursuing effectiveness more indirectly via promotion of good staff morale is better. The results are inconclusive and clearly such a dichotomy will not be clear cut but a matter of emphasis. However, the point is well made that good staff morale is not an end in itself, though desirable, but a means to continuing effective supply of goods and services which are the reason for the existence of the organization and a prerequisite for the manager's own continuing employment in the organization.

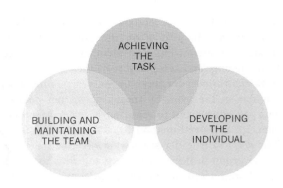

Figure 2   What a leader should do.

Adair (1988) seeks to influence the behaviour of leaders by directing attention to the three topics illustrated in Figure 2.

Change Theory

Change theories provide a theoretical basis for understanding the processes involved in bringing about change. Analogies for the processes of change are frequently used such as unfreezing, moving, refreezing (Lewin, 1951) which presupposes a relatively stable state before and after the change. By contrast, the experience of businesses exposed to rapidly changing competitive situations and technological change may require *ad hoc* innovative manoeuvres to deal with problems as they arise, like a skier on an unfamiliar slope. In the context of this chapter the former, that is the planned change, is the focus of attention though some *ad hoc* actions are likely to be unavoidable in the course of bringing it about.

The impetus to make such a change in an organization usually arises from a mismatch between the organization and its environment. As an example, there has been a change in what women expect from the experience of childbirth and from those who care for them. This has produced a mismatch between this changed expectation and the traditional view of hospital midwifery as processing mothers and babies. Organizations providing midwifery care are reacting to this by initiating new approaches, such as midwife-led care focused on the individual woman, with increased emphasis on integrated schemes of care involving the hospital and community midwifery service for normal, low-risk pregnancies.

Whatever the nature of the change, success in giving effect to it will depend heavily on the quality of the preparatory work to identify all the elements of the new desired configuration and to place them in a time frame for implementation. A substantial change may be viewed as a project and it may be necessary to appoint a project team leader with appropriate staff temporarily seconded to undertake the work of planning and giving effect to the change. There may be merit in selecting team members from groups in which implementation will probably be difficult.

There is likely to be some opposition to the change. For instance, shortage of resources may impose financial constraints which require lower pay rises or fewer staff or poorer facilities for the clients. These are unattractive alternatives and any solution devised by management is unlikely to be readily acceptable to the staff. Chin and Benne (1985) have proposed three types or groups of strategies for overcoming resistance to change and a brief account of these is given below.

STRATEGIES

Empirical–rational strategies

These depend on the belief that people are guided by reason and will calculate rationally where the best interests of themselves and their group lie and act accordingly. As an example, if women can be persuaded of the risks associated with smoking in pregnancy they may give it up in pursuit of better fetal health and outcome of pregnancy.

The calculation need not necessarily be made selfishly but there is likely to be a selfish element in it. It is the task of management to construct arguments which are convincing and where compliance with the change may be calculated to lead to desirable results for key individuals and groups.

Normative re-educative strategies

These strategies relate to attitudes, values and needs rather than reason and seek a wider and deeper change than acceptance of some discrete change in organization or procedure. Maslow (1954) has postulated a hierarchy of needs in which, when lower needs are met, e.g. for food, higher needs supervene. McGregor (1960) argues that existing organizations fixate people in lower motivations and seeks greater self-realization in the development of individuals, leading to greater effectiveness of organizations. Hence strategies are envisaged to change norms of perception, aspiration and behaviour by re-education and self-examination.

Power–coercive strategies

These are strategies of command where, by the use of power to apply sanctions of one kind or another, those involved may be constrained to accept change. These strategies are likely to be applied as a supplement to empirical–rational strategies which, even if successful, are unlikely to persuade everybody. Organizational hierarchies have a range of sanctions available to them from moral pressure to overt action to penalize determined resistance.

Change, like any other activity, demands resources which have to be planned and provided. A change agent, who is counselling staff on a new procedure, is not doing the work of the unit, and staff who are learning to use new documentation are not achieving the task they are there to perform. Taking staff out of their normal roles to plan the change well in advance has the advantage of making them available as extra pairs of hands to resource the change process at the critical time.

Organization of Time

Effectively used time is the main resource in organizations providing direct service to the public and managing time, including their own, is a major responsibility of management. This usually depends more on having the right people in the right place at the right time with appropriate skills, motivation, information, documentation and equipment, than on unremitting hard work; on inspiration rather than perspiration. Time spent effectively is likely to be spent rewardingly for the individual and as McGregor (1960) points out, creativity is widely dispersed throughout the population and is not necessarily the sole province of those in managerial positions. It is important that management time should be well used and this means it must be planned.

There are techniques available to facilitate this which can be applied with advantage, also by others not, or not yet, in managerial positions. These take the form of guidelines for dealing with paperwork, telephones, meetings, office organization, relations with colleagues and staff and all the minutiae of a manager's day. Handbooks such as those by Adair

(1982) and Pernet and Wright (1989) enable the manager to shortcut a great deal of experiential learning in the art of time management.

As with most activities, the central planks for effective management are a clear and complete understanding of what the management task in question is intended to be, analysis of what it is in practice on an hour-by-hour basis and bringing these into conjunction. Thus a manager might proceed as follows:

Research and analyse the personal task   Ensure that all the roles and functions properly appertaining to the post are identified. Put these in a hierarchy of importance, distinguishing between those which must be discharged personally and those which may be delegated. Weed out those for discussion and reallocation which seem incompatible with the task, or unnecessary. Clarify where lines of responsibility and authority are not clear. Take note of regularly occurring events to which deadlines are attached. Produce a rational programme of time allocation to these tasks which reflects their importance and intrinsic time demands. Include the amount of private time which it is intended to devote to work.

Research and analyse actual time usage   Construct suitable log sheets to enable personal use of time to be recorded over a period. Headings may include categories of activity, topics, routine administration, correspondence, interruptions and perhaps marks out of ten for the effectiveness of particular activities. If there are large identifiable tasks such as producing monthly or quarterly returns these may merit separate dedicated log sheets.

The task of reconciling these two tasks is an important test of the ability of the manager and will govern whether he or she is calmly in control or harassed and not coping.

Decision-making

Success depends on making good choices, whether it is in selecting a candidate at interview or a target consumer group in marketing a product. The plans associated with the choice may be well-conceived and executed but success is likely to prove elusive if the initial decision is wrong. A distinguishing feature of decision-making is that it occurs at a discrete moment in time; a choice is made and the other options available are discarded. The timing of the choice is important, neither too early before adequate consideration has been given and valid options identified or too late so that good options have lapsed with the passage of time or progress of work is delayed.

Day-to-day decision-making by managers is the vehicle for evolutionary change of organizations as opposed to relatively large-scale discrete changes discussed earlier in this chapter. It is the task and constant preoccupation of a manager to have a good understanding of policy as it relates to his or her unit, to understand the external relationships of the unit and to have a view on the direction of development of the unit in the context of the development of the organization. This gives the manager a frame of reference for decision-making which is used to respond to requests from the staff for guidance and direction. The summation of these decisions over a period tends to change the operation of the unit; the answers are absorbed into the culture and new questions on the frontiers of that changed culture are formulated and answered. Thus the manager by decision-making is likely to be the leading agent of evolutionary change, but this role is greatly facilitated by the quality of the questions and suggestions which form the main vehicle for change agency by the staff.

Decisions connected with step change rather than evolution tend to originate with senior management, starting with detection of a problem adversely affecting the performance of the organization in meeting its objectives. The sequence of events may be as follows:

1   Detection of the problem.
2   Generation of hypotheses about the cause.
3   Research and analysis to confirm or discredit the hypotheses.
4   Generation of options for action.
5   Evaluation of options by predicting outcomes.
6   Selection of the preferred option.
7   Formal decision-making and authorization.
8   Planning.
9   Implementation.

These activities may be carried out by a single individual, as they would be in a one-man business, by a small group working in strict confidence, or by open consultation.

Management Studies

Many of the ideas in this chapter have their origins in the pioneering work of a relatively small number of influential writers, particularly the following:

Peter Drucker	Elton Mayo
Henri Fayol	Douglas McGregor
Frederick Herzberg	Frederick Taylor
Abraham Maslow	Lyndall Urwick

The large increase in the productivity of labour in the course of the twentieth century which has transformed the lives of ordinary citizens in developed countries is due not only to technology but to development and application of theories of management. F.W. Taylor (1856–1917) has been particularly influential (Pugh and Hickson, 1989).

This work demands some lateral thinking to see its relevance to midwifery management. However, much of it is relevant, justifying study as the following examples show.

Example 1

Elton Mayo was carrying out research on the productivity of a group of workers in a factory in the USA. He made changes in the working environment and observed the results. No matter what he did, apparently good or bad, productivity increased. It was his presence and the fact that someone was taking an interest in what the workers did that produced the effect, not the changes which he was trying to evaluate. This is known as the *Hawthorne effect*, after the Hawthorne factory where the work was done (Mayo, 1949).

Example 2

Our fundamental assumptions and prejudices are challenged by McGregor (1960), who postulates two views of people for our consideration, as a basis for a theory of management. These can be paraphrased as follows:

▶ *Theory X*: The average person is by nature indolent – he works as little as possible. He lacks ambition, dislikes responsibility, prefers to be led. People must be persuaded, rewarded, punished, controlled – their activities must be directed.
▶ *Theory Y*: The motivation, the potential for development, the capacity for assuming responsibility, the readiness to direct behaviour towards organizational

goals are all present in people. It is the responsibility of management to make it possible for people to recognize and develop these human characteristics in themselves.

Clearly, whether a manager holds theory X or Y, or something in between, would influence his or her attitudes and actions.

Ideas such as quality assurance and technological changes such as information technology have been current long enough to alter profoundly the nature of management. Study of published research and up-to-date writing on the subject of management will be particularly important as a new epoch in management theory and practice takes shape. The thoughtful young manager will develop the knowledge, attitudes and skills required for the particular field of operation by choosing role models wisely and selecting those elements in the literature which are relevant to the activity in which he or she is engaged.

References

Adair, J. (1982) *Effective Time Management*. London: Talbot Adair Press.

Adair, J. (1988) *Effective Leadership*. London: Pan.

Chin, R. & Benne, K.D. (1985) General strategies for effecting changes in human systems. In Bennis, W.G., Benne, K.F. & Chin, R. (eds) *The Planning of Change*, 4th edn. New York. Holt Rinehart & Winston.

Drucker, P.F. (1955) *The Practice of Management*. London: William Heinemann.

Drucker, P.F. (1977) *Management*. New York: Harper's College Press.

Drucker, P.F. (1993) *Post Capitalist Society*. Oxford: Butterworth Heinemann.

Fayol, H. (1916) *Administration Industrielle et Generale*. Paris: Dunod.

Lane, E.L. (1991) *The Market Experience*. Cambridge: Cambridge University Press.

Lewin, K., Lippitt, R. & White, R.K. (1939) Patterns of aggressive behaviour in experimentally created social climates. *J. Soc. Psychol.* 10: 271–299.

Lewin, K. (1951) *Field Theory in Social Science*. New York: Harper & Row.

McGregor, D. (1960) *Human Side of Enterprise*. New York: McGraw Hill.

Maslow, A.H. (1954) *Motivation and Personality*. New York: Harper and Row.

Mayo, E. (1949) Hawthorne and Western Electric Co. In Mayo, E. (ed) *The Social Problems of Industrial Civilisation*. London: Routledge.

Pernet, R. & Wright D (1989) *Effective Use of Time*. London: Industrial Society.

Pugh, D.S. & Hickson, D.J. (1989) *Writers on Organisations*, 4th edn. London: Penguin.

Robbins, S.P. (1992) *Essentials of Organisational Behaviour*. New Jersey: Prentice Hall.

93

Quality Assurance

Since the mid-1980s many large organizations in the UK have shown a growing interest in assessing the effectiveness and acceptability of the services they provide. One of the first to develop systems of quality assurance was the Health Service.

The need for quality assurance has increased as a result of the increasing complexity of the way health care is provided, rising expectations of consumers, the need to define standards in health service contracts and to demonstrate the effective use of resources.

A number of factors influence the quality of a health service:

▶ The needs of the population being served.
▶ The values which underpin the purpose of the service.
▶ The resources which are available.
▶ The way the service is organized.

The *needs* of the population include the number of people who require the service, health and social factors, and the presence of any special needs, e.g. interpreters for those with language difficulties.

The *values* of a service influence the range and style

of services to be provided, for example, the ethics and philosophy of a service, the expectations of the public, the professional standards which apply, the laws which govern some of its services, the motivation and commitment of those who deliver the service. Meeting the needs and maintaining the values calls for *resources* which match both. Among resources are included: buildings, equipment, staff, professional knowledge and skill, research, education, heat, light, etc., all of which need adequate and well-used finance.

The fourth item which influences the quality of a service is the way that service is *organized* and how well resources are used. For example, it is no use providing antenatal clinics which are full of highly skilled doctors and midwives at times or in places which make it difficult for women to attend.

What is quality assurance?

The term 'quality assurance' describes a system of management which makes explicit the purpose, standards and objectives of an organization in such a way that the whole operation of a service is geared towards achieving those standards and objectives. Implied within the concept of quality assurance is the need to make it a dynamic and not an academic exercise. Quality assurance has been defined as follows:

> Quality Assessment is the measurement of provision against expectation. Quality Assurance is the same but with the declared intention and ability to correct any demonstrated weaknesses. (Shaw, 1986)

Meeting the Needs and Delivering the Service

Meeting the needs of any population will require both *strategic* and *operational* quality. Strategic quality is concerned with large-scale plans and methods of providing care, while operational quality is concerned with the day-to-day delivery of a particular service.

STRATEGIES FOR MATERNITY CARE

In the United Kingdom a number of strategies have led to the comprehensive service available today, starting with the 1902 Midwives Act which brought the practice of midwifery under statutory control and protection to the recent House of Commons (Winterton) Report on Maternity Services (1992) and Department of Health report *Changing Childbirth* (1993).

The success of those strategies can be seen in the steady reduction in the perinatal, neonatal and maternal mortality rates in this country. Internationally, the World Health Organization has spearheaded the Safe Motherhood Campaign designed to bring a reduction in the high maternal mortality in the developing countries (Maine, 1986).

Uniqueness of maternal services mortality measures

It is important to realize that the way that maternity services have for many years assessed maternal, perinatal and neonatal mortality is unique among health care services. It has not been usual for other services, e.g. surgery, medicine, to evaluate or publish their outcomes, although there is now pressure to do so via clinical audit. Since the 1920s maternity services have measured the efficacy of their care strategies by their mortality statistics and it has been the desire to

improve these that has led to many changes in the provision and delivery of care.

In 1948 a further measure of operational quality was added when it became mandatory for all maternal deaths to be investigated via the Confidential Enquiry into Maternal Deaths. The most recent report (DOH, 1996) shows that maternal mortality has halved every ten years for the last 50 years. It can be claimed, therefore, that the maternity services have led the field in measuring the effectiveness of their care strategies. However, it is in the day-to-day operation of numerous maternity units, departments and staff that such strategic quality is achieved.

OPERATIONAL QUALITY

Operational quality is concerned with the day-to-day operation of a service and most quality assurance initiatives have been developed in this setting. Many different people are involved in providing any service, and as time goes on, there are many changes as new staff arrive, and others leave. The larger the number of people involved the greater is the need to ensure that the standards and objectives of the service are clearly understood and that the service given is acceptable and consistent.

There have been numerous reports which have influenced operational quality in maternity care. The recommendations of the Maternity Services Advisory Committee (1982, 1984, 1985) set standards for all aspects of care. Consumer reports, both local (e.g. by community health councils or branches of the National Childbirth Trust) and national, for example, *The Good Birth Guide* (Kitzinger, 1983) or the *Health Rights Handbook* (Beech, 1987), a good deal of the Winterton Report (House of Commons, 1992) and the *Changing Childbirth* report (DOH, 1993), all address the issue of operational quality in maternity care. So does the research-based and wide-ranging publication *Effective Care in Pregnancy and Childbirth* (Chalmers *et al.*, 1989). The Cumberlege Report (1993) sets clearly defined standards for maternity services together with a time-scale for their implementation within the National Health Service.

Main Components of Quality Assurance Systems

Quality assurance has four main components:

1   Defining the quality to be achieved.
2   Promoting quality via education, guidelines, facilities, etc.
3   Monitoring quality: measuring the performance against expectations.
4   Taking action: acting on the results of an evaluation to acknowledge and praise achievements, to investigate shortfall and setting targets for improvement.

Altogether, these components form the *quality cycle* (Table 1).

DEFINING THE QUALITY TO BE ACHIEVED

This is the most crucial part of the whole process and involves asking fundamental questions about the purpose, nature and expectations of a service. It has many facets and involves all the different levels of an organization. It begins by asking the questions:

▶ What is the purpose of the service?
▶ What type of care or service will best achieve the health outcomes and health benefits which our clients require?

What is the purpose of the service?

Defining the purpose of a service and the values which guide it may take different forms at different levels.

1   *Corporate vision*: This is set by the top management of an organization, and contains a broad grasp of the principles of a service. The *Patient's Charter* and the Cumberledge Report are both examples of statements of corporate vision.
2   *Mission statement*: This may be produced by a health authority, a hospital or a specific care group. For example the mission statement of a maternity service might be as follows:

> Our aim is to enable as many women as possible to achieve their optimum well-being during the process of pregnancy, labour and puerperium, able to play a full role in giving birth to a healthy baby and embarking in strength upon the demands of parenthood.

Table 1   Stages of the quality cycle

1   *Define desired level of quality*   Mission statements, set objectives for care, define standards of practice and performance

2   *Promote quality*   education, research, guidelines, protocols, codes of practice, birth plans, etc.

3   *Assess performance*   Evaluate current performance in relation to the target

4   *Results*   Collate results and identify why current performance is or is not meeting the desired standards

5   *Take action on results and in relation to target:*
   (a)   Acknowledge and applaud achievement of target, and where appropriate use as models of practice for others
   (b)   Improve areas of shortfall, recognizing constraints, setting clear objectives and realistic timetables

5   *Monitor and evaluate results of action*
   (a)   Has action achieved desired standards, improved morale, recognized achievement?

Yes	*No*
continue methods	review methods
	constraints, problems

   (b)   Can better standards be achieved?
         Are standards achievable within current constraints?

6   *Take action on policies, guidelines, changes needed*

7   *Start cycle again, setting new standards*

Where factors in the health of the mother or baby make this more difficult, to provide care in such a way as to reduce the effect of such factors and obtain the best possible outcome.

Once the mission has been stated, then the *standards* and *objectives* of different parts of the service which will help to fulfill that mission can be defined.

Objectives and standards Setting objectives enables different sections of the service to describe the purpose and mission of each department in relation to the overall mission. Standards describe how the objectives are to be achieved and measured. For example, the objectives of an antenatal department may be defined as follows:

1 To ensure that the service reaches those who need it.
2 To provide appropriate, skilled and effective services which will enrich the parenthood experience and reduce the potential for illness or disability in the mother or her infant.
3 To provide care in a way which is convenient and acceptable and meets the needs and expectations of its clients.
4 To ensure that the woman's wishes and preferences for her care in labour and the puerperium are taken account of and recorded.
5 To build mutually satisfactory relationships between the consumers and providers of the service.

The effect of setting such clear and concise objectives ensures that all who come to work in the antenatal department are quite clear about its objectives and that they are expected to work towards their achievement. This is important when one considers how many different people are involved in providing care: doctors, midwives, health care assistants, receptionists, ultrasound technicians, laboratory staff, etc. A further benefit of setting clear objectives is that it lays the ground for the setting of standards. In one maternity unit, midwives setting standards in relation to objective 1 above, found that many young primigravidae did not attend for antenatal care until comparatively late in their pregnancy, mainly because they were not aware of the services available or of the importance of attending early. As a result, one midwife contacted local clothing factories which employed high numbers of women and as a result, was invited to provide health information and to hold a clinic once a month. This resulted in many more young pregnant women receiving advice, care and screening early in their pregnancy.

Setting standards A standard may be described as a 'good model, approved pattern of behaviour, desired level of attainment'. In quality assurance two kinds of standard are set: standards of *practice* and standards of *performance*. A standard of practice describes what is to be achieved, a standard of performance indicates the degree to which the standards should be achieved if the service is giving a good quality service. The Cumberlege Report (1993) sets standards of practice designed to ensure continuity of care, for example 'Every woman should know the midwife who ensures continuity of her midwifery care – the named midwife,' and standards of performance which would indicate whether the desired practice had been achieved, for example 'At least 75% of women should know the person who cares for them during their labour'.

Standards should be written in a way that is clear, unambiguous and which is possible to measure. Wilson (1987) says that standards should be 'RUMBA':

R Relevant
U Understanding
M Measurable
B Behavioural (which means that they can be observed)
A Achievable.

It is important that the setting of standards is not inhibited by caution about what can be achieved. Some standards may not be achievable in the short term, for example, any which require some major change in structure or resource allocation, but they should be kept and used as a future target. One of the difficulties in setting standards and objectives for a service is that of setting only those standards which relate to the present patterns of service rather than defining those which might lead to new or improved ways of achieving the objectives. One way to guard against this is to use a model or framework based upon the literature.

Models for defining quality in healthcare

The two most widely used models are those of Donabedian (1980, 1986) and Maxwell (1984) whose work was expanded by Shaw (1986).

Donabedian: Structure, process and outcome

Donabedian (1980, 1986) defined three aspects of health care which contribute to defining and evaluating the quality of a health care:

1 *Structure* – the physical, financial and organizational resources for health care.
2 *Process* – all the events, interactions and interventions between a service and its clients.
3 *Outcome* – the result of antecedent health care/intervention upon the health status of a client/patient.

Donabedian's model is primarily intended for use as a strategic model, and maintains that the quality of a service depends upon the structure and processes which together affect the outcome. Although this model is valuable it has been somewhat misused in the early development of quality assurance. There was an assumption that using Donabedian meant that all standards should be written to include the structure needed, the processes which should occur and the expected outcome, but this is not always applicable and can result in cumbersome and elongated standards. There is need also to be cautious in the use of the term 'outcome' which Donabedian defines as a change in health status. Frequently the term 'outcome' is used to describe the results of an intervention or process, and although this is understandable, it is not very accurate. There are many processes which do not have a direct effect upon 'outcome' as defined by Donabedian, but which are an integral part of the care process. These have been defined by Buchan *et al.* (1990) as *health benefits*. The term 'health benefits' describes 'information or reassurance or some other aspect of the care process', all of which are relevant to maternity care. Combining the concepts of structure, process, outcome and health benefits makes a useful framework for defining standards of care.

Maxwell's model

The second model is that of Maxwell (1984), who suggested that there are six dimensions of health care which should be addressed when defining and assessing quality:

1 *Access* – the availability of a service, its accessibility, the promptness of its response.
2 *Acceptability* – to its clients; courtesy, choice, comfort, dignity, confidentiality, in short, the *way* in which the service deals with its clients.
3 *Effectiveness* – the degree to which the interaction between the client and the service produces the desired result, outcome or health benefit.
4 *Efficiency* – providing the service in a skilled, competent manner and achieving the desired result without the unnecessary use of resources. This aspect of service is often left out of standard setting, but being efficient enables resources to be more widely spread.
5 *Relevance to need* – ensuring that standards of service meet different patterns of need. This can apply to the range of services provided, or making certain that clients receive care suited to their individual needs. Shaw (1986) used the term 'appropriateness' instead of relevance to need, and this is a useful distinction.
6 *Equity* – ensuring that available resources are fairly distributed among all who have need of them.

Using models in writing standards of care   Both Maxwell's and Donabedian's models are helpful in setting objectives and standards and can be used together, or separately as best suits the situation. Table 2 shows the way these models can be used in setting standards for antenatal care. (Note: there will be many more standards produced than those shown.) Once standards have been defined they can then be used to set in motion the other stages of the quality cycle: promoting and evaluating the quality of a service.

PROMOTING QUALITY

The next stage after setting objectives and standards is to use them in discussions with all the staff concerned in order to gain their commitment and seek ways of achieving them. For example, setting standards may lead to producing new guidelines or stimulate new ideas on ways of working. There are a number of existing methods of promoting the quality of a service which also have a part in quality assurance:

▶ *Professional standards* which control the education and practice of professional staff.
▶ *Codes of practice*, e.g. *Midwives Rules, Patient's Charter*.
▶ *Guidelines and procedures* which lay down the way staff are to deal with certain situations, e.g. dealing with stillbirth.

Table 2   Quality grid for antenatal service

Basis: Maxwell	Standards of practice	Standards of performance	Basis: Donabedian
Access to service	All clients seen as early as possible. Service near to home. Bus route/car park convenient. Crèche. Waiting at clinic kept to minimum	No. and % seen by 12th week; no. and % seen by GP/ community midwife; no. and % attending clinic as requested	Structure Process Issues
Acceptability	Courtesy, personal service. Convenient appointment times for clinics and parentcraft	Client surveys; % who did not attend on follow-up visits	Process
Efficiency	Communications good. All necessary tests undertaken at right time. Minimum waiting time for client	Lack of complaints; good working relationships. Average waiting time in clinic per client	Process
Effectiveness	Oversight/intervention leads to good maternal and neonatal results	No. and % clients with good Hb levels; no and % of normal deliveries at term; no. and % emergencies in pregnancy/ labour	Outcomes
Relevance to needs	Different emphases, arrangements for different groups of clients, e.g. young mothers, multiparae, those with infertility problems, etc.	Guidelines, care plans reflect personalized care. Outcomes analysed by % cared for by consultant, GP or midwives during pregnancy	Structure Process Outcomes
Equity	Available resources shared fairly across all client groups/sites	Success rate on standards is similar for all client groups	Outcome

▶ *Care contracts, birth plans,* by which a client's pre-ferences are sought and recorded for use by all who care for her.

▶ *Research,* making sure that practice is research-based and that care practices are updated in the light of relevant research. Guidelines and standards in maternity care should draw upon such resources as the National Perinatal Epidemiology Unit, MIRIAD, the Royal College of Midwives Publica-tions and MIDIRs.

MEASURING THE QUALITY

Measuring quality will require a mixture of quantita-tive and qualitative techniques. *Quantitative data* are concerned with facts which have a finite range, e.g. 'was the baby offered a breast or bottle feed within one hour of delivery' (Hughes and Goldstone, 1990a,b,c). The answer to this question will be 'yes', 'no' or 'not applicable' (e.g. when baby was too ill or stillborn). If

out of 100 mothers for whom the question was applic-able 85% said 'yes', then that would reflect a good standard of performance.

The familiar perinatal mortality rate is another example of quantitative data. The term *audit* is given to this approach to quality assessment. Valid audit systems must ensure that the question is not ambigu-ous and can be readily answered 'yes' or 'no', and that the sample size is large enough to draw valid conclu-sions.

Most well-written standards can be measured by the audit technique, but there will be other facets of care, expecially in the dimensions of acceptability and appropriateness which will need the *qualitative approach.* For example, a standard might wish to find out how satisfied the clients were with the help they received with feeding the baby. The standard of prac-tice might be that 'all women feel supported in feeding' and the standard of performance might be that 85% of all women responded positively. Measuring this type of standard is best done by presenting the client with a series of statements and inviting her to choose from a range of answers which reflect her experience and to which scores reflecting a rating scale are given. For example,

Statement 1 The midwives were helpful when I was feeding my baby
2 I was made to feel silly when I asked for help in feeding my baby

Responses and scores

Scores for statement 1: Strongly agree (5), agree (4), neither agree nor disagree (3), disagree (2), strongly disagree (1).

It can be seen that the score reflects the positiveness of the response, the higher the score, the more the objective was achieved. However, the score system must be reversed for statement 2 which is negatively phrased. In this case the scores would be

Strongly agree (1), agree (2), neither agree nor disagree (3), disagree (4), strongly disagree (5).

A mean score for each statement can then be produced. For example, if in a sample of 45 women the answers were:

Statement 1 30 agreed, 5 disagreed and 10 strongly disagreed the score would be 30 × 4, 5 × 2, and 10 × 1 = 140/45 = mean score of 3.1 which is not very high.
Statement 2 might provide some of the reason if the scores were 25 strongly agreed, 10 agreed and 10 disagreed = 25 × 1, 10 × 2, 10 × 4 = 90/45 = mean score of 2.

Use of published tools for quality assurance

The process of setting standards is important in promoting quality and should form the basis for evaluation. However, measuring the standards is not an easy task, and it can be useful to use published methods which have been extensively validated, either as the total quality tool or as a model for developing one's own measuring tools. Two methods published specifically for maternity care are: *Midwifery Monitor* (Hughes and Goldstone, 1990a,b,c) which uses an audit approach and the *OPCS Survey Manual* (Mason, 1989) which uses a qualitative method.

TAKING ACTION AND SETTING NEW STANDARDS

As can be seen in Table 1, the final stage of the quality cycle is taking appropriate action once the results of measuring performance have been obtained. This action includes applauding staff for good performance, discussing the reasons for that which is poor, deciding which issues should be addressed and setting a time-scale for improving quality. It may also include setting new standards of practice or performance which are to be achieved at the next evaluation, or producing new guidelines.

Conclusions

Thus the cycle is complete and the process begins again. Most services have an annual quality review, with action to improve and maintain quality being an integral part of the daily pattern of work. Setting quality standards should ideally be undertaken by a group of staff who represent different disciplines and levels of staff and where possible, representatives of the consumers.

Being concerned with providing good-quality care has always been the hallmark of health care. The development of quality assurance systems will help to ensure that all those involved in providing care are clear about the objectives and values of the service and have an opportunity to play their role in achieving high standards of performance.

References

Beech, B.L. (1987) *Who's Having Your Baby? A Health Rights Handbook for Maternity Care*. London: Camden Press.
Buchan, H., Gray, M. & Hill, A. (1990) Needs assessment made simple. *Health Service J.* **100** (5188): 240–241.
Chalmers, I., Enkin, M. & Keirse, M.J.N.C. (eds) (1989)

Effective Care in Pregnancy and Childbirth. Oxford: Oxford University Press.
DOH (Department of Health) (1993) *Changing Childbirth* (Cumberlege Report) Report of the Expert Maternity Group. London: HMSO.

DOH (Department of Health) (1996) *Report on Confidential Enquiries into Maternal Deaths in the United Kingdom 1991–93*. London: HMSO.

Donabedian, A. (1980) *The Definition of Quality Assurance and Approaches to its Measurement*. Ann Arbor: Health Administration Press.

Donabedian, A. (1986) Evaluating the quality of medical care. *Millband Memorial Quarterly* **64**(3): 66–206.

House of Commons (1992) *Maternity Services: Second Report of the Health Committee* (Winterton Report). London: HMSO.

Hughes, D.J.F. & Goldstone, L.A. (1990a) *Midwifery Monitor I; Pregnancy Care; An Audit of the Quality of Midwifery Care in Pregnancy*. Leeds: Poly Enterprises (Leeds) Ltd.

Hughes, D.J.F. & Goldstone, L.A. (1990b) *Midwifery Monitor II; Labour Care; An Audit of the Quality of Midwifery Care in Labour*. Leeds: Poly Enterprises (Leeds) Ltd.

Hughes, D.J.F. & Goldstone, L.A. (1990c) *Midwifery Monitor III; Care after Birth; An Audit of the Quality of Postnatal Midwifery Care*. Leeds: Poly Enterprises (Leeds) Ltd.

Kitzinger, S. (1983) *The New Good Birth Guide*. London: Penguin Paperbacks.

Maine, D. (1986) Maternal mortality: helping women off the road to death. *WHO Chronicle* **40**(5): 175–183.

Mason, V. (1989) *Women's Experience of Maternity Care – A Survey Manual*. London: HMSO.

Maternity Services Advisory Committee (1982) *Maternity Care in Action*. Part I: *Antenatal Care*. London: HMSO.

Maternity Services Advisory Committee (1984) *Maternity Care in Action*. Part II: *Care During Childbirth*. London: HMSO.

Maternity Services Advisory Committee (1985) *Maternity Care in Action*. Part III: *Care of the Mother and Baby*. London: HMSO.

Maxwell, R.J. (1984) Quality assessment in health. *Br. Med. J.* **288**(1): 470–471.

Shaw, C.D. (1986) Introducing quality assurance. King's Fund Project paper no. 64. King's Fund Publishing House, London.

Wilson, C.R.M. (1987) *Hospital-wide Quality Assurance: Models for Implementation and Development*. Canada: W.B. Saunders.

94

Midwifery in an International Context

Contrasts

One of the most striking measurable contrasts between industrialized and non-industrialized (or developing) countries is that of *maternal mortality rates.* On a global scale, it was estimated that half a million women die every year as a result of pregnancy and childbirth. Ninety-nine per cent of these deaths occur in the developing world and rates vary considerably in the different regions of the world (AbouZahr and Royston, 1991). It has recently been acknowledged that previous calculations are now known to be an underestimate and that, in fact, almost 80 000 more maternal deaths occurred in 1990 than was first thought (WHO, 1995). Table 1 presents a summary of the latest estimates available.

The five major causes of maternal death have been identified as (WHO, 1989; AbouZahr and Royston, 1991):

▶ Postpartum haemorrhage.
▶ Puerperal sepsis.
▶ Obstructed labour.
▶ Eclampsia.
▶ Abortion.

Such causes of death are affected by numerous factors. The reasons why women die have been described as 'many layered' (AbouZahr and Royston, 1991). These layers include social, cultural and political factors which determine crucial issues such as the status of women, women's health and fertility and their 'health seeking behaviour'. Other factors which further increase the chance of a woman dying relate to such issues as failures in the health care system and lack of transport.

The global problem of AIDS and HIV-related illness further compounds the situation and is currently adding to the slaughter of young women and their babies.

The average lifetime risk of dying in pregnancy or childbirth will vary according to the number of times a woman becomes pregnant and is significantly dependent upon where she lives (Table 2). It is important to realize that these are average figures and that the actual risk can be much higher. Women living in rural areas who have high fertility rates are particularly vulnerable. For instance, it is estimated that a women in Bali has a lifetime risk of dying of pregnancy related causes of 1 in 32, a woman in Bangladesh 1 in 26 and in rural Africa at least 1 in 15 (WHO, 1987, 1989; AbouZahr and Royston, 1991).

Table 1   Estimates of maternal mortality by United Nations regions (1990)

UN region	Maternal deaths (thousands)	Maternal deaths per 100 000 live births
World	**585**	**430**
More Developed Regions	4	27
Less Developed Regions	581	480
Africa	**235**	**870**
Eastern Africa	97	1070
Middle Africa	31	950
Northern Africa	16	340
Southern Africa	4	260
Western Africa	87	1020
Asia*	**323**	**380**
Eastern Asia*	24	90
South-central Asia	227	560
South-eastern Asia	56	440
Western Asia	16	320
Europe	**3**	**36**
Latin America/Caribbean	**23**	**190**
Caribbean	3	400
Central America	5	140
South America	15	200
Oceania**	**1**	**280**

* (excluding Japan)   ** (excluding Australia and New Zealand)
Source: WHO (1995)

Table 2   Lifetime risk of dying in pregnancy

Industrialized countries	1 in 1750 – 1 in 10 000
Africa	1 in 25
South Asia	1 in 38
Latin America	1 in 90
South East Asia	1 in 870

Source: WHO, 1989

Amongst those most vulnerable to maternal death are teenagers. Studies in Bangladesh and Nigeria illustrate only too graphically that young mothers under 15 years of age have a maternal mortality rate which is five to seven times higher than that for women aged 20–24 years in their respective countries, whilst the death rate for mothers aged 15–19 years in Bangladesh was still double that in the 20–24 year age group. (Chen *et al.*, 1974; Harrison, 1985). This risk is not eliminated for women in the Western world. It has been shown that mothers under 15 years of age in the USA had a mortality rate three times that of women in the 20–24 year age group (Rochat, 1981).

Older women also face increased risk. Studies have shown that women aged 35–39 years were between 85% and 460% more likely to die in a given pregnancy than women aged 20–23 years (Rochat, 1981). Risk is also shown to increase after the third pregnancy (WHO, 1986a), so that increasing parity frequently relates to an ever-increasing risk of death. Causes of maternal death are indeed multifactorial. The birth of children to so many of the world's women may be aptly described as: 'too many, too early, too late and too close together' (WHO, 1989).

Morbidity is less easily measurable. The need to investigate maternal morbidity more thoroughly is evidenced from the fact that the major source of information on this subject is recognized to be a study by Datta *et al.* (1980) who undertook a small survey in an Indian village more than a decade ago and estimated that for every woman who dies, at least a further 16 suffer some disability (WHO, 1990a). These disabilities include horrific injuries such as vesico-vaginal fistulae, recto-vaginal fistulae as well as secondary infertility. In industrialized countries, morbidity has been associated with pelvic floor damage, stress incontinence, dyspareunia and musculoskeletal problems (Chapter 38). Everywhere in the world, childbirth can result in an enormous toll on women's health, even when life itself is not immediately endangered.

It is estimated that 88–98% of all maternal deaths could probably have been avoided (WHO, 1986b). This implies that maternity services have an important function in prevention. In countries where maternal mortality rates are unacceptably high it is increasingly recognized that prevention is a priority if death and morbidity are to be reduced significantly. It is important for the midwife to recognize that this is so wherever in the world she may practise. Active steps must be taken to assess and monitor progress in pregnancy, labour and the puerperium, detect risk and promptly refer the woman for skilled obstetric help when needed.

Skills, Scope and Situations

It is estimated that only about 52% of births are attended by trained personnel (AbouZahr and Royston, 1991). Whilst human resource planning in developing countries has aimed to provide one midwife per 5000 population (Kwast, 1979), this is not a problem easily solved since scattered populations make access to such skilled care the luxury of a few. Midwives carry a heavy burden of responsibility and give care in situations with acute staff shortages, inadequate resources and overcrowding. The World Health Organization estimates that for every 200 normal deliveries each year, one trained midwife is needed to ensure an appropriate quality of care. It is judged that around 1

in 10 births requires the assistance of a specialist, therefore the back up of a practitioner skilled in providing essential obstetric care (Table 3) is required for every nine midwives. Countries are therefore urged to aim to employ one obstetrician and nine midwives for every 2000 births (WHO, 1990b). However, many countries struggle to provide any maternity service at all; for example, in Algeria it is estimated that one midwife is responsible for 1749 deliveries and one obstetrician/gynaecologist is responsible for 4145 deliveries annually (WHO, 1988).

The range of life-saving skills which must be at the fingertips of every midwife will vary and is unique to each country and for regions within each country. For example, in Zaire, midwives are trained to undertake Caesarean section (Duale, 1987). In Cameroon, Ghana, Malawi, Nigeria, the Philippines, Tanzania, Uganda and Zaire midwives and nurses are trained to perform some of the essential obstetric functions (Population Reports, 1988), whilst many countries train nurse anaesthetists. The midwife has the potential to be the key person in providing care and support for women, babies and families. Often, the midwife is the only person available to provide all the necessary professional care. As a team leader she may work with doctors with or without obstetric/paediatric skills, traditional doctors or healers and/or traditional birth attendants (TBAs) whom she may also have responsibility for training. The midwife everywhere has an important role in health promotion. In situations where there may be few basic resources, midwives have to provide the specific help and advice needed in many and varied situations, for example, midwives may need to give advice on growing crops and in rearing livestock before attempting to discuss appropriate nutrition in pregnancy (Figure 1). Cultural

Table 3   Essential obstetric care

Category 1	Surgical obstetrics, e.g. Caesarean section, repair of vaginal and cervical laceration
Category 2	Anaesthesia
Category 3	Medical treatment, e.g. of shock, hypertensive disorders and eclampsia
Category 4	Blood replacement
Category 5	Manual procedures and monitoring labour, e.g. manual removal of placenta, vacuum extraction, partograph
Category 6	Management of women at high risk
Category 7	Family planning support, e.g. tubal ligation, vasectomy, IUD, Norplant
Category 8	Neonatal special care

Source: WHO, 1991a

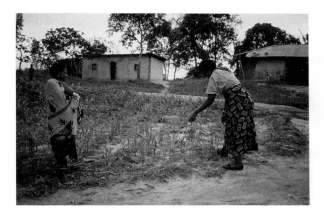

Figure 1   Midwife in Tanzania giving advice about growing crops (photograph courtesy of G.D. Maclean).

issues need to be addressed sensitively and midwives have to consider many traditional practices and taboos. They must, for instance, address issues associated with son preference. This can mean that little girls have less nourishment, less immunizations and less access to medical care when needed, giving them a major health disadvantage from early on in their lives (Graves, 1976; Makinson, 1985a,b; Ware, 1981; Powell and Grantham-McGregor, 1985).

The Safe Motherhood Initiative

Given the enormous death toll associated with childbearing, an international and interdisciplinary effort is underway in order to attempt to reduce the maternal mortality rate by at least 50% by the year 2000 (Table 4).

The Safe Motherhood Initiative is described as:

> a global effort to reduce maternal mortality and morbidity. The target is to reduce maternal deaths by at least half by the year 2000.
>
> The Initiative aims to enhance the quality and safety of girls' and women's lives through the adoption of a combination of health and non-health strategies.
>
> However, the Initiative places special emphasis on the need for better and more widely available maternal health services, the extension of family planning education and services, and effective measures aimed at improving the status of women.

Table 4   Co-sponsors of the Safe Motherhood Initiative

 United Nations Development Programme (UNDP)

 United Nations Children's Fund (UNICEF)

 United Nations Population Fund (UNFPA)

 The World Bank

 World Health Organization (WHO)

 International Planned Parenthood Federation (IPPF)

 The Population Council

Activity within the Initiative may take many forms: increasing awareness of the dimensions of the problem and the need for action; strengthening maternal health services; training of health workers and others; facilitating educational and economic opportunities for women; and research, particularly operational research.

Partners within the Initiative are governments, agencies, non-governmental organizations and other groups and individuals who stimulate and participate in efforts likely to reduce the number of women suffering and dying as a result of pregnancy and childbearing.

(WHO, 1990–94)

This Initiative is giving rise to many and varied activities addressing a complexity of issues which lie at the heart of the problem of maternal death and morbidity. One important project involves the education of midwives. At the WHO/ICM/UNICEF pre-congress workshop held in Kobe, Japan in October 1990, an educational framework was developed by midwife educators and others from more than 20 countries (WHO, 1991b). There was a consensus that current midwifery courses did not adequately prepare practitioners for their roles in order to promote safe motherhood. Subsequently, the World Health Organization has developed learning modules designed specifically to help to educate midwives practising in countries where the maternal mortality rate is unacceptably high (WHO, 1996). There are five modules on:

1 The midwife in the community.
2 Postpartum haemorrhage.
3 Obstructed labour.
4 Puerperal sepsis.
5 Eclampsia.

and a tutor's handbook. These address the five major causes of maternal mortality. The modules are designed initially to meet midwives' needs in continuing education and can be adapted to local situations. A large variety of learning/teaching methods are included and a tutor's handbook provides guidance to assist teachers in using these. Clinical teaching strategies as well as guidance in assessing clinical competence are offered in the modules. The community module provides guidelines for carrying out a community profile. There are also checklists in this first module, identifying what a midwife must know and what she must be

able to do in order to prevent death occurring as a result of postpartum haemorrhage, obstructed labour, puerperal sepsis, eclampsia and abortion. Educational games form an easily detachable portion of each module book and are designed to promote critical thinking and analysis of midwifery practice. These modules have been tested extensively and published in English (WHO, 1996). Some countries are adapting and translating the modules to meet their own needs and situation. The World Health Organization currently plans to translate the literature into other major world languages.

Country Initiatives

Very many countries are undertaking major projects in order to address their maternal mortality rates. Specific needs are often identified through situational analyses, then task forces are formed and action initiated. The country profiles shown in Table 5 give a thumbnail sketch of selected countries and report some initiatives being undertaken in a variety of situations. Each country has specific problems and challenges. These can generate innovative ideas and provide incentive and stimulus to introduce change and sustain efforts

Table 5 Country profiles of selected countries

Botswana		(Non-industrialized)		
Population:		1.2 million (1988)	**GNP/capita:**	US$1050 (1985)
Adult literacy:	**Male:**	73%	**Female:**	69% (1985)
Life expectancy:	**Male:**	53 years	**Female:**	56 years (1980–85)
MMR:	Community Studies (Kalagadi District) (1987): **380**			
	Hospital studies (1982): **90**			

Initiatives include:

A four phase midwifery curriculum review of the basic course:

▶ Phase 1: Preparing the learning environment (clinical teaching and clinical audit, clinical practice update)
▶ Phase 2: Writing the curriculum
▶ Phase 3: Implementation
▶ Phase 4: Evaluation.

The course was extended to 18 months. Safe Motherhood advanced practice skills learned by qualified staff in an intensive short course.

Source: Ministry of Health, Government of Botswana, 1992; University of Botswana, 1994. Personal contact and involvement.

(continued)

Canada   (Industrialized)
Population: 26.5 million (1980–85)   **GNP/capita:**   US$16 960 (1987)
Adult literacy: **Male:**   n.a.   **Female:**   n.a.
Life expectancy: **Male:**   73.3 years   **Female:**   80.3 years (1980–85)
MMR: Latest available figure published 1991: **5**

Initiatives include:

Legislative changes and a variety of education programmes have been introduced. They range from the training of Inuit (indigenous) midwife apprentices nominated by their communities, to part-time inservice education for selected obstetric nurses to enable them to extend their role. A midwifery certificate programme in conjunction with the Master in Nursing Degree aims to prepare midwives who will offer leadership in the profession. Several provinces in Canada are in the process of obtaining midwifery legislation which will strengthen, support and legalize the practice of midwifery.

Source: Relyea, 1992.

For an overview of progress in Canadian midwifery legislation see Herbert, 1995.

China   (Non-industrialized)
Population: 1355 million (1990)   **GNP/capita:**   US$290 (1987)
Adult literacy: **Male:**   82%   **Female:**   56% (1985)
Life expectancy: **Male:**   68 years   **Female:**   71 years (1985–90)
MMR: Community studies (30 provinces) (1989):
          National: **95**   Urban: **50**   Rural: **115**
          Meiyun County: **114**   Jiangsu: **45**   Henan: **147**

          Hospital studies Beijing (1979–83):   **21**
                         Shanghai (1962–71): **11**

Initiatives include:

The reduction of postpartum haemorrhage (PPH). This is the major cause of death and is a particular problem in rural areas compounded by transport difficulties. A major maternal and child health project includes the training of village doctors in techniques to prevent deaths due to PPH. Two manuals concerning the prevention and treatment of PPH have been translated into Chinese and used to reach 200 000 village health workers.

Source: WHO *Safe Motherhood Newletter.*

France   (Industrialized)
Population: 56.1 million (1980–85)   **GNP/capita:**   US$16 090 (1987)
Adult literacy: **Male:**   99%   **Female:**   98%
Life expectancy: **Male:**   71.9 years   **Female:**   80 years (1980–85)
MMR: Latest available figure published 1991: **9**

Initiatives include:

Introduction of a postnatal follow-up home care programme following the example of Holland, England and Switzerland. The mother returns home sooner and has the benefit of care of the same quality as in hospital. Care is adapted to the individual family needs and is described as personalized accompaniment of the mother and child with complete respect of the unique relationship that is established.

Source: Peel-Muracciole, 1990.

(continued)

Indonesia (Non-industrialized)

Population:		180.5 million (1990)	**GNP/capita:**	US$450 (1987)
Adult literacy:	**Male:**	83%	**Female:**	65% (1985)
Life expectancy:	**Male:**	55 years	**Female:**	57 years (1985–90)

MMR: Community studies (national) (1985–86): **450**
Hospital studies (12 teaching hospitals) (1977–80): **390**

Initiatives include:

Major projects to undertake midwifery basic and continuing education. A target to train and place one midwife in each of the country's 67 000 villages has largely been achieved through a three-year programme of direct entry training. After study tours to a range of countries by multidisciplinary teams of government officials, continuing education programmes were planned and legislation relating to the control of midwifery practice has been thoroughly revised. The latter introduces statutory registration of midwives for the first time. The award of travel fellowships has facilitated continuing education programmes for selected senior midwifery teaching personnel in Indonesia and in the UK.

Source: Ministry of Health, Republic of Indonesia, 1991. Personal contact and involvement.

The Netherlands (Industrialized)

Population:		15 million (1980–85)	**GNP/capita:**	US$14 520 (1987)
Adult literacy:	**Male:**	n.a.	**Female:**	n.a.
Life expectancy:	**Male:**	73.5 years	**Female:**	80.2 years (1980–85)

MMR: Latest available figure published 1991: **10**

Initiatives include:

The training and use of home care assistants. Dutch midwives are autonomous practitioners, caring for low-risk mothers and referring high-risk mothers for obstetric care. General medical practitioners can only claim fees if there is no practising midwife in the area. Maternity home care assistants are trained to assist at home births and provide care for mother, baby and family postnatally. The hours worked by the assistants are flexible to meet family needs and this service is used by 73% of mothers in the Netherlands.

Source: Van Teijlingen, 1990.

Nigeria (Non-industrialized)

Population:		105.5 million (1988)	**GNP/capita:**	US$370 (1987)
Adult literacy:	**Male:**	54%	**Female:**	31% (1985)
Life expectancy:	**Male:**	47 years	**Female:**	50 years (1980–85)

MMR: National (1988): **800** (WHO)

Civil registration data/government estimates:
Kaduna, Ogun, Ondo & Oyo states (1981–83): **1500** (MOH)

Initiatives include:

Specific activity of midwives and nurses to discourage female genital mutilation and early marriage of teenage girls which predispose to: 'injury, ill-health, psychological distress, infertility and death.' The National Association of Nigerian Nurses & Midwives has produced two graphically illustrated leaflets to help in their efforts to work with communities to help eradicate these harmful traditional practices.

Sources: WHO, Medical Statistics Division, Ministry of Health, *Safe Motherhood Newsletter of Worldwide Activity*, issue 17, March–June 1995.

(continued)

Pakistan   (Non-industrialized)

Population:		123 million (1990)	**GNP/capita:**	US$350 (1987)
Adult literacy:	**Male:**	40%	**Female:**	19% (1985)
Life expectancy:	**Male:**	57 years	**Female:**	57 years (1985–90)

MMR: Community studies (National) (1988): **270**

Hospital studies (Between 1979 and 1983):
Range from **700 to 5010**

Initiatives include:

Use of a 24-hour flying squad comprising an ambulance equipped and with trained staff able to deal with obstetric emergencies. An educational programme was necessary before the service was used in order to change attitudes of community members and traditional birth attendants. This programme includes open meetings in textile mills, schools, hospitals and clinics to inform about the risks of maternal death and how to prevent it.

Source: WHO *Safe Motherhood Newsletter.*

Sierra Leone   (Non-industrialized)

Population:		3.9 million (1988)	**GNP/capita:**	US$300 (1987)
Adult literacy:	**Male:**	38%	**Female:**	21% (1985)
Life expectancy:	**Male:**	33 years	**Female:**	36 years (1980–85)

MMR: National estimate (1983): **650**
Hospital studies (1986): **342**

Initiatives include:

In Magbil: training of traditional birth attendants, improving the general health of the community and promoting income-generating activities. Here, fetal stethoscopes have been made from local bamboo and cord ligatures from fibres of the palm tree. This makes essential equipment affordable and available to more community health workers. There has been an effort resulting in the recruitment of actors and entertainers into the Safe Motherhood campaign in Bo and Makeni Districts in order to teach local people how to recognize signs of complications in pregnancy and delivery. These all form parts of prevention of maternal mortality projects in the country.

Sources: WHO *Safe Motherhood Newsletters*; Daramy-Kabia, 1993.

Uganda   (Non-industrialized)

Population:		17.2 million (1988)	**GNP/capita:**	US$260 (1985)
Adult literacy:	**Male:**	70%	**Female:**	45% (1985)
Life expectancy:	**Male:**	47 years	**Female:**	51 years (1980–85)

MMR: Hospital studies (1966–67): **397**
National (report by Family Care International) (1989) : **400–700**

Initiatives include:

The training of maternal and child health teams in order to address the 'lack of planning and managerial skills' which are believed to aggravate problems. Training was provided by a multidisciplinary team and carried out in three phases:

▶ Phase 1: Defining problems, setting priorities, collecting and analysing data, writing action plans.
▶ Phase 2: Modification in the light of field experience and implementation.
▶ Phase 3: Evaluation and analysis of the health impact of the project.

The teams work together with community members to address problems.

Source: WHO *Safe Motherhood Newsletter.*

(continued)

Zimbabwe		(Non-industrialized)		
Population:		9.1 million (1988)	GNP/capita:	US$580 (1987)
Adult literacy:	Male:	81%	Female:	67% (1985)
Life expectancy:	Male:	54 years	Female:	58 years (1980–85)
MMR:	Hospital studies (1979): **145**			
	National (government estimates) (1979): **483**			

Initiatives include:

The setting up of 'maternity waiting homes' or 'maternity villages'. These allow women who live some distance from the hospital to stay whilst awaiting the birth of their baby. Women are reported to stay for an average of 18 days and this has been described for many as 'the only holiday of their lives'. During their stay, as well as attending antenatal clinics, mothers also have lectures on fetal development, labour, family planning, AIDS, childcare and other relevant topics. Maternity waiting homes have been shown to reduce the incidence of obstructed labour and ruptured uterus in many countries and are especially useful for women at high risk.

Source: WHO *Safe Motherhood Newsletter*.

to improve services for childbearing women. Exchange of personnel and ideas can be very productive and global networks are increasingly being established to help promote safe motherhood.

The initiatives described in these profiles are illustrative only of some of the activities being undertaken. They by no means describe all that is being attempted within a country, but merely give glimpses of midwifery enterprise in a sample of both industrialized and non-industrialized countries across the world. Innovation frequently results from need identification accompanied by a determination to meet that need, address an issue or overcome a problem.

Internationally, needs and problems vary, but fundamentally midwives everywhere are primarily concerned with enabling women to achieve a safe experience of childbirth. As safety increases there is increased emphasis on making childbirth a satisfying experience, however, safety should never be compromised for the sake of satisfaction and the two aims should not be in conflict. Within each country there is a unique process whereby goals are set, obstacles removed and progress facilitated. This gives rise to many and varied approaches which may include, for example, the introduction of new or amendment of existing legislation (e.g. as in Canada and France), the updating of educational programmes, the introduction of new curricula and provision of continuing education programmes (e.g. as in Botswana and France). These are fundamental to producing necessary changes in midwifery practice. Many countries are

devising strategies to initiate action which improves practice (e.g. China and Uganda). Efforts are also being made to increase the uptake of care by improving the accessibility and acceptability of maternal and child health care through innovation and imaginative thinking. Taking a multidisciplinary approach and involving community members can be crucial steps in achieving these aims (e.g. Indonesia, The Netherlands, France, Nigeria, Pakistan and Sierra Leone).

International Organizations

Numerous international organizations provide assistance for projects within and between countries. Midwifery internationally is able to benefit from provision of resources both human and fiscal which are offered through a variety of schemes. The Safe Motherhood Initiative and its co-sponsors has already been described and is an excellent example of international co-operation. Such organizations may be governmental, intergovernmental or non-governmental. There are also voluntary and religious organizations which offer support and assistance in many countries. A list of useful addresses is included at the end of the chapter but the reader must be aware that these are constantly changing. There is currently an explosion of international aid in a volatile world economy at the end of the twentieth century. Nevertheless there are increasing opportunities and demands for midwives to share their professional expertise and some guidance on this is provided below. Some organizations require special consideration by the midwife. This does not in any way underestimate the valuable contributions of so many others.

World Health Organizations

The World Health Organization (WHO) has the objective of the attainment by all peoples of the best possible level of health. WHO has two main constitutional functions. These are:

1   to act as the directing and co-ordinating authority on international health work; and
2   to encourage technical co-operation for health with member states.

WHO performs its functions through three principal bodies: the World Health Assembly, the Executive Board and the Secretariat. The global headquarters is in Geneva, Switzerland and each of the six world regions has its own regional committee and regional office. The six WHO regions are shown in Figure 2. Increasingly, the policy of decentralization is practised in relation to policy formation and monitoring of regional activities. WHO works closely with other organizations within the United Nations system. It is a constitutional requirement that WHO should 'establish and maintain effective collaboration with the United Nations . . . and provide health services and facilities' (WHO, 1990c). WHO produces technical, professional and educational health information. Major programmes of interest to midwives which are currently underway include the publication of material for the education of midwives, already outlined, the training of traditional birth attendants and a global programme on AIDS which was launched within WHO in 1987. The global strategy of 'Health for all by the year 2000', asserted in the Alma Ata Declaration (WHO, 1978), has been operational since 1981 and has given incentive to make every possible effort to bring health within the reach of every human being. WHO officially designates leading health-related institutions around the world as WHO Collaborating Centres (WHO, 1990c). There are currently more than a thousand WHO Collaborating Centres in the world.

UNICEF

The United Nations Children's Fund (UNICEF) aims to raise public awareness of the needs of children and of strategies to meet those needs and to raise funds for programmes which UNICEF sponsors in 130 countries. The organization provides help and care for women and children, emergency relief and health education in war-torn countries as well as situations of poverty in industrialized and non-industrialized countries. UNICEF has a four-part strategy for the protection of children designated 'GOBI', that is:

G   Growth monitoring
O   Oral rehydration
B   Breastfeeding
I   Immunization.

UNICEF in collaboration with WHO defined a global standard for maternity services described as 'baby friendly care' in 1989. The Baby Friendly Initiative was launched aiming to achieve at least two baby friendly hospitals in each of 12 'lead' countries by February 1992 and as many as possible in all countries by the end of 1992. The initiative involves a global effort with hospitals, health services and parents to focus on the needs of the mother and her newborn and strives to implement the ten steps to successful breastfeeding specified in the initiative (Table 6). In order to help promote breastfeeding on a global scale, the World Alliance for Breastfeeding Action (WABA) was formed at UNICEF headquarters in New York in 1991 and encourages the active participation of indivi-

Table 6   Ten steps to successful breastfeeding (UNICEF/WHO)

1	Have a written breastfeeding policy
2	Train all health staff to implement this policy
3	Inform all pregnant women about the benefits of breastfeeding
4	Help mothers initiate breastfeeding within half an hour of birth
5	Show mothers the best way to breastfeed
6	Give newborn infants no food or drink other than breast milk, unless medically indicated
7	Practice 'rooming in' by allowing mothers and babies to remain together 24 hours a day
8	Encourage breastfeeding on demand
9	Give no artificial teats, pacifiers, dummies or soothers
10	Help start breastfeeding support groups and refer mothers to them

Source: *Take the Baby-Friendly Initiative!* Leaflet UNICEF.

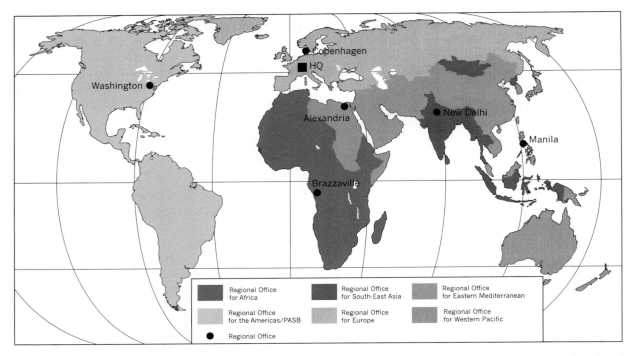

Figure 2   World Health Organization regional offices and the areas they serve. (Reproduced with permission from WHO *Biennial Report 1988–1989*).

duals and organizations in this effort to protect, promote and support breastfeeding.

The World Summit for Children in September 1990 resulted in a commitment by almost all the international community to attain a series of health, nutrition, education and other goals by the end of the decade (UNICEF, 1993).

The International Confederation of Midwives

The International Confederation of Midwives (ICM) is a unique midwifery professional organization. It works to serve the interest of women, their newborn babies and their families through the advancement of midwifery education, practice, management and research worldwide (ICM, 1981). There are four regions of the confederation: Africa, the Americas, Asia Pacific and Europe. The ICM is governed by an International Council which normally meets every three years when an international congress is also held. A Board of Management oversees the management and financial obligations of ICM. An Executive Committee and a Finance subcommittee act as advisory bodies to the

Board of Management and the Council. The Secretary General is the chief executive officer of ICM who is appointed by the Council. The international headquarters are based in London (ICM, 1992).

European Community committees

There are two commitees within the European Union (EU) of special interest to the midwife.

The Midwives' Liaison Committee   This is composed of representatives of the midwives' organizations within the European Community. It was established in 1968 by the International Confederation of Midwives in order to give consideration to the EC Midwives Directives and advise relevant governments of professional views of midwives. The committee looks at the provision of maternity care and midwifery practice issues in all the countries of the European Economic Community.

EU Advisory Committee on the training of midwives   This has been established in accordance with the EU Midwives Directives and advises the

European Commission on all matters relevant to the training of midwives. Midwives from each member country serve on this committee and are drawn from clinical practice, training institutions and the competent authority (EEC, 1977, 1980).

Important Considerations for Midwives Intending to Work Overseas

Midwives practising in any country other than that in which they have been educated, need to consider how they can best prepare and adapt to what may be a vastly different situation.

Midwives who have been educated in an industrialized country and intend to work in a non-industrialized or developing country are best placed if they have considerable experience in clinical practice before leaving their own country. It can be very helpful to learn some advanced clinical skills where this is practicable, for example: vacuum extraction, suturing of cervical and vaginal tears, manual removal of placenta, setting up of intravenous infusions, neonatal intubation, insertion of intrauterine contraceptive devices. Regulations may restrict midwives from acquiring some of these skills, but policy and tradition as well as inadequate preparation may also unnecessarily prevent opportunities. Short courses in tropical medicine and health can be very valuable for midwives expecting to work within these parts of the world and indeed anywhere where there is not ready access to medical services. Discussions with persons who have lived and worked in the intended country of practice can, of course, be invaluable.

Countries will specify their own needs and priorities. Increasingly there is a need for midwives with skills in education and management, but all midwives must be skilled practitioners and able and willing to adapt to local needs. Respect for a different culture and religion is crucial and an ability to speak another language or willingness to learn a new one is a definite asset. It is important for any expatriate worker to appreciate that there are many things in another country which she will never know nor understand, that change must come from within a country and that an 'expert' from another country can best help by demonstrating appropriate knowledge, skills and attitudes

with extreme sensitivity. The midwife must appreciate that without such appropriate attitudes which demonstrate respect, sensitivity, patience, empathy and careful observation of the local situation, knowledge and skills will be impossible either to learn or to share.

Midwives who have been educated in non-industrialized or developing countries and intend working or studying in industrialized countries will probably find that there is much more advanced technology in use than they have previously experienced. They may also find that there is considerably more emphasis on women's choice. The latter must always be balanced with safety and the woman must always be given the opportunity to make an informed choice. This means that the midwife must have a good theoretical and practical understanding of what is involved as well as being aware of popular demand and current thinking. She must keep updating her own knowledge and practice by critically evaluating all innovations in the light of reliable research. There are benefits and hazards associated with both technology and freedom of choice and the midwife will need to carefully evaluate each policy, practice and request from women and their partners in order to consider its advantages and disadvantages.

Midwives who have practised in countries where resources are scarce are often skilled at improvising and can sometimes share ideas and innovations with colleagues who may face different, but none the less significant resource limitations. Midwives who have practised in areas of the world which are remote from medical and obstetric services can also make real to colleagues in industrialized countries the complications which they rarely see but are nevertheless a real threat if appropriate management and referral is not employed. For example, obstructed labour and ruptured uterus can and will occur anywhere that cephalopelvic disproportion exists and septicaemia can and will follow puerperal sepsis. Such complications will result in maternal death anywhere in the world unless there is prompt and appropriate intervention. Thus, meaningful professional dialogue will always be valuable, wherever in the world this takes place between midwives who are ready to learn for the benefit of mothers, babies and families.

It may be seen therefore that midwifery in an international context is a dynamic topic which deserves the consideration of all professional midwives in a world which is ever becoming smaller. International exchange of expertise and ideas should continue to help to promote excellence in professional practice. Everywhere, the needs of childbearing women have a common basic requirement, that of safe motherhood. Everywhere, women are entitled to the best possible professional care which offers respect to them as individuals and for their needs and preferences. Though situations and environments may differ, midwives throughout the world have a vital role in promoting safe motherhood and in so doing becoming the woman's advocate and professional adviser. Few professionals face such a challenge on the brink of the twenty-first century as the target of achieving 'health for all'. The midwife, through her education and practice holds a crucial key to health which can open the door to safe motherhood. Access to this fundamental human right determines not only the health and safety of today's women but also that of tomorrow's global population.

References

AbouZahr, C. & Royston, E. (eds) (1991) *Maternal Mortality: A Global Factbook*. WHO/MCH/MSM91. 3. Genava: WHO.

Chen, L.C., Gesche, M.C., Ahmed, S. *et al.* (1974) Maternal Mortality in rural Bangladesh. *Studies in Family Planning* 5(11): 334–341

Daramy-Kabia, I. (1993) The training of traditional birth attendants for safe motherhood in Magbil, Sierra Leone. In *Book of Proceedings: International Confederation of Midwives 23rd International Congress*. 'Midwives hear the heartbeat of the future', 9–14 May 1993, Vancouver, Canada.

Datta, K.K., Sharma, R.S., Razack, P.M. *et al.* (1980) Morbidity patterns amongst rural pregnant women in Alwar, Rajastan – a cohort study. *Health Population Perspect. Issues* 3: 282–292.

Duale, S.I. (1987) Maternal care breakthrough in Zaire. *People: IPPF review of population & development* 14(3): 16–17.

EEC (1977) The EEC Directives on the activities responsible for general care. *Official J. Eur. Communities* 20 (176) July.

EEC (1980) The EEC Midwives Directives. *Official J. Eur. Communities* 23 (33) February.

Graves, P.L. (1976) Nutrition, infant behaviour and maternal characteristics, a pilot study in West Bengal, India. *Am. J. Clin. Nut.* 29: 305–319.

Harrison, K.A. (1985) Childbearing, health and social priorities: A survey of 22,774 consecutive births in Zaria, Northern Nigeria. *Br J. Obstet. Gynaecol.* Suppl. 5.

Herbert, P. (1995) Midwifery in Canada: the struggle for recognition. *Modern Midwife* 5(2): 11–14.

ICM (1981) Report of the International Confederation of Midwives Council meeting. London: ICM.

ICM (1992) Information leaflet: International Confederation of Midwives v3fd/int.lea, September. London: ICM.

Kwast, B.E. (1979) The role and training of midwives for rural areas. In Philpott, R.H. (ed) *Maternity Services in the Developing World – What the Community Needs*. Proceedings of the 7th Study Group of the Royal College of Obstetricians & Gynaecologists, London.

Makinson, C. (1985a) Age and sex differences in treatment of childhood diarrhoeal episodes in rural Menoufia. Mimeographed document, Cairo Social Research Centre, American University in Cairo.

Makinson, C. (1985b) Sex differentials among children admitted to a Cairo oral rehydration centre. Mimeographed document, Cairo Social Research Centre, American University in Cairo.

Ministry of Health, Government of Botswana (1992): *Safe Motherhood in Botswana: A Situational Analysis*. Prepared on behalf of the Safe Motherhood Task Force by Family Care International, Gaborone, October.

Ministry of Health, Republic of Indonesia (1991) with United Nations Development Programme & WHO. *Safe Motherhood: Executive Summary of Assessment & Recommended National Strategies*, Vol. 4, 17 December.

Peel-Muracciole, B. (1990) A new experience in France: Help at home following a birth. *Book of Proceedings of 22nd ICM, Kobe, Japan*. 7–12 October, pp. 135–137.

Population Reports (1988) Series L, No. 7. September. *Safe Motherhood: A Newsletter of Worldwide Activity* 10.

Powell, C.A. & Grantham-McGregor, S. (1985) The ecology of nutritional status and development in young children in Kingston, Jamaica. *Am. J. Clin Nutrit.* 41: 1322–1331.

Relyea, M.J. (1992) The rebirth of midwifery in Canada: A historical perspective. *Midwifery* 8(4): 355–366.

Rochat, R.W. (1981) Maternal mortality in the United States of America. *World Health Statistics Quarterly* 34: 2–3.

UNICEF (1993) *Annual Report of UNICEF (UK) 1991/1992*.

University of Botswana (1994) *Curriculum for the Diploma in Registered Midwifery*. Institute of Health Sciences, Botswana.

Van Teijlingen, E.R. (1990) The profession of maternity home care assistant and its significance for the Dutch midwifery profession. *Int. J. Nurs. Studies* 27 (4): 355–366.

Ware, H. (1981) Sex differentials in mortality and morbidity. In *Women, Demography and Development*. Canberra: Australian National University.

WHO (World Health Organization) (1978) Primary health care. *Report on the International Conference*, Alma Ata, USSR, 6–12 September 1978. Geneva: WHO.

WHO (1986a) WHO Interregional meeting on prevention of maternal mortality, Geneva, 11–15 November 1985, unpublished report WHE/86.1. In AbouZahr, C. & Royston, E. (eds) *Maternal Mortality: A Global Factbook*. WHO/MCH/MSM/91.3. Geneva: WHO.

WHO (1986b) Maternal mortality: helping women off the road to death. *WHO Chronicle* **40**(5): 175–183

WHO (1987) Fact sheet in: *Maternal Mortality: An Information Kit.* Geneva: WHO

WHO (1988) *World Health Statistics Annual.* Geneva: WHO

WHO (1989) *Preventing Maternal Deaths.* Royston, E. & Armstrong, S. (eds) Geneva: WHO.

WHO (1990a) *Measuring Maternal Morbidity: Report of a Technical Working Group*, 30 August–1 September, 1989. WHO/MCH/90.4. Geneva: WHO.

WHO (1990b) *Human Resource Development for Maternal Health and Safe Motherhood: Report of a Task Force Meeting.* WHO/HRD/90.1. Geneva: WHO.

WHO (1990c) *Facts about WHO.* Geneva: WHO.

WHO (1990–94) *Safe Motherhood Newsletter*, various issues.

WHO (1991a) *Essential Elements of Obstetric Care.* Geneva: WHO.

WHO (1991b) *Midwifery Education: Action for Safe Motherhood: Report of a Collaborative ICM/WHO/UNICEF Precongress Workshop*, Kobe, Japan. 5–6 October 1990. WHO/MCH/91.3. Geneva: WHO.

WHO (1995) Maternal mortality – worse than we thought. *Safe Motherhood: A Newsletter of Worldwide Activity* **19**.

WHO (1996) *Safe Motherhood, Midwifery Education Modules.* Education material for teachers of midwifery. WHO/FRH/MSM/96.1–96.5. Geneva: WHO.

Further Reading

Global issues and safe motherhood

AbouZahr, C. & Royston, E. (eds) (1991) *Maternal Mortality: A Global Factbook.* WHO/MCH/MSM/91.3. Geneva: WHO.

Berer, M. (1992) *Women's Groups, NGOs and Safe Motherhood.* WHO/FHE/MSM/92.3. Geneva: WHO.

Cook, R.J. (1994) *Women's Health and Human Rights.* Geneva: WHO.

Kensington, M. (1994) Safer motherhood – a midwifery challenge. In Alexander, J., Levy, V. & Roch, S. (eds) *Midwifery Practice – A Research-based Approach.* Basingstoke: Macmillan.

Kwast, B.E. (1991) Maternal mortality: the magnitude and the causes. *Midwifery* **7**(1): 4–7.

Kwast, B.E. (1993) Safe Motherhood – the first decade. *Midwifery* **9**(3): 105–123.

Kwast, B.E. & Bentley, J. (1991) Introducing confident midwives: midwifery education – action for safe motherhood. *Midwifery* **7**(1): 8–19.

Rooney, C. (1992) *Antenatal Care and Maternal Health: How Effective Is It?* A review of the evidence by Cleone Rooney of the Maternal & Child Epidemiology Unit of the London School of Hygiene & Tropical Medicine. WHO/MSM/92.4. Geneva: WHO.

Royston, E. & Armstrong, S. (eds) (1989) *Preventing Maternal Deaths.* Geneva: WHO.

WHO (World Health Organization) (1989) *Preventing and Controlling Iron Deficiency and Anaemia through Primary Health Care – A Guide for Health Administrators and Programme Managers.* Geneva: WHO.

WHO (1991a) *Essential Elements of Obstetric Care at First Referral Level – A Guide to Services Needed in Order to Manage Complications of Pregnancy, Labour and the Puerperium.* Order number: 1150364. Geneva: WHO.

WHO (1991b) *Obstetric Fistulae – A Review of Available Information.* WHO/MCH/MSM/91.5. Geneva: WHO.

WHO (1992) *The Prevalence of Anaemia in Women: A Tabulation of Available Information* (includes statistical data of prevalence worldwide), 2nd edn. WHO/MCH/MSM/92.2. Geneva: WHO.

WHO (1993) *Coverage of Maternity Care – A Tabulation of Available Information*, 3rd edn. WHO/FHE/MSM/93.7. Geneva: WHO.

WHO (1994b) *Maternal Health & Safe Motherhood: Research Progress Report, 1987–1992.* WHO/FHE/MSM/94.19. Geneva: WHO.

WHO (1994a) *Indicators to Monitor Maternal Health Goals.* WHO/FHE/MSM/94.14. Geneva: WHO.

WHO (1995) *Directory of Funding Sources for Safe Motherhood Projects.* WHO/FHE/MSM/94.1. Geneva: WHO.

WHO (1996) *Safe Motherhood, Midwifery Education Modules.* Education material for teachers of midwifery. WHO/FRH/MSM/96.1–96.5. Geneva: WHO.

WHO Practical Guides (available free of charge from WHO, Geneva)

   Mother–Baby Package: Implementing Safe Motherhood in Countries. WHO/FHE/MSM/94.11.

   Care of Mother and Baby at the Health Centre. WHO/FHE/MSM/94.2.

   Clinical Management of Abortion Complications. WHO/FHE/MSM/94.1.

   Detecting Pre-eclampsia. WHO/FHE/MSM/92.3.

   Preventing Prolonged Labour: The Partograph. WHO/FHE/MSM/93.8.

   Maternal & Perinatal Infections. WHO/FHE/MSM/91.10.

   Obstetric & Contraceptive Surgery at the District Hospital. WHO/FHE/MSM/92.8.

   Thermal Control of the Newborn. WHO/FHE/MSM/93.2.

   Detecting and Managing Anaemia in Pregnancy (forthcoming).

WHO/UNICEF Statements (available from WHO, Geneva)

   Maternal Care for the Reduction of Perinatal and Neonatal Mortality. WHO/86.

   Traditional Birth Attendants (1992). ISBN 92 4 156150 5.

   Infant Feeding and HIV/AIDS. Available from Documentation Centre, Global Programme on AIDS, WHO, Geneva.

European issues

Holland, W.W. (1991) *European Community Atlas of Avoidable Death*. Oxford: Oxford University Press.

Mead, M. (1993) Midwifery and Europe. *Modern Midwife* 3(3): 22–25 & 28

WHO (World Health Organization) (1986) *Having a Baby in Europe: Report on a Study*. London: WHO/HMSO.

Journals

Adult Education & Development: Journal of adult education in Africa, Asia & Latin America. Available from Institute for International Co-operation of the German Adult Education Association, Obere Wilhelmstrasse 32, D–53225, Bonn, Germany. (Published twice yearly)

Convergence: Journal of the International Council for Adult Education. Available from 720 Bathurst Street, Suite 500, Toronto, Ontario, Canada M5S 2R4. (Published quarterly)

Midwifery: International journal. Available from Churchill Livingstone Medical Journals, Robert Stevenson House, 1–3 Baxter's Place, Leith Walk, Edinburgh EH1 3AF, UK. (Published quarterly)

World Health Organization: *Safe Motherhood Newsletter*. These are issued three times a year and provide information on safe motherhood activities worldwide. Available free of charge on request from the Division of Family Health (WHO), Geneva. Update on resource materials is provided in each issue. An important source of information on new publications.

Useful Addresses

British Council,
10 Spring Gardens, London SW1A 2BN, UK
Center for Population & Family Health
(Prevention of Maternal Mortality) Columbia University, 60 Haven Avenue, B-3, New York, NY 10032, USA.
Centre for International Child Health
30 Guildford Street, London WC1N 1EH, UK
Family Care International
588 Broadway, Suite 510, New York, NY 10012, USA
International Confederation of Midwives
10 Barley Mow Passage, Chiswick, London W4 4PH, UK
International Family Health
1st Floor, Margaret Pyke Centre, 15 Bateman's Buildings, Soho Square, London W1V STW, UK
International Health Exchange
(formerly Bureau for Overseas Medical Service) Africa Centre, 38 King Street, London WC2E 8JY, UK
International Planned Parenthood Federation
Regents College, Regents Park, London NW1 4NS, UK
International Projects Association Services (IPAS)
PO Box 100, Carrboro, NC 27510, USA
Mothercare
John Snow Inc., 1616 N. Fort Myer Drive, Arlington, VA 22209, USA
Overseas Development Administration, UK
94 Victoria Street, London SW1E 5JL, UK

Royal College of Midwives
15 Mansfield Street, London, WIM OBE, UK
Teaching Aids at Low Cost (TALC)
PO Box 49, St Albans AL1 4AX, UK
UNICEF (UK)
55 Lincoln's Inn Fields, London WC2 3NB, UK
Voluntary Service Overseas
(VSO) 317 Putney Bridge Road, London SW15 2PN, UK
World Alliance for Breastfeeding Action
WABA Secretariat, PO Box 1200, 10850 Penang, Malaysia
World Health Organization
International Headquarters, CH-1211 Geneva 27, Switzerland
World Health Organization
Regional Offices:
    Africa PO Box 6, Brazzaville, Congo
    Americas: Pan American Sanitary Bureau, 525 23rd Street, N.W., Washington DC 20037, USA
    Eastern Mediterranean: PO Box 1517, Alexandria–21511, Egypt
    Europe: 8 Scherfigsvej, DK–2100 Copenhagen, Denmark
    South East Asia: World Health House, Indraprastha Estate, Mahatma Gandhi Rd., New Delhi–110002, India
    Western Pacific: PO Box 2392, 1099 Manila, Philippines

Index

Notes: 1. Page numbers for main chapters are **emboldened**. 2. Most references are to the United Kingdom (and England and Wales in particular), except where otherwise indicated. 3. References to women are ubiquitous and therefore *women* has been omitted as an entry

A

AA (Alcoholics Anonymous) 295
AA (arachidonic acid) 803
A/B (systolic/diastolic ratios) in ultrasound 263
A scan 260
abdomen
  abdominal oesophagus 101
  abdominal pregnancy 521–2
  adhesions 694
  antenatal care 220
  circumference determined by ultrasound 262
  enlarged as differential diagnosis of pregnancy 199
  examination 222, 223–30
    attitude 224
    denominator 224
    diagnosis of breech presentation 641
    findings throughout pregnancy 229–30
    labour
    onset of 294
    lie 223–4
    method 226–9
      inspection 227
      palpation 227–9
    position 224–5
    postnatal 486
    presentation 224
    prolonged labour 626
    see also engagement; lie; auscultation
  exercises 322, 325–6, 491–2
  hernia 923
  injuries, birth 910
  massage 273, 274
  muscles 319
  newborn 790, 824
  pain 580
  pendulous 580–1

postnatal care 475
  see also uterus
abnormal moulding 908
abnormalities *see* congenital disorders and abnormalities; *and under* cardiovascular system; gastrointestinal system; genital tract; nervous system; placenta; uterus
ABO blood group system 248
  incompatibility and jaundice 873, 879
  see also rhesus iso-immunization
abortion 512–18
  complete 513
  induced 216, 515–17
    alpha-fetoprotein levels 250
    cervical cancer 247
    chorionic villus sampling 257
    congenital disorders 42, 43, 44
    grief and bereavement 936, 937
    HIV 216
    jaundice 878
    missed 261
    renal disease 546
    rubella 249
    septic 512, 518
    teenage pregnancy 301
    therapeutic 512, 515–17
      criminal 512, 517
      methods 516–17
    toxoplasmosis 251
    vomiting 509
  legislation 249, 301, 515, 936, 1021, 1067
  missed 261, 512, 514
  mortality 1065, 1066, 1067, 1088, 1108
  septic 512, 518, 1066
  spontaneous (miscarriage) 512–15
    antenatal care 216
    causes of 512–13, 514–15

abnormal sperm 178
amniocentesis 252
genetic 37, 46
genital abnormalities 579
infections and medical conditions 174, 897, 898
intercourse 290
preconception care 174, 180
renal disease 546
smoking 180, 293
syphilis 572
travel 291
grief and bereavement 515, 937
inevitable 512, 513–14
missed 512, 514
psychological effects 515
recurrent 514–15
as social phenomenon 994
threatened 513
tubal 521
Abortion Acts 249, 301, 515, 936, 1021, 1067
abrasions 687, 688, 910
abruptio placentae 522, 526–30
causes 526–7
comparison with placenta praevia 525, 528
complications 529–30
hypertensive disorders 536, 545
induction of labour 611
management of 527–9
multiple pregnancy 588
postpartum haemorrhage 704
abscess, breast 724
abstinence syndrome (neonatal) 855, 1052
abused child 971–2
diagnosis 972
management 972
predisposing factors 971–2
warning signs 972
acceleration pattern of fetal heart rate 303–4